Advanced Oncology Nursing Certification Review and Resource Manual

Edited by
Barbara Holmes Gobel, RN, MS, AOCN®
Shirley Triest-Robertson, RN, PhD, AOCNS®
Wendy H. Vogel, MSN, FNP, AOCNP®

Oncology Nursing Society
Pittsburgh, Pennsylvania

ONS Publishing Division

Publisher: Leonard Mafrica, MBA, CAE

Director, Commercial Publishing/Technical Publications Editor: Barbara Sigler, RN, MNEd

Production Manager: Lisa M. George, BA

Staff Editor: Amy Nicoletti, BA

Copy Editor: Laura Pinchot, BA

Graphic Designer: Dany Sjoen

Advanced Oncology Nursing Certification Review and Resource Manual

Library of Congress Control Number: 2008939091

ISBN: 978-1-890504-75-5

Publisher's Note

This book is published by the Oncology Nursing Society (ONS). ONS neither represents nor guarantees that the practices described herein will, if followed, ensure safe and effective patient care. The recommendations contained in this book reflect ONS's judgment regarding the state of general knowledge and practice in the field as of the date of publication. The recommendations may not be appropriate for use in all circumstances. Those who use this book should make their own determinations regarding specific safe and appropriate patient-care practices, taking into account the personnel, equipment, and practices available at the hospital or other facility at which they are located. The editors and publisher cannot be held responsible for any liability incurred as a consequence from the use or application of any of the contents of this book. Figures and tables are used as examples only. They are not meant to be all-inclusive, nor do they represent endorsement of any particular institution by ONS. Mention of specific products and opinions related to those products do not indicate or imply endorsement by ONS. Web sites mentioned are provided for information only; the hosts are responsible for their own content and availability.

ONS publications are originally published in English. Publishers wishing to translate ONS publications must contact the ONS Publishing Division about licensing arrangements. ONS publications cannot be translated without obtaining written permission from ONS. (Individual tables and figures that are reprinted or adapted require additional permission from the original source.) Because translations from English may not always be accurate or precise, ONS disclaims any responsibility for inaccuracies in words or meaning that may occur as a result of the translation. Readers relying on precise information should check the original English version.

Printed in the United States of America

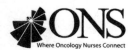

Oncology Nursing Society

Integrity • Innovation • Stewardship • Advocacy • Excellence • Inclusiveness

I would like to acknowledge the love and encouragement of my family—Greg, Megan, and Katie—who supported me through this journey of helping to create a quality oncology nursing book. I would also like to thank the editorial staff at the ONS Publishing Division, particularly Barbara Sigler, whose efforts have made possible the production of this book. Most sincere gratitude goes to the authors of this book who have shared of their time, energy, and expertise. Finally, kudos to Shirley and Wendy for work well done!

—Barbara Holmes Gobel

This book is dedicated to the patience, understanding, and encouragement of Bruce, Jason, Justin, Sally, Gisele, the memory of Jeremy and Albert, and my coeditors, Wendy and Barb. I am indebted to them for allowing me to fulfill a dream.

—Shirley Triest-Robertson

This book is dedicated with my love to Carl, Marlee, and Ben Vogel for their encouragement, understanding and "loving me through" the creation of this book. A special thank you to Sharon Brown for her invaluable assistance with research and to all our authors. To my coeditors, Barb and Shirley . . . the laughter and tears were better because they were shared with you.

—Wendy Vogel

Contributors

Editors

Barbara Holmes Gobel, RN, MS, AOCN®
Oncology Clinical Nurse Specialist
Northwestern Memorial Hospital
Chicago, Illinois
Adjunct Faculty
Rush University College of Nursing
Chicago, Illinois
Chapter 13. Genitourinary, Hepatic, and Pulmonary Toxicities; Chapter 21. Test Questions

Shirley Triest-Robertson, RN, PhD, AOCNS®
Oncology Clinical Nurse Specialist
St. Vincent Hospital
Green Bay, Wisconsin
Chapter 13. Genitourinary, Hepatic, and Pulmonary Toxicities; Chapter 21. Test Questions

Wendy H. Vogel, MSN, FNP, AOCNP®
Oncology Nurse Practitioner
Kingsport Hematology-Oncology Associates
Kingsport, Tennessee
Chapter 10. Pain, Fatigue, and Cognitive Dysfunction; Chapter 13. Genitourinary, Hepatic, and Pulmonary Toxicities; Chapter 21. Test Questions

Authors

Barbara A. Biedrzycki, RN, MSN, CRNP, AOCNP®
Oncology Nurse Practitioner
Sidney Kimmel Comprehensive Cancer Center at Johns Hopkins
Clinical Research Associate
Johns Hopkins University School of Medicine
Baltimore, Maryland
Chapter 9. Clinical Research

Deborah A. Boyle, RN, MSN, AOCN®, FAAN
Magnet Coordinator; Project Leader, Geroncology and Survivorship Nursing Studies Program
Banner Good Samaritan Medical Center
Phoenix, Arizona
Chapter 18. Palliative Care and End-of-Life Care

Heather L. Brumbaugh, RN, MSN, ANP, AOCN®
Nurse Practitioner
Duke University Medical Center
Durham, North Carolina
Chapter 15. Structural Oncologic Emergencies

Nancy Jo Bush, RN, MN, MA, AOCN®
Oncology Nurse Practitioner
Lecturer/Assistant Clinical Professor
School of Nursing
University of California, Los Angeles
Los Angeles, California
Chapter 16. Psychosocial Management

Diane G. Cope, PhD, ARNP-BC, AOCNP®
Oncology Nurse Practitioner
Florida Cancer Specialists
Fort Myers, Florida
Chapter 14. Metabolic Emergencies

Susan A. Ezzone, MS, RN, CNP, AOCNP®
Nurse Practitioner
Arthur G. James Cancer Hospital and Solove
  Research Institute
The Ohio State University Medical Center
Columbus, Ohio
*Chapter 7. Blood and Marrow Stem Cell Trans-
  plantation*

Regina M. Fink, RN, PhD, AOCN®, FAAN
Research Nurse Scientist
University of Colorado Hospital
Aurora, Colorado
Chapter 18. Palliative Care and End-of-Life Care

Tracy K. Gosselin, RN, MSN, AOCN®
Clinical Director, Oncology Services
Duke University Hospital
Clinical Associate
Duke University School of Nursing
Durham, North Carolina
Chapter 6. Radiation Therapy in Cancer Care

Heather Greene, RN, MSN, FNP, AOCNP®
Oncology Nurse Practitioner
Blue Ridge Medical Specialists, P.C.
Bristol, Tennessee
*Chapter 1. Cancer Prevention, Screening, and
  Early Detection*

Jeanne Held-Warmkessel, MSN, RN,
  AOCN®, ACNS-BC
Clinical Nurse Specialist
Fox Chase Cancer Center
Philadelphia, Pennsylvania
*Chapter 12. Cardiac, Gastrointestinal, Neuro-
  logic, and Ocular Toxicities*

Nancy G. Houlihan, RN, MA, AOCN®
Clinical Nurse Specialist, Survivorship
  Program
Memorial Sloan-Kettering Cancer Center
New York, New York
Chapter 17. Cancer Survivorship

Colleen O. Lee, MS, CRNP, AOCN®
Commander, United States Public Health
  Service
Practice Assessment Program Manager
National Institutes of Health, National Can-
  cer Institute
Office of Cancer Complementary and Alter-
  native Medicine
Rockville, Maryland
*Chapter 8. Complementary and Integrative
  Therapies*

Joanne Lester, PhD, CRNP, ANP-BC,
  AOCN®
Associate Director of Nursing Research
Clinical Nurse Scientist
Arthur G. James Cancer Hospital and Solove
  Research Institute
Clinical Assistant Professor, College of Nurs-
  ing
The Ohio State University
Columbus, Ohio
Chapter 5. Surgery

Suzanne M. Mahon, RN, DNSc, AOCN®,
  APNG
Clinical Professor
Internal Medicine Division of Hematology/
  Oncology
Saint Louis University
St. Louis, Missouri
Chapter 2. Genetic Risk

Sandra A. Mitchell, CRNP, PhD, AOCN®
Senior Research Nurse Specialist
Research and Practice Development
Oncology Nurse Practitioner
National Cancer Institute, National Insti-
  tutes of Health
Bethesda, Maryland
*Chapter 19. Roles of the Oncology Advanced
  Practice Nurse*

Jean M. Rosiak, RN, MSN, ANP-BC, AOCNP®
Oncology Nurse Practitioner
Aurora Health Care
Milwaukee, Wisconsin
*Chapter 10. Pain, Fatigue, and Cognitive Dys-
  function*

Kathy Sharp, MSN, FNP-BC, AOCNP®
Oncology Nurse Practitioner
Blue Ridge Medical Specialists, P.C.
Bristol, Tennessee
*Chapter 20. Professional Practice of Advanced
Practice Nurses*

Brenda K. Shelton, MS, RN, CCRN, AOCN®
Clinical Nurse Specialist
The Sidney Kimmel Comprehensive Cancer
Center at Johns Hopkins Hospital
Baltimore, Maryland
Chapter 11. Myelosuppression

Pamela Hallquist Viale, RN, MS, ANP, CS,
AOCNP®
Oncology Nurse Practitioner
Assistant Clinical Professor
University of California, San Francisco,
Department of Physiological Nursing
San Francisco, California
Chapter 3. Cancer Diagnosis and Staging

Gail M. Wilkes, RN, MS, ANP, AOCN®
Oncology Nurse Educator/NP
Boston Medical Center
Boston, Massachusetts
Chapter 4. Chemotherapy and Biotherapy

Contents

Chapter 19. Roles of the Oncology Advanced Practice Nurse 737

Chapter 20. Professional Practice of Advanced Practice Nurses 783

Chapter 21. Test Questions.......... 807

Index.. 849

Preface

The inspiration for writing the *Advanced Oncology Nursing Certification Review and Resource Manual* was in response to requests from past Oncology Nursing Society (ONS) advanced oncology certification review course participants for additional study resources. This book has two timely goals. The first goal is to provide a comprehensive review for oncology advanced practice nurses (APNs) who are preparing to sit for the Oncology Nursing Certification Corporation (ONCC) advanced oncology certified clinical nurse specialist (AOCNS®) or advanced oncology certified nurse practitioner (AOCNP®) examination.

The editors of this book also serve as faculty for the advanced oncology review course at the ONS annual meetings and for the future online review course. This educational experience, feedback from course participants, and the ONCC test bulletins have assisted in developing the content of each chapter. Authors were selected based on expertise in their respective areas, their clinical experience as practitioners, and advanced oncology certification status. This book will provide the foundation for a comprehensive review of advanced oncology nursing content.

Each chapter includes content on an advanced oncology nursing topic, key points to emphasize important concepts for the readers to review, and a case study with questions relevant to the most important topics within the chapter. This approach gives readers an opportunity to affirm their understanding of the content. In addition, practice test questions are offered in Chapter 21. These multiple-choice questions are similar in structure to questions used in the ONCC advanced practice certification exams. The editors believe that these varied methods of instruction address current adult learning principles.

Chapter content is correlated to the weight that ONCC has assigned to the specific topic on the certification exams. Topics are representative of the ONCC blueprints for the advanced oncology certification exams. The number of review questions per topic in Chapter 21 also is reflective of the weight that ONCC has assigned to the topic. These topic percentages may change periodically; therefore, test candidates are advised to refer to the most current test bulletin when preparing for a certification examination.

The most current oncology clinical evidence was used in the preparation of this book. Although it is beyond the scope of any review or resource book to completely cover the entire field of advanced oncology nursing, the editors believe the mastery of the content presented herein will give the readers a broader understanding of advanced oncology nursing. The use of this book does not guarantee successful completion of the advanced oncology nursing examination; however, the readers will be better prepared to identify areas where more in-depth study is required.

The second goal of the *Advanced Oncology Nursing Certification Review and Resource Manual* is to provide a comprehensive clinical resource for oncology APNs. This book will serve as a valuable resource to oncology APNs, graduate nursing students, medical residents, physician assistants, and oncology nurses in clinical practice. To achieve this goal, advanced oncology APN topics have been expanded beyond the scope of a review course to include the most current literature and clinical evidence available at the time of this writing. Certification examination questions generally are developed over a long period of time and may not always reflect the most current evidence. Each chapter contains useful, important, and timely references recommended by the expert and practicing APN authors. The editors believe these recommendations will assist in making this review book a valued resource for oncology clinicians.

It is the editors' hope that the *Advanced Oncology Nursing Certification Review and Resource Manual* will be a timely addition to the oncology nursing literature. We would like to acknowledge and thank our expert authors. We are indebted and grateful to the dedicated ONS Publishing Division staff and the faithful mentorship and friendship of Barbara Sigler, RN, MNEd, director of ONS Commercial Publishing.

Barbara Holmes Gobel
Shirley Triest-Robertson
Wendy H. Vogel

CHAPTER 1

Cancer Prevention, Screening, and Early Detection

Heather Greene, RN, MSN, FNP, AOCNP®

Introduction

In 2008, an estimated 1,437,180 new cases of cancer are expected to be diagnosed in the United States, and 565,650 are not expected to survive (American Cancer Society [ACS], 2008). Two-thirds of these cancer deaths will be related to tobacco use, poor nutrition, physical inactivity, and obesity. All cancer deaths related to tobacco and alcohol abuse are entirely preventable. Additionally, more than one million new cases of skin cancer are expected to be diagnosed this year, and many could be prevented by avoiding overexposure to the sun. Cancers related to viral and/or bacterial infections, such as the hepatitis B virus, human papillomavirus (HPV), HIV, and *Helicobacter,* also can be prevented through changes in lifestyle and use of vaccines or antibiotics (ACS, 2006b).

Deaths related to breast, colorectal, uterine, and cervical cancers could be decreased by greater use of screening tests (ACS, 2006c). Only 55% of women 40 years of age and older reported having had a mammogram within the past year, and 79% of adult women reported having had a Pap smear sometime within the past three years (ACS, 2006c). Fewer than half of all Americans have had recent screening for colorectal cancer, according to ACS (2006c). Half of all new cases of cancer are considered preventable or could be detected at an earlier stage. The five-year survival rate for early-stage cancers is 85%, hence the importance of following established screening and early detection guidelines (ACS, 2006b).

A recent analysis of 2005 data from the National Cancer Institute's (NCI's) Health Information Trends Study, which tracks how Americans obtain and use cancer information, documented that most Americans are aware of the current cancer screening modalities but are unsure of the age at which they need to implement these screening tests. Fifty-seven percent of women were unaware that mammography screening for breast cancer begins at age 40. Sixty-one percent of women were unaware of the correlation between HPV and cervical cancer. Forty percent of Americans surveyed could not name an appropriate screening test for colorectal cancer (NCI, 2005a, 2006b).

In addition to the general knowledge deficits listed here, cultural disparities also were identified in this study. Almost 80% of Hispanic respondents, 75% of African Americans, and 70% of American Indians/Alaska Natives were unaware of the appropriate age at which to begin screening for colorectal cancer, compared to 38% of Caucasians (NCI, 2006b). In general, African American men have higher incidence rates (19%) and higher mortality rates (37%) than Caucasian men (Jemal et al., 2008). African American women have a 6% lower incidence rate but a 17% higher death rate (Jemal et al.). Although part of this disparity is felt to be secondary to various differences in risk factors, knowledge deficits, difficulty with or lack of access to quality screening tests, and delayed diagnosis and treatment also greatly influence ethnic mortality rates (Jemal et al.).

Role of the Advanced Practice Nurse

Given the disparities identified among the general public, oncology advanced practice nurses (APNs) are in a unique position to educate their patients and the public regarding recommended cancer risk reduction and screening guidelines. The scope of practice for nurse practitioners includes an emphasis on health promotion and disease prevention (American Academy of Nurse Practitioners, 2002a, 2002b). The Oncology Nursing Society (ONS) recognizes "screening to prevent illness and promote wellness" as part of the role of the oncology APN (ONS, 2003). Therefore, cancer screening and prevention are clearly responsibilities of the oncology APN required to diagnose cancer at the earliest possible stage, if not prevent some cancers entirely.

It is also the position of ONS, as published in its 2002 position statement *Prevention and Early Detection of Cancer in the United States,* that APNs receive educational preparation in the principles of cancer prevention and early detection. Oncology specialty certification examinations (such as the advanced oncology certified nurse practitioner [AOCNP®] and advanced oncology certified clinical nurse specialist [AOCNS®] examinations) include coverage of this topic. In accordance with their state's scope of practice, nurse practice act, and requirements for educational preparation, oncology APNs must be able to assess, evaluate, and interpret cancer risk assessments and recommend appropriate strategies related to cancer prevention and screening. All oncology nurses must be able to provide culturally sensitive cancer prevention and early detection services and participate in the development of resources that focus on wellness and primary prevention throughout the life span. Evidence-based research on cancer prevention and early detection requires integration into current practice (ONS, 2002).

Cancer Risk Assessment

Cancer risk assessment is a vital part of the oncology APN's role in cancer prevention and early detection. To provide accurate counseling on cancer risk reduction strategies (e.g., tobacco cessation, lifestyle modifications, dietary changes, chemoprevention agents), cancer screening recommendations, and genetic testing (if appropriate), the oncology APN must first perform a comprehensive risk assessment. Cancer risk assessment is an individualized evaluation of a patient's risk for cancer based on a variety of both intrinsic and extrinsic factors and begins with a detailed history. This includes thorough past medical, obstetric/gynecologic, and surgical histories and documentation of recent age-appropriate screening tests, or lack thereof. Family history is a critical part of cancer risk assessment and includes at least a three-generation pedigree, particularly if a hereditary cancer syndrome is suspected (see Chapter 2). Medication history (such as hormone use), dietary history, level of physical activity, environmental exposures, history of tobacco and alcohol use, and other lifestyle choices also are important factors to assess when determining cancer risk. A thorough physical examination concludes the cancer risk assessment and includes a breast, pelvic, and rectal examination.

Some cancer risk assessment tools and models are available to help nurses to convey this risk to patients, such as the Gail model, Claus model, and BRCAPRO for breast cancer risk (Euhus, 2001) and the MMRpro model for hereditary colon cancer risk (Greco, 2007). Each of these tools has its strengths and weaknesses. The Gail model is the most commonly used general breast cancer risk assessment tool and is used to estimate a woman's five-year risk and overall lifetime risk for breast cancer. Scores are calculated based on a variety of risk factors, including age, age at menarche, age at first live birth, race, number of first-degree relatives with breast cancer, and number of previous breast biopsies. The score is based on a comparison to that of a woman of average risk and of the same race and age, with elevated risk considered > 1.7%. However, this model fails to take into account the age at breast cancer diagnosis in affected family members, history of bilateral breast cancer, second-degree relatives affected with breast cancer, and history of ovarian cancer or lobular carcinoma in situ (LCIS). Both the BRCAPRO and Claus models lack accurate risk assessment for minority women and factors other than family history (such as number of previous breast biopsies), and BRCAPRO may fail to identify hereditary breast cancer syndromes that do not conform to *BRCA* mutations (Euhus).

Some cancer risk assessment tools are available online, such as a lung cancer risk assessment tool through Memorial Sloan-Kettering Cancer Center (www.mskcc.org/mskcc/html/12463.cfm), the CancerGene software from the University of Texas Southwestern Medical Center for Breast Care (www.utsouthwestern.edu/utsw/cda/dept47829/files/65844.html), and the NCI's breast cancer risk assessment tool (www.cancer.gov/bcrisktool/default.aspx). The majority of cancers do not have reliable risk assessment tools, and those that do still have weaknesses. Therefore, these models are best used in conjunction with an individualized, comprehensive cancer risk assessment by the APN to best estimate and counsel patients on their overall cancer risk and on interventions to decrease that risk.

Primary Prevention and Risk Reduction

Cancer prevention is achieved through primary, secondary, and tertiary methods. Primary cancer prevention is achieved through two mechanisms: the promotion of health and wellness and reduction of risks known to contribute to cancer development (ONS, 2002). Primary prevention aims to reverse or inhibit the carcinogenic process through modifications in a patient's diet or environment or through pharmacologic mechanisms (Turini & DuBois, 2002). Examples of primary prevention include smoking cessation interventions and chemoprophylaxis in women at high risk for breast cancer. Secondary cancer prevention includes screening and early detection. In general, screening for cancer refers to checking for the presence of disease in populations at risk, and early detection is defined as testing for cancer when no symptoms are present (ONS, 2002). Secondary prevention seeks to detect cancer at the earliest possible stage, when the disease is most likely to be treated successfully. Tertiary cancer prevention is applied to those individuals who have already been diagnosed with a malignancy but are now candidates for screening and early detection of secondary malignancies (ONS, 2002).

Tobacco Use

Smoking has long been established as a detriment to overall health. As early as 1928, studies pointed to smoking and its association with cancer (Koh, Kannler, & Geller, 2001; Lombard & Doering, 1928). Research culminated with the 1964 U.S. Surgeon General's report, which concluded that smoking was the major cause of lung cancer and was associated with oral and laryngeal cancers in men. Since then, more than 60,000 studies and subsequent reports of the Surgeon General have confirmed tobacco's detrimental health effects (Koh et al.). More than 4,000 chemicals have been identified in tobacco products and tobacco smoke, 55 of which are identified as carcinogens by the International Agency for Research on Cancer (IARC). These carcinogens may induce genetic mutations and ultimately lead to cancer development (Koh et al.). Tobacco use is considered a contributing or causative agent in a multitude of malignancies, including oral, laryngeal, lung, renal, bladder, cervical, gastric, and esophageal cancers, in addition to leukemia (Centers for Disease Control and Prevention [CDC], 2004). Smoking is thought to cause up to 90% of lung cancers and is the leading cause of preventable cancer-related and non–cancer-related deaths in the United States (Koh et al.). Lung cancer is estimated to be diagnosed in close to 215,020 Americans in 2008, of which approximately 161,840 will die, encompassing approximately 30% of all cancer deaths (ACS, 2008).

Tobacco abuse and addiction is perhaps one of the greatest public health concerns of our time, particularly as far as cancer is concerned. In 2005, approximately 21% of adult Americans smoked—equal to 45 million people (Mariolis et al., 2006).

Most adult smokers today began smoking in their youth. Experimentation with cigarette smoking often begins early in adolescence and peaks at 13–14 years of age. Although the smoking rates in adults have been declining in the past decade, smoking prevalence in youths has risen dramatically since the 1990s (Fiore et al., 2000). It is estimated that about 4,000 adolescents per day are smoking for the first time, and more than one-fourth of them will become regular users of tobacco (Lindblom & McMahon, 2006). The percentage of high school students smoking declined from 1997 to 2003; however, from 2003 to 2005, the rate of decline slowed, if not stalled (ACS, 2006b; CDC, 2006a). More than 23% of high school–aged adolescents are current smokers (Lindblom & McMahon). Healthy People 2010 includes reducing smoking prevalence among high school students to 16% or less as one of its objectives. These statistics suggest the emergence of a new generation of smokers unless interventions are implemented to cease tobacco use among adolescents (CDC, 2006a).

Given these startling statistics, primary prevention measures for tobacco-related cancers and tobacco deterrent programs must be aimed at children and adolescents. Recent research shows that adolescents are three times more sensitive to tobacco advertising than adults and are more likely to be influenced to smoke by advertisements for cigarettes than by peer pressure (Lindblom & McMahon, 2006). Tobacco prevention efforts include increased tobacco prices and taxes, public smoking restrictions, and anti-tobacco advertisements. Many studies have identified the aforementioned tobacco control efforts as being successful in reducing adolescent smoking rates. In 2000, one study estimated that through large-scale media campaigns and a mere $1 increase in the price per pack of cigarettes, the prevalence of smoking among 18 year olds could be reduced by 26% in the United States and 108,466 lives could be saved (Rivara et al., 2004). This study concluded that efforts to reduce adolescent smoking can affect adult health and mortality. Moreover, continued efforts are needed to focus on implementing statewide tobacco bans; 15 states had done this as of 2006 (ACS, 2006b). Monies to promote tobacco control are also needed—the tobacco industry spent more than $15 billion on marketing in 2003, which is 23 times the amount spent on tobacco control efforts (ACS, 2006b).

Smoking Cessation

Despite the known consequences of tobacco abuse on health and society and the proven benefits of smoking cessation (see Table 1-1), most clinicians fail to identify and counsel patients on this topic (Fiore et al., 2000). Reasons for this include inability to quickly identify current tobacco users and a knowledge deficit about what treatments are effective, how they are delivered, and the associated side effects of treatment. Time constraints and lack of institutional support for tobacco cessation counseling also may contribute to the fact that only 21% of clinic visits with current smokers included smoking cessation counseling (Fiore et al.).

Identification of current tobacco users can be achieved by asking all patients at every visit about their smoking status and whether they are interested in quitting. It also may be beneficial to document tobacco use as the fifth vital sign on the chart. It is estimated that up to 70% of current smokers want to quit, but more than a third of those are never asked about their smoking status or desire to quit (Fiore et al., 2000). Even if patients have attempted smoking cessation in the past and have failed, several attempts at smoking cessation are common before long-term abstinence is achieved (Fiore et al.; Rigotti, 2002).

The U.S. Department of Health and Human Services' (DHHS's) *Treating Tobacco Use and Dependence: Clinical Practice Guideline* (Fiore et al., 2000) is a brief set of instructions

Table 1-1. Health Benefits of Smoking Cessation

Elapsed Time After Smoking Cessation	Health Benefits
2 weeks–3 months	Circulation, skin tone, oral hygiene, and pulmonary function improve.
1–9 months	Ciliary function in the lungs is restored.
12 months	Risk for coronary heart disease is reduced by 50% compared to persistent smokers.
5–15 years	Risk of stroke is decreased to that of nonsmokers.
10 years	Risk of death from lung cancer is reduced by 50% compared to persistent smokers.
15 years	Risk of coronary heart disease is reduced to that of nonsmokers.

Note. Based on information from Fiore et al., 2000.

for clinicians to use in identifying and treating nicotine dependence. ONS (2005) recommends the use of these instructions in all clinical settings in its position *Global and Domestic Tobacco Abuse*. As discussed previously, the first step in treating tobacco dependence is identifying tobacco users. Once identified, smokers can be categorized into one of two groups—those who are interested in making a quit attempt and those who are not. For those patients willing to attempt cessation, the guideline suggests using the "five A's" strategy as listed in Table 1-2 (Fiore et al.).

Table 1-2. The Five A's of Smoking Cessation Counseling

"A"	Intervention
Ask	Ask about tobacco status of every patient at every visit.
Advise	Advise tobacco users to quit in a strong, clear, and personalized manner.
Assess	Assess the patient's readiness to quit.
Assist	Assist in the patient's quit attempt (individualized counseling and pharmacotherapy).
Arrange	Arrange follow-up within one week of the stated quit date.

Note. Based on information from Fiore et al., 2000.

Oftentimes, inadequate knowledge of tobacco cessation therapy inhibits clinicians' ability to assist patients in their quit attempt. Successful smoking cessation interventions contain two components: behavioral counseling and pharmacotherapy. The combined use of these approaches has been shown to improve smoking cessation rates (Fiore et al., 2000; Ranney, Melvin, Lux, McClain, & Lohr, 2006; Rigotti, 2002). Most studies estimate successful smoking cessation rates to be 40%–60% using this combination. This drops to 25%–30% after one year, but it is still higher than the less than 10% of smokers who attain long-term abstinence on their own (Fiore et al.; Rigotti).

Behavioral counseling begins by identifying triggers and stressors unique to each individual smoker. These can be moods, feelings, places, or activities. Some of the most common stressors and triggers include feeling stressed or depressed, talking on the phone or watching television, drinking alcohol or coffee, driving, finishing a meal, managing work and family issues, taking a work break, being with other smokers or seeing someone else smoke, cooling off after a fight, feeling lonely, and having sex (Rigotti, 2002). Making the patient aware of his or her triggers is a valuable method of assisting the patient to stay in control. Once the triggers and stressors have been identified, teaching the patient to cope with these patient-specific triggers involves avoiding these trigger situations and replacing old habits with new ones (Rigotti).

All tobacco users are advised to quit smoking at every encounter (Fiore et al., 2000; Ranney et al., 2006). Even if the individual is uninterested in making a quit attempt at that particular time, discussing the process, benefits, and perceived barriers to smoking cessation can propel the patient closer to seriously contemplating quitting. Therefore, for those who are not willing to attempt cessation, motivational support can be offered using the "five R's," listed in Table 1-3 (Fiore et al.).

In addition to behavioral counseling, pharmacotherapy may benefit all smokers ready to make a quit attempt (with the exception of certain populations, such as ado-

Table 1-3. The Five R's of Smoking Cessation Counseling

"R"	Intervention
Relevance	Encourage personal relevance of smoking cessation (i.e., health status, impact on family members, economic impact).
Risks	Ask the patient to identify risks of continued tobacco use that are pertinent to the patient, including acute (shortness of breath), chronic (cancer, chronic obstructive pulmonary disease), and environmental risks (cancers and lung diseases in the smoker's spouse and children).
Rewards	Ask the patient to identify potential rewards of smoking cessation, including immediate and long term (e.g., improved overall health for individual and family, money saved).
Roadblocks	Ask the patient to identify potential or actual barriers to smoking cessation (e.g., withdrawal symptoms, weight gain).
Repetition	Repeat the five R's at every encounter with the patient. Also, repeated attempts at smoking cessation are common among smokers.

Note. Based on information from Fiore et al., 2000.

lescents, those with specific medical contraindications, and pregnant women) (Fiore et al., 2000; Ranney et al., 2006). Currently, seven U.S. Food and Drug Administration (FDA)-approved first-line therapies are available—five types of nicotine replacement therapy (NRT) (transdermal, oral lozenges, gum, nasal spray, and oral inhaler) and two non-nicotine medications, bupropion sustained release (SR) and varenicline (FDA, 2006a; Fiore et al.; Ranney et al.). Studies show that NRT with or without the use of other FDA-approved medications increases smoking cessation success (Pray & Pray, 2003; Ranney et al.); most studies show a twofold increase in cessation rates with NRT alone over placebo (Fiore et al.; Rigotti, 2002). Most forms of NRT are easy to use and available over the counter, with prices equivalent to or less than cigarettes, depending on the patient's habit. NRT dosing, cost, contraindications, and common side effects are listed in Table 1-4.

Whether through routine office visits or in clinics designed specifically for smoking cessation therapy, several studies have identified the successful role of the APN in smoking cessation interventions (Andrews, Tingen, & Harper, 1999; Christman & Bingham, 1989; Nett & Obrigewitch, 1993; Reeve, Calabro, & Adams-McNeill, 2000). In addition to using the DHHS's guidelines, APNs can take other steps to improve smoking cessation awareness and therapy. For instance, studies have shown that longer, more intensive and individualized interventions for smoking cessation result in higher abstinence rates, up to 40% in some cases (Andrews et al.; Fiore et al., 2000). APNs can have patients set a quit date and sign a smoking cessation contract to facilitate ongoing commitment to their quit attempt. The Fagerstrom Test for Nicotine Dependence (Heatherton, Kozlowski, Frecker, & Fagerstrom, 1991) is a tool used to identify levels of nicotine dependence and thus gear more or less intense interventions accordingly. Oncology APNs are in a unique position to guide patients along the continuum of nicotine dependence—from indentifying tobacco users to providing behavioral counseling and prescriptive and nonprescriptive NRT and aiding in relapse prevention or treatment.

Table 1-4. Nicotine Replacement Therapy

Drug	Dose	Common Side Effects	Precautions/ Contraindications	Cost
Bupropion SR	150 mg every day for 3 days, then bid	Insomnia, dry mouth	History of seizures or eating disorder	~ $3.33/day; prescription
Nicotine gum	2 mg (< 25 cig/day) 4 mg (> 25 cig/day); not to exceed 24 pieces in 24 hours	Dyspepsia, mouth soreness	Dentures may prohibit proper use.	< $7 for 10 of the 2 mg or 4 mg pieces; over the counter
Nicotine inhaler	6–16 cartridges/day	Mouth and/or throat irritation	–	~ $11 for 10 cartridges; prescription
Nicotine lozenges	2 mg and 4 mg; 9–20 lozenges/day	Mouth irritation, nausea, dyspepsia	–	~ $43 for 72-count box
Nicotine nasal spray	8–40 doses/day	Nasal irritation	–	~ $5 for 12 doses; prescription
Nicotine patch	For use > 10 cig/ day: 21 mg every day for 6 weeks, 14 mg every day for 2 weeks, 7 mg every day for 2 weeks	Local skin irritation	–	≤ $4/day; prescription and over the counter
Varenicline (Chantix™, Pfizer Inc.)	0.5 mg once a day for 3 days, then bid for 4 days, then 1 mg bid for total of 12 weeks	Insomnia, nausea	Contraindicated in ages < 18 and during pregnancy or lactation	~ $124/month; prescription; insurance coverage varies.

Note. Based on information from Fiore et al., 2000.

Sun Exposure

Overexposure to the sun is the greatest risk factor for all types of skin cancer, including melanoma and basal and squamous cell cancers (ACS, 2006c; Hegde & Gause, 2005; Wagner & Casciato, 2004). More than one million people are diagnosed with skin cancer each year; 90% of nonmelanoma skin cancers and 65% of melanomas are felt to be directly related to ultraviolet (UV) rays from the sun (U.S. Environmental Protection Agency [EPA], 2006).

UV radiation is a known carcinogen, and two types can affect the skin—UVA and UVB. UVA rays penetrate deeper layers of the skin and are responsible for premature aging effects on the skin, whereas UVB rays mainly affect the epidermis and are the primary cause of sunburn (Brannon, 2007; EPA, 2006). UVB rays vary depending on the season and time of day. Engaging in regular activities to decrease exposure to or protect the skin from UV rays can significantly reduce the risk of skin cancer (ACS, 2006c). Primary prevention of skin cancer includes avoiding UV light as much as possible. ACS (2006c) recommends avoiding exposure to direct sunlight from 10 am to 4 pm, when UV rays are known to be most intense. Avoiding artificial sources of UV light exposure, such as with tanning beds, also is crucial in reducing the risk of skin cancer (ACS, 2006c). According to a recent study, exposure to artificial sunlight increased the risk of basal cell skin cancer by 1.5 and the risk of squamous cell skin cancer by 2.5 (Karagas et al., 2002).

In addition to minimizing exposure to the sun, other sun protective behaviors include protecting the skin with proper clothing and sunscreen. ACS (2007) recommends the following four sun protective measures.

- Slip on a shirt.
- Slop on sunscreen.
- Slap on a hat.
- Wrap on sunglasses.

Wearing hats with wide brims, shirts and pants that adequately cover the extremities, and sunglasses to protect the eyes and covering the rest of exposed skin with sunscreen with a sun protective factor (SPF) of 15 or higher are all pertinent sun protective behaviors (ACS, 2006c, 2006e). Broad-spectrum sunscreens contain ingredients that block or absorb both UVA and UVB rays with chemicals such as avobenzone, titanium dioxide, and zinc oxide (ACS, 2006e; Brannon, 2007; EPA, 2006). The FDA requires that all sunscreens contain an SPF, which correlates to the level of protection from UVB rays. For example, a sunscreen with an SPF of 15 protects against 93% of the sun's UVB rays, and every 15 minutes of wearing sunscreen with an SPF of 15 is equivalent to one minute of UVB exposure without sunscreen (ACS, 2006e; EPA).

In general, use approximately one ounce of sunscreen to cover all exposed areas of skin, enough to form a thin film when first applied (ACS, 2006e; Brannon, 2007). Sunscreen should be applied 30 minutes before exposure to the sun and reapplied every two hours and again after swimming, sweating, or toweling off (ACS, 2006e; Brannon; EPA, 2006). Sunscreens labeled "water resistant" maintain their SPF for 40 minutes of water immersion, and those that are "very water resistant" maintain their SPF for 80 minutes (ACS, 2006e; EPA), but both need routine reapplication. Sunscreen is applied before makeup. When used in combination with insect repellant, sunscreen with a higher SPF should be applied because repellants can reduce sunscreen's effectiveness by up to one-third (ACS, 2006e; Brannon). Most sunscreens expire after one year and should be discarded (ACS, 2006e).

Diet and Exercise

More than 60 million Americans are obese, equal to roughly 30% of the adult population in this country (CDC, 2005). The National Institutes of Health defines obesity in adults older than 20 as having a body mass index higher than 30 (NCI, 2004a). Maintaining a healthy diet and lifestyle is an important way to reduce the risk of a variety of cancers (ACS, 2006c). In 2002, the IARC reported a positive relationship between obesity and the incidence of several cancers, including postmenopausal breast cancer and cancers of the colon, endometrium, esophagus, and kidney (NCI, 2004a, 2007c). Some correlation also has been identified in cancers of the gallbladder, ovaries, and pancreas (NCI, 2004a). In 2002, an estimated 41,000 cases of cancer were related to obesity (Polednak, 2003). Obesity is linked to cancer mortality as well. Obesity is estimated to account for up to one in seven cancer-related deaths in men and one in five cancer-related deaths in women (Calle, Rodriguez, Walker-Thurmond, & Thun, 2003). Obesity increases the risk of dying from cancers of the esophagus, colon, liver, gallbladder, pancreas, and kidney, in addition to non-Hodgkin lymphoma and multiple myeloma (Calle et al.). Obese women have an increased risk of dying from breast, endometrial, cervical, and ovarian cancers, and obese men are at increased risk of dying from prostate and gastric cancers (Calle et al.).

Several reasons account for the drastic increase in the prevalence of obesity in the United States over the past several decades. In general, Americans are eating foods that are higher in calories, fats, and sugars. These foods often are cheaper and marketed more intensely than healthier food choices and are served in large portions by fast-food chains and restaurants (ACS, 2006c). In 2003, the IARC published research showing the cancer-reducing effects of eating a diet high in fruits and vegetables (ACS, 2006c). Studies have shown that regular intake of vegetables decreases the risk of oral, pharyngeal, and laryngeal cancers, in addition to esophageal, gastric, lung, renal, and ovarian cancers (ACS, 2006c). Furthermore, the risk of developing colorectal and bladder cancers is decreased with regular consumption of fruits (ACS, 2006c). Yet, recent reports show that only 23.5% of Americans consume the recommended five servings of fruits and vegetables daily (ACS, 2006c).

While obesity rates are climbing in the United States, levels of physical activity continue to decline, further contributing to the obesity epidemic (ACS, 2008). However, as obesity is linked to increased cancer incidence and mortality, physical activity is associated with a decreased risk of breast, colon, endometrial, lung, and prostate cancers (NCI, 2004b). Unfortunately, more than half of all Americans do not engage in regular physical activity (CDC, 2005). The CDC recommends engaging in moderate physical activity for at least 30 minutes five or more days a week or vigorous activity for at least 20 minutes three or more days per week (CDC, 2006b). ACS also has outlined recommendations for diet and exercise (see Table 1-5) to promote physical activity and combat obesity (ACS, 2006a).

Chemoprevention

Chemoprevention is defined as the use of natural, synthetic, or biologic agents to reverse, suppress, or prevent carcinogenic progression (Tsao, Kim, & Hong, 2004). Chemoprevention primarily is aimed at inhibition or differentiation of cell growth or induction of cell apoptosis (Turini & DuBois, 2002). A variety of agents are being studied, and some have been approved for the prevention of prostate, colon, and breast cancer. To date, no effective chemopreventive agents have been approved for common malignancies such as lung cancer or skin cancer (Tsao et al.). Moreover, certain risks are associated with chemopreventive drugs, such as unwanted side effects and the potential to cause more harm or even higher rates of malignancy, which occurred with the Alpha-Tocopherol, Beta-Carotene Cancer Prevention Trial (ATBC Trial) and the Beta-Carotene and Retinol Efficacy Trial (CARET) (NCI, 1997). In these two studies, no benefit was seen from taking supplements in men at high risk for lung cancer. In fact, in participants taking beta-carotene in the ATBC Trial, 18% more lung cancers were diagnosed, and 8% more deaths occurred. In CARET, 28% more lung cancers were diagnosed, and 17% more deaths occurred in participants taking beta-carotene and vitamin A than in those taking placebos (Clark et al., 1996; Heinonen et al., 1998; NCI, 2006c).

The oncology APN plays an important role in chemoprevention, either through risk assessments that lead to identification of potential candidates for chemopreventive agents, referral to appropriate clinical trials, or referral to qualified colleagues for further evaluation and management. Certain oncology APNs have subspecialized in the area of

Table 1-5. Guidelines on Nutrition and Physical Activity for Cancer Prevention

Topic	Recommendations
Diet	Consume ≥ 5 servings of fruits and vegetables daily. Limit consumption of foods high in fat, such as red meat. Choose whole grains over processed or refined grains and sugars. Limit alcoholic beverages to less than one per day.
Exercise	Adults: Engage in moderate physical activity for at least 30 minutes at least 5 days per week. Children and adolescents: Engage in at least 60 minutes of moderate to vigorous physical activity at least 5 days per week.
Weight control	Balance caloric intake with caloric expenditure. Maintain a healthy weight through the aforementioned diet and exercise guidelines.

Note. Based on information from American Cancer Society, 2006a.

risk assessment, genetics counseling, and chemoprevention and are excellent sources of referral or collaboration (Vogel, 2003).

Tamoxifen and Raloxifene

In 1998, the FDA approved tamoxifen, a selective estrogen receptor modulator (SERM), for the prevention of invasive breast cancer after results from the Breast Cancer Prevention Trial showed a 49% reduction in invasive breast cancer in more than 13,000 high-risk pre- and postmenopausal women (Fisher et al., 2005). Tamoxifen was approved for the prevention of invasive breast cancer for women with a history of noninvasive breast cancer (ductal carcinoma in situ [DCIS] and lobular carcinoma in situ [LCIS]) (Fisher et al.). Tamoxifen is most effective in preventing estrogen receptor–positive breast cancers. Women who benefited most were those with a known genetic predisposition for *BRCA1* or *BRCA2* mutation, history of LCIS, or atypical ductal hyperplasia (Fisher et al.). Additional benefits yielded from the study included a 29% decrease in the risk of osteoporotic bone fractures in women ages 50 and older and a 53% decrease in women younger than 50 (Fisher et al.). Risks associated with tamoxifen use include a higher incidence of thromboembolic events and endometrial cancer (Fisher et al.). Because of these and other risks, the use of tamoxifen is individualized.

Results from the Study of Tamoxifen and Raloxifene recently revealed that raloxifene, a second-generation SERM, has similar effects in reducing invasive breast cancer in high-risk, postmenopausal women as tamoxifen (Vogel et al., 2006). Additionally, fewer cases of uterine cancer, thromboembolic events, and cataracts were seen with raloxifene. Raloxifene was associated with an insignificantly higher number of patients with noninvasive breast cancer compared to tamoxifen (Vogel et al.). Raloxifene is approved for breast cancer risk reduction in postmenopausal women at high risk for invasive breast cancer.

Celecoxib

Aspirin and nonsteroidal anti-inflammatory drugs (NSAIDs) have shown activity in the treatment and prevention of colon cancer; however, their gastrointestinal side effects have limited their applicability (Price, 2002; Turini & DuBois, 2002). Newer NSAIDs, such as celecoxib, selectively inhibit cyclooxygenase-2 (COX-2), a catalytic enzyme in prostaglandin synthesis that is induced in inflammatory conditions, including those involved with tumor proliferation. COX-2 is not normally found in the epithelium of the colon but is overexpressed in a majority of adenocarcinomas and less so in adenomatous polyps of the colon (Price; Turini & DuBois). Celecoxib, at 400 mg bid, has received approval from the FDA for the prevention of adenomatous polyps in patients with familial adenomatous polyposis (FAP) (Price), a hereditary colon cancer syndrome associated with hundreds of thousands of colon polyps and a 100% risk of colorectal cancer if untreated. Celecoxib is not approved for chemoprevention in the general public.

Selenium and Vitamin E

The Selenium and Vitamin E Trial (SELECT) aims to determine the efficacy of these two supplements in preventing prostate cancer. It also aims to identify their effects on lung and colon cancer prevention, although these are not primary end points (NCI, 2005b). Two previous studies alluded to the benefits of selenium and vitamin E on the incidence of prostate cancer, but this was not the studies' primary objective. The Nutritional Prevention of Cancer Trial aimed to determine the relationship between selenium and nonmelanomatous skin cancers. The trial did not do this, but it did identify 60% fewer cases of prostate cancer in men who took selenium for 6.5 years (Clark et al., 1996; NCI, 2005b). In addition to the results of the ATBC Trial discussed earlier, the men taking vitamin E for the prevention of lung cancer were noted to have 32% fewer cases of prostate cancer (Heinonen et al., 1998; NCI, 2005b). SELECT data on more than 35,000 men are expected in 2011 (NCI, 2005b).

Gardasil® Vaccine

In June 2006, the FDA approved Gardasil® (Merck & Co.) (quadrivalent human papillomavirus recombinant vaccine) for the prevention of cervical cancer, precancerous or dysplastic cervical and vaginal lesions, and genital warts associated with HPV types 6, 11, 16, and 18 (FDA, 2006b). This is the first vaccine approved for cervical cancer prevention, and in clinical trials, it showed nearly 100% effectiveness in preventing precancerous cervical, vaginal, and vulvar lesions and genital warts caused by HPV in women who had not yet been infected (FDA, 2006b). Hence, it is important to administer the vaccine in women who have not been exposed to HPV. Gardasil is approved for use in women aged 9–26 years old and is given as a set of three injections over six months (FDA, 2006b). The most common side effects associated with this vaccine included injection site reactions in the form of erythema, pain, edema, fever, nausea, and headache (Saslow et al., 2007). Gardasil is not approved to treat cervical cancer, nor is it intended to replace routine cervical cancer screening (Saslow et al., 2007). Its impact on cervical cancer incidence and mortality will take decades of vaccinations before becoming evident; however, researchers have suggested a possible 70% reduction in cervical cancer incidence worldwide (Saslow et al., 2007).

ACS has recommended routine HPV vaccination in girls aged 11–12 years and also for those aged 13–18 who need to complete the vaccination series and to provide vaccination to those who may have missed the opportunity to be vaccinated previously. ACS does not support routine vaccination of women aged 19–26 years old because of insufficient evidence for this age group (Smith, Cokkinides, & Eyre, 2007).

Secondary Prevention and Screening

According to NCI (2007d), screening for cancer in the general population refers to detecting cancer when no apparent symptoms are present, with an overall goal of decreasing cancer-related morbidity and mortality. For almost all types of cancer, improved outcomes are seen when treatment is initiated at the earliest stage possible (NCI, 2007d), hence the importance of early detection. For example, breast, colorectal, cervical, testicular, oral cavity, and skin cancers—which account for half of all cancer cases diagnosed in the United States each year—collectively have a five-year survival rate of approximately 80% but could be improved to 95% if all Americans adhered to routine screening recommendations (ACS, 2006b).

For cancer screening to be effective, screening tests must meet two criteria. First, the screening test must be able to detect cancer at an earlier stage than if it were detected as a result of the development of symptoms. Second, evidence must support that treatment given at an earlier stage results in improved outcomes (NCI, 2007d). The sensitivity and specificity of all screening tests must be considered. *Sensitivity* refers to the proportion of people with cancer that are found to have a positive test—a higher sensitivity means fewer false negative results. Conversely, *specificity* refers to the proportion of people without cancer that have negative results; in other words, the higher the specificity, the fewer false positive results (NCI, 2006a). Potential harms from screening tests also must be weighed against potential benefits. Some screening tests are invasive, such as colonoscopy for colon cancer, and carry risks associated with any invasive procedure, including some serious if not life-threatening complications (such as bowel perforation with colonoscopy) (NCI, 2007d). Other potential harms include the emotional anxiety associated with false-positive results and the dangers of missing an early malignancy with false-negative test results (NCI, 2007d). The financial cost of different screening tests varies widely. Insurance coverage or lack thereof may prohibit individuals from following recommended screening guidelines. For instance, in 2003, only 29% of women without health insurance had received a mammogram within the past year, compared to almost 60% of women with coverage (ACS, 2005).

Multiple organizations recognized in the oncology community have published screening guidelines for a variety of malignancies, both for average-risk and high-risk populations. The oncology APN must have an understanding of each organization's guidelines and realize the differences among them. However, one may opt to follow and recommend one set of guidelines on a routine basis simply because of familiarity with that set of guidelines and ease of use. No one set of guidelines is superior to the other. In general, consensus exists among screening recommendations for the most common malignancies, including breast, cervical, colorectal, and prostate cancer. Variances in screening intervals and ages of screening initiation and cessation are minute. The recommended routine guidelines from ACS, the American Society of Clinical Oncology (ASCO), ONS, and the National Comprehensive Cancer Network (NCCN) are outlined in Table 1-6.

Breast Cancer

Breast cancer is the most common female malignancy and the second most common cause of cancer death in women (ACS, 2008). In 2008, an estimated 182,460 new cases of breast cancer are expected to be diagnosed (ACS, 2008). The risk of developing breast cancer increases with age and is most common in women; however, approximately 1,990

Table 1-6. Cancer Screening Recommendations for Average-Risk Population

Organization	Breast Cancer	Cervical Cancer	Colorectal Cancer	Prostate Cancer	Skin Cancer
National Comprehensive Cancer Network	For women of average risk between 20–40 years of age: • Clinical breast exam (CBE) every 1–3 years and periodic breast self-exam (BSE) are recommended. For women > 40: • Annual mammogram (MMG) and CBE and periodic BSE are recommended.	Screen with Pap test within 3 years of vaginal intercourse, but starting no later than 21 years of age; continue annually with conventional cervical cytology or every 2 years using liquid-based cytology (vaginal cytology is not indicated in women who have had a total hysterectomy). At age 30, if there have been 3 consecutive normal Pap tests, screening intervals can increase to every 2–3 years. Screening can cease at age 70 with 3 or more consecutive normal Pap tests within the previous 10 years. Continue screening despite age if history of cervical cancer, diethylstilbestrol (DES) exposure, or immunocompromised states. Human papillomavirus (HPV)-positive women continue screening at the discretion of their healthcare providers.	Average risk (age ≥ 50, no history of adenoma, inflammatory bowel disease [IBD], or family history of colon cancer): • Colonoscopy every 10 years is preferred or fecal occult blood test (FOBT) annually and flexible sigmoidoscopy every 5 years or double contrast barium enema (DCBE) every 5 years.	Risk/benefit discussion and offer baseline prostate-specific antigen (PSA) testing and digital rectal exam (DRE) at 40: • PSA ≥ 0.6 ng/ml, or African American, or positive family history: Screen with PSA and DRE annually. • Otherwise, repeat PSA and DRE at age 45. • PSA ≤ 0.6 ng/ml: Begin annual screening at age 50. • PSA > 0.6 ng/ml: Perform annual follow-up.	Not applicable

(Continued on next page)

Table 1-6. Cancer Screening Recommendations for Average-Risk Population *(Continued)*

Organization	Breast Cancer	Cervical Cancer	Colorectal Cancer	Prostate Cancer	Skin Cancer
American Cancer Society	Yearly MMG beginning at age 40 and continuing as long as the woman is in good health CBE every 3 years for women in 20s and 30s and annually if ≥ 40 BSE is optional for women beginning in their 20s.	Pap test annually (or every 2 years with liquid-based Pap test) beginning within 3 years of vaginal intercourse or starting by age 21 At ≥ 30, women with 3 consecutive normal Pap tests continue with Pap test screening every 2–3 years. Women ≥ 70 years old with ≥ 3 consecutive normal Pap tests within the previous 10 years can cease screening. Continue screening despite age if history of DES exposure or immunocompromised states. If woman has had total hysterectomy, may stop screening unless surgery was for cervical cancer or premalignant findings.	At age 50, one of the following tests (with all positive tests followed with colonoscopy): • Yearly FOBT or fecal immunochemical test (FIT) • Flexible sigmoidoscopy every 5 years • Yearly FOBT or FIT, plus flexible sigmoidoscopy (preferred over either alone) • DCBE every 5 years • Colonoscopy every 10 years Discuss early screening if patient has one of the following: • Personal history of colorectal cancer or adenomatous polyps • Family history of colorectal cancer or polyps in first-degree relative < 60 years of age or in two first-degree relatives of any age • Personal history of IBD • Family history of a hereditary colorectal cancer syndrome (familial adenomatous polyposis or hereditary nonpolyposis colorectal cancer)	Annual PSA and DRE beginning at age 50 (if patient has > 10-year life expectancy) High-risk men: • African American men and men with one or more first-degree relatives diagnosed with prostate cancer before age 65: Annual screening at age 45 • Multiple first-degree relatives with prostate cancer at an early age: Consider testing at earlier than age 40; depending on results, may opt to resume screening at age 45.	Not applicable

(Continued on next page)

Table 1-6. Cancer Screening Recommendations for Average-Risk Population *(Continued)*

Organization	Breast Cancer	Cervical Cancer	Colorectal Cancer	Prostate Cancer	Skin Cancer
Oncology Nursing Society	Offer BSE teaching to women older than 20 and the option to perform these monthly. CBE annually beginning at age 20 Annual MMG beginning at age 40	Not applicable	Not applicable	Not applicable	Not applicable
American Society of Clinical Oncology	Monthly BSE and regular physical exam by healthcare provider beginning at age 20 Annual MMG beginning at age 40	Initial Pap test 3 years after beginning sexual intercourse, but starting no later than age 21, and then once every 2–3 years	Beginning at age 50: Annual FOBT, flexible sigmoidoscopy every 5 years, colonoscopy every 10 years, or DCBE every 5 years	Annual PSA and DRE beginning at age 50	Periodic skin self-examination and annual whole body skin examination by healthcare provider, especially after age 40

Note. Based on information from American Cancer Society, 2006a; American Society of Clinical Oncology, 2005; National Comprehensive Cancer Network, 2007a, 2007b, 2007c, 2007d; Oncology Nursing Society, 2002, 2006.

cases of breast cancer are expected to be diagnosed in men in 2008 (ACS, 2008). Other risk factors for breast cancer are linked to reproductive and lifestyle factors (see Figure 1-1). A variety of benign breast lesions also increase the relative risk of breast cancer, depending on the histology (see Table 1-7). Factors that were previously thought to affect risk, but actually do not, include multiparity, lactation, and breast-feeding (Box & Russell, 2004). Factors known to decrease risk include Asian ancestry, early menopause, term pregnancy before age 18, and surgical menopause before age 37 (Box & Russell).

Modifiable Risk Factors
- Recent oral contraceptive use or hormone replacement therapy
- Nulliparity or first birth after age 30
- Postmenopausal obesity
- Sedentary lifestyle
- Consumption of one or more alcoholic beverages per day
- Consumption of diet high in fat and low in fruit and vegetable intake

Irreversible Risk Factors
- Female gender
- Caucasian
- Advanced age
- Inherited genetic mutation *(BRCA1/2)*
- Personal or family history of breast cancer
- Atypical hyperplasia and other benign breast lesions (see Table 1-7)
- History of high-dose radiation to the chest (as with mantle field radiation in Hodgkin lymphoma)
- Early menarche and late menopause

Figure 1-1. Risk Factors for Breast Cancer

Note. Based on information from American Cancer Society, 2006b; Morrow & Jordan, 2003.

Screening guidelines for breast cancer are divided into two populations: those at average risk and those at high risk. The lifetime risk of developing breast cancer in an average-risk woman is one in eight (in North American women up to age 85) (ACS, 2005; Mirshahidi & Abraham, 2005). Breast cancer screening has been shown to decrease mortality from breast cancer (ACS, 2008). As listed in Table 1-6, the general consensus for breast cancer screening in average-risk women includes counseling regarding the technique, benefits, and limitations of monthly breast self-examination (BSE); clinical breast examination (CBE) beginning at various ages and continued at various intervals; and annual mammography beginning at age 40. This table outlines the recommendations and slight variances among the professional organizations' guidelines.

Racial disparities have been documented among Caucasian and African American women with regard to incidence, death rates, and percentage of women who regularly receive mammograms (Jemal et al., 2008). Incidence rates for breast cancer are higher in Caucasian women, in part because of higher rates of mammography, the incidence of hormone replacement therapy use, and older age at first childbirth compared to African American women (Ghafoor et al., 2003; Jemal et al.). Mortality rates from breast cancer are higher in African American women, partly because of the lack of routine mammographic and CBE screening. Thus, this population is more likely to have a more advanced cancer at diagnosis and a corresponding poorer prognosis (Ghafoor et al.). Because screening for breast cancer is known to improve outcomes and decrease mortality, all women need equal access to appropriate screening exams and diagnostics.

Table 1-7. Benign Breast Lesions and Breast Cancer Risk

Type of Lesion	Associated Breast Cancer Risk
Papillomas: Epithelial origin; commonly associated with nipple discharge	Exact risk is debatable but generally is thought to increase risk by 2.3–3.9 times. In younger women, associated with concurrent breast cancer and breast cancer in first-degree relatives
Florid intraductal epithelial hyperplasia: Epithelial origin; most common form of proliferative breast disease	1.5–2-fold elevated risk When associated with papillomas, increases risk by 2.3–3.3-fold
Atypical ductal hyperplasia (ADH): Risk factor for but not a direct precursor of breast cancer; greatest risk is within 10 years of diagnosis	Associated with a 4–5-fold increased risk of breast cancer Relative risk increases to 8.9% when associated with a positive family history of breast cancer.
Atypical lobular hyperplasia: Characterized by changes similar to lobular carcinoma in situ (LCIS), but lack complete criteria	Increases relative risk by 4.3% 8–11-fold increased risk when associated with ADH
Ductal carcinoma in situ: Direct precursor of breast cancer	Relative risk for development of contralateral breast cancer is 2–3-fold.
LCIS: Direct precursor of breast cancer	Relative risk for breast cancer is 5.7 and increases to 8.5 if family history of LCIS exists
Sclerosing adenosis	2.1–2.2-fold increased risk for breast cancer If associated with ADH, 5.3-fold increased risk
Fibroadenomas: Benign tumor most common in women aged 20–30; complex fibroadenomas may have a cystic component, epithelial calcifications, or sclerosing adenosis.	2.17-fold increased relative risk for breast cancer Complex fibroadenomas associated with a higher incidence of breast cancer than simple fibroadenomas

Note. Based on information from Gierach & Vogel, 2004; Morrow & Jordan, 2003; Schnitt et al., 1996.

The CDC initiated the National Breast and Cervical Cancer Early Detection Program in 1990 to improve access for low-income women in need of breast and cervical screening and diagnostic tests (Ghafoor et al.). In 1987, an average of 17% of low-income women age 40 and older had received recent mammography screening, compared to 54.6% in 2003 (ACS, 2005).

BSE has been recommended as part of the triad of screening mechanisms for breast cancer since 1933 (ONS, 2006). However, numerous studies have failed to verify consistent results regarding its efficacy, sensitivity, and specificity (Austoker, 2003). Ku (2001) provided an excellent overview of the history of BSE and cited numerous studies that provide a positive relationship between BSE and breast cancer stage at diagnosis. Conversely, several studies also have identified no relationship between BSE and survival or mortality rates (Ku; NCI, 2007b). Therefore, it is the consensus of all professional organizations to discuss the risks and benefits of BSE and use it in combination with other screening modalities. BSE may be ideal for women who are not yet of age to undergo screening mammography and as a means to continue surveillance between

CBEs (Ku). If a woman decides to perform BSE, proper technique is necessary, an ideal educational task for the oncology APN. Women may be taught proper BSE technique using steps similar to the CBE, as described by ACS (2006d) at www.cancer.org/docroot/CRI/content/CRI_2_6x_How_to_perform_a_breast_self_exam_5.asp.

CBE has a sensitivity range of 40%–69% and specificity of 88%–99%. When CBE is combined with mammography, mortality from breast cancer is reduced by 14%–29% (Humphrey, Helfand, Chan, & Woolf, 2002). A study published in 2005 showed even lower rates of sensitivity (28%–36%) for the community clinician, citing the fact that it often is performed along with other time-consuming tasks during the office visit, such as Pap smear (Fenton et al., 2005). In general, the performance of routine CBE has declined, most likely secondary to the prevalence of screening mammography. One study showed that 95% of women in 1987 had undergone a screening mammogram and CBE within the previous six-month period, plummeting to only 50% in 2004 (Goodson, Grissom, Moore, & Dirbas, 2005). However, studies have shown that CBE is an important part of the screening process for breast cancer, detecting between 4.6%–5.7% of breast cancers alone (McDonald, Saslow, & Alciati, 2004). Figure 1-2 outlines the components of a comprehensive CBE, a requisite skill of the oncology APN.

Visual Inspection	Palpation
Position • View breast from all sides while patient tightly presses hands on hips (to flex pectoralis major muscle) in upright position. Look for and document (using clock face to record location): • Skin retraction, dimpling, or ulceration • Erythema • Skin thickening or peau d'orange • Nipple retraction, inversion, deviation, scaling, or discharge • Scarring • Symmetry.	Position • Infra- and supraclavicular and axillary lymph nodes while upright; breast and nipple in supine position with ipsilateral hand placed behind head (to reduce breast tissue thickness) Palpate • Use pads of first three fingers to make dime-sized, overlapping circular motions. • Apply light, medium, and deep pressure. • Use vertical strip method to cover all tissue in between the midaxillary line and the sternum, and from the inframammary ridge to the clavicle. Document any masses (using clock face to record location) and characteristics: • Size • Shape (round, irregular, linear) • Mobility (mobile or fixed) • Consistency (cystic, hard) • Texture (smooth, irregular) • Nipple discharge (spontaneous or forced; color).

Figure 1-2. Elements of a Comprehensive Clinical Breast Examination

Note. Based on information from Saslow et al., 2004.

Mammography alone results in a 20%–30% reduction in mortality in women who receive regular screening mammograms after age 50 and a 17% reduction in women between 40 and 49 years of age (Mirshahidi & Abraham, 2005). Mammogram specificity is high at 94%–97%, and the sensitivity for annual mammography reaches up to 96% but is lower in younger women (40–49 years old) with denser breasts (Humphrey et al., 2002; NCI, 2007b). According to the Digital Mammographic Imaging Screening Trial, digital mammography proved to be more accurate than film mammography in women with dense breasts who were younger than 50 years of age and who are pre- or perimenopausal (Pisano et al., 2005).

Women at high risk for breast cancer include those with prior radiation therapy to the chest, strong family history of or genetic predisposition to breast cancer (*BRCA1/2* mutations), personal history of LCIS, atypical hyperplasia, or invasive breast cancer (NCCN, 2006). Approximately 5%–10% of all breast cancers can be attributed to germ-line mutations of the *BRCA1* or *BRCA2* genes, which are associated with a 40%–85% risk of breast cancer (Mirshahidi & Abraham, 2005). In general, screening in high-risk women begins at an earlier age and occurs at shorter intervals. NCCN has published screening guidelines for women at high risk for breast cancer, which are summarized in Table 1-8. More comprehensive information regarding screening of women with germ-line mutations and breast cancer is covered in Chapter 2.

Magnetic resonance imaging (MRI) may be superior to mammography in high-risk women (Mirshahidi & Abraham, 2005). Several studies utilizing MRI screening in high-risk populations are ongoing, but as of yet, MRI screening has not been found to reduce mortality in any group of women (NCI, 2007b; Saslow et al., 2007). ACS recently has adopted annual breast screening with MRI as an adjunct to mammography in women with ≥ 20%–25% lifetime risk of developing breast cancer (Saslow et al., 2007). This includes women with a genetic predisposition, significant family history of breast or ovarian cancer, or history of mantle radiation therapy associated with treatment for Hodgkin lymphoma. At present, ACS does not support screening women with other risk factors for breast cancer, including a personal history of breast cancer, DCIS, LCIS, atypical hyperplasia, or dense breast tissue, because of insufficient data (Saslow et al., 2007).

Cervical Cancer

Cervical cancer is the third most common female gynecologic cancer (Posadas & Kotz, 2005). Since the introduction of the Pap smear more than 50 years ago, cervical

Table 1-8. Breast Cancer Screening Guidelines for High-Risk Women

Risk Factor	Screening Recommendation
Prior chest radiation therapy	Age < 25: Annual clinical breast exam (CBE) and periodic breast self-exam (BSE) Age > 25: Annual mammogram (MMG) and CBE every 6–12 months starting 8–10 years after radiation therapy or at age 40
5-year risk of breast cancer ≥ 1.7% per Gail model	Annual MMG and CBE every 6–12 months; periodic BSE
Lobular carcinoma in situ/atypical hyperplasia	Annual MMG and CBE every 6–12 months; periodic BSE
Genetic predisposition or strong family history (See Chapter 2 for more detailed information.)	Age < 25 years: Annual CBE and periodic BSE Age > 25 years: Annual MMG (+/– annual magnetic resonance imaging); CBE every 6–12 months (beginning at age 25 for hereditary breast and ovarian cancer syndrome or 5–10 years earlier than the youngest family member with breast cancer if strong family history); periodic BSE

Note. Based on information from National Comprehensive Cancer Network, 2007a.

cancer incidence and mortality rates have declined steadily (ACS, 2006b; Posadas & Kotz). In 2008, 11,070 new cases of cervical cancer are expected to be diagnosed, and 3,870 deaths from the disease are estimated to occur (ACS, 2008). When detected early, localized cervical cancer is one of the most successfully treated cancers, boasting a five-year survival rate of 92% (ACS, 2008). The lifetime risks for developing and dying from cervical cancer in the United States are 0.88% and 0.29%, respectively (Posadas & Kotz). Cervical cancer is more prevalent in lower socioeconomic classes of women, women of minority populations (Latin American, Native American, and African American), and women with lower education levels (Posadas & Kotz). Caucasian women are more likely to have cervical cancer diagnosed at an earlier stage (53%) compared to African American women (44%) (ACS, 2008).

In addition to these risk factors, other risk factors for cervical cancer include those related to sexual history and gynecologic history, smoking, and immunosuppression (see Table 1-9). However, the most significant risk factor for cervical cancer is HPV infection. HPV, a sexually transmitted disease, is the most common cause of and greatest risk factor for premalignant and malignant cervical lesions. More than 200 types of HPV have been identified, 20 of which have been associated with cancer (Einstein & Goldberg, 2002). Benign cervical lesions (genital warts and cervical intraepithelial neoplasia) are most commonly associated with HPV types 6, 11, 42, 43, and 44. HPV strains 16 and 18 are most commonly associated with cervical cancer and are targeted by the HPV vaccine Gardasil, along with HPV strains 6 and 11 (Dunne et al., 2007). An estimated 26.8% of women ages 14–59 are infected with HPV, according to recent data from the National Health and Nutrition Examination Study (Dunne et al.). HPV infection was highest in women aged 20–24, and 15.2% of women overall were infected with high-risk strains 16 and 18 (Dunne et al.).

Routine screening recommendations for cervical cancer are outlined in Table 1-6, and recommendations generally include initiation of Pap smear by age 21 or within three years of vaginal intercourse. Thus far, routine screening for HPV is not recommended, as clinical outcomes and management of cervical cancer with HPV infection have not changed compared to those cases without (Posadas & Kotz, 2005). Most agree it is acceptable to cease screening women at 70 years and older if certain criteria are met (see Table 1-6) and if individualized risk assessments are discussed between the patient and provider.

Table 1-9. Risk Factors for Cervical Cancer and Associated Relative Risk

Risk Factor	Relative Risk for Cervical Cancer
History of > 6 sexual partners	2.2
Use of oral contraceptive pills > 10 years	2.2
Sexual intercourse before age 18	1.6
Smoking	1.7
Immunosuppression • HIV • History of renal transplantation	 2.5 5.7
Multiparity	1.5

Note. Based on information from Posadas & Kotz, 2005.

Colorectal Cancer

Colorectal cancer (CRC) is the second leading cause of cancer death in the United States and the third most commonly diagnosed cancer in both men and women (ACS, 2008; Kim, Takimoto, & Allegra, 2005). In 2008, an estimated 148,810 new cases of colorectal cancer are expected to be diagnosed, with 49,960 deaths expected to occur (ACS, 2008). The average lifetime risk of developing CRC is 1 in 18 (Kim et al.). Colon cancer is more common in women, whereas rectal cancer is more common in men (Kim et al.). African Americans have a higher incidence of CRC and a 32% increased mortality rate over Caucasians (Kim et al.).

Several known risk factors exist for CRC, although up to 70% of cases have no identifiable risk factors (Kim et al., 2005). The most common risk factor for the development of CRC is age, with more than 90% of cases found in those older than 50 years of age (ACS, 2008; Kim et al.). Other risk factors include lifestyle factors such as physical inactivity, obesity, heavy alcohol intake, and diets high in red meat and low in fiber, fruits, and vegetables (ACS, 2006b). Smoking is associated with a 2.5-fold increased risk of CRC (Kim et al.) and is estimated to account for 5,000–7,000 CRC deaths annually (Alberts & Goldberg, 2004). Other conditions of the colon (e.g., inflammatory bowel disease [IBD], colon adenomas) and a genetic predisposition or hereditary polyposis syndrome increase the risk of CRC (see Table 1-10) (ACS, 2006b; Goldberg, 2000; Kim et al.). Conversely, several factors are known to reduce the risk of colon cancer, such as regular intake of calcium, aspirin, NSAIDs, or 3-hydroxy-3-methylglutaryl coenzyme A reductase inhibitors (i.e., statins) and postmenopausal use of hormone replacement therapy (ACS, 2006b; Alberts & Goldberg; Kim et al.). Only celecoxib has been approved for prevention of adenomatous polyps in FAP (Price, 2002).

The five-year survival rate for CRC detected at a localized stage is 90%; however, because of a lack of appropriate screening, only 39% of cases are diagnosed at this stage (ACS, 2008). As with most malignancies, a more advanced stage at diagnosis of colon cancer is associated with decreased survival (ACS, 2008). The five-year survival rate for locally advanced CRC (involvement of regional lymph nodes) is 68%, and those with distant metastases have even poorer outcomes, with only a 10% five-year survival (ACS, 2008). Studies of large (> 1 cm) untreated colonic polyps have a 2.5% risk of progressing to malignant tumors within 5 years, an 8% risk at 10 years, and a 24% risk at 20 years. On average, a severely dysplastic polyp will take only 3.5 years to evolve into a malignant tumor, whereas a polyp with only mild atypia may take an average of 11.5 years (Alberts & Goldberg, 2004).

The purpose of screening for CRC is to identify adenomatous or precancerous polyps and remove them before they progress to malignancy, thereby resulting in decreased mortality and better outcomes. Polypectomy and subsequent surveillance with colonoscopy can reduce CRC incidence by 90% (Alberts & Goldberg, 2004). Guidelines for screening average-risk populations (age ≥ 50, no history of adenoma or IBD, and negative family history) are outlined in Table 1-6. In general, recommendations include screening beginning at age 50 and either annual fecal occult blood test (FOBT) or fecal immunochemical testing (FIT), sigmoidoscopy or double contrast barium enema every five years, annual FOBT or FIT in combination with sigmoidoscopy every five years, or a full colonoscopy every 10 years. Guidelines for increased-risk or high-risk populations, as recommended by NCCN, are outlined in Table 1-11.

Table 1-10. Diseases of the Colon and Colorectal Cancer Risk

Risk Factor	Risk of Colorectal Cancer (CRC)
Ulcerative colitis	• Causes 1% of all cases of CRC • Increases with age at onset, extent of disease, and duration of active disease • Cumulative risk is 3% at 15 years, 5% at 20 years, and 9% at 25 years.
Crohn disease	• Twofold increased risk of CRC
Polyps	70% of polyps are adenomatous or neoplastic: • 75%–85% tubular adenomas (lowest risk), 10%–25% tubulovillous adenomas (intermediate risk), ≤ 5% villous adenomas (highest risk) • > 1 cm in size: 2–4-fold increased risk of CRC • Multiple polyps: 5–7-fold increased risk • Time to malignant progression: 3.5 years for severely dysplastic polyps and 11.5 years for mild atypia
Family history of CRC	• One first-degree relative: Relative risk increased to 1.72 • Two first-degree relatives: Relative risk increased to 2.75
Hereditary nonpolyposis colorectal cancer	The Lynch syndromes • Lynch I (colonic syndrome) – Autosomal dominant trait associated with proximal mucinous or poorly differentiated synchronous or metachronous colonic tumors – Usual development of CRC by age 50; 75% overall lifetime risk • Lynch II – Associated with extracolonic tumors in the ovaries, endometrium, stomach, small intestine, and genitourinary and hepatobiliary tracts
Familial adenomatous polyposis	• Autosomal dominant inherited syndrome (germ-line mutation in adenomatous polyposis coli gene on chromosome 5q21) consisting of hundreds of colonic polyps developed by late adolescence • 100% lifetime risk of developing CRC

Note. Based on information from Alberts & Goldberg, 2004; Kim et al., 2005.

Prostate Cancer

Prostate cancer is the most commonly diagnosed cancer in American men and the second leading cause of cancer-related death in men (ACS, 2008). In 2008, 186,320 new cases of prostate cancer will be diagnosed, and 28,660 deaths are expected to occur (ACS, 2008). The incidence of prostate cancer has risen steadily with a peak incidence of 191 cases per 100,000 men in 1992, largely as a result of improved detection capabilities with routine prostate-specific antigen (PSA) testing approved by the FDA in 1986 (Gulley & Dahut, 2005; Zisman, Belldegrun, & Figlin, 2000). The most common risk factor for prostate cancer is age; the median age at diagnosis is 72 in Caucasian males (Gulley & Dahut; Zisman et al.). African American males have a lower median age at diagnosis (62 years) and higher incidence and mortality rates (Gulley & Dahut; Zisman et al.).

Screening for early-stage prostate cancer with PSA testing or digital rectal examination (DRE) detects prostate cancer in its earliest stage; however, it is largely debatable as to whether screening asymptomatic men with PSA or DRE reduces mortality (Gulley

**Table 1-11. Screening Recommendations for Colorectal Cancer (CRC)
for High-Risk Populations**

Risk Factor	Screening Recommendations
History of adenoma	Low-risk adenoma • < 3 polyps, < 1 cm, tubular histology • Follow-up colonoscopy every 3–6 years, then every 5 years once normal High-risk adenoma • High-grade dysplasia or carcinoma in situ, > 1 cm, villous histology, or multiple adenomas (> 3 < 10) • Follow-up colonoscopy every 3 years, then every 3–5 years once normal • More than 10 adenomas or > 15 cumulative adenomas in 10 years • Consider polyposis syndrome.
Personal history of CRC	Colonoscopy one year following diagnosis Repeat in 1–3 years if adenoma is identified. If normal, repeat in 2–3 years.
Personal history of ovarian or endometrial cancer < 60 years of age	Colonoscopies beginning at age 40 and repeated every 5 years if no abnormal findings present
Inflammatory bowel disease (ulcerative colitis or Crohn disease)	Colonoscopy beginning within 8–10 years after onset of disease and continue every 1–2 years
Family history	One first-degree relative with CRC < 50 years old at diagnosis, or two first-degree relatives with CRC at any age, or clustering of hereditary nonpolyposis colon cancers, or polyposis in close relatives and does not meet criteria for hereditary syndrome: • Colonoscopy at age 40 or 10 years prior to the age of earliest CRC diagnosis in the family and repeat every 1–5 years One first-degree family member with CRC or two second-degree relatives with CRC at any age: • Colonoscopy at age 40 or 10 years prior to the age of the earliest CRC diagnosis in the family and repeat every 5 years One second-degree relative or any third-degree relative: • Screen according to recommendations of average-risk population with individualized evaluation and risk assessment.

Note. Based on information from National Comprehensive Cancer Network, 2007c.

& Dahut, 2005; NCI, 2007k). Studies have documented that screening for prostate cancer detects disease in some men that would never have caused clinically significant problems, thus resulting in overtreatment in some cases with modalities (e.g., radical prostatectomy and radiation) that carry risks of permanent side effects (Gulley & Dahut; NCI, 2007k). Several studies have demonstrated that more men die with prostate cancer than from it; autopsy data have identified an occult rate of prostate cancer of 75% in men in their 80s (Gulley & Dahut). Despite the controversy, PSA and DRE are widely used in the United States to screen men for prostate cancer.

Most agree that individualized risk assessments and evaluation for screening take place between the patient and provider (ACS, 2006c). Screening guidelines for average-risk and high-risk males (African American heritage, positive family history) are outlined in Table 1-6 and generally consist of initiating PSA screening at age 50 in average-risk individuals and at age 40 in high-risk individuals.

Endometrial Cancer

Endometrial cancer is the most common gynecologic cancer and the fourth most common type of malignancy in females overall, representing 6% of or approximately 40,100 new cases and 7,470 deaths in 2008 (ACS, 2008). Almost all cases are diagnosed in postmenopausal women, with incidence peaking in the sixth and seventh decades of life (Memarzadeh, Farias-Eisner, & Berek, 2004). Less than 5% of all cases of endometrial cancer are diagnosed in women younger than the age of 40, and premenopausal diagnosis usually is associated with Stein-Leventhal syndrome or polycystic ovarian syndrome (Memarzadeh et al.).

Multiple risk factors for endometrial cancer exist, mostly pertaining to unopposed estrogen exposure (both exogenous and endogenous) and reproductive history. These include polycystic ovarian disease, anovulatory ovary disease, granulosa cell tumor of the ovary (or other estrogen-secreting tumors), early menarche and late menopause, irregular menses, infertility, and nulliparity (Annunziasta & Birrer, 2005; Memarzadeh et al., 2004; NCI, 2007e). Nulliparity carries a twofold increased risk for endometrial cancer compared to the risk in women who have had at least one child (Annunziasta & Birrer). Intake of tamoxifen, a weak estrogen administered for treatment and prevention of breast cancer, is thought to carry a twofold increased risk for endometrial cancer (Memarzadeh et al.). Other risk factors include advanced liver disease, hypertension, obesity, and diabetes mellitus (Annunziasta & Birrer; Memarzadeh et al.). Lastly, a family history of endometrial cancer increases the risk for endometrial cancer. A woman's risk is tripled if she has one first-degree relative with endometrial cancer and doubled if she has one first-degree relative with CRC (Annunziasta & Birrer).

As with other cancers, racial disparities exist in endometrial cancer incidence and mortality rates. African American women have a lower incidence of endometrial cancer than Caucasian women yet have a higher mortality rate. Some studies propose that both biologic factors and lower socioeconomic status play a role in this disparity. For instance, lower income has been associated with a lower probability of undergoing potentially curative surgery with hysterectomy. This leads to advanced disease at diagnosis and, thus, lower survival rates (Madison, Schottenfeld, James, Schwartz, & Gruber, 2004).

Routine screening for asymptomatic women is not recommended (Annunziasta & Birrer, 2005; NCI, 2007e). Studies do not support routine transvaginal ultrasound (TVU) or endometrial biopsies, as they have not been proved to reduce mortality. TVU has a low sensitivity and would require additional, more sensitive (and more costly) imaging studies to investigate for the presence of malignancy (NCI, 2007e). Also, endometrial biopsies carry the risk of bleeding and infection, and many endometrial cancers are missed with endometrial sampling (NCI, 2007e).

Screening for endometrial cancer is recommended for certain populations, however. Women with hereditary nonpolyposis colon cancer (HNPCC) carry a 60% lifetime risk of developing endometrial cancer (NCI, 2007e). For these women, routine screening is recommended and consists of TVU and endometrial sampling annually beginning at age 30–35 or 5–10 years earlier than the age at which the first diagnosed case in the family occurred (NCCN, 2007c). Prophylactic surgery with hysterectomy and bilateral salpingo-oophorectomy is an option for women who have completed childbearing (NCCN, 2007c).

Ovarian Cancer

Ovarian cancer is the fifth leading cause of cancer-related death in American women, expected to take 15,520 women's lives of 21,650 diagnosed in 2008 (ACS, 2008). No major improvement in overall survival has been made in more than 30 years (Memarzadeh et al., 2004). Incidence of ovarian cancer increases with age; the average age at diagnosis is 55 years (Memarzadeh et al.). Nulliparity and continuous ovulation also are risk factors. Therefore, conditions or measures that decrease the number of ovulations, such as oral contraceptives, multiparity, and breast-feeding, have a protective effect (Reed & Altaha, 2005).

As with endometrial cancer, routine screening for ovarian cancer in women without known risk factors, such as a known genetic predisposition or strong family history, is not recommended and has not been shown to decrease mortality (NCI, 2007j; Reed & Altaha, 2005). But, studies do support screening in women who are considered high-risk—those women with strong family histories suggestive of a hereditary cancer syndrome such as *BRCA1* or *BRCA2* mutations or HNPCC. Although only 5%–10% of all ovarian cancers are secondary to germ-line mutations, the associated risk of ovarian cancer is 16%–27% with the *BRCA2* gene and as high as 40%–60% with the *BRCA1* mutation (Memarzadeh et al., 2004; NCI, 2002). Ovarian cancer risk associated with HNPCC is two to four times the risk of the general population (Memarzadeh et al.). In these high-risk women, screening with TVU and the tumor assay CA 125 is recommended and is discussed in greater detail in Chapter 2.

Skin Cancer

In 2008, 62,480 cases of malignant melanoma are expected to be diagnosed, in addition to more than one million cases of basal and squamous cell skin cancers (ACS, 2008). Most cases of skin cancer are caused by unprotected and/or excessive exposure of the skin to UV light (ACS, 2008); 90% of all skin cancers occur on sun-exposed areas of the skin (Wagner & Casciato, 2004). UV exposure can come from natural sources or artificial sources, such as tanning beds, and both result in skin damage ranging from wrinkling and premature aging to skin cancer (ACS, 2008). Risk factors for melanoma and basal and squamous cell skin cancers include light skin tone, blue eyes, blond or red hair, personal or family history of skin cancer, overexposure to the sun, history of severe sunburn, and freckles or nevi (ACS, 2008; Hegde & Gause, 2005). The incidence of melanoma in Caucasians is 10 times greater than in African Americans and is slightly higher in females than males (Hegde & Gause).

Melanoma has several risk factors (see Figure 1-3). A family history of melanoma may be indicative of familial melanoma. Familial melanoma consists of multiple melanomas in one family, usually developing at a younger age (< 50), and often is associated with dysplastic nevi. Chromosomal abnormalities also have been recognized in familial melanoma, including loss of chromosome 9p21 (Hegde & Gause, 2005).

ASCO (2005) recommends skin cancer screening in the general population with periodic self skin examinations and annual whole body skin examination by a healthcare provider beginning at age 40. Secondary prevention measures include treatments directed at individual lesions (Wagner & Casciato, 2004). Primary prevention of most skin cancers can be achieved by avoiding excessive sun exposure and using sunscreen.

Precursor Lesions
- Dysplastic nevi
- Congenital nevi
- Acquired melanocytic nevi

Other Risk Factors
- Xeroderma pigmentosum
- Familial atypical mole melanoma syndrome
- Numerous acquired melanocytic nevi
- Immunosuppression
- Chemical exposures
- Trauma
- Ionizing radiation

Figure 1-3. Risk Factors for Melanoma

Note. Based on information from Hegde & Gause, 2005; Wagner & Casciato, 2004.

Lung Cancer

Lung cancer is the most fatal malignancy and the second most commonly occurring cancer in both men and women (ACS, 2008). Despite this, no routine screening recommendations for lung cancer exist for asymptomatic or even high-risk individuals. In 2001, ACS recognized the need for high-risk individuals (smokers and those with occupational exposures) to explore the option of early detection for lung cancer with their healthcare provider (Smith et al., 2007). The U.S. Preventive Services Task Force (USPSTF) cites insufficient evidence to screen asymptomatic people with low-dose computed tomography (LDCT), chest x-ray (CXR), sputum cytology, or a combination of the three (USPSTF, 2004). Several studies have documented earlier detection of lung cancer through one or all of these means but have not shown a decrease in mortality (Bach et al., 2007; NCI, 2007h; USPSTF). Moreover, both NCI (2007h) and USPSTF concluded that CXR, sputum cytology testing, and LDCT have high false-positive rates and would lead to unnecessary and potentially dangerous invasive tests such as lung biopsy (USPSTF). The National Lung Cancer Screening Trial is comparing spiral computed tomography and CXR in 50,000 current or former smokers in an attempt to determine whether a reduction in mortality from lung cancer is achieved by either modality (NCI, 2006c). Results are expected in 2009 (NCI, 2006c).

Other Cancers

Although established screening tests and guidelines exist for several cancers, including three of the most common malignancies—breast, colorectal, and prostate—the majority of malignancies do not have established screening recommendations, as insufficient evidence exists to suggest that screening would affect mortality rates. NCI (2007a, 2007h, 2007i) found inadequate evidence to determine whether screening for bladder or urothelial cancer, lung cancer, and oral cancer would reduce mortality in the United States. Moreover, evidence also suggests that screening for esophageal, gastric, hepatocellular, and testicular cancers would not reduce mortality, and potential side effects of testing outweigh benefits—such as the dangers associated with endoscopy for gastric or esophageal cancers or fine needle aspiration with hepatocellular cancer (NCI, 2006d, 2007f, 2007g). However, clinical trials are ongoing in the search for beneficial screening modalities and recommendations for a majority of malignancies. NCI alone has more than 70 clinical trials dedicated to cancer screening. The National Institutes of Health lists more than 300 clinical trials across the United States that are actively recruiting for cancer screening trial participants.

Implications for Oncology Advanced Practice Nurses

The role of the oncology APN encompasses cancer risk reduction, screening, and early detection. Oncology APNs are able to assess, evaluate, and interpret cancer risk assessments and recommend appropriate interventions. Familiarity with known risk factors for various cancers alerts the APN to patients who would benefit from evidence-based interventions to reduce cancer risk. Guidelines are available to guide APN interventions. Strategies are modified based on individual characteristics, population risk variances, and cultural diversities. It is imperative that the oncology APN masters these topics to provide comprehensive, thorough oncology care that begins with risk assessment to reach the goal of cancer prevention.

Conclusion

Cancer prevention and early detection are integral parts of the cancer care continuum. Ideally, primary cancer prevention in the form of risk reduction is the best way to decrease morbidity and mortality related to cancer. Certain populations are considered to be at high risk for some malignancies, and the screening and management of these populations differ from that of the general population. Risk models are available to assist the APN in assessment for certain cancers. Evidence-based pharmacologic, nonpharmacologic, and behavioral interventions are available. Education of both the individual and populations is crucial. Education encompasses information about exercise, dietary habits, sun exposure, smoking cessation, and recommended screening practices. Early detection achieved by adhering to routine screening guidelines facilitates cancer being diagnosed in the earliest stage of the disease, when it is most likely to be treated successfully and is associated with the best patient outcomes. The oncology APN has an opportunity and an obligation to offer risk reduction care and appropriate screening to both the individual patient and populations.

Case Study

A.J. is a 55-year-old African American female seen in the oncology clinic by the oncology APN for follow-up care for anemia. A.J. states she receives health care at a walk-in clinic only when she is ill and that she had been out of work for some time and had not had insurance to cover routine medical care until recently. Review of her family history confirms colon cancer in her 70-year-old mother, diagnosed at age 65. Her 73-year-old father has heart disease and hypertension and was diagnosed with prostate cancer at age 72. She has two brothers, who also have hypertension. She is married and has no children. She smokes one pack of cigarettes per day and is interested in quitting, but admits she needs help. She denies alcohol use. A.J. works 40–50 hours a week, does not engage in regular exercise, and eats fast food frequently.

Her review of systems is negative except for fatigue and intermittent arthralgia with a previous history of osteoarthritis, for which she takes occasional acetaminophen. She is postmenopausal; her last menstrual cycle was more than two years ago. Other past medical and surgical history is negative. The physical examination (including CBE, pelvic examination, and Pap smear) is also negative, vital signs are stable, and she has no gross abnormalities on examination except for moderate obesity and pale oral mucosal membranes.

1. What risk factors for malignancy can be identified based on this history?
   - Her risks for cancer include tobacco use, sedentary lifestyle, obesity, and poor nutrition. She is nulliparous and has one first-degree relative with a history of colon cancer. Her father's recent diagnosis of prostate cancer at age 72 is noted but does not necessarily affect A.J.'s risk factors at this point.
2. What screening tests does A.J. need, and what cancer risk reduction strategies can the oncology APN discuss with A.J.?
   - As A.J. has not received routine medical care in several years, she has neglected the recommended cancer screening tests. Recommendations include smoking cessation, and because she is willing to make a quit attempt, NRT may be offered in the form of transdermal nicotine. Counseling regarding smoking cessation will increase effectiveness of the intervention. Physical activity of moderate intensity for at least 30 minutes several times per week is a behavioral goal. Dietary counseling is necessary, focusing on eating fewer high-fat foods and consuming at least five servings of fruits and vegetables per day. Counseling on the techniques, benefits, and limitations of BSE will increase her confidence in performing this examination.
   - A screening mammogram is appropriate, as is a referral to a gastroenterologist for a screening colonoscopy. Informational needs include screening recommendations for mammogram and CBE annually, pelvic examination and Pap smear every two to three years, and colonoscopy every five years, given her positive family history (assuming initial colonoscopy results are benign).
3. Before she leaves, A.J. inquires about a television commercial for a vaccine for cervical cancer and wants to know if that is an option for her. How does the oncology APN respond?
   - The oncology APN tells A.J. that Gardasil is a vaccine for prevention of cervical cancer associated with HPV infection and is approved only for administration in females 9–26 years of age. Therefore, A.J. is not a candidate for this vaccination, and the APN recommends she continue with Pap smears for early detection of cervical cancer as discussed previously.

Key Points

- Primary prevention of cancer is achieved through promotion of wellness and reduction of known risks for cancer.
- Cancer risk assessment involves an individualized, comprehensive patient history and examination to provide accurate cancer risk reduction counseling and screening recommendations.

- Major components of cancer risk reduction for the general population include
  - Avoid or cease cigarette smoking.
  - Minimize UV light exposure, and use sunscreen with an SPF ≥ 15 on sun-exposed skin.
  - Maintain an active lifestyle with regular, moderate physical activity.
  - Maintain a healthy weight (avoid obesity).
  - Eat a diet high in fiber, fruits, and vegetables and low in red or processed meats, fats, and sugars.
- Chemoprevention is an option for certain high-risk patients.
- Secondary prevention includes screening and early detection of cancer.
- Screening tests require specificity (few false positives) and sensitivity (few false negatives) for the disease being screened.
- Screening guidelines exist for the general population and for populations at high risk for various cancers, including those with a genetic predisposition for certain cancers.
- Screening for high-risk populations usually begins at an earlier age than screening for the general population and occurs at more frequent intervals.
- Cultural and ethnic disparities exist in almost all malignancies and affect incidence and mortality rates.

Recommended Resources for Oncology Advanced Practice Nurses

- Breast Cancer Risk Assessment Tool (www.cancer.gov/bcrisktool/default.aspx): Computerized tool for the PDA and desktop computer
- CancerGene software (www.utsouthwestern.edu/utsw/cda/dept47829/files/65844 .html): A free computer program that estimates risk for carrying mutation in one of the cancer predisposition genes. Uses BRCAPRO and MMRpro risk models, draws a pedigree, and archives family history and mutation probability.
- CancerPRA™ (Skyscape) (www.collectivemed.com/jump/capra.shtml): PDA tool based on the *Handbook of Cancer Risk Assessment and Prevention* with search capabilities
- Cancer Risk: Understanding the Puzzle (http://understandingrisk.cancer.gov): A Web site from NCI for patients that explains cancer risk and provides tools for patients
- *Handbook of Cancer Risk Assessment and Prevention* (Colditz & Stein, 2004): Handbook of risk factors for the most common cancers, a risk assessment tool, and hints to promote risk-reducing lifestyle changes
- Lung Cancer Risk Assessment Tool (www.mskcc.org/mskcc/html/12463.cfm): A prediction tool from Memorial Sloan-Kettering Cancer Center to assess a long-term smoker's risk of developing lung cancer in the next 10 years
- Melanoma Risk Assessment Tool (www.cancer.gov/melanomarisktool): An interactive tool to estimate a person's absolute risk of developing invasive melanoma
- NCCN Clinical Practice Guidelines in Oncology (www.nccn.org)
  - Breast cancer risk reduction
  - Cervical cancer screening
  - Colorectal screening
  - Genetic/familial high-risk assessment for breast and ovarian cancers

* RiskyDisky: PDA prediction tool that uses the modified Gail, Claus, and Frank models to predict the five-year risk for breast cancer and consequences of five years of tamoxifen therapy

References

Alberts, S.R., & Goldberg, R.M. (2004). Gastrointestinal tract cancers. In D.A. Casciato (Ed.), *Manual of clinical oncology* (5th ed., pp. 185–253). Philadelphia: Lippincott Williams & Wilkins.

American Academy of Nurse Practitioners. (2002a). *Nurse practitioners as an advanced practice nurse role* [Position statement]. Austin, TX: Author.

American Academy of Nurse Practitioners. (2002b). *Scope of practice for nurse practitioners*. Austin, TX: Author.

American Cancer Society. (2005). *Breast cancer facts and figures, 2005–2006*. Atlanta, GA: Author.

American Cancer Society. (2006a). *American Cancer Society guidelines for the early detection of cancer*. Atlanta, GA: Author.

American Cancer Society. (2006b). *Cancer facts and figures, 2006*. Atlanta, GA: Author.

American Cancer Society. (2006c). *Cancer prevention and early detection facts and figures, 2006*. Atlanta, GA: Author.

American Cancer Society. (2006d). *How to perform a breast self-exam*. Retrieved April 22, 2007, from http://www.cancer.org/docroot/CRI/content/CRI_2_6x_How_to_perform_a_breast_self_exam_5.asp?sitearea=

American Cancer Society. (2006e). *Skin cancer protection and early detection*. Atlanta, GA: Author.

American Cancer Society. (2007). *Check and protect your skin*. Atlanta, GA: Author.

American Cancer Society. (2008). *Cancer facts and figures, 2008*. Atlanta, GA: Author.

American Society of Clinical Oncology. (2005). *Cancer prevention and screening: An overview*. Retrieved September 18, 2006, from http://www.asco.org/ASCO/Downloads/Communications/PCGuidelines.pdf

Andrews, J.O., Tingen, M.S., & Harper, R.J. (1999). A model nurse practitioner-managed smoking cessation clinic. *Oncology Nursing Forum, 26*, 1603–1610.

Annunziasta, C.M., & Birrer, H.L. (2005). Endometrial cancer. In J. Abraham, C.J. Allegra, & J. Gulley (Eds.), *Bethesda handbook of clinical oncology* (2nd ed., pp. 237–238). Philadelphia: Lippincott Williams & Wilkins.

Austoker, J. (2003). Breast self examination does not prevent deaths due to breast cancer, but breast awareness is still important. *BMJ, 326*, 1–2.

Bach, P., Jett, J., Pastorino, U., Tockman, M., Swensen, S., & Begg, C. (2007). Computed tomography screening and lung cancer outcomes. *JAMA, 297*, 953–961.

Box, B.A., & Russell, C.A. (2004). Breast cancer. In D.A. Casciato (Ed.), *Manual of clinical oncology* (5th ed., pp. 233–253). Philadelphia: Lippincott Williams & Wilkins.

Brannon, H. (2007). *Proper use of sunscreen*. Retrieved April 13, 2007, from http://dermatology.about.com/cs/skincareproducts/l/blsunscreen.htm

Calle, E., Rodriguez, C., Walker-Thurmond, K., & Thun, M. (2003). Overweight, obesity, and mortality from cancer in a prospectively studied cohort of US adults. *New England Journal of Medicine, 348*, 1625–1638.

Centers for Disease Control and Prevention. (2004). *The health consequences of smoking: A report of the surgeon general*. Atlanta, GA: U.S. Department of Health and Human Services, Centers for Disease Control and Prevention.

Centers for Disease Control and Prevention. (2005, July). *Preventing obesity and chronic diseases through good nutrition and physical activity*. Atlanta, GA: U.S. Department of Health and Human Services, Centers for Disease Control and Prevention.

Centers for Disease Control and Prevention. (2006a, July 7). Cigarette use among high school students—United States, 1991–2005. *Morbidity and Mortality Weekly Report, 55*, 724–726.

Centers for Disease Control and Prevention. (2006b, August 26). *Physical activity for everyone*. Atlanta, GA: U.S. Department of Health and Human Services, Centers for Disease Control and Prevention.

Christman, C., & Bingham, M. (1989). The nurse practitioners' role in smoking cessation. *Journal of the American Academy of Nurse Practitioners, 1*(2), 49–54.

Clark, L.C., Combs, G.F., Turnbull, B.W., Slate, E.H., Chalker, D.K., Chow, J., et al. (1996). Effects of selenium supplementation for cancer prevention in patients with carcinoma of the skin: A randomized controlled trial. *JAMA, 276*, 1957–1963.

Colditz, G.A., & Stein, C.J. (2004). *Handbook of cancer risk assessment and prevention.* Sudbury, MA: Jones and Bartlett.

Dunne, E., Unger, E., Sternberg, M., McQuillan, G., Swan, D., Patel, S., et al. (2007). Prevalence of HPV infection among females in the United States. *JAMA, 297,* 813–819.

Einstein, M.H., & Goldberg, G.L. (2002). Human papillomavirus and cervical neoplasia. *Cancer Investigation, 20,* 1080–1085.

Euhus, D. (2001). Understanding mathematical models for breast cancer risk assessment and counseling. *Breast Journal, 7,* 224–232.

Fenton, J., Barton, M., Geiger, A., Herrinton, L., Rolnick, S., Harris, E., et al. (2005). Screening clinical breast examination: How often does it miss lethal breast cancer? *Journal of the National Cancer Institute, 35,* 67–71.

Fiore, M.C., Bailey, W.C., Cohen, S.J., Dorfman, S.F., Goldstein, M.G., Gritz, E.R., et al. (2000). *Treating tobacco use and dependence: Clinical practice guideline.* Rockville, MD: U.S. Department of Health and Human Services.

Fisher, B., Costantino, J., Wickerham, D.L., Cecchini, R., Cronin, W., Robidoux, A., et al. (2005). Tamoxifen for the prevention of breast cancer: Current status of the National Surgical Adjuvant Breast and Bowel Project P-1 study. *Journal of the National Cancer Institute, 97,* 1652–1662.

Ghafoor, A., Jemal, A., Ward, E., Cokkinides, V., Smith, R., & Thun, M. (2003). Trends in breast cancer by race and ethnicity. *CA: A Cancer Journal for Clinicians, 53,* 342–355.

Gierach, G., & Vogel, V. (2004). Epidemiology of breast cancer. In S.E. Singletary, G.L. Robb, & G.N. Hortobagyi (Eds.), *Advanced therapy of breast disease* (2nd ed., pp. 58–74). Hamilton, Ontario, Canada: B.C. Decker.

Goldberg, R.M. (2000). Gastrointestinal tract cancers. In D.A. Casciato & B.B. Lowitz (Eds.), *Manual of clinical oncology* (4th ed., pp. 182–194). Philadelphia: Lippincott Williams & Wilkins.

Goodson, W.H., Grissom, N.A., Moore, D.H., & Dirbas, F.M. (2005). Streamlining clinical breast examination. *Journal of the National Cancer Institute, 97,* 1476–1477.

Greco, K. (2007). Caring for patients at risk for hereditary colorectal cancer. *Oncology (Williston Park), 21*(Suppl. 2), 29–38.

Gulley, J.L., & Dahut, W.L. (2005). Prostate cancer. In J. Abraham, C.J. Allegra, & J. Gulley (Eds.), *Bethesda handbook of clinical oncology* (2nd ed., pp. 185–202). Philadelphia: Lippincott Williams & Wilkins.

Heatherton, T.F., Kozlowski, L.T., Frecker, R.C., & Fagerstrom, K. (1991). The Fagerstrom test for nicotine dependence: A revision of the Fagerstrom tolerance questionnaire. *British Journal of Addiction, 86,* 1119–1127.

Hegde, U.P., & Gause, B. (2005). Endometrial cancer. In J. Abraham, C.J. Allegra, & J. Gulley (Eds.), *Bethesda handbook of clinical oncology* (2nd ed., pp. 283–285). Philadelphia: Lippincott Williams & Wilkins.

Heinonen, O.P., Albanes, D., Virtamo, J., Taylor, P.R., Huttunen, J.K., Hartman, A.M., et al. (1998). Prostate cancer and supplementation with alpha-tocopherol and beta-carotene: Incidence and mortality in a controlled trial. *Journal of the National Cancer Institute, 90,* 440–446.

Humphrey, L.L., Helfand, M., Chan, B., & Woolf, S.H. (2002). Breast cancer screening: A summary of the evidence for the U.S. Preventive Services task force. *Annals of Internal Medicine, 137,* 347–360.

Jemal, A., Siegel, R., Ward, E., Hao, Y., Xu, J., Murray, T., et al. (2008). Cancer statistics, 2008. *CA: A Cancer Journal for Clinicians, 58,* 71–96.

Karagas, M., Stannard, V., Mott, L., Slattery, M., Spencer, S., & Weinstock, M. (2002). Use of tanning devices and the risk of basal cell and squamous cell skin cancers. *Journal of the National Cancer Institute, 94,* 224–226.

Kim, G.P., Takimoto, C.H., & Allegra, C.J. (2005). Colorectal cancer. In J. Abraham, C.J. Allegra, & J. Gulley (Eds.), *Bethesda handbook of clinical oncology* (2nd ed., pp. 107–109). Philadelphia: Lippincott Williams & Wilkins.

Koh, H.K., Kannler, C., & Geller, A.C. (2001). Cancer prevention: Preventing tobacco related cancers. In V.T. DeVita, S. Hellman, & S.A. Rosenberg (Eds.), *Cancer: Principles and practice of oncology* (6th ed., pp. 549–560). Philadelphia: Lippincott Williams & Wilkins.

Ku, Y. (2001). The value of breast self-examination: Meta-analysis of the research literature. *Oncology Nursing Forum, 28,* 815–822.

Lindblom, E., & McMahon, K. (2006, October 30). *Toll of tobacco in the United States of America.* Retrieved January 8, 2007, from http://tobaccofreekids.org/research/factsheets/index.php?CategoryID=1

Lombard, H.L., & Doering, C.R. (1928). Cancer studies in Massachusetts. *New England Journal of Medicine, 198,* 481–487.

Madison, T., Schottenfeld, D., James, S., Schwartz, A.G., & Gruber, S.B. (2004). Endometrial cancer: Socioeconomic status and racial/ethnic differences in stage at diagnosis, treatment, and survival. *American Journal of Public Health, 94,* 2104–2111.

Mariolis, P., Rock, V.J., Asman, K., Merritt, R., Malarcher, A., Husten, C., et al. (2006). Tobacco use among adults—United States, 2005. *Morbidity and Mortality Weekly Report, 55,* 1145–1148.

McDonald, S., Saslow, D., & Alciati, M.H. (2004). Performance and reporting of clinical breast examination: A review of the literature. *CA: A Cancer Journal for Clinicians, 54,* 345–361.

Memarzadeh, S., Farias-Eisner, R.P., & Berek, J.S. (2004). Gynecologic cancers. In D.A. Casciato (Ed.), *Manual of clinical oncology* (5th ed., pp. 254–285). Philadelphia: Lippincott Williams & Wilkins.

Mirshahidi, H.R., & Abraham, J. (2005). Breast cancer. In J. Abraham, C.J. Allegra, & J. Gulley (Eds.), *Bethesda handbook of clinical oncology* (2nd ed., pp. 155–158). Philadelphia: Lippincott Williams & Wilkins.

Morrow, M., & Jordan, V.C. (2003). *Managing breast cancer risk.* Hamilton, Ontario, Canada: B.C. Decker.

National Cancer Institute. (1997). *Questions and answers about beta-carotene chemoprevention trials.* Retrieved April 2, 2007, from http://www.cancer.gov/cancertopics/factsheet/Prevention/betacarotene

National Cancer Institute. (2002, February 6). *Genetic testing for BRCA1 and BRCA2: It's your choice.* Retrieved April 2, 2007, from http://www.cancer.gov/cancertopics/factsheet/Risk/BRCA

National Cancer Institute. (2004a, March 16). *Obesity and cancer: Questions and answers.* Retrieved April 2, 2007, from http://www.cancer.gov/cancertopics/factsheet/Risk/obesity

National Cancer Institute. (2004b, March 29). *Physical activity and cancer: Fact sheet.* Retrieved April 2, 2007, from http://www.cancer.gov/newscenter/pressreleases/PhysicalActivity

National Cancer Institute. (2005a). *Health information national trends survey.* Retrieved April 2, 2007, from http://hints.cancer.gov/hints

National Cancer Institute. (2005b, June 13). *Selenium and vitamin E cancer prevention trial (SELECT): Questions and answers.* Retrieved April 16, 2007, from http://www.cancer.gov/cancertopics/factsheet/Prevention/SELECT

National Cancer Institute. (2006a). *Dictionary of cancer terms.* Retrieved January 9, 2007, from http://www.cancer.gov/dictionary

National Cancer Institute. (2006b). *Most Americans do not know when or how often to get cancer screening tests.* Retrieved January 8, 2007, from http://www.cancer.gov/newscenter/pressreleases/HINTS

National Cancer Institute. (2006c). *National lung cancer screening trial: Questions and answers.* Retrieved April 2, 2007, from http://www.cancer.gov/cancertopics/factsheet/nlstqa

National Cancer Institute. (2006d). *Testicular cancer screening (PDQ®)* [Health professional version]. Retrieved February 6, 2007, from http://www.cancer.gov/cancertopics/pdq/screening/testicular/healthprofessional

National Cancer Institute. (2007a). *Bladder and urothelial cancers (PDQ®): Screening health professional version.* Retrieved February 6, 2007, from http://www.cancer.gov/cancertopics/pdq/screening/bladder/healthprofessional

National Cancer Institute. (2007b). *Breast cancer screening (PDQ®)* [Health professional version]. Retrieved July 17, 2007, from http://www.cancer.gov/cancertopics/pdq/screening/breast/healthprofessional

National Cancer Institute. (2007c). *Cancer prevention overview (PDQ®)* [Health professional version]. Retrieved January 30, 2007, from http://www.cancer.gov/cancertopics/pdq/prevention/overview/healthprofessional

National Cancer Institute. (2007d). *Cancer screening overview (PDQ®)* [Health professional version]. Retrieved January 29, 2007, from http://www.cancer.gov/cancertopics/pdq/screening/overview/healthprofessional

National Cancer Institute. (2007e). *Endometrial cancer screening (PDQ®)* [Health professional version]. Retrieved February 5, 2007, from http://www.cancer.gov/cancertopics/pdq/screening/endometrial/healthprofessional

National Cancer Institute. (2007f). *Esophageal cancer screening (PDQ®)* [Health professional version]. Retrieved February 6, 2007, from http://www.cancer.gov/cancertopics/pdq/screening/esophageal/healthprofessional

National Cancer Institute. (2007g). *Gastric cancer screening (PDQ®)* [Health professional version]. Retrieved February 6, 2007, from http://www.cancer.gov/cancertopics/pdq/screening/gastric/healthprofessional

National Cancer Institute. (2007h). *Lung cancer screening (PDQ®)* [Health professional version]. Retrieved January 8, 2007, from http://www.cancer.gov/cancertopics/pdq/screening/lung/healthprofessional

National Cancer Institute. (2007i). *Oral cancer screening (PDQ®)* [Health professional version]. Retrieved February 6, 2007, from http://www.cancer.gov/cancertopics/pdq/screening/oral/healthprofessional

National Cancer Institute. (2007j). *Ovarian cancer (PDQ®)* [Health professional version]. Retrieved February 6, 2007, from http://www.cancer.gov/cancertopics/pdq/screening/ovarian/healthprofessional

National Cancer Institute. (2007k). *Prostate cancer screening (PDQ®)* [Health professional version]. Retrieved January 8, 2007, from http://www.cancer.gov/cancertopics/pdq/screening/prostate/healthprofessional

National Comprehensive Cancer Network. (2006). *Genetic/familial high-risk assessment: Breast and ovarian, version 1.2006.* Retrieved January 8, 2007, from http://www.nccn.org/professionals/physician_gls/PDF/genetics_screening.pdf

National Comprehensive Cancer Network. (2007a). *Breast cancer screening and diagnosis, version 1.2007.* Retrieved January 8, 2007, from http://www.nccn.org/professionals/physician_gls/PDF/breast.pdf

National Comprehensive Cancer Network. (2007b). *Cervical cancer screening, version 1.2007.* Retrieved January 8, 2007, from http://www.nccn.org/professionals/physician_gls/PDF/cervical_screening.pdf

National Comprehensive Cancer Network. (2007c). *Colorectal cancer screening, version 1.2007.* Retrieved January 8, 2007, from http://www.nccn.org/professionals/physician_gls/PDF/colorectal_screening.pdf

National Comprehensive Cancer Network. (2007d). *Prostate cancer early detection, version 1.2007.* Retrieved January 8, 2007, from http://www.nccn.org/professionals/physician_gls/PDF/prostate_detection.pdf

Nett, L.M., & Obrigewitch, R. (1993). Nicotine dependency treatment: A role for the nurse practitioner. *Nurse Practitioner Forum, 4*(1), 37–42.

Oncology Nursing Society. (2002). *Prevention and early detection of cancer in the United States* [Position statement]. Pittsburgh, PA: Author.

Oncology Nursing Society. (2003). *The role of the advanced practice nurse in oncology care* [Position statement]. Pittsburgh, PA: Author.

Oncology Nursing Society. (2005). *Global and domestic tobacco use* [Position statement]. Pittsburgh, PA: Author.

Oncology Nursing Society. (2006). *Breast cancer screening* [Position statement]. Pittsburgh, PA: Author.

Pisano, E.D., Gatsonis, C., Hendrick, E., Yaffe, M., Baum, J.K., Acharyya, S., et al. (2005). Diagnostic performance of digital versus film mammography for breast-cancer screening. *New England Journal of Medicine, 353,* 1773–1783.

Polednak, A. (2003). Trends in incidence rates for obesity-associated cancers in the U.S. *Cancer Detection and Prevention, 27,* 415–421.

Posadas, E.M., & Kotz, H.I. (2005). Cervical cancer. In J. Abraham, C.J. Allegra, & J. Gulley (Eds.), *Bethesda handbook of clinical oncology* (2nd ed., pp. 245–247). Philadelphia: Lippincott Williams & Wilkins.

Pray, W.S., & Pray, J.J. (2003, February 15). Nonprescription options for smoking cessation. *U.S. Pharmacist, 28*(2). Retrieved September 12, 2006, from http://www.uspharmacist.com/index.asp?show=article&page=8_1025.htm

Price, A. (2002). Primary and secondary prevention of colorectal cancer. *Gastroenterology Nursing, 26,* 73–81.

Ranney, L., Melvin, C., Lux, L., McClain, E., & Lohr, K.N. (2006). Systematic review: Smoking cessation intervention strategies for adults and adults in special populations. *Annals of Internal Medicine, 45,* 845–856.

Reed, E., & Altaha, R. (2005). Ovarian cancer. In J. Abraham, C.J. Allegra, & J. Gulley (Eds.), *Bethesda handbook of clinical oncology* (2nd ed., pp. 227–228). Philadelphia: Lippincott Williams & Wilkins.

Reeve, K., Calabro, K., & Adams-McNeill, J. (2000). Tobacco cessation intervention in a nurse practitioner managed clinic. *Journal of the American Academy of Nurse Practitioners, 12,* 163–170.

Rigotti, N. (2002). Treatment of tobacco use and dependence. *New England Journal of Medicine, 346,* 506–512.

Rivara, F.P., Ebel, B.E., Garrison, M.M., Christakis, D.A., Wiche, S.E., & Levy, D.T. (2004). Prevention of smoking-related deaths in the United States. *American Journal of Preventive Medicine, 27,* 118–125.

Saslow, D., Hannan, J., Osuch, J., Alciati, M.H., Baines, C., Barton, M., et al. (2004). Clinical breast examination: Practical recommendations for optimizing performance and reporting. *CA: A Cancer Journal for Clinicians, 54,* 327–344.

Saslow, D., Castle, P.E., Cox, J.T., Davey, D.D., Einstein, M.H., Ferris, D.G., et al. (2007). American Cancer Society guideline for human papillomavirus (HPV) vaccine use to prevent cervical cancer and its precursors. *CA: A Cancer Journal for Clinicians, 57,* 7–28.

Schnitt, S.J., Connolly, J.L., Gadd, M., & Houlihan, M. (1996). Benign disorders. In J.R. Harris, M.E. Lippman, M. Morrow, & S. Hellman (Eds.), *Diseases of the breast* (pp. 27–48). Philadelphia: Lippincott-Raven.

Smith, R.A., Cokkinides, V., & Eyre, H.J. (2007). Cancer screening in the United States, 2007: A review of current guidelines, practices, and prospects. *CA: A Cancer Journal for Clinicians, 57,* 90–104.

Tsao, A.S., Kim, E.P., & Hong, W.K. (2004). Chemoprevention in cancer. *CA: A Cancer Journal for Clinicians, 54,* 150–180.

Turini, M., & DuBois, R. (2002). Primary prevention: Phytoprevention and chemoprevention of colorectal cancer. *Hematology/Oncology Clinics of North America, 16,* 811–840.

U.S. Environmental Protection Agency. (2006, September). *Sunscreen: The burning facts.* Washington, DC: Author.

U.S. Food and Drug Administration. (2006a, May 11). FDA approves novel medication for smoking cessation. *FDA News.* Retrieved September 8, 2006, from http://www.fda.gov/bbs/topics/NEWS/2006/NEW01370.html

U.S. Food and Drug Administration. (2006b, June 8). FDA licenses new vaccine for prevention of cervical cancer and other diseases in females caused by human papillomavirus. *FDA News.* Retrieved July 17, 2006, from http://www.fda.gov/bbs/topics/NEWS/2006/NEW01385.html

U.S. Preventive Services Task Force. (2004). Lung cancer screening: Recommendation statement. *Annals of Internal Medicine, 140,* 738–739.

Vogel, V.G., Costantino, J.P., Wickerham, L., Cronin, W.M., Cecchini, R.S., Atkins, J.N., et al. (2006). Effects of tamoxifen vs. raloxifene on the risk of developing invasive breast cancer and other disease outcomes. *JAMA, 295,* 2727–2741.

Vogel, W. (2003). The advanced practice nursing role in a high-risk breast cancer clinic. *Oncology Nursing Forum, 30,* 115–122.

Wagner, R.F., & Casciato, D.A. (2004). Skin cancers. In D.A. Casciato (Ed.), *Manual of clinical oncology* (5th ed., pp. 355–369). Philadelphia: Lippincott Williams & Wilkins.

Zisman, A., Belldegrun, A.S., & Figlin, R.A. (2000). Urinary tract cancers. In D.A. Casciato & B.B. Lowitz (Eds.), *Manual of clinical oncology* (4th ed., pp. 291–298). Philadelphia: Lippincott Williams & Wilkins.

CHAPTER 2

Genetic Risk

Suzanne M. Mahon, RN, DNSc, AOCN®, APNG

Introduction

The evolution of the Human Genome Project has greatly changed the scope of advanced oncology nursing practice. An estimated 10% of all cancers have a hereditary basis (American Cancer Society [ACS], 2008). The field of genetics is rapidly growing with many implications for oncology advanced practice nurses (APNs), including an emphasis on identification of at-risk populations, basic cancer risk assessment, referrals for hereditary cancer evaluation, assistance with implementing cancer prevention and detection measures, and management of psychosocial ramifications of testing (Calzone & Tranin, 2003). The expansion of genetic knowledge will undoubtedly change the focus and priorities in nursing research and nursing education.

Today it is possible, and in many instances routine, to identify individuals who are at increased risk for developing cancer because of an inherited mutated cancer predisposition gene through cancer predisposition genetic testing. Emerging legal ramifications of risk assessment and genetic testing include identifying high-risk individuals and families and informing them about the option for testing; disclosing risks, benefits, and limitations of testing and follow-up; maintaining confidentiality; and warning other relatives who are at risk (American Society of Clinical Oncology [ASCO], 2003). Genetic testing is now readily and commercially available for hereditary breast and ovarian cancer (HBOC), hereditary nonpolyposis colorectal cancer (HNPCC), familial adenosis polyposis (FAP) syndromes, and, most recently, hereditary melanoma. Also, predisposition genes for many unique or rare syndromes exist, and testing is available on a more limited or research basis. Examples of rarer syndromes sometimes encountered in clinical practice include Cowden syndrome, hereditary retinoblastoma, multiple endocrine neoplasia, von Hippel-Lindau syndrome, Wilms tumor, and Li-Fraumeni syndrome. As predisposition testing for malignancy is increasingly available, oncology APNs need a fundamental understanding of the science of genetics and the ramifications of genetic predisposition testing.

Although genetic testing is used more frequently in oncology practice, it is important to remember that genetic testing is best used to help individuals at high risk for developing cancer to make good decisions about cancer screening and prevention strategies. It is not a tool to be used in routine population screening because of the expense of testing and the complex counseling needs associated with it. Because of the increasing availability of testing, individuals with expertise in cancer genetics are needed to educate at-risk individuals about the strengths, limitations, and risks associated with genetic testing. The Oncology Nursing Society (ONS) position *Cancer Predisposition Genetic Testing and Risk Assessment Counseling* (ONS, 2004) emphasizes the need for oncology APNs to provide care and education to at-risk families. The position notes that although many benefits to genetic testing exist, the very process of testing can lead to ethical, legal, and social issues, and nurses need to safeguard patients and families from these potential risks. To provide effective cancer genetics care, oncology nurses need ongoing education in this rapidly changing field.

Definitions

An understanding of basic cancer cell biology is essential when providing cancer genetics care. The evolution of the Human Genome Project led to the development and more widespread use of genetic terms. For many, these terms were not addressed in basic nursing education. An understanding of types of risk, risk assessment strategies, and basic biologic and genetic terms, as well as terms specific to genetic testing, is essential (see Table 2-1). Oncology APNs not only need to understand these terms to read literature and research reports but also must explain this complex and often technical scientific information to patients and families, tailor-

Table 2-1. Definitions of Terms Commonly Used in Cancer Genetics

Term	Definition
Types of Risk	
Absolute risk	Refers to the occurrence of the cancer in the general population (either incidence or mortality)
Attributable risk	Refers to the number of cases of cancer that could be prevented with the manipulation of a known risk factor
Incidence	Refers to the number of cases of cancer that develop in a defined population in a specified period of time (such as one year)
Population	Refers to the number of people in a defined group who are capable of developing cancer
Prevalence	Refers to the actual number of cancers in a defined population at a given time; typically expressed as the number of cases per 100,000 people
Relative risk	Refers to a statistical estimate, which is a comparison of the likelihood of a person with a specific risk factor developing a cancer with the likelihood of a person who does not have the specific risk factor
Risk factor	A trait, characteristic, or lifestyle factor that is associated with a statistically significant increased likelihood of developing a particular cancer

(Continued on next page)

Table 2-1. Definitions of Terms Commonly Used in Cancer Genetics *(Continued)*

Term	Definition
Types of Cancer Prevention	
Primary	Direct measures to avoid carcinogen exposure or implement a healthy practice May include chemoprevention agents or prophylactic surgery
Secondary	Identifying individuals who are at risk for developing a particular cancer and implementing appropriate screening modalities Goal of detecting cancer at the earliest possible stage, when treatment is easiest and most likely to be effective
Tertiary	Monitoring for recurrence and second primary tumors in people who have previously been diagnosed with and treated for cancer
Basic Genetic Terminology	
Allele	One of the various forms of a gene at a particular location on a chromosome
Autosomal dominant	Mendelian inheritance in which an affected individual possesses one copy of a mutant allele and one normal copy A statistical 50% chance exists that the allele and associated disorder or disease will be passed to offspring.
Autosome	Any chromosome other than a sex chromosome Humans have 22 pairs of autosomal chromosomes (46 chromosomes in all).
Chromosome	A thread-like package in the nucleus of the cell that contains genes Humans have 23 pairs of chromosomes; 22 pairs are autosomes, and one pair is a sex chromosome.
Gene	Functional and physical unit of heredity Passed from parent to offspring Contains information necessary for making a specific protein
Genome	The entire DNA contained in an organism
Genotype	Genetic identity May or may not be manifested in outward characteristics
Germ line	Inherited material that comes from the egg or sperm
Heterozygous	Possessing two different forms of a particular gene One is inherited from each parent.
Mutation	A permanent structural change in DNA
Oncogene	Gene that leads to transformation of normal cells into cancer cells
Penetrance	The portion of a population with a particular genotype or mutation that expresses the corresponding phenotype of disorder
Phenotype	Characteristics or traits in an organism that are observable
Proband	Family member who serves as "spokesperson" Risks are calculated based on an individual's relationship to the proband.
Promoter	The part of the gene that contains the information to turn the gene on or off Transcription is initiated in the promoter part of the gene.

(Continued on next page)

Table 2-1. Definitions of Terms Commonly Used in Cancer Genetics *(Continued)*

Term	Definition
Recessive	A trait or disorder that only appears in people who have received two copies of a mutant or altered gene (one from each parent)
Somatic cells	Any cell in the body except the reproductive cells
Tumor suppressor gene	A protective gene that usually limits the growth of tumors; if mutated, it may not be able to keep a cancer from growing, for example, *BRCA* genes.
Terms That Apply to Genetic Testing	
Accuracy	The degree to which a measurement represents the true value of the characteristic being measured
Deletion	A type of chromosomal abnormality in which a piece of DNA is removed or omitted from a gene Results in the disruption of normal structure and function of that gene
DNA sequencing*	Determining the exact order of the base pairs in a segment of DNA
False negative	A test result indicating that the tested person does not have a particular characteristic, but the person actually does have the characteristic Example: a negative mammogram in a woman with early-stage breast cancer
False positive	A test result indicating that the tested person has a particular characteristic, but the person actually does not have the characteristic Example: very suspicious mammogram in a woman who does not have breast cancer
Fluorescence in situ hybridization*	Lab process that involves painting chromosomes or sections of chromosomes with fluorescent molecules Useful technique for identification of chromosomal abnormalities and gene mapping
Insertion	Type of chromosomal abnormality in which an extra piece of DNA is inserted into a gene Results in the disruption of the normal structure and function of that gene
Karyotype	The chromosomal complement of an individual including all chromosomes and abnormalities Also used to refer to a photograph of an individual's chromosomes
Microsatellite	A repetitive short sequence of DNA that is used as a genetic marker to track inheritance in families
Polymerase chain reaction*	Fast, relatively inexpensive means for making an unlimited number of copies of any piece of DNA
Sensitivity	The ability of a screening test to detect individuals with the characteristic being screened for Calculated by dividing the total number of true positives by the total number of the population
Specificity	The ability of a screening test to detect individuals without the characteristic being screened for Calculated by dividing the total number of true negatives by the sum of true negatives and false-positive results

(Continued on next page)

Table 2-1. Definitions of Terms Commonly Used in Cancer Genetics *(Continued)*

Term	Definition
True negative	Test result indicating that the tested person does not have the trait tested for, and the person does not have it Example: A woman has a negative mammogram and does not develop cancer in the next 12–24 months.
True positive	A test result indicating that the tested person has the characteristic tested for, and the person does have it Example: A woman has a suspicious mammogram, and a biopsy demonstrates that the area is a malignancy.
Validity	A measure of how well a test measures what it is supposed to measure

* See Chapter 3 for more information related to diagnostic use of these tests.

Note. Based on information from Greco & Mahon, 2004; Tranin et al., 2003; Trepanier et al., 2004.

ing teaching to meet variable educational and individual needs of patients and families. The biology of cancer and cancer genetics can be overwhelming to patients and families, especially if they have limited education or background in science. Furthermore, many oncology APNs, especially those with expertise in genetics, provide education about hereditary predisposition for developing cancer to other nurses, healthcare providers, and physicians. This education is important to help to ensure that those with a hereditary predisposition for developing cancer are referred for further evaluation. An extensive discussion of genetics and cancer is available in Loescher and Whitesell (2003).

The Genetic Basis of Cancer

Humans carry an estimated 20,000–25,000 genes, which are composed of DNA (Collins, Morgan, & Patrinos, 2003). DNA is composed of four chemicals (adenine [A], thymine [T], cytosine [C], and guanine [G]). The specific order of these chemicals ultimately determines physical characteristics, growth and development, and predisposition for a wide variety of attributes and diseases. Within the human genome, these four chemicals are repeated billions of times in a specific sequence within 23 pairs of chromosomes. Twenty-two of these pairs are autosomes, and one pair is a sex chromosome.

All cancer results from a process of genetic mutations or a change in the arrangement of the four basic chemicals of A, T, C, or G. Mutations that predispose a human to developing a disease such as cancer can occur any time during the lifetime, particularly during growth and development of a tissue or organ (somatic mutations) or at conception in the ova or sperm (germ-line mutations). Hereditary mutations are carried in the DNA of the reproductive cells (germ-line mutations). When reproductive germ cells containing mutations combine to produce offspring, the mutation will be present in all of the offspring's body cells. An accurate family history combined with predisposition genetic testing differentiates between a somatic and germ-line mutation (see Table 2-2). Identifying individuals with germ-line mutations is important because of their increased risk for second primary cancer(s) and the potential risk to other close relatives.

Table 2-2. Differences Between Somatic and Germ-Line Mutations

Characteristic	Somatic Mutations	Germ-Line Mutations
Proportion of cancers	85% of all cancers	10%–15% of all cancers
Type of cancer	Occur in sporadic cancer	Occur in hereditary cancer predisposition syndromes
Timing of mutation	Occur after conception	Occur in the egg or sperm
Transmission of mutation	Cannot be passed to subsequent generations	Can be passed to subsequent generations
Number of cells affected	Affect one cell and the cells that come from that cell's division	Affect all cells in an offspring
Examples	*HER2* amplification in breast cancer, Philadelphia chromosome in chronic leukemia	Mutations in *BRCA1/2, MSH2, MLH1, p16, FAP* genes
Role of genetic testing	Genetic testing may drive treatment decisions. Genetic testing will not help other relatives to determine their risk for developing the cancer.	Genetic testing may alter treatment strategies and often alters prevention and screening strategies. Genetic testing may be able to determine other relatives who are at risk.

Note. Based on information from Calvert & Frucht, 2002; Jeter et al., 2006; Loescher & Whitesell, 2003.

Sporadic cancers occur from multiple somatic mutations in a cell (Calvert & Frucht, 2002). Acquired somatic mutations develop in DNA during a person's lifetime. If the mutation arises in a body cell, copies of the mutation will exist only in descendants of that particular cell. Some mutations are changes in genetic material but do not cause disease or problems; these are referred to as *polymorphisms.* Other mutations, referred to as *deleterious,* can result in disease or other significant changes because of sequence changes that result in alterations of the protein.

As noted, genes come in pairs, with one copy inherited from each parent. Many genes come in a number of variant forms, known as *alleles.* A dominant allele prevails over a recessive allele. A recessive gene becomes apparent if its counterpart allele on the other chromosome becomes inactivated or lost. Not all mutated alleles invariably lead to disease. Even with a dominant allele such as the *BRCA1* breast cancer susceptibility gene, for example, the risk of developing breast cancer by age 65 is 80%, not 100%. An indication of the probability that a given gene mutation will produce disease is referred to as *penetrance.*

A number of mutations occur in malignant cells (Collins et al., 2003). Many malignancies develop as a result of the conversion of proto-oncogenes to oncogenes. Proto-oncogenes regulate normal cell growth, and oncogenes are associated with abnormal cell growth, leading to increased cellular proliferation and uncontrolled growth (Calvert & Frucht, 2002). Other tumors arise because of the inactivation of both alleles of tumor suppressor cells, which play an important role in slowing or stopping abnormal cell growth. Tumor suppressor cells include caretaker genes, which maintain integrity of the genetic material, and gatekeeper genes, which regulate proliferation and cell life. Mismatch repair (MMR) genes repair mistakes that occur during DNA replication. When MMR genes are damaged, genetic stability is altered, and tumor cells replicate. Some mutations interfere with apoptosis (normal programmed cell death). Certain genetic patterns or syndromes occur as a result of some of the mutations described here, and a brief discussion of the more common ones follows.

Common Genetic Cancer Predisposition Syndromes

Oncology APNs will encounter some hereditary cancer predisposition syndromes fairly regularly in their practice. Commercial testing is readily available for these syndromes, which include HBOC, HNPCC, FAP, and hereditary melanoma. It is important to identify families who are at risk for these predisposition syndromes, to know how to refer them for cancer genetics education services, and to provide support for these families as they make complex and often difficult decisions about genetic testing and treatment measures.

Hereditary Breast and Ovarian Cancer Syndromes

An estimated 70% of breast cancer is sporadic, and another 15%–20% is familial, meaning that one or two family members have breast cancer, but no obvious pattern of autosomal dominant transmission is present (Ford et al., 1998). Among women, an estimated 5%–10% of breast cancers and 10%–15% of ovarian cancers are caused by inherited mutations in the *BRCA1* and *BRCA2* genes (Guillem et al., 2006).

The risk of developing cancer in those with *BRCA1/2* mutations has been estimated in many studies. The risk for younger women is estimated to be 33%–50% by age 50 (Daly et al., 2006). For those with mutations in *BRCA1/2,* the cumulative risk for developing breast cancer by age 70 is estimated to be about 87%, and the risk is as high as 44% for ovarian cancer (Lynch, Snyder, Lynch, Riley, & Rubinstein, 2003). The risk of developing a second primary cancer (breast or ovarian) also is elevated. The degree of risk depends on the first primary as well as the age and other comorbidities of the proband (Antoniou et al., 2003). Mutations in the *BRCA1/2* genes also are associated with melanoma and prostate, gastric, pancreatic, and male breast cancers (Debniak et al., 2003; Lynch et al.; Nelson, Huffman, Fu, & Harris, 2005). Key indicators of HBOC syndrome are shown in Figure 2-1.

- Personal and/or family history of breast cancer diagnosed at age 50 or younger
- Personal and/or family history of ovarian cancer diagnosed at any age
- Women of Ashkenazi Jewish ancestry diagnosed with breast and/or ovarian cancer at any age, regardless of family history
- Personal and/or family history of male breast cancer
- Affected first-degree relative with a known *BRCA1* or *BRCA2* mutation
- Bilateral breast cancer, especially if the diagnosis was at an early age
- Breast and ovarian cancer in the same woman

The presence of one or more of these factors in an individual or family history is suggestive of hereditary breast and ovarian cancer syndrome and warrants further evaluation.

Figure 2-1. Key Indicators of Breast and Ovarian Cancer Syndrome

---

Note. Based on information from Guillem et al., 2006; Lynch et al., 2003; Nelson et al., 2005.

Membership in some populations infers increased risk for having a *BRCA1/2* mutation. Founder mutations have been noted in those of Ashkenazi Jewish, Dutch, and Icelandic descent. An estimated 1 in 40 Ashkenazi women carries one of three mutations (185delAG and 5382insc on *BRCA1* and 6174delT on *BRCA2*) (Struewing et al., 1997).

These autosomal dominant genes, which are highly penetrant, predispose individuals to significant risk for developing breast and/or ovarian cancer. The loss of the wild-type allele on chromosomes 17q *(BRCA1)* and 13q *(BRCA2)* suggests that these genes function as tumor suppressor genes (Gudmundsdottir & Ashworth, 2006). *BRCA1* and *BRCA2* are considered caretaker genes and help to maintain genomic stability by recognizing and repairing DNA damage as well as having a role in cell cycle checkpoint control.

Hereditary Nonpolyposis Colorectal Cancer Syndrome

The autosomal dominant syndrome known as HNPCC accounts for 3%–5% of all colorectal cancers (Lynch & de la Chapelle, 2003). It also is associated with endometrial, ovarian, gastric, bile duct, small bowel, renal pelvis, and ureter cancers (Lynch & Lynch, 2006). The majority of mutations responsible for HNPCC syndrome occur in four MMR genes: *MSH2, MLH1, PMS2,* and *MSH6* (Hendriks et al., 2006).

Patients with a mutation in *MLH1* and *MSH2* have an 80% lifetime risk of developing colorectal cancer as compared with a 6% risk in the general population. Women with mutations in these genes have a 60% lifetime risk for developing endometrial cancer and a 12% lifetime risk for developing ovarian cancer (Burt & Neklason, 2005; Lindor et al., 2006).

Individuals with HNPCC-related cancers are more likely to have poorly differentiated tumors with an excess of mucoid and signet-cell features (Lynch & de la Chapelle, 2003). Although not associated with large numbers of polyps, people with HNPCC syndrome who form adenomatous polyps are more likely to do so at an earlier age, are more likely to develop right-sided colon cancer, and tend to exhibit a very rapid progression to malignancy in 1–3 years instead of the 5–10-year pattern seen in the general population (Boland, 2006; Lynch & de la Chapelle).

Risk assessment for HNPCC syndrome is approached in several ways. The Amsterdam and Bethesda criteria assess the number of relatives affected by colorectal cancer or other HNPCC-related cancers with particular emphasis on the age at onset (Umar et al., 2004; Vasen, Watson, Mecklin, & Lynch, 1999). The Bethesda guidelines (see Figure 2-2) assist in identification of tumors that should be tested for microsatellite instability (MSI). The Amsterdam criteria identify tumors that should be considered for immunohistochemical (IHC) testing for one of the four MMR genes (National Comprehensive Cancer Network [NCCN], 2007b).

IHC staining and/or MSI testing may be done to predict an MMR defect and thereby avoid unnecessary, expensive, and time-consuming DNA analyses (Hendriks et al., 2006). IHC staining can be done on tumor tissue from individuals who fulfill the Bethesda criteria to determine the presence or absence of *MLH1, MSH2, MSH6,* and *PMS2* proteins. If IHC is abnormal, this indicates that one of the proteins is not expressed, and an inherited mutation may be present (NCCN, 2007b). Alternatively, an MSI assay could be performed. In HNPCC, mutations in the DNA repair genes result in the phenomenon of MSI. Microsatellites are repeated sequences of DNA that are a defined length for each individual. Because of the accumulation of errors, these sequences can become abnormally longer or shorter, which is referred to as MSI (Umar et al., 2003). An MSI high phenotype is reported in 85%–92% of HNPCC colon cancers and approximately 15% of sporadic cancers (Hendriks et al.). If either of these tests is abnormal, then further testing with DNA analysis would be appropriate. Key indicators of HNPCC syndrome are shown in Figure 2-3.

Revised Amsterdam Criteria II

Three relatives with a cancer associated with HNPCC (colorectal, cancer of endometrium, small bowel, ureter, or renal pelvis)

- One must be a first-degree relative of the other two.
- At least two successive generations must be affected.
- At least one case was diagnosed before age 50.
- Familial adenomatous polyposis should be excluded.
- Tumors are verified by histopathology if possible.

All of the above criteria must be met in order to make a clinical diagnosis of HNPCC and/or to proceed with DNA analysis.

Revised Bethesda Criteria for Testing for Microsatellite Instability (MSI)

- Colorectal carcinoma before age 50
- Presence of synchronous or metachronous HNPCC-related carcinomas, regardless of age*
- Colorectal carcinoma with specific pathologic features before age 60**
- Colorectal carcinoma diagnosed in one or more first-degree relatives with an HNPCC-related tumor, with one before age 50
- Colorectal carcinoma in two or more first- or second-degree relatives with an HNPCC-related tumor, regardless of age

Only one of these criteria must be met to proceed with MSI or immunohistochemical (IHC) testing. If positive by MSI or IHC, then mismatch repair testing may begin.

Figure 2-2. Criteria to Proceed With Microsatellite Instability or Immunohistochemical Testing for Hereditary Nonpolyposis Colorectal Cancer (HNPCC) Syndrome

---

* Colorectal, endometrial, stomach, ovarian, pancreas, ureter and renal pelvis, biliary tract, brain, sebaceous gland, and small bowel carcinomas

** Tumor-infiltrating lymphocytes, Crohn-like lymphocyte reaction, mucinous/signet-ring differentiation, or medullary growth pattern

Note. Based on information from Umar et al., 2004; Vasen et al., 1999.

- Personal history of colorectal and/or endometrial cancer diagnosed before age 50
- First-degree relative with colorectal cancer diagnosed before age 50
- Two or more relatives with colorectal cancer or an HNPCC-associated cancer, which includes endometrial, ovarian, gastric, hepatobiliary, small bowel, renal pelvis, or ureter cancers. The one relative must be a first-degree relative of another.
- Colorectal cancer occurring in two or more generations on the same side of the family
- A personal history of colorectal cancer and a first-degree relative with adenomas diagnosed before age 40
- An affected relative with a known HNPCC mutation

The presence of one or more of these factors in an individual or family history is suggestive of HNPCC syndrome and warrants further evaluation.

Figure 2-3. Key Indicators of Hereditary Nonpolyposis Colorectal Cancer (HNPCC) Syndrome

---

Note. Based on information from Balmana et al., 2006; Lynch & de la Chapelle, 2003; Lynch & Lynch, 2006.

Familial Adenomatous Polyposis Syndromes

FAP, an autosomal dominant trait, is characterized by numerous (usually greater than 100) adenomatous colonic polyps and accounts for about 1% of all cases of colorectal cancer (Lynch & de la Chapelle, 2003). The FAP gene is nearly 100% penetrant; so, if a person is not treated, he or she will develop colorectal cancer because of the sheer number of polyps. The mean age at onset of cancer is 39, although as many as 75% will have developed adenomas by age 20 (Calvert & Frucht, 2002). A less severe form of FAP called attenuated familial adenomatous polyposis (AFAP) is characterized by fewer than 100 polyps (usually about 20) at presentation and later onset of colorectal cancer. More than 800 mutations in the *APC* gene are associated with FAP (Lynch & de la Chapelle). Deleterious mutations in this tumor suppressor gene result in the premature truncation of the APC protein (Jeter, Kohlmann, & Gruber, 2006). An autosomal recessive gene on chromosome 1 also exists, called *MYH*, which is associated with polyposis (Nielsen et al., 2005). Approximately 25% of individuals with FAP have a de novo mutation (Jeter et al.). Figure 2-4 provides an overview of key indicators of FAP and AFAP.

- Patient has a clinical diagnosis of FAP (100 or more polyps).
- Patient has suspected FAP or AFAP (15–99 polyps).
- Patient is a first-degree relative of an individual with FAP or AFAP.
- Patient has an affected relative with a known FAP or *MYH* mutation.
- Patient has any number of adenomas in a family with FAP.

The presence of one or more of these factors in an individual or family history is suggestive of hereditary FAP/AFAP and warrants further evaluation.

Figure 2-4. Key Indicators of Familial Adenomatous Polyposis (FAP) and Attenuated FAP (AFAP)

Note. Based on information from Calvert & Frucht, 2002; Jeter et al., 2006.

Hereditary Melanoma

Hereditary melanoma is an autosomal dominant disease that accounts for about 10% of all melanomas. Germ-line mutations in the tumor suppressor *p16 (CDKN2A)* gene account for 25%–40% of hereditary melanomas (Kefford & Mann, 2003). Mutations in the *p16* gene also have been associated with pancreatic cancer. Those with germ-line mutations in *p16* are at substantial risk for developing melanoma (Hansen, Wadge, Lowstuter, Boucher, & Leachman, 2004). The lifetime risk of developing melanoma approaches 76% (Tsao & Niendorf, 2004). The lifetime risk of developing pancreatic cancer for these individuals approaches 17% (Vasen, Gruis, Frants, van Der Velden, & Hille, 2000). Other genes implicated in hereditary melanoma include the *CDK4* gene (Tsao & Niendorf). Figure 2-5 shows the key indicators of hereditary melanoma.

Indications for Genetic Assessment

Identifying and managing people at risk for hereditary cancer syndromes is now an integral part of oncologic prevention and treatment. With proper assessment, testing,

---

- Three or more primary melanomas in an individual
- A patient with melanoma with three or more melanomas in the family
- Melanoma and pancreatic cancer in an individual and/or family
- First-degree relative of a *p16* mutation carrier

The presence of one or more of these factors in an individual or family history is suggestive of hereditary melanoma and warrants further evaluation.

Figure 2-5. Key Indicators of Hereditary Melanoma

Note. Based on information from Kefford & Mann, 2003; Tsao & Niendorf, 2004.

and implementation of aggressive screening and prevention measures, healthcare providers can significantly affect the future health of patients and their families who have a hereditary risk for cancer. APNs are increasingly assuming responsibility for the management of these families with an emphasis on wellness and cancer prevention.

As many as 10% of people may have a personal or family health history suggestive of a hereditary cancer syndrome (ACS, 2008). In addition to the indicators described in Figures 2-1, 2-3, 2-4, and 2-5, the general factors shown in Figure 2-6 might suggest a person is at risk for a hereditary cancer syndrome. Some family histories do not suggest a specific syndrome such as HBOC or HNPCC but may include a larger number of malignancies than would be expected by chance or that could be explained by environmental exposures. An unusual constellation of cancer types also may be present. When this occurs, it is best to refer to a healthcare provider with expertise in genetics to consider rare syndromes and possible testing strategies or research studies available to help the family to better define their risk (Mahon, 2003).

- A cluster of the same cancer in close relatives
- Cancer occurring at a younger age than expected in the general population
- More than one primary cancer in one person
- Evidence of autosomal dominant inheritance (two or more generations affected, with both males and females affected)
- Bilateral cancer in any paired organ
- Cancers in an organ that are multifocal
- Any pattern of cancer associated with a known cancer syndrome
- Cancers that are occurring more frequently in a family than are expected by chance in the absence of known environmental and lifestyle risk factors

These factors are considered after gathering a family history, and if one or more criteria are present, it may be prudent to refer to a healthcare provider with expertise in cancer genetics.

Figure 2-6. General Indicators of a Hereditary Predisposition for Developing Cancer

---

Note. Based on information from Kefford & Mann, 2003; Tsao & Niendorf, 2004.

Standards for Genetic Testing

Family history and mathematical models are used to calculate a person's risk of developing cancer and carrying a mutation, but ultimately, genetic testing is the only means available to determine who has inherited a germ-line mutation. A number of professional and government agencies have issued position statements regarding genetic testing. Some are more general, but many specify conditions for offering specific cancer predisposition testing, most often *BRCA1/2* testing. These recommendations are updated frequently, and nurses should consult the individual agencies for updates, many of whom post their recommendations and guidelines at the National Guideline Clearinghouse Web site (www.guidelines.gov). A summary of these position statements is shown in Table 2-3. It is important to note that most of the agencies emphasize that testing be done in high-risk people where there is a reasonable likelihood of finding a mutation, where qualified personnel are available to provide informed consent in the context of pre- and post-test counseling, and when the knowledge of mutation status will influence care.

Table 2-3. Standards for Genetic Testing

Agency	Position

American Society of Clinical Oncology	• Genetic testing is offered when
	  1. Personal or family history features suggest a genetic cancer susceptibility condition.
	  2. The test can be adequately interpreted.
	  3. Results will aid in diagnosis or influence the medical or surgical management of the patient and/or at-risk family members.
	• Testing is only done in the setting of pre- and post-test counseling, which includes discussions of possible risks and benefits of cancer early detection and prevention modalities.
	• Efforts should be made to ensure that all individuals at significantly increased risk have access to appropriate genetic counseling, testing, screening, surveillance, and all related medical and surgical interventions, which should be covered without penalty by public and private third-party payers.
	• Providers make direct efforts to protect the confidentiality of genetic information.
	• Educational opportunities for physicians and other healthcare providers are available regarding
	  1. Methods of cancer risk assessment
	  2. Clinical characteristics of hereditary cancer susceptibility syndromes
	  3. Pre- and post-test genetic counseling
	  4. Risk management.

National Society of Genetic Counselors	• Genetic testing for hereditary cancer susceptibility is offered only when
	  1. A client has a significant personal and/or family history of cancer.
	  2. The test can be adequately interpreted.
	  3. The results will affect medical management.
	  4. The clinician can provide or make available adequate genetic education and counseling.
	  5. The client can provide informed consent.
	• Informed consent is a necessary component of genetic testing in both clinical and research settings.
	• The process of informed consent includes
	  1. A thorough discussion of the possible outcomes of testing
	  2. A review of the possible benefits, risks, and limitations
	  3. A discussion of alternatives to molecular testing.

(Continued on next page)

Table 2-3. Standards for Genetic Testing *(Continued)*

Agency	Position

Oncology Nursing Society	• Risk assessment counseling and cancer predisposition genetic testing are essential components of comprehensive cancer care.
	• Healthcare providers offering these services must have educational preparation in both human genetic principles and oncology.
	• Cancer predisposition genetic testing requires informed consent and must include
	  1. Pre- and post-test counseling
	  2. Follow-up by qualified individuals.
	• Legislation exists that provides protection from
	  1. Genetic discrimination in both employment and insurance arenas
	  2. Reimbursement for and access to genetic counseling, cancer predisposition genetic testing services, and appropriate medical management.
	• Ongoing educational resources for healthcare providers, individuals at increased risk, and the lay public are developed, evaluated, and disseminated.

U.S. Preventive Services Task Force	• Fair evidence exists that women with certain specific family history patterns ("increased risk family history") have an increased risk for developing breast or ovarian cancer associated with *BRCA1/2* and may benefit from genetic testing. • These women would benefit from genetic counseling that allows informed decision making about testing and prophylactic treatment. • Counseling is performed by suitably trained healthcare providers.

Note. Based on information from American Society of Clinical Oncology, 2003; Oncology Nursing Society, 2004; Trepanier et al., 2004; U.S. Preventive Services Task Force, 2005.

Provision of Cancer Genetics Education and Counseling

Providing education, counseling, and support are central APN responsibilities when caring for people with a hereditary predisposition for developing cancer. This education is tailored to the individual needs and learning capabilities of each family member. This usually is a labor-intensive process, and families should anticipate at least one to three sessions lasting 60–90 minutes prior to testing to ensure that they truly have informed consent and adequate information to make a good decision that is congruent with their individual needs. Additional counseling sessions following testing also will be needed; how many often depends on the outcome of testing and the person's psychological response to the results.

Assessment of Hereditary Risk

During the assessment for hereditary risk, families are asked to provide detailed information about family history and cancer diagnoses. It often is helpful to inform patients of the need for a detailed family history prior to the appointment. Typically, the proband (the one to be tested) for the family is instructed to gather information about all cancer diagnoses, age at diagnosis, and current age or age at death for all first- and second-degree relatives. This frequently requires the proband to communicate with multiple family members to gather this information. Obtaining this information before the appointment saves time and allows the APN to perform some preliminary risk calculations and identify areas where more information is needed. This usually is organized into a pedigree format as shown in Figure 2-7. This information is confirmed by pathology reports and/or death certificates whenever possible because families often have incomplete or incorrect information about cancer diagnoses. Without accurate information regarding the cancer diagnoses, it is impossible to accurately assess risk and select the correct genetic test to order. This visual presentation also is very helpful for explaining risk to families. A variety of computerized programs are available to facilitate the drawing of these pedigrees. Programs also are available that help to calculate both statistical risk for developing cancer and for carrying a mutation for hereditary predisposition (see Figure 2-8).

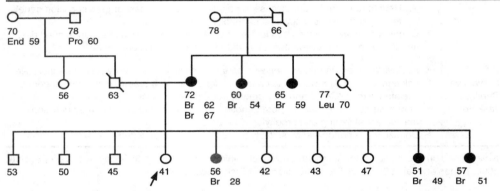

This pedigree represents a typical presentation of family history. Squares represent males, and circles represent females. A slash represents a deceased person. Filled-in circles and squares represent diagnoses confirmed with pathology reports. The family member's current age or age at death is shown as well as the age at any cancer diagnosis. The arrow represents the proband or spokesperson for the family. There are three generations, showing both maternal and paternal sides. If information is known about ethnicity, it can also be included. Ideally, all cancer diagnoses are verified by pathology reports and/or death certificates.

Figure 2-7. Example of a Pedigree

Families deserve basic information on how such risk assessments are completed and what the models imply as well as a summary of their risk. Frequently, this includes a statistical discussion of risk. Patients need to understand the risk for developing the disease in the general population (absolute risk) as well as the relative risk for developing the cancer when compared to people who do not have risk factors. Using relative risk is complicated in people with a family history of cancer. If the individual did not inherit the predisposition gene, the person's relative risk score will overestimate his or her risk. If the individual did inherit the gene, it will probably underestimate the risk (Freedman et al., 2005; Trepanier et al., 2004). Patients need to be informed of these potential and significant limitations.

A risk calculation as to whether the individual has a genetic mutation is necessary. If no testing has been done in a family, this calculation usually is based on the number of family members diagnosed with a specific constellation of cancers, ethnicity, and age at diagnosis (see Figure 2-8). Usually several different models are used, and the patient receives the risk estimate in a range. Each of these methods has distinct strengths and limitations. It is especially important to note that if the family is small with few affected individuals, these models usually will underestimate the risk of having a mutation (Bodmer et al., 2006). In the case of HBOC, additional criteria that may influence a decision to

Gail Model

Purpose: Estimates breast cancer risk in women without a diagnosis of cancer

Target: Women with a minimal to moderate family history of breast cancer

Advantages: Readily available; considers commonly collected risk factors; provides risk estimates for next five years and lifetime

Disadvantage: Does not consider family history of ovarian cancer, age at diagnosis, affected second-degree relatives, or paternal family history

Pedigree Assessment Tool

Purpose: Identifies women at increased risk for hereditary breast or ovarian cancer

Target: Women being seen in primary care settings with multiple family members diagnosed with breast cancer

Advantage: Simple point scoring system based on family history with points weighted according to features associated with *BRCA1/2* mutations

Disadvantage: May over-refer some women for genetic counseling

Claus Model

Purpose: Estimates risk of developing breast cancer over time in 10-year increments

Target: Women with multiple family members diagnosed with breast cancer

Advantage: Considers maternal and paternal history of breast cancer as well as age at diagnosis

Disadvantage: Does not consider history of ovarian cancer or ethnicity

Shattuck-Eidens Model

Purpose: Estimates risk of carrying a *BRCA1* mutation

Target: Women with substantial family history of breast cancer or early-onset breast cancer

Advantage: Considers early-onset breast cancer, bilateral breast cancer, and ovarian cancer history

Disadvantage: Does not consider ethnicity or *BRCA2* mutations

Couch Model

Purpose: Estimates risk of carrying a *BRCA1* mutation

Target: Women with a substantial family history of breast cancer

Advantage: Considers the average age at diagnosis in the family and ethnicity

Disadvantage: Is relatively insensitive in small families or those with few cancers

Berry Model

Purpose: Estimates risk of carrying a *BRCA1* or *BRCA2* mutation

Target: Women with a family history of breast and/or ovarian cancer

Advantage: Considers first- and second-degree relatives, age at diagnosis, and breast and ovarian cancer history

Disadvantage: Has limited utility in some ethnic groups

Frank Model

Purpose: Estimates risk of carrying a *BRCA1* or *BRCA2* mutation

Target: Women diagnosed with breast cancer before age 50

Advantage: Considers first- and second-degree relatives, age at diagnosis, and breast and ovarian cancer history

Disadvantage: May not be as sensitive in families with older age at onset

Manchester Model

Purpose: Estimates risk of carrying a *BRCA1* or *BRCA2* mutation

Target: Non-Jewish women with a family history of breast and/or ovarian cancer

Advantage: Useful in identifying women who have *BRCA2* mutations

Disadvantage: May be less useful in identifying women who have *BRCA1* mutations

Figure 2-8. Risk Models Commonly Calculated for Use When Counseling About Hereditary Cancer Syndromes

(Continued on next page)

Wijnen Model
Purpose: Estimates the risk of carrying an *MSH2* or *MLH1* mutation
Target: People with a family history of colon and/or endometrial cancer
Advantages: Considers history of colon and endometrial cancer; may be more useful when used in conjunction with Amsterdam criteria and microsatellite instability testing
Disadvantage: Does not consider ovarian cancer or other gastrointestinal cancers

PREMM Model
Purpose: Estimates the risk of carrying an *MSH2* or *MLH1* mutation
Target: People with a family history of colorectal and gynecologic cancer
Advantages: Considers both colorectal and gynecologic cancers as well as personal risk factors; easy to complete with a Web-based model
Disadvantage: May not be able to incorporate complex combinations of diagnoses

MMRpro Model
Purpose: Predicts people who may benefit from genetic testing for *MSH2* or *MLH1* mutations
Target: People with a personal and/or family history of colorectal or endometrial cancer
Advantage: May be useful in small families, families with older age at diagnosis, and families that do not meet Bethesda criteria
Disadvantage: Does not consider other cancers associated with hereditary nonpolyposis colorectal cancer

---

Figure 2-8. Risk Models Commonly Calculated for Use When Counseling About Hereditary Cancer Syndromes *(Continued)*

Note. Based on information from Balmana et al., 2006; Berry et al., 1997, 2002; Chen et al., 2006; Claus et al., 1991, 1994; Costantino et al., 1999; Couch et al., 1997; Daly et al., 2006; Evans et al., 2004; Gail et al., 1989; Greco & Mahon, 2004; Hoskins et al., 2006; Lynch et al., 2003; Shattuck-Eidens et al., 1997.

offer testing in a small family might include a diagnosis of both breast and ovarian cancer in one member, male breast cancer, bilateral breast cancer (especially if diagnosed before age 45), ovarian cancer diagnosed before age 40, or breast cancer diagnosed before age 35. Once a mutation is detected in a family, it is possible to offer the statistical risk based on Mendelian patterns of inheritance; in the case of autosomal dominance, first-degree relatives have a statistical 50% chance of having inherited the predisposition gene.

Basic Genetic Information

For families to make an informed decision about testing, a basic background in genetics is required. At the minimum, this includes information about autosomal dominant transmission, penetrance, statistical risks, and the difference between germ-line and somatic mutations. Pictures and diagrams are useful when conveying this information, and the APN or genetic counselor might use a brochure or handout with this information so that the patient can review the information at a later date. A copy of the pedigree is useful to share with the family for better understanding of the principles of autosomal dominant transmission. Other materials that might be shared with families include copies of risk calculations, especially if these calculations help the family to understand how their risk compares with the risk in the general population and estimates of risk over time.

Prevention Strategies

Prior to genetic testing, patients need a clear understanding of the recommendations and guidelines for management of risk if they test positive and if they do not. This anticipatory guidance helps patients to prepare for all potential ramifications so they can make a choice about testing that is congruent with their values and needs.

The area of prevention usually is one in which patients are interested, but it can lead to very difficult choices. For many cancers with a hereditary predisposition, prevention is best achieved by prophylactic surgery such as mastectomy, hysterectomy, colectomy, or oophorectomy. Each of these procedures not only carries the risks associated with surgery and anesthesia but also psychosocial concerns, significant body image changes, and alterations in body function. It is important to explore a patient's feelings, concerns, and openness about these preventive measures prior to testing.

Prevention measures also may include chemoprevention if a strategy exists. In this case, the patient needs to be aware of the risks, side effects, and potential benefits of such an agent. This usually requires a discussion of current research. It is important to explore whether an individual is willing to commit to taking such an agent long term when the effectiveness may not be immediately evident and potential side effects exist.

Finally, prevention measures may include lifestyle measures such as a healthy diet, weight management, exercise, smoking cessation, and application of sunscreen and other measures that protect against ultraviolet light exposure. Patients need more than a simple recommendation. For prevention strategies to be effective, most patients will need specific information, planning, and approaches to such behavior.

Early Detection Strategies

Families and individuals with hereditary predisposition need specific information regarding how to detect cancer in the earliest stages, when treatment is most likely to be effective. This includes signs and symptoms to report promptly, as well as screening measures. For each recommended screening measure, there needs to be a discussion of the sensitivity and specificity of the screening tests, as well as the expected benefits and risks. Guidelines given to the general population may require modification in high-risk families. It is important that families clearly understand that screening will not prevent cancer but rather that it can result in sufficiently early detection for the disease to be treated with limited morbidity and mortality.

Genetic Testing Process

The process of genetic testing is relatively straightforward once the proper test is selected and the patient has been informed of the potential risks, benefits, and limitations of testing. The patient usually must sign a consent to ensure that he or she understands the ramifications of testing and that he or she is not being coerced. A number of agencies, including ASCO, International Society of Nurses in Genetics (ISONG), National Society of Genetic Counselors (NSGC), and ONS, have developed recommendations about the need for informed consent (see Figure 2-9) and consultation with a qualified health professional with expertise in genetics.

Because testing is usually expensive, and insurance reimbursement can vary, preauthorization often is desirable so that a patient understands his or her potential financial responsibilities. Preauthorization frequently requires a letter of medical necessity. Typical components of a letter of medical necessity include the test being ordered, why it is appropriate to order the test, and how the results will influence the care and management of the patient's risk.

- Basic information on the mode of transmission and penetrance
- Genetic test being performed; sensitivity, specificity, and technical aspects of the test
- Likelihood of having a positive test based on risk assessment
- Discussion of how testing may clarify risks in a family
- Implications of a positive test, including prophylactic surgical procedures, chemoprevention, and screening measures
- Benefits of testing an affected person first
- Implications of a negative test if a mutation has not been identified in the family
- Implications of a negative test for a known mutation, including population risks for developing cancer
- Discussion of Mendelian patterns of transmission and risks for children, siblings, and other first-degree relatives
- Discussion of fees for counseling and testing and coverage for prophylactic procedures and screening
- Exploration of feelings about testing
- Discussion of potential negative and positive psychological outcomes associated with testing
- Discussion of potential risks of employer and insurance discrimination as well as risks of loss of privacy, including how confidentiality will be maintained during the testing process
- Discussion of alternatives to testing
- Discussion of policies for storage or reuse of genetic material by the testing laboratory
- Importance of sharing genetic testing results with at-risk relatives and healthcare providers

Figure 2-9. Recommended Components of Informed Consent

Note. Based on information from American Society of Clinical Oncology, 2003; International Society of Nurses in Genetics, 2007; Oncology Nursing Society, 2004; Trepanier et al., 2004.

Once preauthorization has been obtained, a blood specimen is drawn from the patient and sent to the testing laboratory. Some laboratories will hold the specimen until preauthorization is final. Each laboratory has specific rules for collecting and transporting the specimen. In most cases, results are available in three to four weeks. Results are best disclosed in person, and this policy is addressed in pretest counseling. Depending on the outcome, additional sessions may be needed to discuss management strategies.

As genetic testing for a hereditary cancer syndrome has implications for other family members, a clear plan needs to be made prior to testing regarding how other family members will be informed of their risk. Genetic test results are confidential medical information. The proband, or person undergoing testing, will need to inform other at-risk relatives.

A related issue that families sometimes confront deals with testing of minor children. Because testing results may change prevention and screening behaviors, it is important to consider the implications of testing for minor children. In the case of HBOC, HNPCC, and hereditary melanoma testing, knowledge of mutation status will not alter behaviors. Minor children would probably not be candidates for mammography, ultrasonography, or chemoprevention. It would not be necessary to know mutation status to make recommendations regarding a low-fat, high-fiber diet or reduction in ultraviolet exposure. These recommendations would be appropriate for any member of the population. When minors reach an age with maturity to consent and following adequate counseling, they can make their own decision about testing. One exception sometimes encountered in cancer genetics is individuals from families with a known mutation associated with FAP. Because these individuals begin forming polyps early in their teenage years, colonoscopy often is initiated before the individuals reach the legal age to provide consent. In this case, with careful counseling of both the minor child and parents, a decision sometimes is made to test a minor child. In this case, the parents would consent because knowing the results of mutation status may provide support for regular colonoscopy at a young age or may eliminate the need for this invasive screening procedure.

Potential Risks, Benefits, and Limitations of Testing

The biggest risks of testing involve loss of privacy and psychosocial distress. In most cases, pretest counseling aids in the identification of potential problems so that these may be addressed before testing. Efforts need to be made to protect confidentiality. Concerns about confidentiality and potential discrimination often are paramount for patients and, in some cases, make it difficult for patients to even begin to learn about the ramifications of testing. Clearly, these fears keep some individuals and families from seeking genetic services or participating in genetics research (Watson & Greene, 2001). Federal laws exist that are designed to protect the patient's genetic information. The Health Insurance Portability and Accountability Act (1996) specifically addresses genetic discrimination. Group health insurance plans cannot use genetic information to deny or limit eligibility for coverage or to increase premiums, and genetic information cannot be considered a preexisting condition. However, this protection has gaps and does not apply to people who have individual or self-insured plans. The exact extent of genetic discrimination regarding health insurance is not known. Hall and Rich (2000a) reported in an extensive comparative case-study analysis that people with serious genetic conditions who were presymptomatic had little or no difficulty in obtaining health insurance, especially group health insurance. Furthermore, these researchers reported that many insurers were only vaguely aware of state laws that prohibited insurers' use of genetic information in pricing, issuing, or structuring health insurance policies. Hall and Rich (2000b) also noted that the existing state laws have not reduced fears regarding genetic discrimination. This lack of confidence demonstrated by both healthcare providers and the public may stem from the fact that no real test cases of actual enforcement have occurred.

Employment discrimination is a potential risk that needs to be addressed. Legal protection is not completely clear. The Americans With Disabilities Act does not prohibit employers from requesting genetic information from potential employees. Patients need to be counseled about how to manage questions about risk in the workplace.

Prior to testing, patients also are counseled about risks and potential problems with obtaining life or disability insurance. Failure to disclose a genetic condition may result in cancellation of a policy. Some people may opt to purchase or increase coverage prior to testing to avoid possible problems. More controversy exists with life insurance because individuals fear that if they have a mutation and desire increased coverage, it will be unaffordable, which often limits or discourages them from obtaining genetic testing that might provide health benefits. Conversely, life insurance providers argue that they need access to genetic testing information to prevent excessive financial loss (Armstrong et al., 2003).

As part of the informed consent process, patients and families need to understand how their genetic risk and test results will be handled. Some genetics programs will use a specific consent to release genetic information (Greco, 2003). Information about genetic testing is important to many primary care providers and other subspecialists so that they can order proper cancer prevention and early detection measures. As part of the informed consent process, it is important to discuss with patients and families how and whether they intend to release genetic test results to healthcare providers and the implications of these decisions. Many commercial laboratories that perform genetic testing provide a copy of results intended to be given to the patients. Some patients opt to share this directly with their primary healthcare provider rather than having the genetics healthcare provider release the results.

One of the biggest threats to confidentiality is unintentional disclosures from the medical record, such as one healthcare provider dictating a note that the reason for a prophylactic procedure or screening modality was a positive genetic test. That health-care provider inadvertently and unintentionally released confidential information with-out authorization from the patient to whoever reads the note (Greco, 2003). This also occurs when an entire medical record is copied and the genetic testing records also are copied, even if they were not ordered by the healthcare provider.

Patients and families need assurance that their records will be maintained in a con-fidential way. Some practices keep genetic records separate from the regular medical record. Practices vary in how records are stored and copied. If the information is not in the regular medical record, it may be difficult for the healthcare provider to provide proper care and recommendations. Conversely, putting genetic information in the reg-ular medical record increases the risk that it could be disclosed to third parties without proper authorization (Greco, 2003). Genetic records also contain information about other family members, such as pathology reports, medical notes, or death certificates, and these are never to be released to third parties. Any third party desiring this infor-mation needs to go to the source to obtain this information.

Outcomes of Testing

Three outcomes of testing are possible. These include negative results, positive re-sults, or results of a variant of indeterminate significance (see Figure 2-10). Following disclosure, most patients want to know the implications of the results. Recommenda-tions for follow-up, prevention, and early detection are based on the results of testing and, in many cases, the personal and family history. For those individuals who test pos-itive for a mutation, aggressive screening and prevention measures are indicated. For those who test negative for a known mutation in a family, recommendations for screen-ing and prevention that would be appropriate for the general population are given. For those who test negative and there is not a known mutation, recommendations for pre-vention are based on potential risks following a balanced discussion of the potential risks and benefits of such recommendations. These families also may benefit from en-rollment in a hereditary cancer research registry with the hope of identifying a mutation in the family through research. For those who have a variant of indeterminate signifi-cance, results can bring confusion and disappointment because risk has not been clar-ified. Often the laboratory will want to test other family members; if this is an option, testing can be offered to families. Some of these families may be able to enroll in a re-search registry but may not receive useful information in a timely fashion. These fami-lies also will need recommendations for prevention and early detection based on risks with a discussion of the potential risks and benefits of these recommendations.

Psychosocial Concerns

A primary objective of genetic counseling and education is to help each individual and family in weighing the options, risks, and benefits of testing in their unique life sit-uation. Identifying potential psychosocial concerns is a substantial component of the counseling process. Testing is not in itself good or bad, or right or wrong. However, for some people, testing is appropriate and will have positive outcomes, whereas for oth-ers, the risk is significant that the information will result in considerable psychosocial distress (Greco & Mahon, 2004).

Positive Result
- A mutation is detected; individual is at increased risk for developing cancer(s).
- Other relatives can undergo single-site testing to clarify their risk.
- Results do not inform about what cancer or when a cancer will develop, only that the risk is higher.
- Results assist in making informed decisions about cancer prevention and early detection strategies.
- Risks include psychological distress, fears of being isolated, and concerns regarding transmission to offspring.

True Negative Result
- No mutation was detected in a person with a known mutation in family.
- Individual will not need screening greater than that recommended for the general population.
- Patient will not need to consider prophylactic surgery or chemoprevention.
- Patient has a more accurate cancer risk assessment.
- The individual experiences psychological relief regarding risk for developing cancer.
- The individual experiences psychological relief that offspring will not inherit mutation.
- Risks include a false sense of security for the patient that he or she will not develop cancer.
- The individual may feel guilty that he or she "escaped" the mutation (i.e., "survivor guilt").

Negative Result—No Mutation Identified in Family
- No mutation is detected in a family with no known mutations.
- This result usually occurs when the first individual in a family is tested. It may occur because the person did not inherit a mutation, the cancer is due to a different mutation than the one tested, or the cancer seen in the family is due to nonhereditary reasons.
- Results are difficult to interpret and must be considered in conjunction with personal risk factors and family history.
- Testing is not available to other nonaffected members in the family.
- Disappointment that results are inconclusive can occur.
- Uncertainty exists about the usefulness of cancer risk reduction strategies.
- Patient can consider participating in research studies or high-risk registries.

Variant of Indeterminate Significance
- Test identifies a mutation; it is not clear if it is a polymorphism or deleterious.
- Results do not provide meaningful information.
- This result may be anxiety-provoking.
- Meaningful testing will not be available to other family members.
- Uncertainty exists about the usefulness of cancer risk reduction strategies.
- Recommendations for cancer prevention and detection need to be formulated based on personal risk factors and family history with careful information about potential benefits and risks.
- Patient can consider participating in a research study or hereditary cancer registry.

Figure 2-10. Implications of Genetic Testing Results

Note. Based on information from Greco, 2003; Guillem et al., 2006; U.S. Preventive Services Task Force, 2005.

Patients may experience increased anxiety and fear while waiting for their test results (Kausmeyer et al., 2006). Increased support may be needed during this time period. Patients also have reported finding it helpful to have written brochures, a letter summarizing recommendations, and guidance about how to share risk information and testing outcomes with other relatives and healthcare professionals (Hopwood, 2005).

Perceptions of genetic risk are influenced by prior experiences with cancer. People who have experienced loss related to cancer often find it particularly difficult to learn about the risks and benefits of genetic testing (Valverde, 2006). It is important to explore not only the motivations for testing or not testing but also how the individual has coped with past cancer experiences. Individuals who have lost a relative and then test positive often have difficulty coping, as they fear the same outcome and that their children will lose a parent early. For those who test negative after having lost a parent, it often is difficult to accept a negative result because they assume they will have the same outcome. For these patients, it can take time to reframe their personal identity.

Some patients who receive positive results feel empowered and relieved because they can make appropriate decisions about prevention strategies with confidence and feel as though they can exercise some control. Other patients who felt they were prepared for positive results can be overwhelmed by the outcome and require much counseling and support. Many people who test positive are not concerned as much for their own health conditions and fears but rather experience feelings of guilt if a child inherits the gene (Vadaparampil, Wey, & Kinney, 2004).

Those who have a true negative result often feel a huge sense of relief. This is especially true for parents who carry a mutation and learn that a child does not. A true negative result, however, can sometimes be accompanied by a phenomenon referred to as *survivor guilt*. This occurs when the person who tests negative questions and feels guilty as to why he or she was fortunate enough to test negative when another sibling or relative tests positive.

Individuals with a variant of indeterminate significance or an inconclusive negative result may experience a wide range of feelings. Many feel much frustration because they feel they must make decisions about prevention and early detection without clear information. Others with an inconclusive result feel relief because they believe the malignancy may not be related to a hereditary cause.

Overall, research suggests that patients may be slightly distressed immediately following risk communication and genetic testing (Hopwood, 2005). Many patients will experience generalized anxiety during the counseling, testing, and short-term follow-up periods even with counseling (Braithwaite, Emery, Walter, Prevost, & Sutton, 2004). These patients may need more intense psychosocial support during the testing process and in the short term during the follow-up period. Long-term follow-up and support usually are associated with improved knowledge of cancer risks and improved knowledge about testing, which, in most cases, ultimately leads to improved satisfaction with testing decisions and adjustment to risk (Pieterse, van Dulmen, Beemer, Bensing, & Ausems, 2007). These researchers also noted that providing anticipatory guidance prior to the visit is associated with lower feelings of anxiety and an increased sense of control. For patients undergoing prophylactic surgical procedures, the need for psychosocial support may persist longer. Additional support may be required if other members of the family are diagnosed with malignancy. For this reason, many genetic counselors and educators will encourage people to contact them again if questions or concerns arise. Families with children may contact the counselor for additional care as teenagers become old enough to consider their own risks and options for testing. Because of these long-term needs, families may be followed intermittently for years with some periods of more intense service.

Prevention and Screening Strategies for Those With Hereditary Risk

Hereditary Breast and Ovarian Cancer

Because the risks for both breast and ovarian cancer are significant, recommendations for prevention and screening made by the U.S. Preventive Services Task Force

(2005), ASCO (Guillem et al., 2006), and the National Comprehensive Cancer Network (NCCN) (2007c) are summarized in Table 2-4.

Table 2-4. Recommendations for Prevention and Early Detection in Women With a Known Mutation in *BRCA1/2*

Organ	Surveillance	Prevention
Breast	Monthly breast self-exam beginning at age 18 Clinical breast exam every 6 months beginning at age 20 Annual mammography and magnetic resonance imaging beginning at age 25*	Consider prophylactic mastectomy (risk reduction of up to 95%). Consider chemoprevention. Consider prophylactic oophorectomy (risk reduction of up to 50%).
Ovary	Pelvic examination every 6 months beginning at age 25 Transvaginal ultrasound** with color Doppler beginning at age 25 every 6–12 months* Serum CA 125 testing every 6–12 months	Consider prophylactic oophorectomy between ages 35–40 (risk reduction of up to 85%–96%).

* Age to begin screening can vary based on the youngest age at which breast or ovarian cancer was diagnosed in the family.
** Testing in premenopausal women should occur sometime during days 1–10 of the menstrual cycle.

Note. Based on information from Daly et al., 2006; Guillem et al., 2006; Lynch et al., 2003; National Comprehensive Cancer Network, 2007c; Saslow et al., 2007; U.S. Preventive Services Task Force, 2005.

Screening recommendations for those at risk for HBOC are initiated at a much earlier age than in the general population because of the early age at onset seen in this population. Women from these families need education about the signs and symptoms of breast cancer (lump, thickening, change in breast skin or color, nipple direction, or nipple discharge) and ovarian cancer (vague abdominal pain or gastrointestinal symptoms, weight loss, or bloating). Training in breast self-examination (BSE) may offer women some sense of control and ideally begins at age 18. Mammography typically is initiated at age 25. Women need to be clearly instructed on the limitations of mammography in younger age groups because of the density of breast tissue.

Surveillance for ovarian cancer has been shown to be of limited benefit and is not associated with decrease in morbidity or mortality associated with ovarian cancer (Nelson et al., 2005). Current screening recommendations include annual or semiannual concurrent transvaginal ultrasonography and CA 125 level beginning at age 25–35 or 5–10 years earlier than the youngest age at which ovarian cancer was first diagnosed in the family (NCCN, 2007c). The patient needs to clearly understand that these screening procedures are limited in their ability to detect ovarian cancer at a curable stage (Schmeler et al., 2006), and a prophylactic bilateral salpingo-oophorectomy (BSO) should be seriously considered.

Chemoprevention is an option that may be considered by women at risk for HBOC. Recent epidemiologic evidence suggests it may be an appropriate option for all women at risk for HBOC (Guillem et al., 2006). Typically, the oral agent tamoxifen is initiated 5–10 years before the youngest age at onset of breast cancer in the family and is continued for five years. Women who take tamoxifen, especially premenopausal women, need careful counseling about pregnancy prevention, and all women need to be aware of potential side effects, including risk of embolism (Daly et al., 2006; Narod, 2006). In postmenopausal women, raloxifene also may be considered (NCCN, 2007a).

The use of oral contraceptive pills (OCPs) appears to reduce the risk of ovarian cancer by up to 50%, but data are very inconsistent regarding the use of OCPs and breast cancer risk in mutation-positive women (Domchek & Weber, 2006). Given the controversy over breast cancer risk and that oophorectomy often is recommended between ages 35–40, many clinicians are reluctant to use OCPs in this population. If a woman desires to use OCPs, she needs a balanced discussion of the pros and cons of OCPs (Narod, 2006).

Mammography, even when combined with ultrasound, still may be ineffective in detecting breast cancer early in HBOC, especially in women younger than 35 years of age or in women with extremely dense breasts. Recent studies suggest that breast magnetic resonance imaging (MRI) results in higher sensitivity, especially when combined with mammography in high-risk women (Kuhl et al., 2005). The sensitivity of MRI can be as high as 70% in women with HBOC (Kriege et al., 2004). However, screening MRIs are limited if there is not a dedicated breast coil, the ability to perform a biopsy under MRI guidance, and an experienced radiologist to read the test (NCCN, 2007c). When MRI, mammography, and breast ultrasound are used together with clinical breast examination (CBE), sensitivity rises to 95% (Warner et al., 2004). The NCCN (2007c) guidelines recommend that a screening breast MRI and mammography be performed annually on women with a mutated *BRCA* gene. Breast MRI could be offered to patients along with a balanced discussion of potential risks, including an increased number of false-positive readings necessitating biopsy, and benefits, including earlier detection of malignancy (Domchek, Stopfer, & Rebbeck, 2006; Warner & Causer, 2005). An early analysis suggested that breast MRI also might be a cost-effective screening strategy in women with known mutations in *BRCA1/2* (Plevritis et al., 2006). It also may be recommended for individuals considered to be at risk for HBOC even in the absence of a confirmed mutation because of its increased sensitivity (Herrmann & Borelli, 2006).

Prophylactic mastectomy can result in a 90%–95% reduction in breast cancer (Daly et al., 2006; Domchek, Friebel, et al., 2006; Guillem et al., 2006). This is an option for many women, especially those who have already been diagnosed with cancer, have undergone multiple breast biopsies, have abnormalities on CBE or mammography, or have breasts that are difficult to examine clinically or on mammography. Prophylactic mastectomy may lead to significant overall survival in mutation carriers diagnosed with cancer (Van Sprundel et al., 2005). However, it is an irreversible procedure that can be emotionally difficult for many women. In most cases, a prophylactic mastectomy includes total mastectomy without axillary node dissection. Skin-sparing and nipple-sparing procedures sometimes are offered with informed consent that emphasizes that when more breast tissue is left, the effectiveness of the procedure decreases (Guillem et al., 2006). Women who undergo a prophylactic mastectomy can opt for immediate reconstruction with a flap or implant or can choose to use prosthetics. Detailed information about this is available (Casey & Mahon, 2007; Chapman, 2007). This is a difficult decision for a woman and requires much support and education. Some women find the online resources from Facing Our Risk of Cancer Empowered (www.facingourrisk .org) especially helpful. This can allow patients to communicate with women who have made this choice and who can serve as a source of peer support.

Prophylactic BSO may be a prudent choice because the effectiveness of screening for ovarian cancer is limited (Daly et al., 2006). It also has been proved to be a cost-effective measure in this population (Anderson et al., 2006). A BSO is associated with as much as a 90% reduction in risk for ovarian cancer and a 50% reduction in the risk of breast cancer (Guillem et al., 2006). The ideal age seems to be between 35–40 if child-bearing is complete. Approximately 2%–6% of mutation-positive women in this age group will have occult ovarian cancers at the time of prophylactic surgery (Finch et al., 2006). This primary prevention strategy is considered after a careful discussion of the potential benefits of reduced risk of breast and ovarian cancer with the consequences of early menopause associated with increased vasomotor symptoms and potential bone loss (Schmeler et al., 2006). Preliminary data suggest it might be safe to offer short-term hormone replacement therapy following BSO without negating the protective effect of the surgery but decreasing vasomotor symptoms (Rebbeck et al., 2005). Women at substantial risk for cervical and uterine problems and malignancies may want to consider a total abdominal hysterectomy (TAH) (Domchek & Weber, 2006).

Men testing positive for a *BRCA* mutation are recommended to undergo CBE every six months and perform BSE monthly, and mammography can be considered (NCCN, 2007c). Mammography sometimes is offered to men with gynecomastia. Prostate screening, including a digital rectal examination and prostate-specific antigen testing, is initiated at age 40 (ACS, 2008; NCCN, 2007c).

Hereditary Nonpolyposis Colorectal Cancer

Individuals who test positive for an *MSH2* or *MLH1* mutation need a careful plan for screening and prevention of colorectal and gynecologic cancers. Current recommendations are summarized in Table 2-5.

HNPCC is associated with an accelerated carcinogenesis in which polyps can develop into carcinomas in 2–3 years instead of the typical 8–10 years seen in the general population (Lynch & de la Chapelle, 2003). Because of this potentially rapid develop-

Table 2-5. Recommendations for Prevention and Early Detection in People With a Known Mutation in *MLH1* or *MSH2*

Organ	Screening	Prevention
Colon	Perform colonoscopy with prompt removal of polyps annually starting between ages 20–25.* Consider gastroscopy and upper endoscopy. Consider annual urinalysis with cytology and renal imaging.	Consider chemoprevention. Consider colectomy in patients who cannot or will not undergo regular colonoscopy.
Uterus/ovaries	Perform biannual pelvic examination beginning at age 25.* Screen with transvaginal ultrasound with color Doppler beginning at age 30–35* every 6–12 months.** Perform serum CA 125 testing every 6–12 months.	Consider chemoprevention with oral contraceptives. Consider prophylactic hysterectomy including bilateral salpingo-oophorectomy between ages 35–40 or when childbearing is complete.

* Age to begin screening may vary according to youngest age at which cancer was diagnosed in the family.
** Testing in premenopausal women should occur sometime during days 1–10 of the menstrual cycle.

Note. Based on information from Guillem et al., 2006; Levin et al., 2006; Lindor et al., 2006; National Comprehensive Cancer Network, 2007b.

ment of malignancy, colonoscopy is recommended annually after age 20–25 (Levin et al., 2006). Research clearly shows that regular colonoscopy decreases the overall mortality rate by about 65% (Lynch & de la Chapelle).

Because HNPCC also is associated with increased risks to the endometrium and ovaries, females with this mutation require careful surveillance. This usually includes annual or semiannual transvaginal ultrasound of the endometrium and ovaries with concurrent endometrial aspiration for pathologic evaluation and CA 125 testing (Levin et al., 2006). Women need information about the low sensitivity and specificity of ultrasound and CA 125 testing for ovarian cancer (Lynch & de la Chapelle, 2003). Ultrasound also has limited utility in evaluating endometrial thickness in premenopausal women because of cyclic changes (Lu & Broaddus, 2005). Because of this, NCCN (2007b) recommends that transvaginal ultrasound be performed within the first 10 days of the woman's menstrual cycle. Although individuals with HNPCC may be at risk for other cancers, no other standard screening recommendations exist at this time (Lindor et al., 2006). Some families with an increased number of urinary tract malignancies might consider adding ultrasound and urine cytology (Guillem et al., 2006; NCCN, 2007b). Similarly, many clinicians also will recommend upper endoscopy and gastroscopy, but no formal recommendations have been developed (NCCN, 2007b).

Chemoprevention is another strategy sometimes considered in these families. The exact efficacy of nonsteroidal anti-inflammatory drugs (NSAIDs) and aspirin in decreasing incidence of gastrointestinal cancers is not known (Levin et al., 2006; Lindor et al., 2006). These measures are based largely on information gained from people with FAP. Because taking OCPs has been associated with decreased risk of developing ovarian and endometrial cancers, some women will choose to consider this strategy (Lindor et al.). Those people considering chemoprevention strategies for colon or gynecologic cancers need a carefully balanced discussion of the potential benefits and risks associated with the proposed agent. These individuals also may want to consider enrolling in a research study. Similarly, minimal data are available regarding the impact of a healthy diet and exercise in reducing risk of cancer development in people with a mutation in HNPCC (Lindor et al.). Such behaviors, however, may contribute to overall health and well-being and are recommended.

Prophylactic colectomy in HNPCC is controversial. It is not associated with a large increase in life expectancy over annual colonoscopy (Lynch & de la Chapelle, 2003). It generally is reserved for individuals in whom colonoscopy is not technically possible or in individuals who refuse to undergo regular screening (Guillem et al., 2006).

As the risks for endometrial and ovarian cancer are substantial and screening may be ineffective, many women will consider a TAH with BSO at age 35 or older if childbearing is complete (Lindor et al., 2006). These women need to be aware of the risks of premature menopause and that this surgery typically requires four to eight weeks of recuperation.

Familial Adenomatous Polyposis Syndromes

Medical and surgical management of FAP syndromes is complex because the risk of developing colorectal cancer is virtually 100% and the age at onset can occur before age 20. In general, it is recommended that people with FAP begin screening with colonoscopy and often upper endoscopy at puberty and undergo colectomy when symptomatic or when the number of adenomas is considered worrisome or not manageable with polypectomy (Lynch & de la Chapelle, 2003). Some patients will consider a total proctocolectomy with ileal pouch anal anastomosis because the risks of developing rectal cancer after this surgery are small and a permanent stoma is not necessary. This procedure is very complex, requires a temporary stoma, and carries a small risk for bladder and/or sexual dysfunction (Levin et al., 2006). Other patients will choose a total abdominal colectomy with ileorectal anastomosis, but this will require regular endoscopy of the rectum following surgery because of the higher risk of rectal cancer. If many rectal polyps are present prior to surgery, this is not the recommended choice. This surgery carries little to no risk for bowel or bladder dysfunction. A total proctocolectomy with ileostomy is another choice of surgery. However, this choice leaves the patient with a permanent stoma, unlike the first two options. It removes all risk of colorectal cancer, but bladder or sexual dysfunction is a possible result (NCCN, 2007b). Patients and families need much education and support when making decisions about colectomy.

NSAIDs (including the cyclooxygenase-2 [COX-2] inhibitor celecoxib, which has a U.S. Food and Drug Administration indication) and aspirin are sometimes used to prevent or delay polyp formation (Calvert & Frucht, 2002; Lynch & de la Chapelle, 2003). Because COX-2 inhibitors are associated with an increased risk of cardiovascular problems, careful assessment of comorbid conditions is needed. NSAIDs may be particularly useful in patients with ileorectal anastomosis and an increased risk for rectal cancer (Levin et al., 2006).

Hereditary Melanoma

Early detection and prevention measures are critical in families at risk for hereditary melanoma. Currently, no clear consensus exists on the utility of genetic testing in this population because it does not dramatically influence surveillance and prevention measures (Fowler, Wolfe, Chesney, & Schwartzberg, 2006). Early detection of melanoma is particularly important, as the five-year survival rate is 98.5% when the disease is detected in stage I (ACS, 2008). Prevention and early detection measures for skin cancer are listed in Figure 2-11, which are similar to measures recommended for the general population. Individuals from families at risk for hereditary melanoma need to be followed by a dermatologist with expertise in melanoma and biopsy technique. Follow-up must occur on a regular basis (typically every three to six months). It also may be prudent to recommend to those who test positive to consider entering a pancreatic cancer screening trial because of the 17% lifetime risk of developing this disease (Tsao & Niendorf, 2004).

Early Detection
- Perform regular monthly full-body skin self-examination using full-length and handheld mirrors.
- Perform clinical skin examination every six months beginning at age 10. The frequency of this examination may need to be increased during pregnancy and puberty.
- Take full-body photographs every six months to monitor moles for changes.
- Perform prompt biopsy and removal of any suspicious lesions.

Prevention
- Limit ultraviolet light exposure, especially between the hours of 10 am and 3 pm.
- Wear protective clothing when outside. This includes long-sleeved shirts with a dense weave, sunglasses that provide ultraviolet A and B protection, and wide-brimmed hats.
- Use a broad-spectrum sunscreen with ultraviolet A and B protection with a sun protection factor of at least 30 daily and consistently.

Figure 2-11. Recommendations for Prevention and Early Detection in People With a Hereditary Predisposition for Developing Melanoma

Note. Based on information from American Cancer Society, 2008; Kefford & Mann, 2003; Tsao & Niendorf, 2004.

Implications for Oncology Advanced Practice Nurses

Several considerations exist for the APN with expertise in genetics. Specialty credentialing is available through the Genetic Nursing Credentialing Commission (GNCC). The credentialing process involves submission of a professional portfolio that demonstrates advanced nursing education in genetics, as well as evidence of clinical expertise and knowledge submitted in a portfolio format as opposed to taking an examination. Many nurses choose to obtain this credential through GNCC to enhance their credibility and professional practice. To maintain the credential, the APN must pursue continuing education in genetics and develop professional skills in research, publication, and professional and lay presentations. Detailed information about the credentialing process is available at the ISONG Web site at www.isong.org/resources/credentialing .cfm and in the text by Monsen (2005). In addition to ISONG, other opportunities exist for networking with other oncology nurses who are interested in cancer genetics, such as the Cancer Genetics Special Interest Group (SIG) of ONS and the Cancer Genetics SIG of the National Society of Genetic Counselors.

ISONG and the American Nurses Association (ANA) with GNCC have defined roles for basic and advanced practice nurses. ANA and ISONG also have published standards for genetics/genomics nursing (ISONG, 2007). These include roles in risk and physical assessment, diagnostic testing, outcomes identification, planning, implementation, and evaluation of genetics care. These standards address issues related to quality practice indicators, professional and continuing education, collegiality, collaboration, ethics, research, resource utilization, and leadership. APNs who practice in cancer genetics will find these standards to be a valuable resource when developing and improving cancer genetics programs. Table 2-6 provides other helpful resources for patients and healthcare providers.

Table 2-6. Resources for Cancer Genetics

Resource	Patient/ Family	Healthcare Provider
American Medical Association Family History Tools www.ama-assn.org/ama/pub/category/2380.html • Family history form • Sample pedigree • Free online courses		X
Gene Clinics/GeneTests www.geneclinics.org • Directory of inherited diseases • Clinical overview of the diagnosis, management, and genetic counseling of affected or at-risk individuals and families • Medical genetics laboratory directory search engines	X (for patients able to comprehend and who desire more complex information)	X
Genetics Professionals Directory www.cancer.gov/search/genetics_services • National Cancer Institute database of cancer genetics service providers nationwide • Cancer literature and clinical trials search engine		X

(Continued on next page)

Table 2-6. Resources for Cancer Genetics *(Continued)*

Resource	Patient/ Family	Healthcare Provider
International Society of Nurses in Genetics www.isong.org • Educational opportunities for nurses • Links to other genetics-related Web sites • Professional network site for nurses interested in genetics		X
Oncology Nursing Society www.ons.org • Educational resources on cancer genetics • Special interest group for nurses with an interest in cancer genetics • Free and fee-based online courses in genetics		X

National Comprehensive Cancer Network guidelines www.nccn.org
• Downloadable guidelines including
  – Genetics/familial high-risk assessment
  – Breast cancer risk reduction
  – Screening guidelines for breast, colon, melanoma, and other cancers
	X	X

National Institutes of Health Genetics Home Reference http://ghr.nlm.nih.gov • Genetic education modules • Glossary of genetic terms and conditions • Overview of Human Genome Project • Overview of gene therapy • Overview of genetic testing • Resources for healthcare professionals	X	X
BRCAPRO Software www8.utsouthwestern.edu/utsw/cda/dept47829/files/65844.html • Free computer software for computer construction of pedigrees and calculation of statistical models that predict breast and colon cancer risk, as well as risk of carrying other hereditary predisposition mutations		X
MedlinePlus www.nlm.nih.gov/medlineplus • Search engine with numerous topics related to cancer genetics and management of people with a hereditary predisposition for developing cancer	X	X
National Society of Genetic Counselors www.nsgc.org • Searchable directory of professional counselors with expertise in genetics • Educational and other resources on genetics	X	X
Myriad Genetic Laboratories www.myriad.com • Commercial laboratory that provides genetic testing services for common cancer syndromes • Geneticists and other healthcare professionals are available for consultation.	X	X
Facing Our Risk of Cancer Empowered (FORCE) www.facingourrisk.org • Support group for people from families with hereditary breast/ovarian cancer risks	X	

(Continued on next page)

	Patient/ Family	Healthcare Provider
Table 2-6. Resources for Cancer Genetics *(Continued)*		
Resource		
International Society of Nurses in Genetics. (2007). *Genetics/genomics nursing scope and standards of practice.* Silver Spring, MD: Nursesbooks.org		X
Monsen, R.B. (2005). *Genetics nursing portfolios: A new model for credentialing.* Silver Spring, MD: Nursebooks.org.		X
Tranin, A.S., Masny, A., & Jenkins, J. (Eds.). *Genetics in oncology practice: Cancer risk assessment.* Pittsburgh, PA: Oncology Nursing Society.		X

It is important to remember that all oncology APNs, regardless of practice setting, have a responsibility to refer to genetics healthcare providers and understand the influence of genetics in health care. The practice of oncology is greatly influenced by genetics in not only the evaluation and referral of families with a hereditary predisposition, but also in pharmacogenetics and evaluation of tumor characteristics. A growing need and role for oncology APNs also exist in the area of cancer genetics research. Some of these potential areas are summarized in Figure 2-12 and include conducting research,

Risk Assessment and Communication of Risk
- Options for risk estimation with and without genetic testing
- Methods for communicating risk to patients and families
- Patient/family interpretation and ability to understand various risk assessments and ways to enhance understanding of risk assessment
- Development of teaching and risk assessment tools that best utilize the time of genetics professionals, patients, and families

Psychosocial Issues Surrounding Genetic Testing
- Experiences of people who decline testing
- Experiences of people who cannot test because a mutation has not been identified in the family
- Use of telephone and other support groups to facilitate coping in nonaffected people who test positive for a predisposition gene
- Use of support groups for people considering testing and adjusting to the results of testing
- Issues for parents who test positive and how and when they disclose potential risks to their children
- Psychological implication of test results (risks and benefits)

Patterns of Testing and Implementation of Prevention/Detection Strategies
- Patterns of use of genetic testing in geographic areas and practice settings
- Patterns and strategies associated with follow-up with prevention/early detection strategies
- Decisions and satisfaction with prophylactic surgery
- Complications/side effects of prophylactic surgery and/or chemoprevention
- Body image and self-perception issues following genetic testing and/or prophylactic surgery

Professional/Ethical Issues
- Risks of insurance or employer discrimination
- Quantification of amount of clinical time and expertise needed to communicate information about cancer risk and genetic testing
- Ways to enhance referrals for genetics education
- Role delineation for advanced practice nurses

Figure 2-12. Areas for Future Nursing Research

Note. Based on information from American Cancer Society, 2008; Kefford & Mann, 2003; Tsao & Niendorf, 2004.

disseminating findings of research to colleagues, and keeping current with genetics research. Because the field is ever-growing, some APNs may find it helpful to subscribe to a list serve of cancer genetics clinicians available through ISONG or NSGC. These list serves link colleagues who may practice in geographically diverse areas, thereby allowing collaboration on studies and sharing of ideas.

One area in which oncology APNs often participate is referral of families to clinical trials at universities and laboratories studying families who test negative in standard or commercially available testing. Many families desire to participate in such research not only to contribute to science but also in hopes of gaining information about their personal and family risks, especially risk to offspring and siblings. APNs identify such studies for families, assist with the coordination of care, and provide follow-up as needed.

In many cases, oncology APNs will assist in the management of people with hereditary risk after they have undergone genetic testing or consultations with a genetics healthcare professional. Often the APN is responsible for ensuring that recommendations for screening are carried out. They also may assist with the care, education, and support of people who consider prevention measures, especially prophylactic surgery.

Conclusion

In summary, APNs have roles in cancer genetics that include direct care of the patient and family, including risk assessment and interpretation, education regarding testing and treatment options, and provision of psychosocial support. Often, these APNs coordinate complex care with other disciplines and subspecialties along with serving as consultants. APNs also have roles as staff educators, researchers, and administrators of programs that specialize in the care of individuals with a hereditary predisposition for developing cancer. With continuing advances in cancer genetics, this is an ever-growing and challenging area for APNs that requires not only an in-depth understanding of the science of genetics but also patient education skills and psychosocial skills to help patients to manage the risk of hereditary cancer.

Case Study

M.B. presented for education and information about hereditary risk for cancer at the request of her primary care physician. She is a 32-year-old Caucasian female with concerns about her personal risk of cancer. She reports she is certain that she has the "breast cancer gene." She presents with several pathology reports and death certificates from affected family members as requested by the APN prior to the appointment. M.B. is recently married and desires children. She is concerned not only about her personal risks but also about potential risks to her offspring. Additionally, M.B. reports that she had a child at age 24, which she gave up for adoption.

M.B. has three sisters. Two are affected with premenopausal breast cancer; one of these sisters has bilateral breast cancer. A pedigree was constructed (see Figure 2-13). Maternal ethnicity is Irish/English. M.B.'s mother is alive and reported to be healthy. Her only maternal uncle died in a motor vehicle accident. Her maternal grandparents did not have a malignancy. Paternal ethnicity is German/Ashkenazi Jewish. M.B.'s paternal family history is significant for ovarian cancer (paternal aunt), breast cancer (paternal grandmother), prostate cancer (father), and pancreatic cancer (paternal grandfather).

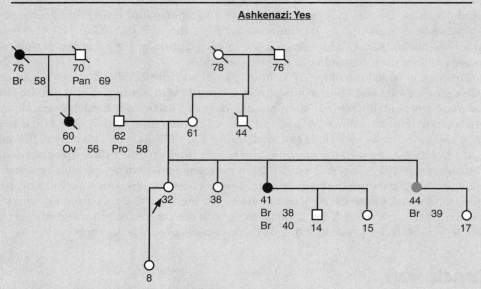

This pedigree shows M.B. as the proband (as designated by the arrow).

Figure 2-13. Pedigree—Case Study

M.B.'s past medical history reports menarche at age 12. She is gravida 1, para 1 (first complete pregnancy at age 24). She reports no hormonal therapy use but reports a past history of more than five years of OCP use from age 24 to about age 30. Her last Pap smear/pelvic examination was within the past three months and negative. She has never had a mammogram. Her last breast examination was negative and was done at the time of the gynecologic examination. She denies having problems with depression or coping with difficult information. M.B. has had two breast biopsies for palpable masses, one at age 26 and one at age 30. The first biopsy was a fibroadenoma; the second one showed ductal hyperplasia with moderate atypia. Both biopsies were confirmed with pathology reports.

M.B. works as an elementary school teacher. She denies use of tobacco or recreational drugs and states she occasionally drinks socially but has less than one or two drinks per month. She walks approximately five miles per day and consumes three to five servings of fruits and vegetables daily. She has disclosed to her husband that she has given up a child for adoption.

M.B. reports being concerned about her personal health as well as risks to potential offspring. She would like to consider prevention strategies and would like recommendations for screening. Her gynecologist recommended that she consider genetic testing, and M.B. believes she will test positive because of her sisters' histories. She has not discussed her desire for testing with her husband. She has discussed it with her affected sisters, who report they have not had testing or counseling for testing.

1. What in M.B.'s history is suggestive of HBOC syndrome?
   - M.B.'s paternal family history is significant for ovarian cancer in a paternal aunt, breast cancer in her paternal grandmother, prostate cancer in her father, and pancreatic cancer in her paternal grandfather. She has two first-degree relatives (sisters) with premenopausal breast cancer, one of which was bilateral. Her father's family is also of Ashkenazi Jewish descent.

2. Which of the risk calculation models would be most appropriate for M.B. (see Table 2-7)?

Table 2-7. Gail and Claus Model Calculations for Case Study (% Risk)

M.B.'s Age	Claus Model	Gail Model	Population	No Risk Factors
37	5.6	2.27	0.3	0.2
42	11.2	5.84	0.6	0.3
52	35.2	15.68	2.3	1.3
62	52	27.42	5.1	2.9
Lifetime	77.8	41.89	13.2	7.6

- The Gail model would underestimate her risk and would not take into account second-degree relatives, ovarian cancer in her family, or age of her relatives at diagnosis. The Claus model is the most appropriate model, as it considers women with multiple family members diagnosed with breast cancer, as well as maternal and paternal history of breast cancer. It also considers age at diagnosis, which is important, considering her sisters were premenopausal at diagnosis. Neither the Claus nor the Gail models consider the history of ovarian cancer. Other models (see Figure 2-8) will provide more information, and each model has disadvantages and advantages. BRCAPRO is a tool that constructs a pedigree and calculates risk using several statistical models that predict breast and colon cancer risk, as well as risk of carrying other hereditary predisposition mutations (see Table 2-6).
- M.B.'s risk of having a mutation in *BRCA1/2* also was calculated. A range of risk figures was provided (see Table 2-8), but almost all are greater than a 10% risk (and most were much higher), suggesting it is appropriate to offer testing. The patient received copies of the pedigree and all risk calculations.

Table 2-8. *BRCA* Mutation Percent Probability Models for Case Study (Based on Ashkenazi Background, 15 Family Members)

Mutation	Proband Probability
BRCA1	
• Couch model	28.6%
• Shattuck-Eidens	39.6%
• BRCAPRO	49.9%
BRCA2 (BRCAPRO)	1.7%
BRCA1 or *BRCA2*	
• Manchester	5.27%
• Frank	28.7%
• BRCAPRO	50.8%

3. Who would be the most appropriate person to test first in this case study?
   - Ideally, the person to test would be the youngest person in the family with cancer that is suspected to be part of a cancer syndrome. In this case, it would be M.B.'s youngest sister with breast cancer. If she tested negative, then most likely this family would not have this hereditary syndrome. If she tests positive, and M.B. then tested negative, that would be considered a true negative, and her risk would then be considered to be that of the general population.
   - M.B.'s sister with bilateral breast cancer decided to test following genetic counseling and discussion of benefits and limitations of testing. She tested positive for a mutation in *BRCA1*. Her other affected sister also tested positive. Both underwent oophorectomy. Her sister with unilateral breast cancer completed a prophylactic mastectomy on the unaffected side. They both began formulating a plan on how to educate their daughters about risks. M.B. underwent testing and also tested positive.
4. Because M.B. tested positive, what screening recommendations could be given?
   - In women with an inherited mutation of *BRCA1* or *BRCA2*, screening recommendations include
     - Monthly BSE
     - CBE every six months
     - Annual mammography and MRI (each alternating every six months)
     - Pelvic examination every six months
     - Transvaginal ultrasound every 6–12 months
     - Serum CA 125 testing every 6–12 months
5. What preventive strategies are available?
   - Prophylactic mastectomy
   - Chemoprevention with tamoxifen
   - Prophylactic oophorectomy between ages 35–40 or after childbearing
6. Would chemoprevention with raloxifene be appropriate?
   - No, raloxifene is only appropriate in postmenopausal women. Tamoxifen could be prescribed for five years following discussion of the benefits of chemoprevention and the risk of toxicities.

M.B. completed prophylactic mastectomies and reconstruction with implants. She hopes to soon become pregnant. She is exploring how to inform the adoption agency about the potential risk to her daughter. She reports that she is gradually adjusting to the changes in her life and is satisfied with her decisions. After childbearing, between ages 35–40, the proband plans to undergo a prophylactic BSO. The proband states that her only regrets are that she is not certain how her adopted child will handle the information and that her nonaffected sister decided not to test. The oncology APN's recommendations were summarized in a letter that M.B. could share with her primary care providers as needed.

Key Points

- Approximately 10% of all cancers are attributable to hereditary predisposition. Genetic testing is increasingly available to identify individuals with this heightened risk.

Genetic testing is readily available for breast and ovarian cancer syndromes, HNPCC, FAP and AFAP, and hereditary melanoma syndromes. Many unusual syndromes have testing available on a more limited or research basis.

- Most agencies recommend that testing be offered when having a positive test is a reasonable likelihood, the knowledge of test results will influence care, and a qualified healthcare provider is available to provide informed consent and psychosocial support in the context of pre- and post-test counseling.
- Risk assessment includes both assessment of risk for developing cancer and risk of carrying a mutation for hereditary risk. Typically, a pedigree is constructed, risk is calculated, and then the risk is interpreted to the patient and family.
- Possible outcomes of testing include a positive result, a true negative result, a negative inconclusive result, and a variant of indeterminate significance.
- Individuals may have a variety of psychosocial responses to test results. Family members are encouraged to share the results of testing with other family members.
- Prevention and early detection measures are based on the outcome of testing, family history, and personal history. Those who test positive often will receive recommendations for prophylactic surgery.
- APNs have professional responsibilities related to cancer genetics, including protecting privacy, conducting further research, and serving as leaders in the field of cancer genetics.

Recommended Resources for Oncology Advanced Practice Nurses

- BRCAPRO software (www8.utsouthwestern.edu/utsw/cda/dept47829/files/65844.html): Free computer software for computer construction of pedigrees and calculation of statistical models that predict breast and colon cancer risk, as well as risk of carrying other hereditary predisposition mutations
- Tranin, A.S., Masny, A., & Jenkins, J. (Eds.). (2003). *Genetics in oncology practice: Cancer risk assessment.* Pittsburgh, PA: Oncology Nursing Society.
- Myriad Genetic Laboratories (www.myriad.com): Commercial laboratory providing genetic testing and services for common cancer syndromes. Geneticists and other healthcare professionals are available for consultation.
- National Institutes of Health Genetics Home Reference (http://ghr.nlm.nih.gov): Genetic education modules and glossary of genetic terms and conditions from the National Library of Medicine
- CancerPRA (www.collectivemed.com/jump/capra.shtml): PDA tool based on the *Handbook of Cancer Risk Assessment and Prevention* (Colditz & Stein, 2004) with search capabilities
- Breast Cancer Risk Assessment Tool (www.cancer.gov/bcrisktool/default.aspx): Computerized tool for the PDA and desktop computer

References

American Cancer Society. (2008). *Cancer facts and figures, 2008.* Atlanta, GA: Author.
American Society of Clinical Oncology. (2003). American Society of Clinical Oncology policy statement update: Genetic testing for cancer susceptibility. *Journal of Clinical Oncology, 21,* 2397–2406.

Anderson, K., Jacobson, J.S., Hetjan, D.F., Zivin, J.G., Hershman, D., Neugut, A.I., et al. (2006). Cost-effectiveness of preventive strategies for women with a *BRCA1* or a *BRCA2* mutation. *Annals of Internal Medicine, 144*, 397–406.

Antoniou, A., Pharoah, P.D., Narod, S., Risch, H.A., Eyfjord, J.E., Hopper, J.L., et al. (2003). Average risks of breast and ovarian cancer associated with BRCA1 or BRCA2 mutations detected in case series unselected for family history: A combined analysis of 22 studies. *American Journal of Human Genetics, 72*, 1117–1130.

Armstrong, K., Weber, B., FitzGerald, G., Hershey, J.C., Pauly, M.V., Lemaire, J., et al. (2003). Life insurance and breast cancer risk assessment: Adverse selection, genetic testing decisions, and discrimination. *American Journal of Medical Genetics, 120a*, 359–364.

Balmana, J., Stockwell, D.H., Steyerberg, E.W., Stoffel, E.M., Deffenbaugh, A.M., Reid, J.F., et al. (2006). Prediction of MLH1 and MSH2 mutations in Lynch syndrome. *JAMA, 296*, 1469–1478.

Berry, D.A., Iversen, E.S., Gudbjartsson, D.F., Hiller, E.H., Garber, J.E., Peshkin, B.N., et al. (2002). BRCAPRO validation, sensitivity of genetic testing of BRCA1/BRCA2, and prevalence of other breast cancer susceptibility genes. *Journal of Clinical Oncology, 20*, 2701–2712.

Berry, D.A., Parmigiani, G., Sanchez, A., Schildkraut, J., & Winer, E. (1997). Probability of carrying a mutation of breast-ovarian cancer gene BRCA1 based on family history. *Journal of the National Cancer Institute, 89*, 227–238.

Bodmer, D., Ligtenberg, M.J.L., van der Hout, A.H., Gloudenmans, S., Ansink, K., Oosterwijk, J.C., et al. (2006). Optimal selection for BRCA1 and BRCA2 mutation testing using a combination of 'easy to apply' probability models. *British Journal of Cancer, 95*, 757–762.

Boland, C.R. (2006). Decoding hereditary colorectal cancer. *New England Journal of Medicine, 354*, 2815–2817.

Braithwaite, D., Emery, J., Walter, F., Prevost, A.T., & Sutton, S. (2004). Psychological impact of genetic counseling for familial cancer: A systematic review and meta-analysis. *Journal of the National Cancer Institute, 96*, 122–133.

Burt, R., & Neklason, D.W. (2005). Genetic testing for inherited colon cancer. *Gastroenterology, 128*, 1696–1716.

Calvert, P.M., & Frucht, H. (2002). The genetics of colorectal cancer. *Annals of Internal Medicine, 137*, 603–612.

Calzone, K.A., & Tranin, A.S. (2003). The scope of cancer genetics nursing practice. In A.S. Tranin, A. Masny, & J. Jenkins (Eds.), *Genetics in oncology practice: Cancer risk assessment* (pp. 13–22). Pittsburgh, PA: Oncology Nursing Society.

Casey, M., & Mahon, S.M. (2007). Breast restoration with prostheses. In S.M. Mahon (Ed.), *Site-specific cancer series: Breast cancer* (pp. 81–89). Pittsburgh, PA: Oncology Nursing Society.

Chapman, D. (2007). Local and regional control. In S.M. Mahon (Ed.), *Site-specific cancer series: Breast cancer* (pp. 63–80). Pittsburgh, PA: Oncology Nursing Society.

Chen, S., Wang, W., Lee, S., Nafa, K., Lee, J., Romans, K., et al. (2006). Prediction of germline mutations and cancer risk in the Lynch Syndrome. *JAMA, 296*, 1479–1487.

Claus, E.B., Risch, N., & Thompson, W.D. (1994). Autosomal dominant inheritance of early-onset breast cancer: Implications for risk prediction. *Cancer, 73*, 643–651.

Claus, E.B., Schildkraut, M.M., Thompson, W.D., & Risch, N. (1996). The genetic attributable risk of breast and ovarian cancer. *Cancer, 77*, 2318–2324.

Colditz, G.A., & Stein, C.J. (2004). *Handbook of cancer risk assessment and prevention.* Sudbury, MA: Jones and Bartlett.

Collins, F.S., Morgan, M., & Patrinos, A. (2003). The Human Genome Project: Lessons from large-scale biology. *Science, 300*, 286–290.

Costantino, J.P., Gail, M.H., Pee, D., Anderson, S., Redmond, C.K., Benichou, J., et al. (1999). Validation studies for models projecting the risk of invasive and total breast cancer incidence. *Journal of the National Cancer Institute, 9*, 1541–1548.

Couch, F.J., DeShano, M.L., Blackwood, M.A., Calzone, K., Stopfer, J., Campeau, L., et al. (1997). BRCA1 mutations in women attending clinics that evaluate the risk of breast cancer. *New England Journal of Medicine, 336*, 1409–1415.

Daly, M.B., Axilbund, J.E., Bryant, E., Buys, S., Eng, C., Friedman, S., et al. (2006). Genetic/familial high-risk assessment: Breast and ovarian. Clinical practice guidelines in oncology, v.1.2006. *Journal of the National Comprehensive Cancer Network, 4*, 156–176.

Debniak, T., Gorski, B., Cybulski, C., Jakubowska, A., Kurzawski, G., Kladny, J., et al. (2003). Increased risk of breast cancer in relatives of malignant melanoma patients from families with strong cancer familial aggregation. *European Journal of Cancer Prevention, 12*, 241–245.

Domchek, S.M., Friebel, T.M., Neuhausen, S.L., Wagner, T., Evans, G., Isaacs, C., et al. (2006). Mortality after bilateral salpingo-oophorectomy in BRCA1 and BRCA2 mutation carriers: A prospective cohort study. *Lancet Oncology, 7,* 223–229.

Domchek, S.M., Stopfer, J.E., & Rebbeck, T.R. (2006). Bilateral risk-reducing oophorectomy in BRCA1 and BRCA2 mutation carriers. *Journal of the National Comprehensive Cancer Network, 4,* 177–182.

Domchek, S.M., & Weber, B.L. (2006). Clinical management of *BRCA1* and *BRCA2* mutation carriers. *Oncogene, 25,* 5825–5831.

Evans, D.G., Eccles, D.M., Rahman, N., Young, K., Bulman, M., Amir, E., et al. (2004). A new scoring system for the chances of identifying a BRCA1/2 mutation outperforms existing models including BRCAPRO. *Journal of Medical Genetics, 41,* 474–480.

Finch, A., Shaw, P., Rosen, B., Murphy, J., Narod, S.A., & Colgan, T.J. (2006). Clinical and pathologic findings of prophylactic salpingo-oophorectomies in 159 BRCA1 and BRCA2 carriers. *Gynecologic Oncology, 100,* 58–64.

Ford, D., Easton, D.F., Stratton, M., Narod, S., Goldgar, D., Devilee, P., et al. (1998). Genetic heterogeneity and penetrance analysis of the BRCA1 and BRCA2 genes in breast cancer families. The Breast Cancer Linkage Consortium. *American Journal of Human Genetics, 62,* 676–689.

Fowler, E.S., Wolfe, K.S., Chesney, T.M., & Schwartzberg, L.S. (2006). Genetic testing for hereditary melanoma: Controversial, standard of care, or somewhere between the two? *Community Oncology, 3,* 158–161.

Freedman, A.N., Seminara, D., Gail, M.H., Hartge, P., Colditz, G.A., Ballard-Barbash, R., et al. (2005). Cancer risk prediction models: A workshop on development, evaluation, and application. *Journal of the National Cancer Institute, 97,* 715–723.

Gail, M.H., Brinton, L.A., Byar, D.P., Corle, D.K., Green, S.B., Shairer, C., et al. (1989). Projecting individualized probabilities of developing breast cancer for white females who are being examined annually. *Journal of the National Cancer Institute, 81,* 1879–1886.

Greco, K. (2003). How to provide genetic counseling and education. In A.S. Tranin, A. Masny, & J. Jenkins (Eds.), *Genetics in oncology practice: Cancer risk assessment* (pp. 189–224). Pittsburgh, PA: Oncology Nursing Society.

Greco, K., & Mahon, S.M. (2004). Common hereditary cancer syndromes. *Seminars in Oncology Nursing, 20,* 164–177.

Gudmundsdottir, K., & Ashworth, A. (2006). The roles of BRCA1 and BRCA2 and associated proteins in the maintenance of genomic stability. *Oncogene, 25,* 5864–5874.

Guillem, J.C., Wood, W.C., Moley, J.F., Berchuck, A., Karlan, B.Y., Mutch, D.G., et al. (2006). ASCO/SSO review of current role of risk-reducing surgery in common hereditary syndromes. *Journal of Clinical Oncology, 24,* 4642–4660.

Hall, M.A., & Rich, S.S. (2000a). Laws restricting health insurers' use of genetic information: Impact on genetic discrimination. *American Journal of Human Genetics, 66,* 293–307.

Hall, M.A., & Rich, S.S. (2000b). Patients' fear of genetic discrimination by health insurers: The impact of legal protections. *Genetics in Medicine, 2,* 214–221.

Hansen, C.B., Wadge, L.M., Lowstuter, K., Boucher, K., & Leachman, S.A. (2004). Clinical germline genetic testing for melanoma. *Lancet Oncology, 5,* 314–319.

Health Insurance Portability and Accountability Act, Pub. L. No. 104-191, 110 Stat. 1936 (1996).

Hendriks, Y.M.C., de Jong, A.E., Morreau, H., Tops, C.M.J., Vasen, H.F., Wijnen, J.T., et al. (2006). Diagnostic approach and management of Lynch syndrome (hereditary nonpolyposis colorectal carcinoma): A guide for clinicians. *CA: A Cancer Journal for Clinicians, 56,* 213–225.

Herrmann, V.M., & Borelli, A.J. (2006). The role of MRI in breast imaging. *Community Oncology, 3,* 727–729.

Hopwood, P. (2005). Psychosocial aspects of risk communication and mutation testing in familial breast-ovarian cancer. *Current Opinion in Oncology, 17,* 340–344.

Hoskins, K.F., Zwaagstra, A., & Ranz, M. (2006). Validation of a tool for identifying women at high risk for hereditary breast cancer in population-based screening. *Cancer, 107,* 1769–1776.

International Society of Nurses in Genetics. (2007). *Genetics/genomics nursing scope and standards of practice.* Silver Spring, MD: Nursesbooks.org.

Jeter, J.M., Kohlmann, W., & Gruber, S.B. (2006). Genetics of colorectal cancer. *Oncology, 20,* 269–276.

Kausmeyer, D.T., Lengerich, E.J., Kluhsman, B.C., Morrone, D., Harper, G.R., & Baker, M.J. (2006). A survey of patients' experiences with the cancer genetic counseling process: Recommendations for cancer genetics programs. *Journal of Genetic Counseling, 15,* 409–431.

Kefford, R.F., & Mann, G.J. (2003). Is there a role for genetic testing in patients with melanoma? *Current Opinion in Oncology, 15,* 157–161.

Kriege, M., Brekelmans, C.T.M., Boetes, C., Besnard, P.E., Zonderland, H.M., Obdeijn, I.M., et al. (2004). Efficacy of MRI and mammography for breast-cancer screening in women with a familial or genetic predisposition. *New England Journal of Medicine, 351*, 427–437.

Kuhl, C.K., Schrading, S., Leutner, C.C., Morakkabati-Spitz, N., Wardelmann, E., Fimmers, R., et al. (2005). Mammography, breast ultrasound, and magnetic resonance imaging for surveillance of women at high familial risk for breast cancer. *Journal of Clinical Oncology, 23*, 8469–8476.

Levin, B., Barthel, J.S., Burt, R.W., David, D.S., Ford, J.M., Giardiello, F.M., et al. (2006). Colorectal cancer screening clinical practice guidelines. *Journal of the National Comprehensive Cancer Network, 4*, 384–420.

Lindor, N.M., Petersen, G.M., Hadley, D.W., Kinney, A.Y., Miesfeldt, S., Lu, K.H., et al. (2006). Recommendations for the care of individuals with an inherited predisposition to Lynch syndrome: A systematic review. *JAMA, 296*, 1507–1517.

Loescher, L.J., & Whitesell, L. (2003). The biology of cancer. In A.S. Tranin, A. Masny, & J. Jenkins (Eds.), *Genetics in oncology practice: Cancer risk assessment* (pp. 23–56). Pittsburgh, PA: Oncology Nursing Society.

Lu, K.H., & Broaddus, R.R. (2005). Gynecologic cancers in Lynch syndrome/HNPCC. *Familial Cancer, 4*, 249–254.

Lynch, H.T., & de la Chapelle, A. (2003). Genomic medicine: Hereditary colorectal cancer. *New England Journal of Medicine, 348*, 919–932.

Lynch, H.T., & Lynch, P.M. (2006). Clinical selection of candidates for mutational testing for cancer susceptibility. *Oncology (Williston Park), 20*(14 Suppl. 10), 29–34.

Lynch, H.T., Snyder, C.L., Lynch, J.F., Riley, B.D., & Rubinstein, W.S. (2003). Hereditary breast-ovarian cancer at the bedside: Role of the medical oncologist. *Journal of Clinical Oncology, 21*, 740–753.

Mahon, S.M. (2003). Cancer risk assessment: Considerations for cancer genetics. In A.S. Tranin, A. Masny, & J. Jenkins (Eds.), *Genetics in oncology practice: Cancer risk assessment* (pp. 77–138). Pittsburgh, PA: Oncology Nursing Society.

Monsen, R.B. (2005). *Genetics nursing portfolios: A new model for credentialing.* Silver Spring, MD: Nursebooks.org.

Narod, S.A. (2006). Modifiers of risk of hereditary breast cancer. *Oncogene, 25*, 5832–5836.

National Comprehensive Cancer Network. (2007a). *NCCN clinical practice guidelines in oncology: Breast cancer risk reduction, version 1.2007.* Retrieved February 25, 2008, from http://www.nccn.org/professionals/physician_gls/PDF/breast_risk.pdf

National Comprehensive Cancer Network. (2007b). *NCCN clinical practice guidelines in oncology: Colorectal cancer screening, version 1.2007.* Retrieved June 8, 2007, from http://www.nccn.org/professionals/physician_gls/PDF/colorectal_screening.pdf

National Comprehensive Cancer Network. (2007c). *NCCN clinical practice guidelines in oncology: Genetic/familial high risk assessment: Breast and ovarian, version 1.2007.* Retrieved June 8, 2007, from http://www.nccn.org/professionals/physician_gls/PDF/genetics_screening.pdf

Nelson, H.D., Huffman, L.H., Fu, R., & Harris, E.L. (2005). Genetic risk assessment and BRCA mutation testing for breast and ovarian cancer susceptibility: Systematic evidence review for the U.S. Preventive Services Task Force. *Annals of Internal Medicine, 143*, 362–379.

Nielsen, M., Franken, P.F., Reinards, T.H., Weiss, M.M., Wagner, A., van der Klift, H., et al. (2005). Multiplicity in polyp count and extracolonic manifestations in 40 Dutch patients with MYH associated polyposis coli (MAP). *Journal of Medical Genetics, 42*(9), e54.

Oncology Nursing Society. (2004). *Cancer predisposition genetic testing and risk assessment counseling* [Position statement]. Pittsburgh, PA: Author.

Pieterse, A.H., van Dulmen, A.M., Beemer, F.A., Bensing, J.M., & Ausems, M.G. (2007). Cancer genetic counseling: Communication and counselees' post-visit satisfaction, cognitions, anxiety, and needs fulfillment. *Journal of Genetic Counseling, 16*, 85–96.

Plevritis, S.K., Kurian, A.W., Sigal, B.M., Daniel, B.L., Ikeda, D.M., Stockdale, F.E., et al. (2006). Cost-effectiveness of screening BRCA1/2 mutation carriers with breast magnetic resonance imaging. *JAMA, 295*, 2374–2384.

Rebbeck, T.R., Friebel, T., Wagner, T., Lynch, H.T., Garber, J.E., Daly, M.B., et al. (2005). Effect of short-term hormone replacement therapy on breast cancer risk reduction after bilateral prophylactic oophorectomy in *BRCA1* and *BRCA2* mutation carriers: The PROSE Study Group. *Journal of Clinical Oncology, 31*, 7804–7810.

Saslow, D., Boetes, C., Burke, W., Harms, S., Leach, M.O., Lehman, C.D., et al. (2007). American Cancer Society guidelines for breast screening with MRI as an adjunct to mammography. *CA: A Cancer Journal for Clinicians, 57*, 75–89.

Schmeler, K.M., Sun, C.C., Bodurka, D.C., White, K.G., Soliman, P.T., Uyei, A.R., et al. (2006). Prophylactic bilateral salpingo-oophorectomy compared with surveillance in women with BRCA mutations. *Obstetrics and Gynecology, 108*(3 Pt. 1), 515–520.

Shattuck-Eidens, D., Oliphant, A., & McClure, M. (1997). BRCA1 sequence analysis in women at high risk for susceptibility mutations: Risk factor analysis and implications for genetic testing. *JAMA, 278,* 1242–1250.

Struewing, J.P., Hartge, P., Wacholder, S., Baker, B.S., Berlin, M., McAdams, M., et al. (1997). The risk of cancer associated with specific mutations of BRCA1 and BRCA2 among Ashkenazi Jews. *New England Journal of Medicine, 336,* 1401–1408.

Tranin, A.S., Masny, A., & Jenkins, J. (Eds.). (2003). *Genetics in oncology practice: Cancer risk assessment.* Pittsburgh, PA: Oncology Nursing Society.

Trepanier, A., Ahrens, M., McKinnon, W., Peters, J., Stopfer, J., Grumet, S.C., et al. (2004). Genetic cancer risk assessment and counseling: Recommendations of the National Society of Genetic Counselors. *Journal of Genetic Counseling, 13,* 83–114.

Tsao, H., & Niendorf, K. (2004). Genetic testing in hereditary melanoma. *Journal of the American Academy of Dermatology, 51,* 803–808.

Umar, A.C., Boland, R., Terdiman, J.P., Syngal, S., de la Chapelle, A., Rüschoff, J., et al. (2004). Revised Bethesda guidelines for hereditary nonpolyposis colorectal cancer (Lynch syndrome) and microsatellite instability. *Journal of the National Cancer Institute, 96,* 261–268.

U.S. Preventive Services Task Force. (2005). Genetic risk assessment and BRCA mutation testing for breast and ovarian cancer susceptibility: Recommendation statement. *Annals of Internal Medicine, 143,* 355–361.

Vadaparampil, S.T., Wey, J.P., & Kinney, A.Y. (2004). Psychosocial aspects of genetic counseling and testing. *Seminars in Oncology Nursing, 20,* 186–195.

Valverde, K.D. (2006). Why me? Why not me? *Journal of Genetic Counseling, 15,* 461–463.

Van Sprundel, T.C., Schmidt, M.K., Rookus, M.A., Brohet, R., van Asperen, C.J., Ruters, E.J., et al. (2005). Risk reduction of contralateral breast cancer and survival after contralateral prophylactic mastectomy in BRCA1 or BRCA2 mutation carriers. *British Journal of Cancer, 93,* 287–292.

Vasen, H.F., Gruis, N.A., Frants, R.R., van Der Velden, P.A., & Hille, E.T. (2000). Risk of developing pancreatic cancer in families with familial atypical multiple mole melanoma associated with a specific 19 deletion of p16 (p16 Leiden). *International Journal of Cancer, 87,* 809–811.

Vasen, H.F., Watson, P., Mecklin, J.P., & Lynch, H.T. (1999). New clinical criteria for hereditary nonpolyposis colorectal cancer (HNPCC, Lynch syndrome) proposed by the International Collaborative Group on HNPCC. *Gastroenterology, 116,* 1453–1456.

Warner, E., & Causer, P.A. (2005). MRI surveillance for hereditary breast cancer risk. *Lancet, 365,* 1747–1749.

Warner, E., Plewes, D., Hill, K., Causer, P., Zubovits, J., Jong, R., et al. (2004). Surveillance of BRCA1 and BRCA2 mutation carriers with magnetic resonance imaging, ultrasound, mammography, and clinical breast examination. *JAMA, 292,* 1317–1325.

Watson, M.S., & Greene, C.L. (2001). Points to consider in preventing unfair discrimination based on genetic disease risk: A position statement of the American College of Medical Genetics. *Genetics in Medicine, 3,* 436–437.

CHAPTER 3

Cancer Diagnosis and Staging

Pamela Hallquist Viale, RN, MS, ANP, CS, AOCNP®

Introduction

A diagnosis of malignancy must be made in order to treat the disease of cancer. Tissues or cells are examined histologically to differentiate malignancy from a benign process (Beahrs, 1991). Therefore, cancer usually is considered a microscopic diagnosis (Compton & Green, 2004). Features such as the macroscopic look of the tissue and the degree of differentiation in the tissue are essential components of the diagnosis. Although degrees of differentiation do not play a specific role in anatomic staging, they do help clinicians to anticipate the behavior of some tumors (Beahrs).

Although not yet standard practice in all tumor types, molecular markers and tumor markers are playing a more significant role in cancer care. Tumor markers generally are substances secreted by the tumor and can be essential in the work-up of many different cancers and play a significant role in staging and diagnosis. Molecular markers in cancer include gene expression levels, structures of proteins, and alterations in gene sequences and can help in shaping specific treatments based on a patient's individual characteristics and in predicting response to therapy (Sidransky, 2002).

Correct staging reflects the burden of the disease at diagnosis, allowing clinicians to determine prognosis and choose the appropriate treatment. Two primary staging periods exist. The first is the pretreatment physical examination of the patient and includes all imaging, laboratory studies, biopsy, or initial surgical findings obtained to determine the initial stage of disease (Beahrs, 1991). The second period of staging is the pathologic staging after the primary surgery (if surgery is done). This staging incorporates the aforementioned data and includes the microscopic evidence obtained from the resected tissue or cells. Restaging occurs at specific intervals in the disease process and is critical, as it allows clinicians to determine subsequent treatment choices for a patient who may have relapsed or progressed during or following initial therapy. Restaging also may determine whether additional treatment is necessary following a favorable response to therapy. For example, restaging may follow neoadjuvant therapy for a nonresectable tumor (as in breast or colon cancer) to determine whether surgical resection is now feasible. Furthermore, in some cases, information obtained from autopsy can contribute to staging (Beahrs).

This chapter will present an overview of the cancer diagnosis and staging process as well as the specific tumor-node-metastasis (TNM) staging systems used for several of the most commonly seen solid tumor types.

Signs and Symptoms of Cancer

A symptom is an indication of disease that may be experienced by an individual, such as prolonged constipation, but is not necessarily noticeable by others. A sign is an indication of disease experienced by an individual that is noted by the healthcare professional, for example, abnormal breath sounds. Cancer causes a multitude of signs and symptoms, depending on the type and location of the cancer, the extent of the disease, and the presence and location of metastases.

Prompt recognition of early signs and symptoms of cancer allows diagnosis when cancer is most curable—in the early stages. As an example, colorectal cancer is not usually considered curable when it has metastasized; however, when the disease is diagnosed early, it has a very favorable outcome. General signs and symptoms exist that may indicate a cancer diagnosis, such as unexplained weight loss, fever, fatigue, pain, or skin changes (Holland et al., 2006). Most symptoms related to cancer are attributed to the effect of a tumor's increasing mass, skin manifestations, or organ dysfunction. Additionally, specific cancer signs and symptoms exist that relate to tumor type as well as physical location of the tumor itself.

History and Physical Examination of Patients With Cancer

Patient History

The clinical evaluation of patients with cancer includes several components. The history includes the chief complaint, related in the patient's own words. The history of the present illness incorporates a chronologic account of the complaint, including symptoms and their manifestations (Bickley & Szilagyi, 2007d; Naumberg, 2007). The family, social, and past medical history is ascertained. When evaluating patients with a potential malignancy, the history includes determining predisposing factors for cancer, prompting the advanced practice nurse (APN) to ask about familial cancers (such as breast, ovarian, prostate, or colorectal cancers), exposure to environmental mutagens (such as smoking cigarettes), alcohol intake, and previous illnesses (as in the example of human papillomavirus infection, which could lead to cervical cancer) (Sherman et al., 2003). This history is critical in the work-up of patients for a suspected cancer. Exploration of symptoms of cancer such as hemoptysis, blood in emesis or stool, abnormal vaginal bleeding, palpable masses or lumps, or any persistent or unexplained pain will be the focus of the physical examination.

Clues obtained in the history can guide the APN toward a diagnosis of malignancy. For example, a history of immunosuppression could lead to the development of cancer (as seen with organ transplant, autoimmune disease, or HIV). A retrospective study of more than 900 patients reported a 40% cancer risk following renal transplant in patients who have received 20 years of immunosuppressive therapy (London, Farmery, Will, Davison, & Lodge, 1995). Chronic infections also have been linked to the development of some cancers, although the connection between these infections and the immune system is not completely understood. Chronic hepatitis C infection has been reported to increase the risk of development of hepatocellular cancer (El-Serag & Mason, 2000). Work history is evaluated for occupational exposure to certain chemicals that have been implicated in the development of specific cancers, such as with benzene exposure and subsequent development of leukemia or lymphoma (Smith, Jones, & Smith, 2007). The patient's drug history is reviewed carefully to determine risk factors for specific cancers. For example, data from randomized controlled trials show that the risk of breast cancer is higher with estrogen-progestin use versus estrogen alone; therefore, a history of estrogen-progestin use could contribute to the development of breast cancer in some patients (Collins, Blake, & Crosignani, 2005; Newcomb et al., 2002).

The Physical Examination

Clues taken from the history will lead to a more focused physical examination. If patients present with specific physical complaints, careful attention is paid to those areas of involvement. Vital signs may provide information that leads to diagnosis. For example, a fever of unknown origin (FUO) often is related to infection or inflammatory disease; however, malignancy also is in the differential diagnosis if fever remains undiagnosed after one week of investigation. Cases of colon cancer have presented as FUO (Agmon-Levin, Ziv-Sokolovsky, Shull, & Sthoeger, 2005).

The skin is carefully inspected, and masses or ulcerations are noted. Enlarged or suspicious moles are examined carefully for signs of skin cancer, including melanoma. All lymphatic areas (including epitrochlear, axillary, infraclavicular, supraclavicular, and cervical) are examined. Enlarged lymph nodes may indicate the presence of lymphoma or metastatic disease.

Examination of the chest includes percussion and auscultation, with specific attention to lung sounds. Coarse breath sounds, wheezing, or rhonchi are assessed. Absence of breath sounds or dullness to percussion could indicate fluid or even a mass (Bickley & Szilagyi, 2007b, 2007d). The breast examination includes inspection of the breast skin and assessment for erythema or thickening, which could indicate an inflammatory carcinoma (Bickley & Szilagyi, 2007b). Changes in the breast contour or appearance of the nipple are noted. Palpation of the entire breast tissue is performed to evaluate for changes, including masses. Although breast cancer is rare in men, this examination is still important but may be of shorter duration.

The abdominal examination includes assessment for hepatomegaly or splenomegaly. Tenderness of the abdominal area is evaluated, and any sign of ascites is noted. Masses in the abdominal area may be harder to discern because of their location (Bickley & Szilagyi, 2007a, 2007b).

Male patients undergo a testicular examination, including assessment for any abnormalities in the scrotum or testicles. Examination of the healthy prostate normally reveals a rubbery, smooth, and nontender gland. Abnormalities of the prostate may manifest as hard nodules that feel irregular (Bickley & Szilagyi, 2007c). The female examination includes inspection of the vulva for any suspicious masses or lesions and a vaginal and adnexal examination, including cervical cytology. Digital rectal examination (DRE) is recommended for both males and females.

The musculoskeletal system is assessed, including range of motion and vertebral percussion tenderness. Pulses and reflexes are evaluated for strength and symmetry. Any clubbing or cyanosis is recorded. Any edema is measured and documented. For appropriate patients, a full neurologic examination may be performed.

Evaluation of Patient Performance Status

Once the history and physical examination are completed, patients may be evaluated by their performance status. Performance status has both prognostic and therapeutic implications. Although performance status grading of patients is standard practice while on clinical trials, routine documentation is rare. By grading patients' baseline performance status, clinicians are able to monitor subsequent changes resulting from disease and therapy. This allows clinicians to make modifications as appropriate to treatment.

The Karnofsky Performance Scale and the Eastern Cooperative Oncology Group (ECOG) scale (also called Zubrod) frequently are used in clinical practice and trials. The Karnofsky scale has been in use since the 1940s, when it was developed by two physicians, David Karnofsky and Joseph Burchenal. The 11 levels evaluate patients and their behaviors, from death to perfect health, with a percentage score (0–100) assigned to each level. The ECOG performance scale was developed by ECOG and has five levels (0–5), with level 0 indicating fully ambulatory and functional, and level 4 indicating fully bedridden and nonfunctional (Mor, Laliberle, & Wiemann, 1984) (see Table 3-1). Modified versions of these scales are available for specific patient populations. For example, the Karnofsky scale was modified by an Australian research group to assess the functional status of patients in palliative care (Abernethy, Shelby-James, Fazekas, Woods, & Currow, 2005).

After evaluation of performance status, diagnostic tests may be ordered to continue the assessment for the presence and extent of cancer. These may include laboratory tests, imaging, and other procedures to facilitate obtaining tissue, tumor markers, molecular markers, and immunohistochemistries.

Table 3-1. Comparison of Eastern Cooperative Oncology Group (ECOG) and Karnofsky Performance Scales

ECOG	Functional Status	Karnofsky
0	Fully functional, no activity restrictions or complaints	100%
1	Only slightly restricted in functional activity; able to continue daily routines with some modifications	80%–90%
2	Activities moderately restricted; out of bed/chair > 50% of the time; unable to perform work but able to perform personal care	60%–70%
3	Activity severely restricted; out of bed/chair < 50% of the time; unable to work; requires assistance with personal care	40%–50%
4	No normal activity; in bed/chair 100% of the time; unable to perform any self-care; may require total care	20%–30%
5	Dead	0%

Note. Based on information from Mor et al., 1984; Oken et al., 1982.

Diagnostic Evaluation

Laboratory Tests

Specific tests are conducted to further assess patients with a suspected malignancy. Initial laboratory tests for patients suspected of cancer usually include complete blood counts (CBCs), chemistry and liver function, coagulation studies, and electrolyte panel with renal function testing. Assessment of blood counts will give valuable information in the work-up of a patient suspected of having a hematologic malignancy along with important baseline information prior to treatment for neoplastic disease. Liver function and coagulation panels can provide important data regarding the functional status of the liver, and electrolyte assessment allows a critical look at the renal system. Specific additional laboratory tests may be required based on patient presentation.

Imaging Tests

Imaging tests such as plain radiographs or x-rays, computed tomography (CT) scans, magnetic resonance imaging (MRI), or positron-emission tomography (PET) scans are ordered to assist clinicians in determining the location and extent of disease, to assist in staging the disease, or to detect recurrence. The selection of the imaging test (or any diagnostic modality) is based on the type of abnormality suspected, including consideration of the value of the information obtained and how it will affect decision making (Patz, 2006). Sensitivity and specificity must be evaluated in reference to the type of suspected cancer. *Sensitivity* refers to the ability of the test to accurately identify a particular disease and is expressed as a percentage. This is calculated by dividing the number of patients who test positive for the disease by the total number of tested patients who actually have the disease. Sensitivity can vary in some diseases based on the stage and/or volume of disease. *Specificity* refers to the ability of the test to accurately identify the absence of a particular disease and also is expressed as a percentage. It is calculated by dividing the number of patients who test negative for the disease by the number of tested patients who do not have the disease. In general, highly sensitive tests are used to rule out a particular suspected disease, and highly specific tests are used to confirm or to eliminate a suspected disease.

Other considerations may include the cost, invasiveness, availability, and safety of the test. APNs may wish to consult with a radiologist if they have questions regarding the appropriateness of a certain imaging study. Although plain radiographs are one of the oldest and most-used imaging tests, many additional imaging tests are useful in the diagnosis and staging of cancer. Some of the more common tests will be discussed in the following section.

Plain radiographs: Although plain radiography exams are not as sophisticated as some of their imaging counterparts, they still play a role in cancer diagnosis. By presenting an image from the different absorption rates of specific tissues, radiographs can show suspicious areas such as in the breast or lung, albeit a two-dimensional image. It is relatively quick and inexpensive. Plain radiographs commonly are used for initial evaluation of osseous malignancies (Cothran & Helms, 2006) but are not as sensitive as bone scan when assessing for bone metastases. If patients present with a new complaint of bone pain, plain radiographs can visualize metastatic disease to the bone and are useful in ruling out impending fractures, as well (see Figure 3-1). Purely lytic bone metastases, such as in multiple myeloma, are best evaluated by plain bone films (skeletal surveys).

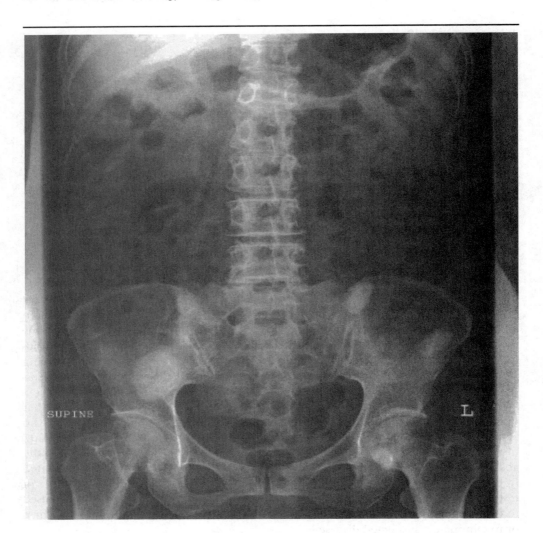

45-year-old female with newly diagnosed metastatic non-small cell lung cancer to the pelvis

Figure 3-1. Plain X-Ray Example of Metastatic Disease

Note. Figure courtesy of Pamela Hallquist Viale.

Plain films also are ideal for evaluating peripheral lung lesions, pneumonias, and intestinal obstructions. A plain radiograph is the first recommended test in the work-up of a soft tissue mass (American College of Radiology [ACR], 2005a). Radiographs of the chest can provide information regarding the size of lesions in the lung, the presence or absence of calcifications, and the growth rate of lung nodules (Ost, Fein, & Feinsilver, 2003). Evaluation of solitary pulmonary nodules and calcifications, which often are reflective of a benign process, is better seen on CT scans; however, plain radiographs have 50% sensitivity and 93% specificity for the identification of calcification (Ost et al.).

Radiography may be limited by patient factors including obesity (reduced contrast image), condition, positioning, and cooperation. Bone film interpretation can be difficult because of benign abnormalities and location of certain bones, such as the sacrum, sternum, and scapula, which have obscured views (Shaffer, 1996).

Ultrasonography: Ultrasound, a method of using sound waves with high frequencies that humans are unable to hear, is a noninvasive diagnostic scan. Using a transducer, which sends sound waves into the body, an image is made from the reflections of those waves back from organs and tissues. Anomalies larger than 2 cm can then be visualized, giving three-dimensional scrutiny (Omerod, 2005). This technique is commonly used for abnormalities of the breast (see the section on breast imaging), thyroid, testes, prostate, liver, biliary, kidneys, ovaries, and vascular system. Ultrasound is helpful in tumor work-up (i.e., biopsy guidance) and staging, as well as in evaluating pleural or pericardial effusions, renal or biliary obstructions, or ascites (Omerod). The use of contrast to enhance ultrasound is superior to conventional sonography in the characterization of lesions, particularly in regard to the degree of tissue perfusion. The use of contrast increases the sensitivity and specificity of this tool by enhancing the functional imaging ability. Delorme and Krix (2006) described contrast-enhanced ultrasound as a potential tool for determining the effects of antiangiogenic treatments in patients. Evidence also has shown that contrast-enhanced sonography improves the detection of thrombotic complications of hepatic malignancies (Rossi et al., 2006).

Endoscopic ultrasonography (EUS) is often used adjunctively to image specific tumor types, including esophageal and gastric cancers. EUS has a reported accuracy of 85% with a sensitivity of 67%–97% for tumors of the esophagus, stomach, and rectum (Montgomery & Ridge, 1998). EUS is an accurate preoperative staging tool for gastric cancer, and in one study, the overall accuracy for identifying T stage was 80%, with individual T stage accuracy determined to be T1, 100%; T2, 71.4%; T3, 87.5%; and T4, 72.7% (Xi, Zhao, & Ren, 2003). EUS showed an overall accuracy of 68.6% for identifying N stages, with sensitivity of 66.7% and specificity of 73.7%. Accurate preoperative staging assists in driving treatment decisions.

One of the best uses of ultrasonography is in guiding interventional procedures. Transrectal ultrasound-guided (TRUS) biopsy has been found to be a helpful technique in the diagnosis of pelvic malignancies, including gastric, cervical, cecal, and prostate cancer (Rinnab, Kufer, Hautmann, & Gottfried, 2006). In fact, TRUS is the most frequently used initial imaging test performed in patients with suspected prostate cancer (Choi, Kaur, Loyer, & Silverman, 2006). If an abnormality is found in the prostate-specific antigen (PSA) level or by DRE, the patient will undergo TRUS biopsy. TRUS provides excellent imaging of the prostate, thus allowing increased accuracy of biopsy, but has limited sensitivity and varied specificity for distinguishing malignant and benign tissue.

Limitations of ultrasound include inability to penetrate through bone or air (bowel or lung) and lack of reproducibility (Hricak et al., 2005). Ultrasound has a lower soft tissue resolution than that of CT or MRI. It also is less useful in deeper tissue evaluations.

Barium studies: Barium studies (e.g., esophagography, upper gastrointestinal [GI] series, lower GI series, barium enema) are conducted to examine the esophagus and small or large bowel (Omerod, 2005). Barium is radiopaque and, therefore, enhances the contrast between tissues. The barium swallow or esophagography is useful in evaluating oropharyngeal and pharyngeal function as well as structural abnormalities. The upper GI series includes the esophagus, duodenum, and anterior jejunum. The barium enema can effectively screen the colon for suspected neoplasms as well as for diverticular disease or irritable bowel disease. The single-contrast barium enema uses low-density barium suspension, whereas the double-contrast (air-contrast) enema uses a high-density barium suspension and air combination. The double-contrast study requires more patient cooperation and time (Shaffer, 1996). Barium is instilled into the colon per rectal tube, and this luminal contrast technique coupled with endoscopy allows for accurate visualization of the large intestine.

However, barium studies have limitations. One limitation is that patients are required to fast and undergo a thorough bowel cleansing. They are contraindicated in patients with intestinal obstructions or those who are pregnant. An important consideration is that a barium study could interfere with other abdominal studies and may need to be done following these other tests. Patients taking narcotics need to be cautioned about a possible increase in constipation and the rare complication of obstruction. Barium studies also may be limited if patients are uncooperative, are obese, or have intractable vomiting.

Computed tomography exams: The CT scan is one of the most common diagnostic imaging techniques in oncology. The CT scan shows abnormalities by sectional views in three dimensions using computer-controlled, multidirectional x-rays to create cross-sectional images of the body (Hricak et al., 2005; Omerod, 2005). This exam may be obtained with or without contrast, although visualization is better with contrast. Contrast may be given orally, rectally, or intravenously. The specificity and sensitivity of CT vary with the type of tumor being evaluated; however, in one review of studies on lung cancer, the sensitivity for CT ranged from 70%–90%, with the specificity ranging from 60%–90% (Shaffer, 1997). In the imaging of oral cancers, the sensitivity rises to 81%–94% (Hurt & Beauchamp, 2006).

Multislice CT (MSCT) has significantly improved the speed of examination, replacing some of the more invasive CT studies used in imaging such as arteriography and other vascular studies (Choi, Kaur, et al., 2006). The spiral or helical CT scan is produced by an x-ray tube that continuously rotates around the patient. It is much faster and increases diagnostic accuracy with reduced radiation exposure. It is especially useful in very young or very old patients and those who are critically ill. It has virtually eliminated image problems caused by inconsistent breath-holding (Hricak et al., 2005).

Multidetector CT allows evaluation of several body processes at one time, such as organ and angiographic imaging. Virtual or CT colonography is an example of multidetector CT. This scan provides axial and endoluminal views of the entire colon in both two-dimensional and three-dimensional images (Hricak et al., 2005). CT colonography has a sensitivity of 81% in the detection of colon polyps greater than 1 cm in size (Choi, Kaur, et al., 2006). In one prospective study evaluating air-contrast barium enema (ACBE), computed tomographic colonography (CTC), and colonoscopy in 614 patients, results showed that colonoscopy was better than the other exams for the detection of colonic polyps and cancers, with a sensitivity of 48% with ACBE, 59% with CTC, and 98% for colonoscopy (Rockey et al., 2005).

CT is the diagnostic imaging tool of choice for the chest. It is considered to be the principal imaging technique for the diagnosis of intra-abdominal lesions; however, contrast must be utilized (Erasmus, Truong, & McAdams, 2006). CT scanning without contrast is optimal for adrenal lesions. Although mammography is considered the diagnostic standard for breast cancer, contrast-enhanced CT has been found to be useful in the diagnosis of local recurrence of the disease, even if lesions were not palpable, with a sensitivity of 91% and a specificity of 85% (Hagay et al., 1997). CT is not ideal for differentiating tissue types in the evaluation of musculoskeletal malignancies (Cothran & Helms, 2006) because the CT may produce image artifact where there is cortical bone. Difficulties in distinguishing between inflammation and neoplastic bone infiltration are present with both CT and MRI techniques (Hurt & Beauchamp, 2006). CT is also used for study of head and neck tumors, esophageal cancers, GI malignancies (including liver tumors), kidney and bladder cancers, and prostate and ovarian cancers and in the evaluation of lymphomas (Choi, Kaur, et al., 2006; Omerod, 2005).

Most CT tables have a weight limit, thus limiting access for some patients. CT scanners are not portable. Patients are required to lie still, sometimes for extended periods. For chest studies, patients must be able to hold their breath. Another limitation is the potential for allergic or anaphylactic reactions to the contrast medium.

Magnetic resonance imaging: MRI may be the exam of choice for many tumor types, especially brain and spinal cord tumors, because of superior spatial resolution and tissue contrast (Hricak et al., 2005). MRI uses radiofrequency waves in the presence of a strong magnetic field, which detects different frequency emissions in the cells of the body (Omerod, 2005). Tumors emit a signal intensity based on their specific chemical makeup, and a true cross-sectional, three-dimensional image will display on a computer screen (Knopp, von Tengg-Kobligk, & Choyke, 2003) (see Figure 3-2). This technique can give valuable information regarding the specific characterization of tissues. Specialized coils are required for detailed views of specific areas of the body (such as the breast and prostate) (Shaffer, 1996). In addition to anatomic data, MRI provides functional, perfusion, and spectroscopic information (Hricak et al.).

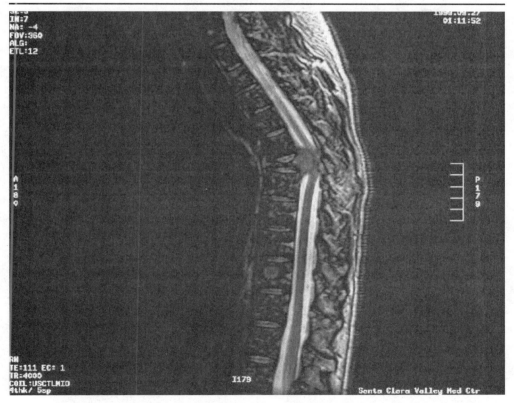

39-year-old male with multiple myeloma who presented with new-onset paraplegia

Figure 3-2. Example of Magnetic Resonance Imaging With Multiple Myeloma to Spine

Note. Figure courtesy of Pamela Hallquist Viale.

As new contrast agents are studied, it is becoming possible to visualize the angiogenic properties of neoplastic lesions with regard to both vascular density and permeability by MRI (Knopp et al., 2003). The dynamic contrast-enhanced functional MRI (DCE-MRI) has the ability to produce a sequence of rapid images, which are particularly useful in oncology, providing information about variations in the structure of the microvascular and pathophysiologic characteristics of individual tumors (Gribbestad et al., 2005). Many types of cancer, such as breast, lung, prostate, and head and neck tumors, have been noted on histopathologic samples to show microvascular density and serve as a sensitive prognostic factor (Gribbestad et al.). As a result, DCE-MRI may be able to show this angiogenic activity in a noninvasive manner, thereby providing advantages over other methods such as tissue sampling.

MRI is more sensitive than CT at determining soft tissue involvement, although MRI may be considered a second-line imaging modality because of its cost and limited availability in some settings (Choi, Kaur, et al., 2006; Omerod, 2005). For individual cancers, MRI is useful in tumors of the thorax, including non-small cell lung cancer (NSCLC), and central nervous system, spinal cord, head and neck, bladder, prostate, and endometrial cancers, and has a role in imaging of breast cancers and abdominal tumors, as well as cancer of unknown primary (Choi, Kaur, et al.; Hurt & Beauchamp, 2006; Shaffer, 2006). MRI is an excellent modality for evaluating musculoskeletal tissue processes. Assessment of the prostate is superior with MRI versus CT.

However, MRI may be somewhat limited in chest and upper abdominal scanning because of respiratory motion artifact. MRI is not portable and may be claustrophobic to some patients. Other limitations include cost, availability, length of time required, uncooperative patients, and small tube size. MRI may be contraindicated in patients with pacemakers or implanted metal devices.

Radionuclide imaging technique: Radionuclide imaging frequently is used in oncology. The technique involves the administration of a radioactive material (or radiopharmaceutical), which is then detected by gamma camera. Images of body tissues that have taken up the radioisotope are produced (Omerod, 2005). Bone scans (or scintigraphy), gallium scans, ProstaScint® (Cytogen Corp.), lymphoscintigraphy, PET scans, and single photon emission computed tomography (SPECT) scans are some of the imaging modalities in this category. Images are useful in terms of functionality but less useful in the description of anatomy. Because of this, these scans often are completed in conjunction with an anatomic scan.

Tumor viability imaging is used for the assessment of breast masses, primary bone tumors (following chemotherapy), thyroid cancer, parathyroid adenomas, and brain tumors (SPECT). Thyroid cancer can be both diagnosed and treated with the use of I131 sodium iodide (Coleman, 2006; Divgi & Larson, 2004). Whole body imaging is performed, and the total uptake is a monitor of the viability of the tumor and effectiveness of treatment (Divgi & Larson).

Positron-emission tomography scans: PET scans involve the injection of a positron-labeled (radioactive) tracer, usually glucose (F-fluorodeoxyglucose or F-FDG). Metabolically active areas, such as tumors, will take up the glucose and will show up as "hot" spots on images produced by gamma camera tomography, giving specific information regarding malignant tissues (Bhalla, 2002; Schrevens, Lorent, Dooms, & Vansteenkiste, 2004). PET scans give prognostic information based on response as well as play an important role in diagnosis and staging of specific tumor types (Schrevens et al., 2004). Certain tissues, such as kidney and brain, take up glucose, thus limiting evaluation by PET scanning. Benign processes, such as muscle uptake after exercise and selective cardiac conditions, can cause physiologic uptake of the FDG; therefore, a positive exam is not completely specific for malignancy (Francis, Brown, & Avram, 2005). Not all malignant tumors will appear "hot" because of limited glucose uptake, as in some slow-growing lesions like bronchoalveolar carcinoma and well-differentiated thyroid carcinomas (Bhalla).

The role of PET scanning is not completely established; however, its use in esophageal carcinoma, melanoma, and lymphoma has improved accuracy of staging for those tumor types (Choi, Kaur, et al., 2006). PET is useful for diagnostic accuracy of stereotactic biopsy of the brain (Omerod, 2005). It also differentiates tissue necrosis from recurrent tumor and between low- and high-grade tumors. Staging accuracy improves when PET scanning is used to assess for metastatic disease. Several tumor types can be diagnosed and staged accurately 80%–98% of the time (Francis et al., 2005). In particular, PET is considered the gold standard for evaluating a solitary pulmonary nodule or mass (Schrevens et al., 2004).

One of the biggest limitations of PET scanning is cost. The Health Care Financing Administration originally approved the use of PET scans in six different cancer types for Medicare patients. The current coverage has since expanded, and Table 3-2 presents information regarding additional tumor types.

Table 3-2. Medicare-Covered Uses of Positron-Emission Tomography Scans

Indication	Covered[1]	Nationally Noncovered[2]	Coverage With Evidence Development[3]
Brain			X
Breast			
• Diagnosis		X	
• Initial staging of axillary nodes		X	
• Staging of distant metastasis	X		
• Restaging, monitoring*	X		
Cervical			
• Staging as adjunct to conventional imaging	X		
• Other staging			X
• Diagnosis, restaging, monitoring*			X
Colorectal			
• Diagnosis, staging, restaging	X		
• Monitoring*			X
Esophagus			
• Diagnosis, staging, restaging	X		
• Monitoring*			X
Head and neck (non-CNS/thyroid)			
• Diagnosis, staging, restaging	X		
• Monitoring*			X

(Continued on next page)

Table 3-2. Medicare-Covered Uses of Positron-Emission Tomography Scans *(Continued)*

Indication	Covered[1]	Nationally Noncovered[2]	Coverage With Evidence Development[3]
Lymphoma			
• Diagnosis, staging, restaging	X		
• Monitoring			X
Melanoma			
• Diagnosis, staging, restaging	X		
• Monitoring*			X
Non-small cell lung			
• Diagnosis, staging, restaging	X		
• Monitoring*			X
Ovarian			X
Pancreatic			X
Small cell lung			X
Soft tissue sarcoma			X
Solitary pulmonary nodule (characterization)	X		
Thyroid			
• Staging of follicular cell tumors	X		
• Restaging of medullary cell tumors			X
• Diagnosis, other staging and restaging			X
• Monitoring*			X
Testicular			X
All other cancers not listed herein (all indications)			X

[1] Covered nationally based on evidence of benefit. Refer to National Coverage Determinations Manual Section 220.6 in its entirety for specific coverage language and limitations for each indication.

[2] Noncovered nationally based on evidence of harm or no benefit.

[3] Covered only in specific settings discussed above if certain patient safeguards are provided. Otherwise, noncovered nationally based on lack of evidence sufficient to establish either benefit or harm or no prior decision addressing this cancer. Medicare shall notify providers and beneficiaries where these services can be accessed, as they become available, via the following:
• Federal Register Notice
• CMS coverage Web site at www.cms.gov/coverage
* Monitoring = monitoring response to treatment when a change in therapy is anticipated.

CNS—central nervous system

Note. From "Positron Emission Tomography (PET) Scans" (pp. 26–27), in *Medicare National Coverage Determinations Manual,* by Centers for Medicare & Medicaid Services, 2006. Reprinted with permission.

Limitations of PET include lesser spatial resolution when compared to CT. PET is expensive, and availability may be restricted. Because of the short half-life of the radiolabeled isotopes, the facility must have its own cyclotron to produce the isotopes. Patients are required to fast for at least eight hours prior to the procedure, and the fasting blood glucose must be within a normal range. Diabetic patients are not to take oral hypoglycemic agents or insulin after midnight. All patients are to avoid vigorous exercise prior to the scan.

Combining PET and CT (PET-CT) scanning gives clinicians precise enough information that cancer can be accurately diagnosed in many patients. PET-CT assists in staging or restaging cancer, as well as in the planning of radiation therapy (Oriuchi et al., 2006). For example, the sensitivity of combination PET-CT is 89% in the imaging of nodal metastases in NSCLC, with a specificity of 94% (Schrevens et al., 2004). The combined PET-CT improves imaging by its ability to show the presence of tumor in normal-sized lymph nodes, locating and characterizing specific functions about the finding. This provides clinicians with important information about both the metabolism and the structure of the anomaly (Francis et al., 2005).

PET-CT is useful in the work-up of a patient with cancer of unknown primary, confirming malignancy in 25%–50% of those patients after conventional imaging and clinical evaluation have failed (Hurt & Beauchamp, 2006). In one study of patients with head and neck cancer (N = 68), the combination test improved accuracy of detection of lesions from 90% to 96%; five lesions were missed by PET alone versus one by PET-CT with FDG (Schoder, Yeung, Gonen, Kraus, & Larson, 2004). In NSCLC, the FDG PET-CT was able to significantly increase the accuracy of tumor staging in a prospective study of 50 patients with the disease (p = .001). The integrated test also improved detection of chest wall involvement, mediastinal invasion, and distant metastases (Lardinois et al., 2003).

For patients with colon cancer, PET-CT improved the overall staging accuracy from 78% to 89% (Cohade, Osman, Leal, & Wahl, 2003). Staging for lymphoma is improved with the use of PET versus CT alone; however, in one study of 27 patients, the combined test significantly improved staging accuracy (sensitivity was 61% with CT; 78% with PET; and 96% with PET-CT) (Freudenberg et al., 2004; Schoder, Larson, & Yeung, 2004). PET-CT is recommended as the modality of choice versus PET alone by some clinicians in the evaluation of malignancies in the abdomen and pelvis following successful experience with the integrated test in ovarian, colon, liver, endometrial, bladder, pancreatic, and cervical tumors (Wahl, 2004).

Single photon emission computed tomography scan: SPECT works similarly to the PET scan by using radioactive tracers and a scanner that provides three-dimensional patient images. Although SPECT imaging exam is less accurate in correction for scatter of the radiation in the body and produces decreased resolution in the detection of lesions compared to the PET scan, SPECT is still used today and may be seen in combination with CT as well (Buscombe & Bombardieri, 2005). The combination of SPECT and CT appears to improve accuracy of tumor detection to 80% (Lee, Sodee, Resnick, & Maclennan, 2005). This method of imaging has been used with some success in the imaging of prostate cancer to detect metastasis (Speight & Roach, 2007). SPECT also may be used in lymphoma.

Scans for Specific Situations

Breast imaging—Mammography, MRI, and sonography: Mammography, which is essentially a plain x-ray of the breast, is the primary tool for breast imaging (Bassett

& Lara, 2006). Mammograms may be either of two types: screening (performed in asymptomatic individuals) or diagnostic (performed when a palpable abnormality is present or when an abnormal screening mammogram indicates the need for additional study). Mammography can identify masses, calcifications, and other signs of malignancy, including architectural distortion or asymmetry. Comparison of new findings to previous mammographic results is important to enhance detection of malignancy (Bassett & Lara). Specialized views, such as spot compression or magnified views, may be necessary for closer evaluation of nodules, architecture, or microcalcifications (Shaffer, 1996).

Mammography detects 85% of all breast malignancies (Box & Russell, 2004). Almost half of all breast cancers can be seen on mammogram before they are palpable. However, a negative mammogram should not exclude biopsy if a palpable mass is present. Mammography may be limited by certain patient factors such as immobility, breast density, ascites, recent upper thoracic surgery, and venous access devices implanted over the upper breast (Shaffer, 1996).

The development of digital mammography may improve accuracy, particularly in younger, premenopausal women and those with dense breasts (Pisano et al., 2005). Digital mammography employs x-rays but collects the x-ray images on computer instead of film, which allows the breast image to be computer-enhanced or magnified.

Ultrasonography is used as an adjunct test for high-risk women with dense breast tissue or when a lesion found on mammography cannot be determined to be cystic or solid. It is appropriate for assisting in the evaluation of a palpable mass, particularly in younger women. An ultrasound is useful for directing accurate biopsy.

MRI of the breast has gained attention, as the American Cancer Society recently revised its recommendations to include the test for high-risk women (Saslow et al., 2007). High-risk women are defined as those having a *BRCA* mutation, a first-degree relative with a *BRCA* mutation, or a lifetime risk of 20%–25% or greater (as defined by BRCAPRO). (See Chapter 1 for more information on MRI breast screening.) MRI also is useful in conjunction with mammography and/or sonography to characterize a breast lesion or to confirm multifocality, multicentricity, or extent of disease (ACR, 2006b).

Detection of bone metastasis: Although plain x-ray can be used to determine the presence of bone metastasis, it is not particularly sensitive, and skeletal scintigraphy (bone scan) generally is considered the exam of choice for many tumor types, including breast (Hamaoka, Madewell, Podoloff, Hortobagyi, & Ueno, 2004). Published reports indicate that 30%–75% of the bone must be lost before plain x-ray can detect bone metastases (Galasko, 1972; Vinholes, Coleman, & Eastell, 1996). Scintigraphy can be used to evaluate the musculoskeletal system and involves the injection of a radiopharmaceutical agent (usually technetium [Tc]-99m methylene diphosphonate) that is taken up by osteoblasts followed by a scan within several hours, which usually reflects osteoblastic activity in the bone (Hendler & Hershkop, 1998) (see Figures 3-3 and 3-4). Bone scans are highly sensitive for bone metastases but are not very specific (Bhalla, 2002). False negatives occur in osteolytic bone metastases, as with multiple myeloma and renal cell carcinoma.

The sensitivity and specificity rates for skeletal scintigraphy range from 62%–100% (Hamaoka et al., 2004). Although this exam is useful in patients with multifocal or extensive disease, patients who have less distinct presentations (as in a single suspicious lesion) might benefit more from other imaging techniques such as x-ray, CT, or MRI (which also can assess for impending fracture) (Hamaoka et al.). CT can show axial bone metastasis, and both CT and MRI show more detail than the scintigraphy exam.

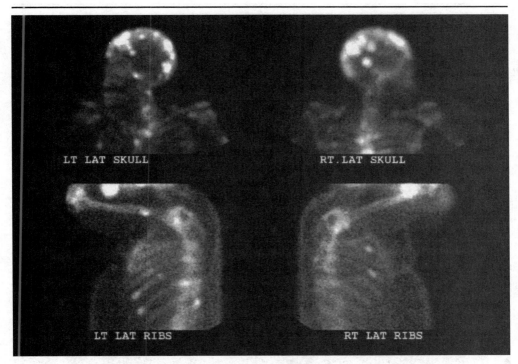

Widespread metastatic breast cancer to the skull, ribs, and spine as
evidenced by brightly lit areas on scan

Figure 3-3. Bone Scan of a Patient With Breast Cancer With Metastatic Disease

Note. Figure courtesy of Pamela Hallquist Viale.

MRI is more helpful in determining marrow disease or spinal cord compression. PET or PET-CT scans can play a role in determining bone metastasis as well (Hamaoka et al.). In addition to its role in diagnosing bone metastasis, scintigraphy has been used in the staging of thyroid tumors, sarcomas, gastroenteropancreatic tumors, laryngeal cancer, and some neuroendocrine tumors.

Gallium scintigraphy in non-Hodgkin lymphoma: The use of gallium-67 citrate scintigraphy in non-Hodgkin lymphoma is helpful for staging, assessing response to therapy, and determining relapse, as well as predicting outcome of disease (Coleman, 2006; Israel et al., 2002). Its usefulness in other cancers (such as lung and melanoma) varies, but its main utility is in lymphoma, although FDG-PET and PET have become the primary modalities in the staging and management of lymphoma in most practice settings (Coleman). PET scanning detects more disease sites above and below the diaphragm (Hricak et al., 2005).

Somatostatin-receptor scintigraphy and metaiodobenzylguanidine (MIBG): The OctreoScan® (Mallinckrodt Inc.) is a scan specific to carcinoid and other tumors that express somatostatin receptors (Coleman, 2006). The OctreoScan scintigraphy exam is able to visualize somatostatin receptors on a variety of neuroendocrine tumors as well as extra-abdominal metastasis. The OctreoScan begins with the injection of radiolabeled

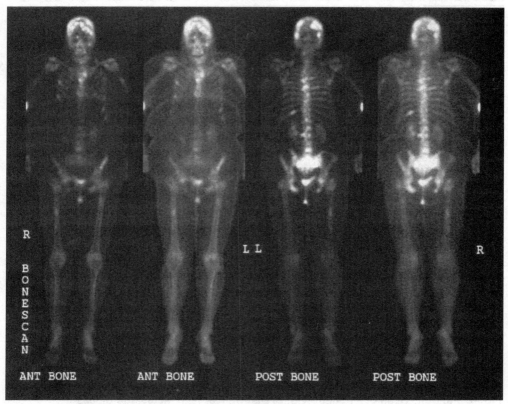

Widespread metastatic breast cancer to the skull, spine, ribs, and femur

Figure 3-4. Bone Scan of a Patient With Breast Cancer With Metastatic Disease

Note. Figure courtesy of Pamela Hallquist Viale.

somatostatin analog substance followed by scans at specific timed intervals (Shi et al., 1998). This technique has been effective in evaluating not only carcinoid but also pancreatic endocrine and medullary carcinoma of the thyroid, as well as other endocrine neoplasms (Shi et al.). The OctreoScan shows sensitivity in NSCLC and meningioma, as well as in other cancers, including breast cancer (Coleman).

MIBG has sensitivity for the detection of pheochromocytomas, carcinoid tumors, and other endocrine tumors when labeled with I123 or I131 and is at least as accurate as OctreoScan (Coleman, 2006). However, when compared to bone scintigraphy for the detection of bone metastases in carcinoid disease, bone scintigraphy exam proves to be more sensitive (Zuetenhorst, Hoefnageli, Boot, Valdes Olmos, & Taal, 2002). It also is used to treat bone metastases of carcinoid or medullary thyroid cancer. Episodes of hypertensive crises following injections of MIBG in patients with pheochromocytoma have been reported (Divgi & Larson, 2004).

Indium-111 capromab pendetide (ProstaScint) in prostate cancer: ProstaScint is a nuclear medicine study in which patients receive an infusion of 5 millicuries (mCi) of a monoclonal antibody labeled with indium-111. This antibody is specific for the prostate-specific membrane antigen that is found in prostate cancer cells (Divgi & Larson, 2004). The infusion is followed in about 30 minutes by SPECT, and SPECT and planar imaging are again conducted four to five days after wash-out of the isotope from the blood vessels and bowel (Taneja, 2004). The ProstaScint has a sensitivity of 63% in the detection of lymph node metastasis at the time of surgery; therefore, its role has been primarily in staging and detection of relapse (Taneja). In the detection of bone metastasis, bone scans were found to be more sensitive than the ProstaScint, and the interpretation is difficult. The usefulness of this exam is dependent on the clinician's ability to interpret the study findings. In one study of 151 men with rising PSA level and a history of prostate cancer, ProstaScint did not significantly correlate with Gleason score, perineural invasion, or pathologic stage (Raj, Partin, & Polascik, 2002). Fusing the ProstaScint with an MRI/CT image may improve the specificity of results (Taneja).

Imaging of bone metastases associated with multiple myeloma: Clinicians have relied upon skeletal radiographs (or skeletal surveys) as the principal method for the diagnosis and assessment of bone lesions associated with multiple myeloma (Angtuaco, Fassas, Walker, Sethi, & Barlogie, 2004). However, in early stages of the disease, the characteristic changes associated with myeloma deposits may not be visualized (Collins, 2005). Other scans useful in the monitoring of disease progression and/or complications may include CT or MRI. The use of multidetector-row CT improves imaging compared to radiographs in detecting lytic lesions, and in combination with MRI, it can help to accurately stage disease and determine the risk of fracture (Angtuaco et al.; Collins). Radiopharmaceuticals also are used to detect bone lesions, although the use of Tc-99m may not detect all lesions because of its decreased sensitivity with osteolytic lesions. Using other agents, such as gallium-67 or thallium-201, or FDG-PET has improved imaging of multiple myeloma lesions as compared to typical bone scanning agents. MRI can determine radiation therapy ports and show responses to treatment of the disease by depicting a decrease or resolution of focal lesions seen on original studies (Angtuaco et al.). MRI is routinely used in this disease because of its high sensitivity. Specific imaging patterns for multiple myeloma can be discerned by MRI, although the specificity is less accurate (Collins).

Diagnostic Procedures

Endoscopy

Multiple studies or procedures may be conducted to facilitate biopsies, including procedures that provide direct visualization and access to suspicious tissue. Upper GI endoscopy, also called upper esophagogastroduodenoscopy (EGD), is the diagnostic procedure of choice for upper GI cancers. EGD uses a thin, easily maneuvered endoscope to visualize and biopsy suspicious lesions of the larynx, upper airways, esophagus, stomach, and upper duodenum (Waxman, 2005). Most patients require only mild sedation. The accuracy of endoscopy with biopsy for upper GI cancers is estimated at 95%. The diagnosis of esophageal cancer often is made by endoscopy with biopsy or can be made by barium-contrast radiography followed by endoscopy and biopsy (Van Dam & Brugge, 1999). However, EUS (as discussed previously) has shown to be much more accurate in the staging of esophageal cancer, even when compared to CT, and can guide fine-needle aspiration (FNA) as well as detect recurrent disease (Brugge, Lee, Carey, & Mathisen, 1997; Van Dam, 1997).

Sigmoidoscopy

Sigmoidoscopies, both rigid and flexible, can be used to visualize the distal colon (Levin, 2002). The modality is both sensitive and specific and can be performed by either physicians or APNs trained in the procedure, with reduced costs associated with APNs (Horton, Reffel, Rosen, & Farraye, 2001). Although not as sensitive as colonoscopy, sigmoidoscopy is 20 times safer than colonoscopy in terms of complications (Levin). It can be used in addition to ACBEs and is considered to be a safe procedure with a low risk of perforation of the colon. However, because of the length of the scope, tumors in the proximal colon will be missed. If an abnormality, such as a polyp, is found on sigmoidoscopy, a follow-up colonoscopy should be performed. Biopsy can be performed during sigmoidoscopy but often is not, as most patients go on to receive colonoscopy (Smith, Duffy, & Eyre, 2006).

Colonoscopy

Colonoscopy can visualize the entire colon with a flexible scope, from the rectum to the cecum, and can facilitate biopsy of any suspicious areas, remove polyps, and collect stool specimens. However, this test is considered to be more invasive and requires total cleansing of the colon as well as sedation during the exam (Smith et al., 2006). Therapeutic colonoscopy can remove entire polyps, and any synchronous polyps can be identified during the exam. Electrocautery follows the removal of the polyp, and the tissue is sent to pathology for assessment. Possible complications of this exam include bowel perforation and hemorrhage. (See Chapter 1 for further information regarding colonoscopy and sigmoidoscopy in screening for colon cancer.)

Contraindications to colonoscopy include acute diverticulitis, significant adhesions in the pelvis or abdomen, acute exacerbations of inflammatory bowel disease, suspected bowel perforation, recent pulmonary embolus or myocardial infarction, and blood coagulation abnormalities.

Laparoscopy

Laparoscopy allows clinicians to visualize areas of the peritoneum, liver, and abdominal lymph nodes, as well as to evaluate for ascites (Hohenberger & Hunerbein, 1996). The practitioner inserts a thin telescope through a small incision or puncture in the anterior abdominal wall while the patient is under local anesthesia and mild sedation. This technique facilitates both esophageal and gastric staging by providing information regarding histology and regional spread of disease (Hohenberger & Hunerbein).

Using this method, intra-abdominal metastases may be diagnosed. This may prevent certain patients from undergoing a major surgery only to find metastatic or unresectable disease (Ko & Lefor, 2005). In one comparison of laparoscopy, ultrasound, and CT scan in detecting intra-abdominal metastases in patients with esophageal and gastric cancer, the sensitivity and accuracy of laparoscopy were better than those of either ultrasound or CT in the evaluation of the liver. Although these imaging studies are less invasive, they are unable to visualize lesions smaller than 1 cm. Neither ultrasound nor CT was able to detect metastases of the peritoneum, but laparoscopy demonstrated a sensitivity of 89% and accuracy of 98% for discovering peritoneal metastases (Watt, Stewart, Anderson, Bell, & Anderson, 1989). In one report of patients presenting with ascites, laparoscopy had an accuracy rate of 87%; other reports have suggested close to 100% accuracy (Herbsman, Gardner, & Alfonso, 1977).

Complications of laparoscopy include bleeding or rare instances of mediastinal emphysema or pneumothorax. Tumor implantation (or port-site implantation) has occurred at the laparoscopy site, although the true incidence is debatable (Ko & Lefor, 2005; Mehta, Griffin, Ganta, Rangraj, & Steichen, 2005). Although once considered routine in the work-up and staging of Hodgkin lymphoma, staging laparotomy has largely been replaced by noninvasive techniques such as PET and CT scans (Ko & Lefor).

Bronchoscopy

Bronchoscopy often is used in diagnosing lung cancer. It allows direct visualization of bronchial tissue and provides a means for obtaining biopsy for further evaluation (Nguyen, Summers, & Finkelstein, 2005). Both rigid and flexible bronchoscopes may be used, although flexible bronchoscopy with a transbronchial needle aspiration (TBNA) is now the preferred diagnostic method, particularly with central lung tumors, carrying a sensitivity of 88% and specificity of 90% (Collins, Haines, Perkel, & Enck, 2007; Rivera, Detterbeck, & Mehta, 2003). Flexible bronchoscopy with or without TBNA for peripheral tumors has a sensitivity of 60%–70%, which is affected by the size of the lesion (Rivera et al.). Patients with early, resectable NSCLC should undergo thoracotomy as their primary exam. Patients with small cell lung cancer (SCLC) or metastatic NSCLC might benefit by bronchoscopy as a convenient and less invasive technique (Collins et al., 2007). Indications for rigid bronchoscopy include endobronchial tumors, removal of foreign bodies, endoluminal stent placement, or management of massive hemoptysis. Rigid bronchoscopy usually requires general anesthesia and is performed in an operating suite (Nguyen et al.).

Complications of bronchoscopy are rare but could include hemorrhage, respiratory failure, or pneumothorax (Nguyen et al., 2005). Transbronchial biopsy appears to incur a higher incidence of adverse events.

Mediastinoscopy

If results from a bronchoscopy and TBNA are nondiagnostic, a mediastinoscopy is appropriate to obtain further information in making the diagnosis (Rivera et al., 2003). Mediastinoscopy is used to obtain information from lymph nodes located in the superior mediastinum for the staging of lung cancer. Information about lymphomas and other conditions can also be gleaned from mediastinoscopy. The exam usually is conducted by a thoracic surgeon while the patient is under general anesthesia. The surgeon makes an incision in the suprasternal area, down to the pretracheal fascia, thus allowing insertion of the mediastinoscope and providing visualization of the superior mediastinum and adjacent areas with opportunity for biopsy (Nguyen et al., 2005).

Complications of mediastinoscopy could include hemorrhage, pneumothorax, recurrent or phrenic nerve injury, tracheal or esophageal injury, wound infection, or difficulties with anesthesia. Overall, it is an extremely safe procedure with low mortality, even if superior vena cava syndrome is present (Nguyen et al., 2005).

Thoracoscopy

Thoracoscopy (also known as pleuroscopy) involves a small incision for the insertion of an open-tube scope for removal of fluid and biopsy of the pleural surface.

Video-assisted thoracoscopy has almost replaced simple thoracoscopy. It is a minimally invasive procedure and is done while the patient is under general anesthesia. It involves the creation of a pneumothorax and allows for visualization of the total visceral and parietal pleural surfaces, as well as biopsy of suspicious areas.

Potential complications include hemorrhage, respiratory failure, prolonged air leak, intercostal neuritis, and port-site metastases (Nguyen et al., 2005). For most patients, excisional biopsies are safe and efficient.

Biopsy and Histopathology

Almost without exception, tissue must be obtained in order for the clinician to make a diagnosis of malignancy. A biopsy of suspicious tissue provides essential information regarding the histology and grade of the tumor before treatment decisions are made (Pollack & Morton, 2006). Unnecessary treatment or diagnostic errors, such as mastectomies on women without sufficient evidence of tumor, occur when adequate diagnostic material is not obtained (Pollack & Morton). Slides of the biopsied material must be reviewed before the administration of therapy, and the resulting histopathology report may determine treatment options (Gillespie, 2005; Omerod, 2005).

Biopsy techniques may vary among differing tumor types. Biopsies can be obtained during a diagnostic imaging procedure as discussed earlier, such as during bronchoscopy or colonoscopy exams (Pollack & Morton, 2006). Certain imaging exams as previously discussed are employed specifically to locate tissue for biopsy. Methods of biopsies are discussed in Chapter 5.

Diagnostic Means

Various methods are used to measure or evaluate tissue retrieved by biopsy. The clinician obtaining the biopsy tissue must ensure that the specimen is adequate in quantity, representative of the suspicious tissue, and well preserved (Omerod, 2005). The role of the surgical pathologist is to evaluate the tissue by various means and determine whether malignancy exists. For most specimens, light microscopy with histochemical stains is adequate to make a diagnosis. However, many other diagnostic means are available that are more sophisticated and less subjective and that improve the diagnostic accuracy and more precisely define prognosis. These diagnostic means may include the use of electron microscopy (EM), immunohistochemistry (IHC), in situ hybridization, flow cytometry, or biomarkers.

Electron Microscopy

Many neoplasms can be identified at the light microscopic level; however, in some instances, more precise identification is needed but cannot be discerned (Fisher, Ramsay, Griffiths, & McDougall, 1985). The EM technique prepares tissue for ultramicroscopic examination, with specimens coming mainly from frozen sectioned tissue. The transmission electron microscope was first developed in the 1930s. It was used for the evaluation of renal biopsies, microorganisms, and cardiac biopsies, but its expanded use occurred in the field of oncology. Some clinicians feel that the use of EM has been supplanted by the use of IHC and is probably not currently as relevant in tumor diagnosis, although this technique may be considered to be underutilized in specific situations by others (Connolly et al., 2006; Mierau, 1999).

EM allows for very detailed examinations, including observation of cellular relations, membrane information, and the patterns of intracellular structures (Fisher et al., 1985; Wick & Swanson, 1997). The detection of these specific organelles is analogous to the detection of markers in IHC (Connolly et al., 2006). Histochemical stains aid in this process by adhering to certain substances in cancer cells, thus improving visualization.

Because the images rendered by EM are extremely specific, this technique often is used in determining the etiology of undifferentiated tumors or in the work-up of a patient with cancer of unknown primary (Connolly et al., 2006). EM can distinguish undifferentiated carcinomas from lymphomas and can be utilized to subclassify tumors. Its limitations include interpreter error and difficulties with improper handling of tissue or inappropriate fixation (Connolly et al.).

Immunohistochemistry

IHC has an expanding role in the diagnosis of cancer and, in conjunction with EM, has enhanced the ability to define tumors more specifically, thereby improving treatment of malignancy (Taylor, 2000). IHC is performed in the pathology laboratory and involves enzymes used in conjunction with specific antibodies directed against certain cancer cell antibodies. The immunologic effect of the recognition of the antigen by the antibody can be viewed under the microscope as a color reaction when certain chemicals are added to the tissue section (Connolly et al., 2006).

IHC helps to determine the site of origin for some tumors. Although microscopy examination can reveal the general histologic type (as in the example of squamous cell carcinoma), further delineation may be difficult. IHC uses specific antibodies for different sites of origin, assisting in the identification of the tumor type and thus affecting treatment decisions (Connolly et al., 2006).

The use of IHC can be important in the identification of undifferentiated tumors (Connolly et al., 2006). Initial identification may be hampered by routine stains of paraffin sections of tumor, which show that a malignancy exists but are unable to provide further etiologic information. The pathologist must use information about the tumor (such as the tumor's appearance histologically or characteristics shown radiographically) to create a differential diagnosis, from which the appropriate antibodies will be selected for testing by IHC (Connolly et al.). At times, a panel of antibodies may be more advantageous than the use of a single antibody, such as in distinguishing undifferentiated carcinoma from lymphoma or melanoma (Connolly et al.). For example, a panel of antibodies may be needed to distinguish between malignant mesothelioma and carcinoma, as well as to provide information to subclassify certain tumors, such as identifying an anaplastic seminoma from an embryonal carcinoma of the testes (by using a stain for the intermediate filament keratin because seminomas are primarily keratin-negative) (Connolly et al.).

IHC also detects antigens that are used in determining important prognostic information, such as estrogen and progesterone receptors (ERs and PRs) in hormonally responsive breast cancers, the identification of oncogenes or other gene products, and markers of proliferative activity (Connolly et al., 2006). Identifying ER and PR status is an essential part of the work-up for patients with breast cancer because positive status not only confers prognostic information but also determines who will benefit from hormonal therapy (Connolly et al.). Ki-67 is a nuclear antigen that exists in all cells that are proliferating; staining for this antigen allows pathologists to determine the growth fraction in a specific tumor sample (Connolly et al.). Both *TP53* and human epidermal growth factor receptor 2 (HER2/neu) may be evaluated by IHC staining and can provide valuable molecular information that guides clinicians in the choice of therapy, although the significance varies for certain tumors and their subtypes (Sawaki et al., 2006). IHC also has proved to be a sensitive method in the detection rate of micrometastases in lymph nodes by the use of specific antibodies against epithelial or tumor-associated lymph nodes (Timar, Csuka, Orosz, Jeney, & Kopper, 2002).

Specific examples of IHC used in clinical practice vary according to tumor types and uses. One common example is testing for epidermal growth factor receptor (EGFR), which may be recommended prior to treating patients with the EGFR inhibitor agents, such as cetuximab or panitumumab. However, although approximately 75% of colorectal cancers overexpress EGFR, little correlation has been shown between the intensity of staining (if any) and response to EGFR inhibitors (Cunningham et al., 2004; Van Cutsem, 2006).

Limitations of IHC can be seen in the significant variability of reagents available and various methods of detection. Variability also may exist in the sensitivity of the different methods as well as in the interpretation of the findings (Taylor, 2000).

In Situ Hybridization

In situ hybridization is a molecular genetic technique that involves DNA probes, thus allowing the visualization of specific nucleic acid sequences. These probes are labeled with different fluorochromes (for example, rhodamine) before hybridization and then are examined with fluorescence microscopy (Willman & Hromas, 2006). An example of a clinical use of in situ hybridization is the detection of excess copies of HER2/neu in women with breast cancer. If IHC testing for HER2/neu is equivocal, further testing by fluorescent in situ hybridization (FISH) may detect overexpression, thus directly affecting treatment decisions. The American Society of Clinical Oncology (ASCO) and the College of American Pathologists recently determined that testing for HER2/neu status is essential for patients diagnosed with invasive breast cancer. Approximately 20% of current testing for HER2 is inaccurate (Wolff et al., 2007). If the IHC score is 2+ rather than 3+ (which represents uniform, intense membrane staining of more than 30% of invasive tumor cells), then FISH is the more accurate test to assess HER2/neu status (Kakar et al., 2000). Clinicians have advocated for adoption of a systematic approach for in situ hybridization methods to improve test performance (Taylor, 2006).

Flow Cytometry

Flow cytometry often is utilized in lymphoma, bladder cancers, and leukemic disorders. The technique provides a rapid and quantitative measurement of cellular characteristics, as well as identification of cell cycle distribution within specific cell populations (Merkel, Dressler, & McGuire, 1987). Measuring the cell cycle distribution (also called the S-phase fraction) helps clinicians to anticipate the behavior or aggressiveness of many tumors and thus plan appropriate treatments (Merkel et al.).

Specimens such as material from surgical or needle biopsies, effusions, bone marrow aspirations, or exfoliative cytology from the bladder can be studied with flow cytometry (Merkel et al., 1987). Flow cytometry, when compared to bone marrow aspirates and bone marrow biopsy in the detection of lymphoid infiltration in B-cell disorders, has higher accuracy than the aspirate and is slightly more sensitive than bone marrow biopsy in the evaluation of this disease (Sah, Matutes, Wotherspoon, Morilla, & Catovsky, 2003).

Cancer Biomarkers

Biomarkers are substances or changes related to a neoplasm and may be correlated with a clinical or biologic outcome (Chui, 2006). These markers can help to identify and measure aspects of malignant growth, contributing to the detection, diagnosis, classification, prognosis, or monitoring of a specific cancer or response to therapy (Chui). Cancer biomarkers (or tumor markers) include proteins, genetic markers (abnormal chromosomes or oncogenes), hormones, hormone receptors, oncofetal antigens, enzymes, or other substances produced by tumor cells or in response to tumor growth (Chui). These biomarkers are measured in the serum or tissue of origin. Recent advances in biomarkers have further defined biomarkers into groups of traits (Chui). Biomarkers are utilized in screening, diagnosis, and prognosis, as well as in the detection of recurrent or metastatic disease (see Table 3-3).

Table 3-3. U.S. Food and Drug Administration–Approved Cancer Biomarkers

Biomarker	Type	Source	Cancer Type	Clinical Use
α-fetoprotein	Glycoprotein	Serum	Nonseminomatous testicular	Staging
Human chorionic gonadotropin-β	Glycoprotein	Serum	Testicular	Staging
CA 19-9	Carbohydrate	Serum	Pancreatic	Monitoring
CA 125	Glycoprotein	Serum	Ovarian	Monitoring
Pap smear	Cervical smear	Cervix	Cervical	Screening
CEA	Protein	Serum	Colon	Monitoring
Epidermal growth factor receptor	Protein	Colon	Colon	Selection of therapy
KIT	Protein (IHC)	Gastrointestinal tumour	GIST	Diagnosis and selection of therapy
Thyroglobulin	Protein	Serum	Thyroid	Monitoring
PSA (total)	Protein	Serum	Prostate	Screening and monitoring
PSA (complex)	Protein	Serum	Prostate	Screening and monitoring
PSA (free PSA %)	Protein	Serum	Prostate	Benign prostatic hyperplasia versus cancer diagnosis
CA 15-3	Glycoprotein	Serum	Breast	Monitoring

(Continued on next page)

Table 3-3. U.S. Food and Drug Administration–Approved Cancer Biomarkers *(Continued)*

Biomarker	Type	Source	Cancer Type	Clinical Use
CA 27-29	Glycoprotein	Serum	Breast	Monitoring
Cytokeratins	Protein (IHC)	Breast tumour	Breast	Prognosis
Oestrogen receptor and progesterone receptor	Protein (IHC)	Breast tumour	Breast	Selection for hormone therapy
HER2/NEU	Protein (IHC)	Breast tumour	Breast	Prognosis and selection of therapy
HER2/NEU	Protein	Serum	Breast	Monitoring
HER2/NEU	DNA (FISH)	Breast tumour	Breast	Prognosis and selection of therapy
Chromosomes 3, 7, 9 and 17	DNA (FISH)	Urine	Bladder	Screening and monitoring
NMP22	Protein	Urine	Bladder	Screening and monitoring
Fibrin/FDP	Protein	Urine	Bladder	Monitoring
BTA	Protein	Urine	Bladder	Monitoring
High molecular weight CEA and mucin	Protein (immunofluorescence)	Urine	Bladder	Monitoring

BTA—bladder tumour-associated antigen; CA—cancer antigen; CEA—carcinoembryonic antigen; FDP—fibrin degradation protein; FISH—fluorescent in-situ hybridization; GIST—gastrointestinal stromal tumour; IHC—immunohistochemistry; NMP22—nuclear matrix protein 22; PSA—prostate-specific antigen

Note. From "Biomarkers in Cancer Staging, Prognosis and Treatment Selection," by J.A. Ludwig and J.N. Weinstein, 2005, *Nature Reviews Cancer, 5,* p. 848. Copyright 2005 by Nature Publishing Group Macmillan Publishers Ltd. Reprinted with permission.

Diagnostic Markers

Serum tumor markers have limited sensitivity and specificity, which, in most cases, limits their use in the early diagnosis of cancer (Chui, 2006). Diagnosis of cancer requires histopathologic evidence of malignancy (Chui); however, tumor markers can help to determine the primary site of malignancy, such as in the case of distinguishing squamous cell carcinoma originating from a head and neck tumor from a squamous cell carcinoma metastatic from the lung, which influences both the prognosis and choice of treatment (Leong et al., 1998; Perkins, Slater, Sanders, & Prichard, 2003). Tumor markers also assist in determining malignant disease from a benign process. The ideal tumor marker would be specific for the suspected malignancy as well as sensitive to changes in tumor growth and response. The use of select tumor markers is routine in specific cancers, such as the use of alpha fetoprotein and beta human chorionic gonadotropin in testicular cancer or CA 125 in ovarian cancer. Tumor markers are very important in those patients who have elevated levels at diagnosis (Chui). However, some tumors might not secrete measurable substances, rendering that marker useless in those cases. Conversely, some individuals may have a positive marker but not have the disease. For example, carcinoembryonic antigen (CEA) is positive in many patients with colorectal cancer but cannot be used as a screening test because other segments of the population may have a positive CEA level without having the disease (Boucher, Cournoyer, Stanners, & Fuks, 1989; Duffy, 2001). Elevated CEA levels also may occur in other types of malignancy, such as breast cancer (Molina et al., 1998).

Prognostic and Response Markers

Biomarkers used for prognosis predict the outcome of a specific tumor type (Chui, 2006). Molecular patterns of tumor tissue are studied to determine the different gene expression patterns of these diseases. Molecular markers may be cellular products detected by a variety of techniques, including immunohistochemically with in situ hybridization (as discussed previously). An example is the assessment of HER2/neu receptor overexpression (Kakar et al., 2000). Another example of a molecular marker is ER/PR hormone receptors (von Knebel-Doeberitz & Syrjanen, 2006).

Prognosis and response markers support the initial choice of neoadjuvant or adjuvant therapy for specific cancers. For example, determining the ER and PR receptor status predicts the response of breast cancer to hormone therapy, thereby guiding the clinician in choice of therapy (Chui, 2006). ER/PR positivity predicts a longer disease-free survival (Sidransky, 2002) as well as a positive response to anthracycline chemotherapy. ASCO guidelines recommend the evaluation of ER/PR status and HER2 expression in all primary breast cancers at diagnosis (Sidransky). Because the TNM staging system is anatomically based, biomarkers can help to further classify the traditional tumor classes into subsets that may perform differently from each other, possibly requiring different therapy in some cases (Ludwig & Weinstein, 2005). Additionally, these markers assist in determining which patients will benefit from a targeted therapy such as imatinib or cetuximab (Ludwig & Weinstein).

Recurrence and Metastasis Markers

Serum tumor markers may be used to determine disease progression or recurrence for several tumor types, including the CA 27-29 in breast cancer, CEA for colorectal cancer, CA 125 in ovarian cancer, and PSA for prostate cancer (Bast et al., 2001). Most serum tumor markers lack the sensitivity and specificity to be useful in screening for primary disease or disease recurrence following primary therapy; however, these are useful in monitoring treatment efficacy and may indicate progression or regression of disease (Chui, 2006).

Selected Molecular Biomarkers in Specific Tumor Types

Colorectal cancer: Some molecular markers of colorectal cancer predict the likelihood of sensitivity to certain treatments, thus helping clinicians to target treatments more effectively. The "ASCO 2006 Update of Recommendations for the Use of Tumor Markers in Gastrointestinal Cancer" includes specific information on molecular markers in this disease (Locker et al., 2006). CEA is the marker of choice for monitoring the response of metastatic disease to treatment. Data are inadequate to recommend routinely using other molecular markers to determine treatment or to predict the effectiveness of therapy for colorectal cancer. Neither CEA nor other molecular markers are recommended for routine screening for colorectal cancer.

Other markers studied in colorectal cancer include *TP53* (tumor suppressor gene), *ras*, CA 19-9, thymidine synthase (TS), dihydropyrimidine dehydrogenase (DPD), thymidine phosphorylase (TP), microsatellite instability (MSI), 18q loss of heterozygosity, or deleted-in-colon-cancer protein. Currently, these are not recommended by ASCO for screening, diagnosis, staging, surveillance, prognostic determination, or treatment monitoring and prognostication, as published data are insufficient (Locker et al., 2006). MSI in colorectal cancer may play a role in the prediction of survival and response. MSI-H (high) is associated with a low frequency of distant metastasis, predicting better response in one study, therefore suggesting a possible protective host reaction that decreases risk for tumor spread (Buckowitz et al., 2005). Another study of 255 patients with sporadic stage C colorectal cancer suggested that MSI-L (low) patients had significantly poorer survival, but the authors suggested that more data are needed to further define the role of MSI in colorectal cancer prognosis (Wright et al., 2005).

If patients undergoing treatment with chemotherapy for colorectal cancer suffer unexpected side effects, it then may be appropriate to test these patients for specific molecular markers indicating increased sensitivity to the toxicities of treatment. For 5-fluorouracil (5-FU), TS overexpression as well as specific gene polymorphisms may lead to drug resistance (Salonga et al., 2000). Low gene expression levels of TP are connected with response and survival of colorectal cancer. Patients with DPD deficiency may develop significant systemic toxicity with 5-FU, as more than 80% of 5-FU is degraded in the liver by DPD (Johnston, Ridge, Cassidy, & McLeod, 1999). Additionally, patients who have low expression of DPD have longer disease-free recurrence and longer survival than their counterparts. For oxaliplatin, increased expression of the excision repair cross-complementing *(ERCC1)* gene and thymidylate synthase gene have been shown to predict decreased response in patients receiving the drug with 5-FU. Additionally, the xeroderma pigmentosum group D (XPD) polymorphism may play a role in the prediction of patient outcome to oxaliplatin (Park et al., 2001; Shirota et al., 2001).

Irinotecan is more toxic in those patients who are homozygous for the UGT1A1*28 allele. These patients have a significantly increased risk for developing severe neutropenia because of a reduced ability to utilize the drug-metabolizing enzyme uridine diphosphate glucuronosyltransferase 1A1 (UGT1A1) (Hahn, Wolff, & Kolesar, 2006). UGT1A1*28, a genetic variant of UGT1A1, is a marker of reduced UGT1A1 activity. Seen increasingly in practice, although not yet the standard of care in all settings, testing for this polymorphism (UGT1A1*28) in patients who suffer unexpected toxicity to irinotecan is appropriate, and a molecular assay is currently available to identify this affected population. For these patients, a reduced dose of irinotecan in the treatment of metastatic colorectal cancer may be clinically sound (Hahn et al.).

Although no commercially available test currently exists in the United States for detection of K-*ras* mutation, recent data have shown that patients with the known mutation do not respond to treatment with EGFR monoclonal antibodies, cetuximab and panitumumab. One study of 30 patients receiving cetuximab showed a response rate of 37% (or 11 patients) (Lievre et al., 2006). A K-*ras* mutation was present in 43% of the tumors and was significantly associated with an absence of response to the agent, prompting the researchers to conclude that these mutations are a predictor of resistance to cetuximab therapy and carry a worse prognosis (Lievre et al., 2006). A more recent study reported in 2008 showed that K-*ras* mutations were associated with resistance to cetuximab and poorer survival as well (Lievre et al., 2008). Eighty-nine patients with metastatic colorectal cancer were enrolled in the study, with 27% of the study participants having a K-*ras* mutation (0% responders noted in the mutated group versus 40% responders in the 65 nonmutated patients) (p < .001). A much larger study of 427 patients randomized to either panitumumab or best supportive care showed 43% with the mutated K-*ras* gene; the study results confirmed that the efficacy of the monoclonal antibody was confined to patients without the mutation, prompting one researcher to conclude that these therapies should be reserved for those patients with wild-type K-*ras* versus the mutated form (Tuma, 2007).

Lung cancer: Currently, no established biomarkers are recommended for routine use in lung cancer (Pfister et al., 2004). Molecular biomarkers may be used to determine tissue of origin in patients with specific types of lung cancer. As previously mentioned, markers identified in squamous cell cancer may allow determination of metastatic disease versus a primary tumor. By observing chromosomal changes and other mutations, researchers can correctly classify the origin of disease, assisting in appropriate treatment selection (Leong et al., 1998). Recent research with gene expression profiling confirms markers for lung cancer that may be used to determine prognosis. A small study of 21 previously untreated patients with NSCLC confirmed two markers (CSNK2A1 and C1-Inh) identified by genomic hybridization that served as independent predictors of survival and outcome in this difficult tumor type (O-charoenrat et al., 2004).

Thyroid transcription factor-1 (TTF-1) is a diagnostic immunohistochemical marker for primary lung cancers. The expression of TTF-1 correlates with the occurrence of lymph node metastases in patients with lung cancer and, therefore, may serve as a predictor marker in this disease (Altaner et al., 2006). Strong TTF-1 expression also was found to be an independent predictor of better survival for patients with NSCLC in one study of 57 patients, although it did not significantly correlate with tumor differentiation (Haque, Syed, Lele, Freeman, & Adeqboyega, 2002). Another use for the TTF-1 marker is to distinguish small cell carcinoma from poorly differentiated squamous cell carcinoma. In one study, a panel of antibodies to TTF-1, *p63*, high-molecular-weight keratin, and *p16* successfully distinguished between the two cancers (Zhang et al., 2005).

Breast cancer: The use of molecular markers in breast cancer is increasing. ASCO last updated its recommendations for circulating and tissue-based tumor markers for this disease in 2007 (Harris et al., 2007). An update committee composed of members from the full panel was convened to review the data published since 1999. The panel examined data regarding CA 15-3, CA 27-29, CEA, ER, PR, human EGFR2, urokinase plasminogen activator, plasminogen activator inhibitor 1, and other multiparameter gene expression assays, finding enough evidence to recommend clinical utility in practice (Harris et al.). However, the panel found insufficient evidence to support routine use of DNA/ploidy by flow cytometry, *TP53*, cathepsin D, cyclin E, proteomics, certain multiparameter assays, detection of bone marrow micrometastases, or circulating tumor cell measurement (Harris et al.). The 2007 recommendation for HER2 evaluation is that HER2 expression and/or amplification should be evaluated in every primary invasive breast cancer at the time of diagnosis or at the time of recurrence to guide clinicians in the choice of therapy with trastuzumab for adjuvant or metastatic breast cancer (Harris et al.). The use of circulating extracellular domain of HER2/neu is not recommended for screening, diagnosis, staging, or routine surveillance in asymptomatic patients. The panel agreed that all patients should be evaluated for ER and PR status and HER2/neu prior to implementation of therapy (Harris et al.; Khatcheressian et al., 2006).

The updated ASCO guidelines comment on the use of multiparameter gene expression analysis for breast cancer and recommend that in newly diagnosed patients with node-negative, ER-positive breast cancer, the Oncotype DX® (Genomic Health, Inc.) assay may be used to help to predict the risk of recurrence for patients treated with tamoxifen as well as to identify patients who are predicted to obtain the most benefit from adjuvant tamoxifen, potentially avoiding adjuvant chemotherapy (Harris et al., 2007). The panel felt that the MammaPrint® (Agendia) assay is still under investigation. The Oncotype DX and MammaPrint tests assist clinicians in determining prognosis in specific patients with breast cancer and in predicting which patients will benefit from further therapy or have increased risk of metastasis. Oncotype DX is a 21-gene panel and recurrence score algorithm (Genomic Health, Inc., n.d.). MammaPrint is a 70-gene assay (Agendia, n.d.).

One retrospective study of 324 patients with stage I–III breast cancer treated with tamoxifen reported evaluation for nine molecular markers. *BCL2, MYC,* and *TP53,* as well as standard hormone receptors ER and PR and growth factor receptor *erbB2,* showed predictive value (Linke, Bremer, Herold, Sauter, & Diamond, 2006). *BCL2* is an antiapoptotic factor; *MYC* is an oncogene; and *TP53* is a tumor suppressor. Another potential use of biomarkers is in the molecular classification of breast cancer. A study of 82 patients with breast cancer showed increased sensitivity to preoperative chemotherapy with paclitaxel and doxorubicin correlating to basal-like and *erbB2*-positive molecular subtypes of breast cancer (Rouzier et al., 2005).

Overview of Staging

Following a thorough work-up, the definitive diagnosis of cancer is made. Following evaluation of performance status, staging of disease occurs. Staging is a process that determines the location and extent of the primary cancer. This information guides the treatment plan and has prognostic value. The physical examination, imaging tests, laboratory tests, tumor and molecular markers, and pathology and surgical reports present the clinician with a picture of the disease. From this information, the cancer can be staged. The goal of staging is to provide a common language for all clinicians to use in the care and treatment of cancer; therefore, accuracy of staging is essential (Greene, 2004).

The TNM system is used for most solid cancers. It was developed and is maintained by the American Joint Committee on Cancer (AJCC) and the International Union Against Cancer. This system undergoes continual evaluation and revision and is currently published in its sixth edition. *T* stands for the original tumor description; *N* depicts the lymph node involvement; and *M* represents the measurement of distant metastases if present (Greene et al., 2002). Staging systems promote comparison of clinical experiences among different centers over a period of time and play an important role in the establishment of specific, uniform criteria for evaluation of patients considering clinical trials (Kotilingam, Lev, Lazar, & Pollock, 2006).

Three different types of staging exist: clinical staging (based on the tests, physical examination, and biopsies), pathologic staging (for patients who have had surgery/biopsy), and restaging (sometimes done to determine the extent of disease once the cancer recurs) (Greene et al., 2002). Once a patient is staged, the original stage usually remains the stage of the disease for the patient's lifetime (see the Case Study).

Neoplasms of the brain and spinal cord are classified according to cell type and grade of the tumor, rather than TNM; and lymphomas and cancers of the blood and bone marrow usually have different staging systems (Greene et al., 2002). For example, the Ann Arbor staging system, which was first developed for Hodgkin disease, is used in non-Hodgkin lymphomas as well (Armitage, 2005).

Although staging of soft tissue sarcomas traditionally includes TNM, it also includes grade, with *a* and *b* designations indicating depth (Kotilingam et al., 2006). Tumor-specific staging systems by the Musculoskeletal Tumor Society stage this disease as well. Clinicians now recognize that accurate staging for soft tissue sarcoma incorporates molecular markers (Kotilingam et al.) and most likely will incorporate them in the future.

The revised melanoma staging system is a good example of a collaborative approach incorporating prognostic factors to create and validate AJCC staging criteria (Balch et al., 2001). This evidence-based approach to staging will continue to evolve and incorporate molecular diagnostic approaches in the evaluation of melanoma (Balch et al., 2004).

As the use of cancer molecular markers expands, questions arise regarding the integration of this information into formal TNM staging and its use in traditional staging systems (Ludwig & Weinstein, 2005). These clinical questions continue to be debated, but as molecular markers play a greater role in the management of specific cancers, their use in formal staging will evolve as well. Collaborative staging is recognized as an attempt to incorporate all the significant features of a specific tumor (which may or may not be used in the original TNM system), including clinical, radiologic, pathologic, biologic, and molecular features (Patel & Shah, 2005). The ideal staging and prognostic system of the future will encompass all of these items.

Work-Up of Common Solid Tumors

Breast Cancer

History

History and current complaints: The work-up for women suspected of having breast cancer consists of the history or discussion of the presenting complaint, including information on the location, method of discovery, size and duration of the lesion (if a palpable mass is present), and symptoms such as tenderness, as well as hormonal status (Osuch, Bonham, & Morris, 2002). Descriptive symptoms are important, such as skin thickening or nipple discharge, including color and consistency (Hortobagyi, Esserman, & Buchholz, 2006). Clear or nonbloody nipple discharge may be a benign sign; all bloody discharges need careful evaluation.

Breast symptoms are common, and recognition and evaluation of these symptoms can result in breast cancer detection. In a study of 2,400 women with breast symptoms (mass, pain, skin or nipple change, or lumpiness) presenting to primary care clinicians over a 10-year period, follow-up exam of 66% of breast symptoms led to 27% of women receiving an FNA or biopsy, with breast cancer diagnosed in 6.2% of patients (Barton, Elmore, & Fletcher, 1999). Although pain is one of the most frequent breast symptoms presenting to clinicians, it is not usually the presenting symptom of cancer and may represent benign findings (Hortobagyi et al., 2006). A mass is the most frequent presenting symptom associated with breast cancer.

The history includes assessment of three important nonmodifiable risks for developing cancer of the breast: female gender, older age (75% of women with breast cancer are older than age 50), and a family history of breast cancer (Draper, 2006; Osuch et al., 2002). Modifiable or lifestyle factors (e.g., not having children, younger age at menarche, heavier alcohol use, obesity, the use of oral contraceptives, postmenopausal hormone therapy [particularly estrogen and progesterone combined]) also are implicated as risks for the development of breast cancer (Vogel & Taioli, 2006). Information is obtained regarding any personal history of breast cancer as well.

Family history: Family history includes information about all relatives (both paternal and maternal) over three generations, documenting all cancer occurrences with a special focus on breast cancer (Kirk, Brennan, Houssami, & Ung, 2006). Depending on the relatives affected and age at diagnosis, the lifetime risk of breast cancer can be significantly increased. Ethnic background also is assessed. Women who have inherited a mutation in the *BRCA1* or *BRCA2* genes are at higher risk (anywhere from 50%–80%) for the development of breast cancer (Brody & Biesecker, 1998). Other hereditary breast cancer syndromes should be considered if appropriate. Although male breast cancer occurs in only 1% of all new cases, the risk may be increased in some individuals with a genetic predisposition. Chapter 2 provides more information about hereditary breast cancers.

Surgical history: Any previous breast biopsies or surgeries are carefully noted. Personal history of proliferative breast disease (fibrocystic masses, moderate epithelial hyperplasia [ductal or lobular]) or atypical epithelial hyperplasia is noted, as these may increase the risk for cancer of the breast twofold and fivefold, respectively (Osuch et al., 2002). (More information on cancer risks with proliferative breast disease may be found in Chapter 1.)

Physical Examination

The clinical breast examination (CBE) ideally is conducted with the patient in both supine and sitting positions. Careful observation of skin contour while the arms are raised is important (Hortobagyi et al., 2006). Breasts are visualized while arms are relaxed and with hands on hips. Dimpling and other changes can be ascertained when the arms are in an elevated position. Clinicians assess skin changes carefully, observing for dimpling, peau d'orange, skin color changes, or ulcers. Nipple position is checked for any asymmetry or retraction. Dryness of the areola area or skin thickness changes may reflect Paget disease (Hortobagyi et al.).

Palpation also is performed in both the sitting and supine positions, although the supine position is better for evaluation of masses. Breast changes can occur during the ovulation cycle, and breast tissue may be nodular and tender during the luteal phase of the cycle (Osuch et al., 2002). Nodularity and thickness of tissue are assessed and documented. Various levels of pressure are used, from light pressure to deep pressure, using the pads of the first three fingers. The entire breast is examined carefully from the second rib to the clavicle, to the sternum, down to the sixth rib, and around to the latissimus dorsi muscle (Osuch et al.). The lymph nodes of the axilla and infraclavicular and supraclavicular regions are assessed. Often, these are best palpated while the patient is in a sitting position. (See Chapter 1 for additional information about CBE.)

If a mass is appreciated, the size and character of the mass are significant. Adequate documentation of the mass utilizes a detailed diagram, noting the size of mass, location, and distance from the nipple (Osuch et al., 2002). Benign lesions may appear smooth with variable density and sometimes move easily within the breast tissue (Hortobagyi et al., 2006). Malignant lesions, in contrast, are harder, less discrete, and less mobile.

Differential Diagnosis

The differential diagnosis includes changes from fibrocystic disease (often symmetric and usually seen in the upper outer quadrants in areas of increased glandular tissue), fibroadenoma, hyperplastic changes with or without atypia, and mammary duct ectasia (Hortobagyi et al., 2006). Any palpable mass, however, is considered cancerous until proved otherwise (Osuch et al., 2002) and is carefully evaluated. Anatomically, breast cancer occurs more frequently in the upper outer quadrant, possibly because tumors are believed to form in the terminal-duct lobular unit, and more of these units exist in that physiologic location (Stacey-Clear et al., 1993).

Diagnostic Tests

Radiologic: A diagnostic mammogram may be ordered and assessed, and if needed, an ultrasound can help to distinguish a cystic mass from a solid mass (Osuch et al., 2002). Additional imaging and special exams or studies may include a digital mammogram, breast MRI, ductal lavage (examining cells obtained from the milk ducts of the breast), scintimammography (adjunct to mammography involving a radioactive tracer followed by nuclear medicine breast imaging), or thermal imaging (adjunct to mammography involving measurement of breast tissue temperature) (Wright & McGechan, 2003). Intriguing new data exist on mammographic breast density playing a role in breast cancer development and whether obtaining serum estradiol might better predict appropriate patients for risk-reduction intervention trials (Vogel & Taioli, 2006; Ziv et al., 2004). This information could influence risk assessments and diagnostic work-ups of breast masses in the future.

Although breast MRI is not considered the standard of care for screening all patients, recent data have reported on the diagnostic advantages of this imaging technique, as it provides a three-dimensional view of tissue with high sensitivity in dense breast tissue. A trial of 969 women with a recent diagnosis of unilateral breast cancer ascertained that MRI can detect cancer in the contralateral breast after clinical and mammographic evaluation showed negative findings (Lehman et al., 2007). The trial results influenced the American Cancer Society to revise its guidelines to recommend MRI in women at high risk because of a strong family history of the disease.

Laboratory studies: Laboratory studies are obtained, including CBC and liver function tests (LFTs). Other laboratory studies are ordered as clinically indicated.

Biopsy: A biopsy is performed to obtain cells for examination and to determine the type of breast cancer. FNA, core needle biopsy, or excisional biopsy are some of the methods used to retrieve cells for pathologic examination in a palpable mass; stereotactic and ultrasound-guided core needle biopsy may be an alternative to excisional biopsy for lesions unable to be appreciated (Hortobagyi et al., 2006; Osuch et al., 2002). (Chapter 5 provides more information regarding biopsies.) The term "triple assessment" indicates the use of imaging, clinical assessment, and pathologic findings in the evaluation of a breast mass (Hortobagyi et al.). FNA has shown to be very useful with a specificity and sensitivity of 99% and 98%, respectively (Hortobagyi et al.). Sentinel lymph node dissection may be used in some patients, following FNA and core biopsy.

Biologic information plays an important role in accurate breast cancer staging. Both DNA ploidy (measurement of the DNA present in breast cancer predicting aggressive behavior or not) and DNA flow cytometry (measurement of the tumor cells' S-phase cells; cell division with high numbers predict more aggressiveness) can be important (Henry & Hayes, 2006; Pusztai, Mazouni, Anderson, Wu, & Symmans, 2006). ER and PR status and HER2/neu status are routinely measured as recommended by ASCO. Data have indicated that HER2/neu and *TP53* are overexpressed in certain types of breast cancer, such as inflammatory breast cancer (Sawaki et al., 2006).

Pathology: The pathologic classification of breast cancer includes the following histologic types: in situ carcinomas (NOS [not otherwise specified], Paget disease, and intraductal); invasive carcinomas (NOS, ductal, inflammatory, medullary [NOS], medullary with lymphoid stroma, mucinous, papillary [predominantly micropapillary pattern], tubular, lobular, and Paget disease); and infiltrating, undifferentiated, squamous cell, adenoid cystic, secretory, and cribriform carcinomas (Greene et al., 2002). Invasive breast carcinomas are graded (except for medullary carcinoma) (Greene et al.). The histologic grade includes GX (grade cannot be assessed), G1 (low combined histologic grade [favorable]), G2 (intermediate combined histologic grade [moderately favorable]), and G3 (high combined histologic grade [unfavorable]) (Greene et al.).

Staging

Recent changes in the AJCC breast cancer staging include the description of the size, number, location, and how regional metastasis to lymph nodes is detected. Other changes focus on new technology and novel diagnostic means used in the diagnosis of breast cancer (Singletary & Connolly, 2006). Clinical staging systems can underestimate the extent of disease (Hortobagyi et al., 2006). Pathologic information is included to improve the accuracy of staging. After a tissue diagnosis is made, other imaging studies may be ordered to complete staging in patients with breast cancer, including chest x-ray, CT, MRI, or bone scan (NCCN, 2008a). The specific test(s) for staging will depend on the individual patient's clinical presentation during the work-up for staging.

The TNM staging for breast cancer is described in Tables 3-4 and 3-5. The grade of breast tumors is scored depending on features such as tubule formation, nuclear pleomorphism, and mitotic count. Grading is in addition to the clinical staging (physical examination of skin, mammary gland, lymph nodes, and imaging) and the pathologic staging (all data from clinical staging and data from surgical specimens and resection and tumor examination, lymph nodes, and metastatic sites) (Greene et al., 2002).

Once patients are diagnosed with breast cancer and staged, the stage of the disease guides the clinician toward treatment. Additional tools are available to help clinicians to individualize therapy by assessing the risk for recurrence more accurately. Adjuvant! Online is a tool to assist clinicians with treatment decisions in patients with invasive breast cancer who have received primary therapy locally and may need systemic adjuvant therapy (Olivotto et al., 2005). By assigning an estimated risk of relapse or breast cancer mortality, the tool estimates effectiveness of selected adjuvant therapy options by calculating the estimated net benefit of these therapies. The tool was validated in a study of 4,083 women with breast cancer and was found to predict outcomes reliably except in a few specific subgroups of patients (Olivotto et al.). Users of Adjuvant! Online assess clinical components such as the patient's age, comorbidities, tumor size, tumor grade, and number of affected lymph nodes, and the tool then calculates an estimate of mortality risk, treatment efficacy, and breast cancer–related mortality. Adjuvant! Online may be accessed online after free registration at www.adjuvantonline.com/index.jsp.

Oncotype DX is a reverse transcriptase-polymerase chain reaction–based multigene assay that provides a quantitative assessment of the likelihood of distant breast can-

Table 3-4. Tumor-Node-Metastasis (TNM) Definitions for Breast Cancer

Primary Tumor (T)

Definitions for classifying the primary tumor (T) are the same for clinical and pathologic classification. If the measurement is made by physical examination, the examiner will use the major headings (T1, T2, or T3). If other measurements, such as mammographic or pathologic measurements, are used, the subsets of T1 can be used. Tumors should be measured to the nearest 0.1 cm increment.

TX	Primary tumor cannot be assessed
T0	No evidence of primary tumor
Tis	Carcinoma *in situ*
Tis (DCIS)	Ductal carcinoma *in situ*
Tis (LCIS)	Lobular carcinoma *in situ*
Tis (Paget's)	Paget's disease of the nipple with no tumor

Note: Paget's disease associated with a tumor is classified according to the size of the tumor.

T1	Tumor 2 cm or less in greatest dimension
T1mic	Microinvasion 0.1 cm or less in greatest dimension
T1a	Tumor more than 0.1 cm but not more than 0.5 cm in greatest dimension
T1b	Tumor more than 0.5 cm but not more than 1 cm in greatest dimension
T1c	Tumor more than 1 cm but not more than 2 cm in greatest dimension
T2	Tumor more than 2 cm but not more than 5 cm in greatest dimension
T3	Tumor more than 5 cm in greatest dimension
T4	Tumor of any size with direct extension to (a) chest wall or (b) skin, only as described below
T4a	Extension to chest wall, not including pectoralis muscle
T4b	Edema (including peau d'orange) or ulceration of the skin of the breast, or satellite skin nodules confined to the same breast
T4c	Both T4a and T4b
T4d	Inflammatory carcinoma

Regional Lymph Nodes (N)
Clinical

NX	Regional lymph nodes cannot be assessed (e.g., previously removed)
N0	No regional lymph node metastasis
N1	Metastasis to moveable ipsilateral axillary lymph nodes
N2	Metastases in ipsilateral axillary lymph nodes fixed or matted, or in clinically apparent* ipsilateral internal mammary nodes in the *absence* of clinically evident axillary lymph node metastasis
N2a	Metastasis in ipsilateral axillary lymph nodes fixed to one another (matted) or to other structures
N2b	Metastasis only in clinically apparent* ipsilateral internal mammary nodes and in the *absence* of clinically evident axillary lymph node metastasis
N3	Metastasis in ipsilateral infraclavicular lymph node(s) with or without axillary lymph node involvement, or in clinically apparent* ipsilateral internal mammary lymph node(s) and in the *presence* of clinically evident axillary lymph node metastasis; or metastasis in ipsilateral supraclavicular lymph node(s) with or without axillary or internal mammary lymph node involvement
N3a	Metastasis in ipsilateral infraclavicular lymph node(s)
N3b	Metastasis in ipsilateral internal mammary lymph node(s) and axillary lymph node(s)
N3c	Metastasis in ipsilateral supraclavicular lymph node(s)

Clinically apparent is defined as detected by imaging studies (excluding lymphoscintigraphy) or by clinical examination or grossly visible pathologically.

(Continued on next page)

Table 3-4. Tumor-Node-Metastasis (TNM) Definitions for Breast Cancer *(Continued)*

Pathologic (pN)[a]

pNX	Regional lymph nodes cannot be assessed (e.g., previously removed, or not removed for pathologic study)
pN0	No regional lymph node metastasis histologically, no additional examination for isolated tumor cells (ITC)

Note: Isolated tumor cells (ITC) are defined as single tumor cells or small cell clusters not greater than 0.2 mm, usually detected only by immunohistochemical (IHC) or molecular methods but which may be verified on H&E stains. ITCs do not usually show evidence of malignant activity e.g., proliferation or stromal reaction.

pN0(i–)	No regional lymph node metastasis histologically, negative IHC
pN0(i+)	No regional lymph node metastasis histologically, positive IHC, no IHC cluster greater than 0.2 mm
pN0(mol–)	No regional lymph node metastasis histologically, negative molecular findings (RT-PCR)[b]
pN0(mol+)	No regional lymph node metastasis histologically, positive molecular findings (RT-PCR)[b]

[a] Classification is based on axillary lymph node dissection with or without sentinel lymph node dissection. Classification based solely on sentinel lymph node dissection without subsequent axillary lymph node dissection is designated (sn) for "sentinel node," e.g., pN0(i+) (sn).

[b] RT-PCR: reverse transcriptase/polymerase chain reaction.

pN1	Metastasis in 1 to 3 axillary lymph nodes, and/or internal mammary nodes with microscopic disease detected by sentinel lymph node dissection but not clinically apparent**
pN1mi	Micrometastasis (greater than 0.2 mm, none greater than 2.0 mm)
pN1a	Metastasis in 1 to 3 axillary lymph nodes
pN1b	Metastasis in internal mammary nodes with microscopic disease detected by sentinel lymph node dissection but not clinically apparent**
pN1c	Metastasis in 1 to 3 axillary lymph nodes and in internal mammary lymph nodes with microscopic disease detected by sentinel lymph node dissection but not clinically apparent.** (If associated with greater than 3 positive axillary lymph nodes, the internal mammary nodes are classified as pN3b to reflect increased tumor burden)
pN2	Metastasis in 4 to 9 axillary lymph nodes, or in clinically apparent* internal mammary lymph nodes in the *absence* of axillary lymph node metastasis
pN2a	Metastasis in 4 to 9 axillary lymph nodes (at least one tumor deposit greater than 2.0 mm)
pN2b	Metastasis in clinically apparent* internal mammary lymph nodes in the *absence* of axillary lymph node metastasis
pN3	Metastasis in 10 or more axillary lymph nodes, or in infraclavicular lymph nodes, or in clinically apparent* ipsilateral internal mammary lymph nodes in the *presence* of 1 or more positive axillary lymph nodes; or in more than 3 axillary lymph nodes with clinically negative microscopic metastasis in internal mammary lymph nodes; or in ipsilateral supraclavicular lymph nodes
pN3a	Metastasis in 10 or more axillary lymph nodes (at least one tumor deposit greater than 2.0 mm), or metastasis to the infraclavicular lymph nodes
pN3b	Metastasis in clinically apparent* ipsilateral internal mammary lymph nodes in the *presence* of 1 or more positive axillary lymph nodes; or in more than 3 axillary lymph nodes and in internal mammary lymph nodes with microscopic disease detected by sentinel lymph node dissection but not clinically apparent**
pN3c	Metastasis in ipsilateral supraclavicular lymph nodes

(Continued on next page)

Table 3-4. Tumor-Node-Metastasis (TNM) Definitions for Breast Cancer *(Continued)*

---

* *Clinically apparent* is defined as detected by imaging studies (excluding lymphoscintigraphy) or by clinical examination.
** *Not clinically apparent* is defined as not detected by imaging studies (excluding lymphoscintigraphy) or by clinical examination.

Distant Metastasis (M)

MX	Distant metastasis cannot be assessed
M0	No distant metastasis
M1	Distant metastasis

DCIS—ductal carcinoma in situ; LCIS—lobular carcinoma in situ

Note. Used with permission of the American Joint Committee on Cancer (AJCC), Chicago, Illinois. From *AJCC Cancer Staging Manual, Sixth Edition* (pp. 227–228), by F.L. Greene, D.L. Page, I.D. Fleming, A. Fritz, C.M. Balch, D.G. Haller, et al. (Eds.), 2002, New York: Springer, www.springeronline.com.

Table 3-5. Tumor-Node-Metastasis (TNM) Stage Grouping for Breast Cancer

Stage	T	N	M
Stage 0	Tis	N0	M0
Stage I	T1*	N0	M0
Stage IIA	T0	N1	M0
	T1*	N1	M0
	T2	N0	M0
Stage IIB	T2	N1	M0
	T3	N0	M0
Stage IIIA	T0	N2	M0
	T1*	N2	M0
	T2	N2	M0
	T3	N1	M0
	T3	N2	M0
Stage IIIB	T4	N0	M0
	T4	N1	M0
	T4	N2	M0
Stage IIIC	Any T	N3	M0
Stage IV	Any T	Any N	M1

---

* T1 includes T1mic

Note. Stage designation may be changed if post-surgical imaging studies reveal the presence of distant metastases, provided that the studies are carried out within 4 months of diagnosis in the absence of disease progression and provided that the patient has not received neoadjuvant therapy.

Note. Used with permission of the American Joint Committee on Cancer (AJCC), Chicago, Illinois. From *AJCC Cancer Staging Manual, Sixth Edition* (p. 228), by F.L. Greene, D.L. Page, I.D. Fleming, A. Fritz, C.M. Balch, D.G. Haller, et al. (Eds.), 2002, New York: Springer, www.springeronline.com.

cer recurrence, while also determining possible benefit of specific chemotherapy options. By performing an assay using formalin-fixed, paraffin-embedded tumor tissue, an analysis of a 21-gene panel provides a Recurrence Score™ (Genomic Health, Inc.), which is reported as a value between 0 and 100. A recurrence score below 18 places the patient in a low-risk range, whereas scores ranging 18–30 constitute the intermediate-risk range. A recurrence score greater than 31 places the patient in a high-risk range (Genomic Health, Inc., n.d.). A calculation of the average rate of distant recurrence at 10 years also is reported (see Figure 3-5). The score can be used with a specific version of Adjuvant! Online, as well. Oncotype DX was validated in several trials, including a population-based study of tumor gene expression and risk of breast cancer death in node-negative patients with breast cancer (Habel et al., 2006; Paik et al., 2006). The test is validated for use in patients who are newly diagnosed with breast cancer, have stage I or II disease, and are node negative and ER positive who will be treated with tamoxifen.

MammaPrint was approved by the U.S. Food and Drug Administration (FDA) in February 2007. The test performs a 70-gene DNA microarray analysis on primary breast tumors, examining cell cycle, invasion, metastasis, and angiogenesis and thus providing prognostic information specifically for the development of distant metastasis. This test is indicated for stage I invasive breast cancer (ER+ or ER– disease) or stage II invasive breast cancer (ER+ or ER–) and lymph node–negative disease. MammaPrint requires a punch biopsy sample of the tumor (at least 3 mm in diameter) (Agendia, n.d.). MammaPrint was validated in a trial of 326 patients with node-negative breast cancer and was found to add independent prognostic information to clinical and pathologic risk information in patients with early-stage breast cancer (Buyse et al., 2006).

Survival and Prognosis

Prognostic factors for breast cancer include hormone receptor status, HER2/neu status, grade and histology of tumor, as well as lymph node status. Women diagnosed with early-stage disease or premalignant ductal carcinoma in situ have up to a 100% five-year survival (Hortobagyi et al., 2006). Using data from 1996–2003, the American Cancer Society statistics for breast cancer in the United States reported five-year survival rates of 98% for localized disease; 84% for women with regional disease; and 27% for those with distant metastases (Jemal et al., 2008).

Cervical Cancer

History

History and current complaints: The work-up for women with suspected cervical cancer begins with a thorough history and description of the current complaint. The clinical symptoms most often seen in carcinoma of the cervix include vaginal bleeding, abnormal vaginal discharge, and pain, although early disease may be asymptomatic (Jhingran, Eifel, Wharton, & Tortolero-Luna, 2006). Symptoms may appear after intercourse or vaginal douching (Eifel, Berek, & Markman, 2005). Once the disease becomes locoregionally invasive, pelvic pain may be prevalent. Flank pain can indicate the presence of hydronephrosis. If the disease spreads to the pelvic wall, patients may present with sciatic pain, leg edema, and hydronephrosis (Eifel et al.). Once the bladder becomes involved, patients may describe a feeling of urinary urgency or frequency; constipation also indicates advanced disease in most cases (Eifel et al.; Jhingran et al.).

The history will focus on specific risk factors for cervical cancer, including multiple sexual partners, early age at first sexual intercourse, and the sexual habits of male part-

Sample Patient Report Form

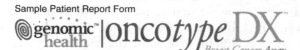

Genomic Health, Inc.
301 Penobscot Drive
Redwood City, CA 94063
Tel (866) ONCOTYPE (866-662-6897)
www.oncotypeDX.com

PATIENT REPORT

Patient: Doe, Jane
Sex: Female
DOB: 01/01/1950
Medical Record/Patient #: 556677771
Date of Surgery: 11/23/2004
Specimen ID: SURG-0001

Requisition: R00003G
Date Received: 12/01/2004
Date Reported: 12/13/2004
Client: Community Medical Center
Treating Physician: Dr. Harry D Smith
Submitting Pathologist: Dr. John P Williams
Additional Physician: Dr. Sally M Jones

ASSAY DESCRIPTION

Oncotype DX™ Breast Cancer Assay uses RT-PCR to determine the expression of a panel of 21 genes in tumor tissue. The Recurrence Score™ is calculated from the gene expression results. The Recurrence Score range is from 0-100.

RESULTS

Recurrence Score = **10**   Test results should be interpreted using the information in the Clinical Experience section below, which applies only to patients consistent with this clinical experience.

CLINICAL EXPERIENCE

Patients with a Recurrence Score of 10 in the clinical validation study had an

Average Rate of Distant Recurrence at 10 years of | **7%** (95% CI: 5%-9%)

The following results are from a clinical validation study with prospectively-defined endpoints involving 668 patients. The patients enrolled in the study were female, stage I or II, node negative, ER-positive, and treated with tamoxifen. *N Engl J Med* 2004; 351: 2817-26.

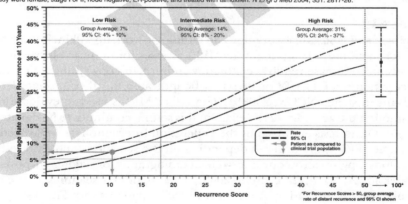

Laboratory Director: Patrick Joseph, MD   CLIA Number 05D1018272

This test was developed and its performance characteristics determined by Genomic Health, Inc. The laboratory is regulated under the Clinical Laboratory Improvement Amendments of 1988 (CLIA) as qualified to perform high-complexity clinical testing. This test is used for clinical purposes. It should not be regarded as investigational or for research. These results are adjunctive to the ordering physician's workup.

301 Penobscot Drive   Redwood City, CA 94063   (866) ONCOTYPE (866-662-6897)   www.oncotypeDX.com
© 2005 Genomic Health, Inc. Oncotype DX and Recurrence Score are trademarks of Genomic Health, Inc.

GHI004 Rev007 06/29/2005

Figure 3-5. Oncotype DX Sample Patient Report

Note. Figure courtesy of Genomic Health, Inc.

ners (Brinton et al., 1987). A history of HIV confers higher rates of cervical abnormalities, as well as larger and higher-grade lesions, when compared with HIV-negative women (Jhingran et al., 2006). However, the most important risk factor for this disease is infection with human papillomavirus (HPV) (Jhingran et al.).

Family history: The relationship between cervical and vaginal dysplasia and prenatal exposure to diethylstilbestrol is well documented; therefore, the history should elicit any information regarding this factor (Robboy et al., 1984). Some studies show familial aggregation in cervical cancer, but it is difficult to separate the hereditary and environmental risk factors involved.

Physical Examination

A thorough physical examination is conducted on a woman with suspected cervical cancer. A complete pelvic examination with bimanual and rectovaginal examination is performed (Eifel et al., 2005). An abdominal examination includes palpation to assess for constipation, blunt percussion to assess for flank pain, and measures to assess for sciatica. Pelvic lymph nodes are carefully assessed. Lower extremities are assessed for lower extremity edema, which could indicate lymphatic and venous obstruction as well as renal failure.

Differential Diagnosis

The differential diagnosis includes cervicitis, endometrial carcinoma, pelvic inflammatory disease, uterine cancer, or vaginitis. Abnormal uterine bleeding could be caused by many benign conditions, including incomplete or missed abortion, ectopic pregnancy, or trophoblastic disease. Other tumors may cause bleeding as well, such as vulvar or vaginal cancers. Infection can mimic symptoms common to cervical cancer, causing bleeding or abnormal vaginal discharge (Brenner, 1996).

Diagnostic Tests

Radiologic and laboratory work-up: The radiologic work-up will include a chest film to assess for metastases. IV pyelography (IVP) assesses for ureteral obstruction by the cancer. Advanced disease requires cystoscopy and proctoscopy (Jhingran et al., 2006). For select patients, a CT/MRI or PET may be indicated to rule out stage IB1 from a more advanced stage (NCCN, 2008b). The CT or MRI is used to evaluate regional nodes, although the accuracy of the exam in this setting continues to be debated (Eifel et al., 2005). Other tests endorsed by the Fédération Internationale de Gynécologie et d'Obstétrique (FIGO) are ordered depending on the specific patient and setting and include colposcopy, hysteroscopy, and skeletal radiography for staging purposes (Benedet, Bender, Jones, Ngan, & Pecorelli, 2000). The use of PET scanning in the imaging of cervical cancer is increasing. A recent study of 22 patients with FIGO stage IB–IVA cervical carcinoma compared MRI and PET-CT examinations prior to lymphadenectomy. PET-CT was more sensitive in the detection of lymph node metastases versus MRI (57.6% and 30.3%, respectively), although no statistical difference was seen in specificity or accuracy (Choi, Roh, et al., 2006).

Laboratory studies: Further evaluation should include laboratory studies with CBC and platelet count as well as LFTs and renal function studies (NCCN, 2008b).

Biopsy: The diagnosis of cervical cancer requires pathologic examination of a tissue specimen obtained from the periphery of the tumor if possible (Jhingran et al., 2006). After an abnormal Pap smear, biopsy procedures for patients with suspected cervical cancer include colposcopy, direct biopsy of the suspected tissue or cone biopsy, and/or endocervical curettage (Eifel et al., 2005; Jhingran et al.).

Pathology: The most common histology of cervical cancer is of epithelial origin with 70%–80% squamous cell cancer (Jhingran et al., 2006). Other types are adenocarcinoma (approximately 20%–25% today versus 5% in the 1950s), small cell carcinoma, melanoma, and lymphomas (Jhingran et al.). The histologic tumor grade is assigned either GX (grade cannot be assessed), G1 (well differentiated), G2 (moderately differentiated), G3 (poorly differentiated), or G4 (undifferentiated).

Staging

Staging of cervical cancer is done by FIGO and classifies the disease by stages 0–IV (see Tables 3-6 and 3-7). Clinical staging is a uniform method of staging, as many patients with cervical cancer are treated with radiation alone and never receive surgical-pathologic staging (Greene et al., 2002). The stage is ascertained before therapy is started and does not change once treatment has started (Eifel et al., 2005). AJCC states that if the actual stage is uncertain, the lesser stage is used to categorize the patient (Greene et al.). Therefore, pathologic staging is not used to change the clinical stage and is recorded as pTNM staging alone (Greene et al.).

Survival and Prognosis

Prognostic factors for cervical cancer include the size of the tumor and extent of disease, lymph node involvement, tumor histology (including grade), and biologic

---

Table 3-6. Tumor-Node-Metastasis (TNM) Staging of Cervical Cancer

---

The definitions of the T categories correspond to the stages accepted by the Fédération Internationale de Gynécologie et d'Obstétrique (FIGO). Both systems are included for comparison.

Primary Tumor (T)

TNM Categories	FIGO Stages	
TX		Primary tumor cannot be assessed
T0		No evidence of primary tumor
Tis	0	Carcinoma *in situ*
T1	I	Cervical carcinoma confined to uterus (extension to corpus should be disregarded)
*T1a	IA	Invasive carcinoma diagnosed only by microscopy. Stromal invasion with a maximum depth of 5.0 mm measured from the base of the epithelium and a horizontal spread of 7.0 mm or less. Vascular space involvement, venous or lymphatic, does not affect classification
T1a1	IA1	Measured stromal invasion 3.0 mm or less in depth and 7.0 mm or less in horizontal spread
T1a2	IA2	Measured stromal invasion more than 3.0 mm and not more than 5.0 mm with a horizontal spread 7.0 mm or less
T1b	IB	Clinically visible lesion confined to the cervix or microscopic lesion greater than T1a/IA2
T1b1	IB1	Clinically visible lesion 4.0 cm or less in greatest dimension
T1b2	IB2	Clinically visible lesion more than 4.0 cm in greatest dimension
T2	II	Cervical carcinoma invades beyond uterus but not to pelvic wall or to lower third of vagina
T2a	IIA	Tumor without parametrial invasion
T2b	IIB	Tumor with parametrial invasion
T3	III	Tumor extends to pelvic wall and/or involves lower third of vagina, and/or causes hydronephrosis or non-functioning kidney
T3a	IIIA	Tumor involves lower third of vagina, no extension to pelvic wall

(Continued on next page)

Table 3-6. Tumor-Node-Metastasis (TNM) Staging of Cervical Cancer *(Continued)*

| T3b | IIIB | Tumor extends to pelvic wall and/or causes hydronephrosis or non-functioning kidney |
| T4 | IVA | Tumor invades mucosa of bladder or rectum, and/or extends beyond true pelvis (bullous edema is not sufficient to classify a tumor as T4) |

* All macroscopically visible lesions—even with superficial invasion—are T1b/IB.

Regional Lymph Nodes (N)

NX		Regional lymph nodes cannot be assessed
N0		No regional lymph node metastasis
N1		Regional lymph node metastasis

Distant Metastasis (M)

MX		Distant metastasis cannot be assessed
M0		No distant metastasis
M1	IVB	Distant metastasis

Note. Used with permission of the American Joint Committee on Cancer (AJCC), Chicago, Illinois. From *AJCC Cancer Staging Manual, Sixth Edition* (p. 260), by F.L. Greene, D.L. Page, I.D. Fleming, A. Fritz, C.M. Balch, D.G. Haller, et al. (Eds.), 2002, New York: Springer, www.springeronline.com.

Table 3-7. Stage Grouping for Cervical Cancer

Stage	T	N	M
Stage 0	Tis	N0	M0
Stage I	T1	N0	M0
Stage IA	T1a	N0	M0
Stage IA1	T1a1	N0	M0
Stage IA2	T1a2	N0	M0
Stage IB	T1b	N0	M0
Stage IB1	T1bl	N0	M0
Stage IB2	T1b2	N0	M0
Stage II	T2	N0	M0
Stage IIA	T2a	N0	M0
Stage IIB	T2b	N0	M0
Stage III	T3	N0	M0
Stage IIIA	T3a	N0	M0
Stage IIIB	T1	N1	M0
	T2	N1	M0
	T3a	N1	M0
	T3b	Any N	M0

(Continued on next page)

Table 3-7. Stage Grouping for Cervical Cancer *(Continued)*

Stage	T	N	M
Stage IVA	T4	Any N	M0
Stage IVB	Any T	Any N	M1

Note. Used with permission of the American Joint Committee on Cancer (AJCC), Chicago, Illinois. From *AJCC Cancer Staging Manual, Sixth Edition* (p. 260), by F.L. Greene, D.L. Page, I.D. Fleming, A. Fritz, C.M. Balch, D.G. Haller, et al. (Eds.), 2002, New York: Springer, www.springeronline.com.

features of tumor vascularity and S-phase fraction, among others (Eifel et al., 2005). Women with HIV have a very poor prognosis and frequently develop rapidly progressive disease (Greene et al., 2002). The current five-year survival for cervical cancer in the United States is reported to be 92% for localized disease, 56% for regional cancer of the cervix, and 17% for distant disease (Jemal et al., 2008). For recurrent cervical cancer, five-year survival rates range from 20%–50% if the patient is deemed a candidate for definitive treatment with surgery or radiation therapy (Jhingran et al., 2006).

Colon Cancer

History

History and current complaints: The most striking risk factor when assessing for colon cancer is age; most cases of colon cancer are found in those older than 50 years of age (Rodriguez-Bigas, Hoff, & Crane, 2006). Nonmodifiable risk factors for colon cancer include a personal history of colon cancer, history of polyps, or history of inflammatory bowel disease (Rodriguez-Bigas et al.). Modifiable risk factors for this disease include a diet high in fat or red meat, lack of exercise, obesity, smoking, and heavy use of alcohol (Rodriguez-Bigas et al.).

Symptoms of colon cancer are variable and may correspond to the physical location of the tumor. Right-sided tumors usually have less associated symptomatology than left-sided or rectal tumors (Rodriguez-Bigas et al., 2006). Often, however, the signs and symptoms are nonspecific, such as vague abdominal discomfort or flatulence, and some patients are essentially asymptomatic (Libutti, Saltz, Rustgi, & Tepper, 2005; Rodriguez-Bigas et al.). General symptoms include unexplained rectal bleeding or blood in the stool; patients might describe a change in their bowel habits or abdominal pain. Unexpected weight loss and anemia also are signs of colon or other cancer and should be evaluated thoroughly (Libutti et al.). Patients may present with partial or complete bowel obstruction or even perforation. These are poor prognostic factors and in patients with stage II disease can be used to determine the need for chemotherapy treatment (NCCN, 2008c). Up to 25% of patients have metastatic disease at presentation (Rodriguez-Bigas et al.).

Family history: Hereditary colorectal cancer syndromes include two major forms: familial adenomatous polyposis and hereditary nonpolyposis colorectal cancer (Lynch & de la Chapelle, 2003) (see Chapter 2 for more comprehensive information). A thorough family history of cancer may assist in identifying a genetic predisposition to the development of colorectal cancer and will focus on the occurrence of any type of cancer or colon polyps, the age at the onset of cancer, multiple primary cancer patterns, and specific phenotypic features that may be related to cancer (Lynch & de la Chapelle). A family history of colorectal cancer in a first-degree relative increases the risk of colorectal cancer. The greater the number of relatives with colorectal cancer and the younger the patient whose risk is being assessed, the higher the risk for developing colon cancer (Fuchs et al., 1994).

Physical Examination

The work-up for patients suspected of colon cancer includes a complete physical examination with rectal exam; however, in early-stage patients, examination may yield no physical findings. As the disease progresses, physical findings may reveal abdominal tenderness or discomfort, a palpable liver mass, adenopathy, hepatomegaly, icterus, jaundice, abdominal mass, bleeding on rectal examination, or the general appearance of cachexia (Libutti et al., 2005). As with presenting symptoms, the clinical findings may vary depending on the location of the cancer. Abdominal distention and constipation may be palpated in patients with sigmoid or left-sided colon cancers. Right-sided colon cancers may not have palpable masses upon examination. Bowel sounds may suggest hypermotility or a bowel obstruction. The liver is palpated carefully to assess for hepatomegaly or metastatic disease. Lymphatics are carefully assessed. Rectal examination might detect an anorectal mass. Female patients also should undergo pelvic examination (Wilkes, 2005).

Differential Diagnosis

The differential diagnosis includes inflammatory or other bowel disease, adenomatous polyps, metastatic disease from another primary cancer, or other tumors of the GI tract (Libutti et al., 2005; Wilkes, 2005).

Diagnostic Tests

Radiologic: Imaging studies depend on the clinical presentation of the patient. If a rectal cancer is present, those patients should receive a TRUS and rigid proctoscopy (Rodriguez-Bigas et al., 2006). When polyps are found, the NCCN guidelines recommend marking of the suspected cancerous polyp site (either at the time of the colonoscopy or within two weeks of polypectomy) (NCCN, 2008c). If the polyps are completely resected and have lower risk features, no further surgery is required. Alternatively, if invasive colon cancer is found, the patient undergoes a colonoscopy, followed by a CT scan of the chest, abdomen, and pelvis. The use of PET is not routinely recommended by NCCN (2008c) unless synchronous metastatic disease exists that is potentially surgically curable. MRI with contrast may be considered for potentially resectable liver disease.

Laboratory studies: Laboratory studies should be drawn (CBC, LFTs, coagulation panel) including a CEA (NCCN, 2008c). The value of obtaining a CEA is most significant in the preoperative phase; however, a poorly differentiated tumor is less likely to result in elevated levels. Elevated CEA is not always reflective of cancer or even disease recurrence. The liver is the site for metabolism of CEA; therefore, benign conditions may cause an elevation in the level (Duffy, 2001). Tumors on the left side of the colon usually have higher CEA levels than their counterparts. Bowel obstruction also can cause higher levels of CEA that drop significantly after decompression (Duffy).

CEA is not useful in detecting early colorectal cancer, thus limiting its use as a screening tumor marker (Duffy, 2001). Serial measurements of CEA are able to detect recurrent colorectal cancer with a sensitivity of approximately 80% and a specificity of 70%

(Duffy). A recent study confirmed the value of CEA as compared to CA 19-9 or *TP53* as a significant prognostic factor for disease-free survival (Gasser et al., 2007). Interestingly, monitoring of CEA level in patients with colorectal cancer can show recurrent cancer with a lead time of five months on average, but the most effective use of this test utilizing serial measurements is for the detection of liver metastasis (Duffy).

Biopsy: Although sigmoidoscopy and barium enema play a role in the diagnosis of colorectal cancer, the colonoscopy remains the gold standard for visualization and biopsy of suspected lesions or masses.

Pathology: The pathology of colorectal cancer is primarily adenocarcinoma (95%) (Rodriguez-Bigas et al., 2006). Most adenocarcinomas are thought to arise from adenomas over a long period of time. Histopathologically, adenocarcinomas may be well, moderately, or poorly differentiated and are classified further as mucin-producing (measurement of how much mucin the tumor is producing) and other characteristics (Rodriguez-Bigas et al.). Other classifications of colorectal tumor include adenosquamous, carcinoid, lymphoma, melanoma, sarcoma, small cell carcinoma, squamous cell carcinoma, or undifferentiated carcinoma (Rodriguez-Bigas et al.). The histologic grade is assigned from GX to G4 (Greene et al., 2002).

Staging

Colon cancer is staged using the TNM staging system, which essentially replaced the historically used Dukes staging system or Astler-Coller modifications (see Tables 3-8 and 3-9). Surgery usually is performed for all patients who can be successfully resected with colectomy and lymphadenectomy; a minimum of 12 lymph nodes should be examined to effectively and accurately stage patients into stage II or more advanced disease where chemotherapy treatments are recommended (Berberoglu, 2004). The number of lymph nodes examined correlates with survival for stage III patients as well (NCCN, 2008c).

Table 3-8. Tumor-Node-Metastasis (TNM) Definitions for Colorectal Cancer

The same classification is used for both clinical and pathologic staging.

Primary Tumor (T)

TX	Primary tumor cannot be assessed
T0	No evidence of primary tumor
Tis	Carcinoma *in situ:* intraepithelial or invasion of lamina propria*
T1	Tumor invades submucosa
T2	Tumor invades muscularis propria
T3	Tumor invades through the muscularis propria into the subserosa, or into non-peritonealized pericolic or perirectal tissues
T4	Tumor directly invades other organs or structures, and/or perforates visceral peritoneum**,***

* *Note:* Tis includes cancer cells confined within the glandular basement membrane (intraepithelial) or lamina propria (intramucosal) with no extension through the muscularis mucosae into the submucosa.
** *Note:* Direct invasion in T4 includes invasion of other segments of the colorectum by way of the serosa; for example, invasion of the sigmoid colon by a carcinoma of the cecum.
*** Tumor that is adherent to other organs or structures, macroscopically, is classified T4. However, if no tumor is present in the adhesion, microscopically, the classification should be pT3. The V and L substaging should be used to identify the presence or absence of vascular or lymphatic invasion.

(Continued on next page)

Table 3-8. Tumor-Node-Metastasis (TNM) Definitions for Colorectal Cancer *(Continued)*

Regional Lymph Nodes (N)

NX	Regional lymph nodes cannot be assessed
N0	No regional lymph node metastasis
N1	Metastasis in 1 to 3 regional lymph nodes
N2	Metastasis in 4 or more regional lymph nodes

Note: A tumor nodule in the pericolorectal adipose tissue of a primary carcinoma without histologic evidence of residual lymph node in the nodule is classified in the pN category as a regional lymph node metastasis if the nodule has the form and smooth contour of a lymph node. If the nodule has an irregular contour, it should be classified in the T category and also coded as V1 (microscopic venous invasion) or as V2 (if it was grossly evident), because there is a strong likelihood that it represents venous invasion.

Distant Metastasis (M)

MX	Distant metastasis cannot be assessed
M0	No distant metastasis
M1	Distant metastasis

Note. Used with permission of the American Joint Committee on Cancer (AJCC), Chicago, Illinois. From *AJCC Cancer Staging Manual, Sixth Edition* (p. 115), by F.L. Greene, D.L. Page, I.D. Fleming, A. Fritz, C.M. Balch, D.G. Haller, et al. (Eds.), 2002, New York: Springer, www.springeronline.com.

Table 3-9. Stage Grouping for Colorectal Cancer

Stage	T	N	M	Dukes*	MAC*
0	Tis	N0	M0	–	–
I	T1	N0	M0	A	A
	T2	N0	M0	A	B1
IIA	T3	N0	M0	B	B2
IIB	T4	N0	M0	B	B3
IIIA	T1–T2	N1	M0	C	C1
IIIB	T3–T4	N1	M0	C	C2/C3
IIIC	Any T	N2	M0	C	C1/C2/C3
IV	Any T	Any N	M1	–	D

---

* Dukes B is a composite of better (T3 N0 M0) and worse (T4 N0 M0) prognostic groups, as is Dukes C (Any T N1 M0 and Any T N2 M0). MAC is the modified Astler-Coller classification.

Note: The y prefix is to be used for those cancers that are classified after pretreatment, whereas the r prefix is to be used for those cancers that have recurred.

Note. Used with permission of the American Joint Committee on Cancer (AJCC), Chicago, Illinois. From *AJCC Cancer Staging Manual, Sixth Edition* (p. 116), by F.L. Greene, D.L. Page, I.D. Fleming, A. Fritz, C.M. Balch, D.G. Haller, et al. (Eds.), 2002, New York: Springer, www.springeronline.com.

Survival and Prognosis

The most important prognostic factor for colorectal cancer is the stage of the disease at diagnosis (Minsky, Mies, Rich, Recht, & Chaffey, 1988). Additional prognostic factors include lymphovascular invasion, inadequate sampling of lymph nodes, high-grade tumors, and presentation with obstruction or perforation (NCCN, 2008c). The five-year survival rate in the United States for colorectal cancer is 90% for patients with localized disease, 68% for patients with regional disease, and 10% for patients with distant metastases (Jemal et al., 2008).

Prostate Cancer

History

History and current complaints: In the work-up of a patient with suspected prostate cancer, various risk factors for the development of prostate cancer are assessed per the patient history. Age is one of the most significant risk factors, as two-thirds of all prostate cancers are found in men older than age 65. In fact, prostate cancer rates increase faster with age than any other cancer (Pienta & Esper, 1993). Data also show that histologic evidence of cancer of the prostate is present in 60%–70% of all men at autopsy (Wynder, Mabuchi, & Whitmore, 1971).

Risk factors other than age that should be considered during the history include family history of prostate cancer, race (occurs more frequently in African American than Caucasian American men), exposure to cadmium, diet (high intake of red meat or high-fat dairy products), and socioeconomic factors. A possible link to vasectomy-induced prostate cancer has been suggested but not proved (Pienta & Esper, 1993).

Family history: Family history has been reported as a consistent risk factor for prostate cancer in all races. Men of African American descent are at higher risk for the disease and also for higher-grade disease. Intriguing research has identified a link between breast and prostate cancer in some African American families (Beebe-Dimmer et al., 2006; Bloom, Stewart, Oakley-Girvans, Banks, & Chang, 2006; Thompson et al., 2006).

Symptoms of prostate cancer are variable and frequently depend on the extent and location of the disease; however, the most common symptoms are urinary problems such as difficulty in voiding or change in the force of the urinary stream (often referred to as *prostatism*), very similar to benign prostatic hypertrophy (BPH) (Ross et al., 2006). Often, symptoms reflect the presence of more advanced disease, and patients complain of perineal pain, problems with sexual performance, or hematuria (Ross et al.).

Physical Examination

PSA and DRE are essential in the work-up for patients suspected of having prostate cancer. Prostate cancer may be nonpalpable, but as most patients do not present with metastatic disease, the DRE may provide the only clinical findings on physical examination (Scher, Leibel, Fuks, Cordon-Cardo, & Scardino, 2005). Although an irregular and firm prostate usually is considered an abnormal rectal finding, symptoms could be the result of an overdistended bladder, lymphedema of the lower extremities, deep vein thrombosis, or even cancer cachexia. Finding areas of induration may indicate direct extension of the disease. DRE is unlikely to find anterior or midline prostate tumors.

Percussion and palpation of the pelvis are performed (Held-Warmkessel, 2005), assessing for bladder distention. Inguinal nodes are assessed carefully as well.

Differential Diagnosis

Although the most common condition in the differential diagnosis is BPH, other reasons could cause patient complaints of pain, bleeding, or change in urinary stream. These include calculi, cysts, and tuberculosis or inflammation of the prostate (Ross et al., 2006). It is important to differentiate prostate cancer from other malignancies such as lymphoma, sarcoma, or metastatic tumors from leukemias, lung cancer, melanoma, and seminoma, among others (Scher et al., 2005).

Diagnostic Tests

Radiologic: Following an abnormal DRE or PSA, the first study ordered usually is a TRUS, which is used to identify biopsy sites. Further studies often are needed to complete staging, including a bone scan, CT scan of the abdomen and pelvis, ProstaScint, or MRI. Endorectal MRI may identify suspicious areas in the prostate and seminal vesicles and has improved staging accuracy (Scher et al., 2005). CT has limited usefulness in staging early disease but may detect soft tissue metastases in advanced disease. ProstaScint may be used to detect areas of metastases. A bone scan is performed in symptomatic patients with at least T1–T2 disease and PSA > 20 ng/ml. The FDG-PET is of limited benefit in this setting at the present time (NCCN, 2007; Ross et al., 2006; Scher et al.).

Laboratory values: Laboratory values include a measurement of PSA. It is a very specific test; however, elevated PSA levels are found in nonmalignant conditions such as BPH or prostatitis (Schatteman, Hoekx, Wyndaele, Jeuris, & Van Marck, 2000; Sturgeon, 2002). Approximately 25% of cancers do not have elevated PSA levels (Held-Warmkessel, 2005). Higher PSA levels are associated with greater tumor burden; however, poorly differentiated tumors may produce less PSA than well-differentiated tumors (Scher et al., 2005). Therefore, the test is not considered to be 100% diagnostic or prognostic. CBC, chemistry panels, and coagulation studies also are needed. An acid phosphatase or alkaline phosphatase level may be obtained to rule out metastatic disease.

Biopsy: A biopsy must be performed to make a definitive diagnosis. In most cases, the tissue is obtained by TRUS-guided systematic or targeted needle biopsy (NCCN, 2007; Ross et al., 2006). Because many of the cancers diagnosed today are not palpable or able to be seen by ultrasound, the standard practice is to obtain samples systematically from areas in the peripheral zone (three on each side). Often, two more core samples are obtained from the transition zone (Ross et al.).

Pathology: Prostate tumors often are multifocal, with approximately 95% adenocarcinomas, arising from the prostatic epithelial cells (Scher et al., 2005). Additional types of prostate cancers include mucinous or signet ring tumors and ductal, transitional cell, carcinoid, and small cell undifferentiated cancers (neuroendocrine appearance). The nonepithelial tumor type examples include sarcoma, lymphoma, and histiocytoma (Ross et al., 2006; Scher et al.). Degrees of differentiation exist within the classification of prostate adenocarcinoma, and the Gleason scoring system was developed to grade this specific tumor type. The pathologist assigns a Gleason score of 1–5 on the two most common growth patterns identified based on the morphology of the specimen and the changes from normal appearance. The final score is the sum of these two numbers (as in the example of 2 + 4 = 6) (Gleason & Mellinger, 1974; Ross et al.; Scher et al.).

The natural history of the disease is poorly understood with variable survival times. Patients with lower-grade tumors may have disease that is slow growing, whereas others with high-grade lesions may progress to metastatic disease quite quickly (Ross et al., 2006). Prostate cancer usually spreads by direct extension, systemically through the lymphatic system in an orderly fashion, or through the blood system (Scher et al., 2005).

Staging

Staging of prostate cancer is completed using the TNM staging system (see Tables 3-10 and 3-11). Staging information includes the PSA level, imaging, and tumor histology (including the TNM stage and Gleason score). This information, along with age, comorbidity, and the long natural history of the disease, helps to predict which patients may be appropriate for surveillance alone and those who have more aggressive features that require treatment (Scher et al., 2005).

Table 3-10. Definition of Tumor-Node-Metastasis (TNM) Staging for Prostate Cancer

---

Primary Tumor (T)

Clinical

TX	Primary tumor cannot be assessed
T0	No evidence of primary tumor
T1	Clinically inapparent tumor neither palpable nor visible by imaging
T1a	Tumor incidental histologic finding in 5% or less of tissue resected
T1b	Tumor incidental histologic finding in more than 5% of tissue resected
T1c	Tumor identified by needle biopsy (e.g., because of elevated PSA)
T2	Tumor confined within prostate*
T2a	Tumor involves one-half of one lobe or less
T2b	Tumor involves more than one-half of one lobe but not both lobes
T2c	Tumor involves both lobes
T3	Tumor extends through the prostate capsule**
T3a	Extracapsular extension (unilateral or bilateral)
T3b	Tumor invades seminal vesicle(s)
T4	Tumor is fixed or invades adjacent structures other than seminal vesicles: bladder neck, external sphincter, rectum, levator muscles, and/or pelvic wall

* *Note:* Tumor found in one or both lobes by needle biopsy, but not palpable or reliably visible by imaging, is classified as T1c.
** *Note:* Invasion into the prostatic apex or into (but not beyond) the prostatic capsule is classified not as T3 but as T2.

Pathologic (pT)

pT2*	Organ confined
pT2a	Unilateral, involving one-half of one lobe or less
pT2b	Unilateral involving more than one-half of one lobe but not both lobes
pT2c	Bilateral disease
pT3	Extraprostatic extension
pT3a	Extraprostatic extension**
pT3b	Seminal vesicle invasion
pT4	Invasion of bladder, rectum

* *Note:* There is no pathologic T1 classification.
** *Note:* Positive surgical margin should be indicated by an R1 descriptor (residual microscopic disease).

(Continued on next page)

Table 3-10. Definition of Tumor-Node-Metastasis (TNM) Staging for Prostate Cancer (Continued)

Regional Lymph Nodes (N)
Clinical

NX	Regional lymph nodes were not assessed
N0	No regional lymph node metastasis
N1	Metastasis in regional lymph nodes(s)

Pathologic

pNX	Regional nodes not sampled
pN0	No positive regional nodes
pN1	Metastases in regional node(s)

Distant Metastasis (M)*

MX	Distant metastasis cannot be assessed (not evaluated by any modality)
M0	No distant metastasis
M1	Distant metastasis
M1a	Non-regional lymph node(s)
M1b	Bone(s)
M1c	Other site(s) with or without bone disease

* *Note:* When more than one site of metastasis is present, the most advanced category is used. pMlc is most advanced.

PSA—prostate-specific antigen

Note. Used with permission of the American Joint Committee on Cancer (AJCC), Chicago, Illinois. From *AJCC Cancer Staging Manual, Sixth Edition* (pp. 310–311), by F.L. Greene, D.L. Page, I.D. Fleming, A. Fritz, C.M. Balch, D.G. Haller, et al. (Eds.), 2002, New York: Springer, www.springeronline.com.

Survival and Prognosis

Prognostic factors in prostate cancer include extent of disease at surgery, PSA levels, Gleason score, and pathologic features of the cancer (Ross et al., 2006; Scher et al., 2005). Nomograms often are used in making an assessment about risk of recurrence and are widely available. The five-year survival rate in the United States for prostate cancer is 100% for patients with localized disease. The prognosis for distant metastasis is 32% at five years (Jemal et al., 2008).

Lung Cancer

History

History and current complaints: The work-up for patients suspected of having lung cancer includes a thorough history and physical examination with special attention to smoking history and other risk factors for lung cancer. Smoking is believed to be responsible for approximately 80%–90% of all cases of lung cancer (Murren, Turrisi, & Pass, 2005; Onn et al., 2006; Schrump et al., 2005). Other risk factors considered in the history include exposure to secondhand smoke, high levels of arsenic, asbestos, radon, or other carcinogens related to occupational exposure (Onn et al.).

During the review of systems, recurrent or persistent infections and any new symptoms or changes in usual ones, such as cough, should be documented (Schrump et al., 2005). Although cough is the most commonly seen symptom, the signs and symptoms

Table 3-11. Stage Grouping for Prostate Cancer

Stage	T	N	M	G
Stage I	Tla	N0	M0	G1
Stage II	Tla	N0	M0	G2, 3–4
	Tlb	N0	M0	Any G
	Tlc	N0	M0	Any G
	T1	N0	M0	Any G
	T2	N0	M0	Any G
Stage III	T3	N0	M0	Any G
Stage IV	T4	N0	M0	Any G
	Any T	N1	M0	Any G
	Any T	Any N	M1	Any G

Histologic Grade (G)

GX	Grade cannot be assessed
G1	Well differentiated (slight anaplasia) (Gleason 2–4)
G2	Moderately differentiated (moderate anaplasia) (Gleason 5–6)
G3–4	Poorly differentiated/undifferentiated (marked anaplasia) (Gleason 7–10)

Note. Used with permission of the American Joint Committee on Cancer (AJCC), Chicago, Illinois. From *AJCC Cancer Staging Manual, Sixth Edition* (p. 311), by F.L. Greene, D.L. Page, I.D. Fleming, A. Fritz, C.M. Balch, D.G. Haller, et al. (Eds.), 2002, New York: Springer, www.springeronline.com.

vary depending on the size and location of the tumor. Central tumors may produce cough, wheezing, and hemoptysis. Tumors resulting in airway obstruction can cause dyspnea, fever, or productive cough (Murren et al., 2005; Onn et al., 2006; Schrump et al.). Small peripheral tumors may be entirely asymptomatic, although some patients may describe chest pain or cough (Onn et al.). Once the disease spreads, the symptoms are related to the location and size of the primary tumor. For example, patients with mediastinal involvement may describe vague chest pains or hoarseness because of entrapment of the recurrent laryngeal nerve (Onn et al.). Intrathoracic spread of tumor also can cause a phenomenon called Pancoast syndrome (with shoulder pain, brachial plexopathy, cutaneous temperature change, and muscle wasting), Horner syndrome (a constellation of signs including ptosis, slow pupillary dilation, and impaired flushing and perspiration on the ipsilateral side of the face), and signs of superior vena cava obstruction (Beckles, Spiro, Colice, & Rudd, 2003). Superior vena cava obstruction is more common in SCLC and may present as facial and upper extremity swelling (particularly in the right upper extremity), dilated neck veins, headache, dizziness, and cough. Pleuritic pain may indicate metastases to the pleura with or without effusion.

Paraneoplastic syndromes can be seen with NSCLC but are more common in SCLC. Some of the paraneoplastic syndromes commonly seen in lung cancer include hypercalcemia, syndrome of inappropriate antidiuretic hormone production, Cushing syndrome, digital clubbing, and hypertrophic osteoarthropathy and other neurologic syndromes, such as Lambert-Eaton myasthenic syndrome or peripheral neuropathy (Beckles et al., 2003).

During the history, clinicians assess patients' weight loss and performance status. These symptoms will affect prognosis and treatment decisions (NCCN, 2008d; Schrump et al., 2005).

Family history: Not all tobacco users develop lung cancer; therefore, a genetic link may be partially responsible for the development of the disease in some individuals. Associations identified between specific markers (including chromosomes 6q and 12) suggest that a genetic component to this disease exists (Onn et al., 2006). Some researchers recommend collection of family history of lung cancer in patients with chronic obstructive pulmonary disease (COPD) and family history of COPD in patients with lung cancer, with notation of age at diagnosis of each member (Schwartz & Ruckdeschel, 2006).

Passive smoking exposure, as well as environmental exposure, also increases the risk of lung cancer death. Gender differences may affect the type of lung cancer developed as well as survival differences (Onn et al., 2006).

Physical Examination

Many patients present with metastatic disease (30%–50%); therefore, the clinical stage may be appreciated on physical examination (Onn et al., 2006). The cervical, supraclavicular, and scalene lymph nodes are examined carefully, and the axillary regions are assessed for masses or signs of adenopathy (Onn et al.). A thorough chest evaluation includes auscultation, percussion, and observation for signs of obstruction or effusions. The abdomen is assessed for pain on palpation and organ enlargement. Because the disease can be metastatic to other sites or may be reflective of metastatic tumor to the lung from other locations, the physical examination includes assessment of the breasts, rectum, and musculoskeletal, neurologic, and genitourinary systems (Onn et al.; Schrump et al., 2005).

Differential Diagnosis

Diagnosis can be difficult because the most common symptoms related to lung cancer (persistent cough, wheeze, hoarseness) may be attributed to other conditions, such as lung infections or other benign processes such as hamartomas, thus delaying the actual diagnosis of malignancy (Bjerager, Palshof, Dahl, Vedsted, & Olesen, 2006). The differential diagnosis of SCLC versus other tumor types includes extrapulmonary small cell carcinoma, Merkel cell tumors, carcinoid tumors, atypical carcinoid tumors, large cell neuroendocrine carcinomas, lymphoma, small cell sarcomas, and other neuroendocrine tumors (NCCN, 2008f).

Diagnostic Tests

Radiologic: A chest radiograph should be obtained and is crucial in the diagnosis of lung cancer. The radiograph guides the clinician in the search for the tumor origin in patients who present with nonspecific symptoms (Beckles et al., 2003). Because of the low sensitivity of chest x-ray and the central location of many lung cancers, other radiologic tests may be needed before lung cancer is ruled out (Schrump et al., 2005). Additional noninvasive radiologic tests ordered depend on the location of the tumor and suspicion for metastatic disease. These tests include a CT scan of the chest and upper abdomen, pulmonary function tests, bone scan, or MRI of the head or vertebral column (NCCN, 2008d, 2008f; Schrump et al.). CT scans can help to determine certain features of benign and malignant lesions but are not always specific enough to totally exclude cancer (Patz, 2000). Therefore, PET is appropriate as an imaging exam to determine benign lesions from malignant disease, with a sensitivity of 83%–100% and a specificity of 80%–100% for tumor type (Dewan, Gupta, Redepenning, Phalen, & Frick, 1993; Gupta et al., 1992). PET scanning is useful in detecting mediastinal lymph node metastases and bone metastases (Schrump et al.). Integrated PET-CT can provide more precise information than just PET alone and may be the superior test (Onn et al., 2006). If neurologic symptoms are present, a CT scan or MRI of the brain is indicated.

Other studies may include sputum cytologic studies, which carry variable accuracy because of sampling errors, processing quality, and observer experience (Onn et al., 2006). Although its positive predictive value can reach 100%, the sensitivity may only be 10%–15% (Onn et al.).

Laboratory studies: Blood count and chemistries are evaluated. Renal function tests, serum lactate dehydrogenase, serum calcium, and serum alkaline phosphatase are recommended (Murren et al., 2005; NCCN, 2008d, 2008f).

Biopsy: Histologic confirmation of malignancy is necessary to rule out other causes of respiratory symptoms (Beckles et al., 2003). A transthoracic needle biopsy guided under CT may obtain adequate cells for diagnosis. Clinicians may use bronchoscopy, mediastinoscopy, or thoracoscopy to obtain tissue for diagnosis. Invasive studies include bronchoscopy, transthoracic percutaneous FNA, and transbronchial FNA (TBNA). FNA shows a 99% sensitivity of diagnosis with 96% specificity (Zarbo & Fenoglio-Preiser, 1992). TBNA has a sensitivity ranging from 14%–50% and specificity of 96%–100% (Onn et al., 2006). Scalene lymph node biopsy may be performed to rule out resection in select patients (Onn et al.).

Molecular studies of the disease have shown amplification of oncogenes and inactivation of tumor suppressor genes, with significant abnormalities noted in H-*ras*, K-*ras*, and N-*ras*, although their role in prognosis is not completely ascertained (Onn et al., 2006). The proto-oncogene *ras* is mutated in 20%–30% of patients with lung cancer, and data have shown that *ras* appears to be a poor prognostic factor in terms of survival (Mascaux et al., 2005; Onn et al.). Research shows that IHC expression of *p54* and Bcl-2, among others, can play a role in determining a more accurate prognosis in some patients with adenocarcinoma of the lung (Carvalho et al., 2000). Almost all SCLCs stain positive for keratin, epithelial membrane antigen, and thyroid transcription factor 1 (TTF-1) (NCCN, 2008f).

Certain molecular features help clinicians to determine treatment for specific cancers (such as with trastuzumab for HER2/neu–positive breast cancers or cetuximab or panitumumab for EGFR-positive colon cancers). Approximately 40%–80% of lung cancer tumors are positive for EGFR (HER1) (Onn et al., 2006). This discovery led to FDA approval for drugs such as erlotinib (Tarceva®, Genentech BioOncology) for NSCLC. Although high levels of EGFR can prognosticate for poorer outcome in some tumor types, the meaning of EGFR overexpression remains controversial in lung cancer (Mendelsohn & Baselga, 2003). HER2 is being studied in lung cancer, but its role is not yet established in this disease (Onn et al.).

Pathology: IHC staining is a valuable tool to differentiate various types of NSCLC. It is used to determine the neuroendocrine status of tumors. This can differentiate between malignant mesothelioma and lung adenocarcinoma (NCCN, 2008f). TTF-1 (along with IHC markers CK7 and CK20) may be used to distinguish primary pulmonary adenocarcinoma from extrapulmonary adenocarcinoma that is metastatic to the lung (Su, Hsu, & Chai, 2006). The use of TTF-1 also may be a valuable prognostic factor for survival in NSCLC, particularly in adenocarcinoma (Berghmans et al., 2006).

Squamous cell carcinoma comprises one-third of all lung cancers, with adenocarcinoma accounting for 45% (Onn et al., 2006). Bronchoalveolar carcinoma (a subtype of adenocarcinoma) accounts for 2%–4% of cases, and large-cell carcinoma (spindle cell is a variant) is found in 9% of patients (Onn et al.). Other subtypes include adenosquamous and pulmonary neuroendocrine neoplasms. The pulmonary neuroendocrine category includes SCLC (which accounts for 10%–15% of all lung cancers and carries a very aggressive course), large-cell neuroendocrine carcinoma, typical carcinoid, and atypical carcinoid (Onn et al.).

The histologic grading for lung cancer ranges from GX to G4 (undifferentiated) (Greene et al., 2002).

Staging

The staging for lung cancer is performed using the TNM system (see Tables 3-12 and 3-13). The Veterans Administration Lung Study Group two-stage system often is used for SCLC. SCLC is classified as limited- or extensive-stage disease (Murren et al., 2005). The majority of patients with SCLC present with extensive-stage disease. However, more recently, because of inconsistencies in SCLC staging and survival outcomes, a revised TNM system may now be used (Greene et al., 2002; Murren et al.; NCCN, 2008f).

Table 3-12. Definition of Tumor-Node-Metastasis (TNM) Staging for Lung Cancer

Primary Tumor (T)

TX	Primary tumor cannot be assessed, or tumor proven by the presence of malignant cells in sputum or bronchial washings but not visualized by imaging or bronchoscopy
T0	No evidence of primary tumor
Tis	Carcinoma *in situ*
T1	Tumor 3 cm or less in greatest dimension, surrounded by lung or visceral pleura, without bronchoscopic evidence of invasion more proximal than the lobar bronchus* (i.e., not in the main bronchus)
T2	Tumor with any of the following features of size or extent: More than 3 cm in greatest dimension Involves main bronchus, 2 cm or more distal to the carina Invades the visceral pleura Associated with atelectasis or obstructive pneumonitis that extends to the hilar region but does not involve the entire lung
T3	Tumor of any size that directly invades any of the following: chest wall (including superior sulcus tumors), diaphragm, mediastinal pleura, parietal pericardium; or tumor in the main bronchus less than 2 cm distal to the carina, but without involvement of the carina; or associated atelectasis or obstructive pneumonitis of the entire lung
T4	Tumor of any size that invades any of the following: mediastinum, heart, great vessels, trachea, esophagus, vertebral body, carina; or separate tumor nodules in the same lobe; or tumor with malignant pleural effusion**

* *Note:* The uncommon superficial tumor of any size with its invasive component limited to the bronchial wall, which may extend proximal to the main bronchus, is also classified T1.

** *Note:* Most pleural effusions associated with lung cancer are due to tumor. However, there are a few patients in whom multiple cytopathologic examinations of pleural fluid are negative for tumor. In these cases, fluid is non-bloody and is not an exudate. Such patients may be further evaluated by videothoracoscopy (VATS) and direct pleural biopsies. When these elements and clinical judgment dictate that the effusion is not related to the tumor, the effusion should be excluded as a staging element and the patient should be staged T1, T2, or T3.

(Continued on next page)

Table 3-12. Definition of Tumor-Node-Metastasis (TNM) Staging for Lung Cancer
(Continued)

Regional Lymph Nodes (N)

NX	Regional lymph nodes cannot be assessed
N0	No regional lymph node metastasis
N1	Metastasis to ipsilateral peribronchial and/or ipsilateral hilar lymph nodes, and intrapulmonary nodes including involvement by direct extension of the primary tumor
N2	Metastasis to ipsilateral mediastinal and/or subcarinal lymph node(s)
N3	Metastasis to contralateral mediastinal, contralateral hilar, ipsilateral or contralateral scalene, or supraclavicular lymph node(s)

Distant Metastasis (M)

MX	Distant metastasis cannot be assessed
M0	No distant metastasis
M1	Distant metastasis present

Note: M1 includes separate tumor nodule(s) in a different lobe (ipsilateral or contralateral).

Note. Used with permission of the American Joint Committee on Cancer (AJCC), Chicago, Illinois. From *AJCC Cancer Staging Manual, Sixth Edition* (p. 171), by F.L. Greene, D.L. Page, I.D. Fleming, A. Fritz, C.M. Balch, D.G. Haller, et al. (Eds.), 2002, New York: Springer, www.springeronline.com.

Table 3-13. Stage Grouping for Lung Cancer

Stage	T	N	M
Occult Carcinoma	TX	N0	M0
Stage 0	Tis	N0	M0
Stage IA	T1	N0	M0
Stage IB	T2	N0	M0
Stage IIA	T1	N1	M0
Stage IIB	T2	N1	M0
	T3	N0	M0
Stage IIIA	T1	N2	M0
	T2	N2	M0
	T3	N1	M0
	T3	N2	M0
Stage IIIB	Any T	N3	M0
	T4	Any N	M0
Stage IV	Any T	Any N	M1

Note. Used with permission of the American Joint Committee on Cancer (AJCC), Chicago, Illinois. From *AJCC Cancer Staging Manual, Sixth Edition* (p. 171), by F.L. Greene, D.L. Page, I.D. Fleming, A. Fritz, C.M. Balch, D.G. Haller, et al. (Eds.), 2002, New York: Springer, www.springeronline.com.

Survival and Prognosis

The five-year survival rate for lung and bronchus cancer (all types) is 49% for localized disease, with only a 15% five-year survival with regional disease (Jemal et al., 2008). Patients diagnosed with distant disease have a five-year survival of just 3% (Jemal et al.). Other prognostic factors indicating a poor response include low performance status, weight loss > 5% preceding diagnosis, male gender, and overexpression or presence of molecular mutations (Murren et al., 2005; Onn et al., 2006).

Almost three-quarters of patients newly diagnosed with SCLC will have extensive disease at diagnosis, affecting overall survival. Although advances occurred in the treatment of this disease in the 1970s, the current therapeutic picture has not changed significantly since then (Pirozynski, 2006). For example, the role of surgery in the treatment of SCLC is not particularly significant, and less than 10% of patients will receive that treatment option after accurate staging (Murren et al., 2005).

The most critical prognostic factor for NSCLC is the stage and extent of disease at diagnosis. This determines resectability and selection of treatment regimens, predicts survival, and is used for the reporting of comparable end results (Onn et al., 2006).

Ovarian Cancer

History

History and current complaints: Specific risk factors to consider while taking the history of a patient with suspected ovarian cancer include age (most ovarian cancers develop after onset of menopause, with only 10%–15% of ovarian cancers occurring in premenopausal patients), obesity, reproductive history (because of the possible connection between number of menstrual cycles and risk of ovarian cancer), or use of fertility or hormone replacement drugs (Cramer, Hutchison, Welch, Scully, & Ryan, 1983; Cramer & Welch, 1983). However, the actual cause of the disease is unknown (Berek & Bast, 2006).

Early diagnosis of this disease does not often occur, as symptoms may be vague and difficult to attribute to cancer in its early stages. Ovarian cancer has been called the "silent killer" because symptoms often occur only when the disease is advanced (Berek & Bast, 2006; Karlan, Markman, & Eifel, 2005). Some of the early symptoms of ovarian cancer, such as GI symptoms or abdominal discomfort, may be due to benign causes (Onn et al., 2006). The most common early symptoms of ovarian cancer are vague abdominal discomfort and bloating (Karlan et al.). Other symptoms include vaginal bleeding and urinary tract symptoms.

Later symptoms may include swelling or bloating of the abdomen or the presence of ascites, abdominal pain, pleural effusion, bowel obstruction, abdominal mass, or even vaginal bleeding (Ozols, Schwartz, & Eifel, 2001). Even later symptoms, however, may be difficult to diagnose as ovarian cancer. One study of 10 patients with pelvic abdominal mass, ascites, and elevated CA 125 found that although patients appeared to have symptoms related to advanced ovarian cancer, further investigation revealed peritoneal tuberculosis (Bilgin, Karabay, Dolar, & Develioglu, 2001).

Family history: Although most epithelial ovarian cancer occurs sporadically, hereditary ovarian cancer occurs in approximately 5%–10% of malignancies (Frank et al., 1998). Certain populations of women with specific family histories (for example, women of Ashkenazi Jewish heritage) have an increased risk of developing ovarian cancer, including those with *BRCA1* and *BRCA2* mutations (Berek & Bast, 2006; Struewing et al., 1997). These cancers occur at earlier ages than the nonhereditary tumors. Patients with a family history of two first-degree relatives with ovarian cancer have a higher risk, as do those with hereditary nonpolyposis colorectal cancer. A three-generation maternal and paternal family history should be taken, assessing for ovarian cancers, breast cancers, a relative with both of these cancers, a relative with colon cancer, early ages at onset of cancer, and males in the family with breast cancer. More information on the hereditary forms of cancer is discussed in Chapter 2.

Physical Examination

Although the pelvic examination is the most widely used examination for a patient suspected of ovarian cancer, it is not very sensitive to early forms of the disease (Karlan et al., 2005; Prorok et al., 2000). A pelvic and bimanual exam with a rectovaginal examination is recommended (Karlan et al.; Walden, 2006). The examination assesses for ascites and a pelvic mass located in the cul-de-sac, which may feel hard and fixed with multiple nodularities (Karlan et al.). Lymph nodes are examined carefully. Breast examination is performed to assess for a possible synchronous breast cancer or metastatic disease. The rest of the physical examination is directed at symptomatology and suspicion of metastatic disease.

Differential Diagnosis

The differential diagnosis includes abdominal or pelvic infections, GI disorders or malignancy, metastases from another primary cancer, pregnancy, ovarian cysts, ectopic pregnancy, or gestational trophoblastic disease, and uterine conditions such as fibroids or benign tumors of the reproductive tract (Berek & Bast, 2006; Karlan et al., 2005; Walden, 2006).

Diagnostic Tests

Radiologic: Transvaginal ultrasound or abdominal/pelvic ultrasound may be used in some settings to evaluate a pelvic mass in the initial work-up for suspected ovarian cancer. Other imaging studies may be obtained and could include chest x-ray, CT of the abdomen and pelvis, or MRI (Berek & Bast, 2006; NCCN, 2008e). These scans are useful in evaluating lymph nodes, peritoneal studding, mesenteric involvement, and omental caking. CTs also may help clinicians to distinguish an ovarian primary cancer from a metastatic pancreatic carcinoma or other possible sites of origin (Berek & Bast; Karlan et al., 2005). CT of the chest is not routinely ordered (NCCN, 2008e). Paracentesis or diagnostic laparoscopy should be used judiciously because these can cause tumor implantation at the site of needle puncture; for this reason, they are not recommended (Berek & Bast; Karlan et al.). For some patients, further testing of the GI system with endoscopy or barium enema may be needed to evaluate for the presence of carcinomatosis or for further evaluation of the rectum or intestinal tract with a finding of occult blood (Berek & Bast; NCCN, 2008e). Mammography may be indicated if a breast mass has been palpated during physical examination (Karlan et al.).

Laboratory studies: Laboratory studies include CA 125 (which may be elevated in approximately one-half of patients with early-stage ovarian cancer but is present in 90% of women with stage II disease), CBC, chemistries, and LFTs (Chu & Rubin, 2006; Jacobs & Bast, 1989; NCCN, 2008e). CA 125 is neither sensitive nor specific enough to use in screening or for a definitive diagnosis. Elevations of CA 125 occur in many benign conditions, such as endometriosis, fibroid tumors, menstruation, ovarian cysts, pancreatitis, pregnancy, hepatitis, cirrhosis, systemic lupus erythematosus, and other malignancies (Jacobs & Bast; Karlan et al., 2005).

Biopsy: Cervical cytology may be performed during pelvic examination, although it is not likely to be positive. Biopsy with FNA or percutaneous biopsy generally is not indicated; instead, most patients proceed directly to a surgical staging laparotomy or laparoscopy (Berek & Bast, 2006). If ascites is present, a diagnostic paracentesis may be performed in select patients. Referral to a gynecologic oncologist is recommended for surgical staging (Karlan et al., 2005; NCCN, 2008e).

Pathology: Ovarian tumors are classified according to the structures of origin within the ovary itself, and histologic findings for ovarian cancer generally show epithelial tumors (85%–90%) (Berek & Bast, 2006). The histologic types of the epithelial tumors include serous (approximately 75%), mucinous, endometrioid, clear cell, Brenner, mixed epithelial, and undifferentiated (Berek & Bast; Karlan et al., 2005). The histologic grade for ovarian cancer is GX to G4 (Greene et al., 2002).

Staging

The staging for ovarian cancer is surgical and follows the FIGO system (see Tables 3-14 and 3-15). The preoperative evaluation excludes the presence of extraperitoneal metastases, and a comprehensive surgical exploration determines the stage of disease and subsequent therapy (Berek & Bast, 2006). A vertical incision is performed with a thorough evaluation of the pelvis and abdominal area, including

Table 3-14. Definition of Tumor-Node-Metastasis (TNM) Staging for Ovarian Cancer

Primary Tumor (T)

TNM Categories	FIGO Stages	
TX		Primary tumor cannot be assessed
T0		No evidence of primary tumor
T1	I	Tumor limited to ovaries (one or both)
T1a	IA	Tumor limited to one ovary; capsule intact, no tumor on ovarian surface. No malignant cells in ascites or peritoneal washings*
T1b	IB	Tumor limited to both ovaries; capsules intact, no tumor on ovarian surface. No malignant cells in ascites or peritoneal washings*
T1c	IC	Tumor limited to one or both ovaries with any of the following: capsule ruptured, tumor on ovarian surface, malignant cells in ascites or peritoneal washings
T2	II	Tumor involves one or both ovaries with pelvic extension and/or implants
T2a	IIA	Extension and/or implants on uterus and/or tube(s). No malignant cells in ascites or peritoneal washings
T2b	IIB	Extension to and/or implants on other pelvic tissues. No malignant cells in ascites or peritoneal washings
T2c	IIC	Pelvic extension and/or implants (T2a or T2b) with malignant cells in ascites or peritoneal washings
T3	III	Tumor involves one or both ovaries with microscopically confirmed peritoneal metastasis outside the pelvis
T3a	IIIA	Microscopic peritoneal metastasis beyond pelvis (no macroscopic tumor)
T3b	IIIB	Macroscopic peritoneal metastasis beyond pelvis 2 cm or less in greatest dimension

(Continued on next page)

Table 3-14. Definition of Tumor-Node-Metastasis (TNM) Staging for Ovarian Cancer *(Continued)*

| T3c | IIIC | Peritoneal metastasis beyond pelvis more than 2 cm in greatest dimension and/or regional lymph node metastasis |

* *Note:* The presence of non-malignant ascites is not classified. The presence of ascites does not affect staging unless malignant cells are present.

Note: Liver capsule metastasis T3/Stage III; liver parenchymal metastasis M1/Stage IV. Pleural effusion must have positive cytology for M1/Stage IV.

Regional Lymph Nodes (N)

NX		Regional lymph nodes cannot be assessed
N0		No regional lymph node metastasis
N1	IIIC	Regional lymph node metastasis

Distant Metastasis (M)

MX		Distant metastasis cannot be assessed
M0		No distant metastasis
M1	IV	Distant metastasis (excludes peritoneal metastasis)

Note. Used with permission of the American Joint Committee on Cancer (AJCC), Chicago, Illinois. From *AJCC Cancer Staging Manual, Sixth Edition* (p. 276), by F.L. Greene, D.L. Page, I.D. Fleming, A. Fritz, C.M. Balch, D.G. Haller, et al. (Eds.), 2002, New York: Springer, www.springeronline.com.

Table 3-15. Stage Grouping for Ovarian Cancer

Stage	T	N	M
Stage I	T1	N0	M0
Stage IA	T1a	N0	M0
Stage IB	T1b	N0	M0
Stage IC	T1c	N0	M0
Stage II	T2	N0	M0
Stage IIA	T2a	N0	M0
Stage IIB	T2b	N0	M0
Stage IIC	T2c	N0	M0
Stage III	T3	N0	M0
Stage IIIA	T3a	N0	M0
Stage IIIB	T3b	N0	M0
Stage IIIC	T3c	N0	M0
	Any T	N1	M0
Stage IV	Any T	Any N	M1

Note. Used with permission of the American Joint Committee on Cancer (AJCC), Chicago, Illinois. From *AJCC Cancer Staging Manual, Sixth Edition* (p. 277), by F.L. Greene, D.L. Page, I.D. Fleming, A. Fritz, C.M. Balch, D.G. Haller, et al. (Eds.), 2002, New York: Springer, www.springeronline.com.

the retroperitoneal spaces and lymph nodes (Karlan et al., 2005). Peritoneal biopsies are taken in specified locations (NCCN, 2008e). Lymphadenectomy is essential to ovarian cancer staging. Examination of peritoneal fluids is important, and careful inspection for intraperitoneal carcinomatosis is required. If no peritoneal fluid is found, the surgeon will irrigate the pelvis and send the fluid for cytology (Karlan et al.). Metastases can be common with ovarian cancers that appear to be early stage (Berek & Bast). FIGO staging is more reflective of disease description than prognosis in ovarian cancer.

Survival and Prognosis

Prognostic factors for ovarian cancer are varied and include the FIGO stage, the histologic subtype and grade, evidence of tumor dissemination, presence of malignant ascites, malignant peritoneal washings, ovarian adhesions, ruptured capsule, or the amount of disease (volume) left behind after cytoreductive surgery. Postoperative levels of CA 125 and age also are recognized as having prognostic significance (Karlan et al., 2005). The five-year survival rate in the United States for ovarian cancer is 92% for localized disease and 71% for regional ovarian cancer. Distant metastasis carries a five-year survival rate of 30% (Jemal et al., 2008).

Implications for Oncology Advanced Practice Nurses

APNs function in varied roles. Many oncology APNs may be directly involved in cancer diagnosis and staging. Accurate diagnosis and staging are essential prior to beginning treatment for cancer. APNs may be involved in the initial examination of the patient with a suspected cancer and/or the ordering of imaging studies, laboratory reports, or biopsies. APNs may review the collected pathologic data and stage the patient once a malignancy is found; restaging may be performed in certain cancers. The APN role may vary among different practice settings, but in every setting, an understanding of diagnosing and staging of cancer is critical to comprehensive, evidence-based care of patients with cancer.

Conclusion

The diagnosis of cancer is made using a variety of tools, including examination techniques, diagnostic and laboratory tests, and histopathologic data. This information gives the clinician data regarding the type, location, and extent of neoplastic disease. The use of biomarkers provides more specific information regarding tumor substances excreted or shed by some tumor types. The role of biomarkers is expected to expand as more is learned about the molecular processes of various cancers. Correct staging is essential to describe the extent of disease so that appropriate treatment options can be considered. APNs are well qualified to participate in the diagnosis and staging of cancer, using these tools and tumor markers or biomarkers for the initial evaluation of a patient suspected of having a cancer. As the science continues to evolve, APNs must keep abreast of the latest information regarding cancer diagnosis and staging in order to provide the most up-to-date and comprehensive care possible.

Case Study

C.M. is a 67-year-old widowed male with complaints of progressively severe obstipation persisting over two weeks. He tried many over-the-counter remedies to treat his bowel complaints, but he was unsuccessful and finally came to the emergency room for management. He states that his bowels have always been "fairly" normal with occasional constipation relieved by prunes or over-the-counter laxatives in the past. He reports new onset of frequent rectal bleeding over the past year and describes this as small amounts of blood on the toilet paper. He has mild abdominal pain, some nausea, and weight loss of 10 pounds over the three years. He admits to increasing fatigue and arthritic complaints over the past year.

Past medical history is significant for acute myocardial infarction at age 58 and subsequent placement of two coronary artery stents. He denies other comorbidities. He walks regularly and gardens in his backyard. He admits to mild alcohol use and denies smoking. C.M.'s family history is negative for colon cancer in his immediate family, but he has a grandfather who was thought to have died of stomach cancer in his 70s. His mother died at age 72 of diabetic complications thought to be cardiac-related, and his father died of an acute myocardial infarction at 54 years of age. He has two healthy children. C.M. denies having any major surgeries. A screening colonoscopy three years ago showed several small noncancerous polyps, which were successfully removed.

On physical examination, C.M. looks generally well and has an ECOG performance status of 0. Chest and abdominal examination are unremarkable except for mild tenderness at the area of the umbilicus with deep palpation. Liver edge is palpable with deep inspiration; the edge is smooth and without nodules. No masses are appreciated during the rectal examination. Stool is trace guaiac positive, and prostate examination reveals slightly enlarged prostate gland with rubbery consistency.

C.M. is scheduled for a colonoscopy, and a large mass is found in his transverse colon as well as several other large (2.2 cm and 1.4 cm) adenomatous polyps in the descending colon. A biopsy reveals moderately differentiated adenocarcinoma of the colon. C.M. has a chest, abdominal, and pelvic CT that shows two metastatic liver lesions. Preoperative CEA is elevated at 77.8.

C.M. undergoes partial colectomy for relief of partial obstruction. Pathology shows moderately differentiated adenocarcinoma of the colon and 4 out of 14 positive lymph nodes. Final staging was determined to be stage IV disease (T4N1M1). Neoadjuvant chemotherapy is considered to enable surgical resection of the liver metastases. FOLFIRI (irinotecan, 5-FU, and leucovorin) with bevacizumab is administered over three months, and serial measurements show a steady decrease in CEA.

Following chemotherapy, C.M. is reevaluated. One liver lesion had completely resolved, and the other was decreased to 2.1 cm. He undergoes successful surgical resection of his liver metastases. The pathology report from this surgery reveals a 2.6 cm poorly differentiated tumor from the right lobe of the liver. No further lymph node involvement is discerned during resection. His postoperative CEA decreases to 7.5 approximately one month after his surgery.

Following liver resection, C.M. receives a total of six months of adjuvant therapy with FOLFIRI and bevacizumab. Three years out from his original diagnosis, he is without evidence of disease, his CEA is 2.0, and scans are negative for recurrence.

1. What further diagnostic testing may be indicated in the work-up of this patient?
   • Staging with CT may not reveal all metastatic lesions. PET scanning is increasingly used in the staging of colorectal cancer. Therefore, an initial PET scan and repeat scanning with PET for follow-up and surveillance may be the optimal imaging choice for this patient.
2. Because the CEA was elevated at diagnosis and decreased following surgery, might this have been a screening tool for him along with colonoscopy?
   • No, although it is considered a poor prognostic factor if elevated following surgery. The CEA may be used as a convenient marker for evaluation of disease recurrence and treatment efficacy, but it is neither sensitive nor specific enough to use in general population screening. However, because it was elevated preoperatively and postoperatively, it should be monitored every three months for the first two years for the assessment of recurrence.
3. If C.M. had undue toxicity while undergoing treatment, what molecular marker testing might be considered?
   • Although evaluation of molecular or genomic markers in the treatment of colorectal cancer is not yet the standard of care, if this patient experienced severe and unexpected toxicity during irinotecan therapy, it could be appropriate to consider testing for UGT1A1* polymorphism. If the patient has been treated with 5-FU and had undue toxicity, consideration of testing for DPD deficiency would be appropriate.
4. What stage would C.M. be three years after diagnosis?
   • Because original staging was stage IV (with metastatic disease to the liver), even though at this time he currently has no evidence of colorectal cancer, he would still be referred to as a stage IV patient who originally presented with a partially obstructing adenocarcinoma of the colon and liver metastasis who underwent successful neoadjuvant chemotherapy with FOLFIRI and bevacizumab with a surgical resection of a solitary liver lesion followed by adjuvant chemotherapy.

Key Points

- Cancer is considered a microscopic diagnosis.
- One of the most important diagnostic tools is the patient history.
- Tumor markers are substances secreted by the tumor and are used in the work-up of many different cancers and play a significant role in staging and diagnosis.
- Molecular markers include expression levels, structures of proteins, and alterations in gene sequences and assist in determining treatments and predicting response to therapy.
- Selection of diagnostic tests is based on the type of abnormality suspected and consideration of the value of information obtained and how it will affect decision making.
- IHC involves enzymes used in conjunction with specific antibodies directed against certain cancer cell antibodies and is viewed under the microscope as a color reaction.
- In situ hybridization is a molecular genetic technique involving DNA probes labeled with a fluorochrome prior to hybridization, allowing visualization of specific nucleic acid sequences.

- Flow cytometry is a rapid and quantitative measurement of cellular characteristics, including cell cycle distribution within specific cell populations
- Cancer biomarkers (tumor markers) include proteins, genetic markers, hormones, hormone receptors, oncofetal antigens, enzymes, or other substances produced by tumor cells or in response to tumor growth.

Recommended Resources for Oncology Advanced Practice Nurses

- ACR (www.acr.org): Offers guidelines on the appropriateness of various imaging tests for the work-up of certain conditions
- ASCO Clinical Practice Guidelines on assays and predictive markers (www.asco.org)
  - ASCO 2006 Update of Recommendations for the Use of Tumor Markers in Gastrointestinal Cancer
  - ASCO Technology Assessment: Chemotherapy Sensitivity and Resistance Assays
  - ASCO 2007 Update of Recommendations for the Use of Tumor Markers in Breast Cancer
  - ASCO-College of American Pathologists Guideline Recommendations for Human Epidermal Growth Factor Receptor 2 Testing in Breast Cancer
- National Guideline Clearinghouse (www.guideline.gov): Public resource for evidence-based clinical practice guidelines, including guidelines for diagnostic testing
- Podoloff, D.A., Advani, R.H., Allred, C., Benson, A.B., III, Brown, E., Burstein, H.J., et al. (2007). NCCN task force report: Positron emission tomography (PET)/computed tomography (CT) scanning in cancer. *Journal of the National Comprehensive Cancer Network, 5*(Suppl. 1), S1–S22.

References

Abernethy, A.P., Shelby-James, T., Fazekas, B.S., Woods, D., & Currow, D.C. (2005). The Australia-modified Karnofsky Performance Status (AKPS) scale: A revised scale for contemporary palliative care clinical practice. *BMC Palliative Care, 4,* 7. Retrieved April 4, 2007, from http://www.pubmedcentral.nih.gov/articlerender.fcgi?tool=pubmed&pubmedid=16283937

Agendia. (n.d.). *About MammaPrint: Sampling instructions.* Retrieved April 4, 2007, from http://www.agendia.com/index.php?option=com_content&task=view&id=80&Itemid=113

Agmon-Levin, N., Ziv-Sokolovsky, N., Shull, P., & Sthoeger, Z.M. (2005). Carcinoma of colon presenting as fever of unknown origin. *American Journal of the Medical Sciences, 329,* 322–326.

Altaner, S., Yoruk, Y., Tokatli, F., Kocak, Z., Tosun, B., Guresci, S., et al. (2006). The correlation between TTF-1 immunoreactivity and the occurrence of lymph node metastasis in patients with lung cancer. *Tumori, 92,* 323–326.

American College of Radiology. (2005a). *ACR appropriateness criteria for soft tissue masses.* Retrieved April 9, 2007, from http://www.acr.org/s_acr/bin.asp?CID=1206&DID=11777&DOC=FILE.PDF

American College of Radiology. (2005b). *ACR practice guideline for the performance of magnetic resonance imaging (MRI) of the breast.* Retrieved February 24, 2008, from http://www.acr.org/Secondary MainMenuCategories/quality_safety/guidelines/breast/mri_breast.aspx

Angtuaco, E.J., Fassas, A.B., Walker, R., Sethi, R., & Barlogie, B. (2004). Multiple myeloma: Clinical review and diagnostic imaging. *Radiology, 231,* 11–23.

Armitage, J.O. (2005). Staging non-Hodgkin lymphoma. *CA: A Cancer Journal for Clinicians, 55,* 368–376.

Balch, C.M., Soong, S.J., Atkins, M.B., Buzaid, A.C., Cascinelli, N., Coit, D.G., et al. (2004). An evidence-based staging system for cutaneous melanoma. *CA: A Cancer Journal for Clinicians, 54,* 131–149.

Balch, C.M., Soong, S.J., Gershenwald, J.E., Thompson, J.F., Reintgen, C.M., Cascinelli, N., et al. (2001). Prognostic factors analysis of 17,600 melanoma patients: Validation of the American Joint Committee on cancer melanoma staging system. *Journal of Clinical Oncology, 19*, 3622–3634.

Barton, M.B., Elmore, J.G., & Fletcher, S.W. (1999). Breast symptoms among women enrolled in a health maintenance organization: Frequency, evaluation and outcome. *Annals of Internal Medicine, 130*, 651–657.

Bassett, L.W., & Lara, O.J. (2006). Imaging the breast. In D.W. Kufe, R.C. Bast, Jr., W.N. Hait, W.K. Hong, R.E. Pollack, R.R. Weichselbaum, et al. (Eds.), *Cancer medicine 7* (pp. 482–487). Hamilton, Ontario, Canada: BC Decker.

Bast, R.C., Ravdin, P., Hayes, D.F., Bates, S., Fritsche, H., Jessup, J.M., et al. (2001). 2000 update of recommendations for the use of tumor markers in breast and colorectal cancer: Clinical practice guidelines for the American Society of Clinical Oncology. *Journal of Clinical Oncology, 19*, 1865–1878.

Beahrs, O.H. (1991). Staging of cancer. *CA: A Cancer Journal for Clinicians, 41*, 121–125.

Beckles, M.A., Spiro, S.G., Colice, G.L., & Rudd, R.M. (2003). Initial evaluation of the patient with lung cancer: Symptoms, signs, laboratory tests, and paraneoplastic syndromes. *Chest, 123*, 97S–104S.

Beebe-Dimmer, J.L., Drake, E.A., Dunn, R.L., Bock, C.H., Montie, J.E., & Cooney, K.A. (2006). Association between family history of prostate and breast cancer among African-American men with prostate cancer. *Urology, 68*, 1072–1076.

Benedet, J.L., Bender, H., Jones, H., Ngan, H.Y., & Pecorelli, S. (2000). FIGO staging classifications and clinical practice guidelines in the management of gynecologic cancers. FIGO Committee on Gynecologic Oncology. *International Journal of Gynaecology and Obstetrics, 70*, 209–262.

Berberoglu, U. (2004). Prognostic significance of total lymph node number in patients with T1-4 N0 M0 colorectal cancer. *Hepatogastroenterology, 51*, 1689–1693.

Berek, J.S., & Bast, R.C., Jr. (2006). Ovarian cancer. In D.W. Kufe, R.C. Bast, Jr., W.N. Hait, W.K. Hong, R.E. Pollack, R.R. Weichselbaum, et al. (Eds.), *Cancer medicine 7* (pp. 1543–1568). Hamilton, Ontario, Canada: BC Decker.

Berghmans, T., Paesmans, M., Mascaux, C., Martin, B., Meert, A.P., Haller, A., et al. (2006). Thyroid transcription factor-1—A new prognostic factor in lung cancer: A meta-analysis. *Annals of Oncology, 17*, 1673–1676.

Bhalla, S. (2002). Oncologic imaging. In R. Govindan & M. Arquette (Eds.), *The Washington manual of oncology* (pp. 533–541). Philadelphia: Lippincott Williams & Wilkins.

Bickley, L.S., & Szilagyi, P.G. (2007a). The abdomen. In L.S. Bickley & P.G. Szilagyi (Eds.), *Bates' guide to physical examination and history taking* (9th ed., pp. 359–410). Philadelphia: Lippincott Williams & Wilkins.

Bickley, L.S., & Szilagyi, P.G. (2007b). Beginning the physical examination: General survey and vital signs. In L.S. Bickley & P.G. Szilagyi (Eds.), *Bates' guide to physical examination and history taking* (9th ed., pp. 89–120). Philadelphia: Lippincott Williams & Wilkins.

Bickley, L.S., & Szilagyi, P.G. (2007c). Male genitalia and hernias. In L.S. Bickley & P.G. Szilagyi (Eds.), *Bates' guide to physical examination and history taking* (9th ed., pp. 411–428). Philadelphia: Lippincott Williams & Wilkins.

Bickley, L.S., & Szilagyi, P.G. (2007d). Overview of physical examination and history taking. In L.S. Bickley & P.G. Szilagyi (Eds.), *Bates' guide to physical examination and history taking* (9th ed., pp. 3–22). Philadelphia: Lippincott Williams & Wilkins.

Bilgin, T., Karabay, A., Dolar, E., & Develioglu, O.H. (2001). Peritoneal tuberculosis with pelvic abdominal mass, ascites and elevated CA 125. *International Journal of Gynecological Cancer, 11*, 290–295.

Bjerager, M., Palshof, T., Dahl, R., Vedsted, P., & Olesen, F. (2006). Delay in diagnosis of lung cancer in general practice. *British Journal of General Practice, 56*, 863–868.

Bloom, J.R., Stewart, S.L., Oakley-Girvans, I., Banks, P.J., & Chang, S. (2006). Family history, perceived risk, and prostate cancer screening among African American men. *Cancer Epidemiology, Biomarkers and Prevention, 15*, 2167–2173.

Boucher, D., Cournoyer, D., Stanners, C.P., & Fuks, A. (1989). Studies on the control of gene expression of the carcinoembryonic antigen family in human tissue. *Cancer Research, 49*, 847–852.

Box, B.A., & Russell, C.A. (2004). Breast cancer. In D.A. Casciato (Ed.), *Manual of clinical oncology* (5th ed., pp. 233–253). Philadelphia: Lippincott Williams & Wilkins.

Brenner, P.F. (1996). Differential diagnosis of abnormal uterine bleeding. *American Journal of Obstetrics and Gynecology, 175*, 766–769.

Brinton, L.A., Hamman, R.F., Huggins, G.R., Lehman, H.F., Levine, R.S., Mallin, K., et al. (1987). Sexual and reproductive risk factors for invasive squamous cell cervical cancer. *Journal of the National Cancer Institute, 79*, 23–30.

Brody, L.C., & Biesecker, B.B. (1998). Breast cancer susceptibility genes. BRCA1 and BRCA2. *Medicine (Baltimore)*, *77*, 208–226.

Brugge, W.R., Lee, M.J., Carey, R.W., & Mathisen, D.J. (1997). Endoscopic ultrasound staging criteria for esophageal cancer. *Gastrointestinal Endoscopy*, *45*, 147–152.

Buckowitz, A., Knaebel, H.P., Benner, A., Blaker, H., Gebert, J., Kienle, P., et al. (2005). Microsatellite instability in colorectal cancer is associated with local lymphocyte infiltration and low frequency of distant metastases. *British Journal of Cancer*, *92*, 1746–1753.

Buscombe, J.R., & Bombardieri, E. (2005). Imaging cancer using single photon techniques. *Quarterly Journal of Nuclear Medicine and Molecular Imaging*, *49*, 121–131.

Buyse, M., Loi, S., van't Veer, L., Viale, G., Delorenzi, M., Glas, A.M., et al. (2006). Validation and clinical utility of a 70-gene prognostic signature for women with node-negative breast cancer. *Journal of the National Cancer Institute*, *98*, 1183–1192.

Carvalho, P.E., Antonangelo, L., Bernardi, F.D., Leao, L.E., Rodrigues, O.R., & Capelozzi, V.L. (2000). Useful prognostic panel markers to express the biological tumor status in resected lung adenocarcinomas. *Japanese Journal of Clinical Oncology*, *30*, 478–486.

Choi, H., Kaur, H., Loyer, E.M., & Silverman, P.M. (2006). Imaging neoplasms of the abdomen and pelvis. In D.W. Kufe, R.C. Bast, Jr., W.N. Hait, W.K. Hong, R.E. Pollack, R.R. Weichselbaum, et al. (Eds.), *Cancer medicine 7* (pp. 474–478). Hamilton, Ontario, Canada: BC Decker.

Choi, H.J., Roh, J.W., Seo, S.S., Lee, S., Kim, J.Y., Kim, S.K., et al. (2006). Comparison of the accuracy of magnetic resonance imaging and positron emission tomography/computed tomography in the presurgical detection of lymph node metastases in patients with uterine cervical carcinoma: A prospective study. *Cancer*, *106*, 914–922.

Chu, C.S., & Rubin, S.C. (2006). Screening for ovarian cancer in the general population. *Best Practice and Research. Clinical Obstetrics and Gynaecology*, *20*, 307–320.

Chui, S. (2006). Cancer biomarkers. In D.W. Kufe, R.C. Bast, Jr., W.N. Hait, W.K. Hong, R.E. Pollack, R.R. Weichselbaum, et al. (Eds.), *Cancer medicine 7* (pp. 199–204). Hamilton, Ontario, Canada: BC Decker.

Cohade, C., Osman, M., Leal, J., & Wahl, R.L. (2003). Direct comparison of 18F-FDG PET and PET/CT in patients with colorectal carcinoma. *Journal of Nuclear Medicine*, *44*, 1797–1803.

Coleman, R.E. (2006). Radionuclide imaging in cancer medicine. In D.W. Kufe, R.C. Bast, Jr., W.N. Hait, W.K. Hong, R.E. Pollack, R.R. Weichselbaum, et al. (Eds.), *Cancer medicine 7* (pp. 488–491). Hamilton, Ontario, Canada: BC Decker.

Collins, C.D. (2005). Problems monitoring response in multiple myeloma. *Cancer Imaging*, *5*(Spec. No. A), S119–S126.

Collins, J.A., Blake, J.M., & Crosignani, P.G. (2005). Breast cancer risk with postmenopausal hormonal treatment. *Human Reproduction Update*, *11*, 545–560.

Collins, L.G., Haines, C., Perkel, R., & Enck, R.E. (2007). Lung cancer: Diagnosis and management. *American Family Physician*, *75*, 56–63.

Compton, C.C., & Greene, F.L. (2004). The staging of colorectal cancer: 2004 and beyond. *CA: A Cancer Journal for Clinicians*, *54*, 295–308.

Connolly, J.L., Goldsmith, J.D., Wang, H.H., Longtine, J.A., Dvorak, A.M., & Dvorak, H.F. (2006). Principles of cancer pathology. In D.W. Kufe, R.C. Bast, Jr., W.N. Hait, W.K. Hong, R.E. Pollack, R.R. Weichselbaum, et al. (Eds.), *Cancer medicine 7* (pp. 437–454). Hamilton, Ontario, Canada: BC Decker.

Cothran, R.L., & Helms, C.A. (2006). Imaging of musculoskeletal neoplasms. In D.W. Kufe, R.C. Bast, Jr., W.N. Hait, W.K. Hong, R.E. Pollack, R.R. Weichselbaum, et al. (Eds.), *Cancer medicine 7* (pp. 479–481). Hamilton, Ontario, Canada: BC Decker.

Cramer, D.W., Hutchison, G.B., Welch, W.R., Scully, R.E., & Ryan, K.J. (1983). Determinants of ovarian cancer risk. I. Reproductive experiences and family history. *Journal of the National Cancer Institute*, *71*, 711–716.

Cramer, D.W., & Welch, W.R. (1983). Determinants of ovarian cancer risk. II. Inferences regarding pathogenesis. *Journal of the National Cancer Institute*, *71*, 717–721.

Cunningham, D., Humblet, Y., Siena, S., Khayat, D., Bleiberg, H., Santoro, A., et al. (2004). Cetuximab monotherapy and cetuximab plus irinotecan in irinotecan-refractory metastatic colorectal cancer. *New England Journal of Medicine*, *351*, 337–345.

Delorme, S., & Krix, M. (2006). Contrast-enhanced ultrasound for examining tumor biology. *Cancer Imaging*, *6*, 148–152.

Dewan, N.A., Gupta, N.C., Redepenning, L.S., Phalen, J.J., & Frick, M.P. (1993). Diagnostic efficacy of PET-FDG imaging in solitary pulmonary nodules. Potential role in evaluation and management. *Chest*, *104*, 997–1002.

Divgi, C., & Larson, S. (2004). Nuclear medicine. In D.A. Casciato (Ed.), *Manual of clinical oncology* (pp. 28–43). Philadelphia: Lippincott Williams & Wilkins.

Draper, L. (2006). Breast cancer: Trends, risks, treatments, and effects. *American Association of Occupational Health Nurses, 54,* 445–451.

Duffy, M.J. (2001). Carcinoembryonic antigen as a marker for colorectal cancer: Is it clinically useful? *Clinical Chemistry, 47,* 624–630.

Eifel, P.J., Berek, J.S., & Markman, M.A. (2005). Cancer of the cervix, vagina, and vulva. In V.T. DeVita, Jr., S. Hellman, & S.A. Rosenberg (Eds.), *Cancer: Principles and practice of oncology* (7th ed., pp. 1295–1397). Philadelphia: Lippincott Williams & Wilkins.

El-Serag, H.B., & Mason, A.C. (2000). Risk factors for the rising rates of primary liver cancer in the United States. *Archives of Internal Medicine, 160,* 3227–3230.

Erasmus, J.J., Truong, M.T., & McAdams, H.P. (2006). Imaging neoplasms of the thorax. In D.W. Kufe, R.C. Bast, Jr., W.N. Hait, W.K. Hong, R.E. Pollack, R.R. Weichselbaum, et al. (Eds.), *Cancer medicine 7* (pp. 468–473). Hamilton, Ontario, Canada: BC Decker.

Fisher, C., Ramsay, A.D., Griffiths, M., & McDougall, J. (1985). An assessment of the value of electron microscopy in tumour diagnosis. *Journal of Clinical Pathology, 38,* 403–408.

Francis, I.R., Brown, R.K., & Avram, A.M. (2005). The clinical role of CT/PET in oncology: An update. *Cancer Imaging, 5*(Spec. No. A), S68–S75.

Frank, T.S., Manley, S.A., Olopade, O.I., Cummings, S., Garber, J.E., Bernhardt, B., et al. (1998). Sequence analysis of BRCA1 and BRCA2: Correlation of mutations with family history and ovarian cancer risk. *Journal of Clinical Oncology, 16,* 2417–2425.

Freudenberg, L.S., Antoch, G., Schutt, P., Beyer, T., Jentzen, W., Muller, S.P., et al. (2004). FDG-PET/CT in restaging of patients with lymphoma. *European Journal of Nuclear Medicine and Molecular Imaging, 31,* 325–329.

Fuchs, C.S., Giovannucci, E.L., Colditz, G.A., Hunter, D.J., Speizer, F.E., & Willett, W.C. (1994). A prospective study of family history and the risk of colorectal cancer. *New England Journal of Medicine, 331,* 1669–1674.

Galasko, C.S. (1972). Skeletal metastases and mammary cancer. *Annals of the Royal College of Surgeons of England, 50,* 3–28.

Gasser, M., Gerstlauer, C., Grimm, M., Bueter, M., Lebedeva, T., Lutz, J., et al. (2007). Comparative analysis of predictive biomarkers for therapeutical strategies in colorectal cancer. *Annals of Surgical Oncology, 14,* 1272–1284.

Genomic Health, Inc. (n.d.). *Oncotype DX.* Retrieved April 4, 2007, from http://www.genomichealth.com/oncotype/default.aspx

Gillespie, T. (2005). Surgical therapy. In C.H. Yarbro, M.H. Frogge, & M. Goodman (Eds.), *Cancer nursing: Principles and practice* (6th ed., pp. 212–228). Sudbury, MA: Jones and Bartlett.

Gleason, D.F., & Mellinger, G.T. (1974). Prediction of prognosis for prostatic adenocarcinoma by combined histological grading and clinical staging. *Journal of Urology, 111,* 58–64.

Greene, F.L. (2004). TNM: Our language of cancer. *CA: A Cancer Journal for Clinicians, 54,* 129–130.

Greene, F.L., Page, D.L., Fleming, I.D., Fritz, A., Balch, C.M., Haller, D.G., et al. (Eds.). (2002). *AJCC cancer staging manual* (6th ed.). New York: Springer.

Gribbestad, I.S., Gjesdal, K.I., Nilsen, G., Lundgren, S., Hjelstuen, M.H.B., & Jackson, A. (2005). An introduction to dynamic contrast-enhanced MRI in oncology. In A. Jackson, D.L. Buckley, & G.J.M. Parker (Eds.), *Dynamic contrast-enhanced magnetic resonance imaging in oncology* (pp. 3–22). Berlin, Germany: Springer.

Gupta, N.C., Frank, A.R., Dewan, N.A., Redepenning, L.S., Rothberg, M.L., Mailliard, J.A., et al. (1992). Solitary pulmonary nodules: Detection of malignancy with PET with 2-[F-18]-fluoro-2-deoxy-D-glucose. *Radiology, 184,* 441–444.

Habel, L., Shak, S., Jacobs, M., Capra, A., Alexander, C., Pho, M., et al. (2006). A population-based study of tumor gene expression and risk of breast cancer death among lymph node-negative patients. *Breast Cancer Research, 8,* R25. Retrieved April 2, 2007, from http://breast-cancer-research.com/content/8/3/R25

Hagay, C., Cherel, P.J.P., de Maulmont, C.E., Plantet, M.M., Gilles, R., Floiras, J.L.G., et al. (1996). Contrast-enhanced CT: Value for diagnosing local breast cancer recurrence after conservative treatment. *Radiology, 200,* 631–638.

Hahn, K.K., Wolff, J.J., & Kolesar, J.M. (2006). Pharmacogenetics and irinotecan therapy. *American Journal of Health-System Pharmacists, 63,* 2211–2217.

Hamaoka, T., Madewell, J.E., Podoloff, D.A., Hortobagyi, G.N., & Ueno, N.T. (2004). Bone imaging in metastatic breast cancer. *Journal of Clinical Oncology, 22,* 2942–2953.

Haque, A.K., Syed, S., Lele, S.M., Freeman, D.H., & Adeqboyega, P.A. (2002). Immunohistochemical study of thyroid transcription factor-1 and HER2/neu in non-small cell lung cancer: Strong thyroid transcription factor-1 expression predicts better survival. *Applied Immunohistochemistry and Molecular Morphology, 10,* 103–109.

Harris, L., Fritsche, H., Mennel, R., Norton, L., Ravdin, P., Taube, S., et al. (2007). American Society of Clinical Oncology 2007 update of recommendations for the use of tumor markers in breast cancer. *Journal of Clinical Oncology, 25,* 5287–5312.

Held-Warmkessel, J. (2005). Prostate cancer. In C.H. Yarbro, M.H. Frogge, & M. Goodman (Eds.), *Cancer nursing: Principles and practice* (6th ed., pp. 1552–1580). Sudbury, MA: Jones and Bartlett.

Hendler, A., & Hershkop, M. (1998). When to use bone scintigraphy. *Postgraduate Medicine Online, 104*(5). Retrieved April 2, 2007, from http://www.postgradmed.com/issues/1998/11_98/hendler.htm

Henry, N.L., & Hayes, D.F. (2006). Uses and abuses of tumor markers in the diagnosis, monitoring, and treatment of primary and metastatic breast cancer. *Oncologist, 11,* 541–552.

Herbsman, H., Gardner, B., & Alfonso, A. (1977). The value of laparoscopy in general surgery. *Journal of Reproductive Medicine, 18,* 235–240.

Hohenberger, P., & Hunerbein, M. (1996). Detection and management of advanced gastric cancer. *Annals of Oncology, 7,* 197–203.

Holland, J.F., Frei, E., Kufe, D.W., Bast, R.C., Jr., Pollock, R.E., Weichselbaum, R.R., et al. (2006). Cardinal manifestations of cancer. In D.W. Kufe, R.C. Bast, Jr., W.N. Hait, W.K. Hong, R.E. Pollock, R.R. Weichselbaum, et al. (Eds.), *Cancer medicine 7* (pp. 3–5). Hamilton, Ontario, Canada: BC Decker.

Hortobagyi, G.N., Esserman, L., & Buchholz, T.A. (2006). Neoplasms of the breast. In D.W. Kufe, R.C. Bast, Jr., W.N. Hait, W.K. Hong, R.E. Pollock, R.R. Weichselbaum, et al. (Eds.), *Cancer medicine 7* (pp. 460–467). Hamilton, Ontario, Canada: BC Decker.

Horton, K., Reffel, A., Rosen, K., & Farraye, F.A. (2001). Training of nurse practitioners and physician assistants to perform screening flexible sigmoidoscopy. *Journal of the American Academy of Nurse Practitioners, 13,* 455–459.

Hricak, H., Akin, O., Bradbury, M., Liberman, L., Schwartz, L., & Larson, S. (2005). In V.T. DeVita, Jr., S. Hellman, & S.A. Rosenberg (Eds.), *Cancer: Principles and practice of oncology* (7th ed., pp. 589–636). Philadelphia: Lippincott Williams & Wilkins.

Hurt, C.J., & Beauchamp, N.J. (2006). Imaging neoplasms of the central nervous system, head, and neck. In D.W. Kufe, R.C. Bast, Jr., W.N. Hait, W.K. Hong, R.E. Pollock, R.R. Weichselbaum, et al. (Eds.), *Cancer medicine 7* (pp. 460–467). Hamilton, Ontario, Canada: BC Decker.

Israel, O., Mor, M., Epelbaum, R., Frenkel, A., Haim, N., Dann, E.J., et al. (2002). Clinical pretreatment risk factors and Ga-67a scintigraphy early during treatment for prediction of outcome of patients with aggressive non-Hodgkin lymphoma. *Cancer, 94,* 873–878.

Jacobs, I., & Bast, R.C. (1989). The CA 125 tumour-associated antigen: A review of the literature. *Human Reproduction, 4,* 1–12.

Jemal, A., Siegel, R., Ward, E., Hao, Y., Xu, J., Murray, T., et al. (2008). Cancer statistics, 2008. *CA: A Cancer Journal for Clinicians, 58,* 71–96.

Jhingran, A., Eifel, P.J., Wharton, J.T., & Tortolero-Luna, G. (2006). Neoplasms of the cervix. In D.W. Kufe, R.C. Bast, Jr., W.N. Hait, W.K. Hong, R.E. Pollack, R.R. Weichselbaum, et al. (Eds.), *Cancer medicine 7* (pp. 1497–1521). Hamilton, Ontario, Canada: BC Decker.

Johnston, S.J., Ridge, S.A., Cassidy, J., & McLeod, H.L. (1999). Regulation of dihydropyrimidine dehydrogenase in colorectal cancer. *Clinical Cancer Research, 5,* 2566–2570.

Kakar, S., Puangsuvan, N., Stevens, J.M., Serenas, R., Mangan, G., Sahai, S., et al. (2000). HER-2/neu assessment in breast cancer by immunohistochemistry and fluorescence in situ hybridization: Comparison of results and correlation with survival. *Molecular Diagnosis, 5,* 199–207.

Karlan, B.Y., Markman, M.A., & Eifel, P.J. (2005). Ovarian cancer, peritoneal carcinoma, and fallopian tube carcinoma. In V.T. DeVita, Jr., S. Hellman, & S.A. Rosenberg (Eds.), *Cancer: Principles and practice of oncology* (7th ed., pp. 1364–1397). Philadelphia: Lippincott Williams & Wilkins.

Khatcheressian, J., Wolff, A., Smith, T., Grunfeld, E., Muss, H., Vogel, V., et al. (2006). American Society of Clinical Oncology 2006 update of the breast cancer follow-up and management guidelines in the adjuvant setting. *Journal of Clinical Oncology, 24,* 5091–5097.

Kirk, J., Brennan, M., Houssami, N., & Ung, O. (2006). An approach to the patient with a family history of breast cancer. *Australian Family Physician, 35,* 43–47.

Knopp, M.V., von Tengg-Kobligk, H., & Choyke, P.L. (2003). Functional magnetic resonance imaging in oncology for diagnosis and therapy monitoring. *Molecular Cancer Therapeutics, 2,* 419–426.

Ko, A.S., & Lefor, A.T. (2005). Laparoscopic surgery. In V.T. DeVita, Jr., S. Hellman, & S.A. Rosenberg (Eds.), *Cancer: Principles and practice of oncology* (7th ed., pp. 253–266). Philadelphia: Lippincott Williams & Wilkins.

Kotilingam, D., Lev, D.C., Lazar, A.J., & Pollock, R.E. (2006). Staging soft tissue sarcoma: Evolution and change. *CA: A Cancer Journal for Clinicians, 56*, 282–291.

Lardinois, D., Weder, W., Hany, T.F., Kamel, E.M., Korom, S., Seifert, B., et al. (2003). Staging of non-small cell lung cancer with integrated positron-emission tomography and computed tomography. *New England Journal of Medicine, 348*, 2500–2507.

Lee, Z., Sodee, D.B., Resnick, M., & Maclennan, G.T. (2005). Multimodal and three-dimensional imaging of prostate cancer. *Computerized Medical Imaging and Graphics, 29*, 477–486.

Lehman, C.D., Gatsonis, C., Kuhl, C.K., Hendrick, E.R., Pisano, E.D., Hanna, L., et al. (2007). MRI evaluation of the contralateral breast in women with recently diagnosed breast cancer. *New England Journal of Medicine, 356*, 1295–1303.

Leong, P.P., Rezai, B., Koch, W.M., Reed, A., Eisele, D., Lee, D.J., et al. (1998). Distinguishing second primary tumors from lung metastases in patients with head and neck squamous cell carcinoma. *Journal of the National Cancer Institute, 90*, 972–977.

Levin, T.R. (2002). Flexible sigmoidoscopy for colorectal cancer screening: Valid approach or short-sighted? *Gastroenterology Clinics of North America, 31*, 1015–1029.

Libutti, S.K., Saltz, L.B., Rustgi, A.K., & Tepper, J.E. (2005). Cancer of the colon. In V.T. DeVita, Jr., S. Hellman, & S.A. Rosenberg (Eds.), *Cancer: Principles and practice of oncology* (7th ed., pp. 1061–1109). Philadelphia: Lippincott Williams & Wilkins.

Lievre, A., Bachet, J.B., Boige, V., Cayre, A., Le Corre, D., Buc, E., et al. (2008). KRAS mutations as an independent prognostic factor in patients with advanced colorectal cancer treated with cetuximab. *Journal of Clinical Oncology, 26*, 374–379.

Lievre, A., Bachet, J.B., Le Corre, D., Boige, V., Landi, B., Emile, J.F., et al. (2006). KRAS mutation status is predictive of response to cetuximab therapy in colorectal cancer. *Cancer Research, 66*, 3992–3995.

Linke, S.P., Bremer, T.M., Herold, C.D., Sauter, G., & Diamond, C. (2006). A multimarker model to predict outcome in tamoxifen-treated breast cancer patients. *Clinical Cancer Research, 12*, 1175–1183.

Locker, G.Y., Hamilton, S., Harris, J., Jessup, J.M., Kemeny, N., Macdonald, J.S., et al. (2006). ASCO 2006 update of recommendations for the use of tumor markers in gastrointestinal cancer. *Journal of Clinical Oncology, 24*, 5313–5327.

London, N.J., Farmery, S.M., Will, E.J., Davison, A.M., & Lodge, J.P. (1995). Risk of neoplasia in renal transplant patients. *Lancet, 346*, 403–406.

Ludwig, J.A., & Weinstein, J.N. (2005). Biomarkers in cancer staging, prognosis, and treatment selection. *Nature Reviews Cancer, 5*, 845–856.

Lynch, H.T., & de la Chapelle, A. (2003). Hereditary colorectal cancer. *New England Journal of Medicine, 348*, 919–932.

Mascaux, C., Iannino, N., Martin, B., Paesmans, M., Berghmans, T., Dusart, M., et al. (2005). The role of RAS oncogene in survival of patients with lung cancer: A systematic review of the literature with meta-analysis. *British Journal of Cancer, 92*, 131–139.

Mehta, P.P., Griffin, J., Ganta, S., Rangraj, M., & Steichen, F. (2005). Laparoscopic-assisted colon resections: Long-term results and survival. *Journal of the Society of Laparoendoscopic Surgeons, 9*, 184–188.

Mendelsohn, J., & Baselga, J. (2003). Status of epidermal growth factor receptor antagonists in the biology and treatment of cancer. *Journal of Clinical Oncology, 21*, 2787–2799.

Merkel, D.E., Dressler, L.G., & McGuire, W.L. (1987). Flow cytometry, cellular DNA and prognosis in human malignancy. *Journal of Clinical Oncology, 5*, 1690–1703.

Mierau, G.W. (1999). Electron microscopy for tumour diagnosis: Is it redundant? *Histopathology, 35*, 99–101.

Minsky, B.D., Mies, C., Rich, T.A., Recht, A., & Chaffey, J.T. (1988). Potentially curative surgery of colon cancer: The influence of blood vessel invasion. *Journal of Clinical Oncology, 6*, 119–127.

Molina, R., Jo, J., Filella, X., Zanon, G., Pahisa, J., Munoz, M., et al. (1998). C-erbB-2 oncoprotein, CEA, and CA 15.3 in patients with breast cancer: Prognostic value. *Breast Cancer Research and Treatment, 51*, 109–119.

Montgomery, R.C., & Ridge, J.A. (1998). Radiologic staging of gastrointestinal cancer. *Seminars in Surgical Oncology, 15*, 143–150.

Mor, V., Laliberle, L., & Wiemann, M. (1984). The Karnofsky performance status scale: An examination of its reliability and validity in a research setting. *Cancer, 53*, 2002–2007.

Murren, J., Turrisi, A.T., & Pass, H.I. (2005). Small cell lung cancer. In V.T. DeVita, Jr., S. Hellman, & S.A. Rosenberg (Eds.), *Cancer: Principles and practice of oncology* (7th ed., pp. 810–843). Philadelphia: Lippincott Williams & Wilkins.

National Comprehensive Cancer Network. (2007). *NCCN clinical practice guidelines in oncology: Prostate cancer, version 2.2007.* Retrieved February 24, 2008, from http://www.nccn.org/professionals/physician_gls/PDF/prostate.pdf

National Comprehensive Cancer Network. (2008a). *NCCN clinical practice guidelines in oncology: Breast cancer, version 2.2008.* Retrieved February 24, 2008, from http://www.nccn.org/professionals/physician_gls/PDF/breast.pdf

National Comprehensive Cancer Network. (2008b). *NCCN clinical practice guidelines in oncology: Cervical cancer, version 1.2008.* Retrieved February 24, 2008, from http://www.nccn.org/professionals/physician_gls/PDF/cervical.pdf

National Comprehensive Cancer Network. (2008c). *NCCN clinical practice guidelines in oncology: Colon cancer, version 1.2008.* Retrieved February 24, 2008, from http://www.nccn.org/professionals/physician_gls/PDF/colon.pdf

National Comprehensive Cancer Network. (2008d). *NCCN clinical practice guidelines in oncology: Non-small cell lung cancer, version 2.2008.* Retrieved February 24, 2008, from http://www.nccn.org/professionals/physician_gls/PDF/nscl.pdf

National Comprehensive Cancer Network. (2008e). *NCCN clinical practice guidelines in oncology: Ovarian cancer, version 1.2008.* Retrieved February 24, 2008, from http://www.nccn.org/professionals/physician_gls/PDF/ovarian.pdf

National Comprehensive Cancer Network. (2008f). *NCCN clinical practice guidelines in oncology: Small cell lung cancer, version 1.2008.* Retrieved February 24, 2008, from http://www.nccn.org/professionals/physician_gls/PDF/sclc.pdf

Naumberg, E.H. (2007). Interviewing and the health history. In L.S. Bickley & P.G. Szilagyi (Eds.), *Bates' guide to physical examination and history taking* (9th ed., pp. 23–64). Philadelphia: Lippincott Williams & Wilkins.

Newcomb, P.A., Titus-Ernstoff, L., Egan, K.M., Trentham-Dietz, A., Baron, J.A., Storer, B.E., et al. (2002). Postmenopausal estrogen and progestin use in relation to breast cancer risk. *Cancer Epidemiology, Biomarkers and Prevention, 11,* 593–600.

Nguyen, D.M., Summers, R.M., & Finkelstein, S.E. (2005). In V.T. DeVita, Jr., S. Hellman, & S.A. Rosenberg (Eds.), *Cancer: Principles and practice of oncology* (7th ed., pp. 643–651). Philadelphia: Lippincott Williams & Wilkins.

O-charoenrat, P., Rusch, V., Talbot, S.G., Sarkaria, I., Viale, A., Socci, N., et al. (2004). Casein kinase II alpha subunit and C1-inhibitor are independent predictors of outcome in patients with squamous cell carcinoma of the lung. *Clinical Cancer Research, 10,* 5792–5803.

Oken, M.M., Creech, R.H., Tormey, D.C., Horton, J., Davis, T.E., McFadden, E.T., et al. (1982). Toxicity and response criteria of the Eastern Cooperative Oncology Group. *American Journal of Clinical Oncology, 5,* 649–655.

Olivotto, I.A., Bajdik, C.D., Ravdin, P.M., Speers, C.H., Coldman, A.J., Norris, B.D., et al. (2005). Population-based validation of the prognostic model ADJUVANT! for early breast cancer. *Journal of Clinical Oncology, 23,* 2716–2725.

Omerod, K.F. (2005). Diagnostic evaluation, classification, and staging. In C.H. Yarbro, M.H. Frogge, & M. Goodman (Eds.), *Cancer nursing: Principles and practice* (6th ed., pp. 153–180). Sudbury, MA: Jones and Bartlett.

Onn, A., Vaporciyan, A.A., Chang, J.Y., Komaki, R., Roth, J.A., & Herbst, R.S. (2006). Cancer of the lung. In D.W. Kufe, R.C. Bast, Jr., W.N. Hait, W.K. Hong, R.E. Pollack, R.R. Weichselbaum, et al. (Eds.), *Cancer medicine 7* (pp. 1179–1224). Hamilton, Ontario, Canada: BC Decker.

Oriuchi, N., Higuchi, T., Ishikita, T., Miyakubo, M., Hanaoka, H., Iida, Y., et al. (2006). Present role and future prospects of positron emission tomography in clinical oncology. *Cancer Science, 97,* 1291–1297.

Ost, D., Fein, A.M., & Feinsilver, S.H. (2003). Clinical practice. The solitary pulmonary nodule. *New England Journal of Medicine, 348,* 2535–2542.

Osuch, J.R., Bonham, V.L., & Morris, L.L. (2002). *Primary care guide to managing a breast mass: Step-by-step workup.* Retrieved November 27, 2006, from http://www.medscape.com/viewarticle/443381_1

Ozols, R.F., Schwartz, P.E., & Eifel, P.J. (2001). Ovarian cancer, fallopian tube carcinoma, and peritoneal carcinoma. In V.T. DeVita, Jr., S. Hellman, & S.A. Rosenberg (Eds.), *Cancer: Principles and practice of oncology* (7th ed., pp. 1597–1632). Philadelphia: Lippincott Williams & Wilkins.

Paik, S., Tang, G., Shak, S., Kim, C., Baker, J., Kim, W., et al. (2006). Gene expression and benefit of chemotherapy in women with node-negative, estrogen receptor-positive breast cancer. *Journal of Clinical Oncology, 24,* 3726–3734. Retrieved April 4, 2007, from http://jco.ascopubs.org/cgi/reprint/JCO.2005.04.7985v1

Park, D.J., Stoehlmacher, J., Zhang, W., Tsao-Wei, D.D., Groshen, S., & Lenz, H.J. (2001). A xeroderma pigmentosum group D gene polymorphism predicts clinical outcome to platinum-based chemotherapy in patients with advanced colorectal cancer. *Cancer Research, 61*, 8654–8658.

Patel, S.G., & Shah, J.P. (2005). TNM staging of cancers of the head and neck: Striving for uniformity among diversity. *CA: A Cancer Journal for Clinicians, 55*, 242–258.

Patz, E.F. (2000). Imaging bronchogenic carcinoma. *Chest, 117*(4 Suppl. 1), 90S–95S.

Patz, E.F. (2006). Principles of imaging. In D.W. Kufe, R.C. Bast, Jr., W.N. Hait, W.K. Hong, R.E. Pollack, R.R. Weichselbaum, et al. (Eds.), *Cancer medicine 7* (p. 455). Hamilton, Ontario, Canada: BC Decker.

Perkins, G.L., Slater, E.D., Sanders, G.K., & Prichard, J.G. (2003). Serum tumor markers. *American Family Physician, 68*, 1075–1082.

Pfister, D., Johnson, D., Azzoli, C., Sause, W., Smith, T., Baker, S., et al. (2004). American Society of Clinical Oncology treatment of unresectable non–small-cell lung cancer guideline: Update 2003. *Journal of Clinical Oncology, 22*, 330–353.

Pienta, K.J., & Esper, P.S. (1993). Risk factors for prostate cancer. *Annals of Internal Medicine, 118*, 793–803.

Pirozynski, M. (2006). 100 years of lung cancer. *Respiratory Medicine, 100*, 2073–2083.

Pisano, E.D., Gatsonis, C., Hendrick, E., Yaffe, M., Baum, J.K., Acharyya, S., et al. (2005). Diagnostic performance of digital versus film mammography for breast-cancer screening. *New England Journal of Medicine, 353*, 1773–1783.

Pollack, R.E., & Morton, D.L. (2006). Principles of surgical oncology. In D.W. Kufe, R.C. Bast, Jr., W.N. Hait, W.K. Hong, R.E. Pollack, R.R. Weichselbaum, et al. (Eds.), *Cancer medicine 7* (pp. 503–516). Hamilton, Ontario, Canada: BC Decker.

Prorok, P.C., Andriole, G.L., Bresalier, R.S., Buys, S.S., Chia, D., Crawford, E.D., et al. (2000). Design of the Prostate, Lung, Colorectal and Ovarian (PLCO) Cancer Screening Trial. *Controlled Clinical Trials, 21*(Suppl. 6), 273S–309S.

Pusztai, L., Mazouni, C., Anderson, K., Wu, Y., & Symmans, W.F. (2006). Molecular classification of breast cancer: Limitations and potential. *Oncologist, 11*, 868–877.

Raj, G.V., Partin, A.W., & Polascik, T.J. (2002). Clinical utility of indium 111-capromab pendetide immunoscintigraphy in the detection of early, recurrent prostate carcinoma after radical prostatectomy. *Cancer, 94*, 987–996.

Rinnab, L., Kufer, R., Hautmann, R.E., & Gottfried, H.W. (2006). Use of transrectal ultrasound-guided biopsy in the diagnosis of pelvic malignancies. *Journal of Clinical Ultrasound, 34*, 440–445.

Rivera, M.P., Detterbeck, F., & Mehta, A.C. (2003). Diagnosis of lung cancer: The guidelines. *Chest, 123*(Suppl. 1), 129S–136S.

Robboy, S.J., Noller, K.L., O'Brien, R.H., Kaufman, D., Townsend, D., Barnes, A.B., et al. (1984). Increased incidence of cervical and vaginal dysplasia in 3980 diethylstilbestrol-exposed young women. Experience of the National Collaborative Diethylstilbestrol Adenosis Project. *JAMA, 252*, 2979–2983.

Rockey, D.C., Paulson, E., Niedzwiecki, D., Davis, W., Bosworth, H.B., Sanders, L., et al. (2005). Analysis of air contrast barium enema, computed tomographic colonography and colonoscopy: Prospective comparison. *Lancet, 365*, 305–311.

Rodriguez-Bigas, M.A., Hoff, P., & Crane, C.H. (2006). Carcinoma of the colon and rectum. In D.W. Kufe, R.C. Bast, Jr., W.N. Hait, W.K. Hong, R.E. Pollack, R.R. Weichselbaum, et al. (Eds.), *Cancer medicine 7* (pp. 1369–1391). Hamilton, Ontario, Canada: BC Decker.

Ross, R.W., Oh, W.K., Hurwitz, M., D'Amico, A.V., Richie, J.P., & Kantoff, P.W. (2006). Neoplasms of the prostate. In D.W. Kufe, R.C. Bast, Jr., W.N. Hait, W.K. Hong, R.E. Pollack, R.R. Weichselbaum, et al. (Eds.), *Cancer medicine 7* (pp. 1431–1461). Hamilton, Ontario, Canada: BC Decker.

Rossi, S., Rosa, L., Ravetta, V., Cascina, A., Quaretti, P., Azzaretti, A., et al. (2006). Contrast-enhanced versus conventional and color Doppler sonography for the detection of thrombosis of the portal and hepatic venous systems. *American Journal of Roentgenology, 186*, 763–773.

Rouzier, R., Perou, C.M., Symmans, W.F., Ibrahim, N., Cristofanilli, M., Anderson, K., et al. (2005). Breast cancer molecular subtypes respond differently to preoperative chemotherapy. *Clinical Cancer Research, 11*, 5678–5685.

Sah, S.P., Matutes, E., Wotherspoon, A.C., Morilla, R., & Catovsky, D. (2003). A comparison of flow cytometry, bone marrow biopsy, and bone marrow aspirates in the detection of lymphoid infiltration in B cell disorders. *Journal of Clinical Pathology, 56*, 129–132.

Salonga, D., Danenberg, K.D., Johnson, M., Metzger, R., Groshen, S., Tsao-Wei, D.D., et al. (2000). Colorectal tumors responding to 5-fluorouracil have low gene expression levels of dihydropyrimidine dehydrogenase, thymidylate synthase, and thymidine phosphorylase. *Clinical Cancer Research, 6*, 1322–1327.

Saslow, D., Boetes, C., Burke, W., Harms, S., Leach, M., Lehman, C., et al. (2007). American Cancer Society guidelines for breast screening with MRI as an adjunct to mammography. *CA: A Cancer Journal for Clinicians, 57,* 75–89.

Sawaki, M., Ito, Y., Akiyama, F., Tokudome, N., Horii, R., Mizunuma, N., et al. (2006). High prevalence of HER-2/neu and p53 overexpression in inflammatory breast cancer. *Breast Cancer, 13,* 172–178.

Schatteman, P.H., Hoekx, L., Wyndaele, J.J., Jeuris, W., & Van Marck, E. (2000). Inflammation in prostate biopsies of men without prostatic malignancy or clinical prostatitis: Correlation with total serum PSA and PSA density. *European Urology, 37,* 404–412.

Scher, H.I., Leibel, S.A., Fuks, Z., Cordon-Cardo, C., & Scardino, P. (2005). Prostate cancer. In V.T. DeVita, Jr., S. Hellman, & S.A. Rosenberg (Eds.), *Cancer: Principles and practice of oncology* (7th ed., pp. 1192–1259). Philadelphia: Lippincott Williams & Wilkins.

Schoder, H., Larson, S.M., & Yeung, H.W. (2004). PET/CT in oncology: Integration into clinical management of lymphoma, melanoma, and gastrointestinal malignancies. *Journal of Nuclear Medicine, 45*(Suppl. 1), 72S–81S.

Schoder, H., Yeung, H.W., Gonen, M., Kraus, D., & Larson, S.M. (2004). Head and neck cancer: Clinical usefulness and accuracy of PET/CT image fusion. *Radiology, 231,* 65–72.

Schrevens, L., Lorent, N., Dooms, C., & Vansteenkiste, J. (2004). The role of PET scan in diagnosis, staging, and management of non-small cell lung cancer. *Oncologist, 9,* 633–643.

Schrump, D.S., Altorki, N.K., Henschke, C.L., Carter, D., Turrisi, A.T., & Gutierrez, M.E. (2005). Non-small cell lung cancer. In V.T. DeVita, Jr., S. Hellman, & S.A. Rosenberg (Eds.), *Cancer: Principles and practice of oncology* (7th ed., pp. 753–810). Philadelphia: Lippincott Williams & Wilkins.

Schwartz, A.G., & Ruckdeschel, J.C. (2006). Familial lung cancer: Genetic susceptibility and relationship to chronic obstructive pulmonary disease. *American Journal of Respiratory and Critical Care Medicine, 173,* 16–22.

Shaffer, K. (1996). Radiologic evaluation of cancer. In A.T. Skarin (Ed.), *Atlas of diagnostic oncology* (2nd ed., pp. 1–25). Barcelona, Spain: Mosby-Wolfe.

Shaffer, K. (1997). Radiologic evaluation in lung cancer: Diagnosis and staging. *Chest, 112,* 235–238.

Sherman, M.E., Lorincz, A.T., Scott, D.R., Wacholder, S., Castle, P.E., Glass, A.G., et al. (2003). Baseline cytology, human papillomavirus testing, and risk for cervical neoplasia: A 10-year cohort analysis. *Journal of the National Cancer Institute, 95,* 46–52.

Shi, W., Johnston, C.F., Buchanan, K.D., Ferguson, W.R., Laird, J.D., Crothers, J.G., et al. (1998). Localization of neuroendocrine tumours with [111In]DTPA-octreotide scintigraphy (Octreoscan): A comparative study with CT and MR imaging. *QJM: A Monthly Journal of the Association of Physicians, 91,* 295–301.

Shirota, Y., Stoehlmacher, J., Brabender, J., Xiong, Y.P., Uetake, H., Danenberg, K.D., et al. (2001). ERCC1 and thymidylate synthase mRNA levels predict survival for colorectal cancer patients receiving combination oxaliplatin and fluorouracil chemotherapy. *Journal of Clinical Oncology, 19,* 4298–4304.

Sidransky, D. (2002). Emerging molecular markers of cancer. *Nature Reviews Cancer, 2,* 210–219.

Singletary, S.E., & Connolly, J.L. (2006). Breast cancer staging: Working with the sixth edition of the AJCC Cancer Staging Manual. *CA: A Cancer Journal for Clinicians, 56,* 37–47.

Smith, M.T., Jones, R.M., & Smith, A.H. (2007). Benzene exposure and risk of non-Hodgkin lymphoma. *Cancer Epidemiology, Biomarkers and Prevention, 16,* 385–391.

Smith, R.A., Duffy, S.W., & Eyre, H.J. (2006). Cancer screening and early detection. In D.W. Kufe, R.C. Bast, Jr., W.N. Hait, W.K. Hong, R.E. Pollack, R.R. Weichselbaum, et al. (Eds.), *Cancer medicine 7* (pp. 389–410). Hamilton, Ontario, Canada: BC Decker.

Speight, J.L., & Roach, M. (2007). Advances in the treatment of localized prostate cancer: The role of anatomic and functional imaging in men managed with radiotherapy. *Journal of Clinical Oncology, 25,* 987–995.

Stacey-Clear, A., McCarthy, K.A., Hall, D.A., Pile-Spellman, E., White, G., Hulka, C.A., et al. (1993). Mammographically detected breast cancer: Location in women under 50 years old. *Radiology, 186,* 677–680.

Struewing, J.P., Hartge, P., Wacholder, S., Baker, S.M., Berlin, M., McAdams, M., et al. (1997). The risk of cancer associated with specific mutations of BRCA1 and BRCA2 among Ashkenazi Jews. *New England Journal of Medicine, 336,* 1401–1408.

Sturgeon, C. (2002). Practice guidelines for tumor marker use in the clinic. *Clinical Chemistry, 48,* 1151–1159.

Su, Y.C., Hsu, Y.C., & Chai, C.Y. (2006). Role of TTF-1, CK20, and CK7 immunohistochemistry for diagnosis of primary and secondary lung adenocarcinoma. *Kaohsiung Journal of Medical Sciences, 22,* 14–19.

Taneja, S.S. (2004). ProstaScint® scan: Contemporary use in clinical practice. *Reviews in Urology, 6*(Suppl. 10), S19–S28.

Taylor, C.R. (2000). The total test approach to standardization of immunohistochemistry. *Archives of Pathology and Laboratory Medicine, 124,* 945–951.

Taylor, C.R. (2006). Standardization in immunohistochemistry: The role of antigen retrieval in molecular morphology. *Biotechnic and Histochemistry, 81,* 3–12.

Thompson, I.M., Ankerst, D.P., Chi, C., Goodman, P.J., Tangen, C.M., Lucia, M.S., et al. (2006). Assessing prostate cancer risk: Results from the prostate cancer prevention trial. *Journal of the National Cancer Institute, 98,* 529–534.

Timar, J., Csuka, O., Orosz, Z., Jeney, A., & Kopper, L. (2002). Molecular pathology of tumor metastasis. *Pathology Oncology Research, 8,* 204–219.

Tuma, R.S. (2007, November 25). KRAS mutation status predicts responsiveness to panitumumab. *Oncology Times,* p. 34. Retrieved February 24, 2008, from http://www.oncology-times.com/pt/re/oncotimes/pdfhandler.00130989-200711250-00010.pdf;jsessionid=HBQdX0vSpklRq6nQxmxfDmcWdZKyN2lDdpv4L5ndtnZCM4QYlVc1!-667243907!181195629!8091!-1

Van Cutsem, E. (2006). Challenges in the use of epidermal growth factor receptor inhibitors in colorectal cancer. *Oncologist, 11,* 1010–1017.

Van Dam, J. (1997). Endosonographic evaluation of the patient with esophageal cancer. *Chest, 112*(Suppl. 4), 184S–190S.

Van Dam, J., & Brugge, W.R. (1999). Endoscopy of the upper gastrointestinal tract. *New England Journal of Medicine, 341,* 1738–1748.

Vinholes, J., Coleman, R., & Eastell, R. (1996). Effects of bone metastases on bone metabolism: Implications for diagnosis, imaging and assessment of response to cancer treatment. *Cancer Treatment Reviews, 22,* 289–331.

Vogel, V.G., & Taioli, E. (2006). Have we found the ultimate risk factor for breast cancer? *Journal of Clinical Oncology, 12,* 1791–1794.

von Knebel-Doeberitz, M., & Syrjanen, K.J. (2006). Molecular markers: How to apply in practice. *Gynecologic Oncology, 103,* 18–20.

Wahl, R.L. (2004). Why nearly all PET of abdominal and pelvic cancers will be performed as PET/CT. *Journal of Nuclear Medicine, 45*(Suppl.), 82S–95S.

Walden, M.S. (2006). Primary care management of dysfunctional uterine bleeding. *Journal of the American Academy of Physician Assistants, 19,* 32–39.

Willman, C.L., & Hromas, R. (2006). Genomic alterations and chromosomal aberrations in human cancer. In D.W. Kufe, R.C. Bast, Jr., W.N. Hait, W.K. Hong, R.E. Pollack, R.R. Weichselbaum, et al. (Eds.), *Cancer medicine 7* (pp. 104–134). Hamilton, Ontario, Canada: BC Decker.

Watt, I., Stewart, I., Anderson, D., Bell, G., & Anderson, J.R. (1989). Laparoscopy, ultrasound and computed tomography in cancer of the oesophagus and gastric cardia: A prospective comparison for detecting intra-abdominal metastases. *British Journal of Surgery, 76,* 1036–1039.

Waxman, I. (2005). Cancer diagnosis: Endoscopy. In V.T. DeVita, Jr., S. Hellman, & S.A. Rosenberg (Eds.), *Cancer: Principles and practice of oncology* (7th ed., pp. 637–651). Philadelphia: Lippincott Williams & Wilkins.

Wick, M.R., & Swanson, P.E. (1997). Principles of diagnostic electron microscopy in oncology. In A.S.-Y. Leong, M.R. Wick, & P.E. Swanson (Eds.), *Immunohistology and electron microscopy of anaplastic and pleomorphic tumors* (pp. 33–58). Cambridge, United Kingdom: Cambridge University Press.

Wilkes, G. (2005). Colon, rectal and anal cancers. In C.H. Yarbro, M.H. Frogge, & M. Goodman (Eds.), *Cancer nursing: Principles and practice* (6th ed., pp. 1155–1214). Sudbury, MA: Jones and Bartlett.

Wolff, A.C., Hammond, M.E., Schwartz, J.N., Hagerty, K.L., Allred, D.C., Cote, R.J., et al. (2007). American Society of Clinical Oncology/College of American Pathologists guideline recommendations for human epidermal growth factor receptor 2 testing in breast cancer. *Journal of Clinical Oncology, 25,* 118–145.

Wright, C.M., Dent, O.F., Newland, R.C., Barker, M., Chapuis, P.H., Bokey, E.L., et al. (2005). Low level microsatellite instability may be associated with reduced cancer specific survival in sporadic Stage C colorectal carcinoma. *Gut, 54,* 103–108.

Wright, T., & McGechan, A. (2003). Breast cancer: New technologies for risk assessment and diagnosis. *Molecular Diagnostics, 7,* 49–55.

Wynder, E.L., Mabuchi, K., & Whitmore, W. (1971). Epidemiology of cancer of the prostate. *Cancer, 28,* 344–360.

Xi, W.D., Zhao, C., & Ren, G.S. (2003). Endoscopic ultrasonography in preoperative staging of gastric cancer: Determination of tumor invasion depth, nodal involvement and surgical respectability. *World Journal of Gastroenterology, 9,* 254–267.

Zarbo, R.J., & Fenoglio-Preiser, C.M. (1992). Interinstitutional database for comparison of performance in lung fine-needle aspiration cytology. A College of American Pathologists Q-Probe Study of 5264 cases with histologic correlation. *Archives of Pathology and Laboratory Medicine, 116,* 463–470.

Zhang, H., Liu, J., Cagle, P.T., Allen, T.C., Laga, A.C., & Zander, D.S. (2005). Distinction of pulmonary small cell carcinoma from poorly differentiated squamous cell carcinoma: An immunohistochemical approach. *Modern Pathology, 18,* 111–118.

Ziv, E., Tice, J., Smith-Bindman, R., Shepherd, J., Cummings, S., & Kerlikowske, K. (2004). Mammographic density and estrogen receptor status of breast cancer. *Cancer Epidemiology, Biomarkers and Prevention, 13,* 2090–2095.

Zuetenhorst, J.M., Hoefnageli, C.A., Boot, H., Valdes Olmos, R.A., & Taal, B.G. (2002). Evaluation of (111)In-pentetreotide, (131)I-MIBG and bone scintigraphy in the detection and clinical management of bone metastases in carcinoid disease. *Nuclear Medicine Communications, 23,* 735–741.

CHAPTER 4

Chemotherapy and Biotherapy

Gail M. Wilkes, RN, MS, ANP, AOCN®

Introduction

This past decade has brought many advances in the treatment of cancer using chemotherapy and biotherapy, including molecular targeted therapy. This chapter will review principles of chemotherapy and biotherapy and implications for the oncology advanced practice nurse (APN).

Cancer is a disease of cellular mutations. The National Cancer Institute (NCI) has declared that by 2015, suffering and death from cancer will be eliminated, in part, by advances in molecular targeted therapy (NCI, 2007). The six hallmarks that result from this genomic instability are self-sufficiency in growth signals, insensitivity to antigrowth signals, tissue invasion and metastases, limitless replication, sustained angiogenesis, and evasion of apoptosis (programmed cell death) (Hanahan & Weinberg, 2000). Chemotherapy has been used for more than 50 years to disrupt genetic functions within the cell and cause cell death (cytotoxic) or alter regulation of growth and division to prevent cell division (cytostatic, such as tamoxifen). As understanding of the many molecular flaws in cancer increases, it is clear that multitargeted therapies are required to more precisely target multiple cancer pathways. The epidermal growth factor receptor is known to be overexpressed in many solid tumors, and a number of agents blocking this pathway have been approved by the U.S. Food and Drug Administration (FDA). Inhibition of this pathway theoretically results in decreased cell proliferation, decreased stimulation of angiogenesis, increased sensitivity to apoptosis, and reduced stimulation of invasion and metastases. Other agents target angiogenesis directly, either by neutralization of the ligand (growth factor or hormone that activates the receptor on the cell membrane) vascular endothelial growth factor (VEGF) or inhibition of the endothelial cell receptor (cell lining the nearest blood vessel) for VEGF. Several targeted biologic agents have been used for many years, such as the monoclonal antibody (mAb) rituximab, a CD20-specific mAb that causes death of CD20-positive lymphocytes. Toxicities related to targeted or biologic therapy are drug and class specific (Rieger, 2001; Zhu, Bohlen, & Witte, 2002).

In contrast, chemotherapy generally is nonspecific, targeting frequently dividing cancer cell populations. Normal, frequently dividing cell populations are more capable of repairing the cellular damage and surviving, but severe, often life-threatening side effects can occur, including febrile neutropenia, thrombocytopenia, and organ damage. Among the few targeted agents under the chemotherapy umbrella are the antiestrogen agents, such as tamoxifen, which are targeted against estrogen receptors in breast cancer cells.

Chemotherapy

General Principles

Chemotherapy is the use of cellular poisons that block cell replication and commonly lead to cell death (apoptosis) in frequently dividing cancer cell populations. Chemotherapy agents are classified by their action during the cell cycle that leads to cell replication, as either cell cycle specific or nonspecific. The cell cycle consists of five phases: G_0, G_1, G_2, S, and M phases (see Figure 4-1). The G stands for *gap*, as scientists were able to see the S and M phases clearly but were not sure what occurred during the times before and after and labeled these phases as G_1, G_2, and G_0 (Weinberg, 2007).

G_0 is the resting phase, where cells that require division will remain until recruited back into the cell cycle. A few cell types remain in G_0 indefinitely, such as neurons. Normal cells have a finite life span, and once the life span is used up, the cells are replaced by new cells. To accomplish this, a certain percentage of cells are recruited into the cell cycle; this is referred to as the growth fraction. Once recruited into the cell cycle, the cell enters G_1. The cell cycle is one of the most highly controlled cellular processes because of key restriction points, or checkpoints, that theoretically would prevent subversion. Unfortunately, in malignancies, mutations are present in the genes that make proteins to control the cell cycle checkpoints. At the G_1 checkpoint, a decision is required for the cell to commit to cell division. The checkpoint determines whether the cell is large enough and whether there is adequate nutrition in the environment (Pardee, 1974). In addition, it determines if the DNA is intact in order to avoid replication of damaged DNA (Merkle & Loescher, 2005). If the conditions are met, the cell commits to cell division, and in late G_1, the nucleus enlarges and the materials needed for DNA duplication are made.

During the S, or synthesis, phase, the cell actively replicates the DNA, forming a complementary set of chromatids (a chromatid is one daughter strand of DNA). During this time, both DNA strands are examined to ensure that they are exact and without errors; if errors are found, they are repaired. If they cannot be repaired, the cell undergoes programmed cell death, or apoptosis, to prevent duplication of mutated DNA. If the DNA strands are intact and pass inspection, they proceed to the G_2 phase. *TP53* is the "guardian of the genome" and is responsible for the checkpoint inspections and ensuring that irreparably damaged DNA is destroyed by apoptosis (Weinberg, 2007). Unfortunately, *TP53* is frequently mutated in solid tumors. In G_2, the cell prepares for mitosis and synthesizes the materials for the mitotic spindle. At the end of the G_2/beginning of the M (mitosis) phase, the cell is inspected again for damaged or unduplicated DNA and unduplicated centrosomes (small areas of cytoplasm next to the nucleus that contain and organize the microtubules), which are key in mitosis (Merkle & Loescher, 2005). If all conditions are met, the cell moves into the M phase.

During the M phase, the chromosomes line up at the centromere (area joining the two chromatids) and are attached by mitotic spindle fibers. An M phase checkpoint delays

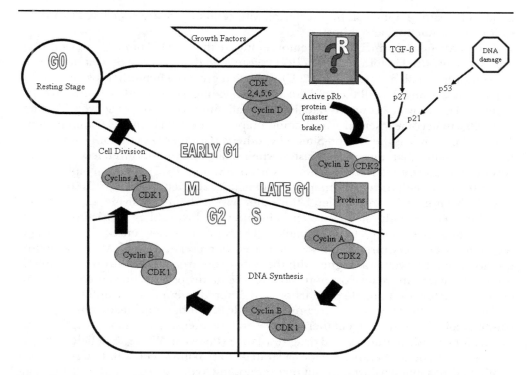

The cell cycle consists of four stages (G1, S, G2, M) that are controlled by proteins called cyclins. The cyclins (D, E, A, B) are activated when complexed with enzymes called cyclin-dependent kinases (CDKs). Upon activation, the cyclin-CDK complex allows the cell to progress through each specific cell cycle stage. Present throughout the cell cycle, the cyclin-CDK complexes serve as checkpoints or monitors of the cell cycle. Inhibitory proteins prevent progression through the cell cycle if DNA damage is present or there is a lack of nutrients or oxygen to support cellular proliferation. Examples of inhibitory proteins include p21 p27, p53. The inhibitory proteins in turn are regulated by the presence of inhibitory growth factors and TGF-β. Once past R (the restriction point) the cell cycle is turned "on" and progression through the cell cycle is inevitable. Cyclin-CDK complexes and pRB (the "master brake") tightly regulate the R point. The stability of the inhibitory proteins and cyclin-CDK complexes are altered in cancer, thereby altering control of the cell cycle and uncontrolled cellular proliferation prevails.

Figure 4-1. Chemotherapy Drug Action During Cell Cycle

Note. From "Biology of Cancer" (p. 15), by C.J. Merkle and L.J. Loescher in C.H. Yarbro, M.H. Frogge, and M. Goodman (Eds.), *Cancer Nursing: Principles and Practice* (6th ed.), 2005, Sudbury, MA: Jones and Bartlett. Copyright 2005 by Jones and Bartlett. Reprinted with permission.

the segregation of chromosomes if they are not attached to the spindle fibers (Merkle & Loescher, 2005), and the cell undergoes metaphase arrest unless it is repaired. Once repaired, the cell can undergo the completion of mitosis, and two identical daughter cells are formed. Depending on the need for additional cells, the daughter cells may enter G_0 or be recruited back into the cycle. In cancer, a mutation often occurs in the M checkpoint, resulting in completion of mitosis, but the daughter cells may have too few or too many chromosomes (aneuploidy) (Kops, Weaver, & Cleveland, 2005).

Cancer chemotherapy is intended to be either cytostatic (preventing cell division) or cytocidal (causing cell death). Most chemotherapy agents are cytocidal and bring about cell death or apoptosis by interfering with cellular processes, such as DNA replication, RNA function, and mitosis.

Two fundamental principles of chemotherapy are the "cell kill model" and Gompertzian tumor growth kinetics. Skipper (1971) postulated that a certain percentage of cancer cells will be killed ("cell kill model") with each cycle of chemotherapy (first-order kinetics), assuming that all the cells are actively dividing, consistently sensitive to treatment, and growing at a constant rate. However, all tumor cells are not actively dividing, and cells can become insensitive to chemotherapy; so, the cell kill model has limitations. A second principle is the Norton-Simon hypothesis (Gompertzian tumor growth kinetics), which states that tumors grow fastest when small, and tumors given less time to recover can be more effectively destroyed (Norton & Simon, 1977). This principle has led to the use of dose-dense chemotherapy that includes shorter cycle intervals so that the actively dividing cells can be killed before they have a chance to divide. In breast cancer, when treatment with standard chemotherapy with doxorubicin (Adriamycin®, Bedford Laboratories) and cyclophosphamide (Cytoxan®, Bristol-Myers Squibb Co.) (AC regimen) given every three weeks was compared with every-two-week AC "dose-dense" therapy, overall survival was higher with the dose-dense treatment (Citron et al., 2003). Although there is more myelosuppression, febrile neutropenia is prevented by the use of growth factors to stimulate production and differentiation of neutrophils.

Factors that affect response to treatment include tumor burden, rate of tumor growth, combination versus single-agent therapy, dose or dose intensity, hormone receptor status in hormone-sensitive tumors, and drug resistance (Polovich, White, & Kelleher, 2005). Combination chemotherapy provides a strategy to maximize cell kill. Drug regimens combine drugs that have synergy but no overlapping toxicities, such as the CHOP regimen: cyclophosphamide, doxorubicin, vincristine, and prednisone. The myelosuppression with cyclophosphamide occurs in 7–10 days, whereas that of doxorubicin occurs in 10–14 days. Vincristine and prednisone are nonmyelosuppressive, but vincristine is neurotoxic, and prednisone causes hyperglycemia and other side effects. The regimens were developed to be given in the ambulatory setting and commonly are dosed on schedules with a cycle every 21 days so that normal cells can recover before the next cycle (Fisher et al., 1993).

Unfortunately, normal, frequently dividing cell populations are affected by chemotherapy as well, including the bone marrow, gastrointestinal (GI) mucosa, gonads, and hair follicles. In addition, chemotherapy agents have drug-specific toxicities, including organ toxicities, such as cardiomyopathy, which are associated with the anthracycline antibiotics. Table 4-1 outlines chemotherapy agents, their activity during the cell cycle, and toxicities. Many of the severe toxicities, including specific organ toxicities and cognitive dysfunction, are discussed in greater detail in other chapters in this manual. Because of the narrow therapeutic window and anticipated toxicities that would not be tolerated with other drugs, it is imperative to employ practices that reduce the chance for prescription error. Errors involving drug overdose, wrong dose, or inappropriate route (e.g., vincristine given intrathecally) have resulted in patient deaths (Schulmeister, 1999).

One strategy to reduce damage to normal cells and improve delivery to malignant cells involves nanotechnology. Liposomal doxorubicin (Doxil®, Alza Corp.) uses stealth technology to evade the immune system and takes advantage of the leaky capillaries supplying tumors so that the drug leaks into the tumor; in addition, the drug has a long half-life of 54 hours (Alza Corporation, 2007). A second example is the use of albumin to wrap paclitaxel, which is preferentially taken up by tumor cells (paclitaxel protein-

Table 4-1. Chemotherapy Agents by Class

Category	FDA-Approved Drugs in the Class	Common Toxicities of the Class
Cell Cycle Nonspecific		
Alkylating agents	Altretamine (Hexalen®, MGI Pharma) BCNU (carmustine, BiCNU®, Bristol-Myers Squibb Co.) Busulfan (Myleran®, GlaxoSmithKline) Carboplatin (Paraplatin®, Bristol-Myers Squibb Co.) Chlorambucil (Leukeran®, GlaxoSmithKline) Cisplatin (Platinol®, Bristol-Myers Squibb Co.) Cyclophosphamide (Cytoxan®, Bristol-Myers Squibb Co.) Dacarbazine (DTIC-DOME®, Bedford Laboratories) Ifosfamide (Ifex®, Bristol-Myers Squibb Co.) Lomustine (CeeNU®, Bristol-Myers Squibb Co.) Mechlorethamine (nitrogen mustard, Mustargen®, Merck & Co., Inc.) Melphalan (Alkeran®, GlaxoSmithKline) Oxaliplatin (Eloxatin®, Sanofi-Aventis) Streptozocin (Zanosar®, Sicor Pharmaceuticals) Temozolomide (Temodar®, Schering Corp.) Thiotepa (Thioplex®, Bedford Laboratories)	Myelosuppression Gonadal suppression (azoospermia, amenorrhea) Nausea and vomiting Alopecia Fatigue Hemorrhagic cystitis (ifosfamide, cyclophosphamide) Neuropathy (cisplatin analogs) Secondary malignancies Comments: Nitrosoureas: Carmustine and lomustine are lipid soluble and cross BBB; temozolomide crosses BBB and is a radiosensitizer. Cisplatin and analogs are radiosensitizers.
Antitumor antibiotics	Actinomycin D (dactinomycin, Cosmegen®, Merck & Co., Inc.) Bleomycin (Blenoxane®, Bristol-Myers Squibb Co.) Mitomycin (Mutamycin®, Bristol-Myers Squibb Co.) Mitoxantrone (Novantrone®, OSI Pharmaceuticals) Anthracycline antibiotics Doxorubicin (Adriamycin®, Bedford Laboratories) Daunorubicin (Cerubidine®, Bedford Laboratories) Epirubicin (Ellence®, Pfizer Inc.) Idarubicin (Idamycin®, Pfizer Inc.) Liposomal doxorubicin (Doxil®, Tibotec Therapeutics) Liposomal daunorubicin (DaunoXome®, Gilead Sciences, Inc.) Valrubicin (Valstar®, Medeva Pharmaceuticals)	Actinomycin D, mitomycin, and anthracycline antibiotics (except for liposomal formulations) are vesicants.* Nausea and vomiting Mucositis Bone marrow suppression (except for bleomycin) Gonadal suppression Alopecia Fatigue Cardiotoxicity (anthracycline antibiotics, dose dependent) Pulmonary fibrosis (bleomycin) Radiation recall
Cell Cycle Specific		
Antimetabolites	Capecitabine (Xeloda®, Roche Pharmaceuticals) Cladribine (Leustatin®, Bedford Laboratories) Clofarabine (Clolar®, Genzyme Corp.) Cytarabine (cytosine arabinoside, Cytosar-U®, Bedford Laboratories) Floxuridine (FUDR®, Bedford Laboratories,) Fludarabine (Fludara®, Sicor Pharmaceuticals) Fluorouracil (5-FU, Adrucil®, Sicor Pharmaceuticals)	Bone marrow suppression Nausea and vomiting Stomatitis, diarrhea Fatigue Anorexia 5-FU and gemcitabine are radiosensitizers.

(Continued on next page)

Table 4-1. Chemotherapy Agents by Class *(Continued)*

Category	FDA-Approved Drugs in the Class	Common Toxicities of the Class
	Gemcitabine (Gemzar®, Lilly Oncology) Hydroxyurea (Hydrea®, Bristol-Myers Squibb Co.) Liposomal cytarabine (DepoCyt®, Chiron Corp.) Mercaptopurine (6-MP, Purinethol®, GlaxoSmith-Kline) Methotrexate (MTX, Mexate®, generic, Bedford Laboratories) Pemetrexed (Alimta®, Lilly Oncology) Pentostatin (Nipent®, SuperGen Inc.) Thioguanine (6-TG, Tabloid®, GlaxoSmithKline) Trimetrexate (Neutrexin®, MedImmune Oncology)	
Miscella-neous agents	Asparaginase (Elspar®, Merck & Co., Inc.) Pegaspargase (Oncaspar®, Enzon Pharmaceuti-cals)	Nausea and vomiting Hypersensitivity reactions includ-ing anaphylaxis (which can be greatly reduced by intramuscu-lar administration) Hyperglycemia Hepatotoxicity Pancreatitis
Mitotic in-hibitors, vinca alkaloids	Vinblastine (Velban®, Bedford Laboratories) Vincristine (Oncovin®, Sicor Pharmaceuticals) Vinorelbine (Navelbine®, Bedford Laboratories)	All agents are vesicants.* Neurotoxicity (vincristine > vin-blastine > vinorelbine) Alopecia Nausea and vomiting, myelosup-pression (vinblastine, vinore-lbine)
Mitotic inhibi-tors, taxanes	Docetaxel (Taxotere®, Sanofi-Aventis) Paclitaxel (Taxol®, Bristol-Myers Squibb Co.) Paclitaxel protein-bound particles (Abraxane®, Abraxis BioScience)	Myelosuppression Sensory-motor peripheral neu-ropathy Arthralgias and myalgias Alopecia Nausea and vomiting Hypersensitivity reactions (pacli-taxel, docetaxel)
Topoisomer-ase I inhibi-tors	Irinotecan (Camptosar®, Pfizer Inc.) Topotecan (Hycamptin®, GlaxoSmithKline)	Myelosuppression Diarrhea Alopecia Nausea and vomiting Cross the BBB
Topoisomer-ase II inhibi-tors	Etoposide (VP-16, VePesid®, Bristol-Myers Squibb Co.) Doxorubicin (Adriamycin®, Bedford Laboratories) Daunorubicin (Cerubidine®, Bedford Laboratories)	Myelosuppression Nausea and vomiting Hypersensitivity Hypotension (See antitumor antibiotics for dox-orubicin and daunorubicin.)

(Continued on next page)

Table 4-1. Chemotherapy Agents by Class *(Continued)*

Category	FDA-Approved Drugs in the Class	Common Toxicities of the Class
	Arsenic trioxide (Trisenox®, Cephalon Oncology)	APL differentiation syndrome (fever, dyspnea, weight gain, pulmonary infiltrates, pleural/pericardial effusions, leukocytosis) QT interval prolongation, with risk of torsades de pointes if serum magnesium, potassium are low Nausea, vomiting, diarrhea Fever, anemia, disseminated intravascular coagulation, bleeding Fatigue Paresthesia, dizziness, tremor, insomnia Comment: Causes degradation of fusion protein PML/RAR alpha, characteristic of acute promyelocytic leukemia
Hormones		
Antiandrogens (nonsteroidal)	Bicalutamide (Casodex®, AstraZeneca) Flutamide (Eulexin®, Schering Corp.)	Hot flashes, gynecomastia, breast tenderness Decreased libido, impotence Nausea Diarrhea or constipation Edema Rare hepatitis
Antiestrogens (nonsteroidal)	Tamoxifen (Nolvadex®, AstraZeneca) Toremifene (Fareston®, GTx, Inc.)	Hot flashes, vaginal bleeding, vaginal discharge, endometrial hyperplasia, increased risk of endometrial cancer (tamoxifen) Hypercalcemia with tumor flare Nausea, vomiting Edema Depression Rare but increased risk of thromboembolic events
Antiestrogen (receptor antagonist)	Fulvestrant (Faslodex®, AstraZeneca)	Given intramuscularly Hot flashes, insomnia, nausea, vomiting Edema Rare but increased risk of thromboembolic events Depression Flu-like syndrome
Antiestrogens (nonsteroidal aromatase inhibitor, reversible)	Anastrozole (Arimidex®, AstraZeneca) Letrozole (Femara®, Novartis Pharmaceuticals Corp.)	Hot flashes, peripheral edema, headache, back or chest pain, nausea, fatigue, dizziness

(Continued on next page)

Table 4-1. Chemotherapy Agents by Class *(Continued)*

Category	FDA-Approved Drugs in the Class	Common Toxicities of the Class
Antiestrogen (steroidal aromatase inhibitor, irreversible)	Exemestane (Aromasin®, Pfizer Inc.)	Hot flashes Nausea Fatigue Diaphoresis
Estrogens	Estradiol (Estrace®, Warner Chilcott) Estramustine (Emcyt®, Pfizer Inc.) Estrogen (Menest®, Monarch Pharmaceuticals, Inc.)	Gynecomastia, breast tenderness Myelosuppression Nausea and vomiting Fluid and sodium retention Hypertension, ischemic heart disease Thrombophlebitis Changes in libido
Luteinizing hormone-releasing hormone analog	Goserelin acetate (Zoladex®, AstraZeneca) Leuprolide acetate (Lupron®, TAP Pharmaceuticals; Viadur®, Alza Corp.)	Hot flashes, gynecomastia Tumor flare, bone pain Edema Decreased libido, erectile impotence Depression Rare anorexia, nausea, vomiting

BBB—blood-brain barrier; FDA—U.S. Food and Drug Administration
* Vesicants cause tissue necrosis if the drug escapes into tissue during IV administration.

Note. This table does not review indications, as they change frequently. Please consult the manufacturer's product information as well as the FDA's Center for Drug Evaluation and Research Web site (www.access data.fda.gov/scripts/cder/drugsatfda/index.cfm) or the Oncology Nursing Society (ONS) e-mail alert that notifies ONS members when a new drug or new indication is approved by the FDA.

Note. Based on information from manufacturers' prescribing information.

bound particles for injectable suspension, Abraxane® [Abraxis BioScience, Inc., and AstraZeneca Pharmaceuticals]).

Drugs that interfere with a specific phase of the cell cycle are called cell cycle–specific agents and include the antimetabolites, antimitotic agents, and topoisomerase inhibitors. Drugs that are active throughout all phases of the cell cycle are called cell cycle–nonspecific agents and include alkylating agents and antitumor antibiotics. Miscellaneous agents include those with indeterminate or unusual activity that are unlike others in its class, such as procarbazine. Because of the extensive scope of this topic, this section will highlight one or two commonly used agents in each class. The reader is referred to chemotherapy texts or the drug package insert for a full discussion of each drug. In addition, please go to the drug or manufacturer Web site to obtain patient and provider resources. All chemotherapy agents pose reproductive hazards, so patients should avoid becoming pregnant and breast-feeding, and nurses should wear personal protective equipment when preparing and administering the drugs and handling patient excreta. Patients receiving home chemotherapy and their families should be instructed in safe handling of hazardous drugs, as well as handling of patient excreta. In addition, they must understand how to use the chemotherapy spill kit provided.

Cell Cycle–Specific Drugs

Antimetabolite agents: These agents prevent the synthesis of the complementary DNA strand during the S phase to make an exact copy of DNA for the daughter cell. Acting as a false cellular nutrient, such as a purine, pyrimidine, or enzyme, when inserted into the DNA strand or when the enzyme tries to function, cell replication is prevented and the cell undergoes apoptosis. In addition, a false metabolite may be inserted in the RNA strand, making it unable to function. Common side effects of antimetabolites include bone marrow depression, with a nadir (lowest blood counts) in 7–10 days after administration and recovery within 21 days, and mucositis (stomatitis, esophagitis, diarrhea) (Tortorice, 2005).

Gemcitabine (Gemzar®, Eli Lilly and Co.) is a prodrug that must be metabolized within the cell into active metabolites, resembling cytosine arabinoside (Cytosar-U®, Bedford Laboratories) in chemical structure. It inhibits DNA synthesis by stopping the enzyme DNA polymerase from making a complementary copy of the DNA strand, thus forcing the cell into apoptosis. It also halts cells as they move from the G_1 phase into the S phase. It is given IV and is metabolized by the liver with drug excretion via the kidneys. This drug should be used cautiously in patients with renal or hepatic insufficiency. This drug is a radiosensitizer. Potential side effects include bone marrow suppression (dose-limiting toxicity), nausea, vomiting, stomatitis, esophagitis (especially in patients with lung cancer receiving radiation therapy to the chest), diarrhea, flu-like symptoms with fever on the day of administration, alopecia, rash, pruritus, and edema. Rarely, pulmonary fibrosis, interstitial pneumonia, or pulmonary edema can occur, as can hemolytic uremic syndrome (Eli Lilly and Company, 2006).

Antimitotic agents: Antimitotic agents are active during the mitosis phase (M phase) and include the plant-derived vinca alkaloids and the taxanes. The vinca alkaloid group includes vincristine, vinblastine, and vinorelbine; all are vesicant agents, causing tissue necrosis if allowed to extravasate outside the vein during administration. Hence, scrupulous technique must be used to administer the drug. If extravasation is suspected, the drug should be stopped, and an IV should be started in another noncontiguous vein to avoid extravasation from the venipuncture hole in the blood vessel proximal to it. The nurse should be familiar with extravasation management, such as aspiration of any remaining drug from the tubing, administration of antidote (recommended hyaluronidase, manufactured by specialty pharmacies, such as Amphadase®, Amphastar Pharmaceuticals), and application of heat at least four times a day, and patients should be reassessed the next day and given specific management instructions (Larson, 1985). The taxanes include paclitaxel and docetaxel. All these agents are given IV and cause differing degrees of peripheral neuropathy because the drugs interfere with microtubular function and the axons are made up of microtubules.

Taxanes: This group affects mitosis in a different way. Whereas the vinca alkaloids prevent the formation of the mitotic spindle, paclitaxel (Taxol®, Bristol-Myers Squibb Co.) promotes early microtubule assembly *and* prevents disassembling, and docetaxel (Taxotere®, Sanofi-Aventis Pharmaceuticals Inc.) stabilizes the microtubules so that they cannot move. Both result in arrest of mitosis and cell death.

Paclitaxel (Taxol) is derived using a semisynthetic process from the Pacific Yew tree *(Taxus brevifolia).* It is extensively protein bound, metabolized in the liver, and excreted in the bile. The solvent used to make the drug soluble in blood, polyoxyethylated castor oil (Cremophor® EL, BASF Corp.), increases the risk of hypersensitivity reactions and requires premedication. Because Cremophor EL can leach the plasticizer di(2-ethylhexyl) phthalate (DEHP) from polyvinyl chloride IV sets, the drug must be administered with non-DEHP tubing and IV bags. This drug should be given by IV infusion following premedication with dexamethasone (usually 20 mg po 12 and 6 hours prior to the infusion), and right before the drug infusion, diphenhydramine and an H_2 antagonist should be administered. Paclitaxel also may be given intraperitoneally. This drug is a radiosensitizer. It causes cardiotoxicity when given concomitantly with either doxorubicin or trastuzumab. Other potential toxicities include bone marrow suppression with nadir in 7–10 days, sensory-motor peripheral neuropathy, hypersensitivity reactions, alopecia, mild nausea and vomiting, diarrhea, stomatitis, hepatotoxicity, hypotension, arrhythmia, fatigue, arthralgia, and myalgia.

Paclitaxel protein-bound particles for injectable suspension albumin-bound (Abraxane) was engineered to take advantage of tumor cells' thirst for albumin. Using nanotechnology, paclitaxel is surrounded by albumin, and the tumor cells preferentially uptake the albumin-bound drug. This obviates the need to use Cremophor EL, so the risk of hypersensitivity is significantly reduced, as is the risk for persistent neurotoxicity. In addition, higher doses of paclitaxel bound to albumin can be given as paclitaxel with Cremophor EL is incorporated into micelles (trapped in Cremophor lipid globule) once a certain dose is reached (Sparreboom et al., 1999), so there is a ceiling effect (Mould, Fleming, Darcy, & Spriggs, 2006). Potential side effects are similar to pac-litaxel; however, the incidence of peripheral neuropathy is higher related to a higher dose of paclitaxel (71% versus 56%) but is more quickly reversible (Abraxis Oncology, 2007).

Topoisomerase inhibitors: Irinotecan, topotecan, doxorubicin, and etoposide are included among the topoisomerase inhibitors. Topoisomerase I and II are critical to allow unwinding and then rewinding of the DNA helix during cell replication so that the DNA can be copied and a complementary strand assembled during the synthesis phase of the cell cycle. Topoisomerase I (makes one strand cut and then subsequent relegation of the DNA break) is inhibited by irinotecan and topotecan, whereas topoisomerase II (causes double-stranded breaks) is inhibited by etoposide and doxorubicin. The action of these agents prevents DNA and RNA synthesis in dividing cells. Topoisomerase I is found in higher-than-normal concentrations in certain malignancies, such as adenocarcinoma of the colon. These drugs are given IV, and topotecan and irinotecan can cross the blood-brain barrier. Doxorubicin (Adriamycin) is a vesicant, causing tissue necrosis if the drug is extravasated (Balazsovits et al., 1989).

Irinotecan (Camptosar®, Pfizer Inc.) is a semisynthetic agent derived from camptothecin, a plant alkaloid. The drug and its active metabolite SN-38 bind to topoisomerase I. Irinotecan is metabolized in the liver to the metabolite SN-38, which then is conjugated by an enzyme UGT1A1 to form a glucuronide metabolite. A UGT1A1*28 polymorphism (variation in a gene copy) exists in 10% of Americans, resulting in impaired metabolism of SN-38. Patients can be tested for this polymorphism, and if positive, they should receive a dose reduction. Otherwise, a higher serum level of SN-38 results with increased toxicity, especially grade 4 febrile neutropenia. In addition, in older adults, the terminal half-life of the drug is longer (6 hours versus 5.5 hours in people younger than 65 years old) (Pfizer Inc., 2006); therefore, patients should be monitored closely for toxicity. Significant drug interactions exist with CYP3A4 inducers (i.e., inducer phenytoin or St. John's wort), as they induce the cytochrome P450 microenzyme system responsible for metabolizing irinotecan; either of these drugs can significantly lower levels of SN-38. These drugs should not be coadministered, and the anticonvulsant should be changed to another, noninteracting agent, two weeks before irinotecan is administered. CYP3A4 inhibitors such as ketoconazole should not be given concurrently and should be stopped one week before irinotecan dosing (Pfizer Inc.).

The dose-limiting drug toxicity is persistent, delayed diarrhea, which can be fatal. Two types of diarrhea exist: One is early, with a cholinergic etiology, manifested as abdominal cramping, diarrhea, diaphoresis, lacrimation, flushing, miosis, and rhinitis during the drug administration. This can be rapidly reversed with IV atropine. The second type, which is delayed from a motility origin, occurs at least 24 hours after the drug is given. This delayed diarrhea is refractory and can lead to dehydration and electrolyte imbalance or sepsis, often simultaneously with nadir. Patients should be taught to take an aggressive regimen of loperamide (Imodium® [McNeil-PPC, Inc.]) 4 mg at the first sign of diarrhea and then 2 mg every two hours until 12 hours have passed without any diarrhea (should not exceed 48 hours of loperamide at these doses) and should be monitored closely. Patients should receive IV hydration if they are unable to maintain oral hydration, should be given antidiarrheals for grade 3 or 4 diarrhea (i.e., octreotide [Sandostatin®, Novartis Pharmaceuticals Corp.], and should be started on antibiotics if the diarrhea persists after 24 hours or if ileus, fever, or neutropenia develop. The drug is emetic, so aggressive antiemetics are given prior to drug administration. Other important side effects are neutropenia, anemia, and, rarely, pulmonary infiltrates. Irinotecan dose must be reduced depending on the severity of side effects experienced (Pfizer Inc., 2006).

Cell Cycle–Nonspecific Agents

Antitumor antibiotics: These are cytotoxic antibiotics that end in the suffix "mycin." All except for bleomycin are vesicant agents (FDA Center for Drug Evaluation and Research, 1999), and bleomycin is the only agent that is cell cycle specific. These drugs often are radiosensitizers.

Doxorubicin (Adriamycin) causes myelosuppression, with nadir in 10–14 days and recovery by day 21. The myofibrils take up the drug, so a key side effect is cardiotoxicity, principally decreased left ventricular ejection fraction (LVEF), with the development of congestive heart failure (CHF) if the drug is continued. A multigated acquisition (MUGA) scan or echocardiogram should be performed to obtain a baseline and periodically during therapy. The drug should be stopped if LVEF decreases to below normal. Common side effects are nausea, vomiting, anorexia, and, less commonly, stomatitis. The drug is red in color, so following administration, the patient's urine is pink for one to two days. In addition, doxorubicin causes darkening of the veins and soft palate, especially in dark-skinned patients. The drug is excreted in the urine and bile; thus, the dose must be modified if the patient has renal or hepatic dysfunction.

Alkylating agents: This class includes many agents, such as nitrogen mustard (Mustargen®, Ovation Pharmaceuticals, Inc.), its derivatives cyclophosphamide (Cytoxan) and ifosfamide (Ifex®, Bristol-Myers Squibb Co.), and others listed in Table 4-1. Included in this class are also the platinum analogs cisplatin (Platinol®, Bristol-Myers Squibb Co.), carboplatin (Paraplatin®, Bristol-Myers Squibb Co.) and oxaliplatin (Eloxatin®, Sanofi-Aventis Pharmaceuticals Inc.) and the nitrosourea carmustine (BiCNU®, Bristol-Myers Squibb Co.), which crosses the blood-brain barrier.

Oxaliplatin (Eloxatin®, Sanofi-Aventis Pharmaceuticals Inc.) is a third-generation platinum analog that is unique in that it has efficacy in colon and rectal cancers. It is synergistic with 5-fluorouracil (5-FU)/leucovorin, and the drug is indicated for the treatment of patients with colorectal cancers in combination with 5-FU/leucovorin by the

FDA. The dose-limiting toxicity is cumulative, persistent peripheral neuropathy that increases in risk at cumulative doses of 750–800 mg/m². This is reversible in many cases but may take a long time. In addition, oxaliplatin causes a very common, reversible, acute neuropathy that lasts less than 14 days and often is precipitated by exposure to cold (Wilkes, 2005). An uncommon manifestation is pharyngolaryngeal dysesthesia, which can be very frightening. The patient senses that no air is being moved into the lungs and becomes anxious (Wilkes). The oncology APN first rules out a hypersensitivity reaction by assessing vital signs, including oxygen saturation. Acute hypersensitivities appear to be related to voltage-gated channelopathy (dysfunction of an ion channel—in this case, calcium) and decreased extracellular calcium. Gamelin et al. (2004) retrospectively reviewed patients who received prophylactic calcium and magnesium infusions before and after oxaliplatin infusion compared to control patients and found that a significant decrease occurred in acute neuropathy symptoms, overall neuropathy, and more rapid recovery from neuropathy. Other common toxicities are neutropenia (very low incidence of febrile neutropenia), nausea and vomiting that is easily preventable with serotonin-antagonist/dexamethasone combinations, diarrhea, and transient, elevated liver transaminases. Anaphylaxis may occur during the infusion but also may occur as a delayed hypersensitivity after 10–12 cycles of therapy, similar to carboplatin.

Hormones: These agents alter the hormonal milieu in tumors that are stimulated by hormones, such as certain breast and prostate cancers. Classes of these agents are summarized in Table 4-1.

Biologic Agents

Biologic therapies offer a targeted approach to treating cancer and, together with an improved understanding of the molecular changes that accompany malignant transformation and growth, have made the 21st century the century of molecular targeted therapy.

Biotherapy may be given alone or in combination with chemotherapy and/or radiotherapy. Biotherapy takes advantage of normal immune mechanisms to stop the growth of or destroy cancer cells. Targeted biotherapy is directed toward an identifiable target on the malignant cell, with the hope of reducing collateral damage to normal cells. In 2003, NCI stated that its 2015 goal of eliminating suffering and death caused by cancer would depend heavily on targeted therapy (Von Eschenbach, 2006). These agents can be reviewed in terms of their classes as well, although some agents fall into more than one class because of their activity. Biologic agents and targeted therapies and their side effects are shown in Table 4-2. Almost all of these agents are fetotoxic or embryotoxic; pregnancy and breast-feeding should be avoided, and in some cases mandatory monitoring is required to prevent pregnancy.

Monoclonal Antibodies

mAbs are antibodies that have been cloned from a single antibody. The mAb was originally made from a hybrid of a myeloma cell (antibody factory) that had lost its ability to make antibody and a healthy B cell that had been exposed to the antigen against which the antibody was to be developed (Margulies, 2005). Today, mAbs are made using DNA recombinant (genetically engineered) technology. As with any antibody, the mAb has an Fc portion, which is responsible for the immune function against the antigen: It can bind to complement and initiate the complement cascade, and it

Table 4-2. Biologic and Targeted Therapies

Drug Class	Target	Drugs	Side Effects
mAb *not* in another category	CD20	Rituximab (Rituxan®, Genentech, Inc.)	• Hypersensitivity reactions during infusion, including anaphylaxis • Rare, fatal infusion reaction within 24 hours of drug infusion (characterized by hypoxia, pulmonary infiltrates, ARDS, MI, VF, or cardiogenic shock). 80% occur after first infusion. • Fever, chills • In new patients, tumor lysis syndrome may occur following rapid lysis of lymphoma cells. • Severe mucocutaneous (e.g., Stevens-Johnson syndrome) reactions; reactivation of hepatitis B and fulminating hepatitis • Posterior leukoencephalopathy syndrome (headache, lethargy, confusion, seizure, visual changes)
	CD52	Alemtuzumab (Campath®-1H anti-CD52, Genzyme Corp.)	• Humanized IgG1 • Infusion reactions (rash, fever, rigors, hypotension) require premedication. • Myelosuppression • Pain, asthenia, peripheral edema, headache, dysesthesia, dizziness
mAb conjugated to a cytotoxic antibiotic	CD33	Gemtuzumab ozogamicin (Mylotarg®, Wyeth Pharmaceuticals, Inc.)	• Acute hypersensitivity reactions (including anaphylaxis, pulmonary edema); fever, neutropenia, thrombocytopenia, diarrhea, nausea, vomiting, chills, headache; dyspnea • Hypokalemia, stomatitis, abnormal LFTs, hepatotoxicity (including VOD)
mAb conjugated with radioisotope	CD20	^{90}Y ibritumomab tiuxetan (Zevalin®, Biogen Idec Inc.) Two-step administration (1) Infusion of 250 mg/m^2 rituximab preceding a fixed dose of 5 mCi Zevalin administered as a 10-minute IV push (2) 7–9 days later, infusion of 250 mg/m^2 of rituximab prior to 0.4 mCi/kg of ^{90}Y Zevalin administered as a 10-minute IV push	• Rare, fatal infusion reactions reported within 24 hours of rituximab infusion (hypoxia, pulmonary infiltrates, ARDS, MI, VF, cardiogenic shock); 80% occurred during first infusion of rituximab. • Prolonged and severe cytopenias; severe cutaneous and mucosal reactions (e.g., Stevens-Johnson syndrome); fetotoxicity (avoid pregnancy) • Rare secondary malignancies (AML, MDS) • Contraindicated: > 25% bone marrow occupied by lymphoma, impaired bone marrow reserve • Hypersensitivity reaction to murine antibody; altered biodistribution

(Continued on next page)

Table 4-2. Biologic and Targeted Therapies *(Continued)*

Drug Class	Target	Drugs	Side Effects
	CD20	Tositumomab and I131 tositumomab (Bexxar®, GlaxoSmithKline) Two-step administration: (1) Dosimetry testing (after having received three doses of iodine [SSKI, Lugol's or potassium iodide tablet]) (2) Therapeutic dose 7–14 days later	• Hypersensitivity reactions including anaphylaxis; prolonged and severe cytopenias; nausea, vomiting, diarrhea; rash; arthralgia, myalgia • Fetotoxicity (avoid pregnancy) • Hypothyroidism • Secondary malignancy (MDS, AML) • Contraindicated: hypersensitivity reaction to murine antibody
TKI, not otherwise classified (small molecule, oral)	Bcr-Abl, *c-kit*	Imatinib mesylate (Gleevec®, Novartis Pharmaceuticals Corp.)	• Neutropenia, anemia, thrombocytopenia • Fluid retention, edema • GI irritation if not taken with food; nausea, vomiting, muscle cramping; diarrhea • Rash, headache, myalgia • Bullous dermatologic reactions • Teratogenicity (avoid pregnancy) • Rare hemorrhage, hepatotoxicity
Antiangiogenesis agents	VEGF (ligand) Type of agent: mAb	Bevacizumab (Avastin®, Genentech, Inc.)	• Hypertension, bleeding (epistaxis, rare GI bleeding), rare hemorrhage, delayed wound healing (do not give within 28 days of major surgery, until wound has healed), rare proteinuria, rare arterial thromboembolic complications, rare CHF in patients who have received anthracyclines, rare nasal septum perforation, rare reversible posterior leukoencephalopathy syndrome (headache, lethargy, confusion, seizure, visual changes), teratogenicity (avoid pregnancy)
Multi-targeted	Bcr-Abl, *c-kit*, PDGFR-β	Dasatinib (Sprycel®, Bristol-Myers Squibb Co.)	• Severe myelosuppression • Fluid retention (including pleural and pericardial effusions) • Edema • Nausea, vomiting, diarrhea • Pain, headache, fatigue, arthralgia, fatigue • QT interval prolongation • Teratogenicity and embryotoxicity/fetotoxicity (avoid pregnancy)
	VEGFR1, 2, 3; PDGFR-α, PDGFR-β, FLT3, *c-kit*, others Type of agent: TKIs (small molecule, oral)	Sunitinib (Sutent®, Pfizer Oncology)	• Bleeding, hypertension, fatigue, diarrhea, nausea, mucositis/stomatitis, altered taste, rash, vomiting, constipation, skin discoloration, hypertension, anorexia, dyspnea, hand-foot syndrome, peripheral neuropathy, risk of adrenal insufficiency, rare decreased LVEF with risk for developing CHF, rare hypothyroidism

(Continued on next page)

Table 4-2. Biologic and Targeted Therapies *(Continued)*

Drug Class	Target	Drugs	Side Effects
	VEGFR2, PDGFR-ß, Raf kinase	Sorafenib (Nexavar®, Bayer HealthCare and Onyx Pharmaceuticals)	• Bleeding, hypertension, elevated serum lipase and amylase, reduced serum phosphate, rash, hand-foot reaction, alopecia, pruritus, diarrhea, nausea, anorexia, vomiting, constipation, stomatitis, mucositis, sensory neuropathy, rare MI, GI hemorrhage, teratogenicity (avoid pregnancy)
EGFR1 inhibitors	EGFR1-mAbs	Cetuximab (Erbitux®, ImClone Systems, Inc., and Bristol-Myers Squibb Co.)	• Sterile, inflammatory rash that may be severe; increased hair growth of eyelashes and eyebrows; alopecia; hypomagnesemia; 3% severe hypersensitivity reaction (90% occur during first infusion); nausea, vomiting, diarrhea, stomatitis; rare ILD
		Panitumumab (Vectibix™, Amgen Inc.)	• Rash (which may be severe), severe infusion reactions (1%), paronychia, pruritus, diarrhea, nausea, vomiting, stomatitis, hypomagnesemia and hypocalcemia, rare ILD • Do not give with IFL regimen, as severe diarrhea may result.
	EGFR1-TKIs (small molecule, oral)	Gefitinib (Iressa®, AstraZeneca Pharmaceuticals)	• Diarrhea, rash, acne, dry skin, nausea, vomiting, rare ILD, fetotoxicity (avoid pregnancy)
		Erlotinib (Tarceva®, OSI Pharmaceuticals, Inc., and Genentech, Inc.)	• Rash, diarrhea, conjunctivitis, eye dryness, mucositis, anorexia; rare ILD; in pancreatic CA trial, rare MI, cerebrovascular accident, microangiopathic hemolytic anemia with thrombocytopenia; may be embryotoxic/fetotoxic (avoid pregnancy)
EGFR2 inhibitors	EGFR2 (HER2/ neu receptor)	Trastuzumab (Herceptin®, Genentech, Inc.)	• Decreased LVEF and cardiomyopathy (increased risk when receiving anthracycline chemotherapy); infusion reactions, some severe (dyspnea, hypotension); increased risk of neutropenia and anemia when receiving chemotherapy; increased risk thrombotic events; diarrhea; rare pulmonary toxicity (e.g., pneumonitis, ARDS), especially in patients with lung disease or pulmonary metastases; rare nephritic syndrome
Combined EGFR1 and 2	EGFR1, EGFR2	Lapatinib ditosylate (Tykerb®, GlaxoSmith-Kline)	• Rash, fatigue, diarrhea

(Continued on next page)

Table 4-2. Biologic and Targeted Therapies *(Continued)*

Drug Class	Target	Drugs	Side Effects
Proteasome inhibitors	Proteasome	Bortezomib (Velcade®, Millennium Pharmaceuticals)	• Peripheral neuropathy; hypotension; nausea, diarrhea, constipation, vomiting; thrombocytopenia; neutropenia; psychiatric disorders; decreased appetite; rare hepatic failure; rare CHF; rare pulmonary disease; rare reversible posterior leukoencephalopathy syndrome; fetotoxicity (avoid pregnancy)
Immuno-modulatory agents	Tumor microenvironment; antiangiogenesis activity	Thalidomide (Thalomid®, Celgene Corp.)	• Teratogenicity (avoid pregnancy): special prescribing requirements required (STEPS® program); increased risk of DVT and PE; constipation; peripheral neuropathy; confusion; hypokalemia; edema; dyspnea; rash/desquamation; somnolence
		Lenalidomide (Revlimid®, Celgene Corp.)	• Teratogenicity (avoid pregnancy): special prescribing requirements required (RevAssist®); neutropenia, thrombocytopenia; DVT and PE; constipation; insomnia; muscle cramps; diarrhea; fatigue; anemia; pyrexia; edema; headache; dizziness; rash
Miscellaneous	Primitive promyelocytes in acute promyelocytic leukemia; promoting maturation followed by repopulation of the bone marrow and peripheral blood with normal myeloid cell line in patients who achieve a CR	Tretinoin (all-trans-retinoic acid, ATRA, Vesanoid®, Roche Laboratories) (IV formulation, liposomal tretinoin [Atragen®, Aronex Pharmaceuticals], is investigational.)	• Retinoic acid-APL syndrome (rapid leukocytosis, fever, dyspnea, weight gain, pulmonary infiltrates, effusions, which may be fatal; treated with high-dose steroids), vitamin A toxicity (headaches, fever, skin/mucous membrane dryness, bone pain, nausea, vomiting, rash, mucositis, pruritus, diaphoresis, visual disturbances, skin changes, alopecia), arrhythmia, flushing, earache, hypercholesterolemia and/or hypertriglyceridemia; teratogenicity and embryotoxicity (avoid pregnancy); rare pseudotumor cerebri
	Retinoid X receptor: selectively binds and activates retinoid X receptor (RXRα, RXRβ, RXRγ), thus inhibiting transcription factors that regulate gene expression controlling differentiation and proliferation	Bexarotene (Targretin®, Ligand Pharma)	• Clinical hypothyroidism; cataracts; elevated fasting triglycerides, cholesterol; LFT abnormalities; leukopenia, diarrhea, fatigue/lethargy, headache, rash, pancreatitis, nausea, anemia, muscle spasm; rare teratogenicity and embryotoxicity (avoid pregnancy)

(Continued on next page)

Table 4-2. Biologic and Targeted Therapies *(Continued)*

Drug Class	Target	Drugs	Side Effects
Hypo-methylating agents (reverse epigenetic silencing of tumor suppressor genes)	Methylation groups with DNA	Decitabine (Dacogen®, MGI Pharma)	• Neutropenia (including febrile neutro-penia), thrombocytopenia, anemia, nausea, diarrhea, constipation, hyper-glycemia, cough, pyrexia • Teratogenicity (avoid pregnancy)
		Azacitidine (Vidaza®, Pharmion Corp.)	• Neutropenia, thrombocytopenia, ane-mia, nausea, vomiting, diarrhea, pyrexia, injection site reactions, constipation, fatigue, dyspnea, weakness, rigors, anorexia
Fusion protein	Interleukin-2 receptors with a CD25 component (activated T and B lymphocytes, macrophages)	Denileukin diftitox (On-tak®, Seragen Inc.)	• Acute hypersensitivity reactions (hy-potension, back pain, dyspnea, vasodi-lation, rash, chest pain/tightness, chills/fever, tachycardia with rare anaphylaxis); vascular leak syndrome, which is re-duced by saline hydration and steroid premedication; hypoalbuminemia; edema; nausea, vomiting, diarrhea, an-orexia; loss of visual acuity with loss of color vision • Avoid pregnancy, as fetotoxicity tests have not been done.

AML—acute myeloid leukemia; ARDS—acute respiratory distress syndrome; CA—carcinoma; CD—cluster of differentiation antigen on lymphocytes; CHF—congestive heart failure; CR—complete remission; DVT—deep vein thrombosis; EGFR1—epidermal growth factor receptor 1; EGFR2—epidermal growth factor receptor 2, also known as HER2/neu; GI—gastrointestinal; IFL—bolus irinotecan, 5-FU, leucovorin regimen for colorectal cancer; IF-α—interferon-α; ILD—interstitial lung disease; LFTs—liver function tests; LVEF—left ventricular ejection fraction; mAbs—monoclonal antibodies; MDS—myelodysplastic syndrome; MI—myocardial infarction; PDGFR—platelet-derived growth factor receptor; PE—pulmonary embolus; TKIs—tyrosine kinase inhibitors (small molecule, oral); VEGF—vascular endothelial growth factor; VEGFR—vascular endothelial growth factor receptor; VF—ventricular fibrillation; VOD—veno-occlusive disease

Note. This table does not review indications, as they change frequently. Please consult the manufacturer's product information as well as the U.S. Food and Drug Administration (FDA) Center for Drug Evaluation and Research Web site (www.accessdata.fda.gov/scripts/cder/drugsatfda/index.cfm) or the Oncology Nursing Society (ONS) e-mail alert that notifies ONS members when a new drug or new indication is approved by the FDA.

Note. Based on information from manufacturers' prescribing information.

can bind to receptors on immunomodulatory cells such as macrophages, resulting in phagocytosis as well as stimulation of cytokine release that orchestrates the immune response, leading to destruction of the cell expressing the antigen (Muehlbauer, Cusack, & Morris, 2006). The fragment, antigen-binding (Fab) portion is variable and will bind to only one antigen (Muehlbauer et al.). The core of the mAb theoretically makes a difference. mAbs derived from IgG1 are believed to have the strongest antibody-dependent cell-mediated cytotoxicity (ADCC) effect, and they also have complement activation compared to IgG2 mAbs, which bind with weaker activation of host immune function (Adams & Weiner, 2005). IgG1 mAbs include bevacizumab, cetuximab, rituximab, trastuzumab, and yttrium-90 ibritumomab tiuxetan, whereas pani-tumumab is an IgG2 mAb.

mAbs are made to be totally human (human, suffix -umab), mostly human and only a small part mouse (humanized, suffix -zumab), some mouse and some human (chimeric, suffix -ximab), or from mouse protein (murine, suffix -momab) (see Figure 4-2). Although murine antibodies are better at finding their target because their Fab portion of the antibody is more efficient than the human Fab, significant difficulties exist as well. These include hypersensitivity reactions and development of neutralizing antibodies against the mouse antibody (human antimouse antibodies). mAbs differ from chemotherapy in a number of ways, including the fact that they may have long half-lives. For example, rituximab (Rituxan® [Biogen Idec Inc. and Genentech, Inc.]) can still be found in the blood six months after the dose was administered (Muehlbauer et al., 2006).

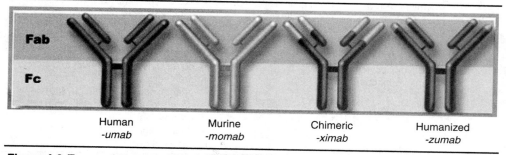

Figure 4-2. Types of Monoclonal Antibodies

Note. From *Biomolecular Targeted Therapies in Cancer Treatment* [Slide kit], by Oncology Education Services, Inc., 2003, Pittsburgh, PA: Author. Copyright 2003 by Oncology Education Services, Inc. Reprinted with permission.

mAbs can be unconjugated (naked) or conjugated (attached to a toxin or radionucleotide). The unconjugated mAb kills tumor cells by first attaching to the antigen, such as the CD20 B lymphocyte. It then has five biologic activities that can injure or kill the cell (Muehlbauer et al., 2006).

- Direct interference with cell signaling of target cell (cytostatic)
- ADCC: Cytokines recruit phagocytes, T cells, and natural killer cells, which destroy the target cell.
- Complement-dependent cytotoxicity (CDC): Complement system is activated to destroy the target cell.
- Direct induction of apoptosis (programmed cell death) in antibody-bound cell
- Release of inhibitory checkpoints so that target cell is attacked by immune system (antibodies against cytotoxic T-lymphocytic antigen-4, antibodies against T-regulatory cells)

Unconjugated Monoclonal Antibodies

This category of naked mAbs includes rituximab (Rituxan), alemtuzumab (Campath®, Genzyme Corp.), trastuzumab (Herceptin®, Genentech, Inc.), cetuximab (Erbitux®, ImClone Systems Inc. and Bristol-Myers Squibb Co.), panitumumab (Vectibix™, Amgen Inc.), and bevacizumab (Avastin®, Genentech, Inc.). Rituximab is perhaps the most well known, as it was the first mAb approved for treatment of cancer and has found application in a number of non-oncology settings, such as rheumatoid arthritis (see Table 4-2 for indications).

Rituximab (Rituxan): Rituximab is an IgG1 mAb that targets the CD20 antigen, found on both malignant and normal B lymphocytes. Cell death occurs by induction of ADCC; activation of the complement that coats the antigen-bearing cell, causing cell lysis; inhibition of cell growth; and induction of apoptosis (Smith, 2003). It is used in the treatment of CD20 antigen–positive non-Hodgkin lymphoma (NHL), including low-grade follicular lymphoma, diffuse large cell lymphoma (in combination with CHOP), and refractory lymphoma (see Table 4-2 for full indications). The drug has a long half-life, which is initially 76.3 hours but with subsequent infusions increases to 205.8 hours (Berinstein et al., 1998). The NHL dose is 375 mg/m^2 as a weekly IV infusion for four to eight doses, whereas for rheumatoid arthritis, the dose is 1,000 mg IV infusion every two weeks for two doses, together with glucocorticoid premedication (Genentech, Inc., 2008b). Rituximab also is given in combination with yttrium-90 ibritumomab tiuxetan (Zevalin®, Biogen Idec Inc.) or other chemotherapy regimens such as CHOP. Potential side effects include infusion reactions (chills, rigors, severe hypersensitivity reaction of hypotension, bronchospasm, and anaphylaxis requiring emergency intervention) and rare severe mucocutaneous reactions. An increased risk of tumor lysis syndrome exists in newly diagnosed patients with lymphoma with a high tumor burden because of the dramatic lysis of lymphocytes during their first rituximab treatment. Rarely, the drug has been associated with bowel obstruction and perforation, renal failure, cardiac arrhythmias, and hepatitis B reactivation with fulminant hepatitis. Most recently, rituximab has been implicated in rare sudden death within 24 hours of receiving the drug (symptom constellation includes hypoxia, pulmonary infiltrates, acute respiratory distress syndrome [ARDS], myocardial infarction, ventricular fibrillation, or cardiogenic shock); 80% occur after the first infusion. If this occurs, the drug must be stopped and life-saving treatment begun. In addition, fatal progressive multifocal leukoencephalopathy has been reported after the off-label use of rituximab for systemic lupus erythematosus, which may be related to reactivation of viral infection caused by John Cunningham virus (referred to as the JC virus), a type of human polyomavirus (FDA, 2006).

A number of mAbs block the epidermal growth factor receptor (EGFR) or the human epidermal receptor (HER). The EGFR family is made up of four receptors: EGFR1 (HER1), EGFR2 (HER2), EGFR3, and EGFR4 (see Figure 4-3). EGFR1 and EGFR2 may be mutated or overexpressed in a number of solid tumors. Figure 4-4 depicts the activity of the EGFRs when overexpressed, leading to cell survival (avoidance of apoptosis), growth and proliferation, release of VEGF to begin angiogenesis, and metastases. Blocking the receptor results in interruption of signal transduction, so the message for the cell to proliferate, make VEGF become invasive, and ignore death signals (apoptosis) never reaches the cell nucleus. EGFR inhibitors represent a powerful group of agents in molecular targeted therapy (O'Reilly, 2002).

Trastuzumab (Herceptin): Trastuzumab is an IgG1 mAb that targets the HER2 receptor, or EGFR2. The HER or EGFR family has four receptors, as shown in Figure 4-3. The HER2 receptor has extracellular, transmembrane, and intracellular domains; trastuzumab targets the extracellular domain, which is overexpressed in 20%–30% of breast cancers (i.e., too many copies of the HER2 gene are present) (Muehlbauer et al., 2006). Although HER2 overexpression confers a more aggressive disease with a less favorable prognosis, success with trastuzumab has improved survival, especially in the adjuvant setting. In a number of adjuvant studies, the relative risk of recur-

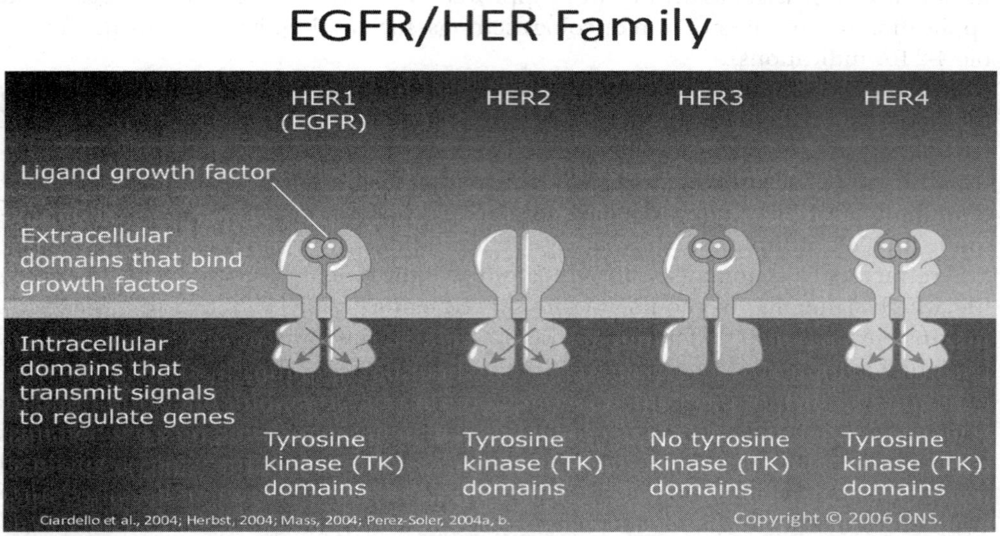

EGFR/HER Family

Figure 4-3. Epidermal Growth Factor Receptor Family of Receptors

Note. From *Clinical Breakthroughs in EGFR Inhibition: Applying the Science to Your Clinical Practice* (Slide 14), by T. Knoop, M. Morse, and L. Tyson, May 2006. Presentation given at the Oncology Nursing Society 31st Annual Congress, Boston, MA. Copyright 2006 by Oncology Nursing Society. Reprinted with permission.

rence decreased by 52% when trastuzumab was added to chemotherapy, and the absolute difference in disease-free survival was 12% at three years and 18% at four years in favor of the trastuzumab-plus-chemotherapy group (Baselga, Perez, Pienkowski, & Bell, 2006; Romond et al., 2005). However, up to a 4.1% incidence of cardiotoxicity was found in the group receiving trastuzumab (Baselga et al.). Once trastuzumab binds to the HER2 receptor on the cell surface, it is believed to interrupt dimerization (two surface receptors must come together or dimerize to initiate the signal for proliferation), thus bringing about G_1 phase cell cycle arrest, decreased cell proliferation, antiangiogenic factor release, suppression of VEGF secretion, and enhancement of ADCC immune function (Sliwkowski et al., 1999). Patients must have significant overexpression of HER2 to benefit from trastuzumab, so National Comprehensive Cancer Network (NCCN) guidelines recommend confirming immunohistochemistry 2+ findings (borderline positive, with weak to moderate tissue staining in > 10% of tumor cells) with fluorescence in situ hybridization (NCCN, 2008). Accurate HER2 testing is critical to effectively plan therapy for women who are HER2 positive. In January 2007, NCCN and the Research Advocacy Network created an online report for patient teaching about the significance and importance of HER2 testing (Carlson et al., 2006).

Once a patient has been determined to be HER2 positive, discussion about treatment with an HER2 receptor antagonist takes place. Trastuzumab is the most well-studied agent to date. The drug is given weekly, with a 4 mg/kg IV loading dose given over 90 minutes, and if well tolerated, subsequent weekly doses of 2 mg/kg IV given over 30 minutes. If the patient develops mild to moderate infusion reactions, the infusion rate should be reduced and the drug administered over a longer time. Signs of infusion re-

Anti-EGFR Antibodies

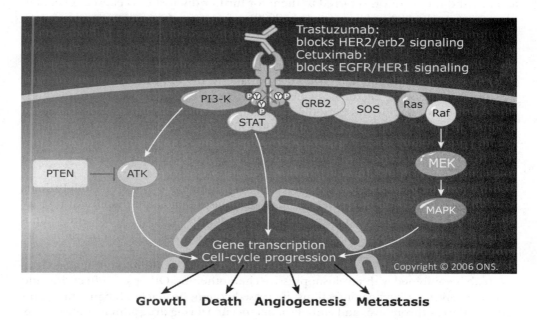

Growth   Death   Angiogenesis   Metastasis

A growth factor (ligand) binds to the EGFR, causing dimerization or pairing of receptors, and this initiates the signaling cascade telling the nucleus what to do. Many pathways to reach the nucleus exist: shown in this slide are the mitogen-activated protein kinase (MAPK) pathway and the PI3-K/ATK pathway (phosphoinositide 3 kinase/protein kinase B). The monoclonal antibody cetuximab blocks the EGFR1 from initiating a message, while trastuzumab blocks the HER-2 receptor from initiating the signal. This prevents the signaling cascade and subsequent proliferation and angiogenesis and encourages the cell to die.

Figure 4-4. Trastuzumab and Cetuximab Mechanism of Action as Anti-Epidermal Growth Factor Receptor (EGFR) Antibodies

ATK—protein kinase B; GRB2—growth factor receptor-binding protein 2; MAPK—mitogen-activated protein kinase; MEK—Map erk kinase; P—phosphorylation of EGFR tyrosine kinase; PI3-K—phosphoinositide 3 kinase; PTEN—phosphatase and tensin homolog; Raf—protein kinase that is a Ras effector (carries out its work); Ras—protein product from *ras* family of oncogenes; SOS—son of sevenless protein; STAT—signal transducer and activator of transcription; Y—yes, phosphorylation occurs and the signal activates the indicated pathways

Note. From *Clinical Breakthroughs in EGFR Inhibition: Applying the Science to Your Clinical Practice* (Slide 29), by T. Knoop, M. Morse, and L. Tyson, May 2006. Presentation given at the Oncology Nursing Society 31st Annual Congress, Boston, MA. Copyright 2006 by Oncology Nursing Society. Reprinted with permission.

action characteristically include fever and chills, which respond to acetaminophen, diphenhydramine, and meperidine. Less commonly, nausea, vomiting, pain (related to tumor), headache, dizziness, dyspnea, hypotension, rash, and asthenia also may occur. Rarely, more serious infusion reactions may include bronchospasm, hypoxia, dyspnea, and severe hypotension, which may develop during or immediately following drug infusion. For these responses, the drug should be interrupted until symptoms completely resolve. If severe or life-threatening infusion reactions occur, such as anaphylaxis, angioedema, pneumonitis, or ARDS, the drug should be discontinued (Genentech, Inc., 2008a). There are reports of successful desensitization protocols for hypersensitivity reactions, and the reader is referred to them for further discussion (Feldweg, Lee, Matulonis, & Castells, 2005; Markman et al., 2000).

The incidence of cardiomyopathy is 3%–7% with trastuzumab (Herceptin) as a single agent, but the risk increases to 27% in patients receiving concomitant anthracycline and cyclophosphamide-containing chemotherapy regimens (Seidman et al., 2002). Among adjuvant clinical trials, one trial had 16% of patients discontinue therapy because of cardiac dysfunction or decreases in LVEF. Baseline LVEF should be determined just before treatment begins and periodically during treatment using an echocardiogram or MUGA scan. Normal baseline LVEF is 50%–55%. The drug should be discontinued if a significant drop in LVEF occurs, and patients should be followed for possible further decline in LVEF. In addition, mural thrombosis with subsequent stroke has been reported (Genentech, Inc., 2008a).

Pulmonary toxicity has been reported with trastuzumab and has been fatal. Patients with existing lung disease or extensive lung metastases that cause dyspnea at rest appear to be at risk. Toxicity includes dyspnea, pneumonitis, hypoxia, ARDS, and pulmonary fibrosis, which may occur during or after the infusion as part of an infusion reaction (Genentech, Inc., 2008a).

More pronounced neutropenia, especially febrile neutropenia, may occur when trastuzumab is combined with myelosuppressive chemotherapy. Other side effects include nausea, vomiting, diarrhea, infections, increased cough, headache, fatigue, rash, and myalgia. Rarely, thrombosis and embolism may occur. During drug administration, only normal saline should be used in order to avoid incompatibilities with 5% dextrose solutions (Genentech, Inc., 2008a).

Cetuximab (Erbitux): This agent is a mAb that targets the extracellular domain of EGFR1, as shown in Figure 4-4. Cetuximab is FDA-approved for treatment of patients with advanced colorectal cancer (CRC) or head and neck cancer as described in Table 4-2. The initial loading dose is 400 mg/m^2 IV over two hours, followed by weekly maintenance treatments of 250 mg/m^2 over 60 minutes. Premedications before each treatment are H$_1$ antagonists such as diphenhydramine. Cetuximab is a chimeric mAb that may cause infusion reactions, including severe reactions in 3% of patients, such as symptomatic bronchospasm, hypotension, and anaphylaxis. Ninety percent of these reactions occur during the first infusion (ImClone Systems, Inc. & Bristol-Myers Squibb Co., 2007). EGFRs are located in the skin, hair follicles, and gastric mucosa; therefore, toxicity is manifested in these areas and includes a sterile, inflammatory skin rash (follicular or maculopapular); alopecia; increased hair growth on face, eyebrows, and eyelashes; paronychia and skin fissures; xerosis (dry skin); pruritus; diarrhea; hypomagnesemia and hypocalcemia because EGFR receptors are located in the renal loop of Henle where magnesium and calcium are resorbed; and, rarely, interstitial lung disease (ILD).

Managing skin toxicity is a major challenge, as few evidence-based interventions exist and the available grading scales are inadequate to fully characterize the rash or its subjective effect on the patient. The rash typically is on the face, back, and chest. It is hypothesized that EGFR inhibition results in abnormal proliferation, migration, and differentiation of keratinocytes, leading to disruption of skin integrity and recruitment of inflammatory cells (Lacouture, 2006; Peus, Hamacher, & Pittelkow, 1997; Woodworth et al., 2005). Initial skin changes are erythema, sensory changes, and edema that is similar to sunburn. The next phase is the papulopustular stage, which begins within

7–10 days of starting therapy and is most prominent in sun-exposed areas. Over time, the pustules crust over, followed by healing and formation of telangiectasias (dilated capillaries), as well as dry skin and itching. The skin becomes thin and loses its ability to retain moisture. Within several months of starting therapy, changes in the hair and nails occur: Diffuse, reversible alopecia may occur, along with increased growth (hypertrichosis) with distortion of facial hair and eyelashes (trichomegaly). The long eyelashes may irritate and cause conjunctivitis. Periungual irritation (paronychia) may result in crusting on the nail folds and nails, especially on the thumbs, which can become tender and interfere with function. Severe paronychia may require treatment with oral doxycycline (Shu, Kindler, Medenica, & Lacouture, 2006). Finally, skin fissures may occur on the fingers.

Management recommendations include the following (Lacouture, Basti, Patel, & Benson, 2006; O'Keefe, Parrilli, & Lacouture, 2006; Perez-Soler et al., 2005; Rhee, Oishi, Garey, & Kim, 2005; Sapadin & Fleischmajer, 2006; Shu et al., 2006). Please refer to these articles for a more in-depth discussion.

- Use water-based moisturizing creams for skin, and teach the patient to stay well hydrated.
- Teach the patient to avoid sun exposure and use sunscreen with a sun protection factor (SPF) of at least 30 that contains zinc or titanium.
- Control and prevent itching, as rash may become infected; use skin emollients and topical or systemic agents to prevent itch.
- Teach the patient to use zinc pyrithione shampoo, such as Head and Shoulders® (Procter & Gamble), to wash hair and scalp to prevent scalp dryness.
- Use tetracycline analogs such as doxycycline for the anti-inflammatory effect.
- Culture any lesion that looks suspicious (e.g., vesicular rash, oozing, yellow crusting), and treat the patient based on culture and sensitivity.
- Steroid tape may be prescribed for painful paronychia or fissures in the skin.
- Refer the patient to a dermatologist when the rash is progressive or treatment is ineffective; refer the patient to an ophthalmologist for conjunctivitis related to long, irritating eyelashes and to trim the eyelashes as needed.

If the patient develops rapid-onset dyspnea, hold the infusion and rule out ILD. If chest computed tomography (CT) and pulmonary function tests confirm ILD, treatment involves high-dose steroids, oxygen therapy, bronchodilator therapy, and hospitalization as needed (Higenbottam, Kuwano, Nemery, & Fujita, 2004). Finally, serum magnesium and calcium levels should be assessed before each treatment and repleted as needed.

Bevacizumab (Avastin): A humanized mAb directed against the ligand VEGF (see Figure 4-4), bevacizumab is the first antiangiogenesis agent to demonstrate a survival advantage in patients with advanced CRC (Hurwitz et al., 2004). This drug is given by IV infusion with a dose of 5 mg/kg with irinotecan, 5-FU, and leucovorin (IFL) or 10 mg/kg with oxaliplatin, leucovorin, and 5-FU (FOLFOX) every two weeks for treatment of advanced CRC, or 15 mg/kg every three weeks for treatment of nonsquamous non-small cell lung cancer. The tumor cannot grow larger than 1–2 mm, the diffusion distance of oxygen, without developing a new blood supply. The tumor cells must then release VEGF, and as mentioned earlier, EGFR overexpression stimulates the release of VEGF as it drives cell proliferation. By binding to VEGF, bevacizumab effectively halts angiogenesis as the growth factor is unable to bind to the endothelial VEGF receptors. Nitric oxide is necessary for normal relaxation of blood vessels, and it depends upon VEGF to function.

The most serious but uncommon side effects of bevacizumab are hemorrhage, gastrointestinal perforation, arterial thrombotic events, and delayed wound healing. Fatal hemorrhage occurred during a study of patients with squamous cell lung cancer, thus making the drug contraindicated in this patient population. The half-life of bevacizumab is 20 days, so this drug should not be given sooner than 28 days after major surgery, or until healing has occurred (Genentech, Inc., 2007). In addition, the incidence of more severe neutropenia, febrile neutropenia, and infection is increased in patients receiving both bevacizumab and chemotherapy. More common side effects are mild and easily managed, including epistaxis, asthenia, hypertension, constipation or diarrhea, and headache. Less commonly experienced side effects include proteinuria and nephritic syndrome, reversible posterior leukoencephalopathy syndrome, CHF in patients who have previously received anthracycline chemotherapy, and perforation of the nasal septum.

Hypertension with VEGF inhibition is a class effect of antiangiogenesis agents. Fortunately, the resulting hypertension develops over time and generally is well controlled with available antihypertensives such as diuretics, angiotensin-converting enzyme (ACE) inhibitors, or calcium channel blockers as recommended by the Joint National Committee 7 guidelines (Chobanian et al., 2003; Kozloff et al., 2007; van Heeckeren, Ortiz, Cooney, & Remick, 2007). Some clinicians assert that ACE inhibitors may be preferable, as these drugs also help to manage proteinuria (Dincer & Altundag, 2006). Patients in clinical trials were excluded if they had brain metastases. Clinical trials are ongoing to study the safety of bevacizumab in this population.

Conjugated Monoclonal Antibodies

These mAbs have an attached toxin or radioisotope. The Fab portion recognizes the target antigen and brings the attached toxin or radioisotope to the target cell to destroy it. Examples of conjugated mAbs are two radioisotope conjugated mAbs that are directed against the CD20 antigen on malignant B lymphocytes: yttrium-90 ibritumomab tiuxetan (Zevalin) and tositumomab and iodine-131 tositumomab (Bexxar®, GlaxoSmithKline), both of which are murine mAbs with an attached radioisotope. Gemtuzumab ozogamicin (Mylotarg®, Wyeth Pharmaceuticals) is a mAb targeted against the CD33-positive lymphocytes found in acute myeloid leukemia.

Gemtuzumab ozogamicin (Mylotarg): A humanized IgG4 mAb, attached by a linker molecule to the potent poison calicheamicin, a cytotoxic antitumor antibiotic. It targets the CD33 antigen expressed on leukemic blast cells and immature normal myelomonocytic cells, but not stem cells. Once the Fab portion of the mAb attaches to this antigen, it is internalized into the cell, bringing with it the poison, much like a Trojan horse. The calicheamicin binds to DNA, causes double-stranded breaks, and causes the cell to undergo apoptosis. Following premedication with diphenhydramine 50 mg orally and acetaminophen 650–1,000 mg orally, the initial dose of 9 mg/m² IV infusion is given over two hours, followed by a repeated dose in 14 days even if the bone marrow has not recovered. If the patient's white blood cell (WBC) count is more than 30,000/mm³, then the patient should be leukoreduced with hydroxyurea or leukapheresis to bring the count to less than 30,000/mm³ to minimize the risk of pulmonary leukostasis and tumor lysis syndrome (Wyeth Pharmaceuticals, 2007). Measures to prevent hyperuricemia and tumor lysis syndrome should be instituted (e.g., hydration, allopurinol), and the patient should be monitored during and following the infusion for at least four hours. Acute infusion reactions, including anaphylaxis, may occur. The drug should be interrupted if the patient develops dyspnea or severe hypotension and, in general, should be discontinued if the patient develops anaphylaxis, pulmonary edema, or ARDS. Acute pulmonary events are uncommon but may occur, especially in individuals with ILD and who have a WBC count of more than 30,000/mm^3. Acute pulmonary events that could arise include dyspnea, pulmonary infiltrates, pleural effusions, noncardiogenic pulmonary edema, hypoxia, and ARDS. A postinfusion reaction characterized by chills and fever and, less commonly, hypotension and/or dyspnea, may occur within 24 hours of the drug infusion. Most commonly, reaction occurs soon after the infusion is completed and resolves with diphenhydramine, acetaminophen, and fluids. The reaction is less common after the second drug dose.

As expected, gemtuzumab causes severe myelosuppression. Other side effects include nausea, vomiting, and, rarely, hepatotoxicity including veno-occlusive disease (VOD). VOD is evidenced by rapid weight gain, right upper quadrant pain, hepatomegaly, ascites, and elevated bilirubin and/or liver enzymes.

Epidermal Growth Factor Receptor Inhibitors

EGFR inhibitors include both mAbs and tyrosine kinase inhibitors (TKIs) (small molecules given orally). The EGFR is a receptor to tyrosine kinase that regulates cell growth and differentiation. When it is mutated or overexpressed, or when an overabundance of the ligand EGF exists, EGFR leads to cell proliferation, angiogenesis, and resistance to apoptosis, invasion, and metastasis. The aberrant signaling can be blocked at the extracellular domain by the mAbs cetuximab and panitumumab as previously discussed or by inhibiting the intracellular domain by TKIs. Normally, the message (cell signal) reaches the tyrosine kinase just inside the cell membrane. The tyrosine kinase phosphorylates or adds a phosphate group from adenosine triphosphate (ATP), and this sends the message along to the next signaling molecule in the pathway like a "bucket brigade" until it reaches the nucleus to bring about DNA transcription. This leads to protein synthesis, which directs cell growth and other functions. Protein kinases regulate cell signaling pathways in all cells and commonly are mutated in cancer (Weinberg, 2007). TKIs block the ATP binding domain so that phosphorylation, and hence signal transduction, cannot occur. Names of TKIs have a suffix that ends in "inib." Compared to EGFR inhibitor mAbs, rash that occurs with TKIs is less severe in general, but diarrhea tends to be more frequent and severe. These agents, side effects, and indications are shown in Table 4-2.

Erlotinib (Tarceva®, OSI Pharmaceuticals, Inc. and Genentech, Inc.): The bioavailability of the oral agent erlotinib increases from 60% to about 100% when taken with food; thus, the drug should be taken one hour before or two hours after a meal. The usual dose is 150 mg once a day. Studies showed no advantage when given together with chemotherapy (OSI Pharmaceuticals, Inc. & Genentech, Inc., 2007). The drug is metabolized by the CYP3A4 microenzyme system in the liver and thus has potential drug interactions. Inducers increase metabolism (e.g., rifampin, phenytoin, phenobarbital, St. John's wort, carbamazepine, rifapentine, rifabutin); therefore, the dose may need to be increased. Inhibitors may decrease metabolism (e.g., ketoconazole, itraconazole, grapefruit or grapefruit juice, clarithromycin, metronidazole, isoniazid, telithromycin, voriconazole), and as such, the dose may need to be decreased. Interaction with warfarin may increase international normalized ratio (INR), so this should be monitored closely.

Other Kinase Inhibitors

Many redundant cell signaling pathways exist, most of which are regulated by tyrosine kinases, and several FDA-approved multitargeted TKIs are available.

Imatinib mesylate (Gleevec®): This designer drug inhibits Bcr-Abl tyrosine kinase, which is mutated in Philadelphia-positive chronic myeloid leukemia. In addition, the drug inhibits c-kit, which is mutated in gastrointestinal stromal tumor, as well as tyrosine kinases for platelet-derived growth factor (PDGF) and stem cell factor. Dasatinib (Sprycel®, Bristol-Myers Squibb Co.) is a multitargeted TKI that targets a number of kinases, including Bcr-Abl, c-kit, and PDGF-beta.

Imatinib mesylate (Gleevec®, Novartis Pharmaceuticals Corp.) has a variety of doses for its many indications. It is metabolized by the cytochrome P450 microenzyme system, especially CYP3A4, and has a number of potential drug interactions. Drugs that may increase imatinib concentrations (substrates) are ketoconazole, itraconazole, erythromycin, and clarithromycin. Drugs that may decrease imatinib concentrations are St. John's wort, dexamethasone, phenytoin, carbamazepine, rifampin, and phenobarbital (inducers). In addition, a number of drugs may have their plasma concentrations altered, including warfarin; if patients require anticoagulation, they should receive either low-molecular-weight heparin or unfractionated heparin (Novartis Pharmaceuticals Corp., 2006).

Dasatinib (Sprycel): This agent is able to overcome imatinib mesylate resistance. It is also metabolized by CYP3A4. Potential drug interactions include inducers, which decrease dasatinib plasma concentration and include dexamethasone, phenytoin, carbamazepine, rifampin, and pentobarbital, and substrates, which alter concentrations of alfentanil, cisapride, cyclosporine, fentanyl, pimozide, quinidine, sirolimus, tacrolimus, and ergotamine. Patients should avoid concurrent administration with St. John's wort, antacids, and proton pump inhibitors. The usual dose is 70 mg orally twice a day, taken in the morning and evening, because of the drug's short half-life (average terminal half-life is three to five hours) (Bristol-Myers Squibb Co., 2006).

Angiogenesis Inhibitors

Agents that can block either the ligand VEGF or the receptor tyrosine kinase on the endothelial cell can theoretically prevent tumor growth. Bevacizumab (Avastin) was the first angiogenesis inhibitor to be approved, and it has been followed by two multitargeted kinase inhibitors, sorafenib (Nexavar®, Bayer HealthCare Pharmaceuticals and Onyx Pharmaceuticals, Inc.) and sunitinib (Sutent®, Pfizer Inc.). It is hypothesized that the improved response and patient survival rates with angiogenesis inhibitors when combined with chemotherapy are attributable to normalization of tumor vasculature, permitting entrance of chemotherapy into tumor cells (Hurwitz et al., 2004; Jain, 2001). Tumor blood vessels have multiple structural and functional aberrations, making them leaky, with some vessels dilated and others constricted or even dead-ended, thus preventing distribution of chemotherapy into the tumor (Baluk, Hashizume, & McDonald, 2005).

Hypertension is a class effect for this type of drug. Normal blood pressure depends upon nitric oxide for vasodilation, which depends upon VEGF. It is postulated that antiangiogenesis agents block nitric oxide, leading to vasoconstriction and a class effect of hypertension (Pande et al., 2006). In addition, angiogenesis is necessary for healing, so inhibition will lead to delayed wound healing. Finally, bleeding (i.e., epistaxis, but with risk of hemorrhage) and possible GI perforation also are class effects.

Sorafenib (Nexavar): The oral agent sorafenib targets the VEGF1, 2, and 3 receptors on the endothelial cell, as well as PDGF (both alpha and beta), FLT3, and c-kit. It is both antiangiogenic and antiproliferative and is the first FDA-approved multikinase inhibitor. Drug interactions include CYP2C9 substrates (e.g., warfarin [monitor INR closely]), CYP3A4 inducers (e.g., rifampin, St. John's wort, phenytoin, phenobarbital, dexamethasone [expect decreased serum levels of sorafenib]), and antineoplastic agents (e.g., doxorubicin, irinotecan [do not coadminister]). The usual dose is 400 mg orally twice a day, taken one hour before or two hours after eating.

Sunitinib (Sutent): This oral agent targets multiple kinases and, similar to sorafenib, inhibits both angiogenesis and cell proliferation. Drug interactions are possible: CYP3A4 inhibitors (e.g., ketoconazole, itraconazole, clarithromycin, indinavir and others, telithromycin, voriconazole, grapefruit or grapefruit juice [do not coadminister, if possible]) and CYP inducers (e.g., rifampin, dexamethasone, phenytoin, phenobarbital, St. John's wort [avoid coadministration, if possible]). Drug dose is 50 mg orally once a day for four weeks followed by two weeks off.

Cytokines

Cytokines are substances released from activated lymphocytes that communicate between immune cells or affect the behavior of other immune cells. This group includes interleukins, interferons, tumor necrosis factor, and colony-stimulating factors. These agents are summarized in Table 4-3.

Table 4-3. Cytokines in Cancer Treatment

Drug Class	Mechanism of Action	Drug	Side Effects and Comments
Cytokines			
Interleukin-2	Produced by T cells after antibody-antigen reaction to amplify the immune response	Aldesleukin (Proleukin®, Chiron Therapeutics)	Flu-like syndrome (chills, rigors, fever, headache, myalgia, arthralgia, malaise, anorexia, asthenia); hypotension with high dose (HD); capillary leak syndrome with HD; nausea, vomiting, diarrhea; hepatotoxicity; renal dysfunction; anemia, thrombocytopenia; rash
Interferon (IF) alfa	IF-α: stimulated by viruses and tumor cells; antiviral activity > antiproliferative > immunomodulatory activity; there are at least 20 subtypes	IF-α: IF alfa-2a (Roferon®-A, Roche Pharmaceuticals) IF-α-2b (Intron® A, Schering Corp.)	Fever, chills, headache, myalgias, fatigue, nausea, vomiting, anorexia, diarrhea, depression, suicidal ideation, alopecia, blood disorders, increased liver function tests; injection site discomfort
IF beta	IF-ß: stimulated by viruses; equal antiviral, antiproliferative, and immunomodulatory activity; two subtypes	IF-ß-1a (Avonex®, Biogen Idec Inc.)	Flu-like symptoms (fever, chills, diaphoresis, myalgias, fatigue), depression, hepatotoxicity, allergic reactions

(Continued on next page)

Table 4-3. Cytokines in Cancer Treatment *(Continued)*

Drug Class	Mechanism of Action	Drug	Side Effects and Comments
IF gamma	IF-γ: produced by activated T cells and natural killer cells, involved in regulating immune and inflammatory response	IF-γ-1b (Actimmune®, InterMune, Inc.)	Neutropenia, thrombocytopenia, hepatotoxicity, decreased mental status, unsteady gait, dizziness, flu-like symptoms, worsening of cardiac dysfunction
Colony-Stimulating Factors (CSFs)			
Erythropoietin	Stimulates erythropoiesis in the same way that endogenous erythropoietin does	Darbepoetin alfa (Aranesp®, Amgen Inc.) Epoetin alfa (Procrit®, Ortho Biotech)	Uncommon headache, diarrhea, risk of thrombosis if hemoglobin > 12 g/dl; rare red cell aplasia
Granulocyte-CSF Neutrophil cell line stimulation	Stimulates proliferation, differentiation, end-cell activation of neutrophil cell line	Filgrastim (Neupogen®, Amgen Inc.)	Bone pain, rare allergic reaction, rare splenic rupture, rare acute respiratory distress syndrome (ARDS) in neutropenic patients with sepsis
		Pegfilgrastim (Neulasta®, Amgen Inc.)	Bone pain, rare allergic reaction, rare splenic rupture, rare ARDS in neutropenic patients with sepsis
Myeloid progenitors Granulocyte macrophage–CSF	Stimulates production and differentiation of myeloid progenitor cells, including macrophages and neutrophils	Sargramostim (Leukine®, Berlex)	Flu-like syndrome, bone pain, rash, injection site reaction; rare dyspnea, supraventricular arrhythmias, renal and hepatic dysfunction

Note. This table does not review indications, as they change frequently. Please consult the manufacturer's product information, as well as the U.S. Food and Drug Administration (FDA) Center for Drug Evaluation and Research Web site (www.accessdata.fda.gov/scripts/cder/drugsatfda/index.cfm) or the Oncology Nursing Society (ONS) e-mail alert that notifies ONS members when a new drug or new indication is approved by the FDA.

Note. Based on information from manufacturers' prescribing information.

Gene Therapy

As cancer is a disease of cellular mutations, gene therapy offers the promise of normalization of mutated oncogenes, tumor suppressor genes, and mismatch repair genes, as well as significant genes such as *TP53* and cell cycle genes. However, this work is still investigational (NCI, 2006).

Resources

The Oncology Nursing Society (ONS) has established standards for oncology nurses who are administering chemotherapy and caring for patients receiving chemotherapy or biotherapy in the *Chemotherapy and Biotherapy Guidelines and Recommendations for Practice* (Second Edition) (Polovich et al., 2005). This comprehensive resource should be used for principles of drug administration, specific chemotherapy and biotherapy drug toxicities, and assessment and management of patients receiving these agents. ONS also has developed Putting Evidence Into Practice® (PEP) cards, which are a valuable resource in summarizing the evidence for the management of fatigue, sleep disturbances, nausea and vomiting, infection, caregiver strain and burden, constipation, depression, dyspnea, peripheral neuropathy, mucositis, pain, bleeding, anorexia, anxiety, diarrhea, and lymphedema (ONS, n.d.; see www.ons.org/outcomes/index.shtml). The American Society of Clinical Oncology (n.d.) provides practice guidelines (e.g., antiemetic use in oncology, use of WBC and erythropoietin growth factors, use of chemotherapy protectants) and quality care initiatives. NCCN has consensus-developed evidence-based guidelines that include chemotherapy and biotherapy and each tumor type and location, as well as supportive care. These guidelines are frequently updated to reflect changing practice standards.

In terms of personal protection in administering hazardous drugs, the following guides provide the national standard. The Occupational Safety and Health Administration *OSHA Technical Manual,* Section VI, Chapter 2, "Controlling Occupational Exposure to Hazardous Drugs" (1995), identifies recommended personal protective safety guidelines and a list of some hazardous drugs. However, this list does not include any new targeted therapies or most mAbs. ONS also publishes *Safe Handling of Hazardous Drugs* (Polovich, 2003). Finally, the National Institute for Occupational Safety and Health (2004) publishes *Preventing Occupational Exposure to Antineoplastic and Other Hazardous Drugs in Health Care Settings.*

Patient and Family Education

Chemotherapy has a very narrow therapeutic window. Therefore, toxicities are anticipated that would not be tolerated by patients receiving any other medications. As a result, oncology APNs have successfully developed patient and family education plans (and materials that can be individualized) for those receiving chemotherapy, as the evidence base for prevention and management of side effects becomes clearer. These include self-assessment and self-care measures to minimize infection, bleeding, fatigue, nausea and vomiting, diarrhea, cognitive dysfunction, hand-foot syndrome, and injury from peripheral neuropathy, to name a few. In addition, the APN must ensure that the patient has the knowledge required to make an informed decision to undergo therapy. Often the APN, through knowledge of the science and clinical trial data, as well as the individual strengths of the patient, can best help the patient to make a decision about which chemotherapy regimen to select when all other factors are equal, such as in patients with newly diagnosed advanced CRC. The reader is referred to specific chapters within this book that discuss in detail the patient teaching in each of these areas.

With the rapidly progressing evolution of targeted therapies, anecdotal reports form the basis for many patient and family education materials. Nurses need to work together to conduct prospective trials of potential prevention and intervention strategies to establish evidence-based practice. Skin rash and other skin complications from EGFR inhibitors are probably among the most challenging symptoms.

Implications for Oncology Advanced Practice Nurses

The APN is recognized by the patient and family as a key member of the healthcare team, advocating for the patient and family and ensuring that they understand discussions with the physician about the disease, treatment, and care planning goals. The APN prescribing chemotherapy or managing patients receiving chemotherapy must understand the potential toxicities and preassessment criteria, such as baseline bone marrow, renal, hepatic, and, depending on the drug, cardiac and other organ functions. In addition, most patients receive chemotherapy in an ambulatory care setting, with most toxicities occurring while the patient is at home. Patients must be able to self-assess and provide self-care or rely on a competent family member to do this. The APN must be able to use knowledge of differential diagnoses to evaluate patient complications between scheduled visits and work collaboratively with the triage nurse. As molecular targeted treatments become more numerous, the APN will not only have to maintain a knowledge base of this rapidly exploding field but also must be able to simplify the mechanism of action, potential side effects, and self-care measures so that patients can make informed decisions about treatment choices and management. The APN must be active in establishing the evidence base for interventions to prevent or minimize symptoms and provide structure and monitoring, as patients will be on these therapies for the rest of their lives. As these agents become approved by the FDA and are more commonly used, new toxicities will emerge that perhaps were not recognized during clinical trials of patients with very good performance status. The APN must ensure that this information is communicated to the appropriate agencies and to oncology APN colleagues. The future has never been brighter in oncology care.

Conclusion

This chapter has reviewed principles of chemotherapy and biotherapy and identified general toxicities of agents. As the understanding of malignant transformation and molecular flaws in cell signaling and function develops, this new paradigm in cancer diagnosis and treatment will continue to change. Already, genetic fingerprints of different tumor types of breast cancer have been identified (O'Shaughnessy, 2006; van't Veer et al., 2002), leading to individualized treatment planning. This has paved the way for similar study in lymphoma and colorectal, lung, and prostate cancers. Nanotechnology will allow precise, rapid diagnosis, real-time monitoring of response, and treatment. The APN must take steps to ensure knowledge and understanding of these developments in order to translate them to patients and their families and provide competent care. APNs also must take a leadership role in undertaking nursing research to provide the evidence base for new side effect prevention and management as new targeted agents are approved by the FDA.

Case Study

J.C. is a 48-year-old patient with metastatic CRC who is coming in for her first cycle of infusional FOLFOX (5-FU, leucovorin, and oxaliplatin) and bevacizumab. She had a history of bright red blood per rectum for four months but thought it was related to hemorrhoids. When she started feeling tired and lost her appetite, she went to the emergency department for evaluation, as she had no primary care provider. Her computed tomography (CT) scan showed a questionable obstructing lesion in her ascending colon, along with liver and lung metastases. She underwent a hemicolectomy to prevent obstruction. Her labs were within normal limits (WNL) except for carcinoembryonic antigen preoperatively that was 240 ng/dl, and postoperatively it was 50 ng/dl (normal < 5); alkaline phosphatase was slightly elevated at 300 u/L (normal 70–230); and her lactate dehydrogenase was 175 u/L (normal 90–190). She has no known drug allergies.

J.C. is divorced, and her two children are married and live nearby. She works as a housekeeper for a family in the nearby city. She does not smoke. She has a past medical history of type II diabetes that is well controlled by metformin 1 g po bid, exercises "in her work," and has a history of alcoholism. She goes to Alcoholics Anonymous regularly. She has a family history of cardiovascular disease but has no family history of cancer in either her mother's or father's family.

On physical examination, the APN notes a young-appearing African American woman who is in no acute distress. Her blood pressure is 120/80. Her incision is well-healed. She is appropriately sad about her diagnosis but hopeful that the treatment will "slow the cancer" so she can "live to see her grandchildren born."

J.C. has tolerated the treatment well except for acute cold-induced neuropathy that has subsequently been prevented by calcium and magnesium infusions immediately before and after the oxaliplatin infusion. Her nadir blood counts are absolute neutrophil count of 1,200/mm^3, platelet count of 100,000/mm^3, and hemoglobin of 12 g/dl. Her serum electrolytes, including magnesium and calcium, and renal and liver function tests are WNL. She has a urinalysis for protein every month, and today has trace protein in her urine. Her recent CT has shown a 50% reduction in measurable disease. She receives dexamethasone plus a serotonin antagonist to prevent nausea and vomiting. She has grade 0–1 persistent peripheral neuropathy characterized by paresthesias of fingertips and toes.

J.C. experiences a hypersensitivity reaction to her FOLFOX. After she has been stabilized, she is admitted and observed overnight. The next day, the oxaliplatin is restarted to infuse over six hours following premedication with diphenhydramine, famotidine, and dexamethasone. She tolerates the infusion without further hypersensitivity reaction. She then continues to receive six more biweekly cycles of FOLFOX and then on follow-up CT shows disease progression. She is begun on FOLFIRI (5-FU, leucovorin, and irinotecan) for three cycles, but no interval improvement is shown on CT. Her chemotherapy regimen is changed to irinotecan plus cetuximab.

1. As the APN prepares to complete an assessment prior to the patient beginning FOLFOX chemotherapy, what are five key factors to assess?
    * She is receiving oxaliplatin, which has as a cumulative dose-limiting toxicity of peripheral neuropathy. It is very important, given her past history of alcoholism and type II diabetes, that the APN does a complete neurologic examination, paying close attention to sensory peripheral neuropathy, especially that of the large fiber nerves, for position and vibration. Second, bevacizumab can cause hypertension over time, so the APN would want to know her blood pressure status. She is normotensive, and the APN would monitor this

before each treatment. Third, the clinician would assess her GI status, as she will be at risk for developing diarrhea from the 5-FU, leucovorin, and oxaliplatin. She is at risk for nausea and vomiting from the oxaliplatin, but the APN will use aggressive antiemetics to prevent this. Fourth, as she is receiving bevacizumab and has a history of diabetes, she is at risk for proteinuria. Thus, the APN would want to check a baseline urinalysis for protein and monitor this at least monthly during her treatment. Fifth, the APN would want to do a baseline nasal septum evaluation because, rarely, bevacizumab can cause nasal septum perforation.

2. She complains of a feeling of chest tightness during the oxaliplatin infusion, slight shortness of breath, and feeling very cold. Her blood pressure is 100/70 (baseline 118/80), heart rate is 120 (baseline 82), respiratory rate is 24 (baseline 13), and O_2 saturation is 92% (baseline 99%). What would the APN suspect, and how would he or she manage this?
   - Delayed hypersensitivity can occur with oxaliplatin, usually about cycle 8–12. The APN would stop the drug, provide oxygen, and reassess. If it was severe, with symptomatic bronchospasm and/or severe hypotension, the APN would give epinephrine 1:1000 IM, as well as IV saline for hypotension. The patient has already received dexamethasone, so the APN would also give her IV hydrocortisone. Patients have been successfully desensitized (Gammon, Bhargava, & McCormick, 2004), and given J.C.'s success with the current regimen, the APN would discuss this with her oncologist as well as the patient and family.

3. Prior to her first cycle of FOLFIRI, the APN reviews the potential side effects of this regimen, including potential toxicity and self-care measures with irinotecan. What areas would he or she cover in teaching the patient about cetuximab?
   - The APN would teach her that although uncommon, hypersensitivity reaction may occur during the first infusion (3% incidence, and 90% occur during the first infusion). The APN reassures her that she will be closely monitored during the infusion. The APN also tells her about possible skin changes, including rash.

4. What specific teaching would the APN give her about skin changes?
   - The APN would teach her about skin changes, which include
     (1) She may develop a sunburn-like skin effect initially, which she may not feel because she has dark skin. To manage this, she should use skin emollients to keep the skin moist and well hydrated.
     (2) The rash may get worse at about 15 days after the first treatment but will improve over time. It is very important for her not to scratch her face, as that may lead to infection. She should continue to use moisturizers and keep out of the sun, as sun exposure makes the rash worse. (She is African American and may or may not have the rash.) If she needs to go out in the sun, she should use a zinc-based sunscreen with SPF 30 or higher. She should call for anti-itch medication if an itch develops that cannot be controlled by a moisturizer.
     (3) The rash will crust over. She needs to assess her skin for the formation of blisters (vesicles), yellow crusting, or drainage. These should be reported immediately to the healthcare provider, as they may be an indication of

> infection. She may receive antibiotics (tetracycline-class antibiotic, topical and/or systemic depending upon the severity).
>
> 5. The APN also would teach her about changes in her hair and fingers. What specifically would the APN tell her?
>   - The APN would teach her that she may develop hair changes, such as thinning of the hair, scalp dryness, and lengthening of her eyelashes. It is important that J.C. notify the healthcare provider if she develops conjunctivitis or eye irritation, and she will be referred to an ophthalmologist for evaluation. Additionally, the APN teaches her that she may develop paronychia or fissures on her fingers. She should wear gloves when working around the house or doing dishes, and she needs to let the healthcare provider know if this occurs and is difficult to manage. The APN will then advise her about and may prescribe steroid tape if this becomes uncomfortable.

Key Points

- Advances in the development of chemotherapy include nanotechnology.
- Major advances have occurred in the understanding of cancer and biologic pathways, resulting in targeted agents that are changing the paradigm of cancer care.
- Chemotherapy most often interferes with frequently dividing normal cell populations, including bone marrow, gonads, hair follicles, and GI mucosa, with resulting potential problems of myelosuppression, infertility, alopecia, and mucositis (including diarrhea).
- Biotherapy and targeted therapy require vigilance to prevent and/or intervene rapidly and efficiently if hypersensitivity reactions occur.
- Antiangiogenesis agents have class effects including hypertension and bleeding.
- EGFR inhibitors have class effects including sterile, inflammatory rash, diarrhea, hypomagnesemia (mAbs), and ILD.
- Advances in targeted therapy are occurring frequently. APNs must understand cell physiology, cell signaling, angiogenesis, and other vital cell functions to be able to prepare patients for treatment.

Recommended Resources for Patient Teaching

- American Society of Clinical Oncology: People Living With Cancer "Managing Side Effects" Web page (see www.plwc.org)
- CancerCare: *Managing Rash and Other Skin Reactions to Targeted Treatments,* by R.S. Herbst, L.P. Fox, C.S. Viele, and C. Messner, 2007. Available from CancerCare at www.cancercare.org/pdf/booklets/ccc_managing_rash.pdf. This organization offers many other self-empowering resources related to chemotherapy side effects at www.cancercare.org/about_us/connect_booklets.php.
- ONS: Symptom management information (www.cancersymptoms.org; Ask an Oncology Nurse: www.cancersymptoms.org/questions); "NeutroPhil" neutropenia patient education booklet (www.ons.org/patiented/symptom/documents/booklet.pdf)

Recommended Resources for Oncology Advanced Practice Nurses

- FDA Center for Drug Evaluation and Research Oncology Tools Web site: www.fda .gov/cder/cancer/index.htm
- ONS mailing list: ONS offers a subscription e-mail list that members can join to be notified when a new drug or new drug indications have been approved by the FDA. See www.ons.org/fda/archives.shtml for a list of archived FDA messages regarding new cancer drug approvals and updates, and a link for ONS members to join the list serve.

References

Abraxis Oncology. (2007, May). Abraxane [Package insert]. Los Angeles: Author.

Adams, G.P., & Weiner, L.M. (2005). Monoclonal antibody therapy of cancer. *Nature Biotechnology, 23,* 1147–1153.

Alza Corporation. (2007, December). Doxil [Package insert]. Mountain View, CA: Author.

American Society of Clinical Oncology. (n.d.). *Supportive care and quality of life practice guidelines.* Retrieved January 29, 2007, from http://www.asco.org/portal/site/ASCO/menuitem.509189bfd2c2bf5ca7ffa 807320041a0/?vgnextoid=04d61f886024a010VgnVCM100000ed730ad1RCRD

Balazsovits, J.A., Mayer, L.D., Bally, M.B., Cullis, P.R., McDonell, M., Ginsberg, R.S., et al. (1989). Analysis of the effect of liposome encapsulation on the vesicant properties, acute and cardiac toxicities, and antitumor efficacy of doxorubicin. *Cancer Chemotherapy and Pharmacology, 23,* 81–86.

Baluk, P., Hashizume, H., & McDonald, D.M. (2005). Cellular abnormalities of blood vessels as targets in cancer. *Current Opinion in Genetics and Development, 15,* 102–111.

Baselga, J., Perez, E.A., Pienkowski, T., & Bell, R. (2006). Adjuvant trastuzumab: A milestone in the treatment of HER-2-positive early breast cancer. *Oncologist, 11*(Suppl. 1), 4–12.

Berinstein, N.L., Grillo-Lopez, A.J., White, C.A., Bence-Bruckler, I., Maloney, D., Czuczman, M., et al. (1998). Association of serum rituximab (IDEC-C2B8) concentration and anti-tumor response in the treatment of recurrent low-grade or follicular non-Hodgkin's lymphoma. *Annals of Oncology, 9,* 995–1001.

Bristol-Myers Squibb Co. (2006, July). Sprycel [Package insert]. Princeton, NJ: Author.

Carlson, R.W., Moench, S.J., Hammond, M.E., Perez, E.A., Burstein, H.J., Allred, D.C., et al. (2006). HER2 testing in breast cancer: NCCN Task Force report and recommendations. *Journal of the National Comprehensive Cancer Network, 4*(Suppl. 3), S1–S22.

Chobanian, A.V., Bakris, G.L., Black, H.R., Cushman, W.C., Green, L.A., Izzo, J.L., Jr., et al. (2003). The seventh report of the Joint National Committee on prevention, detection, evaluation, and treatment of high blood pressure: The JNC 7 report. *JAMA, 289,* 2560–2572.

Citron, M.L., Berry, D.A., Cirrincione, C., Hudis, C., Winer, E.P., Gradishar, W.J., et al. (2003). Randomized trial of dose-dense versus conventionally scheduled and sequential versus concurrent combination chemotherapy as postoperative adjuvant treatment of node-positive primary breast cancer: First report of Intergroup Trial C9741/Cancer and Leukemia Group B Trial 9741. *Journal of Clinical Oncology, 21,* 1431–1439.

Dincer, M., & Altundag, K. (2006). Angiotensin-converting enzyme inhibitors for bevacizumab-induced hypertension. *Annals of Pharmacotherapy, 40,* 2278–2279.

Eli Lilly and Company. (2006, July). Gemzar [Package insert]. Indianapolis, IN: Author.

Feldweg, A.M., Lee, C.W., Matulonis, U.A., & Castells, M. (2005). Rapid desensitization for hypersensitivity reactions to paclitaxel and docetaxel: A new standard protocol used in 77 successful treatments. *Gynecologic Oncology, 96,* 824–829.

Fisher, R.I., Gaynor, E.R., Dahlberg, S., Oken, M.M., Grogan, T.M., Mize, E.M., et al. (1993). Comparison of a standard regimen (CHOP) with three intensive chemotherapy regimens for advanced non-Hodgkin lymphoma. *New England Journal of Medicine, 324,* 1002–1006.

Gamelin, L., Boisdron-Celle, M., Delva, R., Guerin-Meyer, V., Ifrah, N., Morel, A., et al. (2004). Prevention of oxaliplatin-related neurotoxicity by calcium and magnesium infusions. *Clinical Cancer Research, 10*(12, Pt. 1), 4055–4061.

Gammon, D., Bhargava, P., & McCormick, M.J. (2004). Hypersensitivity reactions to oxaliplatin and the application of a desensitization protocol. *Oncologist, 9,* 546–549.

Genentech, Inc. (2007, September). Avastin [Package insert]. South San Francisco, CA: Author.

Genentech, Inc. (2008a, January). Herceptin [Package insert]. South San Francisco, CA: Author.

Genentech, Inc. (2008b, January). Rituxan [Package insert]. South San Francisco, CA: Author.

Hanahan, D., & Weinberg, R. (2000). The hallmarks of cancer. *Cell, 100,* 57–70.

Higenbottam, T., Kuwano, K., Nemery, B., & Fujita, Y. (2004). Understanding the mechanisms of drug-associated interstitial lung disease. *British Journal of Cancer, 91*(Suppl. 2), S31–S37.

Hurwitz, H., Fehrenbacher, L., Novotny, W., Cartwright, T., Hainsworth, J., Heim, W., et al. (2004). Bevacizumab plus irinotecan, fluorouracil, and leucovorin for metastatic colorectal cancer. *New England Journal of Medicine, 350,* 2335–2342.

ImClone Systems, Inc. & Bristol-Myers Squibb Co. (2007, November). Erbitux [Package insert]. Branchburg and Princeton, NJ: Authors.

Jain, P.K. (2001). Normalizing tumor vasculature with antiangiogenic therapy: A new paradigm for combination therapy. *Natural Medicine, 7,* 987–989.

Kops, G.J., Weaver, B.A., & Cleveland, D.W. (2005). On the road to cancer: Aneuploidy and the mitotic checkpoint. *Nature Reviews Cancer, 5,* 773–785.

Kozloff, M., Hainsworth, J., Badarinath, A., Cohn, P.J., Flynn, W., Dong, S., et al. (2007). Management of hypertension (HTN) in patients (pts) with metastatic colorectal cancer treated with bevacizumab (BV) plus chemotherapy. *American Society of Clinical Oncology, 2007 Gastrointestinal Cancers Symposium,* Abstract 364. Retrieved February 18, 2008, from http://www.asco.org/ASCO/Abstracts

Lacouture, M.E. (2006). Mechanisms of cutaneous toxicities to EGFR inhibitors. *Nature Reviews Cancer, 6,* 803–812.

Lacouture, M.E., Basti, S., Patel, J., & Benson, A. (2006). The SERIES clinic: An interdisciplinary approach to the management of toxicities of EGFR inhibitors. *Journal of Supportive Oncology, 4,* 236–238.

Larson, D.L. (1985). What is the appropriate management of tissue extravasation by antitumor agents? *Plastic and Reconstructive Surgery, 75,* 397–405.

Margulies, D.H. (2005). Monoclonal antibodies: Producing magic bullets by somatic cell hybridization. *Journal of Immunology, 174,* 2451–2452.

Markman, M., Kennedy, A., Webster, K., Kulp, B., Peterson, G., & Belinson, J. (2000). Paclitaxel-associated hypersensitivity reactions: Experience of the gynecologic oncology program of the Cleveland Clinic Cancer Center. *Journal of Clinical Oncology, 18,* 102–105.

Mass, R.D. (2004). The HER receptor family: A rich target for therapeutic development. *International Journal of Radiation Oncology, Biology, Physics, 58,* 932–940.

Merkle, C.J., & Loescher, L.J. (2005). Biology of cancer. In C.H. Yarbro, M.H. Frogge, & M. Goodman (Eds.), *Cancer nursing: Principles and practice* (6th ed., pp. 3–26). Sudbury, MA: Jones and Bartlett.

Mould, D.R., Fleming, G.F., Darcy, K.M., & Spriggs, D. (2006). Population analysis of a 24-h paclitaxel infusion in advanced endometrial cancer: A gynaecological oncology group study. *British Journal of Clinical Pharmacology, 62,* 56–70.

Muehlbauer, P.M., Cusack, G., & Morris, J.C. (2006). Monoclonal antibodies and side-effect management. *Oncology (Williston Park), 20*(10, Suppl. Nurse Ed.), 11–27.

National Cancer Institute. (2006). *Gene therapy for cancer: Questions and answers.* Retrieved February 1, 2007, from http://www.cancer.gov/cancertopics/factsheet/Therapy/gene

National Cancer Institute. (2007, January). *The NCI strategic plan for leading the nation to eliminate the suffering and death due to cancer.* Retrieved January 19, 2007, from http://strategicplan.nci.nih.gov/pdf/nci_2007_strategic_plan.pdf

National Comprehensive Cancer Network. (2008). *NCCN clinical practice guidelines in oncology: Breast cancer v. 2.2008.* Retrieved February 18, 2008, from http://www.nccn.org/professionals/physician_gls/PDF/breast.pdf

National Institute for Occupational Safety and Health. (2004, September). *Preventing occupational exposure to antineoplastic and other hazardous drugs in health care settings* [NIOSH Publication No. 2004-165]. Retrieved February 1, 2007, from http://www.cdc.gov/niosh/docs/2004-165

Norton, L., & Simon, R. (1977). Tumor size, sensitivity to therapy, and design of treatment schedules. *Cancer Treatment Reports, 61,* 1307–1317.

Novartis Pharmaceuticals Corporation. (2006, June). Gleevec [Package insert]. East Hanover, NJ: Author.

Occupational Safety and Health Administration. (1995). *OSHA technical manual, section VI, chapter 2: Controlling occupational exposure to hazardous drugs.* Retrieved January 29, 2007, from http://www.osha.gov/dts/osta/otm/otm_vi/otm_vi_2.html

O'Keefe, P., Parrilli, M., & Lacouture, M.E. (2006). Toxicity of targeted therapy: Focus on rash and other dermatologic side effects. *Oncology (Williston Park), 20*(13, Suppl. Nurse Ed.), 25–30.

Oncology Nursing Society. (n.d.). *Outcomes resource area: Putting evidence into practice.* Retrieved April 15, 2007, from http://www.ons.org/outcomes/index.shtml

O'Reilly, M.S. (2002). Targeting multiple biological pathways as a strategy to improve the treatment of cancer. *Clinical Cancer Research, 8,* 3309–3310.

O'Shaughnessy, J.A. (2006). Molecular signatures predict outcomes in breast cancer. *New England Journal of Medicine, 355,* 615–617.

OSI Pharmaceuticals, Inc. & Genentech, Inc. (2007, May). Tarceva [Package insert]. Melville, NY, and South San Francisco, CA: Authors.

Pande, A.U., Lombardo, J.C., Fakih, M., Wong, M.K., Iyer, R.V., Kuvshinoff, B.W., et al. (2006). Bevacizumab (BV) induced hypertension (HT): A manageable toxicity. *Journal of Clinical Oncology, 2006 ASCO Annual Meeting Proceedings (Post-Meeting Edition), 24*(18S), Abstract 13539.

Pardee, A.B. (1974). A restriction point for control of normal animal cell proliferation. *Proceedings of the National Academy of Sciences, 71,* 1286–1290.

Perez-Soler, R., Delord, J.P., Halpern, A., Kelly, K., Krueger, J., Sureda, B.M., et al. (2005). HER1-EGFR inhibitor associated rash: Future directions for management and investigation outcomes from the HER1/EGFR inhibitor rash management forum. *Oncologist, 10,* 345–356.

Peus, D., Hamacher, L., & Pittelkow, M.R. (1997). EGF-receptor tyrosine kinase inhibition induces keratinocyte growth arrest and terminal differentiation. *Journal of Investigational Dermatology, 109,* 751–756.

Pfizer Inc. (2006, June). Camptosar [Package insert]. New York: Author.

Polovich, M. (Ed.). (2003). *Safe handling of hazardous drugs.* Pittsburgh, PA: Oncology Nursing Society.

Polovich, M., White, J.M., & Kelleher, L.O. (Eds.). (2005). *Chemotherapy and biotherapy guidelines and recommendations for practice* (2nd ed.). Pittsburgh, PA: Oncology Nursing Society.

Rhee, J., Oishi, K., Garey, J., & Kim, E. (2005). Management of rash and other toxicities in patients treated with epidermal growth factor receptor-targeted agents. *Clinical Colorectal Cancer, 5,* 101–106.

Rieger, P.T. (2001). Biotherapy: An overview. In P.T. Rieger (Ed.), *Biotherapy: A comprehensive overview* (2nd ed., pp. 3–23). Sudbury, MA: Jones and Bartlett.

Romond, E.H., Perez, E.A., Bryant, J., Suman, V.J., Geyer, C.E., Davidson, N.E., et al. (2005). Trastuzumab plus adjuvant chemotherapy for operable HER-2 positive breast cancer. *New England Journal of Medicine, 353,* 1673–1684.

Sapadin, A.N., & Fleischmajer, R. (2006). Tetracyclines: Nonantibiotic properties and their clinical applications. *Journal of the American Academy of Dermatology, 54,* 258–265.

Schulmeister, L. (1999). Chemotherapy medication errors: Descriptions, severity, and contributing factors. *Oncology Nursing Forum, 26,* 1033–1042.

Seidman, A., Hudis, C., Pierri, M.K., Shak, S., Paton, V., Ashby, M., et al. (2002). Cardiac dysfunction in the trastuzumab clinical trials experience. *Journal of Clinical Oncology, 20,* 1215–1221.

Shu, K.Y., Kindler, H.L., Medenica, M., & Lacouture, M.E. (2006). Doxycycline for the treatment of paronychia induced by the epidermal growth factor receptor inhibitor cetuximab. *British Journal of Dermatology, 154,* 191–192.

Skipper, H.E. (1971). Kinetics of mammary tumor cell growth and implications for therapy. *Cancer, 28,* 1479–1499.

Sliwkowski, M.X., Lofgren, J.A., Lewis, G.D., Hotaling, T.E., Fendly, B.M., & Fox, J.A. (1999). Nonclinical studies addressing the mechanism of action of trastuzumab (Herceptin). *Seminars in Oncology, 26*(Suppl. 12), 60–70.

Smith, M.R. (2003). Rituximab (monoclonal anti-CD20 antibody): Mechanisms of action and resistance. *Oncogene, 22,* 7359–7368.

Sparreboom, A., van Zuylen, L., Brouwer, E., Loos, W.J., de Bruijn, P., Gelderblom, H., et al. (1999). Cremophor EL-mediated alteration of paclitaxel distribution in human blood: Clinical pharmacokinetic implications. *Cancer Research, 59,* 1454–1457.

Tortorice, P.V. (2005). Chemotherapy: Principles of therapy. In C.H. Yarbro, M.H. Frogge, & M. Goodman (Eds.), *Cancer nursing: Principles and practice* (6th ed., pp. 315–350). Sudbury, MA: Jones and Bartlett.

U.S. Food and Drug Administration. (2006, December 18). *FDA warns of safety concern regarding Rituxan in new patient population.* Retrieved January 29, 2007, from http://www.fda.gov/bbs/topics/NEWS/2006/NEW01532.html

U.S. Food and Drug Administration Center for Drug Evaluation and Research. (1999, April). *FDA oncology tools product label details for administration of bleomycin.* Retrieved April 21, 2007, from http://www.accessdata.fda.gov/scripts/cder/onctools/administer.cfm?GN=bleomycin

van Heeckeren, W.J., Ortiz, J., Cooney, M.W., & Remick, S.C. (2007). Hypertension, proteinuria, and antagonism of vascular endothelial growth factor signaling: Clinical toxicity, therapeutic target, or novel biomarker? *Journal of Clinical Oncology, 25,* 2993–2995.

van't Veer, L.J., Dai, H., van de Vijver, M.J., He, Y.D., Hart, A.A., Mao, M., et al. (2002). Gene expression profiling predicts clinical outcome of breast cancer. *Nature, 415,* 530–536.

Von Eschenbach, A. (2006). Progress with a purpose: Eliminating suffering and death due to cancer. *Oncology, 20,* 1691–1696.

Weinberg, R.A. (2007). *The biology of cancer.* New York: Garland Science.

Wilkes, G.M. (2005). Therapeutic options in the management of colon cancer: 2005 update. *Clinical Journal of Oncology Nursing, 9,* 31–44.

Woodworth, C.D., Michael, E., Marker, D., Allen, S., Smith, L., & Nees, M. (2005). Inhibition of the epidermal growth factor receptor increases expression of genes that stimulate inflammation, apoptosis, and cell attachment. *Molecular Cancer Therapeutics, 4,* 650–658.

Wyeth Pharmaceuticals. (2007, January). Mylotarg [Package insert]. Philadelphia: Author.

Zhu, Z., Bohlen, P., & Witte, L. (2002). Clinical development of angiogenesis inhibitors to vascular endothelial growth factor and its receptors as cancer therapeutics. *Current Cancer Drug Targets, 2,* 135–156.

CHAPTER 5

Surgery

Joanne Lester, PhD, CRNP, ANP-BC, AOCN®

Introduction

Surgical oncology is a branch of medicine that deals with the management and eradication of malignant neoplasms. Surgery, as an intervention, is the oldest treatment modality for cancer. Today, surgical intervention remains an integral component in the care of patients with cancer. Adequate surgical resection of solid tumors is an important strategy and mainstay in the cure of many cancers (Lopez, 2005).

Surgical oncology involves the prevention of cancer occurrence, diagnosis of a primary or metastatic site, surgical resection as a primary or secondary treatment, postoperative care, surgical access for administration of therapy, rehabilitation with reconstructive procedures, surveillance for recurrence and second primaries, and palliation with symptom management. Oncologic emergencies also may necessitate a surgical procedure for resolution. The advanced practice nurse (APN) is an integral member of the surgical oncology healthcare team throughout the cancer trajectory. Surgical oncology, together with medical and radiation oncology, constitute the framework of the oncology healthcare team and are the mainstays of cancer care (Lester, 2007).

The history of cancer treatment has progressed to multiple modalities, adding and subtracting interventions in a hierarchal and logical process. A single modality approach is unlikely to provide the optimum outcome for most patients. Surgery is one of several interventions used for cancer control, with recommendations based on studies matching patients related to disease status and characteristics and use of prior therapies. This methodical approach is necessary to obtain the highest yield for each patient with the lowest toxicity possible (Wagman, 2007).

This chapter outlines current surgical oncology evidence-based interventions and management of common cancers. It discusses innovative interventional radiology techniques and minimally invasive surgical procedures, all aimed at patient comfort and cure. The APN is adjunct to the cancer experience using evidence-based practice for nursing-sensitive patient outcomes regarding cancer and symptom management.

Surgical Oncologic Strategies

Surgery is central to the care of the patients, providing strategies in cancer prevention, diagnosis, resection, postoperative care, access, rehabilitation, surveillance, and palliation (see Figure 5-1). The surgical healthcare team consists of physicians, APNs, RNs, ancillary staff, and support personnel. This team is a common thread throughout the cancer trajectory, offering expert assessment, psychosocial support, education, symptom management, and prevention of complications. The *prevention* of cancer in high-risk patients results from improvements in the understanding of cancer biology, thus enabling risk assessment, screening, and potentially life-saving interventions, including prophylactic surgical procedures. The surgical *diagnosis* of cancer employs innovative techniques for cancer discovery to allow treatment at its earliest stage with expectation of cure. The surgical *resection* of cancer allows for removal of cancerous tissue and accurate staging of disease. Today, less invasive surgical procedures are possible because of advances in bioengineering and biotechnology and utilization of interventional approaches. *Postoperative care* involves maintenance or reestablishment of homeostasis, with prevention of complications related to surgical intervention. Surgically implanted *access* devices provide necessary routes for nutrition, medications, and chemotherapy, while affording additional comfort to the patient. *Rehabilitation* after the cancer diagnosis employs surgical procedures that repair or reconstruct to enhance function and well-being. *Surveillance* of patients with cancer and their family provides screening and periodic observation to detect recurrent cancer, hereditary syndromes, or subsequent primary cancers. Finally, surgical *palliation* utilizes interventions in tumor control and symptom management for patients with recurrent or metastatic disease or in cancers that challenge a curative surgical approach.

This model, as illustrated in Figure 5-1, is an effective framework to enable collaborative relationships between APNs and other members of the surgical oncology healthcare team (hereafter, surgical team). These strategies of the surgical trajectory can undergo expansion, repetition, reversal, or omission based on individual characteristics of patients and families. APN interventions in colorectal cancer illustrate application of the model (see Table 5-1).

Prevention and Early Detection

The surgical team often is involved in the screening, early detection, and prevention of cancer. A thorough medical history is important to obtain information that can reduce the incidence, morbidity, and mortality of certain cancers. An accurate personal and family history identifies patterns related to familial and genetic predispositions, with genetic counseling referral as indicated. Information about health behaviors, risks, and personal habits can target behaviors that affect cancer occurrence, such as smoking, alcohol intake, dietary patterns, and exercise habits. Discussion of risk reduction strategies enables adjustment of behaviors to reduce the overall cancer risk (Vogel, 2003).

Routine screening practices potentially reduce the incidence, morbidity, and mortality of common cancers such as breast, cervical, colorectal, prostate, and skin. Investigation of the absence or presence of cancer can involve physical examination, radiographic and serum studies, screening interventions (such as colonoscopy), and/or tissue sampling. Screening for asymptomatic or unrecognized cancers and/or subsequent evaluation of abnormal screening results often are responsibilities of the surgical team

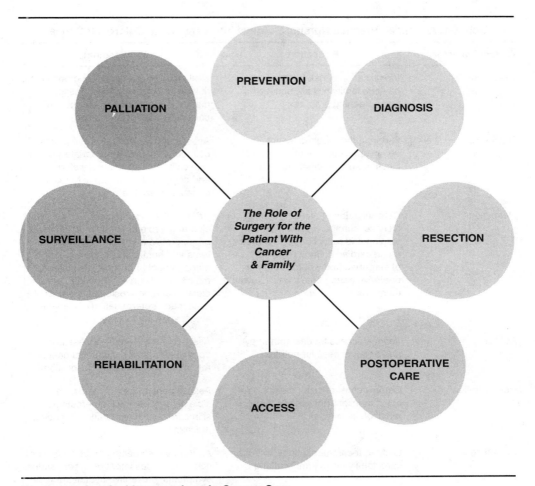

Figure 5-1. Surgical Interventions in Cancer Care

(Duffy, McCann, Godward, Gabe, & Warwick, 2006; Port, Park, Borgen, Morris, & Montgomery, 2007). Surgeons frequently are the primary provider of health care, especially in otherwise healthy patients. As such, these surgical visits must include education for patients and families about genetic risk factors and potential occurrence of related cancers or familial involvement.

Another fundamental responsibility of the surgical team is individual risk assessment with evaluation of patient eligibility for prophylactic surgical interventions. Patients identified as having a significantly increased risk of cancers such as testicular, colon, thyroid, breast, and ovarian may benefit from removal of the nonvital organ. In-depth discussion about the cancer risk, as opposed to the risk and morbidity of surgery, often arises. Possible chemoprevention strategies also deserve exploration and discussion (Morrow & Jordan, 2006). The surgical team needs to remain current with evidence-based practice for chemoprevention. These surgical and chemoprevention strategies must be tailored to the specific cancer and individual based on the patient's personal health history, risk profile, lifestyle, goals, and possible options.

Table 5-1. Advanced Practice Nursing Surgical Interventions in Colorectal Cancer

Cancer Trajectory	Education	Management
Prevention	Identification of risk factors and behaviors, family history, genetic risk, and screening practices	Evaluation of risk factors and behaviors, colonoscopy, genetic counseling, dietary interventions, and control of coexisting colorectal disease
Diagnosis	Ordering the required testing to obtain specimen; identification of location and extent of disease	Assessment of signs and symptoms of colorectal disease, appropriate work-up with colonoscopy, radiology studies and computed tomography to rule out metastatic disease
Resection	Determination of the extent of disease; surgical intervention for staging and resection, pain management, cardiac/pulmonary toilet, type of surgery/ostomy potential, postoperative care, home care, adjuvant therapies	Preoperative assessment with surgical clearance, role of neoadjuvant therapy, perioperative management of body systems and homeostasis, postoperative management to prevent infection and maximize outcomes, consultation with dietitian and enterostomal therapist, if necessary; determination of disease stage, adjuvant therapy
Access	Venous access for chemotherapy and/or gut access for nutrition	Assessment of venous access and options for therapy, nutritional needs related to oral intake/gut absorption
Rehabilitation	Ostomy care/reversal, dietary habits, colon function, post-chemotherapy/radiation care	Assessment of current status, possible ostomy reversal, enterostomal/skin care, elimination patterns, coping mechanisms
Surveillance	Lifetime recommendations, follow-up care, family history implications	Appropriate screening and colonoscopy schedule, assessment of current status, symptoms, preventive healthcare maintenance, screening of family members
Palliation	Diagnosis of recurrent disease, pain and symptom management, nutritional status, end-of-life issues	Assessment of signs and symptoms of recurrent disease, pain and symptom management

Note. Based on information from Lester, 2007.

Early detection and prevention strategies in surgical oncology provide unique opportunities for involvement of APNs. Discussion of personal risk profiles with avoidance of risky behaviors requires time, a reasonable plan of action, and subsequent evaluation. Detailed documentation of historical events is vital for *accurate* individual assessments of relative and actual risks of cancer development. Often, this requires repetitive and reframed questions to provide clarification. A prime example lies in patient descriptions of gynecologic cancers (i.e., confusion regarding cervical intraepithelial neoplasia versus cervical cancer versus uterine cancer versus ovarian cancer). Obtaining a copy of the pathology reports for placement in the patient's medical record is ideal. (Additional information on cancer screening and prevention is available in Chapter 1.)

Diagnosis

A confirmatory diagnosis of cancer relies on tissue acquisition for pathologic, cytologic, and possibly histologic review. When a malignancy is suspected, consultation with the surgical team typically occurs. A potential cancer diagnosis must be distinguished from other diseases, with a systematic comparison of signs and symptoms. Information obtained from an individualized approach with review of documented history, physical examination, objective observation, radiology and laboratory review, and patient subjective interview is invaluable. This prediagnostic summary guides the development of the surgical plan for appropriate tissue acquisition.

Knowledge about the natural history of various cancers and their presentation is integral to the differential diagnosis process and appropriate work-up. After the initial consultation is complete, the surgical team discusses the suspected cancer origin, appropriate type of biopsy, timing, and further staging. If another discipline, such as radiology, receives the diagnostic consult, clinicians must be sure to apply this same scrutiny to the overall diagnostic assessment. The APN commonly is the coordinator of care, providing continuity between services and relaying updates to patients and families.

A variety of biopsy techniques are available that can provide sufficient tissue for the pathologic and histologic diagnosis of a suspected cancer (see Table 5-2). The surgical team selects the appropriate tissue sampling technique based on information gained from the initial consultation. A fine-needle aspiration (FNA) biopsy, utilizing a 20-gauge needle and 10 ml syringe, can obtain cells from a palpable mass for identification of the presence or absence of malignant cells in the sample. FNA does not indicate histologic differences necessary for treatment; therefore, patients typically require a more definitive tissue biopsy. Procurement of additional pathologic markers may be imperative, as when neoadjuvant chemotherapy is under consideration, to obtain adequate information for cancer care throughout the trajectory. A larger-gauge core needle biopsy (CNB) may be an appropriate method to obtain additional tissue that provides a diagnosis with histologic detail. The benefits of needle biopsy include easy access, minimal or no scarring, and minimal discomfort. In the hands of a skillful clinician, needle biopsies are reliable methods of obtaining tissue for diagnosis (Carroll, 2006; Mack & Pasieka, 2007; Sabel, 2007).

All needle biopsies carry a word of caution: A negative biopsy reading obtained by FNA or CNB does not ensure a benign lesion. If a lesion is highly suspect for malignancy and a needle biopsy yields negative or inconclusive results, an open biopsy is necessary in order to obtain enough tissue to verify a diagnosis. In the case of precursor neoplastic findings, as in lobular carcinoma in situ of the breast, a needle biopsy is insufficient for diagnosis and management. A follow-up surgical excision removes additional tissue for pathologic examination to exclude adjacent malignant cells (Elsheikh & Silverman, 2005).

Open biopsies, otherwise known as incisional or excisional, are performed through a skin incision and are used in certain masses relative to size, location, and the suspected malignancy type. An incisional biopsy removes part of the visible mass for pathologic review, whereas an excisional biopsy removes visible components of the mass in its entirety. Imaging studies may be of benefit to localize lesions, especially in the case of nonpalpable lesions or areas of microcalcification in the breast. Needle localization biopsy combines radiographic guidance with a small gauge and flexible wire to isolate the lesion or area of concern. Radiology guidance may be done through ultrasound, mammography, computed tomography, or magnetic resonance imaging (MRI), depending on the location of the suspect lesion, ease of access, and anticipated accuracy. Preoperative placement of a thin needle relative to the area of concern marks the

Table 5-2. Biopsy Techniques

Biopsy Types	Advantages	Disadvantages	Common Cancer Use
Fine-needle aspiration biopsy • Obtains cellular material with 20- or 21-gauge needle and syringe	Is easy for patients Can be performed in ambulatory setting/office Requires minimal preparation Is less invasive Is inexpensive Produces quick results Leaves no scar Can be done with ultrasound guidance Can be performed with local skin/tissue anesthesia Allows patients to resume activities immediately	Can be painful Requires experienced practitioners and pathologists Yields minimal pathologic information, as it is based on cellular material only Can cause development of problematic hematoma at biopsy site May still require core needle or open biopsy	Palpable masses Breast masses Skin lesions Palpable lymph nodes in neck, clavicle, and axillae Groin areas
Core needle biopsy • Obtains core(s) of tissue via spring-loaded device with 14- or 16-gauge core of tissue *Stereotactic biopsy* • Obtains core(s) of tissue using stereotactic machine via 12- or 14-gauge needle; usually vacuum-assisted *Vacuum-assisted core needle biopsy* • Utilizes suction through probe to draw multiple samples of tissue	Can be used on palpable masses Is somewhat easy for patients Can be performed in ambulatory setting/office Requires minimal preparation Is less invasive Is less expensive Leaves only a tiny nick/scar Retractable needle contains tissue fragments Can be performed by several disciplines Can be combined with radiographic guidance, including ultrasound, magnetic resonance imaging (MRI), computed tomography, or stereotactic imaging Provides pathologic and histologic information Can be performed with local skin/tissue anesthesia Allows patients to resume activities the next day	Can be painful Can be performed as a "procedure only" by other disciplines without evaluation or examination of patients Can cause development of problematic hematoma at biopsy site Requires removal of needle track if malignant May still require open biopsy Stereotactic biopsy of the breast requires prone position.	Palpable soft tissue masses Breast masses, microcalcifications Prostate masses Brain lesions Palpable lymph nodes
Mammotome® (Johnson & Johnson Ethicon Endo-Surgery, Inc.) • Obtains core(s) of tissue using stereotactic guidance via vacuum-assisted device that rotates and cuts tissue	Is fairly easy for patients Can be performed in ambulatory setting/office Is less invasive Leaves a small scar with one or more sutures Needle "contains" tissue Can be performed by several disciplines Can be performed with ultrasound, mammography, or MRI	Can be painful Can be performed as a "procedure only" by other disciplines without evaluation or examination of patients Can cause development of problematic hematoma at biopsy site Requires removal of needle track if malignant	Breast masses, microcalcifications

(Continued on next page)

Table 5-2. Biopsy Techniques *(Continued)*

Biopsy Types	Advantages	Disadvantages	Common Cancer Use
	Provides pathologic and histologic information Allows small lesions/nodules to be completely removed Can be performed with local skin/tissue anesthesia Allows patients to resume activities the next day	May still require an open biopsy for margins Is an understudied procedure for breast cancer removal (i.e., without additional surgery)	
Incisional biopsy • Removes part of tumor mass via small skin incision	Can be performed on an outpatient basis or, less often, in the office Provides pathologic and histologic information Can be performed with local skin/tissue anesthesia Can be performed with flexible fiber-optic instrument	Is more involved for patients Can be painful Is more invasive Requires small incision/leaves scar with sutures May require sedation or anesthesia Is not intended to obtain clean margin of tissue Will require further treatment if malignant May delay patients' return to daily activities	Any mass
Excisional biopsy • Removes all of tumor mass via small skin incision *Needle localization* • Uses tiny wire with hooked end to mark nonpalpable masses for open biopsy	Can be performed on an outpatient basis/same-day surgery Provides pathologic and histologic information Can be performed under local skin/tissue anesthesia Can be performed with flexible fiber-optic instrument	Is more involved for patients Can be painful Is more invasive Requires small incision/leaves scar with sutures May require sedation or anesthesia Will require further treatment if malignant Is not intended to obtain clean margin of tissue May delay patients' return to daily activities	Any mass

Note. Based on information from Carroll, 2006; Lester, 2007.

site to be biopsied. As the placement needle is withdrawn, a fine wire with a hooked end remains to localize the area or mass of concern that requires tissue sampling. Wire removal occurs at the time of biopsy; the wire typically is attached to the biopsy specimen as it exits the body.

All tissue biopsies require adherence to the following principles in anticipation of identification of a malignancy: (a) mark a suitable anatomic plane and position for needle tracks and incisions before tissue removal, (b) avoid contamination of adjacent tissue planes, (c) avoid hematoma formation by providing adequate hemostasis, (d) meticulously mark the orientation of the specimen to ensure proper identification of tissue fragments, and (e) obtain adequate tissue for subsequent clinical or surgical decision making (Sabel, 2007). Lack of attention to these details can be deleterious to the patient and can create situations that may compromise decision making throughout the cancer trajectory.

APNs, depending on the practice setting, may make the decision regarding biopsy type and approach, arrange the procedure, and assist with the biopsy. They may even perform less invasive biopsies such as FNA and CNB, depending on institutional and state regulatory guidelines. Prior to assuming this independent role, the nurse must meet core competencies, including performing an agreed-upon number of physician-mentored procedures without complication. Communication between the surgical team and radiology is essential, along with possible concomitant radiology film review for clarification. Often, APNs bridge this gap with knowledge about the clinical *and* radiographic presentation of the patient.

Pathology and Staging

Correlation of the pathologic information obtained from the tissue biopsy with radiology studies, physical examination, and the patient's history is crucial to accurate identification of a malignancy. The surgical team often performs this critical role to establish an accurate, site-specific diagnosis. If further clarification is warranted, additional testing or tissue sampling may be necessary. APNs employ intuitive skills to assemble the diagnostic pieces of cancer presentations, such as in the preparation of clinically relevant cases for tumor board meetings.

Clinical Stage

The healthcare team assesses the presenting clinical stage using professional judgment, physical examination and assessment, and radiologic reports to determine clinical evidence of malignancy at primary or metastatic site(s) and estimate the size (Johnson, 2007). All malignancies, regardless of planned surgical interventions, have an initial intuitive "clinical" estimation of stage. This clinical stage is particularly prudent when administration of neoadjuvant chemotherapy precedes definitive surgery. The APN, as a clinical provider, often is responsible for accurate documentation of clinical stage prior to and throughout neoadjuvant therapy.

Upon completion of neoadjuvant therapy, primary surgical removal of the tumor typically occurs with pathologic examination of excised tissue. If a complete remission has occurred (i.e., no pathologic evidence exists of malignancy in tissue removed from the primary and/or regional nodal surgical sites), the clinical stage stands as the only means of documentation of the presenting cancer stage. True pathologic staging cannot occur, as the specimen may show limited evidence of disease. Therefore, an accurate clinical stage *prior* to neoadjuvant therapy is essential to provide the most accurate estimation of disease stage *at the time of cancer diagnosis*. Often, this is the only accurate objective measurement of a patient's cancer stage.

Surgical Staging

Surgical staging is an invasive assessment, using laparoscopic or open surgical procedures that enable the surgeon to visualize structures, assess the visible extent of disease, and obtain necessary tissue for pathologic examination. The surgical team assesses the cancer from a surgical standpoint, noting tumor size, enlarged lymph nodes, and possible metastatic sites. All surgically removed tissue undergoes pathologic examination. Adequate tissue sampling must occur for the pathologist to derive the most accurate pathologic stage of the tumor. Surgical oncology APNs, armed with clinical and surgical staging assessments, must verify that identifying information and tissue are provided to the pathology team.

Pathologic Staging

Pathologic staging derives its information from gross and microscopic examination of provided tissue (Johnson, 2007). Pathologic staging defines a cancer as related to the organ or organs of origin, stating the tumor size, lymph node status, and metastatic sites. Additional histologic data, including differentiation, mitotic rate, receptors, and special stains, often are requisite to a better understanding of the biology of the specific cancer.

Ideally, surgical and pathologic staging correlate, thus validating that excision of all suspicious sites occurred with subsequent pathologic examination. The surgical team is responsible for marking tissue with regard to orientation and margins. At some institutions, the pathologist enters the operating room to view and receive the tissue specimens and to verify orientation of the specimen with the surgeon.

Ultimately, the site or origin of the malignancy and information derived from clinical, surgical, and pathologic staging provide the information needed to devise, or revise, the treatment plan. Additional surgery may be necessary to secure clear tissue margins around the primary or metastatic site. The surgical oncology APN must be familiar with cancer types and staging, with an understanding of tumor markers and characteristics as well as possible sites of metastasis. Identification of metastatic disease in another organ or distant organs may alter the treatment plan but retains the original pathologic diagnosis (i.e., the etiology of the malignancy itself does not change). For example, lung cancer (that originates in the lung) is a "lung cancer." Lung cancer that metastasizes to the liver pathologically remains a "lung cancer"; it does not become "liver cancer." Therefore, pathologic examination of a cancerous lesion in the liver can essentially confirm a primary lung cancer diagnosis. This concept often is confusing to patients and families and requires explanation and education from the APN to avoid misinterpretation of information.

Oncogene Typing

Oncogene typing can provide adjunct information to the pathologic findings, thereby allowing for improved stratification of prognostic factors. This study of gene expression in combination with clinical markers and biomarkers can suggest potential target genes for treatment as well as aid in the prediction of progression of the cancer and clinical outcomes. Subsequently, implementation of individually tailored systemic treatments may occur with avoidance of over- or undertreatment of patients. Surgical APNs must be familiar with the basic concepts of the rapidly expanding field of oncogene typing, as this information may guide treatment decisions (Buyse et al., 2006; Dunkler, Michiels, & Schemper, 2007; James, Quinn, Mullan, Johnston, & Harkin, 2007; Jiang & Zhao, 2006; Sun, Goodison, Li, Liu, & Farmerie, 2007).

Staging Systems

The tumor-node-metastasis (TNM) anatomic system from the American Joint Committee on Cancer (AJCC) and the Surveillance Epidemiology and End Results program reports the pathologic staging of tumors based on tissue received by the pathologist. The TNM system divides cancers into stages with numerical markings of 0–IV. In this system, higher numbers indicate more disease. Unfortunately, no standardized system exists that includes all tumor characteristics such as histologic grade, estrogen and progesterone receptors, HER2/neu status, biologic markers, and molecular and genetic information, which are all inherent to definitive staging with accurate prognostic outcomes. The astute clinician must carefully combine all information to create a prognostic profile, as the TNM system cannot fulfill this requirement in current cancer care. Ongoing clinical trials will aid in the establishment of future staging systems (Greene, 2006; Greene et al., 2002; Sabel, 2007). Further information on diagnosis and staging may be found in Chapter 3.

APNs often are the team members who explain these difficult concepts to surgical patients and their families to promote understanding of the disease process and treatment. The presumed tumor stage stated at the initial consultation may change based on final pathologic findings. Alteration of previously discussed treatment plans may occur, resulting in confusion and frustration for patients and families. APNs provide continuity and reassurance throughout this difficult and stressful time.

Resection—Preoperative Phase

The surgical treatment of cancer involves decision making on the part of the patient as well as the surgical team. Patients require information about cancer risk or a specific cancer, with related treatment trajectory, anticipated outcome, and long-term prognosis. Involvement of the patient's family and support system is inherent to achieving successful outcomes, including discharge planning and short- and long-term care. Information about possible neoadjuvant and/or adjuvant therapies is important to patients, as many may be unaware of the concept of micrometastasis and the potential need for further systemic treatment. APNs play vital roles as patient navigator, educator, and advocate during this difficult process.

Surgical APNs must be knowledgeable about related modalities of cancer therapy and need to inform patients and families of all available treatment options that may, in turn, influence their decision-making processes. Certain cancer types have a planned trajectory with few options. Other cancer types, especially breast cancer, have multiple options that require continuing explanation to enable an informed patient choice. Surgical APNs may facilitate interdisciplinary consultations necessary for disease or health status evaluation and often become "interpreters" for both healthcare professionals and patients. APNs as patient advocates and navigators provide the continuity that patients and families seek as they strive to synthesize massive amounts of information resulting in difficult treatment decisions.

Surgical resection is an integral part of cancer treatment, as detailed in Table 5-3. Additional modalities such as radiation, chemotherapy, and biologic therapies may be given at the time of surgery to increase the therapeutic effects. The potential combinations of cancer modalities and their approach for each cancer type are too lengthy to list, especially with the added variability of patient and tumor characteristics. These

Table 5-3. Surgical Interventions by Cancer Type

Cancer/Indications	Oncologic Surgical Procedures
Breast cancer	Lumpectomy/segmental mastectomy, with sentinel lymph node biopsy (SLNB), possible axillary node dissection (AND) Total mastectomy with SLNB, possible AND (if AND performed, essentially modified radical mastectomy (MRM) with or without reconstruction MRM with or without reconstruction Reconstruction following mastectomy, immediate or delayed; performed with autologous tissue, synthetic implants, or combination Transverse rectus abdominis myocutaneous flap—pedicled or free
Melanoma	Wide local excision, with or without SLNB/AND Possible skin graft, split or full thickness, autologous tissue
Nonmelanoma skin cancer	Excision with clean margin Mohs micrographic surgery Curettage and cautery/electrodessication
Bone, soft tissue sarcoma	Wide local excision; with or without regional lymphadenectomy; if intra-abdominal, complete surgical resection with or without regional lymph-adenectomy
Brain cancer	Craniotomy, with or without spiral computed tomography imaging and/or ro-botic assistance
Head and neck cancer	Surgical resection; possible skin graft; possible reconstruction; possible lymphadenectomy, possible SLNB
Thoracic malignancies	Pneumonectomy versus parenchyma-conserving lobectomy; wedge resec-tion; segmentectomy; possible mediastinal node dissection; possible video-assisted thoracoscopic surgery
Esophageal carcinoma	Surgical resection, often after neoadjuvant chemotherapy (i.e., subtotal esophagectomy); total esophagectomy with reconstruction Possible laser therapy, possible fiber-optic–guided resection
Gastric cancer	Surgical resection, total gastrectomy versus subtotal gastrectomy; regional lymphadenectomy; fiber-optic–guided resection, laparoscopy
Small bowel/carcinoid	Wide excision, ranging from local excision to pancreaticoduodenectomy
Colon cancer	Right hemicolectomy; extended right hemicolectomy with or without trans-verse colostomy; left hemicolectomy; low anterior resection; subtotal colec-tomy; total abdominal colectomy; abdominoperineal resection; laparoscopic approach for resection
Rectal cancer	Resection with clear margin with or without regional lymph nodes; abdomino-perineal resection, low anterior resection, laparoscopic resection; coloanal anastomosis, transanal approach, trans-sacral approach; sphincter pres-ervation; colonic J pouch; ileal pouch-anal anastomosis; ileorectal anas-tomosis; proximal diversion; transanal excision; posterior proctotomy; total proctocolectomy
Hepatobiliary cancer	Resection of mass; orthotopic liver transplantation, cryosurgery, radiofre-quency ablation

(Continued on next page)

Table 5-3. Surgical Interventions by Cancer Type *(Continued)*

Cancer/Indications	Oncologic Surgical Procedures
Pancreatic cancer	Cattell-Braasch maneuver; Kocher maneuver; portal dissection; resection of stomach, jejunum with or without reconstruction; regional pancreatectomy with retroperitoneal and hepatoduodenal lymphadenectomy; pancreaticoduodenectomy
Endocrine tumors and multiple endocrine neoplasia	Excision; distal pancreatectomy; pancreaticoduodenectomy
Adrenal tumors	Resection; laparoscopy
Thyroid, parathyroid	Thyroidectomy—thyroid lobectomy with isthmectomy versus total thyroidectomy; with or without unilateral/bilateral neck dissection; modified radical neck dissection; parathyroidectomy
Hematologic tumors/ spleen	Splenectomy for hypersplenism
Genitourinary cancers	Prostate: radical prostatectomy with or without regional lymph nodes: open versus laparoscopic, robotic-assisted surgery Bladder: bladder-sparing surgery; radical cystectomy with pelvic lymphadenectomy; orthotopic ureter diversion with ileal segment Renal: surgical excision; radical nephrectomy; resection of renal vein/artery; laparoscopy Testicular: radical orchiectomy with or without retroperitoneal lymph node dissection
Gynecologic cancers	Vulvar: wide local excision; radical vulvectomy with or without inguinal lymph node dissection Vaginal: radical hysterectomy with pelvic lymph node dissection Cervical: conization; simple hysterectomy; radical hysterectomy with pelvic lymph node dissection Endometrial: simple hysterectomy; radical hysterectomy with pelvic lymph node dissection Ovarian: cytoreduction with multiple biopsies; total abdominal hysterectomy with bilateral salpingo-oophorectomy; omentectomy, appendectomy, pelvic and para-aortic lymph node dissection; occasional second-look surgery (seldom performed) Low malignant potential: fertility-sparing surgery with unilateral salpingo-oophorectomy
Oncologic emergencies	Spinal cord compression; pericardial tamponade; central venous catheter sepsis; intestinal obstruction; intestinal perforation; biliary obstruction; hemorrhage
Implantable port placement	Guide wire–assisted cephalic vein

Note. Based on information from Azzoli, 2006; Baxter et al., 2007; Chapman, 2007; Crane-Okada & Loney, 2007; Ellsmere et al., 2006; Feig et al., 2003; Gee & Rattner, 2007; Greene et al., 2007; Guillem, 2007; Kocak et al., 2007; Law et al., 2007; Liang et al., 2007; Matthews et al., 2006; Ota & Nelson, 2007; Pare, 2006; Poon, 2007; Schlaerth & Abu-Rustum, 2006; Slattery & Sahani, 2006; Starnes & Sims, 2006a, 2006b; Vanderveen et al., 2007; Yokomizo et al., 2007; Zerey et al., 2006.

potential treatment combinations are specific to individual cancer types but share the same overall principles of surgical resection and local tumor control that are inherent in the treatment of solid tumors. Liquid tumors, such as lymphoma and leukemia classifications, seldom use surgery as the primary interventional treatment because of the characteristics that are inherent to these tumor types. Nevertheless, a role for surgery does exist for liquid tumors, including access device placement and palliative surgical interventions for symptom management (Cai et al., 2007; Mack & Pasieka, 2007).

The goals of cancer surgical therapy should be reviewed with the patient and family. These goals include (a) maximizing potential for control or cure of cancer, (b) minimizing comorbidities, and (c) retaining active participation of patients and families. A cancer diagnosis is challenging in itself, but the enormous amount of information given in a short time span by multiple providers can be even more difficult for patients and family members to manage as they prepare for surgical intervention. APNs hold a pivotal role in the balance of these three goals and are the constant throughout the patient's disease course, reprioritizing as necessary with explanation to the patient and family.

Colorectal cancer surgery is one example that illustrates the importance of consistent verbal and written communication. Patients must complete bowel sterilization and adjust their diet two to three days before surgery; undergo a bowel preparation that typically consists of a combination of laxatives and enemas; and take oral antibiotics. Failure to comply with instructions may result in postponement of surgery because of inadequate cleansing of the bowel. Older adults and debilitated patients may suffer from nausea and vomiting, abdominal distention, and electrolyte imbalance. If a colostomy is indicated, referral to an enterostomal therapist is ideal for marking the stoma site. Ideally, the patient is able to see the stoma with avoidance of skin creases, folds, previous scars, bony prominences, and the belt line (Williams, 2007). Psychological support related to the cancer diagnosis and possible ostomy is necessary to ensure that adequate support systems are in place (Murphy, 2007).

Preoperative Assessment

Preoperative assessment and evaluation are integral to safe completion of the surgical intervention and decrease in postoperative complications. The surgical team determines the operative risk, weighing potential benefits against risks of the cancer-related surgical interventions with the examination of past and current health history and current physical status. Surgery is demanding of the body's homeostatic mechanisms. Identification and resolution of problems that may increase morbidity and mortality risk are essential to optimal outcomes. Attention to concomitant diagnoses is important in providing efficient, effective surgical care. Consultations with other services such as cardiology, pulmonology, or endocrinology are best done in the preoperative phase, prior to the stress of surgery. If the benefits of surgery outweigh the identified risks, a thorough preoperative work-up alerts the anesthesia and surgical teams to possible difficulties during the intra- and postoperative periods. APNs play a critical role in patient evaluation as well as in communication within and between teams (Backman, Bondy, Deschamps, Moore, & Schricker, 2006).

Attention to preexisting medical conditions with possible adverse outcomes is crucial in the preoperative evaluation. APNs must perform a thorough assessment that includes previous medical, surgical, and psychosocial histories; nutritional status; medications; laboratory and imaging studies; and teaching needs. Appropriate management of comorbid diseases, especially those related to mental health, endocrinology disease or diabetes, heart disease, or pulmonary, renal, and gastrointestinal function, as well as safety issues, must occur concomitantly with cancer care (Lester, 2007).

Statistics show that certain comorbid conditions may increase the risk of adverse events during the surgical procedure as well as during the postoperative period. In general, a personal history of congestive heart failure leads to a 12% increase in hospital stay, and a history of hypertension allows a twofold increase in the intraoperative risk of a cardiac event. A history of asthma allows for a five-time increase in the risk of respiratory events such as bronchospasms, and smoking is responsible for a fourfold increase in postoperative respiratory difficulties. Obesity is responsible for a fourfold increase in intraoperative and postoperative respiratory events, and a history of uncontrolled reflux allows for an eightfold increase in intubation events including aspiration (Backman et al., 2006). APNs are responsible for obtaining a thorough history and physical and have the opportunity to improve a patient's outcome from surgery with consideration of the aforementioned criteria. Comorbid conditions must be medically controlled to prevent additional complications; if not, the surgery may be postponed until greater control is achieved.

Preoperative Assessment of Infection Risk

Surgical site infection (SSI) is a major cause of patient morbidity and mortality as well as increased healthcare costs and length of hospital stay. Several factors create the infection matrix, including the patient's health status, the physical environment of the surgery, clinical risks, patient selection, preparation for surgery, antibiotic prophylaxis, hand hygiene of the surgical team, and the facility's use of universal precautions. Bacterial sources can be endogenous or exogenous, with myriad potential carriers (McCay & Farley, 2006; Meakins & Masterson, 2006). APNs are responsible for preemptively identifying infection risk factors and for preventing or eliminating as many of these factors as possible.

Critical examination of the clinical risks of infection relative to each patient is important to predict potential infection risk. Review of concomitant illnesses or diagnoses, age, preoperative nutritional status, and smoking habits provide baseline information that allows APNs to intervene. Suboptimal nutritional states increase the risk of infection. Nutritional supplements and possibly enteral feedings may be necessary to prepare the body for surgery and to improve nitrogen balance and protein stores. Patients suffering from significant malnutrition caused by a catabolic state or inability to ingest adequate nutrition may require parenteral feedings prior to a major surgery (Mirtallo & Ezzone, 2006). Control of metabolic disease such as diabetes is imperative in order to arm the body with necessary defenses. Tight control of serum blood sugars with sliding scale insulin may improve the infection threshold. Attention to drug use, especially recent chemotherapy, chronic steroid use, and immunosuppressive drugs, may offer additional avenues for intervention. Although smoking cessation is desired, abstinence from smoking for as little as one week before surgery can make a positive impact on tissue oxygenation. Appropriate preoperative skin and bowel preparations reduce bacterial flora, especially endogenous bacteria. Avoidance of a preoperative admission may decrease nosocomial bacterial exposure, as the rate of nosocomial infections is reduced in same-day admissions versus preoperative admissions to the hospital unit (Fakhry, Rutherford, & Sheldon, 2006; Meakins & Masterson, 2006).

Review of the patient's health status and personal hygiene habits with a focus on potential acute and chronic infections may identify additional interventions. Appropriate antibiotic use preoperatively for acute infection can reduce bacterial load and potentially eliminate postoperative infection from host bacteria. Cultures of acute infection and serum titers of administered antibiotics may be helpful to target bacteria and ascertain systemic absorption of antibiotics. Culturing of chronic infection sites, such as skin ulcers, is not helpful, as normal skin flora and secondary organisms typically contaminate the specimen. Examination of bodily fluids such as urine and sputum may enable the APN to troubleshoot harboring bacteria that could cause a catheter-induced bladder infection or pneumonia (Malangoni & McHenry, 2006; McCay & Farley, 2006; Smith et al., 2004).

Unlike elective, planned surgeries, the timing of a cancer surgery often does not allow for correction of preexisting comorbidities. APNs should involve the patient and family in recommended changes in the immediate pre- and postoperative periods, as well as long-term lifestyle changes. Modifications that can immediately affect surgical outcomes are smoking cessation, increase in dietary protein, control of serum glucose, and engagement in aerobic and pulmonary exercise with deep breathing. The patient and family are dealing with the cancer diagnosis itself, making it difficult to address poor personal habits and lifestyle choices.

Medications Affecting Surgery

Attention to preoperative drug dosing and/or discontinuation of certain medications is important to avoid anesthesia-related complications or excessive bleeding. Detailed personal or family history of difficulties with anesthesia is crucial information to obtain preoperatively, specifically in regard to anesthesia-induced hyperthermia. This condition, known as malignant hyperthermia (termed *malignant* but is unrelated to cancer), is a rare and often hereditary condition that occurs after exposure to certain anesthetic agents, such as volatile gases or muscle relaxants. Symptoms range from an increased fever to hypoxia, to circulatory collapse and death. If the patient or family has a history of malignant hyperthermia, this information must be communicated to the anesthesia team. The anesthesia team will perform a more in-depth preoperative assessment and discuss a plan of care with the patient, family, and surgeon.

Avoidance of abrupt changes to the following medications is prudent in the preoperative period in order to avoid withdrawal or a rebound effect: beta-blockers, alpha agonists, barbiturates, and opioids. Other medications that require adjustment, especially in the pre- and perioperative period, include oral hypoglycemics, insulin, corticosteroids, angiotensin-converting enzyme inhibitors, and calcium channel blockers. If possible, discontinuation of monoamine oxidase inhibitors should occur several days preoperatively. Table 5-4 lists some of the common medications that require discontinuation before surgery. Special attention to these medications may prevent patients with cancer from experiencing unnecessary side effects during the pre-, peri-, and postoperative periods (Backman et al., 2006). APNs are responsible for reviewing all medications, including over-the-counter drugs, for possible interaction or reaction with the cancer diagnosis and pending surgical procedure. Alterations in medication type, brand, or dosage optimally occur prior to the surgery to ascertain the patient's tolerance to the adjustment.

Drugs that alter platelet aggregation or prolong bleeding should be evaluated several weeks before surgery, if possible, to ensure proper dosage adjustments. These drugs include herbal remedies and antithrombolytic and antiplatelet agents. Discontinuation of these drugs may be required to avoid unnecessary bleeding, hemorrhage, or hematoma formation in the peri- or postoperative period (see Table 5-4). In reviewing patient anticoagulant use, attention to underlying health conditions is necessary to investigate the clinical reason for anticoagulation, such as a history of hypercoagulable

Table 5-4. Drugs and Their Interfering Properties in the Preoperative Setting

Name of Drug	Interfering Properties	Preoperation (Preop) Discontinuation
Angiotensin-converting enzyme inhibitors	Intensify hypotension, effects of anesthesia	Individual consideration; 24 hours preop
Angiotensin receptor blockers	Intensify hypotension	Individual consideration; 24 hours preop
Calcium-channel blockers	Intensify hypotension, effects of anesthesia	Individual consideration; 24 hours preop
Aspirin Clopidogrel Ticlopidine Tirofiban (Aggrastat®, Medicure Pharma) Eptifibatide (Integrilin®, Millennium Pharmaceuticals)	Antiplatelet effect	7–10 days preop
Celecoxib (Celebrex®, Pfizer Inc.) Naproxen	Antiplatelet effect	72 hours preop
Ketorolac	Antiplatelet effect	24 hours preop
Fenoprofen	Antiplatelet effect	12 hours preop
Monoamine oxidase inhibitors	Fatal drug reaction with anesthetic agents	2 weeks preop
Tricyclic antidepressants	Cardiac arrhythmias, hypotension	Individual consideration; cessation probably not necessary; norepinephrine is drug of choice
Selective serotonin-reuptake inhibitors Benzodiazepines	Withdrawal effects	Important **not** to alter preoperatively
Herbals: garlic, ginseng, ginkgo, ginger, kava, valerian, St. John's wort	Antiplatelet, anticoagulation effect	2 weeks preop
Warfarin	Anticoagulation effect	Individual consideration; 3–5 days preop; may consider heparin bridge
Heparin	Anticoagulation effect	Just prior to surgery

Note. Based on information from Backman et al., 2006; Pass & Simpson, 2004.

state, significant cardiac valvular disease, artificial cardiac valves, atrial fibrillation, and thrombotic events such as deep vein thrombosis (DVT) or pulmonary embolism (PE). In these serious hypercoagulable states, maintenance of anticoagulation with short-acting heparin may be implemented during the time the patient is unable to take routine anticoagulation medication. Hospital admission for this bridge therapy with heparin may be necessary to avoid thromboembolytic events (Backman et al., 2006; Pass & Simpson, 2004). APNs provide continuity among the primary care physician, the surgical team, and the house staff and often direct the stop of oral or subcutaneous (SC) anticoagulants, the start of IV heparin, the stop of heparin on the day of surgery, anticoagulant orders in the postoperative phase, and the transition to oral and SC anticoagulation with serum monitoring in the home setting.

Resection—Perioperative Phase

The scope of this chapter does not allow for sufficient discussion of issues relevant to potential APN roles in the perioperative phase of cancer surgery. Intraoperative APNs, such as certified registered nurse anesthetists, receive certification by boards outside of oncology nursing and may not be the largest audience of this text. Nevertheless, the perioperative phase includes issues relevant to the surgery itself, anesthesia, safety, blood products, fluid management, infection, electrolyte balance, cardiac hemostasis, pulmonary function, oxygenation, and positioning. Other chapters in this book include additional information about these topics. Information related to perioperative anesthesia, infection, and positioning follows.

Anesthesia

A number of anesthesia types are possible for cancer surgeries: general, regional, or local. The selection is decided upon between the surgical team, anesthesiologist, and patient. General anesthesia induces a reversible state of loss of consciousness and provides the surgeon with a controlled, motionless operating field and a secure airway, with total unawareness for the patient. General anesthesia can produce analgesia, amnesia, muscle relaxation, unconsciousness, and inhibition of reflexes. IV agents such as ultra-short-acting barbiturates or tranquilizers frequently are used to obtain a rapid onset of unconsciousness. A number of inhaled anesthetic agents also can be used, which provide a safe form of anesthesia in combination with narcotics and muscle relaxants. Although these side effects may be desirable, general anesthesia carries risks, including the potential for cardiac dysfunction with myocardial infarction, arrhythmias, and cerebral vascular accident. Other negative side effects include nausea and vomiting, headache, blurred vision, disorientation, sore throat secondary to intubation, respiratory paralysis, muscle pain, a feeling of cold and shivering, dizziness, and drowsiness (Arora, Dhar, & Fahey, 2006; Backman et al., 2006).

Local and regional anesthesias involve a reversible blockage of pain perception. Topical/skin anesthesia occurs after application of topical anesthetic agents to the skin or mucous membranes. Local anesthesia of a specified anatomic area occurs through injection of anesthetic agents directly into the operative field. These methods can involve short-acting or long-acting drugs, depending on the blockage time interval desired. Peripheral nerve blocks achieve pain blockage to a regional area of nerve trunks, thus providing anesthesia to an entire anatomic area, such as the arm or leg. These approaches are administered alone or in combination with general anesthesia (Arora et al., 2006; Backman et al., 2006).

Potential alternatives to general anesthesia include epidural or spinal anesthesias. These methods produce numbness of the area below the injected nerve roots. Epidural anesthesia, either short- or long-term, can be achieved by depositing analgesic or anesthetic drugs into the extradural space of the spinal canal using a spinal needle. A catheter may be left in place for continued, intermittent interjection of either set of drugs, even after the surgical procedure has been completed. Epidural anesthesia, in combination with general anesthesia, is a common approach for intensely painful surgeries, such as thoracic procedures. Drugs can be delivered directly to the injured nerves to optimize pain control and to minimize systemic side effects. Spinal anesthesia is induced with an injection of local anesthetic agents into the cerebrospinal fluid after puncture of the dural sac between the L2 and L4 vertebrae. This provides anesthesia to the lower abdomen and extremities without the side effects of general anesthesia, thereby allowing the patient to remain in a semiconscious or awake state with spontaneous breathing (Backman et al., 2006). APNs are responsible for ascertaining appropriate patient education for methods of anesthesia.

Infection Risk

The risk of SSI is a systems issue requiring diligent attention to asepsis and infection control guidelines. To maintain the patient's host defense mechanisms, the physical environment of surgery is controlled. This includes preoperative surgical decisions, timing of surgery, surgical technique, use of blood products, control of blood loss, duration and extent of surgery, perioperative glucose control, adequate tissue oxygenation, normothermia, normovolemia, pain control, and sterility (Lafreniere et al., 2006; Meakins & Masterson, 2006).

Preparation of the skin overlying the surgical site requires use of an antibacterial scrub and removal of body hair that is adjacent to the incision line. Clipping of the hair is preferred. If complete removal of body hair surrounding the surgical site is necessary, removal just prior to the skin incision in surgery is preferred in deference to hours prior to surgery. This reduces potential areas of inflammation and subsequent superficial infection caused by trauma to the skin. Use of depilatory products for the surgical patient is not advisable because of the risk of skin inflammation (Meakins & Masterson, 2006).

The administration of preoperative and intraoperative antibiotics occurs depending on individual patient risk factors, type of surgery, anatomic location of surgery, and length of surgical time. The risk of infection increases as surgery time lengthens, although SSIs can establish several hours after exposure to an endogenous or exogenous pathogen. Administration of antibiotics before contamination reduces the risk of subsequent infection. Proper choice of an antimicrobial and timing of administration are crucial to effective prophylaxis.

Antibiotics are not indicated for patients undergoing short (less than two hours) surgical procedures in tissues outside of the alimentary tract (designated as "clean" cases). Exception to this guideline occurs in patients with a known infection, immunocompromised state, significant cardiac valvular disease, or artificial valves or joints or if surgical time may extend beyond two hours. These cases may benefit from administration of an IV broad-spectrum antibiotic just prior to skin incision.

Cases involving the alimentary tract, including oral and digestive organs (designated as "dirty" cases), abscess drainage, or overt infections require preoperative and intraoperative administration of antibiotics. Surgical procedures involving the upper or lower digestive tracts (e.g., colon resection) also may require preoperative sterilization with multiple doses of oral agents. Surgical placement of vascular access devices requires prophylactic antibiotic administration just prior to the skin incision because of the possible introduction of skin flora into the circulatory system, as well as the placement of a foreign body that can trap organisms (Lafreniere et al., 2006; Meakins & Masterson, 2006; Smith et al., 2004).

Positioning

Patient positioning during surgery is imperative to the prevention of postoperative complications related to muscular and neuropathic injury and compartmental syndromes. Attention to deficits from coexisting conditions such as osteoarthritis, artificial joints, spinal disorders, and rheumatoid diseases can potentially decrease postoperative discomfort and time to ambulation. Well-documented information on the surgical chart by the APN can alert surgical personnel to preexisting physical conditions. Care can include simple interventions such as ensuring proper alignment, placing pillows under the knees, avoiding abduction/adduction movements, taking special care during transfers, and padding for lithotomy positioning. Avoidance of unnatural positioning can decrease unnecessary myalgias and avoid neuropathic injuries.

Of added importance are the gravitational effects of positioning on the circulatory and pulmonary systems. Supine positioning increases the cardiac output because of enhanced return of lower extremity venous blood to the heart. The supine lithotomy position can create an even greater cardiac return secondary to elevation of the lower extremities. Supine positioning can alternatively decrease functional lung capacity. Perfusion changes related to a decreased flow of blood to the lung bases can negatively affect oxygenation status. Trendelenburg positioning, as noted in abdominal surgeries, can increase the pressure of abdominal contents on diaphragmatic movement and alter pulmonary expansion (Lafreniere et al., 2006).

Operative Procedure

The role of surgery in cancer treatment is dependent upon the presentation of the cancer and complications that ensue throughout the cancer trajectory. Knowledge of cancer development and progression is essential in understanding the disease and resulting surgical recommendations. Cancers possess characteristics that drive the surgical approach, and patients present with individual characteristics that direct surgical options. For example, a woman newly diagnosed with breast cancer with a previous history of upper chest wall radiation therapy for the treatment of Hodgkin lymphoma is unable to choose between the standard treatment options of a lumpectomy plus radiation versus a mastectomy, as she is unable to receive radiation therapy to the chest wall again. Therefore, she must have a total mastectomy to treat her breast cancer.

Success with minimally invasive approaches to cancer surgery is heartening, as these techniques offer a significant reduction in surgical-related morbidities and postoperative recovery. Advances in screening and early detection enable cancers to be found in their earliest stage, with the accompanying benefit of less invasive measures of resection. Unfortunately, not all cancers are amenable to these improved surgical approaches, nor are all cancers found in an early stage. Thus, the radical en bloc resection of a cancer and surrounding organs remains a discouraging reality with its associated disfigurement and morbidity.

Resection of Malignancy

Resection remains the primary therapy to eradicate solid tumors and involves removal of the tumor with adequate margins of normal tissue. The goal of every surgeon is to remove the cancer with as little tissue as necessary to remove the primary tumor source and avoid local recurrence. In most cancer surgeries, negative pathologic margins provide quantification of surgical clearance of local tumor evidence. Adequate margins vary from cancer to cancer; the important work of clinical trials serves to document what constitutes a "negative" or adequate margin with each individual cancer. Unfortunately, most cancers initiate their invasive growth many years before detection. As a result, micrometastatic disease is a possibility, indicating probable systemic disease that is not evident in the preoperative assessment. Therefore, the phrase "we got it all" can only theoretically apply to local surgical therapy and seldom indicates a "cure" of the cancer.

Neoadjuvant chemotherapy and/or radiation therapy may precede surgery in an effort to decrease the overall size of the tumor and potentially allow a less aggressive surgical approach. In some examples of neoadjuvant chemotherapy, systemic treatment of the cancer may simultaneously provide treatment of micrometastasis. Intraoperative radiation therapy (i.e., administered during the surgical procedure) also may be a treatment option with the application of concentrated doses of radiation directly to the tumor bed after the surgical team completes initial resection of obvious disease (Sabel, 2007). Consideration of these multimodality approaches to cancer optimally occurs *prior* to surgery, with involvement and education of the patient and family (Wagman, 2007).

Surgical intervention to debulk the tumor involves the surgical removal of visible or palpable tumor to decrease overall tumor burden in advanced presentations. The goal is not necessarily to achieve clean margins or remove all microscopic evidence of disease. Instead, debulking aims to improve quality of life and enhance the ability of systemic therapy to treat advanced cancer.

Surgical resection of metastatic sites may be a surgical strategy for patients with advanced cancer. This approach resects cancers confined to one metastatic organ, typically colorectal cancer with metastasis to the liver or osteogenic soft-tissue sarcomas with metastasis to the lung. With respect to each individual case, surgical excision of these metastatic sites can improve overall survival for five years by 25%–40% (Sabel, 2007; Wagman, 2007). Research is ongoing regarding the resection of metastatic cancer, although most cancer types are not amenable to this approach because of the malignant potential from systemic, micrometastatic disease.

Surgical Procedures

The surgical algorithm and subsequent interventions are dependent upon the specific cancer, presentation, symptoms, and characteristics inherent to each individual patient. The specific surgical approach varies according to the skill level of the surgical team, equipment availability, and regional practices that affect decision making. The science of surgery originates from evidence-based practice, with the art of surgery arising from the skill and experience of the surgical team. Emerging innovations and advancements in technology and instrumentation have transformed operative procedures, with the surgical oncologist, interventional radiologist, and endoscopist often working in concert. At times, the roles blur, yet the goal is always to provide the highest level of care with the least invasive approach and side effect profile, and optimized recovery. This multimodality approach and the potential combination of interventions enable creation and tailoring of the surgical approach to individuals with cancer.

The surgical approach includes assessment and evaluation of the individual patient. Only then can surgical planning begin, with revision as needed. Table 5-3 outlines common surgical interventions for specific cancers; this is a broad summary of standard surgical approaches *without* the necessary corresponding knowledge of the individual patient and/or operative and management skill sets of the surgical team. The surgical approach may be minimally invasive, traditional open, or combined, depending on specific factors individual to each patient, disease presentation, and surgical team.

Lymph Node Evaluation

Regional lymph nodes are the most common site of metastasis for the majority of solid tumors. Surgical resection of regional lymph nodes generally is part of the staging work-up of the cancer, even if visible tumor is not evident in the lymph nodes. If visible tumor is evident, or if intraoperative pathology verifies microscopic tumor, a lymph node dissection is performed to provide regional control of the cancer. In some cancers—for example, breast cancer—it is uncertain whether a full lymph node dissection plays a role in eliminating future sites of systemic metastasis. Elective lymph node resection (i.e., without evidence of disease or positive results with lymph node biopsy) bears skepticism, as aggressive removal of micrometastatic disease may not improve mortality rates but rather may increase morbidity. These concepts support the notion that many solid tumors undergo years of transformational growth with micrometastatic seeding via the lymphatic and hematologic pathways, which occurs many years before actual detection of the cancer. Treatments such as systemic chemotherapy, hormonal therapy, or biologic therapy may be sufficient to eradicate the disease in clinically benign lymph nodes without an extensive resection (Sabel, 2007).

Sentinel lymph node biopsy (SLNB) is a surgical approach to evaluate regional lymph nodes, specifically in breast cancer and melanoma. On the day of surgery, injections of a radioactive tracer and/or vital blue dye occur, directed at the tumor bed and lymph supply (Povoski et al., 2006). These provide the surgeon with visible and radioactive maps to the first node or nodes that drain the tumor. After the visual identification of blue dye and measurement of in vivo gamma-ray counts, excision of the node or nodes occurs with intraoperative pathologic evaluation. If the lymph node is pathologically negative for tumor, often a node dissection does not occur, and the surgery proceeds to removal of the primary malignancy only. If the lymph node is pathologically positive, surgery to remove regional lymph nodes often commences along with the scar of the prior tumor. Clinical trials continue to validate the use of SLNB in various cancers and its overall reliability in identifying occult lymph node involvement. The identification of micrometastasis in regional lymph nodes may be adequate to indicate the stage of disease and guide appropriate systemic treatment, with ultimate avoidance of lymph node dissection even if the sentinel node is positive (Bilchik, 2006; Harlow, Krag, Reintgen, Moffat, & Frazier, 2006; Hsueh, Hansen, & Giuliano, 2000; Karakousis et al., 2007).

The role of SLNB in gastroesophageal carcinoma is under investigation as a method to detect micrometastasis without extensive surgical resection. Difficulty arises in gastroesophageal carcinoma with regard to retrospective analysis of anatomic skip metastasis in a large number of esophageal cancers and, to a lesser extent, gastric cancers. Breast cancer and melanoma tend to present an orderly progression of lymph node metastasis, but the same uniform patterning is not necessarily found in gastroesophageal cancers. In addition, difficulty with the blue dye method occurs in esophageal cancers because of pigmentation of regional lymph nodes of the thoracic esophagus. Therefore, a radio-guided procedure is standard for SLNB in esophageal cancer, with injection to the submucosal layer of the primary lesion via an endoscopic puncture needle. For gastric cancer, use of the standard dual-tracer method with radioactive colloid and dye occurs, with possible laparoscopic detection, thus allowing for minimally invasive surgery (Kitagawa & Kitajima, 2006).

Minimally Invasive Surgery

Minimally invasive surgery is surgery performed with small incisions (less than 1 cm), typically via laparoscopic access with specialized techniques. The type of minimally invasive surgery depends on which body part requires access (i.e., organ, body space, joint, and/or bone). Instead of using a large incision to gain access to the body part, small portholes provide access for passage of laparoscopes. Visualization of the inside of the body is accomplished via miniature cameras with microscopes, tiny fiber-optic flashlights, and high-definition monitors. Instruments pass through the laparoscopes, enabling surgeons to perform a number of surgical techniques.

Generally, minimally invasive surgery is advantageous over an open procedure because it causes lesser degrees of trauma to the body, less blood loss from the surgery, smaller surgical scars, less overall surgical pain, and decreased postoperative stay. Most patients who undergo minimally invasive surgery are able to leave the hospital sooner with quicker return to normal activities as compared to patients who undergo surgery with a conventional open incision. Nevertheless, one must remember that essentially the patient undergoes the same surgical procedure internally, with a modified external approach. The body must still heal. The APN must often remind patients of this need to heal, as well as the realization of the side effects of prolonged anesthesia resulting from longer procedures with the laparoscopic approach. Disadvantages for the surgeon related to minimally invasive surgery compared to traditional open surgery include decreased depth perception, lack of tactile feedback with the surgical field (although removed tissue can still be palpated once outside the body), and decreased intracavitary ease of suturing (Schlaerth & Abu-Rustum, 2006).

Minimally invasive surgery typically is reserved for early-stage cancer surgical procedures, although research continues to study uses in more advanced presentations. It is used widely in diagnostic and staging procedures, second-look procedures, diagnosis of recurrent disease, and palliative care. For example, in a woman who is clinically and radiographically diagnosed with stage II ovarian cancer, her surgical procedure may start with a diagnostic and exploratory laparoscopy. Tissue can be obtained for intraoperative confirmation of ovarian cancer, and the lower abdomen can be explored for evidence of disseminated disease, allowing an intraoperative decision as to the surgical approach. Another example is in the patient with pancreatic cancer. If an exploratory laparoscopy reveals widespread disease, an en bloc procedure may be aborted, thus sparing the patient the morbidity and healing that accompany a large abdominal incision. The use of diagnostic laparoscopy in cancer surgery may prevent the traditional "open and close" approach, or more importantly, unwarranted exenterative procedures. The opportunity to begin systemic treatment is not complicated by the delays related to surgical morbidity and healing. The role of minimally invasive surgery in the management of cancer continues to expand with the emergence of new techniques that are safe and reasonable options in cancer care (Plante & Roy, 1998; Schlaerth & Abu-Rustum, 2006).

Video-assisted thoracoscopic surgery: Video-assisted thoracoscopic surgery (VATS) is a minimally invasive approach that allows visualization of the chest and access for biopsies of the pleura, diaphragm, and pericardium. Pulmonary wedge resection using the VATS approach is a standard method of obtaining tissue for pathologic diagnosis of small, indeterminate pulmonary nodules. VATS also is useful for the diagnosis and treatment of pleural effusions, allowing for biopsies and pleurodesis. Robotic VATS can aid in mediastinal lymph node dissection, esophagectomy, and cardiac windows. VATS is not a minor surgery, but it is a minimally invasive approach to complex intrathoracic procedures (Flores, Park, & Rusch, 2007).

Robotic surgery: Robotic surgery takes minimally invasive surgery to yet another level with the use of an intuitive robotic system, such as ZEUS™ or, most recently, the da Vinci® Surgical System (Intuitive Surgical, Inc.). The robot itself is a programmable and multifunctional machine that manipulates and performs a variety of tasks through the surgical team's guidance. Robotic assistance in minimally invasive surgery bridges the gap between standard laparoscopic procedures and the traditional open approach, providing extensive manipulation, motion tracking, and three-dimensional imaging. This set of operative equipment includes the surgeon's console, a computerized control system, two instrument robotic arms, and a fiber-optic camera. The traditional laparoscope approach is used, and the robot "holds" the ports, with insertion of robotic instruments through the port openings. These instruments together provide controls for the surgeon to micro-manipulate the robot, which in turn copies the movements made by the surgeon. This allows a full range of motion similar to the surgeon's hands and wrists beyond what is possible in standard laparoscopy. The pictures emitted on the screen are high definition and three-dimensional, unlike with traditional laparoscopic surgery, in which images are less distinct and are two-dimensional. This method of computer-aided surgery can overcome some of the drawbacks of traditional minimally invasive laparoscopic surgery, allowing improved access and visualization and precise dissection, especially around arteries, veins, and nerves (Hashizume, 2007).

As with traditional minimally invasive surgery, robotic surgery has the potential advantages of reduced pain and trauma, minimal blood loss, less postoperative pain, reduced infection risk, shorter hospital stay, improved recovery, and reduced scarring. Unfortunately, robotic-assisted laparoscopy surgery often can take 1.5 times longer than traditional open surgery. Appropriate patient selection is important to avoid additional surgical and anesthesia time. APNs play a pivotal role in identifying appropriate patients for robotic surgery with appropriate preoperative clearance. Additional education is necessary for the patient and family, as well as staff members, related to new equipment, procedures, preoperative and postoperative care of the patient, and cultural, environmental, and social issues that require attention for the patient undergoing robotic surgery (Starnes & Sims, 2006a, 2006b).

Endoluminal instrumentation: Endoluminal instrumentation is yet another form of minimally invasive surgery that enables endoscopists to perform a variety of procedures, including suturing, dissecting, and ligating. The endoscopy approach can be more advantageous than laparoscopy, as procedures can be done with the patient under conscious sedation, as an outpatient, and without abdominal wounds. These advantages result in less pain, improved cosmetic result, faster recuperation, and reduced costs. Examples of the endoluminal approach include a snare polypectomy (versus transabdominal colotomy for polypectomy); procedures performed to inject, cauterize, or clip lower or duodenal bleeding (versus transabdominal approach for duodenectomy); ligation and transjugular intrahepatic portosystemic shunting (versus transabdominal portal systemic shunt for variceal bleeding); percutaneous endoscopic gastrostomy (versus transabdominal approach for placement of a feeding tube); endoscopic retrograde cholangiopancreatography (versus transabdominal approach of common bile duct exploration); endoluminal suturing (versus Nissen fundoplication); and endoscopic mucosal resection (Ellsmere, Jones, Pleskow, & Chuttani, 2006).

Transluminal endoscopic surgery: Transluminal endoscopic surgery, or natural orifice transluminal endoscopic surgery (NOTES), is an emerging alternative to conventional surgery that combines minimally invasive endoscopic and laparoscopic techniques to diagnose and treat intra-abdominal disease. In this procedure, the surgeon inserts the endoscope through a natural orifice, such as the mouth, anus, urethra, or vagina, and enters the peritoneal cavity via a transvisceral incision. This potential means of access to the abdominal cavity from the lumen of hollow viscera can eliminate multiple laparoscopic or larger incisions that traverse through skin and muscle, thus reducing complications such as wound infection, hernia, pain, and adhesions (McGee et al., 2006).

Some of the more common uses of NOTES include the external insertion of percutaneous feeding tubes with endoscopic lighted access, sphincter access, and balloon dilation methods. Although these procedures are common, this passage from the lumen of hollow viscera into the abdominal cavity awaits additional research with translation of animal to human studies and perfection of adequate closure of the viscerotomy (McGee et al., 2006).

Adjuncts to Surgical Resection

Radiofrequency ablation: Radiofrequency ablation (RFA) is a method of tissue removal through the application of high-frequency radio waves that provide local destruction of tumor, either primary or metastatic. Uses of RFA for the primary treatment of cancers continue to be under scientific investigation, such as in breast cancer and hepatocellular carcinoma. Most often, RFA is used for control of metastatic liver disease, typically if patients have failed conventional control of their disease. RFA employs percutaneous, laparoscopic, or open surgical access to tumors, with subsequent destruction of targeted tumor. Often, noninvasive surgical approaches are successful and cause minimal discomfort to the patient (Chow et al., 2006; Ryan, 2006; Siperstein et al., 2000).

Cryosurgery: Cryosurgery utilizes liquid nitrogen to destroy malignant tissue and provide local control of tumor growth. A variety of cryosurgical delivery methods exist to provide external or internal death of tissue, which may result in semipermanent or permanent cell death. Cryoablation and cryolocalization are methods undergoing study for use in the treatment and diagnosis of breast disease. Salvage cryosurgery for locally recurrent prostate cancer following radiotherapy may be an alternative to salvage radical prostatectomy (Ahmed, Lindsey, & Davies, 2005).

Unlike RFA, as discussed earlier, patients potentially may better withstand cryoablation because cold is analgesic in nature, whereas heat can be more uncomfortable. Cryoablation, as a freezing technique, produces necrosis and local destruction of tissue. However, margins are difficult to ascertain; therefore, it remains most useful in benign disease such as fibroadenomas. Cryolocalization can create a well-delineated mass of frozen tissue around a tumor and may provide an alternative approach to needle-localization for surgical removal of a breast mass. Additional research is necessary in this field of cryotechnology before it replaces surgical excision for removal of malignant tissue (Tafra et al., 2006; Whitworth & Rewcastle, 2005).

Radioimmunoguided surgery: Radioimmunoguided surgery (RIGS) employs a radioactive tracer to identify possible malignant tissue. Intraoperatively, a neoprobe localizes radioactivity, guiding resection with the potential of identifying areas of malignancy distant from the main primary and reduction of operating time. Examples include SLNB as previously described, radioguided parathyroidectomy, and RIGS-intraoperative radiotherapy. Studies continue to identify labeled radiographic tracers specific for various cancer types and subtypes that successfully guide the surgeon to malignant tissue (Nag, Martinez-Monge, Neiroda, & Martin, 1999; Nichol et al., 2003).

Light amplification by stimulated emission: Light amplification by stimulated emission of radiation (known as *laser*) employs an intense, narrow beam, enabling precise surgery for removal of precancerous or cancerous lesions. Laser also can enable procedures that relieve symptoms of cancer. Different types of laser approaches and instrumentation exist that allow direct application of laser therapy through an open incision or endoscopic instruments. As with most minimally invasive techniques, the use of laser with endoscopic assistance results in less bleeding and damage than with other resection methods. Photodynamic therapy is another laser therapy technique that uses an injectable photosensitizing agent followed by targeted laser therapy to destroy malignant cells. Laser-induced interstitial thermotherapy is another laser modality that utilizes laser light to heat and kill malignant cells. This procedure may have more benefit if used in conjunction with arterial embolization, as in the case of liver metastases. These laser techniques offer additional approaches to destroy cancer cells, although the benefit does not typically persist (Butani, Arbesfeld, & Schwartz, 2005; Ritz et al., 2007).

Postoperative Care

Evaluation of patients with cancer and their family and caregivers during the preoperative phase of surgery minimizes the stress of the operative procedure and thus promotes a prompt return to a state of health during the postoperative phase. Criticism surrounds shorter lengths of hospital stays with concern that patients are not well enough to return home or have not remained in the hospital long enough to heal from their procedures. In fact, shorter lengths of stay have led patients to be active sooner after surgery, leading to decreased levels of postoperative pain, enhanced mobility and exercise capacity, and improved enteral intake soon after surgery (Kehlet, 2006). Body measurements such as temperature, pulse, respiration, blood pressure, weight, and intake and output of fluids/urine remain important indices upon which to measure postoperative stability and progress. Additionally, results of postoperative laboratory studies, specifically renal function, hematologic status, oxygenation, and electrolyte balance, enable APNs to augment surgical outcomes and minimize complications.

Preexisting comorbid conditions such as cardiac, pulmonary, renal, and hepatic disease present additional postoperative challenges in balancing metabolic disease with the stress of surgery. Appropriate volume resuscitation with isotonic fluids is required to maintain intravascular volume and adequate hydration. Vital signs and urine output provide guides for adjustments in volume and fluid type. Control of peripheral capillary permeability prevents unwanted effects that lead to uncomfortable peripheral edema causing limited movement and ineffective ambulation. Those patients with inadequate renal or cardiac function may require diuretics, but otherwise, a natural diuresis will occur postoperatively as fluid mobilizes from the periphery into vascular spaces (Fakhry et al., 2006). A variety of perioperative and postoperative symptoms can occur in patients, including electrolyte imbalances, anemia, mental status change, and acid-base disorders. Various chapters throughout this text contain information regarding management of some of these conditions. In healthy surgical patients, pain, nausea and vomiting, and infection are the three largest threats to homeostasis and will be addressed here.

Pain

Postoperative pain is a constellation of unpleasant experiences precipitated by surgical injury that can be acute or chronic in nature. These sensory, emotional, and mental experiences in turn are associated with autonomic, psychological, and behavioral responses. The control of postoperative pain aims to provide subjective comfort and inhibit blunt trauma–induced nociceptive impulses. Management of these autonomic and somatic reflex responses to pain enables restoration of function with early ambulation accompanied by objective and subjective improvement (Kehlet, 2006). APNs have a compendium of analgesics to reduce or eliminate postoperative pain. In addition, nonpharmaceutical interventions with attention to mechanical positioning often are successful in reducing overall pain.

Special attention is required for patients with a history of chronic pain requiring management with narcotics who then experience acute pain related to a surgical procedure. APNs are responsible for assessing patients' pain management strategies prior to surgery and the change in level of pain after surgery. In some cases, the surgical procedure actually may reduce pain that was caused by compression, thereby resulting in less overall pain for the postoperative patient. In other cases, incisional pain may increase overall pain needs, requiring narcotic dosages greater than usual doses. APNs must ascertain that appropriate pain management techniques and dosages are in place with frequent reassessment and must educate those involved in the care of these compromised patients.

Of all cancer surgeries, the thoracotomy and major abdominal procedures are potentially the most painful. A combination approach to pain management often is required with consideration of local anesthetics and opioids through an epidural catheter, systemic nonsteroidal anti-inflammatory drugs (NSAIDs) or cyclooxygenase-2 inhibitors, and systemic opioids. The combination of these agents provides both synergistic and additive effects. Abdominal procedures also can present challenges related to decreased bowel motility and ileus. If possible, use of systemic opioids is minimal until bowel motility returns as evidenced by flatus and passage of stool. Often, the addition of IV NSAIDs provides enhanced pain relief with smaller doses of narcotics when compared to the use of narcotics alone. Use of patient-controlled analgesia is one method to monitor pain medication requirements if only the patient is requesting the medication through activation of the pump (Hudcova, McNicol, Quah, Lau, & Carr, 2006; Wuhrman et al., 2007).

Epidural pain management can be effective for major mid-chest, abdominal, and lower extremity surgeries. Epidural medications are difficult to administer for head, neck, upper chest, and upper extremity surgeries, as the location of the epidural catheter with concomitant administration of pain medication may compromise respiratory function. Epidural pain management requires close monitoring of appropriate drug, dosage, and infusion rate because of the concentration of drug. Frequent assessment by the entire surgical team of bladder distention, lower extremity motor loss, and skin integrity is essential, as patients are unlikely to accurately report these signs and symptoms because of a lack of sensation. APNs can be effective in optimizing pain management for patients undergoing these surgeries by including potential epidural pain management, as well as anesthesia when appropriate, in their discussion with the surgical team. APNs often are responsible for adequate postoperative pain management and must be prepared to alter the pain regimen as needed.

Nausea and Vomiting

Nausea and vomiting are common in postoperative patients and are responsible for unplanned hospital admission of ambulatory surgery patients, delay in discharge, significant discomfort, and patient dissatisfaction. Risk factors for postoperative nausea and vomiting include female sex, pediatric patient, prior history of nausea and vomiting with anesthesia, history of motion sickness, ingestion of food too quickly after surgery, side effects of pain medication, duration of surgery, and ear, nose, throat, and breast augmentation procedures. APNs often coordinate preoperative care and therefore are responsible for obtaining and synthesizing the history as well as a list of the patient's current medications, smoking history, and perceived barriers to nausea and vomiting management. With this information, the anesthesia team then may modify commonly used drugs and avoid the use of emesis-inducing agents such as fentanyl, nitrous oxide, and other volatile inhalational gases (Iverson & Lynch, 2006).

The receptor systems for nausea and vomiting in postoperative patients are similar to those related to chemotherapy (see Chapter 4 for further explanation). In most cases, stimulation of receptors in the brain from anesthetic agents induces nausea and vomiting, as opposed to chemical irritation of the stomach itself. Concomitantly, once vomiting begins, the epigastric muscles experience spasms that exacerbate symptoms. Therefore, interventions for both sources of nausea and vomiting often are necessary, with the use of a serotonin antagonist and a smooth muscle relaxant. Serotonin antagonists are effective and safe drugs with minimal side effects. Smooth muscle relaxants often cause somnolence but otherwise are well tolerated. An additional preventive approach can be used to decrease stimulation of histamine receptors in the brain with the application of a scopolamine patch several hours before surgery, especially in patients with a history of motion sickness. The control of postoperative nausea and vomiting begins in the operating room and includes a multimodal approach with serotonin antagonists and other antiemetic agents (Iverson & Lynch, 2006).

Fever and Infection

Fever in the postoperative setting is common and often is not associated with an infectious process. Typically, fever of noninfectious origin occurs early in the postoperative period and resolves, whereas fever related to an infection occurs days after surgery and persists. Fever generally increases in the evening and decreases in the morning. It is important to remember that the absence of fever does not rule out infection. This is especially true in immunocompromised patients, whose host defense mechanisms, including temperature response, are altered. Disease processes, including cancer, can also cause persistent temperatures. These are typically low-grade in nature (< 100.5°F [38°C]) but can exhibit fevers as high as 103°F (39.4°C) (Ezzone, 2006; Fakhry et al., 2006).

Physical examination is the most useful tool in the differential diagnosis of an infectious process. The most common sites of postoperative fever arise in the pulmonary system, urinary tract, or operative site and also can be related to medications or occur as a result of phlebitis. Bacterial infections in postoperative patients can be endogenous or exogenous and can originate from preexisting conditions, the surgical procedure, or nosocomial risk from rotating staff. In seriously ill individuals, one or more sources of infection can exist at the same time or secondarily as a result of stress on the immune system. Single-room occupancy is desirable, if possible, to reduce potential nosocomial infection through direct contact with other patients and family (Bracco, Dubois, Bouali, & Eggimann, 2007; Fakhry et al., 2006). Infection surveillance is extremely important throughout the postoperative phase.

SSIs can occur in a variety of anatomic locations: superficial incision, deep incision, and organ space. An SSI occurs in the first 30 days after surgery. Infections occurring after 30 days are not termed SSIs and are not attributable to the surgical procedure or immediate postoperative phase. One exception is surgical implants; infections up to one year following the operation can be attributable to the surgical procedure. Superficial incision SSI occurs in the skin layers and subcutaneous tissues related to the incision. Deep incisional SSI involves the deep soft tissues. Organ space SSI occurs in adjacent organ space, regardless of whether the organ remains (Lafreniere et al., 2006).

Surgical drain placement often is necessary for intracavitary drainage of the surgical bed to prevent pooling of bodily fluids that inadvertently delay wound healing, yet these drains also are a source of infection. The number of drains placed, the duration of placement, and the type of drainage apparatus are all factors related to possible SSI. Closed suction apparatus are preferred to minimize contamination from airborne sources. Prompt removal of drains is desirable to reduce the potential of surgical wound infections, although this cannot occur until intracavitary fluid accumulation slows. Removal of drains can occur as soon as two to three days after surgery, or they may remain in place for many weeks, pending decrease in accumulated fluid drainage. Any external tube is a portal for infection to the inside of the body. These tubes can colonize with bacteria, allowing yet another source of infection (Fakhry et al., 2006).

Pneumonia can occur when normal host mechanisms of defense are unable to prevent pathogenic invasion. A number of factors are involved in the development of postoperative pneumonia, including the cancer diagnosis, intubation for general anesthesia, nosocomial exposure, inactivity, and a host of risk factors. APNs must assess patient-specific risk factors, monitor clinical signs and symptoms, observe patient progress, and preemptively intervene as needed to maintain pulmonary health. Expedient recovery and prevention of additional complications related to infection rely on implementation of evidence-based nursing interventions relative to the care of the patient with pneumonia as well as postoperative mobilization (Brungs & Render, 2006; Kennedy, 2006; Zitella et al., 2006).

Additional Complications

A number of postoperative cardiac and pulmonary conditions can occur related to preexisting conditions or resulting from the physical stress of surgery. Treatment of these conditions with evidence-based interventions specific to the cardiac or pulmonary event can prevent further serious adverse events. APNs can address these common adverse events in surgical patients to improve healing and avoid deleterious events. For example, postoperative hypertension commonly is caused by surgical pain or hypoxia; thus, adequate pain control and oxygenation are necessary. Use of various monitoring devices to measure oxygenation is warranted, as adequate oxygenation is necessary for tissue healing. Treatment of persistent hypertension is essential to prevent cardiac events, such as myocardial infarction, arrhythmias, and cerebral vascular accident. Respiratory complications, including atelectasis, aspiration, and pneumonia, often are preventable with therapeutic interventions, especially in high-risk patients. Upright positioning and early ambulation are essential to mobilization of secretions and prevention of pneumonia.

Diabetes mellitus is a preexisting, chronic condition that can necessitate acute attention during the postoperative phase. Diabetic patients require close management with careful avoidance of hypoglycemia or hyperglycemia and associated complications of diabetic ketoacidosis and dehydration. Diabetes can have a significant negative impact on wound healing and may require tight control with sliding scale insulin to maximize outcomes.

Thromboembolism, presenting as PE or DVT, is another serious potential side effect of surgery because of stasis of blood. Risk factors include age greater than 40 years, obesity, immobilization, hypercoagulable states, Virchow triad, venous access devices, varicosities, pregnancy, history of malignancy, hormonal drugs, history of prior thromboembolus, and complicated, lengthy surgery (Heit, 2006; Owings, 2006). A variety of prophylactic measures are available, such as elevation of the legs with knee flexion, mobilization, pneumatic boots, leg exercises, elastic stockings, and anticoagulation with heparin (Leonardi, McGory, & Ko, 2007). Interventions by APNs must aim at prevention as well as primary and secondary treatment.

Access Devices

The infusion of chemotherapy and blood products often requires reliable and easy venous access, ensuring safety and maximum comfort for patients with cancer. Totally implantable access ports are widely used, with insertion by the surgical team or radiology interventionalists. Typically, either a cephalic vein cutdown or subclavian vein puncture technique is used. Additional venous access devices are discussed in *Access Device Guidelines: Recommendations for Nursing Practice and Education* (Second Edition), published by the Oncology Nursing Society (Camp-Sorrell, 2004). APNs are instrumental in identifying those patients who may benefit from the insertion of venous access devices, as well as in educating the healthcare team to anticipate this need for their patients.

Rehabilitation

Comprehensive rehabilitation of patients with cancer is a responsibility of all members of the oncology healthcare team, including surgical oncology. Rehabilitation begins in the hospital setting based on discussion with patients and families in the preoperative setting. Survival rates for most cancers continue to improve, yet life-altering treatments may be necessary to bring life-saving results. The goals of cancer rehabilitation include improvements in quality of life and reduction in handicaps from cancer and its related treatments. All cancers share common rehabilitation goals, but each cancer brings its own set of challenges (Olsson, Bosaeus, Svedlund, & Bergbom, 2007; Yadav, 2007).

Wounds

Acute Wounds

Acute surgical wound management is the interaction of appropriate surgical closure, postoperative healing, and preexisting or acquired comorbid conditions. Initially, most cancer wounds are a result of mechanical trauma resulting from surgery. Primary closure of the wound occurs at the time of surgery with internal suturing and external suturing/staples, creating an incision line that heals as a scar. Secondary closure occurs if a surgical incision has opened or if the incision was intentionally left open at the time of surgery, and the body heals by secondary intent (i.e., from the inside out). Tertiary closure involves mechanical or natural closure of the wound after a period of secondary healing. The goal of acute wound management is to facilitate healing with the scar being as minimally apparent as possible (Lawrence, Bevin, & Sheldon, 2007).

Cancer wounds can occur because of surgical intervention or from the cancer itself with erosion of surrounding healthy tissue causing fistula formation, abscess, edema, or vascular changes. Superficial wounds involve the epidermis; partial-thickness wounds involve the dermis; and full-thickness wounds involve all layers of the skin, subcutaneous tissue, muscle, and/or bone. Treatment centers on the control or elimination of causative factors, as well as pressure, shearing force, friction, moisture, circulation, and neuropathy (Taylor, 2007).

In patients with comorbid conditions, additional interventions may be necessary to maximize wound healing and prevent skin breakdown. Assessment of factors revolving around nutritional status, preexisting cancer, diabetes, uremia, liver function/jaundice, advanced age, systemic corticosteroids, use of chemotherapeutic agents, previous radiation therapy, and alcoholism is imperative. Prophylactic antibiotics are indicated for contaminated wounds, patients who are immunocompromised or diabetic, patients with cardiac valvular disease, and patients with artificial prostheses such as valve and joint replacements. Lymphedematous extremities are particularly prone to cellulitis and are of priority when performing surgery on these limbs. Patients who have stool-contaminated wounds or those having contact with gastrointestinal contents typically are treated with prophylactic antibiotics (Lawrence et al., 2007).

Smoking impairs tissue oxygenation, stimulates vasoconstriction, and contributes to factors of chronic atherosclerosis and vascular disease. All these conditions potentially can affect tissue and wound healing. Smoking cessation is ideal in the preoperative phase and *imperative* after surgery for maximal wound healing. Nutritional and fluid support is necessary with a balanced diet and adequate hydration to provide the body with appropriate nutrients for healing. Attention to nitrogen and protein balance is essential to wound healing and often can be improved with dietary interventions. Frequently, patients with cancer require nutritional supplements to boost the natural healing process, such as supplemental protein shakes, dietary supplements, and in some cases, total parenteral nutrition (Lawrence et al., 2007).

The avoidance and prevention of surgical wound dehiscence is paramount in cancer surgical care. Recognition of risk factors is essential, and elimination of mechanical stress on the incision is necessary to prevent wound dehiscence. A dehisced wound may require immediate surgical intervention or may heal by secondary intent. APNs recognize those patients who are at risk for wound dehiscence and provide added surveillance with the surgical team.

Soft tissue infections can involve the skin and underlying subcutaneous tissue, fascia, or muscle. These infections are divided into necrotizing and non-necrotizing categories: non-necrotizing infections are resolved primarily with antibiotic therapy, whereas necrotizing infections or skin/tissue death may also require operative debridement followed by antibiotics. Blood cultures rarely are positive and are only recommended when the patient exhibits concomitant high fever and chills. Other debridement techniques may be used instead of or after surgery, such as high-pressure, mechanical irrigation or wet-to-dry dressings. Vacuum-assisted closure therapy may be helpful in wound healing, especially for deep, chronic wounds of moderate to high exudate. This technique creates topical negative pressure with improved blood flow, decreased edema, and removal of excessive fluid from the wound bed. Improved tissue perfusion and oxygenation results with increased tissue granulation and regeneration. The hypoxic environment across the wound surface prevents survival of aerobic bacteria (Ford-Dunn, 2006; Lawrence et al., 2007).

Chronic Wounds

Chronic wounds are distinguished from acute wounds by their healing characteristics and etiology and can persist for months or years. The most common chronic wound etiologies include changes related to burns, vasculitis, or dermatitis and complications related to delays in surgical wound healing, fistulae, manifestation of cancer to the skin, and tissue damage or death from radiation therapy. Although wound healing typically occurs in an orderly fashion, impediment of this process can occur in the patient with cancer. Chronic wound classification related to etiology, wound depth, or degree of tissue damage is important, but accurate assessment of the wound and resulting healing is imperative to the plan of care.

Wound Assessment

Wound status must be assessed throughout the treatment period, which is a responsibility of APNs and the surgical team. Item descriptors from the Bates-Jensen Wound Assessment Tool are helpful for quantitative assessment, with attention to anatomic characteristics of the wound: size, depth, edges, undermining, necrotic tissue type, necrotic tissue amount, exudate type, exudate amount, skin color surrounding the wound, peripheral tissue edema, peripheral tissue induration, granulation tissue, and epithelialization (Bates-Jensen, 1999; McNees, 2006). Education of staff members, patients, and families augments wound management and partnership in wound rehabilitation.

Risk assessment and prevention of pressure ulcers are essential in the care of patients with cancer. Conditions for skin breakdown are ideal because of the cancer itself, suboptimal nutrition, fatigue, and immunosuppression. Multiple comorbid risk factors also exist that contribute to development of pressure ulcers. Preventive measures with meticulous skin assessment are necessary, focusing on the individual patient's risk assessment, skin care, fluid balance, and nutrition. If a pressure wound is apparent, early intervention may avoid progression of tissue damage and ultimate surgical debridement (Lyder, 2006).

Malignant Wounds

Malignant fungating wounds can present in advanced cancer as a result of local invasion by the primary tumor or metastatic disease. Unless treated, the tumor spreads and creates additional tissue destruction with resulting skin ulceration. Vascular and lymphatic supplies may change, leading to edema, exudates, bleeding, and tissue necrosis. The tumor mass may extend above the skin surface, presenting as an erosive and ulcerative lesion or a cauliflower-like growth. The wound bed typically consists of friable or necrotic tissue with fragile surrounding skin. Tissue necrosis and underlying infection are responsible for significant malodor. Management of odor occurs by decreasing local bacterial colonization, cleansing the wound, and debriding the wound. Dressing needs vary as to the location of the wound, amount of exudates, and ability to secure the dressing to surrounding healthy skin. Adequate pain management is essential to maintaining patient comfort. Education and emotional support with attention to cosmesis and odor control potentially can improve quality of life for patients and caregivers (Seaman, 2006).

Wound Care Management

Multiple (more than 800) wound care products are available to aid in delayed wound healing and fungating masses. These include but are not limited to hydrocolloids, impregnated gauze, hydrogels, alginates, film dressings, foam, hydrofibers, creams, ointments, sprays, enzymatic agents, powders, skin sealants, collagen matrix products, biologic or skin substitutes, and accessory products. Basic principles of wound assessment and management are key to guide the treatment plan and dressing selection. APNs play an important role in wound management related to cancer therapy and may be consulted in the initial assessment phase. Enterostomal therapists are valuable resources for wound management and selection of wound care products specific to each patient (Taylor, 2007).

Stoma Care

A stoma is a mouth-like opening created surgically on the skin surface for access to underlying organs. Stoma openings are necessary in cancer surgery to divert normal internal lumen and to provide an alternative airway or method of elimination for urine or feces. The most common cancers requiring stoma are those related to the oropharynx/larynx, small and large bowel, and urinary system. The decision to create a stoma is relevant to the location and extent of a cancer along with concomitant issues such as infection or comorbid conditions (e.g., chronic obstructive pulmonary disease, scar tissue from previous surgeries).

Skin complications can occur as a result of irritation from surface contact with digestive fluids, poor skin integrity, excessive moisture, and restrictive appliances. External drainage apparatus containing bile or digestive products require attention to skin integrity maintenance caused by degradation of the skin surfaces that are in frequent contact with digestive enzymes. Various products exist to improve stoma fit and to shield the skin from contact, thus preventing skin breakdown. Careful planning and education during the preoperative and postoperative phases are integral to successful adaptation of the body and patient to a stoma. The enterostomal therapy nurse and wound, ostomy, and continence nurses are key resources for appliance fit and skin interventions (Williams, 2007).

Skin Grafting

The extent of surgery, deformity, loss of function, and cosmetic result are factors to consider regarding skin grafting. If possible, skin grafting occurs at the time of tumor resection to maximize use of the anesthesia time and minimize postoperative colonization of endogenous and exogenous bacteria. Often, the decision of whether to graft is made at the time of surgery and can be difficult to predict because of potential unknown circulatory deficits. Assumed circulation to surrounding tissue and appropriate dressings may preclude the necessity of grafting, given adequate surface skin for closure. Delayed surgical graft placement can occur if healing does not progress, although closure of the wound by secondary intent or natural means often is preferred at this point. Skin grafting can be necessary in any surgery, given the amount of removed subcutaneous tissue and skin, but the more common cancer types requiring grafting include head and neck, melanoma, and limb (i.e., amputation).

Skin graft healing is concomitant with wound healing, as the skin graft with its own architecture covers the wound. Skin graft revascularization occurs as blood and lymphatic vessels begin to grow from the surgical site into the graft and as preexisting vessels connect between the two sites. Blood and lymphatic flow to the graft approaches near-normal levels about seven days postoperatively. Maturity of the vascular supply continues and often is near normal by day 21 (Lawrence et al., 2007).

Reconstruction

Reconstruction of body parts altered by cancer surgical treatment continues to evolve with choices of immediate reconstruction (performed at the time of the cancer surgery) and delayed reconstruction (performed in a separate procedure after the cancer surgery). Reconstructive techniques include procedures such as tissue expansion, pedicled flaps, myocutaneous flaps, and free tissue transfer. The most common areas of reconstruction are the head and neck, breast, vagina, and extremities (Cordeiro, 2006). The goal of reconstructive surgery in cancer is to eliminate suffering, decrease the deformity caused by cancer surgery, and restore wholeness.

An increasing number of patients with breast cancer receive adjuvant radiation therapy after a mastectomy, with or without a reconstructed breast mound. Unsatisfactory results of conventional immediate reconstruction techniques when followed by radiation therapy have led to the formation of new algorithms. Questions arise as to the best method, timing, and outcomes for women undergoing immediate and delayed breast reconstruction *without* prior knowledge of the need for radiation therapy. Unfortunately, nodal status often is unknown during the decision-making phase for the type of breast surgery and possible type of reconstruction. The lack of this important information can lead to complications in the plastic surgery trajectory when postoperative radiation therapy is submitted for consideration *after* the definitive surgery has been performed (Pomahac, Recht, May, Hergrueter, & Slavin, 2006).

The scope of this chapter does not permit detailed discussion of various reconstructive procedures. APNs have a responsibility to identify patients who will have significant morbidity secondary to their cancer surgery and to tailor a personalized plan for their surgical care. Patients choose reconstruction to restore their removed body part and achieve symmetry, balance, weight replacement, and functionality. Reconstruction is an important component of restoring cosmesis and self-esteem (Chapman, 2007). The plastic surgery team is responsible for restoring wholeness after the surgical team removes the cancer. Guiding patients and families through this trajectory can pose challenges that require ongoing revision, both physically and psychologically.

Surveillance

All patients with cancer require ongoing surveillance for the unique medical needs related to their cancer diagnosis. Monitoring for possible local tumor recurrence as well as disseminated disease is necessary, including periodic interaction with the patient and updated history and physical examinations. Patients may be at risk for recurrence of their primary tumor, at risk for the development of a second or related primary tumor because of genetic susceptibility, or at risk for development of a second primary tumor resulting from the cancer treatment. Unfortunately, in most cancers, extensive batteries of laboratory and imaging studies do not improve survival benefit. Specific surveillance tests that describe tumor-specific management provide long-term follow-up in this group of patients with diverse physical and psychosocial needs. (See Chapter 17 for more information on cancer surveillance following treatment.) The surgical team often maintains an ongoing relationship with patients with cancer and their families, thus assuming responsibility for appropriate surveillance testing with integral interventions.

APNs must take a leadership role in primary care of the cancer survivor to promote effective cancer screening, healthy lifestyle choices, and continuing rehabilitation of the known cancer. Attention to the prevalence of multiple cancers is necessary, with review of genetic predisposition, environmental exposure, tobacco use, and aging. The spectrum of needs of cancer survivors and their families is extensive, requiring awareness of pertinent issues such as cancer-specific tumor biology, surveillance, genetic counseling and testing, second primaries, complications related to treatment, physiologic alterations, altered lifestyle, and psychosocial challenges. APNs often fulfill the role of advocate, attending to the best interests of patients and families (Mariotto, Rowland, Ries, Scoppa, & Feuer, 2007).

Palliation

Palliation from a surgical perspective begins at the cancer diagnosis for all cancers. The goal is to maximize life and minimize side effects and disability, with the hope that the cancer will not recur locally or systemically. Although a few cancers can claim "cure" following a designated time period after surgery, the potential characteristics of most solid tumors do not avail a *guarantee* of cure with surgery alone. Prolongation of life is not the only measure of success in cancer treatment. Palliation accomplished by surgical procedures is measured by disease-free intervals and the degrees of freedom from distress, rather than merely duration of earthly life.

Each surgical intervention has risks and benefits. Surgical decisions, made together by the surgical team and patient, occur after thorough and thoughtful review of the patient's presentation, comorbid disease states, extent of disease, and wishes of the patient. Consideration of age alone as a factor is not relevant to decision making about palliative care, as older people are heterogeneous in terms of physical and psychological functioning. Discussion about goals, expectations, and physical cost of the intervention must be weighed against the potential negative side effects and complications, all in concert with personal belief systems, ethics, and end-of-life desires (Duggleby & Raudonis, 2006; Galante et al., 2005).

Surgical interventions to relieve symptom distress caused by side effects from metastatic cancer and to improve quality of life are becoming more common *prior* to the debilitating presence of life-threatening complications. Surgeons, endoscopists, interventional radiologists, anesthesiologists, and APNs all offer surgical expertise in controlling cancer-related symptoms. The rapid expansion of minimally invasive surgical approaches significantly decreases postoperative morbidity and hastens an improved outcome from the surgical intervention itself. Patient and procedure selection together require scrutiny in an effort to improve quality of life, sustain quantity of desired length of life, and maximize the side effect profile. And, as with all phases of medicine and the human body, no guarantees for outcome exist.

Conclusion

The role of surgery for patients with cancer and their families occurs throughout the cancer continuum, from prevention to diagnosis, from surgical resection through postoperative care, from access and rehabilitation to surveillance, and finally in palliative care. Members of the surgical healthcare team, including APNs, play a vital role in the education, support, and care of patients with cancer and their families.

Case Study

M.F. is a 33-year-old African American female with a family history of breast cancer in her mother (age 48) and sister (age 37). M.F. has a personal history of a benign left breast biopsy performed at age 31. M.F. was referred to the high-risk breast clinic by her gynecologist.

1. How would the APN staffing this clinic proceed?
   - The APN would interview the patient to obtain a complete history, including family history of cancer, personal breast history, imaging studies, breast self-examination findings, age at menarche, parity/age at birth of first child, endogenous hormonal status including menstrual history, exogenous hormone use, and patient's perception of breast cancer risk. If possible, the APN may review prior imaging studies (including films) and pathology results (including slides). A clinical breast examination is performed.
   - M.F.'s physical examination is within normal limits for a premenopausal woman; no abnormalities are noted. She is scheduled for a bilateral mammogram and bilateral MRI of the breasts, which are indicated for age- and risk-appropriate surveillance. These studies indicate dense fibrous tissue bilaterally but are within normal limits. M.F. is scheduled for a genetic consultation.
   - M.F. was lost to follow-up in the high-risk breast clinic and presents today in the abnormal breast clinic. Previous appointment reminder letters from the high-risk breast clinic were returned as "addressee unknown"; these dated letters and envelopes are noted in the chart. M.F. states that she re-

cently noted her bra was tighter, specifically on the right side. She saw her gynecologist who noted a right breast mass; M.F. was referred for further work-up.

- M.F.'s personal and family history is unchanged from her office visit four years ago. She is currently 37 years old. A recent right mammogram indicates a 3.5 cm suspicious mass in the upper outer quadrant of the right breast. Her physical examination confirms a fixed, irregular, 3 cm dominant mass in the right upper outer quadrant. The skin overlying the mass is erythematous and dimpled. Several palpable 1–2 cm nodes are noted in the right axilla and supraclavicular region. The left breast and axilla are within normal limits.

2. What would the APN discuss with M.F. regarding these clinical findings?
   - The APN would discuss with M.F. the concern that these radiographic and physical findings are highly suspicious for a locally advanced breast cancer with regional lymph node involvement. These findings would be discussed with the collaborating surgical oncologist, and the APN would prepare M.F. for a CNB of the right breast. A mammogram of the left breast would be ordered. If the biopsy shows cancer, then staging scans of the head, chest, and abdomen, as well as a bone scan, are ordered to rule out distant metastasis, which is a concern based on findings of supraclavicular node involvement.
   - M.F. returns to the breast cancer clinic after completing several months of neoadjuvant chemotherapy for breast cancer. Her physical examination reveals a normal left breast and axilla and marked reduction in size of the right breast mass. Bilaterally, no axillary or supraclavicular adenopathy is noted. A recent MRI of the right breast indicates a 1.5 cm mass.
   - M.F. undergoes a right modified radical mastectomy. Pathology reports a 1.7 cm, poorly differentiated, infiltrating lobular carcinoma that is estrogen and progesterone receptor negative and HER2/neu negative. The right axillary contents reveal 0/29 positive lymph nodes. Margins are free of cancer involvement. Three weeks after the operation, M.F. calls, stating that she has noted some redness around her chest wall incision. She also complains of frequent urination the past several days and is very thirsty. She denies a temperature elevation.

3. What are the differential diagnoses of the right chest wall erythema?
   - The source of the erythema is unknown at present; physical examination is necessary. Differential diagnoses for the erythema include skin reaction to suture material and SSI, with possible underlying diabetes. Recurrent breast cancer to the chest wall also is considered but is not likely at this time, given the most recent pathology report. Most likely, the erythema represents a local SSI aggravated by underlying diabetes.
   - Two years later, M.F. presents to the clinic, stating that she recently underwent a metastatic work-up that indicated diffuse bony metastasis. She complains of right hip pain that increases with ambulation. The bone scan report shows increased intensity in the right acetabulum. The APN obtains a plain right hip film that confirms hairline fractures in the proximal right femur and acetabulum. An orthopedic consultation is arranged for today.

4. M.F. asks what the orthopedist will discuss. What would the APN tell her?
   • The APN will explain that most likely the orthopedist will recommend surgery with insertion of hardware to stabilize the bones. The concept of palliative care with surgical intervention for symptom management is common in this setting.

Key Points

- Surgery is the oldest modality for cancer treatment and today is still the only means of cure in many cancers. It is used in every aspect of oncology care, including cancer prevention, diagnosis, resection, postoperative care, access, rehabilitation, surveillance, and palliation. Surgery involves removal of the tumor with adequate margins of normal tissue. Adequate margins vary from cancer to cancer.
- A diagnosis of cancer relies on tissue acquisition for pathologic, cytologic, and possibly histologic review. Information obtained from the history, physical examination, observation, and diagnostic testing guides the surgical plan for tissue acquisition. Correlation of pathologic information obtained from the tissue biopsy with radiology studies, physical examination, and the patient's history is necessary for accurate diagnosis.
- A negative needle biopsy (fine or core needle) does not ensure that a lesion is benign. If suspicion for malignancy is high and the needle biopsy is negative or inconclusive, an open biopsy is necessary to verify a diagnosis.
- Surgical APNs often serve as navigators or interpreters for patients and families by explaining available treatment options that may influence patients' decision-making processes, facilitating interdisciplinary consultations, and providing continuity of care as patients transition to other care settings.
- The goals of cancer surgical therapy are to (a) maximize potential for control or cure of cancer, (b) minimize comorbidities, and (c) retain active participation of patients and families.
- The preoperative assessment includes medical, surgical, and psychosocial history, nutritional status, medication review, laboratory and imaging studies, teaching needs, and risk of postsurgical infection. Potential surgical benefits are weighed against the risks of the cancer-related surgical interventions.
- Regional lymph nodes, the most common site of metastasis for most solid tumors, often are resected as part of the staging work-up of the tumor, even if visible tumor is not evident. If visible tumor is evident (or is confirmed by intraoperative pathology), then lymph node dissection is performed for regional control of the cancer. Sentinel lymph node biopsy is a surgical approach to evaluate regional lymph nodes by using a radioactive tracer and/or dye directed at the tumor bed and lymph supply that enables the surgeon to visualize the first node or nodes draining the tumor. If the first lymph node is pathologically negative for tumor, node dissection often is not performed, thus saving the patient from unnecessary surgery.
- Surgical resection of metastatic sites removes cancers that are confined to one metastatic organ, improving overall five-year survival by 25%–40% (depending on the cancer and metastatic site). However, most cancer types are not amenable to this approach because of the malignant potential caused by systemic, micrometastatic disease.

- Minimally invasive surgery lessens the degree of trauma and blood loss and involves smaller surgical scars, less overall surgical pain, and decreased postoperative stays. It typically is reserved for early-stage cancer and is widely used in diagnostic and staging procedures, second-look procedures, diagnosis of recurrent disease, and palliative care.

Recommended Resources for Oncology Advanced Practice Nurses

- Greene, F.L., Page, D.L., Fleming, I.D., Fritz, A., Balch, C.M., Haller, D.G., et al. (Eds.). (2002). *AJCC cancer staging manual* (6th ed.). New York: Springer.
- National Comprehensive Cancer Network Clinical Practice Guidelines in Oncology (www.nccn.org)
- Rosenberg, S. (2005). Principles of surgical oncology. In V.T. DeVita, Jr., S. Hellman, & S. Rosenberg (Eds.), *Cancer: Principles and practice of oncology* (7th ed., pp. 243–266). Philadelphia: Lippincott Williams & Williams.

References

Ahmed, S., Lindsey, B., & Davies, J. (2005). Salvage cryosurgery for locally recurrent prostate cancer following radiotherapy. *Prostate Cancer and Prostatic Diseases, 8,* 31–35.

Arora, N., Dhar, P., & Fahey, T.J. (2006). Seminars: Local and regional anesthesia for thyroid surgery. *Journal of Surgical Oncology, 94,* 708–713.

Azzoli, C.G. (2006). Management of patients with resectable stage IIIA (N2) NSCLC. *Journal of Surgical Oncology, 94,* 551–552.

Backman, S.B., Bondy, R.M., Deschamps, A., Moore, A., & Schricker, T. (2006). Perioperative consideration for anesthesia. In W.W. Souba, M.P. Fink, G.J. Jurkovich, L.R. Kaiser, W.H. Pearce, J.H. Pemberton, et al. (Eds.), *ACS surgery: Principles and practice 2006* (pp. 46–59). New York: WebMD Professional Publishing.

Bates-Jensen, B.M. (1999). Chronic wound assessment. *Nursing Clinics of North America, 34,* 799–845.

Baxter, N.N., Whitson, B.A., & Tuttle, T M. (2007). Trends in the treatment and outcome of pancreatic cancer in the United States. *Annals of Surgical Oncology, 14,* 1320–1326.

Bilchik, A.J. (2006). Novel insights into the diagnosis and treatment of melanoma. *Surgical Oncology Clinics of North America, 15*(2), xv–xvi.

Bracco, D., Dubois, M.J., Bouali, R., & Eggimann, P. (2007). Single rooms may help to prevent nosocomial bloodstream infection and cross-contamination of methicillin-resistant *Staphylococcus aureus* in intensive care units. *Intensive Care Medicine, 33,* 836–840.

Brungs, S.M., & Render, M.L. (2006). Using evidence-based practice to reduce central line infections. *Clinical Journal of Oncology Nursing, 10,* 723–725.

Butani, A., Arbesfeld, D.M., & Schwartz, R.A. (2005). Premalignant and early squamous cell carcinoma. *Clinics in Plastic Surgery, 32,* 223–235.

Buyse, M., Loi, S., van't Veer, L., Viale, G., Delorenzi, M., Glas, A.M., et al. (2006). Validation and clinical utility of a 70-gene prognostic signature for women with node-negative breast cancer. *Journal of the National Cancer Institute, 98,* 1169–1171.

Cai, S., Cannizzo, F., Jr., Bullard Dunn, K.M., Gibbs, J.F., Czuczman, M., & Rajput, A. (2007). The role of surgical intervention in non-Hodgkin's lymphoma of the colon and rectum. *American Journal of Surgery, 193,* 409–512.

Camp-Sorrell, D. (Ed.). (2004). *Access device guidelines: Recommendations for nursing practice and education* (2nd ed.). Pittsburgh, PA: Oncology Nursing Society.

Carroll, C.M. (2006). Sorting out breast biopsy options. *Nursing 2006, 36*(3), 70–71.

Chapman, D.D. (2007). Local and regional control. In S.M. Mahon (Ed.), *Site-specific cancer series: Breast cancer* (pp. 63–80). Pittsburgh, PA: Oncology Nursing Society.

Chow, D.H.F., Sinn, L.H.Y., Ng, K.K., Lam, C.M., Yuen, J., Sheung, T.F., et al. (2006). Radiofrequency ablation for hepatocellular carcinoma and metastatic liver tumors: A comparative study. *Journal of Surgical Oncology, 94,* 565–571.

Cordeiro, P.G. (2006). Forward of reconstruction. *Seminars in Surgical Oncology, 94,* 439–440.

Crane-Okada, R., & Loney, M. (2007). Breast cancers. In M.E. Langhorne, J.S. Fulton, & S.E. Otto (Eds.), *Oncology nursing* (5th ed., pp. 101–124). St. Louis, MO: Mosby.

Duffy, S.W., McCann, J., Godward, S., Gabe, R., & Warwick, W. (2006). Some issues in screening for breast and other cancers. *Journal of Medical Screening, 13,* 28–34.

Duggleby, W., & Raudonis, B.M. (2006). Dispelling myths about palliative care and older adults. *Seminars in Oncology Nursing, 22,* 58–64.

Dunkler, D., Michiels, S., & Schemper, M. (2007). Gene expression profiling: Does it add predictive accuracy to clinical characteristics in cancer prognosis? *European Journal of Cancer, 43,* 745–751.

Ellsmere, J., Jones, D., Pleskow, D., & Chuttani, F. (2006). Endoluminal instrumentation is changing gastrointestinal surgery. *Surgical Innovation, 13,* 145–151.

Elsheikh, T.M., & Silverman, J.F. (2005). Follow-up surgical excision is indicated when breast core needle biopsies show atypical lobular hyperplasia or lobular carcinoma in situ. *American Journal of Surgical Pathology, 29,* 534–543.

Ezzone, S.A. (2006). Fever. In D. Camp-Sorrell & R.A. Hawkins (Eds.), *Clinical manual for the oncology advanced practice nurse* (2nd ed., pp. 979–998). Pittsburgh, PA: Oncology Nursing Society.

Fakhry, S.M., Rutherford, E.J., & Sheldon, G.F. (2006). Routine postoperative management of the hospitalized patient. In W.W. Souba, M.P. Fink, G.J. Jurkovich, L.R. Kaiser, W.H. Pearce, J.H. Pemberton, et al. (Eds.), *ACS surgery: Principles and practice 2006* (pp. 90–110). New York: WebMD Professional Publishing.

Feig, B.W., Berger, D.H., & Fuhrman, G.M. (Eds.). (2003). *The M.D. Anderson surgical oncology handbook* (3rd ed.). Philadelphia: Lippincott Williams & Wilkins.

Flores, R.M., Park, B., & Rusch, V.W. (2007). Video-assisted thoracic surgery. In W.W. Souba, M.P. Fink, G.J. Jurkovich, L.R. Kaiser, W.H. Pearce, J.H. Pemberton, et al. (Eds.), *ACS surgery: Principles and practice 2006* (pp. 373–396). New York: WebMD Professional Publishing.

Ford-Dunn, S. (2006). Use of vacuum-assisted closure therapy in the palliation of a malignant wound. *Palliative Medicine, 20,* 477–478.

Galante, J.M., Bowles, T.L., Khartri, V.P., Schneider, P.D., Goodnight, J.E., & Bold, R.J. (2005). Experience and attitudes of surgeons toward palliation in cancer. *Archives of Surgery, 140,* 873–880.

Gee, D.W., & Rattner, D.W. (2007). Management of gastroesophageal tumors. *Oncologist, 12,* 175–185.

Greene, F.L. (2006). A cancer staging perspective: The value of anatomical staging. *Journal of Surgical Oncology, 95,* 6–7.

Greene, F.L., Kercher, K.W., Nelson, H., Teigland, C.M., & Boller, A.M. (2007). Minimal access cancer management. *CA: A Cancer Journal for Clinicians, 57,* 130–146.

Greene, F.L., Page, D.L., Fleming, I.D., Fritz, A., Balch, C.M., Haller, D.G., et al. (Eds.). (2002). *AJCC cancer staging manual* (6th ed.). New York: Springer.

Guillem, J.G. (2007). Hereditary colorectal cancer and polyposis syndromes. In W.W. Souba, M.P. Fink, G.J. Jurkovich, L.R. Kaiser, W.H. Pearce, J.H. Pemberton, et al. (Eds.), *ACS surgery: Principles and practice 2006* (pp. 562–571). New York: WebMD Professional Publishing.

Harlow, S.P., Krag, D.N., Reintgen, D.S., Moffat, F.L., & Frazier, T.G. (2006). Lymphatic mapping and sentinel lymph node biopsy. In W.W. Souba, M.P. Fink, G.J. Jurkovich, L.R. Kaiser, W.H. Pearce, J.H. Pemberton, et al. (Eds.), *ACS surgery: Principles and practice 2006* (pp. 278–288). New York: WebMD Professional Publishing.

Hashizume, M. (2007). MRI-guided laparoscopic robotic surgery for malignancies. *International Journal of Clinical Oncology, 12,* 94–98.

Heit, J.A. (2006). The epidemiology of venous thromboembolism in the community: Implications for prevention and management. *Journal of Thrombosis and Thrombolysis, 21,* 23–29.

Hsueh, E.C., Hansen, N., & Giuliano, A. (2000). Intraoperative lymphatic mapping and sentinel lymph node dissection in breast cancer. *CA: A Cancer Journal for Clinicians, 50,* 279–291.

Hudcova, J., McNicol, E., Quah, C., Lau, J., & Carr, D.B. (2006). Patient controlled opioid analgesia versus conventional opioid analgesia for postoperative pain. *Cochrane Database of Systematic Reviews 2006,* Issue 4. Art. No.: CD003348. DOI: 10.1002/14651858.CD003348.pub2.

Iverson, R.E., & Lynch, D.J. (2006). Practice advisory on pain management and prevention of postoperative nausea and vomiting. *Plastic and Reconstructive Surgery Journal, 118,* 1060–1069.

James, C.R., Quinn, J.E., Mullan, P.B., Johnston, P.G., & Harkin, D.P. (2007). BRCA1, a potential predictive biomarker in the treatment of breast cancer. *Oncologist, 12,* 142–150.

Jiang, D., & Zhao, N. (2006). A clinical prognostic prediction of a lymph node negative breast cancer by gene expression profiles. *Journal of Cancer Research in Clinical Oncology, 132,* 579–587.

Johnson, G.B. (2007). Cancer diagnosis and staging. In M.E. Langhorne, J.S. Fulton, & S.E. Otto (Eds.), *Oncology nursing* (5th ed., pp. 70–77). St. Louis, MO: Mosby.

Karakousis, G.C., Gimotty, P.A., Czerniecki, B.J., Elder, D.E., Elenitsas, R., Ming, M.E., et al. (2007). Regional nodal metastatic disease is the strongest predictor of survival in patients with thin vertical growth phase melanomas: A case for SLN staging biopsy in these patients. *Annals of Surgical Oncology, 14,* 1596–1603.

Kehlet, H. (2006). Postoperative pain. In W.W. Souba, M.P. Fink, G.J. Jurkovich, L.R. Kaiser, W.H. Pearce, J.H. Pemberton, et al. (Eds.), *ACS surgery: Principles and practice 2006* (pp. 75–89). New York: WebMD Professional Publishing.

Kennedy, M.M. (2006). Pneumonia. In D. Camp-Sorrell & R.A. Hawkins (Eds.), *Clinical manual for the oncology advanced practice nurse* (2nd ed., pp. 195–208). Pittsburgh, PA: Oncology Nursing Society.

Kitagawa, Y., & Kitajima, M. (2006). Gastroesophageal carcinoma: Individualized surgical therapy. *Surgical Oncology Clinics of North America, 15,* 793–802.

Kocak, E., Al-Saif, O., Satter, M., Bloomston, M., Abdessalam, S.F., Mantil, J., et al. (2007). Image guidance during abdominal exploration for recurrent colorectal cancer. *Annals of Surgical Oncology, 14,* 405–410.

Lafreniere, R., Berguer, R., Seifert, P.C., Belkin, M., Roth, S., Williams, K.S., et al. (2006). Preparation of the operating room. In W.W. Souba, M.P. Fink, G.J. Jurkovich, L.R. Kaiser, W.H. Pearce, J.H. Pemberton, et al. (Eds.), *ACS surgery: Principles and practice 2006* (pp. 13–26). New York: WebMD Professional Publishing.

Law, W.L., Lee, Y.M., Choi, H.K., Seto, C.L., & Ho, J.W. (2007). Impact of laparoscopic resection for colorectal cancer on operative outcomes in survival. *Annals of Surgery, 245*(1), 1–7.

Lawrence, W.T., Bevin, A.G., & Sheldon, G.F. (2007). Acute wound care. In W.W. Souba, M.P. Fink, G.J. Jurkovich, L.R. Kaiser, W.H. Pearce, J.H. Pemberton, et al. (Eds.), *ACS surgery: Principles and practice 2006* (pp. 111–134). New York: WebMD Professional Publishing.

Leonardi, M.J., McGory, M.L., & Ko, C.Y. (2007). A systematic review of deep venous thrombosis prophylaxis in cancer patients: Implication for improving quality. *Annals of Surgical Oncology, 14,* 929–936.

Lester, J. (2007). Surgery. In M.E. Langhorne, J.S. Fulton, & S.E. Otto (Eds.), *Oncology nursing* (5th ed., pp. 337–345). St. Louis, MO: Mosby.

Liang, J.T., Lai, H.S., & Lee, P.H. (2007). Laparoscopic pelvic autonomic nerve-preserving surgery for patients with lower rectal cancer after chemoradiation therapy. *Annals of Surgical Oncology, 14,* 1285–1287.

Lopez, M.J. (2005). The evolution of radical cancer surgery. *Surgical Oncology Clinics of North America, 14*(3), xiii–xv.

Lyder, C.H. (2006). Assessing risk and preventing pressure ulcers in patients with cancer. *Seminars in Oncology Nursing, 22,* 178–184.

Mack, L.A., & Pasieka, J.L. (2007). An evidence-based approach to the treatment of thyroid lymphoma. *World Journal of Surgery, 31,* 978–986.

Malangoni, M.A., & McHenry, C.R. (2006). Soft tissue infection. In W.W. Souba, M.P. Fink, G.J. Jurkovich, L.R. Kaiser, W.H. Pearce, J.H. Pemberton, et al. (Eds.), *ACS surgery: Principles and practice 2006* (pp. 224–237). New York: WebMD Professional Publishing.

Mariotto, A.B., Rowland, J.H., Ries, L.A.G., Scoppa, S., & Feuer, E.J. (2007). Multiple cancer prevalence: A growing challenge in long-term survivorship. *Cancer Epidemiology, Biomarkers and Prevention, 16,* 566–571.

Matthews, E., Snell, K., & Coats, H. (2006). Intra-arterial chemotherapy for limb preservation in patients with osteosarcoma: Nursing implications. *Clinical Journal of Oncology Nursing, 10,* 581–589.

McCay, M., & Farley, M. (2006). Infection control circle of safety. *Canadian Operating Room Nursing Journal, 24*(4), 20–24, 41–42.

McGee, M.F., Rose, M.J., Marks, J., Onders, R.P., Chak, A., Faulx, A., et al. (2006). A primer on natural orifice transluminal endoscopic surgery: Building a new paradigm. *Surgical Innovation, 13,* 86–93.

McNees, P. (2006). Skin and wound assessment and care in oncology. *Seminars in Oncology Nursing, 22,* 130–143.

Meakins, J.L., & Masterson, B.J. (2006). Prevention of postoperative infection. In W.W. Souba, M.P. Fink, G.J. Jurkovich, L.R. Kaiser, W.H. Pearce, J.H. Pemberton, et al. (Eds.), *ACS surgery: Principles and practice 2006* (pp. 27–45). New York: WebMD Professional Publishing.

Mirtallo, J.M., & Ezzone, S.A. (2006). Total parenteral nutrition ordering and monitoring. In D. Camp-Sorrell & R.A. Hawkins (Eds.), *Clinical manual for the oncology advanced practice nurse* (2nd ed., pp. 1137–1143). Pittsburgh, PA: Oncology Nursing Society.

Morrow, M., & Jordan, C. (2006). The current status of breast cancer chemoprevention: A star is born. *Journal of Surgical Oncology, 95,* 4–5.

Murphy, M.E. (2007). Colorectal cancers. In M.E. Langhorne, J.S. Fulton, & S.E. Otto (Eds.), *Oncology nursing* (5th ed., pp. 125–140). St. Louis, MO: Mosby.

Nag, S., Martinez-Monge, R., Neiroda, C., & Martin, E., Jr. (1999). Radioimmunoguided-intraoperative radiation therapy in colorectal carcinoma: A new technique to precisely define the clinical target volume. *International Journal of Radiation Oncology, Biology, Physics, 44,* 133–137.

Nichol, P.F., Mack, E., Bianco, J., Hayman, A., Starling, J.R., & Chen, H. (2003). Radio-guided parathyroidectomy in patients with secondary and tertiary hyperparathyroidism. *Surgery, 134,* 713–719.

Olsson, U., Bosaeus, I., Svedlund, J., & Bergbom, I. (2007). Patients' subjective symptoms, quality of life and intake of food during the recovery period 3 and 12 months after upper gastrointestinal surgery. *European Journal of Cancer Care, 16,* 74–85.

Ota, D., & Nelson, H. (2007). The surgeon and adjuvant therapy for stage II colon cancer. *Annals of Surgical Oncology, 14,* 272–273.

Owings, J.T. (2006). Venous thromboembolism. In W.W. Souba, M.P. Fink, G.J. Jurkovich, L.R. Kaiser, W.H. Pearce, J.H. Pemberton, et al. (Eds.), *ACS surgery: Principles and practice 2006* (pp. 955–973). New York: WebMD Professional Publishing.

Pare, J. (2006). Laparoscopic radical prostatectomy: A less invasive approach. *Canadian Operating Room Nursing Journal, 24*(3), 31–37.

Pass, S.E., & Simpson, R.W. (2004). Discontinuation and reinstitution of medications during the perioperative period. *American Journal of Health-System Pharmacy, 61,* 899–912.

Plante, M., & Roy, M. (1998). Operative laparoscopy prior to a pelvic exenteration in patients with recurrent cervical cancer. *Gynecologic Oncology, 69,* 94–99.

Pomahac, B., Recht, A., May, J.W., Hergrueter, C.A., & Slavin, S.A. (2006). New trends in breast cancer management: Is the era of immediate breast reconstruction changing? *Annals of Surgery, 244,* 282–288.

Poon, R.T. (2007). Optimal initial treatment for early hepatocellular carcinoma in patients with preserved liver function: Transplantation or resection? *Annals of Surgical Oncology, 14,* 541–547.

Port, E.R., Park, A., Borgen, P.I., Morris, E., & Montgomery, L.L. (2007). Results of MRI screening for breast cancer in high-risk patients with LCIS and atypical hyperplasia. *Annals of Surgical Oncology, 14,* 1051–1057.

Povoski, S.P., Olsen, J.O., Young, D.C., Clarke, J., Burak, W.E., Walker, M.D., et al. (2006). Prospective randomization comparing intradermal, intraparenchymal, and subareolar injection routes for sentinel lymph node mapping and biopsy in breast cancer. *Annals of Surgical Oncology, 13,* 1412–1421.

Ritz, J.P., Lehmann, K.S., Zurbuchen, U., Wacker, F., Brehm, F., Isbert, C., et al. (2007). Improving laser-induced thermotherapy of liver metastasis: Effects of arterial microembolization and complete blood flow occlusion. *European Journal of Surgical Oncology, 33,* 608–613.

Ryan, D.P. (2006). Nonsurgical approaches to colorectal cancer. *Oncologist, 11,* 999–1002.

Sabel, M.S. (2007). Principles of surgical therapy. In M.S. Sabel, V.K. Sondak, & J.J. Sussman (Eds.), *Surgical foundations: Essentials of surgical oncology* (pp. 39–64). Philadelphia: Mosby.

Schlaerth, A.C., & Abu-Rustum, N.R. (2006). Role of minimally invasive surgery in gynecologic cancers. *Oncologist, 11,* 895–901.

Seaman, S. (2006). Management of malignant fungating wounds in advanced cancer. *Seminars in Oncology Nursing, 22,* 185–193.

Siperstein, A., Garland, A., Engle, K., Rogers, S., Berber, E., String, A., et al. (2000). Laparoscopic RFA of primary and metastatic liver tumors: Technical considerations. *Surgical Endoscopy, 14,* 400–405.

Slattery, J.M., & Sahani, D.V. (2006). What is the current state-of-the-art imaging for detecting and staging of cholangiocarcinoma? *Oncologist, 11,* 913–922.

Smith, R.L., Bohl, J.K., McElearney, S.T., Friel, C.M., Barclay, M.M., Sawyer, R.G., et al. (2004). Wound infections after elective colorectal resection. *Annals of Surgery, 239,* 599–605.

Starnes, D.N., & Sims, T.W. (2006a). Care of the patient undergoing robotic-assisted prostatectomy. *Urologic Nursing, 26,* 129–136.

Starnes, D.N., & Sims, T.W. (2006b). Robotic prostatectomy surgery. *Urologic Nursing, 26,* 138–140.

Sun, Y., Goodison, S., Li, J., Liu, L., & Farmerie, W. (2007). Improved breast cancer prognosis through the combination of clinical and genetic markers. *Bioinformatics, 23,* 30–37.

Tafra, L., Fine, R., Whitworth, P., Berry, M., Woods, J., Ekbom, G., et al. (2006). Prospective randomized study comparing cryo-assisted and needle-wire localization of ultrasound visible breast tumors. *American Journal of Surgery, 192,* 462–470.

Taylor, D. (2007, April). *Wounds secondary to the occurrence or removal of cancer lesions.* Presentation at the Central Ohio Oncology Nursing Society Spring Conference, Columbus, OH.

Vanderveen, K.A., Paterniti, D.A., Kravitz, R.L., & Bold, R.J. (2007). Diffusion of surgical techniques and early stage breast cancer: Variables related to adoption and implementation of sentinel lymph node biopsy. *Annals of Surgical Oncology, 14,* 1662–1669.

Vogel, W.H. (2003). The advanced practice nursing role in a high-risk breast cancer clinic. *Oncology Nursing Forum, 30,* 115–122.

Wagman, L.D. (2007). More tools, new strategies: Enlarging the therapeutic scope for the patient with liver metastasis from colorectal cancer. *Journal of Surgical Oncology, 95,* 1–3.

Whitworth, P.W., & Rewcastle, J.C. (2005). Cryoablation and cryolocalization in the management of breast disease. *Journal of Surgical Oncology, 90,* 1–9.

Williams, J.G. (2007). Intestinal stomas. In W.W. Souba, M.P. Fink, G.J. Jurkovich, L.R. Kaiser, W.H. Pearce, J.H. Pemberton, et al. (Eds.), *ACS surgery: Principles and practice 2006* (pp. 803–815). New York: WebMD Professional Publishing.

Wuhrman, E., Cooney, M.F., Dunwoody, C.J., Eksterowicz, N., Merkel, S., & Oakes, L.L. (2007). Authorized and unauthorized ("PCA by proxy") dosing of analgesic infusion pumps: Position statement with clinical practice recommendations. *Pain Management Nursing, 8,* 4–11.

Yadav, R. (2007). Rehabilitation of surgical cancer patients at University of Texas M.D. Anderson Cancer Center. *Journal of Surgical Oncology, 95,* 361–369.

Yokomizo, H., Yamane, T., Hirata, T., Hifumi, M., Kawaguchi, T., & Fukuda, S. (2007). Surgical treatment of pT2 gallbladder carcinoma: A reevaluation of the therapeutic effect of hepatectomy and extrahepatic bile resection based on the long-term outcome. *Annals of Surgical Oncology, 14,* 1366–1373.

Zerey, M., Burns, J.M., Kercher, K.W., Kuwada, T.S., & Heniford, B.T. (2006). Minimally invasive management of colon cancer. *Surgical Innovation, 13*(1), 5–15.

Zitella, L.J., Friese, C.R., Hauser, J., Gobel, B.H., Woolery, M., O'Leary, C., et al. (2006). Putting evidence into practice: Prevention of infection. *Clinical Journal of Oncology Nursing, 10,* 739–750.

CHAPTER 6

Radiation Therapy in Cancer Care

Tracy K. Gosselin, RN, MSN, AOCN®

Introduction

Radiation therapy (RT) is an integral component of cancer treatment. This treatment modality has experienced advancement, refinement, and greater biologic understanding in the past 20 years. RT may be used alone or in combination with other therapies in the neoadjuvant, adjuvant, and palliative care settings. Approximately 50%–60% of patients with cancer will receive RT at some point in their disease trajectory (American College of Radiology, 2000). What is unique about RT compared to other cancer treatments is the variety of treatments that can be offered as well as the population receiving treatment. In many RT centers, adult and pediatric patients receive treatment in the same facility, thus requiring healthcare providers to have additional knowledge and skills related to the care of all patient populations.

The advanced practice nurse (APN) role is a newer role in radiation oncology. Several publications in the 1980s and 1990s were related to the role of nursing in radiation oncology. Since 1999, descriptive studies also have included the role of the APN. Depending upon the practice setting, APNs may have administrative, clerical, patient care, and research responsibilities. This chapter will provide an overview of RT for the APN, including indications for treatment, patient and family education, and implications for practice. A list of common terms used in RT can be found in Table 6-1, and the minimal and maximal tissue doses are noted in Table 6-2.

Indications

General

RT can be used for cure, control, palliation, and prophylaxis of disease in a variety of disease sites (see Table 6-3). In the curative setting, RT commonly is used to treat skin

Table 6-1. Common Radiation Therapy Definitions

Term	Definition	Comments
Acute toxicity	This type of side effect arises during the course of radiation therapy (RT) and typically subsides within weeks once treatment is completed. Patients experience these effects at the treatment site but also may experience global symptoms such as fatigue. When the symptoms persist following treatment, they are referred to as *late effects*.	Common acute effects include nausea, diarrhea, mucositis, xerostomia, esophagitis, and skin reaction.
Boost	This term commonly is used to describe a smaller field within the larger field of radiation that typically is treated at the end of radiation.	Women who undergo a lumpectomy may receive external beam RT to the entire breast, followed by a boost to the surgical scar to minimize the risk of recurrence.
Brachytherapy	This therapy involves the use of radioactive seeds or liquids. Seeds may be placed on or near a tumor while liquids may be given intravenously or orally. Treatment can be either high-dose rate (HDR) or low-dose rate (LDR). Sources may be left in place permanently (e.g., prostate LDR) or temporarily (e.g., cervix HDR, prostate HDR, sarcoma LDR, cervix LDR).	–
Chemoradio-therapy	Chemotherapy is given daily, weekly, or as a continuous infusion while the patient is undergoing RT for a synergistic effect.	Diseases treated with chemoradiotherapy include breast, lung, head and neck, gastrointestinal, and gynecologic cancers. This is based upon pathology and staging of disease.
Dose-volume histogram (DVH)	A DVH is a graphical representation of the amount and percentage of RT that is given to the planned treatment volume and other surrounding anatomic structures.	–
Dosing	Dosing is broken down from a total dose (gray [Gy]) to individual doses (centigray [cGy]); this commonly is referred to as *fractionation*.	If the total dose is 54 Gy, this equals 5,400 cGy. If a patient is to receive 30 treatments, this becomes the denominator and divides into 5,400, giving us a daily treatment dose of 1.8 Gy or 180 cGy.
Fractionation	The total dose of RT is divided into equal fractions. This is one of the most common methods of delivering RT, as treatments are given once daily, Monday through Friday, for a prescribed number of weeks.	–

(Continued on next page)

Table 6-1. Common Radiation Therapy Definitions *(Continued)*

Term	Definition	Comments
GliaSite® Radiation Therapy System (Cytyc Corp.)	GliaSite is used in the treatment of malignant brain tumors. A balloon with a catheter is inserted into the resected tumor cavity, and iodine-125 is inserted into the catheter to give an LDR of RT over three to seven days.	–
Hyperfraction-ation	When RT is given twice a day, separated by six hours, it is referred to as *hyperfraction-ation.* The total dose of treatment often is increased, while the dose per fraction is decreased.	Treatment may be given this way in certain cases of head and neck and pediatric cancers. This also may be used in breast brachytherapy as well as in patients requiring total body irradiation for the purposes of stem cell transplantation.
Hypofractionation	The dose of RT per fraction is increased, and the total dose and treatment time are decreased. This type of fractionation has changed how many patients with bone metastasis are treated, in that they receive a higher daily dose over a shorter amount of time.	–
Intensity-modulated radiation therapy (IMRT)	IMRT is an advanced form of RT whereby the intensity of the dose can be controlled within each treatment field by small beam-lets. This allows the patient to receive more or less of a dose to a certain part of the treatment field based upon tumor characteristics, anatomy, and physiology.	–
Late effects	These are side effects that persist months to years after treatment has been completed or effects that arise months to years later at the site of treatment.	Common late effects include fibrosis, enteritis, xerostomia, telangiectasia, and vaginal stenosis.
Particulate radiation	Particulate radiation consists of different particles that are used in different ways to treat cancer. • Alpha particles—Large, positively charged particles that have poor penetration and are emitted during the decay of radioactive sources • Electrons—Small, negatively charged particles that are accelerated to high energies and do not penetrate deeply • Beta particles—Electrons that are emitted during the decay of radioactive sources • Protons—Large, positively charged particles that penetrate deeply and have a stopping point • Neutrons—Large, uncharged particles	Electrons commonly are used to treat cutaneous T-cell lymphoma (mycosis fungoides) and also commonly are used during a boost treatment. Proton therapy is provided only at select centers across the United States because of the cost of equipment and facilities needed to operate. Brachytherapy and radioimmunotherapy are types of alpha, beta, and gamma rays.

(Continued on next page)

Table 6-1. Common Radiation Therapy Definitions *(Continued)*

Term	Definition	Comments
Radiobiology	This is the study of the effect of absorbed ionizing radiation on cells and is composed of the four R's: repair, redistribution, repopulation, and reoxygenation. • Repair—Key in normal cells, this allows for the cells to repair themselves between doses of RT. This also may happen in tumor cells. • Redistribution—Cell kill increases as cells move through the cell cycle. As cells are delayed in each cycle, cell kill increases as DNA damage occurs. • Repopulation—This is key in normal cells to minimize acute and late effects. In cancer cells, this rarely happens as the cells attempt to divide due to the multiple RT treatments. • Reoxygenation—As the tumor shrinks, it becomes better oxygenated and more sensitive to the effects of RT.	–
Radiosensitivity	Radiosensitivity is concerned with how sensitive tumor cells and other structures and tissues respond to the radiation. It is an important consideration, as acute and late toxicities are related to this concept. Cells in the late G_2 and M phases are most sensitive to RT, whereas those in the S phase are more resistant to RT.	–
Respiratory gating	A small, lightweight, reflective block is placed on the patient's chest that tracks to an infrared camera in the ceiling; this camera monitors the patient's breathing cycle and can turn the beam on and off based upon the patient's breathing cycle. This technique assists in minimizing treatment to normal healthy tissue.	This may be used in patients with breast, thoracic, and abdominal malignancies.
Simulation	Part of the treatment planning process that may take one to two hours depending on the patient. Fluoroscopy is used to visualize anatomy. Patients may or may not receive IV contrast, and a positioning device is typically made for treatment positioning.	This may take place on a conventional simulator or a computed tomography (CT)–based simulator. This is done prior to the initiation of treatment.
Stereotactic radiosurgery	This is a type of treatment used to treat tumors that are intracranial or extracranial, and primary or metastatic in origin. It typically is one large dose of radiation that uses multiple arcs/beams to treat a focal area.	This treatment can be used in patients with metastatic disease to the brain, lung, and spinal cord and may be used as a primary treatment for prostate cancer using more than one treatment.

(Continued on next page)

Table 6-1. Common Radiation Therapy Definitions *(Continued)*

Term	Definition	Comments
Stereotactic radiotherapy	This is a type of treatment used to treat intracranial lesions that may or may not be malignant. Treatments are fractionated and may use multiple arcs/beams.	–
Teletherapy	Teletherapy is also known as external beam RT; often the acronym EBRT is used. This treatment is given on a linear accelerator or with a cobalt unit.	–
Three-dimensional (3-D) conformal RT	Use of computer-based treatment planning and CT during the planning process to develop a 3-D image of the tumor that then allows for a tighter margin around the tumor.	–
Tolerance dose	The dose of radiation that can be given that will still allow the tissue and/or organ to function is called the tolerance dose (see Table 6-2).	–
Total body irradiation	This is a type of photon treatment that is given to the whole body in patients undergoing stem cell transplantation.	–

Note. Based on information from Gosselin-Acomb, 2005; Ma, 2005.

cancer, prostate cancer, and early-stage Hodgkin disease. This also is referred to as *definitive RT.* In this setting, the disease is confined to a particular area and/or organ. When the goal of treatment is that of control, patients typically present with advanced disease. The goal is to provide a symptom-free interval for patients. Palliative RT often is a shorter course of treatment that focuses on providing comfort when cure is not possible. Treatment also is given to minimize pain in patients with metastatic disease to the bone and to stop bleeding in patients whose tumors are friable. Furthermore, RT is used to treat structural oncologic emergencies (see Chapter 15), including increased intracranial pressure from brain metastases, spinal cord compression, and superior vena cava syndrome. Lastly, RT is used for prophylaxis in patients with small cell lung cancer who are at high risk for brain metastases. These patients receive prophylactic whole brain radiation therapy.

The next section will focus on breast, colorectal, non-small cell lung, and prostate cancer and palliative radiation treatments, as these are some of the most common indications for RT.

Breast Cancer

Treatment of breast cancer with RT has undergone rapid evolution over the past 35 years. The studies conducted by the National Surgical Adjuvant Breast and Bowel Project (NSABP) have made breast-conserving treatment (BCT) a standard of care in this country that provides patients with the option of breast preservation. Ongoing research continues to look at different types of treatment for breast cancer using RT.

Table 6-2. Minimal and Maximal Tissue Tolerance to Radiotherapy Dose

Tissue	Dose-Related Injury	Minimal Tolerance Dose (TD) 5/5[a] (Gy)	Maximal TD 50/5[b] (Gy)	Amount of Tissue Treated (Field Size or Length)
Eye	Blindness			
	• Retina	55	70	Whole
	• Cornea	50	> 60	Whole
	• Lens	5.0	12	Whole
Bone marrow	Aplasia, pancytopenia	2.5	4.5	Whole
		30	40	Segmental
Liver	Acute and chronic hepatitis	25	40	Whole
		15	20	Whole (strip)
Stomach	Perforation, ulcer, hemorrhage	45	55	100 cm²
Intestine	Ulcer, perforation, hemorrhage	45	55	400 cm²
		50	65	100 cm²
Brain	Infarction, necrosis	60	70	Whole
Spinal cord	Infarction, necrosis	45	55	10 cm
Heart	Pericarditis, pancarditis	45	55	60%
		70	80	25%
Lung	Acute and chronic pneumonitis	30	35	100 cm²
		15	25	Whole
Kidney	Acute and chronic nephroscle-rosis	15	20	Whole (strip)
		20	25	Whole
Uterus	Necrosis, perforation	> 10	> 200	Whole
Vagina	Ulcer, fistula	90	> 100	Whole
Fetus	Death	2.0	4.0	Whole

[a] TD 5/5 = minimal tolerance dose; the dose, given to a population of patients under a standard set of treatment conditions, that will result in no more than a 5% rate of severe complications within five years after treatment.

[b] TD 50/5 = maximal tolerance dose; the dose, given to a population of patients under a standard set of treatment conditions, that will result in a 50% rate of severe complications within five years after treatment.

Note. Based on information from Bentel et al., 1989; Rubin et al., 1975.
From *Manual for Radiation Oncology Nursing Practice and Education* (3rd ed., p. 19), by D.W. Bruner, M. Haas, and T.K. Gosselin-Acomb (Eds.), 2005, Pittsburgh, PA: Oncology Nursing Society. Copyright 2005 by Oncology Nursing Society. Reprinted with permission.

Breast cancer is one of the top diseases treated in RT departments; therefore, a comprehensive knowledge base about treatment options regarding this disease is critical. Radiation may be used after lumpectomy, after mastectomy, and in the setting of metastatic disease. Patients who present with large tumors also may undergo RT and/or chemotherapy prior to surgery (neoadjuvant therapy). Radia-

Table 6-3. Common Disease Sites/Diseases Treated With Radiation Therapy

Disease Site	Radiation Therapy Technique That May Be Used
Brain	External beam radiation therapy, stereotactic radiosurgery, stereotactic radiotherapy, GliaSite® Radiation Therapy System (Cytyc Corp.)
Head and neck	External beam radiation therapy, high-dose rate brachytherapy, low-dose rate brachytherapy
Breast	External beam radiation therapy, high-dose rate brachytherapy
Lung	External beam radiation therapy, high-dose rate brachytherapy, whole brain radiation therapy in small cell lung cancer
Gastrointestinal	External beam radiation therapy, intraoperative radiation therapy
Prostate	External beam radiation therapy, high-dose rate brachytherapy, low-dose rate brachytherapy
Gynecologic	External beam radiation therapy, high-dose rate brachytherapy, low-dose rate brachytherapy
Skin	External beam radiation therapy
Leukemia	Total body irradiation
Lymphoma	External beam radiation therapy
T-cell lymphoma	Total skin external beam therapy
Nonmalignant (keloids, heterotopic bone)	External beam radiation therapy
Metastatic disease to bone, brain, spinal column	External beam radiation therapy, stereotactic radiosurgery (for intracranial and extracranial metastasis)

Note. External beam radiation therapy includes the use of parallel fields, three-dimensional conformal therapy, and intensity-modulated radiation therapy.

tion usually is delivered via external beam or brachytherapy with the use of photons and electrons.

Patients who are to receive BCT may have a diagnosis of ductal carcinoma in situ (DCIS) or invasive breast cancer. RT should only be given after careful review of radiologic studies, pathologic findings, and surgical procedures (Morrow et al., 2002). Figure 6-1 reviews contraindications related to RT use in patients undergoing BCT. Recently, Joslyn (2006) found that women who underwent breast-conserving surgery and RT had a significantly lower risk of death compared to women who were treated with BCT alone. These results are similar to those found by Bijker et al. (2006), who demonstrated that at 10-year follow-up, women who underwent local excision plus RT had a higher local recurrence-free survival (85%) versus those who received local excision (74%). Treatment of DCIS with RT continues to be controversial, and factors that affect the decision to use RT include age at diagnosis, tumor grade, tumor size, and comedo histology. Women should be educated on their treatment options and factors that may increase the risk of recurrence.

Contraindications for breast-conserving therapy requiring radiation therapy include:

Absolute:
- Prior radiation therapy to the breast or chest wall
- Radiation therapy during pregnancy
- Diffuse suspicious or malignant appearing microcalcifications
- Widespread disease that cannot be incorporated by local excision through a single incision that achieves negative margins with a satisfactory cosmetic result.
- Positive pathologic margin

Relative:
- Active connective tissue disease involving the skin (especially scleroderma and lupus)
- Tumors > 5 cm (category 2B)
- Focally positive margin
- Women ≤ 35 y or premenopausal women with a known BRCA 1/2 mutation:
  – May have an increased risk of ipsilateral breast recurrence or contralateral breast cancer with breast conserving therapy
  – Prophylactic bilateral mastectomy for risk reduction may be considered. (See NCCN Breast Cancer Risk Reduction Guidelines.)

Figure 6-1. Special Considerations to Breast-Conserving Therapy Requiring Radiation Therapy

Note. Reproduced with permission from the NCCN 1.2007 Breast Cancer Guideline, *The Complete Library of NCCN Clinical Practice Guidelines in Oncology* [CD-ROM]. Jenkintown, Pennsylvania: © National Comprehensive Cancer Network, March 2007. To view the most recent and complete version of the guideline, go online to www.nccn.org

These Guidelines are a work in progress that will be refined as often as new significant data become available.

The NCCN Guidelines are a statement of consensus of its authors regarding their views of currently accepted approaches to treatment. Any clinician seeking to apply or consult any NCCN guideline is expected to use independent medical judgment in the context of individual clinical circumstances to determine any patient's care or treatment. The National Comprehensive Cancer Network makes no warranties of any kind whatsoever regarding their content, use or application and disclaims any responsibility for their application or use in any way.

These Guidelines are copyrighted by the National Comprehensive Cancer Network. All rights reserved. These Guidelines and illustrations herein may not be reproduced in any form for any purpose without the express written permission of the NCCN.

    The treatment planning process for the management of breast cancer includes computed tomography (CT) and simulation. Both of these are used together to develop a three-dimensional (3-D) treatment plan. A treatment positioning device is made, with the patient's arm being raised above the head on the side that is being treated. During the treatment planning process, a dose-volume histogram (DVH) also is constructed to show the dose to the breast as well as to other anatomic structures. In patients with breast cancer, it is common to look at the dose to the head of the clavicle, heart, lung, and stomach because of anatomy and treatment beam arrangement. Surgical clips that are placed at the time of surgery also may assist in identifying the treatment area. If a patient is at risk for cardiac exposure, a heart block may be placed to minimize the RT dose. Intensity-modulated radiation therapy (IMRT) is not used as commonly as 3-D conformal RT in patients with breast cancer.

    Common RT treatment fields to the whole breast include tangential fields (medial and lateral fields that are directed obliquely at the breast) and a variety of additional fields if nodal involvement exists. These fields may include the axilla, intramamma-ry, and supraclavicular nodal areas. It is critical that these fields do not overlap, as the patient may be at higher risk in that area for acute and late effects. A small part of the lung volume also may be included, but efforts should be taken to minimize any poten-tial heart exposure. Patients typically are prescribed a dose of 46–50 gray (Gy) that is divided into daily doses of 1.8–2 Gy; this is then administered five days a week over the course of five weeks (Moore-Higgs, 2006). This dose range is similar for patients who require nodal irradiation.

Patients undergoing BCT commonly receive treatment to what is known as a boost field. This field usually is treated alone once the patient has completed treatment to the entire breast. This treatment field is around the surgical scar, and treatment is aimed at local tissues, as this area has a high chance of recurrence. This treatment is common-ly delivered with electrons as opposed to photons, which are used to treat the whole breast, and a patient typically receives 2 Gy a day for a total of six to eight treatments. The boost treatment at some institutions is delivered via brachytherapy. Patients typi-cally receive a total of 30–33 treatments. If delivered via brachytherapy, catheters are placed into the breast, and treatment is delivered by high-dose radiation. Patients go home with the catheters in place until the treatment is complete.

Partial-breast irradiation (PBI) commonly is referred to as *accelerated partial-breast irradi-ation* and can be performed using the MammoSite® (Cytyc Corp.) treatment device (sin-gle catheter), on a linear accelerator, or via high-dose rate (HDR) brachytherapy (multi-ple catheters). The MammoSite treatment device comes in a spherical as well as an ellip-tical shape and can be placed into the lumpectomy cavity at the time of surgery or post-operatively with a trocar. Patients receive a total of 10 treatments over the course of five days. Each day, the patient typically receives two treatments separated by six hours. The catheter is attached to the HDR after-loader machine, and treatment is accomplished with iridium-192. This type of treatment decreases dosage to the heart and lung, while giving the most dose to the area at greatest risk of recurrence. Small studies report a benefit with the use of MammoSite. Many studies do not have long-term follow-up (greater than five years) because this technology is relatively new. The American Society of Breast Sur-geons (2005) has a consensus statement for accelerated PBI that can be accessed online to guide providers. The total dose of PBI is 34 Gy with a daily dose of 3.4 Gy. Currently, the NSABP and the Radiation Therapy Oncology Group are conducting a clinical trial to evaluate the feasibility of this type of treatment in select patients with breast cancer. The National Comprehensive Cancer Network (NCCN, 2007a) recommends that PBI should only be used within the confines of a prospective clinical trial.

Side effects of MammoSite include pain, seroma, infections, erythema, discoloration, subcutaneous tissue changes, skin contour changes, and late skin changes (Chao et al., 2007; Jeruss et al., 2006). Late effects, contralateral breast disease, and local recurrence are all issues that one should be prepared to discuss with a patient who is considering PBI. Until long-term follow-up studies are able to document the pros and cons as they have with whole breast RT, practitioners need to continue to be aware of the current treatment recommendations by NCCN and the American Society of Breast Surgeons.

Patients who require RT after mastectomy typically have similar fields and treatment doses as those who elect to undergo BCT. Patients may require the use of bolus doses along the scar to provide enhanced dosing during part of the treatment. Photons and electrons also are used during this treatment.

Patients undergoing RT for breast cancer are at risk for developing a variety of acute and late effects. The two most common acute side effects related to RT for breast cancer are fatigue and skin reaction (dermatitis). Fatigue is a common side effect in patients with breast cancer undergoing RT and can occur in up to 100% of patients (Mock et al., 1997).The onset and duration of fatigue are different for each patient, and a baseline assessment prior to the initiation of RT is warranted. Patients who have received prior treatment and have not fully recovered may come into RT with a baseline measure of fatigue that is higher than a patient who has not had prior treatment.

Skin reactions are a common side effect of RT and are treatment site and dose dependent. Typically, the skin reaction occurs the second week of treatment and is dose and time dependent. This side effect may initially start as a dry, flaky, pruritic rash that may then progress into erythema, dry desquamation, and lastly, moist desquamation. Hair loss within the treatment field also may be noted, as well as skin pigmentation changes based upon the individual's complexion. A variety of factors affect the development of an acute skin reaction, including prior RT, age, weight, breast size, bony prominence, nutritional status, concurrent chemotherapy, and type of energy used (photons or electrons) (Harper, Franklin, Jenrette, & Aguero, 2004). Additionally, certain medical conditions such as collagen vascular disease and diabetes affect a patient's risk, as do lifestyle behaviors such as smoking.

No standard management exists for these acute reactions. Many products used to treat these reactions can be purchased over the counter and/or have been approved by the U.S. Food and Drug Administration as a medical device, making the determination of the best product challenging for the healthcare provider and patient. Patients should be encouraged to keep the skin clean and dry and to use a non–alcohol-based moisturizer to minimize dryness. Pruritus may be managed with topical steroids, oatmeal-based products, and cornstarch, although controversy exists about the use of cornstarch, as it can promote a yeast infection in patients who have desquamation of the skin (Moore-Higgs, 2005). A variety of ointments, creams, and gels are available, with many having been evaluated in small studies with mixed results. Commonly used products include Biafine® (OrthoNeutrogena), Jeans Cream® (Jeans Cream), and a variety of gels and creams with aloe vera. For women with large breasts and those receiving treatment to the axilla, patients must keep the area as dry as possible to minimize breakdown in the skin folds. Patients also should avoid trauma and sun exposure to the treatment area. Skin products should be applied no sooner than four hours prior to treatment, although this varies from institution to institution. The concern is that certain skin products can create a bolus effect to the skin, resulting in a higher dose of radiation being administered.

Patients experiencing moist desquamation may benefit from the use of a hydrocolloid dressing to minimize the risk of infection, promote healing, and enhance comfort. Patients should be cautioned against the use of cornstarch to manage moisture, as once an area develops moist desquamation, this product can lead to a yeast infection. The literature is mixed regarding the use of Silvadene® cream (King Pharmaceuticals), and petroleum jelly should also be avoided because it is not water permeable. These two products often can be difficult to remove and cause additional trauma to the area when the patient bathes. A systematic review of the literature concluded that gentle skin washing should be encouraged, and evidence is insufficient to support or refute the use of topical agents (Bolderston, Lloyd, Wong, Holden, & Robb-Blenderman, 2006).

Patients who have a MammoSite catheter in place or multiple brachytherapy catheters should be taught catheter care to minimize the risk of infection. Catheter care can be developed institutionally, as no current standard exists. Pain assessment and management in these patients also is important because the catheters may cause some level of discomfort.

Late effects of RT to the skin include atrophy, scaling, fibrosis, telangiectasia, necrosis, and pigmentation changes (Archambeau, Pezner, & Wasserman, 1995; Davis et al., 2003). These side effects arise months to years after treatment, typically are not reversible, and occur with dose ranges of 2.5–3 Gy per day. They affect the ultimate cosmetic outcome and should be discussed with the patient prior to initiation of RT.

Follow-up care for each patient is individualized but should include physical examination, clinical breast examination, and mammograms based on recommended guidelines from NCCN. Practitioners also should closely examine the treated breast for changes related to RT as well as the scar. Women may verbalize changes they have noticed since treatment and should be encouraged to perform breast self-exams, as their treated breast tissue will change over time. Patients receiving hormonal therapy also should be evaluated regularly by a gynecologist.

Colorectal Cancer

Colorectal cancer (CRC) is divided into two treatment areas; the first treatment area is the colon, and the second is the rectum, with the latter being more commonly treated with RT. RT typically is not used alone but rather is used in the neoadjuvant (preoperative) or adjuvant setting (postoperative or after the primary treatment) with chemotherapy. The goal of treatment in the neoadjuvant setting for CRC is to reduce tumor burden (generally done with rectal tumors), thus making the tumor more resectable and sparing healthy tissue at the time of resection, and to down-stage the tumor to reduce the patient's chance of requiring a permanent colostomy (Gosselin, 2001). Sphincter preservation is another goal of neoadjuvant RT. In the adjuvant treatment setting, RT is used to minimize the risk of local recurrence.

Radiation can be delivered via external beam and/or with an intraoperative RT (IORT) approach, which is given while the patient is in the operating room. Neoadjuvant RT typically is given over the course of five to six weeks. A total dose of 45–50.4 Gy usually is prescribed and given as a daily dose of 1.8 Gy for a total of 25–28 treatments with photons. Patients with CRC typically have three to four treatment fields, and IMRT may be used to minimize toxicity in high-risk situations where the bowel and/or other organs or tissues may be in the treatment field, although 3-D treatment planning may be used. A three-field treatment approach incorporates the use of a posterior-anterior field, right lateral, and left lateral. A four-field treatment approach uses all of the same fields as the three-field approach but has an anteroposterior field in addition that is delivered from the front of the patient versus the back. Postoperative RT plus chemotherapy has been shown to have better disease control and survival when compared with surgery alone and surgery plus irradiation (Gunderson, Haddock, & Schild, 2003). Advantages of postoperative RT include that the stage of the cancer is known, which spares 10%–15% of early-stage patients having to undergo RT, and a more accurate outline of the surgical bed during RT planning with surgical clips in place (Minsky, 1997). Endocavitary RT also may be used in select patient populations (patients with small, mobile lesions) for sphincter preservation (Aumock et al., 2001).

Patients receiving RT need to undergo careful treatment planning to minimize the amount of small bowel in the treatment field, as this is the dose-limiting organ and can cause significant side effects. During simulation, a positioning device is made, and a rectal tube, vaginal marker, and BBs or wires (on the skin) may be used to outline the anatomy during the planning process. Some patients may be placed in the prone position on a belly board that allows for the bowel to fall away from the treatment field to minimize side effects during treatment. A DVH constructed during the planning phase will show doses to the planning target volume (PTV), including the femoral heads, bladder, and rectum. Treatment fields should include the tumor bed, a 2–5 cm margin, and the presacral and internal iliac nodes (NCCN, 2007d). A treatment boost also may be given to patients with CRC to the tumor or tumor bed, with the dose and number of fractions varying based upon preoperative or postoperative status. A treatment boost typically is performed once the patient reaches 45 Gy and includes anywhere from three to five fractions to the tumor bed.

IORT may be considered in patients with large tumors or with recurrent disease and also may be given in combination with external beam radiation therapy, with or without chemotherapy and surgical resection (Willett, Czito, & Tyler, 2007). This particular type of therapy can be performed by two different methods, depending on the treating facility. If performed in the operating suite, the room may have a linear accelerator in the suite, or an HDR unit may be brought to the suite to perform the treatment during the surgical procedure. The surgical room requires special shielding, and staff members need to be trained in radiation safety. The other option is for the patient to be transported to the radiation department during the operation to receive treatment. The latter option has multiple challenges related to patient transport and safety. During this treatment, the patient receives radiation to the surgical bed and surrounding areas that the surgical and radiation teams deem necessary.

Patients receiving RT for CRC are at risk for developing a variety of acute and late toxicities related to treatment (see Table 6-4). Many of these side effects are RT specific, but many also can be attributed to the role that chemotherapy plays in treating this disease. For example, myelosuppression is not common in patients receiving RT alone but may be seen more frequently in patients receiving RT plus chemotherapy. Many patients undergoing RT for CRC also receive concurrent 5-fluorouracil (5-FU). Coordination of this therapy, including management of an ambulatory infusion pump and understanding of the side effects, is critical to patient care and compliance with treatment. Common side effects of RT alone and with chemotherapy for CRC include fatigue, nausea, diarrhea, and skin reactions.

The APN must assess for chemotherapy-related side effects in the RT setting with patients receiving combined modality therapy. Complete blood cell counts should be evaluated throughout treatment. Nausea should be assessed, as this symptom is not common with RT but can develop with chemotherapy. The American Society of Clinical Oncology, the Multinational Association of Supportive Care in Cancer, and NCCN have developed evidence-based guidelines for the management of nausea and vomiting in patients receiving chemotherapy and RT.

Diarrhea is a dose-limiting toxicity of 5-FU, and the small bowel is a dose-limiting factor in RT. Diarrhea occurs as a result of cell death in the crypt epithelium, which results in insufficient replacement of the crypt cells and atrophy of the villi with breakdown of the mucosal barrier (Hauer-Jensen, Wang, & Denham, 2003). This then results in a loss of absorptive function and diarrhea. Patients will need to be educated early in their treatment about this side effect and what to expect. Diarrhea typically occurs one to two weeks into treatment and can worsen with the administration of chemotherapy. The amount and duration of diarrhea are patient dependent and should be routinely assessed. Dietary modifications, such as a low-residue diet, and over-the-counter and prescription medications may be necessary, and IV fluids may be required depending on the patient's vital signs at the time of assessment. Common medications used to manage the diarrhea associated with RT to the small bowel include Imodium® A-D

Table 6-4. Common Acute and Late Toxicities of Colorectal Treatment With Radiation Therapy and Chemotherapy

Symptom	Acute	Late
Allergic reaction	X	
Alopecia	X	
Anorexia	X	X
Cholinergic syndrome	X	
Diarrhea	X	X
Cystitis, dysuria, hematuria	X	
Enteritis		X
Fever	X	
Hand-foot syndrome	X	
Mucositis	X	
Myelosuppression	X	
Nausea, vomiting	X	
Peripheral neuropathy	X	X
Proteinuria	X	
Skin erythema, desquamation	X	
Skin fibrosis		X
Sterility		X
Tenesmus		X
Urgency, incontinence	X	
Vaginal dryness, dyspareunia, stenosis	X	X
Vascular effects	X	

Note. From "Colorectal Cancer" (p. 154), by T.K. Gosselin-Acomb in K.H. Dow (Ed.), *Nursing Care of Women With Cancer*, 2006, St. Louis, MO: Mosby. Copyright 2006 by Elsevier Health Sciences. Reprinted with permission.

(McNeil) and Lomotil® (Pfizer Inc.). Sandostatin® (Novartis Pharmaceuticals) is not used as frequently but is used in select patients who are not controlled on other medications (Stern & Ippoliti, 2003; Yavuz, Yavuz, Aydin, Can, & Kavgaci, 2002). Some patients also may complain of rectal discharge or tenesmus (feeling of incomplete defecation), which usually results from inflammation or scarring of the bowel. Patients should be encouraged to use absorbent pads or briefs if this condition occurs.

Skin reactions typically arise in the perianal area about two to three weeks into treatment, depending on the location of the treatment field. The most common areas at risk for skin reactions are the gluteal folds and the perineal area. Patients initially present with erythema that can progress into dry and then moist desquamation over the course of treatment. Patients are instructed to use a mild skin cleanser and to apply a moisturizing protective cream. Haisfield-Wolfe and Rund (2000) developed a perineal-rectal skin care protocol (see Table 6-5) to be used in clinical practice to manage this often uncomfortable side effect, which can be exacerbated by diarrhea. Good hygiene during this time is essential to alleviate and reduce the risk of infection and pain associated with this side effect.

Table 6-5. Perineal-Rectal Skin Care Protocol

Routine Care

During morning care and after each episode of urination or defecation, the patient will receive the following care.

- Gently cleanse skin with tepid water or a mild cleansing agent followed by gently patting areas dry **or** cleanse with tepid to cool sitz baths.
- If open lesions are present, cleanse with a wound cleanser or normal saline solution and treat.
- Apply a moisturizing cream.
- Recommend cotton undergarments; avoid restrictive clothing.
- Perform a full assessment of the perineal-rectal skin.
- Perform a nutrition assessment followed by nutrition consult, if needed.
- Consult an enterostomal therapy or wound-care nurse as needed.

Assessment	Recommendations for Care
Erythema signs and symptoms Pink Tenderness	Gently cleanse using a mild cleansing agent (perineal skin cleansers). Apply a moisturizing, protective cream. If cleanser is not accessible and soap must be used, use a soap without perfumes and thoroughly rinse all soap residues from the skin. Avoid lotions or creams containing perfume and talc (if receiving radiation therapy to area, avoid products containing metals or ointments or cleanse area prior to receiving radiation therapy). Frequency of skin care: Daily and after toileting
Dry desquamation signs and symptoms Scaling Flaking Pruritus Pain	Cleanse with tepid water or a wound cleanser. Apply a protective cream. Assess for pruritus, if present. • Apply topical antihistamine creams. • Take a cool shower or bath. • Consider analgesics or antihistamines. Assess for fungal infection, if present. • Treat with topical antifungal or systemic antifungal agent. Frequency of skin care: Twice a day/as needed after toileting

---

(Continued on next page)

Table 6-5. Perineal-Rectal Skin Care Protocol *(Continued)*

Moist desquamation signs and symptoms

Pain	Recommend sitz bath, shower, whirlpool as needed.
Weeping	
Sloughing	Cleanse with a wound cleanser as needed.
Abscess	Apply a protective cream that will adhere to open skin.
	Apply an adhesive peripad or a pantyliner without deodorant to the undergarments.
	Assess need for analgesics, pain medications.
	If desquamation worsens, apply a wound hydrogel.
	Frequency of skin care: Twice a day/as needed after toileting

Possible complications of moist desquamation

Vesicles	Consult with physician or advanced practice nurse for treatment and systematic antibiotics.
Furuncle	
Carbuncles	If vesicles are present, rule out herpes and treat appropriately.
Abscess formation	

Report to Physician	Documentation
Worsening of skin alteration	Anatomical area involved
Increase in inflammation	Size of involvement
Appearance of furuncle, carbuncles, abscess	• Area may be difficult to measure because of the perineal-rectal anatomy.
Appearance of vesicles	
Pain or increase in pain, change in character of pain	• Attempt to record in centimeters.
	• Measure from where the normal skin stops to where it begins again (use a disposable ruler). If open areas develop, measure width, length, and depth.
	• Record daily in acute care or weekly in home or long-term care.
	Changes in skin or wound conditions
	Colors of skin
	Drainage (i.e., amount, odor, color, consistency)
	Presence of sloughing or necrosis
	Presence and intensity of pain or pruritus
	Patient outcomes

Note. From "Nursing Protocol for the Management of Perineal-Rectal Skin Alterations," by M.E. Haisfield-Wolfe and C. Rund, *Clinical Journal of Oncology Nursing, 4,* p. 19. Copyright 2000 by Oncology Nursing Society. Reprinted with permission.

Late effects of RT in this population may include enteritis and sexuality issues. Enteritis is characterized by dysmotility (changes in movement through the bowel) and malabsorption that may need further diagnostic evaluation (Hauer-Jensen et al., 2003). These side effects take months to years to develop, and patients may experience adhesions, fibrosis, fistulas, and obstruction (Hauer-Jensen et al.). Mild cases of enteritis may require dietary modification with a low-residue diet, whereas more severe cases may require additional fiber to assist in stool formation and over-the-counter or prescription medications.

Sexuality issues related to dyspareunia, vaginal dryness, and vaginal stenosis may arise in women, and men may experience weakened orgasm and erectile dysfunction resulting from the effect of RT on the tissues. Patients must understand the risks of these symptoms as well as the interventions that may be used to assist them in maintaining intimacy in their relationship. Interventions for women may include the use of hormone therapy, vaginal dilators, and moisturizers and lubricants to keep the vagina open for sexual intercourse as well as for pelvic examinations (Bruner, 2001). For men, pharmacologic and nonpharmacologic interventions may be used, including vasoactive agents and penile prostheses (Bruner). The American Cancer Society (ACS, 2001a, 2001b) publishes two brochures, one for women and one for men, titled *Sexuality and Cancer* that can be provided and reviewed with patients. Female patients also may require education and instruction related to the use of a vaginal dilator.

Follow-up care for each patient is individualized but should include physical examination, carcinogenic embryonic antigen monitoring, and colonoscopy. NCCN recommends that a physical exam and blood work should be performed every three to six months for two years and then every six months for a total of five years. Colonoscopy should be performed the first year after treatment and, if abnormal, repeated in a year. If no polyps are present, then the test should be repeated in three years and then every five years (NCCN, 2007d).

Non-Small Cell Lung Cancer

RT can be used in the treatment of non-small cell lung cancer (NSCLC) in the curative or palliative treatment setting. Patients should be evaluated by the multidisciplinary team and should complete appropriate imaging studies before final treatment plans are developed. NCCN (2007b) recommends that RT should be offered in the following situations: in patients with stage I and II disease who are inoperable, in postoperative patients with negative margins and positive mediastinal nodes, and in postoperative patients with positive margins. Patients also may receive adjuvant or concurrent chemotherapy. For patients with advanced disease, RT is used for palliation of the symptoms associated with the primary tumor or sites of metastatic disease.

Treatment planning should include a CT scan and simulation; in some institutions, positron-emission tomography (PET) and CT scans will be done. Patients will have a treatment positioning device made to help position their arms above their head. Three-dimensional (3-D) treatment planning then will take place, and a DVH will be constructed to identify doses to the PTV, including the lung, heart, and other tissues of concern. Planning the fields for this treatment can often be complex because of the anatomy of the chest, which includes the heart, stomach, and esophagus, and if nodal fields are involved, including the hilar, mediastinal, and supraclavicular areas. Multiple fields and oblique beams may be used to provide adequate dosing as well as opposed fields (left and right laterals) in some cases. Total doses of RT may range from 44–45 Gy in the preoperative setting to 50 Gy in the postoperative setting, with supplemental dosing to extranodal sites (NCCN, 2007b). In the curative chemoradiation setting, total doses may range from 60–66 Gy (NCCN, 2007b). Higher total doses have been reported in clinical trials with chemotherapy (Hayman et al., 2001; Marks et al., 2004), ranging from 63–86 Gy. Daily doses usually are 1.8–2 Gy, and treatment usually is delivered over five to six weeks. Some patients may undergo respiratory gating with each treatment, which requires additional time on the linear accelerator machine each day. IMRT as well as HDR brachytherapy also may be used in select cases.

Acute side effects of RT for treatment of NSCLC include cough, fatigue, skin reactions, and esophagitis/pharyngitis. A baseline assessment of symptoms that the patient may be experiencing needs to be obtained before initiating RT. Patients may be experiencing cough, dyspnea, anorexia, and weight loss related to the disease itself and not the treatment. If patients are receiving concurrent chemotherapy, assessment of the effect of combination therapy is important.

Esophagitis typically arises during the second or third week of therapy and is caused by the RT irritating the esophagus. This side effect may appear sooner if the patient is receiving concurrent chemotherapy. Patients will complain of dysphagia and the feeling of a lump in the throat. They also may report heartburn and occasional chest pain. Dietary modification should include eating soft, moist foods and consuming liquids with foods, so that swallowing is made easier. Medications that coat the irritated area as well as pain medications may be beneficial. Use of the World Health Organization ladder for pain management or the NCCN Adult Cancer Pain Guidelines may help as well. The provider also will want to rule out an oral *Candida* infection, as this often can arise early in treatment and can be confused with esophagitis. *Candida* infection usually is treated with Diflucan® (Pfizer Inc.). Some patients may require IV fluids if their vital signs and fluid status demonstrate dehydration.

A skin reaction will appear about two to three weeks into treatment and is characterized by pruritus, dry skin, and erythema. Patients also will experience temporary hair loss on the chest within the treatment field and should be encouraged to use a moisturizing lotion that is alcohol free. Patients may have an additional area of pruritus at the exit site of the radiation beam, based on the beam arrangement. This occurs when the beam is exiting the body on the posterior side.

A cough can arise during treatment, which usually is caused by irritation of the tissues from the treatment and typically subsides with the use of antitussive therapy with or without codeine. Fatigue is common in patients being treated for lung cancer. NCCN and the Oncology Nursing Society both have guidelines that provide pharmacologic and nonpharmacologic recommendations for the management of fatigue. Pneumonitis can be both an acute and late side effect of RT and can be attributed to the total dose of radiation, volume of lung treated, fractionation schedule, and use of concomitant chemotherapy. Patients with pneumonitis usually present with a cough, tachycardia, low-grade fever, and shortness of breath (Marks et al., 2003). Treatment generally includes short-term bed rest, oxygen, bronchodilators, and corticosteroids. Antibiotics typically are not used unless an associated infection is present. Fibrosis is a late effect of RT in which patients present with cough, dyspnea, and tachypnea. Management is similar to that of patients with pneumonitis.

Follow-up care for each patient is individualized but should include physical examination and diagnostic tests based on recommended guidelines from NCCN. Specific recommendations for follow-up are different for patients with stage I–IIIA disease than for patients with stage IIIB and IV disease. Patients should undergo a physical examination and chest x-ray every four months in the first two years, then every six months for two years, and then annually. Spiral CT scans also may be used in the follow-up phase. Patients should be referred to smoking cessation programs as needed (NCCN, 2007b).

Prostate Cancer

Prostate cancer can be treated with a variety of RT approaches as well as with watchful waiting, hormone therapy, surgery, and chemotherapy. Cryosurgery has seen recent improvements and also can be used to treat localized prostate cancer (Hogle, 2007). Treatment controversy still exists regarding the pros and cons as to whether radical prostatectomy or radiation is superior both as a treatment and in relation to acute or late effects that may arise. Initial treatment decisions should focus on the extent of the tumor: both surgery and RT can be used when the tumor is confined to the prostate. Other factors related to the initial treatment decision include the patient's age, comorbid conditions, general health status, and pretreatment bowel, bladder, and sexual function. Men who decide to undergo RT may receive external beam RT, brachytherapy, or a combination of the two in select populations.

Simulation for men undergoing external beam RT includes the development of a positioning device, the placement of rectal and urethral catheters, and the use of a penile clamp to stop the flow of contrast during the planning session. The urethral catheter is used to delineate the prostate base, whereas the rectal catheter shows the contour of the rectum. A planning CT also will be performed in patients who are to receive 3-D conformal or IMRT treatment. A variety of treatment techniques have been employed in treating prostate cancer. These include a four-field technique, a six-field approach, 3-D conformal therapy, and IMRT, with the latter two being the more popular choices today because they minimize toxicity (Luxton, Hancock, & Boyer, 2004). Some patients may have fiducials or markers placed in the prostate to assist with treatment planning. The DVH would include the amount and percentage of radiation to the prostate, femoral heads, bladder, rectum, and seminal vesicles.

Based on NCCN guidelines (2007c), patients with low-risk cancers should receive doses of 70–75 Gy given in 35–41 fractions, whereas those with intermediate- or high-risk disease should receive doses of 75–80 Gy. Each of these risk categories (see Table 6-6) factors in staging, Gleason score, and prostate-specific antigen (PSA) level, which are used together to determine what type of treatment may be best for the patient. Daily doses typically are 1.8 Gy, and patients with intermediate- or high-risk disease also may receive treatment to the pelvic lymph nodes to a dose of 50 Gy. Men receiving IMRT will have more treatment fields and a tighter margin around the PTV to minimize side effects. If a boost dose is going to be given with brachytherapy, then the total dose from external beam will be approximately 40–50 Gy.

Brachytherapy can be used as a monotherapy or in addition to external beam treatment as a boost. As a monotherapy, it is used in patients with early-stage disease. Brachytherapy is used with other therapies for patients with higher-grade tumors. Patient convenience, costs, and short recovery time factor into why men may choose brachytherapy over external beam therapy. Contraindications for brachytherapy include a large prostate (> 60 g) or small prostate (< 15–20 g), symptoms of bladder outlet obstruction (International Prostate Symptom Score > 15), or a previous transurethral resection of the prostate (NCCN, 2007c). This treatment can be given at a low-dose rate (LDR) or HDR (see Table 6-1). Factors determining HDR use include minimization of

Table 6-6. Prostate Cancer Risk			
Diagnosis Components	**Low**	**Intermediate**	**High**
Staging	T1–2a	T2b–T2c	T3a
Gleason score	2–6	7	8–10
Prostate-specific antigen	< 10 ng/ml	10–20 ng/ml	> 20 ng/ml

Note. Based on information from Carroll et al., 2005; National Comprehensive Cancer Network, 2007c.

underdosing areas of the gland, physician and staff training, and decreased source exposure for staff members (Hogle, 2007).

Treatment planning for LDR brachytherapy includes a CT scan one to two weeks before starting RT. This scan assists the physician in determining optimum placement of the permanent seeds. LDR is accomplished while the patient is receiving general or spinal anesthesia. While the patient is in a lithotomy position, a perineal template and a transrectal ultrasound (TRUS) probe are placed. The TRUS allows visualization of the needles and seeds as they are placed, and the template provides stabilization of the needles into the prostate. The seeds can be preloaded in the needle or placed once the needles are in place. A total of 18–30 needles and 75–150 tiny seeds may be placed, depending on prostate volume. Once the seeds are placed, the needles are removed and the patient is sent to the postoperative holding area. With patients going home the same day, discharge teaching is a critical component of care. Discharge instructions should include contact numbers in the event of acute urinary retention, information about expected side effects (e.g., pain, seed migration, sexuality issues, skin and urinary changes), safety precautions related to the radioactive seeds, and follow-up appointments. Safety precautions include straining urine for seeds and using condoms during intercourse. Additionally, maximizing the distance between the patient and family members, pregnant or possibly pregnant women, and young children also should be reviewed with the patient and family.

Iodine-125 (^{125}I) and palladium (^{103}Pd) seeds commonly are used in LDR because they have a short range, slow dose rate, and low energy source; can give adequate dose levels to the prostate; and can avoid radiation to the bladder and rectum. However, side effects from LDR are more prolonged than those from HDR because of the half-life of the isotopes used. Abel et al. (1999) provides an overview of the patient management related to LDR brachytherapy that discusses the symptoms as well as nonpharmacologic and pharmacologic interventions.

In patients receiving HDR, the setup is done the same way as it is with LDR, except the perineal template is sutured into the perineum. The needles or flexiguides are left in place because they will be attached to the after-loading machine for treatment. After CT-based treatment planning, several high-dose fractions ranging from 4–6 Gy are administered over an interval of 24–36 hours (Hogle, 2007). Iridium-192 (^{192}I) is the source of radiation, and each treatment takes approximately 20–30 minutes. Patients will remain on bed rest until all fractions are given and will be transported to the radiation department for each fraction. Typically, two fractions are given each day, with each fraction separated by six hours. Patients will have a urinary catheter in place and could potentially have a continuous bladder irrigation running to keep the urine clear. Patients also will be put on a clear liquid diet and will receive parenteral analgesics for pain and other supportive care medications. Antidiarrheals may be used so that the patient does not need to have a bowel movement during this period of two to three days. Pain management is critical in these patients. After each treatment, the seeds are returned to the after-loader; therefore, the patient is not radioactive between treatments or at the time of discharge. When the needles and template are removed, the patient may experience perineal bleeding and swelling. A pressure dressing should be applied following treatment, and side effects including perineal bleeding and swelling and urinary and bowel changes should resolve in two to four weeks. Some patients may receive this treatment during external beam RT and may receive HDR more than once.

Acute and late toxicities of RT to the prostate include bowel and urinary changes, fatigue, sexual dysfunction, and skin reactions. A baseline symptom assessment should be conducted before the start of treatment so that changes can be documented over time. Bowel changes are more prevalent in patients undergoing 3-D conformal treatment than those receiving IMRT. Patients may experience diarrhea a few weeks into treatment. Many patients can be managed on a low-residue diet and Imodium A-D or Lomotil. Proctitis is another side effect that may occur. It is characterized by inflammation of the rectal lining and causes pain, bleeding, and a mucous or purulent discharge. This side effect can occur months to years after treatment and may require laser treatment. Patients should be encouraged to use a psyllium-based supplement so that they have well-formed stools that can easily pass through the rectum. Narcotics and topical Proctofoam® HC (Schwarz Pharma), which is a combination of a topical corticosteroid and local anesthetic, may be used to minimize discomfort.

Patients may experience perianal hair loss as well as skin changes from external beam RT. Men may experience mild erythema and desquamation, although desquamation is less common in these patients. For patients who experience skin breakdown, use of the perianal guidelines, such those seen in Table 6-5, would be beneficial.

Urinary side effects of RT to the prostate may include dysuria, frequency, hematuria, hesitancy, nocturia, and urgency. Patients must understand that these are expected side effects of treatment that result from the effects of radiation on the tissue and should be reported so that appropriate symptom management can be initiated. Ruling out bladder obstruction and infection is essential to the management of these symptoms. Patients should drink plenty of fluids throughout the day and decrease their intake in the evening. A variety of pharmacologic medications, including ibuprofen, oxybutynin chloride, phenazopyridine, tamsulosin hydrochloride, terazosin hydrochloride, and doxazosin, can be used to manage urinary symptoms (Hogle, 2005).

Sexual dysfunction is a common side effect of prostate cancer therapy. As with other side effects, patients' pretreatment sexual function must be understood. Sexual dysfunction related to RT of the prostate includes impotence, premature ejaculation, and retrograde ejaculation. Treatment for dysfunction may include counseling and use of the ACS brochure *Sexuality for Men and Their Partners.* Medications such as vardenafil, tadalafil, and sildenafil may be used in men who are experiencing erectile dysfunction (Donatucci & Greenfield, 2006; Stephenson et al., 2005). Vasoactive agents, such as intracavernosal injections and intraurethral suppositories, as well as vacuum devices and penile prostheses, may be beneficial for patients who cannot achieve or maintain an erection (Hogle, 2007).

Follow-up care for each patient is individualized but should include physical examination, digital rectal examination (DRE), and PSA monitoring based on recommended guidelines from NCCN. PSA may be done as frequently as every three months, whereas DRE may be performed every six months. Patients also should be evaluated for erectile dysfunction, as this is a common side effect of treatment (NCCN, 2007c).

Radiation Therapy With Palliative Intent

Patients with advanced disease often present with pain, bleeding, neurologic changes, and other symptoms that invoke distress to the patient and caregiver. In patients with advanced disease, a prompt history and physical are essential, including attaining a thorough understanding of prior cancer therapies that the patient may have received. Prior RT treatment fields, dose, and volume treated are important in determining the potential for overlap of treatment fields if the patient is to receive RT, which may lead to unacceptable toxicities in patients with advanced disease. For example, a patient with NSCLC may complain of pain in the mid-back and undergo magnetic resonance imaging (MRI) that confirms spinal cord compression. The patient then would be started on steroids to reduce edema in the spinal cord and receive 30 Gy of RT in 10 fractions. The goal of therapy is not to cure but rather to palliate the symptom of pain and enhance patient comfort. The patient also may require pain medications. A course of palliative RT is much shorter than a curative course, usually by several weeks. Pain assessment and management will be critical during this time as well, and a referral to hospice should be made if the patient is an appropriate candidate. Ongoing dialogue with caregivers also is important, as they may need to bring the patient back and forth or may require the use of ambulance services.

Pediatric Considerations

Pediatric patients undergoing RT and their families often have unique treatment considerations. One of the primary concerns in the treatment of children is the ability of these patients to remain still during treatment. Typically, patients younger than age three or four may require sedation for simulation and treatment. This requires patients to be evaluated by the anesthesia staff. Consultation with child life experts to work with patients and families is critical in minimizing the use of sedation by doing play therapy with the positioning device, although cognitive impairment related to disease may affect patients' ability to forgo sedation. Parents need to be educated about dietary restrictions if their child is to undergo daily or hyperfractionated RT with anesthesia. Other potential areas of education include the use of growth hormone, fertility issues, and secondary malignancies. Growth hormone deficiency is a common disorder in children who have received RT to the hypothalamus and can occur months to years after treatment. Fertility issues arise when the testes or ovaries receive RT, and an example of a secondary malignancy would be the development of breast cancer in later life in a woman who underwent RT for Hodgkin disease as a teenager. It is important that as the child continues to grow and develop that the parents understand the need for life-long follow-up and surveillance.

Geriatric Considerations

Caring for older patients who are receiving RT potentially can pose logistical issues depending on their functional status and activities of daily living. Patients with impaired vision may require a driver for their daily treatment appointments. Also, older adults are at an increased risk for skin reactions because of the natural aging and thinning of the skin. Care coordination with family and friends is critical in this population. Kagan and Garrett (2007) provided a framework for working with older clients who are undergoing RT.

Standards

Standards of care and standards of professional performance are outlined in the *Manual for Radiation Oncology Nursing Practice and Education* (Third Edition) (Bruner, Haas, & Gosselin-Acomb, 2005). The standards of care pertain to interaction between the provider and patients and families, whereas standards of professional performance relate to how the provider looks to enhance his or her professional development and patient outcomes. Eight standards exist related to professional practice, and each will be interpreted in relation to the role of the APN in radiation oncology.

1. Quality of care—APNs should systematically evaluate and document the effectiveness of clinical care. This documentation includes completion and dictation of patients' history and physical examination, ordering of laboratory and radiology tests, performance of procedures, and documentation of weekly treatment and follow-up visits. APNs may prescribe supportive care medications (with appropriate prescriptive privileges) and should evaluate the medication's effectiveness in patient care. Additionally, APNs may review nursing practice and make recommendations regarding documentation tools as well as serve on safety and quality committees. Furthermore, they may assume "on-call" responsibilities, evaluating patients at the emergency room or rounding on hospitalized patients on weekends and holidays (Carper & Haas, 2006).

2. Accountability—The APN will educate medical staff in defining the APN role, understanding the privileges that are set forth by the state, and establishing any competencies.

3. Education—APNs entering into the field of radiation oncology will need to evaluate their current level of radiation knowledge in comparison to what is required on the job, as the role varies with practice setting. APNs will develop a self-education plan as well as an education plan for other professionals in the department, may facilitate education sessions, and may provide education to healthcare professionals outside of the department. APNs should review and develop patient education materials as well as conduct support groups.

4. Leadership—APNs may serve as the manager of nurses in the department and, therefore, should serve as a role model. This may require interviewing, hiring, performance management, budgetary functions, and oversight for staff and patient programs. APNs will be involved with both departmental and facility committees.

5. Ethics—APNs ensure that patient needs are met regardless of background and incorporate diversity and sensitivity into practice. APNs must be aware of role limitations. This area also involves serving as a resource for staff members who are having difficulty in managing a particular care situation.

6. Collaboration—APNs are part of the multidisciplinary team and assist in care coordination across the continuum. They develop symptom management plans and communicate significant findings and issues to others on the team. Barriers to practice may exist, and APNs may need to educate colleagues about the role as well as develop the scope and standards of the role (Moore-Higgs et al., 2003).

7. Research—APNs translate research into practice but also are able to develop research studies to enhance patient care and outcomes. They may develop studies investigating symptom management, patient education, palliative care, and acute and late side effects. APNs should look at the role of technology in care and how it can assist both patients and providers and should examine how the role of the APN affects patient care and satisfaction.

8. Resource utilization—APNs understand the resource needs of both patients and the larger community. APNs will serve primarily in a clinical role and will see patients in the inpatient and outpatient setting as well as in multidisciplinary clinics.

Patient and Family Education

RT is a unique treatment, and most patients are unfamiliar with the planning process, technology, and highly technical aspects of care, thus making patient and family education a critical component of the APN role. APNs can assist in minimizing the anxiety of patients and families by providing education to meet patient and family learning needs. In a 2003 survey, 93% of APN respondents indicated that they provided education related to expectations of RT and specific symptom management strategies (Moore-Higgs et al., 2003). A variety of materials are available for APNs to use in practice that can assist in supplementing verbal instruction regarding RT (see Table 6-7).

Patient education starts at the time of consultation, once it is determined that the patient will receive RT. APNs should educate the patient about the goals of treatment, the treatment planning process, treatments, and weekly treatment check, as well as acute and late side effects of treatment. This is often an overwhelming amount of information provided in one session, so CD-ROMs, DVDs, and written materials should be used to supplement the verbal instruction. Educational media also are helpful in educating patients who are not able to read. Written consent also may be appropriate at this time or when the patient returns for the simulation appointment.

Simulation and Treatment Planning

During most simulations, the patient will be asked to wear a hospital gown, and the patient needs to know that the area that is to receive treatment will be exposed. Patients must understand this prior to treatment, as it can cause emotional distress. Patients need to understand how long the procedure will take and that a body mold or mask may be made to assist in positioning and the reproducibility of the treatment field,

Table 6-7. Sample of Available Patient Education Materials

Type of Education	Resources	Organization
General	*Radiation Therapy and You*	National Institutes of Health and National Cancer Institute
	Understanding Radiation Therapy: A Guide for Patients and Families	American Cancer Society
Site specific	Breast, colorectal, lung, prostate, and 28 other disease-site booklets	National Cancer Institute
	Brochures on bladder, brain, breast, colorectal, gynecologic, head and neck, lung, prostate, and skin cancers and Hodgkin and non-Hodgkin lymphoma	American Society for Therapeutic Radiology and Oncology
	Guidelines on bladder, breast, colon and rectum, lung, ovarian, and prostate cancers, melanoma, and non-Hodgkin lymphoma	National Comprehensive Cancer Network
Symptom management	*Sexuality for Women and Their Partners*	American Cancer Society
	Sexuality for Men and Their Partners	American Cancer Society
	Guidelines on fatigue, pain, distress, nausea, and vomiting	National Comprehensive Cancer Network

as well as the need for them to remain still during this time. Certain patients may need placement of an IV for contrast administration, urinary catheter, rectal tube, or vaginal marker. Simulation can be completed on a variety of different machines, such as a conventional simulator and a CT simulator. During this time, marks may be made on the patient's skin (using a marker) to outline the treatment area, and patients should not remove these until instructed to do so.

Patients also may be required to undergo additional tests, including PET scans, MRI, and CT scans, to provide an understanding of anatomic and physiologic information to be used for the development of the treatment plan. The treatment plan will then be developed, and in most cases where cure is the goal of therapy, it may take anywhere from one to two weeks before the patient starts treatment.

Treatment

Patients undergoing daily RT can expect to be in the RT department anywhere from 30–90 minutes. Conventional RT and 3-D conformal treatments typically take an average of 15 minutes of treatment time, whereas IMRT treatments can take up to 30–45 minutes. The addition of onboard imaging, which allows for visualization of the treatment site and ensures beam accuracy as well as respiratory gating, will require more time. Patients who are receiving hyperfractionated RT will need to come twice a day, and the feasibility of this schedule needs to be determined at the time of consultation/simulation. The radiation therapist will make permanent tattoos on the patient's skin once therapy has been initiated; once these tattoos are made, the markings made during simulation can be removed.

The treatment team will evaluate the patient at least once a week. This will include checking the patient's weight and vital signs and providing an opportunity for the patient to address any concerns related to the care and treatment. The healthcare provider will review the treatment prescription, evaluate any expected and unexpected acute effects, and provide evidence-based symptom management strategies. Patients may be seen more frequently because of toxicity and put on a treatment break if needed, although treatment breaks are not favored in RT because of concerns about cell repopulation.

Planning for Follow-Up

As patients are preparing to complete treatment, they must be educated on the follow-up plan of care, including the frequency of appointments, laboratory and radiology studies, and cancer screenings as defined by NCCN and the ACS. Patients also should be educated about the resolution of their symptoms and what to expect over the next two to four weeks as their symptoms subside.

Implications for Oncology Advanced Practice Nurses

The American Society for Therapeutic Radiology and Oncology conducted a descriptive survey in 1997 on the role of nonphysician providers (Kelvin & Moore-Higgs, 1999). The survey received a total of 76 APN respondents (45 clinical nurse specialists [CNSs] and 31 nurse practitioners [NPs]). Based upon the nurse's role, the researchers found that CNSs and NPs completed a patient history at the time of consultation (63% and 57% of the time, respectively), during treatment visits (67% and 80%), or during fol-

low-up (62% and 58%). Physical examination completion for CNSs and NPs was identified at the time of consult (19% and 42%), on treatment (36% and 74%), and during follow-up (26% and 57%). They found that CNSs were more likely than NPs to develop patient education materials, lead patient education programs, and participate in
planning new programs. NPs were found to be more involved with ordering laboratory studies and radiology studies and prescribing medications. Involvement with simulation also was reported, but not by practice role (Kelvin & Moore-Higgs).

In a survey of 1,000 APN members of the Oncology Nursing Society, only 6% of respondents listed RT as their primary specialty (Lynch, Cope, & Murphy-Ende, 2001).
All respondents identified that patient care and education were the most common activities that they performed in their role. Lastly, in a smaller sample of 28 NPs who work
in RT, it was found that the top three activities performed by the respondents included performing symptom management, conducting weekly treatment visits, and seeing
patients at follow-up visits (Carper & Haas, 2006).

In another study comparing the roles of staff nurses in RT, nurse managers, and APNs,
it was found that APNs spent the majority of their time in direct patient care and education (Moore-Higgs et al., 2003). APNs also were involved with triage, research, and
consultations. One interesting finding from this study was that all roles studied reported involvement with patient education. The APN role is still in development in this specialty. APNs may see patients at time of consultation, during weekly treatment for symptom management, or during the follow-up care. Depending upon the practice setting,
APNs may provide informed consent for patients, assist in treatment planning, and assist in the development of plans of care. Collaboration with the medical and surgical
oncology teams is critical for APNs in RT, as many patients are receiving combined modality treatment and may require additional treatment following RT. Telephone triage
and on-call responsibilities also may be part of the APN role (Carper & Haas, 2006).
Furthermore, APNs may use other resources to improve the quality of care for patients
receiving RT, such as dietitians, financial counselors, and social workers. Issues such as
housing, transportation, out-of-pocket costs and insurance, child care, and support systems may all affect a patient's compliance with the prescribed treatment.

APNs play a critical role in symptom assessment and management. Issues related to
contrast reactions, allergies, pregnancy, and sexuality during treatment are all important topics that often may go unaddressed. APNs should be able to manage both acute
and late effects of treatment. Collaboration with the team is essential when a patient is
experiencing significant side effects and is in need of a treatment break.

In planning for discharge and follow-up, APNs may develop survivorship care plans
and guidelines for routine screening and follow-up for patients. Lambert (2007) provides additional detail about what APNs may want to consider when they enter the field
of radiation oncology.

Conclusion

The role of the APN in the radiation oncology setting is one of excitement and opportunity. APNs have tremendous opportunity in this field to showcase their knowledge and expertise to other healthcare providers as well as to be a pivotal provider of
patient care services. APNs should look to develop programs that improve patient outcomes and satisfaction with care. These types of programs may include development
and coordination of a fast-track symptom management program, development of a sur-

vivorship clinic, and establishment of palliative programs to support patients and families. The growing need to provide the right care at the right time is fundamental to the APN role in radiation oncology.

Case Study

Harriet is a 54-year-old postmenopausal woman diagnosed with a T1N0M0 breast cancer. In December 2006, a screening mammogram showed an abnormality in the lateral left breast. A biopsy on February 1, 2007, was positive for adenocarcinoma that was estrogen/progesterone–receptor positive, human epidermal growth factor receptor-2 negative, and epidermal growth factor receptor-negative. Surgery later that month revealed a 1.5 cm invasive ductal carcinoma. Surgical margins were negative, and one sentinel node was negative. She has recovered well from surgery and presents today for evaluation and discussion about her treatment options. Upon entry into the room, you notice that Harriet is anxious and alone. You quickly assess the situation and ask if anyone is with her. You explain to her the purpose of her visit today, and that based upon her surgical report, she had clean margins. Harriet breathes a sigh of relief, and you begin taking a history. You note that Harriet is a mother of two children, ages 16 and 18. Your review of systems is negative, except for her breast scar, and Harriet reports that she has had sharp, shooting pains intermittently in her left lateral breast and axilla since surgery.

You make an appointment for Harriet to return in three days for simulation. You review with her what simulation is and what will occur during this time. You then discuss treatment, weekly visits while under treatment, and the acute and late effects of RT.

On the day of her simulation, the therapists tell Harriet, "We are going to remove the gown over your breast." Harriet states, "What do you mean?" The therapists tell her that they will need to be able to make appropriate marks on her skin and that no one else can see her except for them. Harriet takes a breath and closes her eyes. The therapists ask her if she would like to listen to some music. She responds yes.

Treatment planning is completed, and Harriet starts treatment five days later. She is going to receive 23 treatments for a total dose of 46 Gy, with a boost to the surgical area for eight additional treatments at 200 centigray (cGy) a day, bringing her total dose to 62 Gy. Later that week, you see her for her weekly treatment check. Her blood counts are fine, and she has no complaints.

The next two weeks are uneventful. She is reporting minor fatigue but attributes it to taking care of her kids and her home. At the end of week three, she reports that she has been experiencing some redness and itching of her breast. She tells you she just does not like the way she looks right now. You discuss her concerns with her and ask if there is anything else you can do. She tells you no and thanks you for listening.

During the fourth week of treatment, Harriet has dry desquamation and asks for treatment recommendations. She tells you she has heard about a variety of different products from others who have gone through this treatment and shows you a cream that she has bought that has a nice floral scent. You recommend a moisturizing product such as Aquaphor® (Beiersdorf) and tell her not to use the product she bought because it contains alcohol.

The final two weeks of treatment are uneventful for Harriet. She continues to use Aquaphor, and her fatigue continues to be low. On her final day before treatment, you meet and review her discharge instructions and follow-up care. You tell her that her skin reaction will resolve within the next two to four weeks and that her fatigue also should improve.

1. At the time of the history taking, the patient asks you why she has to come back in before starting treatment. You respond by telling her which of the following statements?
   • CT and simulation (treatment planning) need to occur.
   • She will need lab work to make sure that she is ready for treatment.
   • She needs to return to ensure that her insurance covers the full cost of the treatment.
   • A tour of the facility is planned so that she will feel more comfortable during treatment.

   A CT and simulation always are performed prior to treatment to set up the precise treatment field that is required for RT.

2. The patient wants to know again the acute effects of radiation that she is going to experience from the treatment. You tell her which of the following?
   • Fatigue and alopecia
   • Fatigue and skin changes to the breast
   • Alopecia and skin changes to the breast
   • Nausea, vomiting, and myelosuppression

   Because radiation therapy is a local therapy, side effects generally will occur related to the areas of the body that have been treated. The patient will likely experience fatigue and skin changes to the breast, including erythema and dry desquamation, which can lead to moist desquamation.

3. A boost treatment is used to do which of the following?
   • Treat the entire breast.
   • Provide prophylaxis treatment to the contralateral breast.
   • Provide a "boost" of radiation to the surgical site prior to radiation of the entire breast.
   • Provide a "boost" of radiation to the surgical site, including the area around the surgical scar.

   A boost treatment is used to provide a "boost" of radiation to the surgical site at the completion of the radiation to the entire breast. The treatment field includes the area around the surgical scar (as this area has a high chance of developing a recurrence).

4. Which recommendation do you provide to Harriet when she is experiencing dry desquamation?
   • Any moisturizer will help to provide relief related to her symptoms.
   • Apply any skin product at least one hour before any radiation treatment.
   • Apply a moisturizer with an air-occlusive dressing over the site for at least four hours a day.
   • Although no standard treatment exists, the patient should keep the skin clean and dry and use a nonalcohol moisturizer.

   No standard of care exists for the management of skin changes of the breast related to RT. Best practice dictates keeping the skin clean and dry along with using nonalcohol moisturizers. The patient also should be taught to avoid sun exposure to the site that has been radiated.

Key Points

- Radiation oncology is a rapidly evolving field with new treatment modalities.
- Patient treatment is customized and requires careful planning to outline critical structures and anatomy.
- For the majority of patients, a curative course of RT is five to six weeks of treatment.
- Radiation side effects are treatment site dependent versus systemic.
- Acute and late effects of RT are influenced by the type of radiation used, the volume of tissue irradiated, the total dose and daily dose of radiation, the radiosensitivity of the organ or site, and the use of concurrent chemotherapy.
- Patients across all age groups are treated in RT departments; therefore, staff competencies and skill sets need to be current in relation to the diverse age groups.
- Appropriate discharge instructions should be provided to patients outlining their required follow-up plans.
- The role of the APN in radiation oncology is evolving; therefore, APNs should look to develop programs to support patients throughout the care continuum.

Recommended Resources for Oncology Advanced Practice Nurses

- Bruner, D.W., Haas, M.L., & Gosselin-Acomb, T.K. (Eds.). (2005). *Manual for radiation oncology nursing practice and education* (3rd ed.). Pittsburgh, PA: Oncology Nursing Society.
- Bruner, D.W., Moore-Higgs, G., & Haas, M. (2001). *Outcomes in radiation therapy: Multidisciplinary management.* Sudbury, MA: Jones and Bartlett.
- Chao, K.S., Perez, C.A., & Brady, L.W. (2001). *Radiation oncology: Management decisions* (2nd ed.). Philadelphia: Lippincott Williams & Wilkins.
- Haas, M.L., Hogle, W.P., Moore-Higgs, G., & Gosselin-Acomb, T.K. (Eds.). (2007). *Radiation therapy: A guide to patient care.* St. Louis, MO: Elsevier.
- Oncology Nursing Society. (2006). *Radiation oncology nurses enhancing excellence (RONEE)* [CD-ROM set]. Pittsburgh, PA: Oncology Nursing Society.
- *Pocket Guide of Commonly Prescribed Medications in Radiation Oncology* from Texas Oncology P.A., US Oncology

References

Abel, L.J., Blatt, H.J., Stipetich, R.L., Fuscardo, J.A., Miller, S.E., Dorsey, A.T., et al. (1999). Nursing management of patients receiving brachytherapy for early stage prostate cancer. *Clinical Journal of Oncology Nursing, 3,* 7–15.

American Cancer Society. (2001a). *Sexuality and cancer: For the man who has cancer and his partner.* Atlanta, GA: Author.

American Cancer Society. (2001b). *Sexuality and cancer: For the woman who has cancer and her partner.* Atlanta, GA: Author.

American College of Radiology. (2000, September 7). *Introduction to cancer therapy (radiation oncology).* Retrieved January 2, 2007, from http://www.radiologyinfo.org/en/info.cfm?pg=intro_onco

American Society of Breast Surgeons. (2005, December 8). *Consensus statement for accelerated partial breast irradiation.* Retrieved April, 14, 2007, from http://www.breastsurgeons.org/apbi.shtml

Archambeau, J.O., Pezner, R., & Wasserman, T. (1995). Pathophysiology of irradiated skin. *International Journal of Radiation Oncology, Biology, Physics, 31,* 1171–1185.

Aumock, A., Birnham, E.H., Fleshman, J.W., Fry, R.D., Gambacorta, M.A., Kodner, I.J., et al. (2001). Treatment of rectal adenocarcinoma with endocavitary and external beam radiotherapy: Results for 199 patients with localized tumors. *International Journal of Radiation Oncology, Biology, Physics, 51,* 363–370.

Bentel, G.C., Nelson, C.E., & Noell, K.T. (1989). *Treatment planning and dose calculation in radiation oncology.* Elmsford, NY: Pergamon Press.

Bijker, N., Meijnen, O., Peterse, J.L., Bogaerts, J., Hoorebeck, I.V., Julien, J.P., et al. (2006). Breast conserving treatment with or without radiotherapy in ductal carcinoma-in-situ: Ten year results of European Organisation for Research and Treatment of Cancer randomized phase III trial-10853—A study by the EORTC breast cancer cooperative group and EORTC radiotherapy group. *Journal of Clinical Oncology, 24,* 3381–3387.

Bolderston, A., Lloyd, N.S., Wong, R.K.S., Holden, L., & Robb-Blenderman, L. (2006). The prevention and management of acute skin reactions related to radiation therapy: A systematic review and practice guideline. *Supportive Care in Cancer, 14,* 802–817.

Bruner, D.W. (2001). Maintenance of body image and sexual function. In D.W. Bruner, G. Moore-Higgs, & M. Haas (Eds.), *Outcomes in radiation therapy: Multidisciplinary management* (pp. 611–631). Sudbury, MA: Jones and Bartlett.

Bruner, D.W., Haas, M.L., & Gosselin-Acomb, T.K. (Eds.). (2005). *Manual for radiation oncology nursing practice and education* (3rd ed.). Pittsburgh, PA: Oncology Nursing Society.

Carper, E., & Haas, M. (2006). Advanced practice nursing in radiation oncology. *Seminars in Oncology Nursing, 22,* 203–211.

Carroll, P.R., Carducci, M.A., Zietman, A.L., & Rothaermel, J.M. (2005). *Report to the nation on prostate cancer: A guide for men and their families.* Santa Monica, CA: Prostate Cancer Foundation.

Chao, K.K., Vicini, F.A., Wallace, M., Mitchell, C., Chen, P., Ghilezan, M., et al. (2007). Analysis of treatment efficacy, cosmesis, and toxicity using the MammoSite® breast brachytherapy catheter to deliver accelerated partial-breast irradiation: The William Beaumont hospital experience. *International Journal of Radiation Oncology, Biology, Physics, 69,* 32–40.

Davis, A.M., Dische, S., Gerber, L., Saunders, M., Leung, S.F., & O'Sullivan, B. (2003). Measuring postirradiation subcutaneous soft-tissue fibrosis: State-of-the-art and future directions. *Seminars in Radiation Oncology, 13,* 203–213.

Donatucci, C.F., & Greenfield, J.M. (2006). Recovery of sexual function after prostate cancer treatment. *Current Opinion in Urology, 16,* 444–448.

Gosselin, T.K. (2001). Radiation therapy. In D. Berg (Ed.), *Contemporary issues in colorectal cancer* (pp. 135–156). Sudbury, MA: Jones and Bartlett.

Gosselin-Acomb, T.K. (2005). Principles of radiation therapy. In C.H. Yarbro, M. Goodman, & M.H. Frogge (Eds.), *Cancer nursing: Principles and practice* (6th ed., pp. 229–249). Sudbury, MA: Jones and Bartlett.

Gunderson, L.L., Haddock, M.G., & Schild, S.E. (2003). Rectal cancer: Preoperative versus postoperative irradiation as a component of adjuvant treatment. *Seminars in Radiation Oncology, 13,* 419–432.

Haisfield-Wolfe, M.E., & Rund, C. (2000). A nursing protocol for the management of perineal-rectal skin alterations. *Clinical Journal of Oncology Nursing, 4,* 15–21.

Harper, J.L., Franklin, L.E., Jenrette, J.M., & Aguero, E.G. (2004). Skin toxicity during breast irradiation: Pathophysiology and management. *Southern Medical Journal, 97,* 989–993.

Hauer-Jensen, M., Wang, J., & Denham, J.W. (2003). Bowel injury: Current and evolving management strategies. *Seminars in Radiation Oncology, 13,* 357–371.

Hayman, J.A., Martle, M.K., Ten Haken, R.K., Normolle, D.P., Todd, R.F., Littles, J.F., et al. (2001). Dose escalation in non-small cell lung cancer using three-dimensional conformal radiation therapy: Update of a phase I trial. *Journal of Clinical Oncology, 19,* 127–136.

Hogle, W.P. (2005). Male pelvis. In D.W. Bruner, M.L. Haas, & T.K. Gosselin-Acomb (Eds.), *Manual for radiation oncology nursing practice and education* (3rd ed., pp. 132–141). Pittsburgh, PA: Oncology Nursing Society.

Hogle, W.P. (2007). Male genitourinary cancers. In M.L. Haas, W.P. Hogle, G. Moore-Higgs, & T. Gosselin-Acomb (Eds.), *Radiation therapy: A guide to patient care* (pp. 234–266). St. Louis, MO: Elsevier.

Jeruss, J.S., Vicini, F.A., Beitsch, P.D., Haffty, B.G., Quiet, C.A., Zannis, V.J., et al. (2006). Initial outcomes for patients treated on the American Society of Breast Surgeons MammoSite clinical trial for ductal carcinoma-in-situ of the breast. *Annals of Surgical Oncology, 13,* 967–976.

Joslyn, S.A. (2006). Ductal carcinoma in situ: Trends in geographic, temporal, and demographic patterns of care and survival. *Breast Journal, 12,* 20–27.

Kagan, S.H., & Garrett, M.L. (2007). Geriatric considerations in radiation oncology nursing. In M.L. Haas, W.P. Hogle, G. Moore-Higgs, & T. Gosselin-Acomb (Eds.), *Radiation therapy: A guide to patient care* (pp. 684–698). St. Louis, MO: Elsevier.

Kelvin, J.F., & Moore-Higgs, G.J. (1999). Description of the role of nonphysician practitioners in radiation oncology. *International Journal of Radiation Oncology, Biology, Physics, 45,* 163–169.

Lambert, C.K. (2007). Advanced practice nurses in radiation oncology. In M.L. Haas, W.P. Hogle, G. Moore-Higgs, & T. Gosselin-Acomb (Eds.), *Radiation therapy: A guide to patient care* (pp. 641–663). St. Louis, MO: Elsevier.

Luxton, G., Hancock, S.L., & Boyer, A.L. (2004). Dosimetry and radiobiologic model comparison of IMRT and 3D conformal radiotherapy in treatment of carcinoma of the prostate. *International Journal of Radiation Oncology, Biology, Physics, 59,* 267–284.

Lynch, M.P., Cope, D., & Murphy-Ende, K. (2001). Advanced practice issues: Results of the ONS Advanced Practice Nursing survey. *Oncology Nursing Forum, 28,* 1521–1530.

Ma, C. (2005). Practice of radiation therapy. In D.W. Bruner, M.L. Haas, & T.K. Gosselin (Eds.), *Manual for radiation oncology nursing practice and education* (3rd ed., pp. 12–18). Pittsburgh, PA: Oncology Nursing Society.

Marks, L.B., Garst, J., Socinski, M.A., Sibley, G., Blackstock, A.W., Herndon, J.E., et al. (2004). Carboplatin/paclitaxel or carboplatin/vinorelbine followed by accelerated hyperfractionated conformal radiation therapy: Report of a prospective phase I dose escalation trial from the Carolina Conformal Therapy Consortium. *Journal of Clinical Oncology, 22,* 4329–4339.

Marks, L.B., Yu, X., Vujaskovic, Z., Small, W., Folz, R., & Anscher, M.A. (2003). Radiation-induced lung injury. *Seminars in Radiation Oncology, 13,* 333–345.

Minsky, B.D. (1997). The role of adjuvant radiation therapy in the treatment of colorectal cancer. *Hematology/Oncology Clinics of North America, 11,* 679–697.

Mock, V., Dow, K.H., Meares, C.J., Grimm, P.M., Dienemann, J.A., Haisfield-Wolfe, M.E., et al. (1997). Effects of exercise on fatigue, physical functioning, and emotional distress during radiation therapy for breast cancer. *Oncology Nursing Forum, 24,* 991–1000.

Moore-Higgs, G. (2005). Breast. In D.W. Bruner, M. Haas, & T.K. Gosselin-Acomb (Eds.), *Manual for radiation oncology nursing practice and education* (3rd ed., pp. 98–109). Pittsburgh, PA: Oncology Nursing Society.

Moore-Higgs, G. (2006). Radiation options for early stage breast cancer. *Seminars in Oncology Nursing, 22,* 233–241.

Moore-Higgs, G.J., Watkins-Bruner, D., Balmer, L., Johnson-Doneski, J., Komarny, P., Mautner, B., et al. (2003). The role of licensed nursing personnel in radiation oncology part A: Results of a descriptive study. *Oncology Nursing Forum, 30,* 51–58.

Morrow, M., Strom, E.A., Bassett, L.W., Dershaw, D.D., Fowble, B., Giuliano, A., et al. (2002). Standard for breast conservation therapy in the management of invasive breast carcinoma. *CA: A Cancer Journal for Clinicians, 52,* 277–300.

National Comprehensive Cancer Network. (2007a). *NCCN clinical practice guidelines in oncology: Breast cancer, version 1.2007.* Retrieved January 26, 2007, from http://www.nccn.org/professionals/physician_gls/PDF/breast.pdf

National Comprehensive Cancer Network. (2007b). *NCCN clinical practice guidelines in oncology: Non-small cell lung cancer, version 1.2007.* Retrieved January 26, 2007, from http://www.nccn.org/professionals/physician_gls/PDF/nscl.pdf

National Comprehensive Cancer Network. (2007c). *NCCN clinical practice guidelines in oncology: Prostate cancer, version 1.2007.* Retrieved January 26, 2007, from http://www.nccn.org/professionals/physician_gls/PDF/prostate.pdf

National Comprehensive Cancer Network. (2007d). *NCCN clinical practice guidelines in oncology: Rectal cancer, version 1.2007.* Retrieved January 26, 2007, from http://www.nccn.org/professionals/physician_gls/PDF/rectal.pdf

Rubin, P., Cooper, R., & Phillips, T.L. (1975). *Radiation biology and radiation pathology syllabus, set RT 1: Radiation oncology.* Chicago: American College of Radiology.

Stephenson, R.A., Mori, M., Hsieh, Y.C., Beer, T.M., Stanford, J.L., Gilliland, E.D., et al. (2005). Treatment of erectile dysfunction following therapy for clinically localized prostate cancer: Patient reported use and outcomes from the Surveillance, Epidemiology, and End Results Prostate Cancer Outcomes Study. *Journal of Urology, 174,* 646–650.

Stern, J., & Ippoliti, C. (2003). Management of acute cancer treatment-induced diarrhea. *Seminars in Oncology Nursing, 19*(Suppl. 3), 11–16.

Willett, C.G., Czito, B.G., & Tyler, D.G. (2007). Intraoperative radiation therapy. *Journal of Clinical Oncology, 25,* 971–977.

Yavuz, M.N., Yavuz, A.A., Aydin, F., Can, G., & Kavgaci, H. (2002). The efficacy of octreotide in the therapy of acute radiation-induced diarrhea: A randomized controlled study. *International Journal of Radiation Oncology, Biology, Physics, 54,* 195–202.

CHAPTER 7

Blood and Marrow Stem Cell Transplantation

Susan A. Ezzone, MS, RN, CNP, AOCNP®

Introduction

More than a hundred years ago, researchers investigated the use of bone marrow infusions to treat diseases and to promote bone marrow recovery. Beginning in the 19th century, bone marrow was used as a treatment for a variety of diseases such as anemia, leukemia, and chlorosis. The first attempts at using bone marrow for the treatment of disease involved feeding or injecting bone marrow or spleen extract into patients. Although some benefit seemed to occur with the administration of bone marrow, the reasons were not well understood (Quine, 1896). In the 1950s, the radioprotective benefits of marrow infusion to replace the hematopoietic system after lethal irradiation was demonstrated (Ford, Hamerton, Barnes, & Loutit, 1956). Dr. E. Donnall Thomas subsequently attempted to treat human leukemia using high-dose cyclophosphamide and syngeneic (identical twin) marrow transplantation in 1959 (Thomas, Lochte, Cannon, Sahler, & Ferrebee, 1959). Over the next several years, much was learned regarding the hematologic and immunologic benefits of bone marrow stem cell infusion. In 1986, a nuclear reactor accident in Chernobyl, Russia, occurred that led to the use of marrow infusions to assist with hematologic recovery (Baranov et al., 1989). Today, much advancement has occurred in the use of marrow and blood stem cells for the treatment of hematologic and nonhematologic diseases. Although much has been learned, new and improved strategies of blood and marrow stem cell transplantation (BMT) continue to be discovered.

Conditions Treated

The recognized clinical indications for use of stem cell transplantation as a treatment option have expanded over the years and include both malignant and nonmalignant

&s; 261 &s;

conditions. The most common indications for stem cell transplantation include leukemia, lymphoma, and multiple myeloma. Examples of conditions treated with transplantation are listed in Table 7-1.

Table 7-1. Hematologic and Nonhematologic Conditions Treated With Hematopoietic Stem Cell Transplantation

Type of Transplant	Malignant Conditions	Nonmalignant Conditions
Allogeneic	Hematologic disease • Acute lymphocytic leukemia • Acute myeloid leukemia • Chronic lymphocytic leukemia • Chronic myeloid leukemia • Hodgkin disease • Multiple myeloma • Myelodysplastic syndrome (preleukemia) • Non-Hodgkin lymphoma	Hematologic disorders • Aplastic anemia • Diamond-Blackfan anemia • Fanconi anemia • Sickle cell anemia • Beta thalassemia major • Chediak-Higashi syndrome • Chronic granulomatous disease • Congenital neutropenia • Reticular dysgenesis Congenital immunodeficiencies • Severe combined immunodeficiency • Wiskott-Aldrich syndrome • Functional T-cell deficiency Mucopolysaccharidoses • Hurler disease • Hunter disease • Sanfilippo syndrome • Morquio syndrome Lipidoses • Adrenoleukodystrophy • Metachromatic leukodystrophy • Gaucher disease Miscellaneous • Osteopetrosis • Langerhans cell histiocytosis • Lesch-Nyhan syndrome • Glycogen storage diseases
Autologous	Hematologic disease • Multiple myeloma • Non-Hodgkin lymphoma • Hodgkin disease • Acute myeloid leukemia Solid tumors • Neuroblastoma/glioma • Ovarian cancer • Germ cell tumors • Sarcoma • Melanoma • Lung cancer • Breast cancer	Amyloidosis Autoimmune diseases

Types of Transplantation

In hematopoietic stem cell transplant (HSCT), the hematopoietic stem cell is transferred from one person to another or is collected, stored, and reinfused to the same individual following a predetermined treatment plan or conditioning regimen. Three types of bone marrow and peripheral stem cell transplantation have been defined: autologous, allogeneic, and syngeneic. The goal of HSCT is to promote bone marrow recovery following a conditioning regimen that includes some combination of chemotherapy and immunosuppressive therapy, with or without total body irradiation (TBI).

Autologous Transplantation

The process of autologous transplantation involves steps to mobilize and then collect stem cells from an individual and later reinfuse the stem cells to the same person to allow for marrow recovery. Mobilization of stem cells consists of causing the stem cell to move from the bone marrow to the peripheral blood for collection through an apheresis procedure. Stem cell mobilization may be accomplished through the administration of a variety of chemotherapy agents and colony-stimulating factors (CSFs) or CSFs alone. The most common CSFs used for stem cell mobilization include granulocyte colony-stimulating factor (G-CSF) and granulocyte macrophage–colony-stimulating factor (GM-CSF). Clinical trials have evaluated the use of additional growth factors in mobilizing stem cells. The use of AMD3100 plus filgrastim (Neupogen®, Amgen Inc.) has demonstrated improved mobilization of peripheral blood stem cells (PBSCs) in autologous recipients in comparison to Neupogen alone in clinical trials (Flomenberg et al., 2005). A transient increase in circulating stem cells occurs following administration of CSFs, allowing collection of PBSCs by apheresis (blood cell separation). Following chemotherapy plus CSFs, apheresis of stem cells begins 10–16 days after chemotherapy, once the blood counts begin to recover. Many chemotherapy regimens have been used to mobilize stem cells, and the most common chemotherapy agent used is cyclophosphamide. When mobilization is initiated with CSFs alone, apheresis usually begins on the fourth or fifth day of CSF administration. Research efforts continue to evaluate optimal methods and new agents to mobilize PBSCs for collection. Venous access may be accomplished through peripheral veins or central venous catheters as indicated. If peripheral access is determined to be inadequate, a central venous catheter is placed for apheresis of stem cells for autologous, allogeneic, or unrelated donors. Apheresis for stem cell collection is done daily until sufficient stem cells are collected, and each apheresis procedure may take four to six hours. Following collection, stem cells are cryopreserved with dimethyl sulfoxide (DMSO), frozen, and stored. Stem cells are reinfused following a myeloablative conditioning regimen (Schmit-Pokorny, 2004).

Allogeneic Hematopoietic Stem Cell Transplantation

Allogeneic HSCT refers to the use of a donor for the source of stem cells. Bone marrow, blood, or umbilical cord stem cells may be collected from donors who are related or unrelated to the recipient. To identify an acceptable donor, human leukocyte antigen (HLA) typing is performed on the recipient and all potential donors. Usually, related donors are siblings, but other family members may be used if adequate HLA matching is determined. In general, the chance of identifying a fully HLA-matched donor among siblings is about one in four. Unrelated donors may be identified through the National Marrow Donor Program (NMDP). Ideally, finding a fully HLA-matched donor is preferred, but an HLA mismatch donor may be used in some settings when other treatment options are not available. The International Blood and Marrow Transplant Registry (IBMTR) reports similar overall survival outcomes in related versus unrelated HSCT (Loberiza, 2003). Allogeneic donors undergo PBSC mobilization with CSFs alone followed by PBSC collection through apheresis.

For many years, allogeneic transplantation was performed using myeloablative conditioning regimens with significant treatment-related toxicities. However, since the late 1990s, increasing interest has been directed at the use of nonmyeloablative conditioning regimens for allogeneic transplantation. The goal of nonmyeloablative stem cell transplant (NMSCT) is to decrease regimen-related toxicities and mortality by administering a less toxic conditioning regimen. Common terms used to describe NMSCT include "mini"-transplant or reduced-intensity transplant. *Minitransplant* usually refers to a nonmyeloablative regimen that is intended to reduce hematologic and nonhematologic toxicity. Patients who undergo NMSCT may experience treatment-related toxicities such as nausea, vomiting, diarrhea, mucositis, and hair loss, but to a lesser degree than with fully myeloablative regimens. Patients who otherwise are ineligible for allogeneic HSCT because of preexisting comorbid conditions or increased age may be offered NMSCT with potential curative effects (Schmit-Pokorny, 2007).

Syngeneic Hematopoietic Stem Cell Transplantation

Syngeneic HSCT uses an identical twin donor for the source of stem cells for transplantation. The procedure involves a conditioning regimen followed by infusion of the donated stem cells from an HLA-identical twin donor. Although the patient is at risk for conditioning regimen–related toxicities, no risk of graft-versus-host disease (GVHD) (a common complication of allogeneic transplant) exists because the identical twin donor is considered to be genetically identical to the recipient, and immunosuppression therefore is not indicated (Niess & Duffy, 2004). As no risk of GVHD is present with syngeneic transplant, patients do not benefit from the graft-versus-leukemia (GVL) effect. In a study that compared the survival data of syngeneic transplant with autologous and allogeneic transplant for the treatment of high-grade non-Hodgkin lymphoma, no significant difference existed in relapse rates among the types of transplant (Bierman et al., 2001).

Factors that have been used to predict when to initiate stem cell collection include measurement of the white blood cell (WBC) count, mononuclear cell count, and $CD34^+$ antigen count (Schmit-Pokorny, 2004, 2007). The $CD34^+$ antigen or hematopoietic stem cell marker is used to determine adequate collection of stem cells to promote engraftment. A variety of $CD34^+$ cell collection targets have been reported. An adequate stem cell collection has been described to be at least $2–4 \times 10^6$ $CD34^+$ cells/kg, or 2 million to 4 million cells. This number is considered adequate for autologous or allogeneic transplant and results in neutrophil and platelet engraftment (Cottler-Fox et al., 2003).

Sources of Stem Cells

Three sources of stem cells used in transplantation include bone marrow, peripheral blood, and umbilical cord blood (UCB). For many years, bone marrow was used as the source of stem cells and in some cases may still be used if adequate PBSCs are not collected or upon request of the NMDP. This method of stem cell collection involves multiple needle aspirations from the posterior iliac crest to collect adequate stem cells directly from the bone marrow for transplantation. The procedure is usually performed with the donor under general anesthesia in the operating room. Donors tolerate the procedure well but may require pain medications or red blood cell transfusions for supportive care.

The use of PBSCs for transplantation has been evolving for more than 20 years and has nearly replaced the use of stem cells collected directly from the bone marrow. Advantages for using stem cells collected from the peripheral blood include more rapid hematologic recovery, decreased morbidity of the recipient, and avoidance of general anesthesia for the donor. Donors generally experience no pain related to the procedure because of the less invasive approach of collecting stem cells by apheresis. Peripheral blood CD34$^+$ cell counts are monitored to determine when apheresis should be started to collect stem cells (Demirer et al., 2002). Thresholds of CD34$^+$ cell counts vary according to institutional practice and research protocols. PBSCs may be collected from allogeneic donors as well as autologous transplant patients by a large or standard volume apheresis procedure of the donor or autologous patient (Gasova, Marinov, Vodvarkova, Bohmova, & Bhuvian-Ludvikova, 2005).

Because stem cells live in the bone marrow, methods to mobilize stem cells into the peripheral blood must be used. Options for stem cell mobilization include administration of chemotherapy, chemotherapy and CSFs, CSFs alone, or investigational agents (Schmit-Pokorny, 2007). Allogeneic or unrelated donors receive CSFs, most commonly filgrastim, for stem cell mobilization. The timing of apheresis for stem cell collection may vary according to institutional standards of practice or specific research protocols, but apheresis usually occurs on the fifth day of filgrastim administration. In autologous transplantation, when chemotherapy is given with or without CSFs for stem cell mobilization, apheresis begins when the patient's blood counts recover. When CSFs are used for stem cell collection, stem cells are forced out of the bone marrow into the blood, thus allowing for collection of large numbers of CD34$^+$ cells (Chouinard & Finn, 2007). Additional growth factors that have been studied for stem cell mobilization include pegylated G-CSF, PIXY321 (Immunex Corp.), recombinant human stem cell factor, recombinant Mpl ligands, and the FLT3 ligand (Bishop et al., 1996; Dawson et al., 2005; Fruehauf et al., 2007; Huang et al., 2006; Piacibello et al., 1998).

The umbilical cord contains a rich source of stem cells that may be HLA typed, collected, and used for autologous, allogeneic, or unrelated stem cell transplant. Cord blood stem cells are collected at birth and may be used immediately or may be cryopreserved, frozen, and stored for later use. The dose of stem cells collected from the umbilical cord may be small and considered adequate only for infants or small children. The successful use of UCB transplantation in children and adults has been described (Ballen, 2005). In some cases, the use of two UCB products for transplantation in adults has been implemented (Laughlin, 2005). Umbilical cord stem cell storage banks can be used for cryopreservation and storage of stem cells but may be cost prohibitive because of fees charged for indefinite storage of stem cells. Several cord blood banks are available, and the costs of cord blood storage vary. Newborn Blood Banking, Inc. (2007) lists costs to include a registration fee, cryopreservation, a licensing fee, and an annual fee.

Process of Blood and Marrow Stem Cell Transplantation

Understanding the process of HSCT has become more challenging over the years as the science and clinical practice of transplantation continue to evolve. Although many of the basic principles remain the same, the steps of the transplantation process have become more complex for each type of transplant. During the transplant process, a specialized team of physicians, advanced practice nurses (APNs), physician assistants, nurses, pharmacists, dietitians, research personnel, transplant coordinators, and other healthcare workers are needed to manage patient care activities.

Patient Eligibility

Many factors are considered regarding patient eligibility for transplantation. Some of these include disease status, response to chemotherapy, comorbid medical conditions, and identification of a donor for an allogeneic or unrelated donor transplant. Before the transplant, candidates undergo an extensive clinical evaluation to determine their eligibility and appropriateness to proceed with transplantation.

Clinical evaluation of the pretransplant candidate involves completion of diagnostic tests to determine baseline organ function and infectious comorbidities. Figure 7-1 describes the common diagnostic tests ordered for pretransplant evaluation. A complete history is obtained to document the history of present illness; past medical, surgical, and family history; allergies and medications; gynecologic history for female patients; vaccinations; history of blood transfusions; and travel history. A psychosocial assessment also is obtained to identify family, social, or financial issues that need to be addressed before and during the transplant process. A thorough physical examination is completed to evaluate general health status and identify physical findings that are important to follow during the transplant process. It is important to document abnormal physical findings regarding examination of the heart, lungs, abdomen, neurologic system, lymph nodes, skin, and oral cavity.

Human Leukocyte Antigen Typing

The major histocompatibility complex (MHC) gene is located on the short arm of chromosome 6 and encodes the glycoprotein HLA that is capable of recognizing self from nonself for each individual (Roitt, Brostoff, & Male, 1996; Williams, 2004). HLA testing, or tissue typing, is done by serologically testing HLA protein expression on the WBC. Molecular testing also may be performed to more specifically identify the HLA type. Technology to determine HLA typing continues to become more sophisticated and now can be accomplished by using noninvasive techniques such as the use of cells obtained from the hair or buccal mucosa. Patients who are identified as candidates for allogeneic transplantation and all potential donors should undergo HLA typing immediately to avoid delays in initiating the transplant process. In most cases, insurance companies pay for HLA typing of the recipient and potential sibling donors. On occasion, insurance companies deny payment for HLA typing if transplantation is not considered an appropriate treatment option. Insurance benefits do not pay volunteer donors to enter the NMDP registry. Volunteer donor drives often are sponsored for reduced or no charge, with the sponsoring group paying the expenses of tissue typing.

Laboratory Data
- Hepatic panel
- Pregnancy test
- Creatinine clearance
- Blood urea nitrogen, creatinine
- Complete blood count with differential
- Electrolytes, magnesium, calcium, phosphorus
- Infectious disease titers
  - HIV
  - Cytomegalovirus
  - Epstein-Barr virus
  - Herpes simplex virus
  - Hepatitis C antibody
  - Hepatitis B core antibody
  - Hepatitis B surface antigen
  - Human T-cell lymphotropic virus
- ABO/Rh typing
- Tissue typing (allogeneic only)
- Prothrombin time/international normalized ratio/partial thromboplastin time

Diagnostic Studies/Consults
- Chest radiograph
- Electrocardiogram
- Dental examination
- Social work evaluation
- Pulmonary function test
- Psychological evaluation
- Multigated acquisition scan/echocardiogram

Disease Staging Studies (as appropriate)
- Lumbar puncture
- Myeloma survey
- Computed tomography
- Magnetic resonance imaging
- 24-hour urine protein, creatinine
- Bone marrow biopsy and aspirate
- Myeloma blood and urine studies
- Positron-emission tomography or gallium scan

Figure 7-1. Pretransplant Clinical Evaluation

Note. Based on information from Niess & Duffy, 2004; Schmit-Pokorny, 2007.

Three classes of MHC genes or loci have been identified: class I, class II, and class III. Class I and II genes are the HLA genes and are used to determine HLA typing of recipients and donors in HSCT. Class I HLA genes are expressed on all nucleated cells in the body and have been identified on the A, B, and C loci of the MHC; therefore, they are called HLA-A, -B, and -C. The class II genes are expressed on B cells, macrophages, and activated T cells and are identified as HLA-DR, -DP, and -DQ. Class II genes are involved in immunity and histocompatibility. Class III MHC genes are involved in immunity but do not have a role in histocompatibility. In addition, antigens considered to be minor histocompatibility antigens may have a significant effect on transplant outcomes, but their functions are not well described (Morishima et al., 2002; Snustad & Simmons, 2000).

Numerous HLA alleles have been identified for each class I and class II gene or locus. HLA alleles are recognized markers used in HLA typing that identify the unique serologic or molecular identification of individuals. Naming of the HLA alleles is complex and involves use of the HLA region, name of the HLA gene or locus, group number of alleles that encode an antigen, and the number of the specific allele. The specific HLA allele may be serologically or molecularly identified for each HLA gene or loci. Williams (2004) listed Internet resources for recognized HLA alleles. Internet resources may be used as an up-to-date reference to identify currently recognized HLA alleles. In the practice setting, use of these resources may be helpful when determining HLA typing for patients and donors. Some HLA alleles are common in particular ethnic groups, and others are common in all populations. One set of HLA genes is inherited from each parent and is called a haplotype. Siblings may inherit the same or different haplotype from their parents. In general, siblings have a one in four chance of inheriting the same haplotype from each parent, called haploidentical (see Figure 7-2).

The NMDP guidelines for HLA matching for unrelated transplants suggest specific optimal matching that may be associated with overall survival. Recommended donors are matched at all four alleles for HLA-A, -B, -C, and -DRB1, but donors who are partially matched are not contraindicated. Differences are documented regarding the effect of HLA mismatching on overall survival. In 2003, the NMDP HLA matching guidelines reported that an HLA mismatch at HLA-A, -B, -C, and -DRB1 may affect survival outcomes. In addition to HLA match, other factors that should be considered when selecting a donor include age, gender, cytomegalovirus (CMV) serology, ABO compatibility, body weight, and matched race. None of these factors are used as definitive exclusion criteria, but they must be considered when choosing a donor. In general, CMV seronegative donors should be used for CMV seronegative recipients if possible. An increased risk of chronic GVHD may arise when using multiparous female donors (Hurley et al., 2003).

When a suitable HLA identical sibling donor is not identified, a search for an unrelated donor may be initiated through the NMDP. The NMDP was founded in 1986 and is the largest of several unrelated donor programs throughout the world. The NMDP coordinates the search for unrelated donors worldwide and the process of collecting and delivering stem cells to the designated transplant center. The amount of time it takes to find an HLA donor varies but may take four to six weeks or longer.

Transplant Center Selection

Several important factors have been identified to assist with the selection of a transplant center. Patients and families will determine the pros and cons of each factor when choosing a transplant center. In some circumstances, patients and families may need to temporarily relocate to an area closer to the transplant center, and the availability of affordable and acceptable housing arrangements becomes an important issue to consider. Issues related to the experience of the transplant team are critical for evaluating a transplant center. Patients and families must identify how long the transplant center has been open, the number and type of transplants performed per year, mortality rates, incidence of complications, and overall success rates. Careful evaluation of the treatment plan should include the proposed preparative regimen, immunosuppressive agents, infectious prophylaxis, infection control guidelines, posttransplant care guidelines, patient education, support groups, and investigational protocols offered. In some circumstances, the financial coverage allotted by the insurance company for transplantation may determine the transplant center of choice for individual patients.

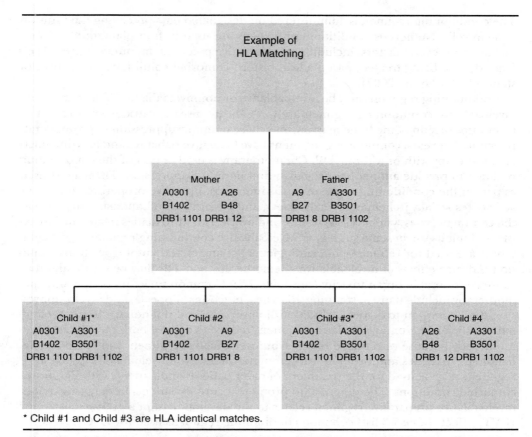

* Child #1 and Child #3 are HLA identical matches.

Figure 7-2. Example of Human Leukocyte Antigen (HLA) Typing and Matching of Siblings

Note. Based on information from Niess & Duffy, 2004; Schmit-Pokorny, 2007.

Determining the mix of staff involved with the transplant program also may be helpful, including years of experience, number and ratio of physicians, nurse practitioners, clinical nurse specialists, nurses, and transplant coordinators. Ancillary staff that is important to inquire about includes additional nursing personnel, social workers, pharmacists, dietitians, chaplains, and financial counselors. A description of the transplant unit is helpful in understanding whether it is a designated unit, the number of transplant beds, and a description of outpatient facilities. Many institutions are utilizing APNs to provide direct patient care and collaborate with the interdisciplinary team. APNs may be responsible for managing a set of patients on the inpatient transplant unit as well as in the outpatient setting. APNs perform many procedures, including but not limited to bone marrow biopsy and aspirate, lumbar puncture, Ommaya reservoir tap, intrathecal chemotherapy, and skin biopsies (Schmit-Pokorny, 2007).

Conditioning Regimens

The pretransplant conditioning regimen or preparative regimen consists of various combinations of chemotherapy, radiation therapy, and immunosuppressive therapy.

The conditioning regimen is administered on designated days preceding the infusion of stem cells. Numerous conditioning regimens are used in transplantation and may be based on several factors, including myeloablative potential, immunosuppressive effects, disease being treated, past medical history, comorbid conditions, and source of stem cells (Poliquin, 2007).

Conditioning regimens may be myeloablative or nonmyeloablative. The goals of the myeloablative conditioning regimen are to eradicate disease, cause myeloablation or myelosuppression of the bone marrow, and cause immunosuppression to prevent graft rejection. For years, conditioning regimens have been myeloablative and have included chemotherapy with or without TBI. Chemotherapy is used as part of the conditioning regimen to provide antineoplastic activity and immunosuppression. TBI may be used as part of the conditioning regimen for its immunosuppressive properties, antitumor activity (especially in hematologic diseases), and penetration of sanctuary sites such as the central nervous system (CNS), testes, and ovaries. Many toxicities related to TBI exist and limit its use in some situations. Myeloablative conditioning regimens most commonly are used for refractory hematologic malignancies and autologous transplantation. Adverse effects of myeloablative chemotherapy and TBI may be severe and may cause considerable organ toxicity (see Table 7-2). Common toxicities of TBI and chemotherapy include nausea, vomiting, diarrhea, mucositis, alopecia, and myelosuppression. Less common toxicities include cardiomyopathy and pulmonary, hepatic, or renal insufficiency. Nonmyeloablative regimens reduce toxicity of both the TBI and chemotherapy because of reduced doses. Nonmyeloablative regimens minimize the hematologic toxicities and promote earlier engraftment. Nonmyeloablative preparative regimens may be used for the treatment of older patients and patients with significant comorbid conditions. The potential to promote a cure in patients undergoing a nonmyeloablative preparative regimen relates to the development of a graft-versus-tumor (GVT) effect. Table 7-3 lists common conditioning regimens used for HSCT.

Infusion of Stem Cells

Infusion of stem cells occurs on a designated day following the conditioning regimen and is given the label of "day zero" or transplant day. Autologous stem cells previously were cryopreserved, frozen, and stored prior to transplantation or reinfusion. Adverse effects of stem cell infusion occur related to the preservative DMSO, red blood cell contamination, or the volume of cells infused and usually resolve within 24–48 hours. Common adverse effects include fever, chills, cough, nausea, vomiting, diarrhea, dyspnea, tachypnea, abdominal cramps, facial flushing, hypertension, cardiac arrhythmias, chest tightness, hemoglobinuria, and garlic-like taste (related to the DMSO). Patients may receive IV hydration to promote renal perfusion and minimize hemolysis that may be caused by the DMSO. Symptomatic treatment of adverse effects usually is effective, but occasionally the stem cell infusion may need to be slowed or stopped briefly. Premedications prior to the infusion may include an antiemetic, acetaminophen, and diphenhydramine. Emergency equipment, oxygen, and cardiac monitoring equipment should be readily available (McAdams & Burgunder, 2004).

Allogeneic stem cells most often are infused fresh, and patients experience fewer immediate side effects. Adverse effects may include symptoms that occur during blood transfusions such as hives, chills, rash, fever, nausea, vomiting, flushing, shortness of breath, hypotension, hypertension, tachycardia, chest pain or tightness, or anaphylaxis. Symptomatic treatment usually is adequate to relieve symptoms. Premedica-

Table 7-2. Side Effects of Preparative Regimens by Agent and System

System	Cyclophosphamide	Busulfan	Carboplatin	Thiotepa	Melphalan	Carmustine	Cytarabine	Etoposide	Fludarabine	Mitoxantrone	ATG	TBI
Hematopoietic												
Anemia	X	X	X	X	X	X	X	X	X	X	X	X
Leukopenia	X	X	X	X	X	X	X	X	X	X	X	X
Thrombocytopenia	X	X	X	X	X	X	X	X	X	X	X	X
Gastrointestinal												
Nausea/vomiting	X	X	X	X	X		X	X	X		X	X
Anorexia	X			X	X		X	X			X	X
Mucositis/stomatitis	X	X	X	X	X		X	X	X	X	X	X
Diarrhea	X		X	X	X		X	X	X			X
Constipation												
Hepatotoxicity	X					X	X					
Genitourinary												
Hemorrhagic cystitis	X							X			X	
Nephrotoxicity	X	X	X	X		X					X	
Electrolyte imbalances	X	X	X					X				
Cardiovascular												
Cardiotoxicity	X									X		
Hypo- or hypertension												
Pulmonary												
Fibrosis	X		X		X	X			X			X
Pneumonitis	X								X			X
Reproduction												
Infertility	X		X	X	X	X						X
Gynecomastia		X										
Integumentary												
Dermatitis	X		X	X	X	X	X	X			X	X
Hyperpigmentation	X			X				X				X

(Continued on next page)

Table 7-2. Side Effects of Preparative Regimens by Agent and System *(Continued)*

System	Cyclophosphamide	Busulfan	Carboplatin	Thiotepa	Melphalan	Carmustine	Cytarabine	Etoposide	Fludarabine	Mitoxantrone	ATG	TBI
Alopecia	X		X	X	X	X	X			X	X	X
Erythema			X	X		X	X	X				X
Immunologic												
Fever/chills				X			X	X	X		X	
Hypersensitivity/allergic reaction/anaphylaxis		X	X	X				X	X		X	X
Neurologic												
Ototoxicity			X									
Peripheral neuropathy			X			X	X					
Seizures		X				X	X	X				
Headache/altered mental status	X			X			X	X				
Miscellaneous												
Secondary malignancy	X										X	X
Cataracts												X
Nasal congestion	X											
Conjunctivitis						X	X					
Parotitis												X

ATG—antithymocyte globulin; TBI—total body irradiation

Note. Based on information from Ezzone, 1997; Ezzone & Camp-Sorrell, 1994; Gross & Johnson, 1994. From "Transplant Course" (p. 45), by F.W. McAdams and M.R. Burgunder in S. Ezzone (Ed.), *Hematopoietic Stem Cell Transplantation: A Manual for Nursing Practice,* 2004, Pittsburgh, PA: Oncology Nursing Society. Copyright 2004 by Oncology Nursing Society. Reprinted with permission.

Table 7-3. Common Preparative Regimens and Indications[a]

Abbreviation	Regimen/Agents	Indications/Disease
Cy/TBI	Cyclophosphamide/total body irradiation	AML, MDS, ALL, CML, CLL, MM, HD, NHL
TBI/VP	Total body irradiation/etoposide	AML, ALL, NHL, HD
Bu/Cy	Busulfan/cyclophosphamide	AML, MDS, ALL, CML, CLL, MM, HD, NHL
Bu/Cy/VP	Busulfan/cyclophosphamide/etoposide	AML, MDS, ALL, CML, CLL, MM, HD, NHL
Cy	Cyclophosphamide	Severe aplastic anemia
Cy/ATG	Cyclophosphamide/antithymocyte globulin	Severe aplastic anemia
TBI/Mel	Total body irradiation/melphalan	MM
Mel	Melphalan	MM, nonmyeloablative SCT[b]
CTCb	Cyclophosphamide/thiotepa/carboplatin	Breast cancer
CT	Cyclophosphamide/thiotepa	Breast cancer
CEC	Cyclophosphamide/etoposide/carboplatin	Breast cancer, solid tumors
CBV	Cyclophosphamide/carmustine/etoposide	NHL, HD
BEAM	Carmustine/etoposide/cytarabine/melphalan	NHL, HD
MCC	Mitoxantrone/carboplatin/cyclophosphamide	Ovarian cancer
TBI	Total body irradiation	Nonmyeloablative SCT[b]
Fludara/Bu/ATG	Fludarabine/busulfan/antithymocyte globulin	Nonmyeloablative SCT[b]
Fludara/Cy	Fludarabine/cyclophosphamide	Nonmyeloablative SCT[b]
Fludara/Cy/ATG	Fludarabine/cyclophosphamide/antithymocyte globulin	Nonmyeloablative SCT[b]
Fludara/Mel	Fludarabine/melphalan	Nonmyeloablative SCT[b]

[a] This list is not all-inclusive and serves only as examples of preparative regimens.
[b] These agents are currently used in clinical trials.

ALL—acute lymphocytic leukemia; AML—acute myeloid leukemia; CLL—chronic lymphocytic leukemia; CML—chronic myeloid leukemia; HD—Hodgkin disease; MDS—myelodysplastic syndrome; MM—multiple myeloma; NHL—non-Hodgkin lymphoma; SCT—stem cell transplant

Note. Based on information from Armitage & Antman, 1992; Ezzone, 1997; Mangan, 2000.
From "Transplant Course" (p. 44), by F.W. McAdams and M.R. Burgunder in S. Ezzone (Ed.), *Hematopoietic Stem Cell Transplantation: A Manual for Nursing Practice,* 2004, Pittsburgh, PA: Oncology Nursing Society. Copyright 2004 by Oncology Nursing Society. Reprinted with permission.

tions may include antiemetics, acetaminophen, and diphenhydramine. Emergency equipment, oxygen, and cardiac monitoring should be available during the infusion of stem cells (McAdams & Burgunder, 2004). Immediate or delayed immune hemolysis may occur in ABO mismatch transplantation and should be monitored for approximately four months following transplant because the life span of the red blood cell is approximately 120 days. Immune hemolysis may occur resulting from ABO incompatible HSCT between the donor and recipient. Immune hemolysis or passenger lymphocyte syndrome (PLS) is caused by the production of donor B lymphocytes against recipient red blood cell antigens (Reed, Yearsley, Krugh, & Kennedy, 2003). Management of PLS may include transfusion of ABO compatible red blood cells, use of corticosteroids, exchange transfusion, and maintenance of renal perfusion. Over time, the recipient's red blood cell type converts to the donor's red blood cell type, and the risk of hemolysis resolves. Blood work studies for ABO titers of the recipient are monitored to detect when the transition to donor blood type occurs. During this time, patients receive type O blood products to minimize the risk of transfusion-related hemolysis.

Engraftment and Recovery

Engraftment refers to the hematopoietic and immunologic recovery that occurs after HSCT. Factors that affect the rate of engraftment include the source of stems cells used for transplantation, the type of transplant, the conditioning regimen, use of CSFs during PBSC mobilization, use of CSFs post-transplant, and the occurrence of infection or GVHD. Following the conditioning regimen, the nadir of blood counts generally occurs five to seven days after HSCT. Engraftment may be delayed in patients who develop GVHD or infections, particularly viral infections.

In autologous HSCT, engraftment using CSF-mobilized stem cells derived from the peripheral blood occurs approximately one week earlier than with stem cells collected from the bone marrow (Korbling & Anderlini, 2001). Collection and infusion of greater than 2.0×10^6 CD34+ cells per kilogram is recommended (Montgomery & Cottler-Fox, 2007). Engraftment is accelerated by the use of CSFs during PBSC mobilization and collection, and the use of CSFs post-transplant speeds engraftment by three to five days. Following autologous PBSC transplant, engraftment occurs more quickly than with use of bone marrow stem cells, with the recovery of granulocytes to 500/mm³ occurring by day 12 and recovery of platelets to 20,000/mm³ occurring by day 14 (Korbling & Anderlini).

Engraftment after myeloablative allogeneic HSCT is more variable but also has been demonstrated to occur earlier with the use of PBSCs than with the use of bone marrow stem cells. Bensinger et al. (2001) described recovery of blood counts to occur with neutrophils greater than 500/mm³ at day 16 and platelets greater than 20,000/mm³ at day 13 following allogeneic PBSC transplant. Using stem cells derived from the bone marrow, engraftment occurred more slowly and was reported as neutrophils greater than 500/mm³ at day 21 and platelets greater than 20,000/mm³ at day 19 post-transplant.

Following nonmyeloablative HSCT, the nadir of blood counts may not be as low, and the duration of myelosuppression is shorter because the conditioning regimen is myelosuppressive rather than myeloablative. The WBC count recovers more quickly, and transfusion of red blood cells and platelets sometimes is avoided. Engraftment after umbilical cord stem cell transplant occurs more slowly than with the use of PBSCs or marrow stem cells. A high concentration of stem cells is present in the UCB, but recovery of blood counts occurs at approximately day 28 for neutrophils and day 60 for platelets.

In some cases, the number of CD34+ cells collected may not be sufficient for an adult recipient (Gluckman, Rocha, & Chastang, 2000; Rocha et al., 2001).

Post-Transplant Follow-Up

Historically, the process of transplantation has occurred during an inpatient hospitalization. However, in recent years, transplant centers increasingly perform the acute phase of transplantation, including the conditioning regimen and infusion of stem cells, and the post-transplant care in the outpatient setting. Preparation of the transplant center to successfully coordinate care in the outpatient setting involves many factors, including the availability of adequate lodging, homecare resources, and outpatient care facilities. Family members or significant others are trained as caregivers to assist patients with activities of daily living, basic hygiene, meal preparation, medication administration, central venous catheter care, and transportation to outpatient appointments. Regardless of whether the acute phase of transplantation occurred in the inpatient or outpatient setting, the duration of post-HSCT outpatient care at the transplant center varies. Variability may depend on the type of transplant, steps of recovery, the patient's clinical condition, and the transplant center's routine practice. In general, autologous transplant recipients are referred back to their primary oncologist sooner than recipients who underwent allogeneic transplant.

Post-transplant follow-up appointments focus on adherence to standard guidelines for routine care and disease evaluation, tapering of immunosuppressive medications, and adherence to clinical research protocol requirements. Clinical trial requirements for medication adjustments, disease evaluation, and donor lymphocyte infusion must be followed as appropriate. The Centers for Disease Control and Prevention (CDC) has published recommendations for vaccination for both autologous and allogeneic transplant recipients (CDC, Infectious Diseases Society of America, & American Society of Blood and Marrow Transplantation, 2000). In general, revaccination is initiated when the immune system has recovered and the immunosuppressive medications have been discontinued (see Table 7-4).

Chimerism and Donor Lymphocyte Infusions

Chimerism (a term used to describe the balance of donor and host lymphohematopoietic cells) studies often are performed following allogeneic or unrelated HSCT to determine conversion to donor cells. An allogeneic stem cell transplant recipient is considered to have converted to full chimerism if all of the patient's hematopoietic cells and lymphoid cells are derived from the allogeneic donor. Methods to document chimerism include cytogenetic analysis for XX/XY chromosomes in sex-mismatch transplant, as well as cytogenetic or molecular pathology analysis to identify the presence of specific disease abnormalities. In addition, chimerism studies may be performed to quantitate the presence of donor versus recipient cells by CD3+ (T lymphocyte) or CD33+ (myeloid cell) antigens. Conversion to donor chimerism is intended to be achieved post-transplant. If achievement of donor chimerism is delayed or relapse of disease occurs, donor lymphocyte infusions (DLIs) may be given to promote conversion to donor cells and/or to achieve a GVT effect. The dose of donor cells infused for DLI varies according to institutional practice or research protocols. In some cases, additional lymphocytes are obtained at the time of stem cell collection and are frozen, stored, and saved for infusion post-HSCT to trigger GVHD, leading to the GVT or GVL effect. Related

Table 7-4. Centers for Disease Control and Prevention Vaccination Recommendations for Autologous and Allogeneic Hematopoietic Stem Cell Transplant Recipients

Vaccine	Time Post-Transplant		
	12 Months	14 Months	24 Months
Tetanus-diphtheria toxoid (Td)[ab]	X	X	X
Haemophilus influenzae type b (Hib) conjugate	X	X	X
Hepatitis B (high-dose—40 mg/dose)	X	X	X[c]
23-valent pneumococcal polysaccharide	X		
Influenza	Starting six months after transplant, yearly at the start of influenza season		
Inactivated polio (IPV)	X	X	X
Measles-mumps-rubella (MMR)[d]			X[e]

[a] Only applies to people ≥ 7 years of age
[b] Should continue to be revaccinated every 10 years, as recommended for all adults
[c] Serum titer should be checked 1–2 months after third dose. If antibody not present, series of three vaccinations should be repeated.
[d] Live attenuated vaccine—administer only to patients assumed to be immunocompetent.
[e] A second dose is recommended 6–12 months later. If an outbreak of a disease occurs, the second dose can be administered four weeks after the initial dose.

Note. Based on information from Centers for Disease Control and Prevention et al., 2000.
From "Post-Transplant Follow-Up" (p. 210), by L. Williams in S. Ezzone (Ed.), *Hematopoietic Stem Cell Transplantation: A Manual for Nursing Practice,* 2004, Pittsburgh, PA: Oncology Nursing Society. Copyright 2004 by Oncology Nursing Society. Reprinted with permission.

or unrelated donors may be asked to donate additional lymphocytes. The effectiveness of DLI in promoting antitumor activity has been described to be most effective for the treatment of persistent chronic myeloid leukemia following HSCT (Huff et al., 2006; Luznik & Fuchs, 2002).

Quality-of-Life Issues

Psychosocial concerns pertaining to people undergoing HSCT are necessary to consider. Several authors have described measures to assess and define quality of life after transplant. A quality-of-life transplant model with four domains—physical, psychosocial, social, and spiritual well-being—has been described (Ferrell et al., 1992). Each of the domains identifies specific issues that may affect quality of life during the transplant process. Quality-of-life issues may be significant within the first year after transplant because of many factors, including separation from home and family, financial burdens, and a prolonged post-HSCT recovery process. In addition, people with long-term complications may experience psychological and physical problems that interfere with overall functioning and lead to disability. Further research is needed to better define quality of life, initiate assessment strategies, and develop interventions to promote quality of life for post-transplant patients.

Complications of Hematopoietic Stem Cell Transplantation

Graft-Versus-Host Disease

GVHD is a unique complication of allogeneic HSCT that may occur in 30%–60% of cases and, if severe, may lead to a 50% mortality rate (Antin, 2002). The incidence of GVHD has been reported to occur less frequently with the use of umbilical cord stem cells because of the lower number of T cells in the product. GVHD occurs more often with the use of PBSCs and with the use of unrelated or mismatched donors (Anders & Barton-Burke, 2007; Dean & Bishop, 2003). Although much progress has been made in understanding GVHD as well as its prophylaxis and management, it remains a complex complication of allogeneic transplant that is challenging and has limited treatment options.

Pathophysiology of graft-versus-host disease: GVHD is an immune reaction that occurs between the recipient cells and the immunologically competent donor T lymphocytes. It is an immune-mediated process that consists of several steps involving MHC and T-cell activation (Erlich, Oelz, & Hansen, 2001). The HLA antigens or genes that currently determine tissue typing include the class I antigens (HLA-A, -B, and -C) and class II antigens (DR, DP, and DQ). Class I HLA-C antigen matching decreases the incidence of GVHD in unrelated transplants (Petersdorf et al., 2001). Matching of HLA antigens of the recipient and donor decreases the risk of developing GVHD. An increased risk of developing GVHD exists in the setting of an HLA mismatched HSCT. In addition, minor histo-incompatible differences may exist despite HLA typing and can lead to the development of GVHD.

The immune system of the allogeneic recipient must be incompetent so that the recipient cells do not recognize donor cells as foreign. Conversely, the donor T lymphocytes must be immunologically competent to recognize and attack the defined target organs of the recipient. Induction of acute GVHD begins by administration of the myeloablative conditioning regimen that results in recipient immune system ablation and tissue damage to many organ systems, including the skin, gastrointestinal (GI) tract, and liver, causing cytokine release. The donor T lymphocytes proliferate, recognize, and attack target organs of the recipient. Additional cytokines are released as tissue damage continues to perpetuate the clinical sequelae of GVHD (Anders & Barton-Burke, 2007). The pathophysiology of chronic GVHD is not well understood but has been described as an alloreactivity of T cells, dysfunctional immune recovery, or similar to an autoimmune disorder with development of autoantibodies. Alloreactivity of T cells occurs between the recipient and donor usually as a result of immune dysfunction (Biedermann et al., 2002; Kataoka et al., 2001; Vogelsang, Lee, & Bensen-Kennedy, 2003).

The benefits of GVHD following allogeneic transplant primarily are the result of promotion of the attack on residual tumor or leukemic cells by donor T lymphocytes. GVT or GVL effect often is considered beneficial following nonmyeloablative transplant. Maintaining post-transplant remission or disease control due to occurrence of GVHD resulting in GVT or GVL effect has been reported for many treated conditions. Post-transplant, DLI may be given to trigger a GVT or GVL effect in patients who relapse or who have persistent mixed chimerism (donor and recipient cells). Conversion to full donor chimerism (donor cells) and occurrence of GVHD are predictive of reaching a complete remission.

Risk factors for the development of graft-versus-host disease: Many risk factors have been identified for the development of GVHD. Risk factors may include histo-incompatibilities, HLA disparities, unrelated allogeneic transplant, cumulative blood transfusions, increasing age, and cytokine mobilized PBSCs (Dean & Bishop, 2003). The existence of acute GVHD increases the risk for development of chronic GVHD. Reports regarding the occurrence of GVHD with the use of bone marrow cells versus PBSCs are conflicting. Authors have suggested that the incidence of GVHD with the use of PBSCs versus bone marrow may increase, decrease, or remain the same (Cutler et al., 2001; Dean & Bishop).

Clinical manifestations of graft-versus-host disease: Acute GVHD is defined as occurring from the time of engraftment until approximately day +100 post-transplant, and late-onset chronic GVHD is that occurring after day +100. Symptoms of acute GVHD also may occur following DLI. The common clinical manifestations of acute GVHD involve the skin, mucous membranes, GI tract, and liver and are described in Figure 7-3. Symptoms of cutaneous acute GVHD include an erythematous rash and itching. The oral mucosa may become erythematous with blister-type lesions. GI symptoms may involve some combination of nausea, vomiting, diarrhea, and abdominal cramping. Abnormal liver

---

Clinical Manifestations

Acute graft-versus-host disease (GVHD)
- Mouth—erythema, lesions
- Skin—maculopapular rash
- Gastrointestinal (GI)—nausea, vomiting, diarrhea, oral lesions
- Liver—elevated liver enzymes, hyperbilirubinemia

Chronic GVHD
- Skin—macular, erythematous eruption; thickened, tight, sclerotic patches; lichen planus–type features
- GI—nausea, vomiting, diarrhea, malabsorption, esophageal strictures
- Mouth—erythema, lichen-type hyperkeratosis, ulcerations, xerostomia, sensitivities, leukoplakia, lichenoid appearance, dry mouth
- Liver—elevated alkaline phosphatase, hyperbilirubinemia, cholestasis
- Ocular—dry eyes, reduced tear flow
- Neuromuscular—joint motion affected in patients with scleroderma; muscle cramping, fasciitis, joint stiffness
- Pulmonary—bronchiolitis obliterans
- Hematologic—cytopenias, autoimmune, eosinophilia, decreased platelet count
- Reproductive—lichen planus, dry skin–type features; women may have inflammation, mucosal dryness, adhesions, vaginal stenosis; men may have impotence, erectile dysfunction

Diagnostic Evaluation
- Skin biopsy
- Schirmer's test
- Open lung biopsy
- Endoscopy with biopsy
- Colonoscopy with biopsy
- Pulmonary function tests
- High-resolution computed tomography of the chest

Figure 7-3. Clinical Manifestations of Graft-Versus-Host Disease

---

Note. Based on information from Anders & Barton-Burke, 2007; Filipovich et al., 2005; Mitchell, 2004.

function tests include an elevated total bilirubin with jaundice and hepatomegaly. Diagnosis of acute GVHD often is made by clinical evaluation, but skin, GI tract, or liver biopsies may be necessary and helpful to obtain a diagnosis.

The grading and staging of acute GVHD have been described by Glucksberg et al. (1974), Thomas et al. (1975), and the IBMTR (Przepiorka et al., 1995) as involving three organ systems—the skin, liver, and GI tract. Cahn et al. (2005) evaluated the use of the Glucksberg and IBMTR grading systems in 607 patients to compare scoring systems for acute GVHD. Both scoring systems were found to be similar in predicting long-term survival outcomes based on the maximum grade of acute GVHD. The Rule of Nines (see Figure 7-4) is used to describe the extent of skin involvement that correlates with the stage of cutaneous involvement. A human body diagram is used to describe the percentage of skin involvement with GVHD. A new, improved grading system is needed to predict prognosis and consider histologic and immunologic parameters in both myeloablative and nonmyeloablative allogeneic transplant. The Glucksberg et al. and IBMTR staging and grading systems for acute GVHD are described in Table 7-5.

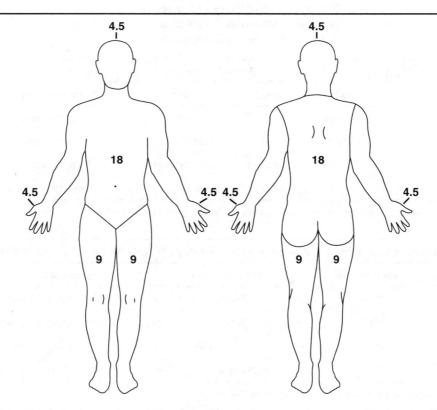

The Rule of Nines body surface area diagram is used to estimate the percentage of body surface involved with graft-versus-host disease of the skin.

Figure 7-4. Rule of Nines

Table 7-5. Staging and Grading Systems for Acute Graft-Versus-Host Disease (GVHD)

Consensus Criteria for Clinical Staging and Grading of Acute GVHD		
Organ	**Grade**	**Description**
Skin	+1	Maculopapular eruption over < 25% of body area
	+2	Maculopapular eruption over 25%–50% of body area
	+3	Generalized erythroderma
	+4	Generalized erythroderma with bullous formation and often with desquamation
Liver	+1	Bilirubin 2–3 mg/dl
	+2	Bilirubin 3.1–6 mg/dl
	+3	Bilirubin 6.1–15 mg/dl
	+4	Bilirubin > 15 mg/dl
Gut	+1	Diarrhea > 500 ml/day or > 30 ml/kg
	+2	Diarrhea > 1,000 ml/day or > 60 ml/kg
	+3	Diarrhea > 1,500 ml/day or > 90 ml/kg
	+4	Diarrhea > 2,000 ml/day or > 120 ml/kg

Overall Stage				
Stage	**Skin**	**Liver**	**Gut**	**Performance Status**
I	+1 to +2	0	0	No decrease
II	+1 to +3	+1	and/or +1	Mild decrease
III	+2 to +3	+2 to +3	and/or +2 to +3	Marked decrease
IV	+2 to +4	+2 to +4	and/or +2 to +4	Extreme decrease

If no skin disease is present, the overall grade is the higher, single organ stage.

Criteria for International Bone Marrow Transplant Registry Severity Index for Acute GVHD						
Index*	**Extent of Rash**		**Total Bilirubin**		**Volume of Diarrhea**	
A	< 25%	or	< 2 mg/dl	or	> 500 ml/day or 30 ml/kg	
B	25%–50%	or	2–6 mg/dl	or	> 1,000 ml/day or 60 ml/kg	
C	> 50%	or	6.1–15 mg/dl	or	> 1,500 ml/day or 90 ml/kg	
D	Bullae	or	> 15 mg/dl	or	> 2,000 ml/day or 120 ml/kg	

* Index assigned based on maximum organ involvement.

Note. Based on information from Glucksberg et al., 1974.
From "Graft Versus Host Disease" (p. 92), by S. Mitchell in S. Ezzone (Ed.), *Hematopoietic Stem Cell Transplantation: A Manual for Nursing Practice,* 2004, Pittsburgh, PA: Oncology Nursing Society. Copyright 2004 by Oncology Nursing Society. Adapted with permission.

Chronic GVHD occurs from day +100 to years after transplant and has been described as a multiorgan system condition involving the mouth, eyes, skin, liver, lungs, GI tract, and hematopoietic system (Pavletic, Lee, Socie, & Vogelsang, 2006). Clinical manifestations related to organ systems involved in chronic GVHD are described in Table 7-6. Dryness of the eyes, skin, and mouth are common. GI tract symptoms may include nausea, vomiting, diarrhea, and malabsorption. Limited or extensive involvement of the liver and lungs may occur in severe cases. Bronchiolitis obliterans or chronic GVHD of the lungs is a late complication that is often fatal because of pulmonary failure (Dudek, Mahaseth, DeFor, & Weisdorf, 2003). Diagnostic studies to evaluate chronic GVHD of the lungs include pulmonary function tests and computed tomography (CT). Diagnosis of

Table 7-6. Complications of Hematopoietic Stem Cell Transplantation

Complication	Risk Factors/Causes	Clinical Sequelae	Diagnostic Findings
Bleeding	Anemia Thrombocytopenia Altered coagulation factors Altered mucosal barriers Veno-occlusive disease Failed or delayed engraftment ABO-incompatible transplant	Petechiae, ecchymosis, easy bruising Hematuria, menorrhagia Bloody stool or emesis Epistaxis, hemoptysis Headache, change in pupil response or mental status	Platelet count < 10,000–20,000/mm^3 Hemoglobin < 8 g/dl Elevated prothrombin time/international normalized ratio/partial thromboplastin time Chemstick reveals blood. Guaiac-positive stool, emesis Computed tomography (CT) of the head—intracranial bleed
Cardiac	Cardiomyopathy—previous exposure to anthracyclines; administration of cyclophosphamide; total body irradiation (TBI)	Pulmonary edema, poor peripheral perfusion, systemic edema	Electrocardiogram (ECG)—decreased voltage Echocardiogram—cardiomegaly, decreased ejection fraction
	Cardiac arrhythmias	Palpitations, chest discomfort, anxiety, abnormal heart sounds, hypotension	ECG findings specific to type of arrhythmia
	Cardiac infections—endocarditis related to bacteremia	Nonspecific symptoms of fever, chills, malaise, night sweats Arrhythmias	ECG conduction or rhythm disturbances Echocardiogram—valvular vegetations, decreased ventricular function
Pulmonary	Idiopathic pneumonia syndrome (IPS)—TBI used in preparative regimen, graft-versus-host disease (GVHD), methotrexate for GVHD prophylaxis	IPS—fever, dyspnea, nonproductive cough, hypoxemia, respiratory failure	IPS—chest radiograph (CXR) and CT diffuse or multilobular interstitial or alveolar infiltrates, thickened deep and superficial interlobular septa, nodules of varying sizes

(Continued on next page)

Table 7-6. Complications of Hematopoietic Stem Cell Transplantation *(Continued)*

Complication	Risk Factors/Causes	Clinical Sequelae	Diagnostic Findings
	Diffuse alveolar hemorrhage (DAH)—radiation prior to transplantation, age > 40, solid tumors, severe mucositis, granulocyte recovery, fever, renal insufficiency, acute GVHD	DAH—dyspnea, cough, hemoptysis, hypoxemia, respiratory failure	DAH—CXR unilateral or bilateral infiltrates, diffuse alveolar pattern; bronchial alveolar lavage bloody fluid and hemosiderin-laden macrophages, diffuse alveolar damage
	Pulmonary toxicity—chemotherapy induced, radiation therapy induced	Pulmonary toxicity—nonproductive cough, dyspnea, decreased exercise tolerance	Pulmonary toxicity—lung biopsy with interstitial fibrosis, decreased diffusing capacity of the lung for carbon monoxide (DLCO) < 60% with symptoms and < 50% without symptoms; CXR and chest CT interstitial and alveolar infiltrates, ground glass appearance, hazy pulmonary markings
	Pulmonary edema—sepsis, chemotherapy, radiation therapy, heart failure, pericarditis, infusion of large volumes of IV fluids or stem cell infusion	Pulmonary edema—fluid overload, dyspnea, tachypnea, cough, weight gain, bibasilar rales, hypoxemia	Pulmonary edema—CXR cardiac enlargement, vascular redistribution
	Bronchiolitis obliterans (BO)—chronic GVHD	BO—progressive dyspnea, wheezing, nonproductive cough	BO—CXR normal or hyperinflation, pneumothorax, pneumomediastinum; pulmonary function tests reveal airflow obstruction, decreased forced expiratory volume in one second, reduced vital capacity, increased residual lung volume, normal DLCO
	Infections—bacterial, viral (cytomegalovirus, herpes simplex virus, respiratory syncytial virus), fungal *(Aspergillus, Fusarium, Mucor)*, protozoal *(Pneumocystis carinii)*, mycobacterial	Infection—fever, productive or nonproductive cough, rhinitis, nasal congestion, sore throat, pneumonia	Sputum culture CXR diffuse infiltrates, diffuse air space disease, solitary or multiple pulmonary modules CT scan of chest ground-glass opacities, lung nodule, consolidations, cavitations; bronchoscopy; open lung biopsy

(Continued on next page)

Table 7-6. Complications of Hematopoietic Stem Cell Transplantation (Continued)

Complication	Risk Factors/Causes	Clinical Sequelae	Diagnostic Findings
Renal insufficiency	Hypovolemia Dehydration Septic shock Nephrotoxic drugs Prolonged ischemia Hemorrhagic cystitis Tumor lysis syndrome Acute tubular necrosis Congestive heart failure	Doubling of baseline creatinine Oliguria Fluid and electrolyte imbalance Pulmonary edema Cardiac compromise Multiple organ failure	Urinalysis Fluid balance Blood chemistries
Veno-occlusive disease	Hepatitis prior to transplant Repeated courses and higher doses of chemotherapy Hepatotoxic radiation therapy Immunosuppressive agents Elevated liver function tests prior to transplant Infection/sepsis Estrogen or progesterone therapy	Azotemia Ascites Weight gain Hepatomegaly Encephalopathy Fluid balance intake > output	Hyperbilirubinemia Elevated alkaline phosphatase Elevated serum aspartate aminotransferase and alanine aminotransferase Elevated prothrombin time Liver biopsy

chronic GVHD often is sought by obtaining biopsy of the skin, liver, lungs, or GI tract. A Schirmer's test may be done by ophthalmology to evaluate dry eyes. Shulman et al. (1978) published the first attempt to describe chronic GVHD and develop a staging system. Since that time, many transplant centers have tried to better describe chronic GVHD using staging systems and response criteria. Limited and extensive chronic GVHD have been described based on the extent of organ involvement. This description of chronic GVHD has limited usefulness in describing the full spectrum of clinical sequelae that may occur. In June 2004, the first meeting of the chronic GVHD consensus project of six working groups met to begin developing recommendations for diagnosis, scoring, prognostic indicators, and measurement of response to treatment. In 2005, the National Institutes of Health Consensus Development Project published guidelines for diagnosis and staging of GVHD. A chronic GVHD clinical scoring system was developed using a 0–3 scale (Filipovich et al., 2005). The scoring system is complex and includes all organ systems that may be affected. Guidelines for treatment suggest that local therapies may be indicated for mild chronic GVHD. Systemic therapy is recommended if three or more organs are involved or if a score of 2 or higher is present in any organ system (Filipovich et al.).

Prophylaxis and management of graft-versus-host disease: Pharmacologic approaches to prevent acute GVHD include administration of a combination of systemic immunosuppressive medications. Cyclosporine A (CSA) or tacrolimus along with methotrexate (MTX) commonly is used and is initiated days before the transplant. Monitoring of drug levels and side effects of these drugs is necessary to anticipate toxicities that may occur. Suggested therapeutic drug levels for CSA blood are > 200 mcg/ml, and levels for tacrolimus are 5–15 mcg/ml, but these levels may vary according to institutional practices or research protocols. Numerous drug interactions may occur that increase or decrease tacrolimus or CSA levels. Some drugs that may alter tacrolimus or CSA levels include calcium channel blockers, antifungal agents, antibiotics, prokinetic agents, and anticonvulsants (Mitchell, 2004). Common adverse drug effects related to these immunosuppressive medications include renal, metabolic, neurologic, GI, cardiovascular, hematologic, cutaneous, and infusion-related toxicities (Mitchell). Renal insufficiency and electrolyte abnormalities that may occur include increased creatinine, hyperglycemia, hypomagnesemia, and hyperkalemia. Seizure activity and change in mental status have been reported. Nausea, vomiting, hirsutism, hypertension, and gum hypertrophy have been described (Anders & Barton-Burke, 2007). Immunosuppressive medications are tapered gradually over a few months after the transplant, according to institutional guidelines or research protocols. Other pharmacologic agents used to prevent or treat GVHD include steroids, antithymocyte globulin (ATG), infliximab, daclizumab, and pentostatin. Research is ongoing to determine the most effective method to prevent and treat GVHD. Nonpharmacologic approaches used to prevent acute GVHD include phototherapy, T-cell or lymphocyte depletion of the stem cell product pretransplant, or total lymphoid irradiation (Anders & Barton-Burke; Mitchell). Figure 7-5 lists common options for the prevention and treatment of GVHD.

Hematologic Complications

In addition to GVHD, many other complications may occur post-transplant; these are listed in Table 7-6. Profound pancytopenia and immune suppression following HSCT result from the effects of the conditioning regimen and the immunosuppressive agents used in allogeneic transplant to prevent GVHD. Myeloablative conditioning regimens eradicate hematopoietic function, thus resulting in severe anemia, neutropenia, and thrombocytopenia. Most patients require red blood cell and platelet transfusions during the post-transplant course if their hemoglobin is < 8 g/dl and platelet count is < 10,000/mm^3. Diagnostic studies used to assess bleeding may include guaiac of stool and emesis, urinalysis, and a CT scan of the head to evaluate for intracranial hemorrhage. Because nonmyeloablative conditioning regimens are less toxic, suppression of blood counts may not be as severe and blood counts usually recover quicker, thereby minimizing the need for transfusions. The duration of neutropenia is dependent on several factors, including the stem cell source, type of transplant, and CSFs used for stem cell mobilization and during the post-transplant course (Burcat & McAdams, 2007).

Infection

The risk of infection related to HSCT is present during three phases of the transplant process—the pre-engraftment phase, the early postengraftment phase, and the late postengraftment phase. Viral, bacterial, fungal, and protozoan infections occur at predicted phases following transplant as described in Table 7-7. Common viral infections described include herpes simplex virus (HSV), cytomegalovirus (CMV), Epstein-Barr virus (EBV), enteric viruses, echoviruses, varicella zoster, and respiratory syncytial virus (RSV). Gram-positive and gram-negative bacterial infections have been documented at all phases during the post-transplant process. During the early post-transplant phase, the most common fungal infections described are of the *Candida* species. Invasive fungal infections, including *Aspergillus,* mucormycosis, coccidioidomyco-

Systemic Immunosuppression
- Corticosteroids
- Cyclosporine
- Tacrolimus
- Mycophenolate mofetil
- Methotrexate
- Rapamycin

Polyclonal or Monoclonal Antibody–Based Therapies
- Antithymocyte globulin
- Daclizumab
- Infliximab
- Etanercept
- Alemtuzumab

Other Systemic Therapies
- IV immunoglobulin
- Thalidomide
- Octreotide
- N-acetylcysteine
- Pentoxifylline
- Beclomethasone
- Hydroxychloroquine

Phototherapy
- 8-methoxypsoralen plus ultraviolet A irradiation (PUVA)
- UVB phototherapy
- Extracorporeal photopheresis

Local and Topical Therapy
- Topical corticosteroids
- Intralesional steroid injections (mouth only)
- Topical tacrolimus
- Corticosteroid mouthwash
- Vaginal cyclosporine or tacrolimus ointment/gel
- Ophthalmic cyclosporine

Other
- T cell depletion pretransplant
- Total lymphoid irradiation

Figure 7-5. Options for Graft-Versus-Host Disease Prevention and Treatment

Note. From "Graft Versus Host Disease" (p. 99), by S. Mitchell in S. Ezzone (Ed.), *Hematopoietic Stem Cell Transplantation: A Manual for Nursing Practice,* 2004, Pittsburgh, PA: Oncology Nursing Society. Copyright 2004 by Oncology Nursing Society. Reprinted with permission.

sis, and *Cryptococcus neoformans* may occur later following transplant. Common protozoan infections include *Pneumocystis carinii* pneumonia (PCP) and *Toxoplasma gondii.*

Various measures can reduce the risk of infection, including protective isolation, positive air pressure rooms, air filtration systems such as HEPA filtration or laminar airflow rooms, hand washing, limited visitation, low bacterial diet, and other institution-specific guidelines. Despite a variety of preventive measures used, hand washing is the most effective practice to minimize the risk of infection (Boyce & Pittet, 2002). The risk of infection in allogeneic transplantation is complex because of the profound immunosuppression induced by both the conditioning regimen and the medications used to prevent or treat GVHD. Risk of infection after allogeneic transplant is greatest during the early postengraftment phase but also may occur in later months following transplant as

Table 7-7. Infectious Complications and Occurrence in Hematopoietic Stem Cell Transplantation Recipients

Organism	Common Sites	Treatment
First Month Post-Transplant		
Viral		
Herpes simplex virus (HSV)	Oral, esophageal, skin, gastro-intestinal (GI) tract, genital	Acyclovir, famciclovir
Respiratory syncytial virus (RSV)	Sinopulmonary	Aerosolized ribavirin
Epstein-Barr virus (EBV)	Oral, esophageal, skin, GI tract	Treatment usually is not indicated.
Bacterial		
Gram + (*S. epidermidis, S. aureus, Streptococci*)	Skin, blood, sinopulmonary	Third- and fourth-generation cepha-losporins, quinolones, aminoglyco-sides, vancomycin
Gram – (*E. coli, P. aeruginosa, Klebsiella*)	GI, blood, oral, perirectal	
Fungal		
Candida species (*C. albicans, glabrata, krusei*)	Oral, esophageal, skin	Fluconazole, voriconazole, itracon-azole, amphotericin B, liposomal amphotericin
Aspergillus (fumigata, flavum)	Sinopulmonary	
One to Four Months Post-Transplant		
Viral		
Cytomegalovirus (CMV)	Pulmonary, hepatic, GI	Ganciclovir, foscarnet, valacyclovir, acyclovir
Enteric viruses (rotavirus, Coxsackie, adenovirus)	Pulmonary, urinary, GI, hepatic	No specific treatment
RSV	Sinopulmonary	Aerosolized ribavirin
Parainfluenza	Pulmonary	Possibly ribavirin, but no standard treatment
Bacterial		
Gram +	Sinopulmonary	Third- and fourth-generation cepha-losporins, quinolones, aminoglyco-sides, vancomycin
Fungal		
Candida species	Oral, hepatosplenic, integu-ment	Fluconazole, voriconazole, itracon-azole, amphotericin B, liposomal amphotericin
Aspergillus species	Sinopulmonary, central ner-vous system (CNS)	
Mucormycosis	Sinopulmonary	
Coccidiomycosis	Sinopulmonary	
Cryptococcus neoformans	Pulmonary, CNS	

(Continued on next page)

Table 7-7. Infectious Complications and Occurrence in Hematopoietic Stem Cell Transplantation Recipients *(Continued)*

Organism	Common Sites	Treatment
Protozoan		
Pneumocystis carinii	Pulmonary	Standard is trimethoprim-sulfamethoxazole (TMP-SMZ) Pentamidine, atovaquone may be used if allergic to sulfa
Toxoplasma gondii	Pulmonary, CNS	Pyrimethamine and sulfonamides may be combined with clindamycin and spiramycin, especially if sulfa allergy
4–12 Months Post-Transplant		
Viral		
CMV, echoviruses, RSV, varicella zoster (VCV)	Integument, pulmonary, hepatic	CMV—ganciclovir, foscarnet, valacyclovir, acyclovir RSV—aerosolized ribavirin VCV—acyclovir, valacyclovir, famciclovir Echoviruses—no specific treatment, IVIG
Bacterial		
Gram + (*S. pneumoniae, H. influenzae, Pneumococci*)	Sinopulmonary, blood	Third- and fourth-generation cephalosporins, quinolones, aminoglycosides, vancomycin
Fungal		
Aspergillus	Sinopulmonary	Fluconazole, voriconazole, itraconazole, amphotericin B, liposomal amphotericin
Coccidiomycosis	Sinopulmonary	
Protozoan		
Pneumocystis carinii	Pulmonary	Standard is TMP-SMZ. Pentamidine, atovaquone may be used if allergic to sulfa.
Toxoplasma gondii	Pulmonary, CNS	Pyrimethamine and sulfonamides may be combined with clindamycin and spiramycin, especially if sulfa allergy.
Greater Than 12 Months Post-Transplant		
Viral		
VZV	Integument	Acyclovir, valacyclovir, famciclovir
Bacterial		
Gram + (*Streptococci, H. influenzae,* encapsulated bacteria)	Sinopulmonary, blood	Third- and fourth-generation cephalosporins, quinolones, aminoglycosides, vancomycin

Note. Based on information from Barnes, 1998a, 1998b; Prentice et al., 1998; Riley, 1998; Shapiro et al., 1997; Westmoreland, 1998.
From "Hematologic Effects" (pp. 136–137), by G.B. Johnson and K. Quiett in S. Ezzone (Ed.), *Hematopoietic Stem Cell Transplantation: A Manual for Nursing Practice,* 2004, Pittsburgh, PA: Oncology Nursing Society. Copyright 2004 by Oncology Nursing Society. Reprinted with permission.

a result of prolonged immunosuppression as described in Table 7-7. Following autologous HSCT, the risk of infection is greatest during the early postengraftment period because of neutropenia. For both autologous and allogeneic transplants, patients are at greatest risk for the development of infection while neutropenic, with an absolute neutrophil count $< 500/mm^3$. Neutrophil engraftment is described as a neutrophil count $> 500/mm^3$ (CDC et al., 2000). Medications recommended for infection prophylaxis posttransplant include antibacterial, antiviral, and antifungal agents (see Table 7-8).

Risk factors for the development of bacterial infections in transplant recipients include central venous catheters, altered oral mucosa, and altered GI tract because of bacterial translocation. Bacterial infections following transplant most commonly are caused by gram-positive organisms such as *Staphylococcus aureus, Staphylococcus epidermidis,* and *Streptococci* species or gram-negative organisms such as *Escherichia coli, Klebsiella pneumoniae,* and *Pseudomonas aeruginosa* (Johnson & Quiett, 2004). The CDC does not recommend specific guidelines for antibacterial prophylaxis for afebrile transplant recipients (CDC et al., 2000). Institutional guidelines for antibacterial prophylaxis are based on commonly occurring infections, resistant organisms, and antibiotic susceptibilities. Antibiotic regimens for the empiric treatment of neutropenic or febrile transplant recipients may include third- and fourth-generation cephalosporins, quinolones, aminoglycosides, and vancomycin. If cultures remain negative, vancomycin should be discontinued because of the risk of vancomycin-resistant *Enterococcus* (CDC et al.).

Table 7-8. Centers for Disease Control and Prevention Recommendations for Infection Prophylaxis

Pathogen	Recommendations
Pneumocystis	Alternative therapy includes dapsone, pentamidine, or atovaquone.
Toxoplasma gondii	Trimethoprim-sulfamethoxazole double strength, 1 pill three times per week
	Alternative therapy includes clindamycin plus pyrimethamine, plus leucovorin.
	Begin therapy after engraftment and continue until 6 months after hematopoietic stem cell transplant (HSCT) and off immunosuppressive medications.
Herpes simplex virus	Acyclovir 200 mg po tid or 250 mg/m²/dose every 12 hours from beginning of conditioning regimen until engraftment or mucositis resolves
	Alternative therapy: valacyclovir (Valtrex®, GlaxoSmithKline) 500 mg by mouth daily
	Prophylaxis for seropositive allogeneic HSCT recipients
Cytomegalovirus	Ganciclovir 5 mg/kg/dose IV every 12 hours for 5–7 days; followed by 5–6 mg/kg IV for 5 days per week from time of engraftment until day 100 post-HSCT.
	Alternative therapy includes foscarnet.
Fungal—*Candida* species	Fluconazole 400 mg by mouth or IV daily
	Begin at the day of transplant and continue until engraftment or until 7 days after the ANC > 1,000 cells/mm³.

Note. Based on information from Centers for Disease Control and Prevention et al., 2000.

Common viral infections that may reactivate during the early post-transplant period include HSV I and II, HHV-6, and CMV. Pretransplant viral serologic testing is performed to determine past exposure to viral infections of the transplant recipient and donor. Prophylactic use of antiviral medications such as acyclovir, valacyclovir, or famciclovir is common practice during the transplant process. HSV most commonly is associated with oral mucositis. Risk factors for the development of CMV infections include CMV seropositivity prior to transplant, infusion of CMV seropositive blood products to CMV seronegative patients, GVHD, and the use of immunosuppressive agents. Another measure for prevention of viral infections includes the use of leukocyte filters for blood product transfusions (Johnson & Quiett, 2004; van Burik & Weisdorf, 1999). Antigen detection techniques to test for CMV should be performed until day +60 after autologous transplant and day +100 after allogeneic transplant. Because of profound immunosuppression after allogeneic transplant, patients are at risk for developing EBV infections. Screening for EBV may be done weekly using the polymerase chain reaction test. Treatment of EBV may include administration of rituximab (Park et al., 2002). Local or disseminated varicella zoster virus infections may occur as a result of prolonged immunosuppression at 4–12 months post-transplant or later and require treatment with high-dose acyclovir or valacyclovir.

Fungal infections may occur during the post-transplant period and commonly include *Candida* species or *Aspergillus*. Prophylactic antifungal agents may include fluconazole, itraconazole, or voriconazole. Oral antifungal agents may be used to prevent oral candidiasis caused by mucositis (Zitella et al., 2006). Invasive fungal infections have been reported including *Aspergillus, Fusarium,* and *Mucor.* Prolonged antifungal therapy may be necessary with amphotericin, caspofungin, itraconazole, voriconazole, or posaconazole.

Many other infections may occur following transplant. These may include PCP, *Toxoplasma gondii,* and *Clostridium difficile.* The use of prophylactic sulfonamides to prevent PCP has nearly eliminated this post-transplant infectious complication (Johnson & Quiett, 2004). Toxoplasmosis infections have occurred in transplant recipients because of profound immunosuppression. The most effective treatment for toxoplasmosis infections is the use of combination therapy including pyrimethamine and sulfonamides (Roemer et al., 2001). *Clostridium difficile* may develop post-transplant in patients who are treated with antibiotics allowing for GI overgrowth of other organisms. GI symptoms that are associated with colitis, such as diarrhea, nausea, and vomiting, usually are present. Treatment with oral vancomycin or metronidazole is preferred to allow for GI absorption of the medications.

Bleeding

Thrombocytopenia and anemia commonly occur post-transplant as a result of the profound myelosuppressive effects of the conditioning regimen. Institutional guidelines for transfusion of blood products should be used to develop a standard of practice. Transfusion needs must be individualized for each patient based on signs and symptoms of bleeding, presence of red blood cell or platelet antibodies, response to transfusions, and the presence of refractoriness to blood products. General guidelines for transfusions in patients who underwent HSCT are to transfuse red blood cells if the hemoglobin is less than 8 g/dl and to transfuse platelets if platelets are less than 10,000/mm³. In a study that compared prophylactic platelet transfusions at 10×10^9 versus 30×10^9 cells/kg, the number of platelet transfusions and cost associated with transfusions were reduced using the lower platelet threshold. The risk of bleeding, or significant bleeding events, was not increased by giving prophylactic platelet transfusion for a level of 10 x

10^9 (Diedrich, Remberger, Shanwell, Svahn, & Ringden, 2005). The American Society of Clinical Oncology published guidelines that recommend platelet transfusions for a level of 10,000/mm³. Platelet transfusions may be necessary at higher levels if signs of bleeding, coagulation abnormalities, rapidly falling platelet count, or invasive procedures are involved (Schiffer et al., 2001). In critically ill patients, a hemoglobin level of 7–9 g/dl should be maintained (Hebert et al., 1999). Fresh frozen plasma and cryoprecipitate may be given for coagulation abnormalities as needed. In ABO mismatched allogeneic transplant, the ABO type of the recipient will change to the ABO type of the donor in approximately three to four months. The ABO titer of the recipient must be monitored to detect when this change occurs so that blood transfusions can be adjusted appropriately. Type O blood products usually are used for transfusion until the recipient's blood type completely changes to the donor ABO type.

Gastrointestinal Complications

GI complications after autologous and allogeneic transplant are common and may have multiple etiologies. Post-transplant GI complications include nausea, vomiting, mucositis, dysphagia, diarrhea, anorexia, dry mouth, perirectal abscess, taste alterations, and nutritional compromise resulting from the conditioning regimen, infections, or GVHD. Mucositis may occur during the time of neutropenia with or without colonization of the oral cavity with fungal infection. Prophylactic fluconazole, pain medications, and oral hygiene are used to treat oral and pharyngeal mucositis. Mucosal damage caused by the preparative regimen also may occur to the stomach, esophagus, small intestine, and colon, therefore resulting in nausea, vomiting, diarrhea, esophagitis, and perirectal abscess. Use of antiemetics, antidiarrheal medications, and analgesics can manage symptoms. Attention to the perirectal area to assess for abscess formation is important. The occurrence of abscesses may require surgical intervention for drainage and wound care. A dietary consultation may be needed to assist with management of nutritional support. Daily weight, calorie counts, and intake and output measurements are helpful to monitor nutritional and fluid status (Stevens, 2004; Warnick & Rust, 2007).

Hepatic Complications

Liver abnormalities following transplant have been reported to occur in 77%–84.2% of allogeneic recipients and 44.8%–52% of autologous recipients (Kim et al., 2000; Ozdogan et al., 2003). Liver damage may occur after transplant for many reasons, including veno-occlusive disease (VOD), hepatitis B infection, hepatitis C infection, iron overload, gallbladder disease, and drug toxicity (Douglas & Shelton, 2007). Multiorgan system consequences may occur as a result of liver dysfunction and may include ascites, hypotension, coagulopathies, hyponatremia, hypoalbuminemia, encephalopathy, impaired renal insufficiency, fluid overload, pleural effusion, and pulmonary edema. Management of VOD involves adjusting dosages of medications that are metabolized by the liver and symptomatically treating the organ dysfunction that results from the liver insufficiency.

Pulmonary Complications

Many pulmonary complications following HSCT can arise. Idiopathic pneumonia syndrome (IPS) may occur 50–100 days after transplant in about 15% of patients (Veys & Owens, 2002). IPS is more common in patients with a hematologic malignancy, with the presence of GVHD, with the use of MTX for GVHD prophylaxis, and with the use of TBI in the conditioning regimen. The treatment of IPS is supportive care, and the mortality rate associated with IPS has been reported at 60%–70% (Veys & Owens). Corticosteroids have been used to treat IPS, but available data are inadequate to determine the benefits of corticosteroid use with IPS (Crawford, 1999).

Diffuse alveolar hemorrhage occurs in approximately 21% of both allogeneic and autologous transplant recipients near the time of engraftment and has a very poor prognosis (Kreit, 2000; Lewis, DeFor, & Weisdorf, 2000). Treatment of diffuse alveolar hemorrhage includes supportive care, such as transfusion of platelets to minimize thrombocytopenia, treatment of associated renal failure, mechanical ventilation, and high-dose corticosteroid therapy.

Pulmonary toxicity associated with drug or radiation effects can occur in the autologous or allogeneic transplant setting. Treatment of pulmonary toxicity related to drug or radiation effects involves administration of systemic and inhaled corticosteroids. Pulmonary edema that commonly occurs in the early transplant period may be associated with many factors, such as fluid retention, acute renal failure, and VOD. Increased capillary permeability that leads to pulmonary edema has been reported to occur as a result of chemotherapy or radiation exposure. Bronchiolitis obliterans is a unique pulmonary complication of allogeneic transplant and is associated with chronic GVHD. Progressive shortness of breath results from obstructive airway disease causing occlusion of the bronchioles. Treatment consists of corticosteroids, but no proven benefit has been clearly described (Marcellus & Vogelsang, 2000).

Numerous pulmonary infections can develop following transplant, including bacterial, viral, fungal, protozoan, and parasitic infections. Bacterial pneumonia may be caused by both gram-positive and gram-negative organisms. The most common gram-positive organisms responsible for pulmonary infections include *Staphylococcus aureus*, *Staphylococcus epidermidis*, and *Streptococcus pneumoniae*. Gram-negative organisms may include *Klebsiella* and *Pseudomonas* species. Prolonged immunosuppression caused by chronic GVHD may be a risk factor for pneumococcal pneumonia.

Late pulmonary infections have been described in people with chronic GVHD and may include *Legionella, Chlamydia, Mycobacteria,* and *Mycoplasma* (Veys & Owens, 2002). Viral pneumonia post-transplant most commonly is caused by CMV (Veys & Owens). The most significant risk factors for CMV pneumonia include prior CMV exposure and the immunosuppression used during the transplant process. RSV also may result in pneumonia and is very contagious. Protective precautions are necessary to avoid the spread of RSV to other patients. Additional viruses reported to cause pneumonia in transplant recipients include adenovirus, parainfluenza virus, influenza virus, and human herpes virus 6. Parasitic infections such as PCP also may lead to pneumonia in transplant recipients. Trimethoprim-sulfamethoxazole often is given after allogeneic HSCT following engraftment for prophylaxis against PCP and is continued until immunosuppression therapy is stopped. Several fungal infections have been reported in transplant recipients, including *Aspergillus, Candida, Cryptococcus neoformans, Fusarium, Penicillium,* and *Mucor.* Fungal prophylaxis for pneumonia may include fluconazole, itraconazole, voriconazole, and more recently, posaconazole.

Cardiac Complications

Cardiac complications following HSCT are uncommon and occur because of the cardiotoxic effects of chemotherapy and radiation therapy given prior to transplant or as part of the conditioning regimen. Chemotherapeutic agents with well-described cardiac toxicity include anthracyclines and cyclophosphamide, both of which may cause cardiomyopathy. TBI and total lymphoid irradiation have been reported to cause cardiac toxicity in rare cases. Cardiac arrhythmias have been reported during the transplant course. Cardiac infections are rare but most commonly are associated with endocarditis in the presence of bacteremia (Burgunder, 2007). Fungal organisms, such as *Aspergillus,* also have been found to be associated with the development of endocarditis (Keller, 2004).

Renal Complications

Renal compromise is a common complication after HSCT and may occur in approximately 40%–50% of patients early post-transplant (Parikh et al., 2002). Drug-induced toxicity and infection account for the etiology of renal insufficiency in most patients, which may lead to acute renal failure. Administration of medications such as CSA and tacrolimus for GVHD prophylaxis is challenging because of the renal toxicity of these immunosuppressive medications. Many other medications that are necessary after transplant also may cause renal toxicity, such as antibacterial, antiviral, and antifungal agents. Management of renal insufficiency may include administration of IV fluids, avoidance of nephrotoxic drugs, and implementation of hemodialysis.

Neurologic Complications

Several neurologic complications may occur following transplant and generally are related to side effects of TBI, chemotherapy, immunosuppressive agents, anti-infective medications, CNS infections, CNS hemorrhage, supportive medications, encephalopathy, or immune-mediated toxicities (Shelton, 2007; Warnick, 2004). Symptoms of the various neurologic toxicities may be similar, and determining the cause of the adverse effect can be difficult. Examples of post-transplant neurologic toxicities include seizures, tremors, confusion, drowsiness, ataxia, hallucinations, dysarthria, hearing loss, cognitive dysfunction, mood disturbances, visual disturbances, and symptoms of peripheral neuropathy. Management of neurologic toxicity is directed at the specific complication and symptoms experienced. Figure 7-6 summarizes the common neurologic toxicities that may occur after HSCT.

Late Effects After Hematopoietic Stem Cell Transplantation

Many late effects following transplant are associated with delayed toxicities of the preparative regimen, the occurrence of GVHD, or the administration of steroids. Careful and diligent evaluation for late effects is essential to the overall well-being and recovery of patients after transplant. The etiology of several late complications is described in Figure 7-7. Development of ophthalmologic late effects can include cataracts caused by TBI or steroid use and dry eyes in people who develop chronic GVHD. Possible pulmonary complications include recurrent infections such as bronchitis, pneumonia, or sinusitis; bronchiolitis obliterans; pulmonary fibrosis; IPS; and hepatopulmonary syndrome. Chronic GVHD may cause bronchiolitis obliterans, and late effects of the preparative regimen may lead to pulmonary fibrosis. Cardiac dysfunction post-transplant has not been clearly described but is thought to be related to the effects of the preparative regimen and may include left ventricular dysfunction or conduction abnormali-

Chemotherapy agents
- Cisplatin
- Busulfan
- Etoposide
- Paclitaxel
- Ifosfamide
- Cytarabine
- Carmustine
- Methotrexate

Total body irradiation

Immunosuppressive agents
- Steroids
- Tacrolimus
- Cyclosporine

Anti-infectives
- Acyclovir
- Imipenem
- Ganciclovir
- Cephalosporins
- Aminoglycosides

Central nervous system (CNS) infections
- Bacterial—*Streptococcus epidermidis, Staphylococcus aureus, Pseudomonas aeruginosa, Haemophilus influenzae,* pneumococcus
- Fungal—*Aspergillus, Candida*
- Viral—human herpes virus 6, cytomegalovirus, Epstein-Barr virus, varicella zoster
- Protozoan—toxoplasmosis

CNS hemorrhage or stroke

Encephalopathy
- Leukoencephalopathy
- Metabolic encephalopathy

Immune-mediated toxicities
- Polymyositis
- Myasthenia gravis
- Inflammatory demyelinating polyneuropathy

Figure 7-6. Common Etiology of Neurologic Complications

ties. Infertility, thyroid dysfunction, and growth hormone deficiency are the most common endocrine late effects that may occur. Late renal dysfunction is not well understood but may be related to the effects of the preparative regimen and other nephrotoxic agents used during the transplant process. Possible GI complications include effects of GVHD, such as dry mouth, gastritis, esophagitis, gallstones, hepatitis, CMV, and impaired oral health. The most common musculoskeletal disorders following transplant include avascular necrosis, diminished bone density, and osteochondromas. Use of steroids post-transplant for treatment of GVHD predisposes individuals to develop avascular necrosis, which may lead to the need for a surgical joint replacement. Immune function recovery may be delayed for a year or longer with prolonged use of immunosuppressive medications and can increase the risk of developing late infections. Cognitive and psychological effects of cancer therapy have been described in both adults and children (Ruble, 2007).

Ophthalmologic
- Cataracts
- Sicca syndrome

Pulmonary
- Chronic bronchitis
- Pulmonary fibrosis
- Bronchiolitis obliterans
- Hepatopulmonary syndrome
- Idiopathic pneumonia syndrome

Cardiac
- Conduction abnormalities
- Left ventricular dysfunction

Endocrine
- Infertility
- Thyroid dysfunction
- Gonadal dysfunction
- Growth hormone deficiency

Renal
- Renal insufficiency

Gastrointestinal
- Hepatitis
- Gallstones
- Cytomegalovirus
- Gastritis/esophagitis
- Oral health impairment
- Graft-versus-host disease

Musculoskeletal
- Osteochondromas
- Avascular necrosis
- Diminished bone density

Immune reconstitution
- Late infections
- Returned by one year after transplant or longer

Neurocognitive
- Cognitive function abnormalities
- Psychological function abnormalities

Secondary malignancy
- Myelodysplasia
- Acute myeloid leukemia
- Post-transplant lymphoproliferative disorders

Figure 7-7. Late Effects of Hematopoietic Stem Cell Transplantation

---

Note. Based on information from Ruble, 2007.

Secondary Malignancies

The most common post-transplant secondary malignancies reported in the literature are post-transplant lymphoproliferative disorder (PTLD), myelodysplastic syndrome (MDS), and acute myeloid leukemia (AML). Risk factors for PTLD include HLA mismatched transplant, positive EBV serology, and splenectomy prior to transplant. In a study by Sundin et al. (2006), the rate of PTLD occurrence was 0.26% with no risk factors, 8.2% with one risk factor, and 35.7% with two risk factors. PTLD also has been reported to occur in solid organ transplant. Presence of EBV, proliferation of B lymphocytes, and clinical features of lymphadenopathy are common findings associated with PTLD. The mortality rate of PTLD is high, and treatment options include use of rituximab, an anti-B-lymphocyte antibody. Strategies to predict the risk of PTLD and careful monitoring of EBV after transplant are important considerations.

MDS and AML have occurred following therapy using alkylating agents and topoisomerase II inhibitors in HSCT recipients and patients with cancer (Andre et al., 1998; Pedersen-Bjergaard, Anderson, & Christiansen, 2000). The rationale for development of MDS or AML is related to the adverse effects of chemotherapy on bone marrow.

Standards of Care

Several organizations have developed standards of care for HSCT programs. National and international organizations have developed guidelines for various aspects of transplant program development and the clinical care of the transplant recipient (Ezzone, Fliedner, & Sirilla, 2007). In the 1970s, the IBMTR was formed to serve as a site to collect and analyze data from all participating transplant centers. The Autologous Blood and Marrow Transplant Registry (ABMTR) was formed in 1990 to accomplish similar goals in the autologous transplant setting. The Center for International Blood and Marrow Transplant Research (CIBMTR) was formed to unite the IBMTR, the ABMTR, and the NMDP. The purpose of the CIBMTR is to design and conduct clinical research to promote clinical expertise in the field of transplantation. In 1996, the Foundation for the Accreditation of Cellular Therapy (FACT) formed to promote quality medical and laboratory practice related to HSCT. FACT accreditation is sought by many transplant centers. FACT standards have been developed for all aspects of the HSCT clinical program, including hematopoietic progenitor cell collection and processing, as well as the acute transplant phase of HSCT. Specific standards for each category have been developed and guide transplant centers in program development and maintenance (FACT, 2008).

Implications for Oncology Advanced Practice Nurses

Over the years, the role of APNs and staff nurses working in HSCT has grown tremendously. In many settings, APNs have taken on more clinical and direct patient care responsibilities that traditionally have been delegated to physicians, such as residents and interns. The daily assessment and management of patients during the inpatient hospital stay and at outpatient visits often is coordinated by APNs. APNs must maintain current knowledge in all aspects of transplantation in order to provide expert care.

Conclusion

Much advancement has occurred in the field of HSCT as a treatment for malignant and nonmalignant diseases. Although much has been learned and has positively affected both medical and nursing practice, the basic concepts of transplantation have remained the same over the years. Myeloablative and nonmyeloablative preparative regimens are used to treat a variety of diseases. Nonmyeloablative regimens offer less toxicity and mortality, thus enabling older patients and people with some comorbid conditions to undergo transplantation. Ongoing research continues on strategies for mobilization of stem cells, use of immunosuppressive agents, prophylactic anti-infective medications, donor lymphocyte infusions, and treatment of GVHD. Nursing management of transplant recipients remains complex and challenging. The multidisciplinary transplant team must work together to provide education to physicians, APNs, staff nurses, and other staff members to keep up to date on changes in practice related to transplantation.

Case Study

B.J. is a 44-year-old white male who is day +196 after a one-antigen mismatch allogeneic stem cell transplant from a sex- and ABO-mismatch donor for treatment of acute lymphocytic leukemia using the TBI and etoposide preparative regimen. B.J. has had an uneventful post-transplant course and has not experienced any complications. Today, B.J. presents to the outpatient clinic for his scheduled every-other-month visit for routine evaluation. Upon walking into the clinic, the nurse notices that B.J. has mild dyspnea. During the initial interview, the nurse questions B.J. about symptoms of dyspnea. B.J. reports that for about a month he has had shortness of breath with climbing stairs and walking long distances. He also reports dry mouth, eyes, and skin. On physical examination, significant findings include dry mouth, skin, and conjunctiva of the eyes; loss of skin turgor and sclerotic changes of the arms and back; and diminished breath sounds with poor inspiratory effort. Vital signs are temperature = 97.8°F (36.6°C), heart rate = 104, respiratory rate = 32, blood pressure = 140/82, and oxygen saturation = 89% on room air. B.J. is currently on no medications and has been off of immunosuppressive drugs for two months.

Diagnostic studies
- WBC = 4.2 K/ul
- Hemoglobin = 12.6 g/dl
- Platelets = 148,000 K/ul
- Absolute neutrophil count = 3.2 K/ul
- Eosinophils = 18%
- Chest x-ray = normal
- Pulmonary function tests
  Diffusing capacity of the lung for carbon monoxide (DCLO) = 48%
  Forced expired volume in one second (FEV_1) = 46%
  Pattern of obstructive ventilatory defect

1. As an APN seeing this patient in follow-up, what are the differential diagnoses to consider?
   • Pneumonia, because of complaints of shortness of breath, diminished breath sounds, poor inspiratory effort, respiratory rate = 32, oxygen saturation = 89%, status post-allogeneic stem cell transplant
   • Pulmonary embolism, because of complaints of shortness of breath, diminished breath sounds, poor inspiratory effort, respiratory rate = 32, oxygen saturation = 89%
   • Chronic GVHD, because of status post-allogeneic stem cell transplant (day +196); complaints of shortness of breath; diminished breath sounds; poor inspiratory effort; respiratory rate = 32; oxygen saturation = 89%; dry mouth, eyes, and skin; loss of skin turgor and sclerotic changes of arms and back; DLCO = 48%; FEV_1 = 46%; pattern of obstructive ventilatory defect
2. What other diagnostic studies could be ordered to further evaluate the patient's pulmonary condition?
   • CT of chest
   • Arterial blood gases
   • Open lung biopsy
3. What treatment options would be initiated for chronic GVHD of the lungs, skin, mouth, and eyes?
   • Initiate immunosuppressive therapy with corticosteroids or other immunosuppressive agents.
   • Perform a skin biopsy to confirm chronic GVHD of the skin.
   • Apply steroid skin cream (i.e., triamcinolone cream).
   • Refer patient for an ophthalmology consult.
   • Apply eye drops/ointment (i.e., Refresh® [Allergen, Inc.] tears, Restasis® [Allergen, Inc.] eye drops, Duratear® [Alcon Laboratories] ointment).
   • Provide supportive care as needed, such as home oxygen.

Key Points

• The types of transplants discussed in the chapter include autologous, allogeneic, and syngeneic HSCT. Types of allogeneic HSCT include sibling donor, unrelated donor, and umbilical cord, as well as myeloablative and nonmyeloablative transplant.
• The three sources of stem cells used in HSCT are derived from the bone marrow, peripheral blood, or umbilical cord.
• Malignant diseases (e.g., leukemia, lymphoma, multiple myeloma) and nonmalignant diseases are treated with HSCT.
• The process of peripheral blood stem cell mobilization and collection was described, including chemotherapy, chemotherapy and CSFs, CSFs alone, and investigational agents.
• The steps of infusion of stem cells and side effects were discussed.
  -- Autologous cells are cryopreserved, frozen, and stored prior to transplant.
  -- Adverse effects of autologous stem cell infusion are related to the preservative DMSO, red blood cell contamination, or the volume of cells infused.

- Common adverse effects include fever, chills, cough, nausea, vomiting, diarrhea, dyspnea, tachypnea, abdominal cramps, facial flushing, hypertension, cardiac arrhythmias, chest tightness, hemoglobinuria, and garlic-like taste.
  - Allogeneic stem cells generally are reinfused fresh.
  - Adverse effects include hives, fever, chills, rash, nausea, vomiting, flushing, shortness of breath, hypotension, hypertension, tachycardia, chest pain or tightness, and anaphylaxis.
  - Emergency equipment, oxygen, and cardiac monitoring equipment should be readily available during infusion of marrow.
  - The day of infusion is day 0.
- Complications of HSCT include GVHD, infection, bleeding, organ toxicities (GI, hepatic, pulmonary, cardiac, renal, neurologic), late effects, and secondary malignancies.
- Acute and chronic GVHD clinical manifestations, prevention, and treatment were described.
  - GVHD is an immune reaction that occurs between the recipient cells and immunologically competent donor T lymphocytes.
  - Acute GVHD can occur from time of engraftment until approximately day +100 following transplant.
    * Acute GVHD affects primarily the skin, liver, mucous membranes, and GI tract.
    * Pharmacologic approaches to prevent acute GVHD include administration of a combination of systemic immunosuppressive medications.
  - Chronic GVHD can occur after day +100 following transplant.
    * Chronic GVHD is a multiorgan system condition involving the mouth, eyes, skin, GI tract, liver, lungs, and hematopoietic system.
    * Pharmacologic (as used for acute GVHD) and nonpharmacologic approaches (e.g., phototherapy, T-cell depletion pretransplant, total lymphoid irradiation) are used to treat chronic GVHD.
- DLI may be given to promote conversion of recipient cells to donor cells and to achieve a GVT effect. The dose of DLI varies according to institutional practice or research protocols.
- Chimerism studies often are performed following allogeneic or unrelated HSCT to determine conversion to donor cells.
  - Stem cell transplant recipients are considered to have converted to full chimerism if all of their hematopoietic cells and lymphoid cells are derived from the allogeneic donor.
  - Full chimerism is a good prognostic sign in patients who have undergone allogeneic or unrelated HSCT.

Recommended Resources for Oncology Advanced Practice Nurses

Many references are available on various topics on HSCT. The following suggested references may be easily used in the clinical practice setting. Internet resources are very helpful for obtaining current information on HSCT.
- ASBMT: www.asbmt.org

- CIBMTR: www.ibmtr.org
- National Comprehensive Cancer Network: www.nccn.org
- Newborn Blood Banking, Inc.: www.newbornblood.com
- NMDP: www.nmdp.org

References

Anders, V., & Barton-Burke, M. (2007). Graft versus host disease: Complex sequelae of stem cell transplantation. In S. Ezzone & K. Schmit-Pokorny (Eds.), *Blood and marrow stem cell transplantation: Principles, practice and nursing insights* (3rd ed., pp. 147–181). Sudbury, MA: Jones and Bartlett.

Andre, M., Henry-Amar, M., Blaise, D., Colombat, P., Fleury, J., Miliped, N., et al. (1998). Treatment-related deaths and second cancers risk after autologous stem cell transplantation for Hodgkin's disease. *Blood, 92,* 1933–1940.

Antin, J. (2002). Clinical practice: Long-term care after hematopoietic-cell transplantation in adults. *New England Journal of Medicine, 347,* 36–42.

Armitage, J.O., & Antman, K.H. (Eds.). (1992). *High-dose cancer therapy: Pharmacology, hematopoietins, stem cells.* Baltimore: Williams & Wilkins.

Ballen, K.K. (2005). New trends in umbilical cord blood transplantation. *Blood, 105,* 3786–3792.

Baranov, A., Gale, R.P., Guskova, A., Piatkin, E., Selidovkin, G., Muravyova, L., et al. (1989). Bone marrow transplantation after the Chernobyl nuclear accident. *New England Journal of Medicine, 321,* 205–212.

Barnes, R.A. (1998a). Fungal infections. In J. Barrett & J.G. Treleaven (Eds.), *The clinical practice of stem cell transplantation, vol. 2* (pp. 723–740). St. Louis, MO: Mosby.

Barnes, R.A. (1998b). Other infections. In J. Barrett & J.G. Treleaven (Eds.), *The clinical practice of stem cell transplantation, vol. 2* (pp. 741–744). St. Louis, MO: Mosby.

Bensinger, W.J., Martin, P., Storer, B., Clift, R., Forman, S.J., Negrin, R., et al. (2001). Transplantation of bone marrow as compared with peripheral-blood cells from HLA-identical relatives in patients with hematologic cancers. *New England Journal of Medicine, 344,* 175–181.

Biedermann, T., Schwarzler, C., Lametschwandtner, G., Thoma, G., Carballido-Perrig, N., Kund, J., et al. (2002). Targeting CLA/E-selectin interactions prevents CCR4-mediated recruitment of human Th2 memory cells to human skin in vivo. *European Journal of Immunology, 32,* 3171–3180.

Bierman, P.J., Sweetenham, J., Loberiza, F., Zhang, M., Lazarus, H., Van Besien, K., et al. (2001). Syngeneic hematopoietic stem cell transplantation for non-Hodgkin lymphoma (NHL): Comparison with allogeneic and autologous transplants suggests a role for purging [Abstract 15]. *Proceedings of the 2001 ASCO Annual Meeting, 20,* 187.

Bishop, M.R., Jackson, J.D., O'Kane-Murphy, B., Schmit-Pokorny, K., Vose, J.M., Bierman, P.J., et al. (1996). Phase I trial of recombinant fusion protein PIXY321 for mobilization of peripheral-blood cells. *Journal of Clinical Oncology, 14,* 2521–2526.

Boyce, J.M., & Pittet, D. (2002). Guideline for hand hygiene in health-care settings: Recommendations of the Healthcare Infection Control Practices Advisory Committee and the HICPAC/SHEA/APIC/IDSA Hand Hygiene Task Force. *Infection Control and Hospital Epidemiology, 23*(Suppl. 12), S3–S40.

Burcat, S., & McAdams, F. (2007). Hematologic effects of transplantation. In S. Ezzone & K. Schmit-Pokorny (Eds.), *Blood and marrow stem cell transplantation: Principles, practice and nursing insights* (3rd ed., pp. 183–205). Sudbury, MA: Jones and Bartlett.

Burgunder, M.R. (2007). Pulmonary and cardiac effects. In S. Ezzone & K. Schmit-Pokorny (Eds.), *Blood and marrow stem cell transplantation: Principles, practice and nursing insights* (3rd ed., pp. 245–262). Sudbury, MA: Jones and Bartlett.

Cahn, J.Y., Klein, J.P., Lee, S.J., Milpied, N., Blaise, D., Antin, J.H., et al. (2005). Prospective evaluation of 2 acute graft-versus-host (GVHD) grading systems: A joint Société Française de Greffe de Moëlle et Thérapie Cellulaire (SFGM-TC), Dana Farber Cancer Institute (DFCI), and International Bone Marrow Transplant Registry (IBMTR) prospective study. *Blood, 108,* 1495–1500.

Centers for Disease Control and Prevention, Infectious Diseases Society of America, & American Society of Blood and Marrow Transplantation. (2000). Guidelines for preventing opportunistic infections among hematopoietic stem cell transplant recipients. *Biology of Blood and Marrow Transplantation, 6,* 659–733.

Chouinard, M.S., & Finn, K.T. (2007). Understanding hematopoiesis. In S. Ezzone & K. Schmit-Pokorny (Eds.), *Blood and marrow stem cell transplantation: Principles, practice and nursing insights* (3rd ed., pp. 29–58). Sudbury, MA: Jones and Bartlett.

Cottler-Fox, M.H., Lapidot, T., Petit, I., Kollet, O., DiPersio, J.F., Link, D., et al. (2003). Stem cell mobilization. *Hematology: The Education Program of the American Society of Hematology*, pp. 419–437.

Crawford, S.W. (1999). Noninfectious lung disease in the immunocompromised host. *Respiration, 66*, 385–395.

Cutler, C., Giri, S., Jeyapalan, S., Paniagua, D., Viswanathan, A., & Antin, J. (2001). Acute and chronic graft versus host disease after allogeneic peripheral blood stem cell and bone marrow transplantation: A meta-analysis. *Journal of Clinical Oncology, 19*, 3685–3693.

Dawson, M.A., Schwarer, A.P., Muirhead, J.L., Bailey, M.J., Bollard, G.M., & Spencer, A. (2005). Successful mobilization of peripheral blood stem cells using recombinant human stem cell factor in heavily pretreated patients who have failed a previous attempt with a granulocyte colony-stimulating factor-based regimen. *Bone Marrow Transplantation, 36*, 389–396.

Dean, R.M., & Bishop, M.R. (2003). Graft-versus-host disease: Emerging concepts in prevention and therapy. *Current Hematology Reports, 2*, 287–294.

Diedrich, B., Remberger, M., Shanwell, A., Svahn, B.M., & Ringden, O. (2005). A prospective randomized trial of prophylactic platelet transfusion trigger of 10×10^9 per L versus 30×10^9 per L in allogeneic hematopoietic progenitor cell transplant recipients. *Transfusion, 45*, 1064–1072.

Demirer, T., Ilhan, O., Ayil, M., Arat, M., Dagli, M., Ozcan, M.H., et al. (2002). Monitoring of peripheral blood CD34+ cell counts on the first day of apheresis is highly predictive for efficient CD34+ cell yield. *Therapeutic Apheresis, 6*, 384–389.

Douglas, T.T., & Shelton, B.K. (2007). Renal and hepatic effects. In S. Ezzone & K. Schmit-Pokorny (Eds.), *Blood and marrow stem cell transplantation: Principles, practice and nursing insights* (3rd ed., pp. 263–295). Sudbury, MA: Jones and Bartlett.

Dudek, A.Z., Mahaseth, H., DeFor, T.E., & Weisdorf, D.J. (2003). Bronchiolitis obliterans in chronic graft-versus-host disease: Analysis of risk factors and treatment outcomes. *Biology of Blood and Marrow Transplantation, 9*, 657–666.

Erlich, H.A., Oelz, G., & Hansen, J. (2001). HLA DNA typing and transplantation. *Immunity, 14*, 347–356.

Ezzone, S.A. (Ed.). (1997). *Peripheral blood stem cell transplantation: Recommendations for nursing education and practice*. Pittsburgh, PA: Oncology Nursing Society.

Ezzone, S.A., & Camp-Sorrell, D. (Eds.). (1994). *Manual for bone marrow transplant nursing: Recommendations for practice and education*. Pittsburgh, PA: Oncology Nursing Society.

Ezzone, S., Fliedner, M., & Sirilla, J. (2007). Transplant networks and standards of care: International perspectives. In S. Ezzone & K. Schmit-Pokorny (Eds.), *Blood and marrow stem cell transplantation: Principles, practice and nursing insights* (3rd ed., pp. 441–461). Sudbury, MA: Jones and Bartlett.

Ferrell, B., Grant, G., Schmidt, M., Rhiner, M., Whitehead, C., Fonbuena, P., et al. (1992). The meaning of quality of life for bone marrow transplant survivors. Part 1. The impact of bone marrow transplant on quality of life. *Cancer Nursing, 15*, 153–160.

Filipovich, A.H., Weisdorf, D., Pavletic, S., Socie, G., Wingard, J.R., Lee, S.J., et al. (2005). National Institutes of Health consensus development project on criteria for clinical trials in chronic graft-versus-host disease: I. Diagnosis and staging working group report. *Biology of Blood and Marrow Transplantation, 11*, 945–956.

Flomenberg, N., Devine, S.M., DiPersio, J.F., Liesweld, J.L., McCarty, J.M., Rowley, S.D., et al. (2005). The use of AMD3100 plus G-CSF for autologous hematopoietic progenitor cell mobilization is superior to G-CSF alone. *Blood, 106*, 1867–1874.

Ford, C.E., Hamerton, J.L., Barnes, D.W., & Loutit, J.F. (1956). Cytological identification of radiation-chimaeras. *Nature, 177*, 452–454.

Foundation for the Accreditation of Cellular Therapy. (2008). *Hematopoietic progenitor cell collection, processing, and transplantation: Accreditation manual* (3rd ed.). Omaha, NE: Author.

Fruehauf, S., Klaus, J., Huesing, J., Veldwijk, M.R., Buss, E.C., Topaly, J., et al. (2007). Efficient mobilization of peripheral blood stem cells following CAD chemotherapy and a single dose of pegylated G-CSF in patients with multiple myeloma. *Bone Marrow Transplantation, 39*, 743–750.

Gasova, Z., Marinov, I., Vodvarkova, S., Bohmova, M., & Bhuvian-Ludvikova, Z. (2005). PBPC collection techniques: Standard versus large volume leukapheresis (LVL) in donors and in patients. *Transfusion and Apheresis Science, 32*, 167–176.

Gluckman, E., Rocha, V., & Chastang, C. (2000). Allogeneic cord blood hematopoietic stem cell transplants in malignancies. In J.O. Armitage & K.H. Antman (Eds.), *High-dose cancer therapy: Pharmacology, hematopoietins, stem cells* (3rd ed., pp. 211–220). Philadelphia: Lippincott Williams & Wilkins.

Glucksberg, H., Storb, R., Fefer, A., Buckner, C.D., Neiman, P.E., Clift, R.A., et al. (1974). Clinical manifestations of graft versus host disease in human recipients of marrow from HLA-matched sibling donors. *Transplantation, 18*, 295–304.

Gross, J., & Johnson, B.L. (Eds.). (1994). *Handbook of oncology nursing.* Sudbury, MA: Jones and Bartlett.

Hebert, P.C., Wells, G., Blajchman, M.A., Marshall, J., Martin, C., Pagliarello, G., et al. (1999). A multicenter randomized, controlled clinical trial of transfusion requirement in critical care. *New England Journal of Medicine, 340,* 409–416.

Huang, Y., Kucia, M., Rezzoug, F., Ratajczak, J., Tanner, M.K., Ratajczak, M.Z., et al. (2006). Flt3-ligand-mobilized peripheral blood, but not Flt3-ligand-expanded bone marrow, facilitating cells promote establishment of chimerism and tolerance. *Stem Cells, 24,* 936–948.

Huff, C.A., Fuchs, E.J., Smith, D., Blackford, A., Garrett-Mayer, E., Brodsky, R.A., et al. (2006). Graft-versus-host reactions and the effectiveness of donor lymphocyte infusions. *Biology of Blood and Marrow Transplantation, 12,* 414–421.

Hurley, C.K., Baxter Lowe, L.A., Logan, B., Karanes, C., Anasetti, C., Weisdorf, D., et al. (2003). National Marrow Donor Program HLA-matching guidelines for unrelated marrow transplants. *Biology of Blood and Marrow Transplantation, 9,* 610–615.

Johnson, G.B., & Quiett, K. (2004). Hematologic effects. In S. Ezzone (Ed.), *Hematopoietic stem cell transplantation: A manual for nursing practice* (pp. 133–145). Pittsburgh, PA: Oncology Nursing Society.

Kataoka, Y., Iwasaki, T., Kuroiwa, T., Seto, Y., Iwata, N., Kaneda, Y., et al. (2001). The role of donor T cells for target organ injuries in acute and chronic graft versus host disease. *Immunology, 103,* 310–318.

Keller, C.A. (2004). Cardiopulmonary effects. In S. Ezzone (Ed.), *Hematopoietic stem cell transplantation: A manual for nursing practice* (pp. 177–189). Pittsburgh, PA: Oncology Nursing Society.

Kim, B., Chung, K., Sun, H., Suh, J., Min, W., Kang, C., et al. (2000). Liver diseases during the first post-transplant year in bone marrow transplantation recipients: Retrospective study. *Bone Marrow Transplantation, 26,* 193–197.

Korbling, M., & Anderlini, P. (2001). Peripheral blood stem cell versus bone marrow allotransplantation: Does the source of hematopoietic stem cells matter? *Blood, 98,* 2900–2908.

Kreit, J.W. (2000). Respiratory complications. In E.D. Ball, J. Lister, & P. Law (Eds.), *Hematopoietic stem cell therapy* (pp. 563–577). New York: Churchill Livingstone.

Laughlin, J. (2005). Transplantation of 2 UCB units in adults. *Blood, 105,* 915–916.

Lewis, I.D., DeFor, T., & Weisdorf, D.J. (2000). Increasing incidence of diffuse alveolar hemorrhage following allogeneic bone marrow transplantation: Cryptic etiology and uncertain therapy. *Bone Marrow Transplantation, 26,* 539–543.

Loberiza, F. (2003). Report on state of the art in blood and marrow transplantation—Part 1 of the IBMTR/ABMTR summary slides with guide. *IBMTR/ABMTR Newsletter, 10*(1), 7–10.

Luznik, L., & Fuchs, E.J. (2002). Donor lymphocyte infusions to treat hematologic malignancies in relapse after allogeneic blood or marrow transplantation. *Cancer Control, 9,* 123–137.

Mangan, K.F. (2000). Choice of conditioning regimens. In E.D. Ball, J. Lister, & P. Law (Eds.), *Hematopoietic stem cell therapy* (pp. 403–413). New York: Churchill Livingstone.

Marcellus, D.C., & Vogelsang, G.B. (2000). Chronic graft versus host disease. In E.D. Ball, J. Lister, & P. Law (Eds.), *Hematopoietic stem cell therapy* (pp. 514–624). New York: Churchill Livingstone.

McAdams, F.W., & Burgunder, M.R. (2004). Transplant course. In S. Ezzone (Ed.), *Hematopoietic stem cell transplantation: A manual for nursing practice* (pp. 43–49). Pittsburgh, PA: Oncology Nursing Society.

Mitchell, S. (2004). Graft versus host disease. In S. Ezzone (Ed.), *Hematopoietic stem cell transplantation: A manual for nursing practice* (pp. 85–131). Pittsburgh, PA: Oncology Nursing Society.

Montgomery, M., & Cottler-Fox, M. (2007). Mobilization and collection of autologous hematopoietic progenitor/stem cells. *Clinical Advances in Hematology and Oncology, 5,* 127–136.

Morishima, Y., Sasazuke, T., Inoko, H., Juji, T., Akaza, T., Yamamoto, K., et al. (2002). The clinical significance of human leukocyte antigen (HLA) allele compatibility in patients receiving a marrow transplant from serologically HLA-A, HLA-B, HLA-DR matched unrelated donors. *Blood, 99,* 4200–4206.

Newborn Blood Banking, Inc. (2007). *Storing life blood.* Retrieved April 29, 2007, from http://www.newbornblood.com

Niess, D., & Duffy, K.M. (2004). Basic concepts of transplantation. In S. Ezzone (Ed.), *Hematopoietic stem cell transplantation: A manual for nursing practice* (pp. 13–21). Pittsburgh, PA: Oncology Nursing Society.

Ozdogan, O., Ratip, S., Al Ahdab, Y., Dane, E., Al Ahdab, H., Imeryuz, N., et al. (2003). Causes and risk factors for liver injury following bone marrow transplantation. *Journal of Clinical Gastroenterology, 36,* 421–428.

Parikh, C.R., McSweeney, P.A., Korular, D., Ecder, T., Merouani, A., Taylor, J., et al. (2002). Renal dysfunction in allogeneic hematopoietic cell transplantation. *Kidney International, 62,* 566–573.

Park, S., Noguera, M.E., Briere, J., Feuillard, J., Cayuela, J.M., Sigaux, F., et al. (2002). Successful rituximab treatment of an EBV-related lymphoproliferative disease arising after autologous transplantation for angioimmunoblastic T-cell lymphoma. *Hematology Journal, 3,* 317–320.

Pavletic, S.Z., Lee, S.J., Socie, G., & Vogelsang, G. (2006). Chronic graft-versus-host disease: Implications of the National Institutes of Health consensus development project on criteria for clinical trials. *Bone Marrow Transplantation, 38,* 645–651.

Pedersen-Bjergaard, J., Anderson, M.K., & Christiansen, D.H. (2000). Therapy-related acute myeloid leukemia and myelodysplasia after high dose chemotherapy and autologous stem cell transplantation. *Blood, 95,* 3273–3279.

Petersdorf, E.W., Hansen, J.A., Martin, P.J., Woolfrey, A., Malkki, M., Gooley, T., et al. (2001). Major-histocompatibility-complex class I alleles and antigens in hematopoietic-cell transplantation. *New England Journal of Medicine, 345,* 1794–1800.

Piacibello, W., Sanavio, F., Garetto, L., Severino, A., Dane, A., Gammaitoni, L., et al. (1998). The role of c-Mpl ligands in the expansion of cord blood hematopoietic progenitors. *Stem Cells, 16*(Suppl. 2), 243–248.

Poliquin, C. (2007). Conditioning regimens in hematopoietic stem cell transplantation. In S. Ezzone & K. Schmit-Pokorny (Eds.), *Blood and marrow stem cell transplantation: Principles, practice and nursing insights* (3rd ed., pp. 109–146). Sudbury, MA: Jones and Bartlett.

Prentice, G., Grundy, J.E., & Kho, P. (1998). Cytomegalovirus. In J. Barrett & J.G. Treleaven (Eds.), *The clinical practice of stem cell transplantation, vol. 2* (pp. 697–707). St. Louis, MO: Mosby.

Przepiorka, D., Weisdorf, D., Martin, P., Klingemann, H.G., Beatty, P., Hows, J., et al. (1995). 1994 consensus conference on acute GVHD grading. *Bone Marrow Transplantation, 15,* 825–828.

Quine, W.E. (1896). The remedial application of bone marrow. *JAMA, 26,* 1012–1013.

Reed, M., Yearsley, M., Krugh, D., & Kennedy, M. (2003). Severe hemolysis due to passenger lymphocyte syndrome after hematopoietic stem cell transplantation from an HLA-matched related donor. *Archives of Pathology and Laboratory Medicine, 127,* 1366–1368.

Riley, U. (1998). Bacterial infections. In J. Barrett & J.G. Treleaven (Eds.), *The clinical practice of stem cell transplantation, vol. 2* (pp. 690–696). St. Louis, MO: Mosby.

Rocha, V., Cornish, J., Sievers, E.L., Filipovich, A., Locatelli, F., Peters, C., et al. (2001). Comparison of outcomes of unrelated bone marrow and umbilical cord blood transplants in children with acute leukemia. *Blood, 97,* 2962–2971.

Roemer, E., Blau, I.W., Basara, N., Kiehl, M.G., Bischoff, M., Gunzelmann, S., et al. (2001). Toxoplasmosis, a severe complication in allogeneic hematopoietic stem cell transplantation: Successful treatment strategies during a 5-year single-center experience. *Clinical Infectious Diseases, 32,* E1–E8.

Roitt, I., Brostoff, J., & Male, D. (Eds.). (1996). *Immunology* (4th ed.). London: Mosby.

Ruble, K. (2007). Late effects of bone marrow transplant. In S. Ezzone & K. Schmit-Pokorny (Eds.), *Blood and marrow stem cell transplantation: Principles, practice and nursing insights* (3rd ed., pp. 327–338). Sudbury, MA: Jones and Bartlett.

Schiffer, C.A., Anderson, K.C., Bennett, C.L., Bernstein, S., Elting, L.S., Goldsmith, M., et al. (2001). Platelet transfusion for patients with cancer: Clinical practice guidelines of the American Society of Clinical Oncology. *Journal of Clinical Oncology, 19,* 1519–1538.

Schmit-Pokorny, K. (2004). Stem cell collection. In S. Ezzone (Ed.), *Hematopoietic stem cell transplantation: A manual for nursing practice* (pp. 23–42). Pittsburgh, PA: Oncology Nursing Society.

Schmit-Pokorny, K. (2007). Bone marrow transplantation: Indications, procedure, process. In S. Ezzone & K. Schmit-Pokorny (Eds.), *Blood and marrow stem cell transplantation: Principles, practice and nursing insights* (3rd ed., pp. 1–27). Sudbury, MA: Jones and Bartlett.

Shapiro, T.W., Davison, D.B., & Rust, D.M.A. (1997). *Clinical guide to stem cell and bone marrow transplantation.* Sudbury, MA: Jones and Bartlett.

Shelton, B. (2007). Neurologic complications of hematopoietic stem cell transplantation. In S. Ezzone & K. Schmit-Pokorny (Eds.), *Blood and marrow stem cell transplantation: Principles, practice and nursing insights* (3rd ed., pp. 297–325). Sudbury, MA: Jones and Bartlett.

Shulman, H.M., Sale, G.E., Lerner, K.G., Barker, E.A., Weiden, P.L., Sullivan, K., et al. (1978). Chronic cutaneous graft-versus-host disease in man. *American Journal of Pathology, 91,* 545–570.

Snustad, D.P., & Simmons, M.J. (2000). *Principles of genetics* (2nd ed.). New York: Wiley.

Stevens, M.M. (2004). Gastrointestinal complications of hematopoietic stem cell transplantation. In S. Ezzone (Ed.), *Hematopoietic stem cell transplantation: A manual for nursing practice* (pp. 147–165). Pittsburgh, PA: Oncology Nursing Society.

Sundin, M., LeBlanc, K., Olle, R., Barholt, L., Omazic, B., Lergin, C., et al. (2006). The role of HLA mismatch, splenectomy and recipient Epstein-Barr virus seronegativity as risk factors in post-transplant lymphoproliferative disorder following allogeneic hematopoietic stem cell transplantation. *Haematologica, 91,* 1059–1067.

Thomas, E.D., Lochte, H.L., Jr., Cannon, J.H., Sahler, O.D., & Ferrebee, J.W. (1959). Supralethal whole body irradiation and isologous marrow transplantation in man. *Journal of Clinical Investigation, 38,* 1709–1716.

Thomas, E.D., Storb, R., Clift, R.A., Fefer, A., Johnson, F.L., Neiman, P.E., et al. (1975). Bone marrow transplantation. *New England Journal of Medicine, 292,* 895–902.

van Burik, J.A., & Weisdorf, D.J. (1999). Infections in recipients of blood and marrow transplantation. *Hematology/Oncology Clinics of North America, 13,* 1065–1089.

Veys, P., & Owens, C. (2002). Respiratory infections following haemopoietic stem cell transplantation in children. *British Medical Bulletin, 61,* 151–174.

Vogelsang, G.B., Lee, L., & Bensen-Kennedy, D.B. (2003). Pathogenesis and treatment of graft-versus-host disease after bone marrow transplant. *Annual Review of Medicine, 54,* 29–52.

Warnick, E. (2004). Neurologic complications. In S. Ezzone (Ed.), *Hematopoietic stem cell transplantation: A manual for nursing practice* (pp. 191–199). Pittsburgh, PA: Oncology Nursing Society.

Warnick, E., & Rust, D. (2007). Gastrointestinal effects. In S. Ezzone & K. Schmit-Pokorny (Eds.), *Blood and marrow stem cell transplantation: Principles, practice and nursing insights* (3rd ed., pp. 207–243). Sudbury, MA: Jones and Bartlett.

Westmoreland, D. (1998). Other viral infections. In J. Barrett & J.G. Treleaven (Eds.), *The clinical practice of stem cell transplantation* (Vol. 2, pp. 709–721). St. Louis, MO: Mosby.

Williams, L. (2004). Comprehensive review of hematopoiesis and immunology: Implications for hematopoietic stem cell transplant recipients. In S. Ezzone (Ed.), *Hematopoietic stem cell transplantation: A manual for nursing practice* (pp. 1–12). Pittsburgh, PA: Oncology Nursing Society.

Zitella, L., Friese, C., Gobel, B.H., Woolery-Antill, M., O'Leary, C., Hauser, J., et al. (2006). *Putting evidence into practice (PEP®): Prevention of infection.* Pittsburgh, PA: Oncology Nursing Society.

CHAPTER 8

Complementary and Integrative Therapies

Colleen O. Lee, MS, CRNP, AOCN®

Introduction

Complementary and alternative medicine (CAM) is a broad domain of resources that surrounds the modalities, practices, and health belief systems and their associated theories that are other than those of the surrounding society or culture within a historical period of time (Committee on the Use of Complementary and Alternative Medicine by the American Public, Institute of Medicine of the National Academies, 2005). Complementary medicine modalities are used alongside conventional medicine, whereas alternative medicine modalities are used instead of conventional medicine. Some modalities are considered both complementary and alternative. *Conventional medicine* is medicine that is practiced by medical doctors, osteopaths, and allied health professionals and also is termed *allopathic* or *Western* medicine. Conventional approaches, known as *standard, traditional,* or *biomedical* approaches, are those that historically have seen broad application in the United States since the 1800s. *Quackery* is the scientifically unfounded positive assurances of disease control or cure that remain, although diminished, today (Karnofsky, 1959; Winnick, 2005).

The major domains of CAM are (a) alternative medical systems, (b) energy therapies (including biofield and electromagnetic-based therapies), (c) exercise therapies (formerly movement therapies), (d) manipulative and body-based methods, (e) mind-body interventions, (f) nutritional therapeutics, (g) pharmacologic and biologic treatments (including the subcategory of complex natural products), and (h) spiritual therapies (National Cancer Institute [NCI] Office of Cancer Complementary and Alternative Medicine, 2007). Characterizations of these domains and examples are listed in Table 8-1.

Integrative medicine combines conventional and CAM modalities for which high-quality evidence of safety and effectiveness exists and is an emergent healthcare approach with the development of centers nationwide (National Institutes of Health [NIH] Na-

Table 8-1. Complementary and Alternative Medicine Modalities in Clinical Trials

Domain	Definition	Examples	Examples of Modalities Studied in Clinical Trials
Alternative medical systems	Systems built upon well-developed systems of theory and practice	Traditional Chinese medicine (acupuncture), Ayurveda, homeopathy, naturopathy, Tibetan medicine	Traditional Chinese medicine (acupuncture), acupressure, homeopathy (Traumeel S®, Heel Co.)
Energy therapies	Therapies involving the use of energy fields	Qigong, Reiki, therapeutic touch, pulsed fields, magnet therapy	Qigong, Reiki, therapeutic touch
Exercise therapies	Modalities used to improve patterns of bodily movement	Tai Chi, Feldenkrais, hatha yoga, Alexander technique, dance therapy, Rolfing, Trager method, applied kinesiology	Tai Chi, hatha yoga
Manipulative and body-based methods	Methods based on manipulation and/or movement of one or more parts of the body	Chiropractic, therapeutic massage, osteopathy, reflexology	Therapeutic massage, reflexology
Mind-body interventions	Techniques designed to enhance the mind's capacity to affect bodily function and symptoms	Meditation, hypnosis, art therapy, biofeedback, mental healing, imagery, relaxation therapy, support groups, music therapy, cognitive-behavioral therapy, psychoneuroimmunology, aromatherapy, animal-assisted therapy	Meditation, art therapy, imagery, relaxation therapy, music therapy, cognitive-behavioral therapy, aromatherapy, animal-assisted therapy, narrative medicine
Nutritional therapeutics	Assortment of nutrients, non-nutrients, and bioactive food components that are used as chemopreventive agents, and the use of specific foods or diets as cancer prevention or treatment strategies	Dietary regimens such as macrobiotics, vegetarian, Gerson therapy, Kelley/Gonzalez regimen, vitamins, dietary macronutrients, supplements, antioxidants, melatonin, selenium, coenzyme Q10, ephedrine, orthomolecular medicine	Selenium, curcumin, soy isoflavones, genistein, lycopene, omega-3 fatty acids, L-carnitine, alpha-lipoic acid, glutamine, coenzyme Q10, zinc, Gonzalez regimen
Pharmacologic and biologic treatments	Drugs, complex natural products, vaccines, and other biologic interventions not yet accepted in mainstream medicine; off-label use of prescription drugs	Antineoplastons, 714-X, low-dose naltrexone, Met-enkephalin, immunoaugmentive therapy, Laetrile, hydrazine sulfate, Newcastle virus, ozone therapy, thymus therapy, enzyme therapy, high-dose vitamin C	Antineoplastons, ascorbic acid

(Continued on next page)

Table 8-1. Complementary and Alternative Medicine Modalities in Clinical Trials
(Continued)

Domain	Definition	Examples	Examples of Modalities Studied in Clinical Trials
Complex natural products	Subcategory of pharmacologic and biologic treatments consisting of an assortment of plant samples (botanicals), extracts of crude natural substances, and unfractionated extracts from marine organisms used for healing and treatment of disease	Herbs and herbal extracts, mixtures of tea polyphenols, shark cartilage, Essiac tea, cordyceps, Sun Soup, MGN-3, products from honey bees, mistletoe	Green tea extract, Essiac tea, mistletoe, valerian, noni fruit extract, licorice root, *Boswellia serrata*
Spiritual therapies	Interventions geared toward connection with or source of ultimate meaning (Silverman & Schneider, 2006)	Intercessory prayer, spiritual healing	Prayer

Note. From "Clinical Trials in Cancer Part 1: Biomedical, Complementary, and Alternative Medicine: Finding Active Trials and Results of Closed Trials," by C.O. Lee, 2004, *Clinical Journal of Oncology Nursing, 8,* p. 534. Copyright 2004 by Oncology Nursing Society. Adapted with permission.

tional Center for Complementary and Alternative Medicine [NCCAM], 2007c). Integrative oncology expands the conventional focus of cancer care in several ways: It (a) considers body, mind, soul, and spirit within cultural groups, (b) renews the focus of medicine back to its foundational guiding principles, (c) expands the goal of intervention to include translational, preventive, and supportive medicine, and (d) develops recommendations based on therapy goals and individual risk-benefit analyses (Mumber, 2006b).

Although a formal definition has not been established, CAM practitioners generally are thought to be individuals who deliver CAM modalities as part of or all of their practice. They may hold state, national, or certifying body licensure and practice across multiple settings. CAM researchers, likewise, generally are thought to be individuals who embrace an interest in developing theoretical frameworks and sound methodology for the investigation of CAM modalities in preclinical and clinical settings as a part of or all of their research endeavors.

Complementary and Integrative Therapy Use in the United States

The use of CAM and surveys measuring its use has been increasing steadily in recent decades in the United States. Topics significant in understanding CAM utilization are prevalence (the frequency with which use occurs), motive (the reasons for using CAM), and patient characteristics (the people who use it). Data from the 2002 National Center for Health Statistics (NCHS) indicated that 62% of adults in the United

States had used some form of CAM therapy during the previous 12 months (Barnes, Powell-Griner, McFann, & Nahin, 2004). Back or neck pain, colds, joint pain and stiffness, anxiety, and depression were the most common conditions for which individuals sought CAM therapies. Specifically in the oncology population, studies conducted since 2000 (N ≥ 100) found that 25%–80% of adults had used CAM (Ashikaga, Bosompra, O'Brien, & Nelson, 2002; Bernstein & Grasso, 2001; Maskarinec, Shumay, Kakai, & Gotay, 2000; Richardson, Sanders, Palmer, Greisinger, & Singletary, 2000; Sparber et al., 2000; Swisher et al., 2002).

Adults who used CAM reportedly were more likely to do so because they believed that combining CAM with conventional therapy would be beneficial, interesting to try, or in agreement with their health and life beliefs (Astin, 1998; Barnes et al., 2004). These data support the findings of previously published, well-known national surveys (Eisenberg et al., 1998; Kessler et al., 2001). Survey data to date have not yet captured the frequency to which patients with cancer choose to *forgo* conventional therapy in favor of conventional therapy, but a recent small study (N = 31) that took place in Canada described four potential predisposing factors: (1) negative prior experiences with conventional medicine, (2) experiences of family members who died under the care of conventional medicine, (3) use of CAM therapies prior to cancer diagnosis, and (4) strong belief system of the value of mind-body healing versus conventional medicine (Verhoef & White, 2002).

According to the NCHS survey, CAM use spans all ethnic backgrounds and was found to be greater in women, individuals with higher education levels, individuals who have been hospitalized in the past year, and former smokers versus current smokers or those who never smoked (Barnes et al., 2004). In a recent survey of patients with cancer (N = 100) and caregivers (N = 80), higher patient education level was associated with a predetermined selection of an increased number of CAM therapies from one therapy to two or three therapies (Kozachik, Wyatt, Given, & Given, 2006).

Despite the increasing number of surveys, comparatively little is known about what patients expect from CAM therapy versus what is experienced, characteristics differentiating the use of one versus more than one therapy, the relationship between health status and CAM use, patterns of use over time, reasons for participating in clinical trials involving CAM, reasons for referral (or lack of referral), and more specific use among patients with cancer. Recent inquiry is attempting to address some of these areas (Goldstein et al., 2005; Kozachik et al., 2006; Richardson, Masse, Nanny, & Sanders, 2004).

Complementary and Integrative Therapies Research

In tandem with increasing interest in and use of CAM in the United States, a growing amount of research dollars is being dedicated to the prevention, diagnosis, and treatment of acute and chronic conditions (and their related symptoms) through the use of CAM. Between 1999 and 2005, NIH sponsored CAM research expenditures across all institutes, which more than doubled from $116 million to $303 million dollars (NIH NCCAM, 2007a). In fiscal year 2005, NCI supported approximately $121,077,000 in the form of grants, cooperative agreements, supplements, or contracts representing more than 400 projects related to cancer CAM (NCI, 2006).

Levels of evidence in CAM are developed in the same manner as in conventional medicine, starting with clinical trials for prevention, supportive care, and treatment. The positive or negative clinical trial results form the foundation for a meta-analysis and systematic review that, in turn, affect the development of evidence-based practice, research utilization, evidence-based health care, and practice guidelines. Levels of evidence are used regularly by organizations such as NCI (n.d.) for clinical trials and the Oncology Nursing Society (ONS) in its Priority Symptom Management project (Ropka & Spencer-Cisek, 2001) and Putting Evidence Into Practice® resources (ONS, n.d.). Levels of evidence also are used in databases such as the Natural Medicines Comprehensive Database (www.naturaldatabase .com) and the Natural Standard databases (www.naturalstandard.com).

Meta-analyses and systematic reviews compile the best available knowledge in their respective content areas and are vital in facilitating public policy, practice decision making, and integration into cancer care. The Cochrane Collaboration, a premier source for systematic reviews in CAM, contains more than 200 completed systematic reviews, some of which include cancer CAM (Cochrane Library, n.d.; University of Maryland Complementary Medicine Program, n.d.). Meta-analyses and systematic reviews are not available for all areas in cancer CAM; thus, clinical trial results, unpublished data (e.g., dissertations), and case reports can be found in biomedical, social science, and nursing journals (either print or electronic). Finally, NCI's Physician Data Query (PDQ®) offers clinical trial results for closed trials in the "status of trial" option in the advanced search mechanism (www.cancer.gov/Search/SearchClinicalTrialsAdvanced.aspx) and in the PDQ cancer information summaries on CAM (www.cancer.gov/cancertopics/pdq/cam).

Complementary and Integrative Therapies Standards

Dietary Supplement Health and Education Act of 1994

CAM's influence on individuals, the public, hospitals, managed care plans, schools of nursing and medicine, and pharmacies is considerable; however, much remains unknown in terms of the safety and efficacy of most therapies. For those therapies that are not provider-based, such as nutritional therapies or dietary supplements, the U.S. Food and Drug Administration (FDA) gives oversight through the Dietary Supplement Health and Education Act (DSHEA) of 1994. The DSHEA allows manufacturers to use various statements on a product label that do not need preapproval, but claims must not be made about the diagnosis, prevention, treatment, or cure for a specific disease. The DSHEA grants the FDA the authority to develop good manufacturing practices governing preparation, packing, and holding of products (FDA, n.d.). The NIH Office of Dietary Supplements (ODS) also was created as a result of the DSHEA to promote, collect, and compile research and maintain a database on supplements and individual nutrients (NIH ODS, n.d.). From a consumer standpoint, the DSHEA allows for over-the-counter access to an array of products without the prerequisite of stringent requirements for manufacturing, product characterization, safety and efficacy data, and benefit claim as required for conventional medicines (Kinsel & Straus, 2003).

White House Commission on Complementary and Alternative Medicine

In 2000, the White House Commission on CAM (WHCC) was assembled at the request of the president of the United States and Congress to explore scientific policy and practice questions regarding CAM utilization. Several guiding principles emerged from these discussions: (a) deliver high-quality health care of the whole person, (b) use science to generate evidence that protects and promotes public health, (c) support the right to choose freely among safe and effective approaches and qualified practitioners, (d) promote partnerships and teamwork in integrated health care among patients, healthcare professionals (HCPs), and researchers committed to creating healing environments and respecting diversity of healthcare traditions, (e) disseminate comprehensive, timely evidence about CAM systems, practices, and products, and (f) obtain input from informed consumers for incorporation in proposing priorities for health care, research, and policy decisions (U.S. Department of Health and Human Services, 2002).

Federation of State Medical Boards

In April 2002, the Special Committee for the Study of Unconventional Health Care Practices of the Federation of State Medical Boards approved the Model Guidelines for the Use of Complementary and Alternative Therapies in Medical Practice. This model is used in educating and regulating physicians and those who co-manage patients, such as advanced practice nurses (APNs), who use CAM in their practices but may not be currently licensed by a governing body with licensed or state-regulated CAM providers. The guidelines affirm that all HCPs have a duty to avoid harm and a duty to act in a patient's best interest. The initiative encourages the medical community to adopt clinically responsible and ethically appropriate standards that promote public safety while at the same time educating HCPs on safeguards to ensure that services are provided within professional practice boundaries. Seven central areas are patient evaluation, treatment planning, consultation and/or referral to licensed or state-regulated HCPs, medical records documentation, education, selling of health-related products, and conformance to ethical standards when conducting clinical investigations. The ultimate emphasis is on balancing evidence-based practice while remaining compassionate and respectful of patient autonomy and dignity (Committee on the Use of Complementary and Alternative Medicine by the American Public, Institute of Medicine of the National Academies, 2005).

The WHCC guiding principles and Institute of Medicine model guidelines are the only existing framework on a national level at the present time. Although these documents provide an excellent framework for a societal, academic, and healthcare approach to CAM utilization, they are void of specific recommendations for nursing. The American Holistic Nurses Association (AHNA) and ONS have well-developed position statements that provide guidance and minimal competency expectations for nurses at all levels of practice. AHNA (n.d.-a) has published its *Position on the Role of Nurses in the Practice of Complementary and Alternative Therapies,* and ONS's (2006) position is titled *The Use of Complementary, Alternative, and Integrative Therapies in Cancer Care.* Several individual state boards of nursing have addressed the use of CAM and offered guidance to nurses, such as the Maryland Board of Nursing (www.mbon.org/main .php?v=norm&p=0&c=practice/therapies.html) and the California Board of Nursing (www.rn.ca.gov/pdfs/regulations/npr-b-28.pdf). CAM associations, schools, and domain-focused CAM centers have varying levels of guidelines and competency expectations. A searchable guide to CAM associations, centers, and institutes by domain is available through the National Library of Medicine Directory of Health Organizations (http://sis.nlm.nih.gov/dirline.html).

Complementary and Integrative Therapies Indications

Surveys, secondary analyses, systematic reviews, and studies support that CAM use is pervasive in all areas of oncology care, including prevention, supportive care (symptom management, palliative care, and end-of-life care), and treatment (Fouladbakhsh, Stommel, Given, & Given, 2005; Lafferty, Downey, McCarty, Standish, & Patrick, 2006; Lengacher et al., 2006; Yates et al., 2005). Use, however, does not signify efficacy or safety. Applying CAM modalities to any of the areas of cancer care today ultimately is a patient's choice, and the patient may or may not involve an oncology APN in the decision process. Some CAM modalities, however, can be safely used and have sufficient clinical research findings to support evidence-based recommendations.

Complementary and Alternative Medicine Modalities in Cancer Prevention

Multiple mechanisms such as genetics, environment, lifestyle, current and past health habits, and psychosocial attributes may have a role in cancer development (Offit & Siddiqui, 2004; Strickland & Kensler, 2004). Thus, cancer prevention using CAM modalities is multimodal in approach. Critical appraisal of the quality of CAM approaches in cancer prevention is available for a limited number of modalities at this time because of evolving approaches and impending clinical trials. Examples of CAM modalities that have evidence of effectiveness for cancer prevention are presented in Table 8-2.

Table 8-2. Prevention and Treatment Modalities for Common Cancers

Cancer Site	Complementary and Alternative Medicine Modalities
Breast	*Strong/good evidence:* No modality has been tested sufficiently yet to determine if strong evidence of efficacy exists. *Unclear or conflicting evidence:* Prevention—lycopene, soy; treatment—coenzyme Q10, evening primrose, flaxseed, resveratrol, vitamin B_{12}, vitamin E
Cervical	*Strong/good:* No modality has been tested sufficiently yet to determine if strong or good evidence of efficacy exists. *Unclear or Conflicting:* Dehydroepiandrosterone
Colorectal	*Strong/good:* No modality has been tested sufficiently yet to determine if strong or good evidence of efficacy exists. *Unclear or conflicting:* Prevention—calcium, omega-3 fatty acids, soy, vitamin E; treatment—protein-bound polysaccharide (PSK, adjuvant), psyllium
Gastric	*Strong/good:* No modality has been tested sufficiently yet to determine if strong or good evidence of efficacy exists. *Unclear or conflicting:* PSK
Leukemia	*Strong:* The prescription drug all-trans-retinoic acid is a vitamin A derivative that is an established treatment for acute promyelocytic leukemia.

(Continued on next page)

Table 8-2. Prevention and Treatment Modalities for Common Cancers *(Continued)*

Cancer Site	Complementary and Alternative Medicine Modalities
Lung	*Strong:* No modality has been tested sufficiently yet to determine if strong evidence of efficacy exists. *Good:* Probiotics *Unclear or conflicting:* Prevention—lycopene
Prostate	*Strong:* No modality has been tested sufficiently yet to determine if strong evidence of efficacy exists. *Good:* Prevention—selenium *Unclear or conflicting:* Prevention—vitamin E, lycopene, soy; treatment—green tea, PC-SPES, red clover, vitamin D

Note. This table comprises information available in the Natural Standard Database (www.naturalstandard .com) at the time of writing, September 20, 2007, as summarized by Shirley Triest-Robertson, and does not cover all types of cancer or cancer-related conditions. Natural Standard does not recommend specific therapies or practitioners. The Natural Standard grading scale is validated, reproducible, proprietary, and trademarked. Grading of evidence is per the Natural Standard scale as follows:

- Strong: Statistically significant evidence of benefit from > 2 randomized controlled trials *or* one properly conducted randomized controlled trial and one properly conducted meta-analysis. Strong evidence also may include evidence from several randomized controlled trials with evidence of benefit and supporting evidence in basic science, animal data, or theories.
- Good: Statistically significant evidence of benefit from 1–2 randomized controlled trials or evidence from ≥ 1 properly conducted meta-analysis or > 1 case-controlled or nonrandomized trials and supportive evidence from basic science, animal data, or theories.
- Unclear or conflicting: Evidence of benefit from ≥ 1 randomized controlled trial that may not have adequate size, power, or statistical significance, or conflicting evidence from multiple randomized controlled trials without evidence of benefit or ineffectiveness, or evidence of benefit from ≥ 1 case-controlled trial and without supporting evidence in basic science, animal data, or theories. This category also may include evidence of efficacy only from basic science, animal data, or theories.

Examples of CAM therapies that have been used in prevention trials include selenium, curcumin, soy isoflavones, green tea, genistein, probiotics, folate, grape seed extract, fish oil supplement, broccoli sprout extract, lycopene, and zinc (NCI, n.d.).

Complementary and Alternative Medicine Modalities in Symptom Management

Symptom management spans the precancer diagnosis to the survivorship spectrum. Tremendous advances have occurred in offering relief from symptoms associated with the disease process, its treatment, and the possible physical, emotional, spiritual, and psychological long-term consequences. The popularity and availability of CAM therapies have enhanced conventional approaches to symptom management in the past several years. An evidence-based review of both conventional and CAM modalities for common symptoms associated with cancer and its treatment was compiled recently (Decker, Lee, & Krebs, in press). Examples of effective CAM modalities for common cancer-related symptoms appear in Table 8-3.

Examples of CAM modalities in supportive care trials include omega-3 fatty acids, L-carnitine, valerian, alpha-lipoic acid, pet therapy, acupressure bracelets, auricular

Table 8-3. Evidence of Effective Complementary and Alternative Medicine Modalities for Common Cancer-Related Symptoms

Symptom	Complementary and Alternative Medicine Modalities
Anemia	*Strong:* For specific anemias • Folate: Megaloblastic anemia caused by folate deficiency • Iron: Iron-deficiency anemia and anemia of chronic disease • B_{12}: Megaloblastic anemia caused by B_{12} deficiency, pernicious anemia • B_6: Hereditary or sideroblastic anemia *Unclear or conflicting:* Iron, taurine, vitamin A (for iron-deficiency anemia), betel nut, riboflavin (B_2), vitamin E (for general anemia); antineoplastons, prayer/distant healing, vitamin B_{12} (for sickle-cell anemia); wheatgrass, zinc (for beta-thalassemia)
Anorexia/cachexia	*Strong evidence:* Soy and soy isoflavones (as a dietary source of protein); replacement of biotin, calcium, copper, folate, iodine, iron, niacin, pantothenic acid, phosphorus, riboflavin, vitamins A, B_{12}, B_6, C, D, E, and K in the setting of deficiency *Good evidence:* Vitamins B_1, C *Unclear or conflicting evidence:* Bromelain, devil's claw, hydrazine sulfate, safflower, taurine, zinc
Constipation	*Strong:* Aloe (aloe components have laxative properties) *Good:* Flaxseed, psyllium *Unclear or conflicting:* Ayurveda, barley, cascara, iodine, massage, probiotics, rhubarb
Depression	*Strong:* Music therapy (for mood enhancement), St. John's wort (for depressive disorders) *Good:* 5-hydroxytryptophan, dehydroepiandrosterone (DHEA), psychotherapy, yoga *Unclear or conflicting:* Acupressure, acupuncture, art therapy, Ayurveda, *Coleus forskohlii,* folate, ginkgo biloba, guarana, healing touch, kundalini yoga, lavender, massage, melatonin, omega-3 fatty acids, psychotherapy, Qi gong, Reiki, relaxation therapy, vitamin B_2, Tai Chi, vitamin B_6
Diarrhea	*Strong: Saccharomyces boulardii* (a probiotic that reduces the incidence of antibiotic-associated diarrhea) *Good:* Probiotics, psyllium *Unclear or conflicting:* Arrowroot, berberine, bilberry, colonic irrigation, goldenseal, *Lactobacillus acidophilus, Saccharomyces boulardii* (*Clostridium difficile*), slippery elm, soy, vitamin A
Fatigue	*Strong/good:* No modality has been tested sufficiently yet to determine if strong or good evidence of efficacy exists. *Unclear or conflicting:* Shiatsu acupressure, acustimulation (used by patients undergoing hemodialysis), betel nut, ginseng, glyconutrients, kiwi, physical therapy, selenium, taurine, vitamin B_{12}, yoga; for chronic fatigue syndrome: DHEA, evening primrose oil, and folate
Menopausal symptoms	*Strong:* No modality has been tested sufficiently yet to determine if strong evidence of efficacy exists. *Good:* Calcium (for premenstrual symptoms), soy (for menopausal hot flashes) *Unclear or conflicting:* Acupuncture, black cohosh, bilberry, chiropractic, flaxseed and flaxseed oil, gamma linolenic acid, gamma oryzanol, ginseng, green tea, hypnotherapy, kudzu, maca, red clover, relaxation therapy, St. John's wort, traditional Chinese medicine, wild yam

(Continued on next page)

Table 8-3. Evidence of Effective Complementary and Alternative Medicine Modalities for Common Cancer-Related Symptoms *(Continued)*

Symptom	Complementary and Alternative Medicine Modalities
Mucositis	*Strong:* No modality has been tested sufficiently yet to determine if strong evidence of efficacy exists. *Unclear or conflicting:* Chamomile, zinc, Traumeel S® (Heel Co.), oral cryotherapy (ice chips), chamomile, povidone (Betadine®, Alcon, Inc.)
Nausea	*Strong:* No modality has been tested sufficiently yet to determine if strong evidence of efficacy exists. *Good:* Acupuncture and acupuncture-related interventions (electroacupoint stimulation, acupressure and acustimulation wrist bands, electroacupuncture), ginger *Unclear or conflicting:* Aromatherapy (for postoperative nausea), ginger (for postoperative nausea), transcutaneous electrical nerve stimulation (TENS) (for postoperative nausea)
Neuropathy	*Strong:* No modality has been tested sufficiently yet to determine if strong evidence of efficacy exists. *Good:* Gamma linolenic acid (omega-6 fatty acid to treat diabetic neuropathy) *Unclear or conflicting:* For peripheral neuropathy: acupuncture, TENS; for diabetic neuropathy: evening primrose, magnet therapy, physical therapy, zinc
Pain	*Strong:* No modality has been tested sufficiently yet to determine if strong evidence of efficacy exists. *Good:* Guided imagery, hypnotherapy, music therapy, physical therapy, therapeutic touch; acupuncture (for endoscopy), bromelain (for inflammation) *Unclear or conflicting:* Postoperative: Acupressure, acupuncture, healing touch, TENS Chronic pain: Acupuncture, healing touch, massage, Qi gong Localized pain: Acupuncture, chiropractic, TENS Dental pain: Propolis Postherpetic pain: Reishi mushroom Cancer pain: Acupuncture, TENS Burning pain: Acupuncture, TENS Inflammation: Clove, coleus, dandelion, euphorbia, eyebright, turmeric, vitamin D (immunomodulator) Nonspecific pain: Acupressure, acustimulation, focusing, lavender, psychotherapy, Reiki, relaxation therapy, shark cartilage Phantom limb pain: TENS
Sleep changes	*Strong:* Melatonin (for jet lag) *Good:* Melatonin (used for insomnia in older adults, sleep enhancement in healthy people); music therapy, valerian *Unclear or conflicting:* Acupuncture, Ayurveda, guided imagery, hypnotherapy, kundalini yoga, relaxation therapy, and yoga (for insomnia); chiropractic (for jet lag); 5-hydroxytryptophan (for sleep disorders); aromatherapy, chamomile, and lemon balm (used as sleep aids)
Taste changes	*Strong/good:* No modality has been tested sufficiently yet to determine if strong or good evidence of efficacy exists. *Unclear or conflicting:* Zinc

(Continued on next page)

Table 8-3. Evidence of Effective Complementary and Alternative Medicine Modalities for Common Cancer-Related Symptoms *(Continued)*

Symptom	Complementary and Alternative Medicine Modalities
Xerostomia (psycho-tropic drug induced)	*Strong/good:* No modality has been tested sufficiently yet to determine if strong or good evidence of efficacy exists. *Unclear or conflicting:* Acupuncture, yohimbe (for dry mouth)

Note. This table comprises information available in the Natural Standard Database (www.naturalstandard .com) at the time of writing, September 20, 2007, as summarized by Shirley Triest-Robertson, and does not cover all types of cancer or cancer-related conditions. Natural Standard does not recommend specific therapies or practitioners. The Natural Standard grading scale is validated, reproducible, proprietary, and trademarked. Grading of evidence is per the Natural Standard scale as follows:
- Strong: Statistically significant evidence of benefit from > 2 randomized controlled trials *or* one properly conducted randomized controlled trial and one properly conducted meta-analysis. Strong evidence also may include evidence from several randomized controlled trials with evidence of benefit and supporting evidence in basic science, animal data, or theories.
- Good: Statistically significant evidence of benefit from 1–2 randomized controlled trials or evidence from ≥ 1 properly conducted meta-analysis or > 1 case-controlled or nonrandomized trials and supportive evidence from basic science, animal data, or theories.
- Unclear or conflicting: Evidence of benefit from ≥ 1 randomized controlled trial that may not have adequate size, power, or statistical significance, or conflicting evidence from multiple randomized controlled trials without evidence of benefit or ineffectiveness, or evidence of benefit from ≥ 1 case-controlled trial and without supporting evidence in basic science, animal data, or theories. This category also may include evidence of efficacy only from basic science, animal data, or theories.

acupuncture, healing touch, Reiki/energy therapy, meditation, garlic, ginger, Pycnogenol® (Horphag Research), mindfulness meditation, Tai Chi, massage, glutamine, hatha yoga, coenzyme Q10, narrative medicine, soy, and music therapy (NCI, n.d.).

Complementary and Alternative Medicine Modalities in Cancer Treatment

The prevention and conventional treatment of cancer are complex disciplines and characteristically involve a multimodality approach. CAM prevention and treatment approaches for cancer in the United States, for the most part, remain under study. Table 8-2 lists examples of CAM modalities with evidence of effectiveness for cancer prevention and treatment.

Examples of CAM modalities in treatment trials include curcumin, coenzyme Q10, antineoplastons, genistein, fruit and vegetable extracts, calcitriol, green tea extract, selenium, *Boswellia serrata,* isoflavones, licorice root, beta-glucan, noni fruit extract, ascorbic acid, Essiac, mistletoe extract *(Viscum album),* and pomegranate juice (NCI, n.d.).

Complementary and Integrative Therapies Clinical Decision Making

Licensure and Credentialing

Legal experts explain that the doctrines that usually apply in healthcare law, such as malpractice and informed consent, are applicable to the practice and integration of CAM (Cohen, 2001). The requirements for professional practice vary by CAM modality. For example, acupuncture training leading to certification and licensure may take several years, whereas certification in therapeutic touch may take several months. Professional licensure is governed by state law, which leaves states able to regulate the health, safety, and welfare of citizens via a medical licensing statute. This statute prohibits the unlicensed practice of medicine. In most states, CAM providers who lack a medical license could be viewed as diagnosing and treating patients and as practicing medicine unlawfully. To provide a frame of reference, as reported in 2002: Chiropractors are licensed in all states; physician acupuncturists are licensed in 31 states (some exclusions apply); nonphysician acupuncturists are licensed in 42 states; naturopathic doctors are licensed in 11 states; massage therapists are licensed in 25 states; and homeopathic physicians are licensed in 3 states (Eisenberg et al., 2002). Training, internship/residency, and other educational requirements vary by state.

Certification for Nurses

AHNA is the sole nursing body that offers an inclusive certification in the area of CAM. New York University School of Nursing offers an APN practitioner program that is endorsed by AHNA and provides a program of study based on the standards of practice for holistic nursing (AHNA, n.d.-b). Many nurses choose to undergo training in specific areas of CAM, such as bodywork or aromatherapy, but these certifications focus on a specific modality versus the broad field. With increasing access to multiple sources, APNs can select preferred modes of learning and, over a period of time, develop baseline knowledge of CAM. An ongoing area of pursuit for many APNs, once they are certified and practicing in the CAM specialty, is reimbursement.

Third-Party and Medicare Coverage

Slowly, insurance companies and Medicare are recognizing CAM as a reimbursable expense via established billing codes for patients who choose these modalities for supportive care and/or treatment. The number and scope of current procedural terminology (CPT) codes for the billing of CAM services have increased in recent years. CAM services that do not yet have CPT codes are not considered covered. CAM-specific codes were proposed to document services rendered by CAM providers so that billing for these services would be more accurate. The coding system received initial attention but was later rejected by the Centers for Medicare and Medicaid Services (Alternative Link, 2007). Thus, CAM providers may opt to designate an office visit in which a CAM modality was delivered under a designation that is not CAM-specific. The coding selection may not be approved by the insurance company, and the patient potentially may need to pay out of pocket for the visit. The lack of reimbursable services poses a challenge for patients and conventional medicine and CAM providers who desire to offer integrative care. Current regulations require APNs to inform patients when potential services are not covered and to document patient awareness of these outstanding costs (Mumber, 2006a).

Core Competencies

A principal question arises as to what degree oncology APNs are responsible and accountable for baseline knowledge of CAM when patients choose to integrate conventional medicine with CAM. Compelling reasons to develop baseline knowledge are (a) patients use CAM, often without provider knowledge, so the topic must be addressed in the provider-patient relationship, (b) safe and effective CAM modalities exist for some common conditions, and oncology APNs need to be familiar with these modalities so that they can suggest options for a comprehensive approach to clinical problems, and (c) known or suspected interactions may occur between some CAM modalities and conventional care, and APNs need to avoid and recognize these interactions in a timely manner.

The development of clinical core competencies and curricula to teach core competencies is a sequential progression for oncology APNs in the attainment of baseline knowledge in CAM. This knowledge could be achieved through the completion of a smaller curriculum program or a larger fellowship program that teaches the established core competencies. Oncology APNs could then augment baseline knowledge and obtain nationally recognized certification. Ideally, the development of baseline knowledge would be simpler if nationally recognized practice guidelines governing the use of CAM were established and widely disseminated; however, as discussed earlier, these guidelines are not yet available.

CAM core competencies are fundamental skills, abilities, and expertise in the area of CAM and integrated medicine as applied to clinical scenarios versus the skills and abilities to deliver CAM interventions. In conceptualizing core competencies, general end points should be developed. Decker and Lee (2005) offered the following end points for nurses in cancer CAM.
- Expand baseline knowledge.
- Provide high-quality education regarding safety and efficacy.
- Facilitate partnerships between patients, HCPs, and CAM providers.
- Seek proper training and credentials if practicing a CAM therapy.
- Require informed consent if delivering a CAM therapy.
- Guarantee credentialing of a provider if referring a patient.
- Establish standards of practice for the use of CAM within specified patient groups.
- Document consent procedures and response to therapy.
- Assist in the design or maintenance of any preexisting integrated program.
- Develop a working knowledge of cost issues and reimbursement.
- Assist in the design of methodologically sound, rigorous research.
- Contribute to the body of knowledge through publications and presentations.

Burman (2003) developed similar specific core competencies for family nurse practitioners with many implications for nurse educators.

Curriculum Development

Through the Consortium of Academic Health Centers for Integrative Medicine (2006), programs integrating biomedicine and CAM train APNs as integrative medicine fellows. Nursing leaders and educators also are actively seeking content and developing curricula in CAM and integrated care (Halcon, Chlan, Kreitzer, & Leonard, 2003; Sofhauser, 2002). Continuing education not culminating in certification is offered by several government and industry sponsors (American Botanical Council, 2007; Center for Mind-Body Medicine, 2007; NIH NCCAM, 2007b). For self-paced learning, Lee (2005a) provides a thorough review of reliable written sources of high-quality CAM information that includes conventional and alternative medicine journals, electronic media and resources, full-text databases, and newsletters.

Conducting an Integrative Assessment and Advising Patients

Integrative assessments conducted by trained oncology APNs can elicit pertinent information regarding past and current use of CAM for various conditions as well as the potential for future use of CAM for cancer-related symptoms or treatment. A well-conducted integrative assessment by the oncology APN could potentially communicate an openness to learn the value and significance of CAM to patients. This, in turn, allows patients to express their willingness and desire to be involved in decision processes or to "take the lead" in affecting their care. Open dialogue can lead to an increased level of confidence on the part of patients in knowing that oncology APNs are interested in their viewpoints and concerns; possible identification of safe and effective modalities for specific symptoms; education regarding unsafe and ineffective modalities; and recognition of potential interactions between conventional and CAM modalities as care continues. Although no standard integrative assessment tool has been published, sources agree on the inclusion of several critical aspects.

- Health history basics: Demographics (including insurance), chief complaint, history of present illness, past medical history, medications (including adherence), allergies, social history, immunizations and travel, family history, review of systems, labs, diagnostics
- Integrative assessment basics: Comprehensive medication assessment (Lee, 2005b), previous and current CAM therapies (use, duration, reason, benefit, provider, cost, location, side effects), general well-being, nutrition, physical activity/exercise, stress management, spirituality, personal image, view toward illness state and recommended conventional therapies, and anticipated CAM use (or desire for more information) (Chong, 2006; Kenner, 2002; Maizes, Koffler, & Fleishman, 2002)
- Treatment plan basics (Jonas, Linde, & Walach, 1999): Is a safe and effective conventional therapy available? Is receiving a conventional therapy desirable to the patient? Is a safe and effective CAM therapy available? Is the population studied similar to the patient? Is there a strong belief or agreement in the rationale of the CAM therapy between the APN and patient? Is the CAM therapy affordable? Can the patient be monitored during the treatment period? Are interactions between the conventional and CAM therapies a risk? Has a plan for consistent follow-up been established?

A comprehensive guide to decision making in integrative oncology for nurses has not yet been developed, although many APNs are functioning daily in conducting assessments as described previously, advising patients about CAM, and developing integrative plans for cancer care. APNs who are in a position to refer or are functioning in roles that facilitate integrative care are cognizant of the challenges posed by risk management assessment, referral practices, billing audits, and required medical record documentation, all while overseeing the safe and effective delivery of both conventional and CAM practices. Attention to detail in proper communication and documentation of interactions among APNs is critical to this aspect of practice.

Herbal Products and Cytotoxic Agents

A discussion on advising patients in selecting CAM would be remiss without addressing the need to recognize and communicate potential drug interactions between herbal products and cytotoxic drugs. When herbs and cytotoxic drugs are taken simultaneously, the pharmacologic dynamics are not well understood and may not be realized in the short term. Overdosing or underdosing of cytotoxic agents can greatly affect a patient's course of care. APNs can perform an evaluation of interactions with the assistance of a pharmacist and known drug databases and communicate potential concerns with the patient and other HCPs.

Patient Disclosure and Motivation for Complementary and Alternative Medicine Use

A survey examining conversations between patients and their physicians regarding CAM use revealed that in spite of the high known use of CAM among people age 50 or older, 69% of those individuals do not talk to their physicians about it (AARP & NCCAM, 2007). According to a telephone survey of 1,559 respondents age 50 or older, most often patients did not discuss their CAM use with physicians because the provider never asked (42%); the patients did not know that they should discuss it (30%); or patients did not have enough time during the office visit to discuss it (19%). Personal responsibility for one's health and obtaining health care has led patients to seek interventions, including CAM. Patients may consider CAM to be beneficial to maintaining wellness, treating symptoms, or perhaps even treating an acute or chronic disease state. In many settings, such as managed care, consumerism is encouraged, with the intended outcome that adopting wellness behaviors or more consistent symptomatic relief may decrease overall healthcare costs for insurers and the insured (Rizzo & Xie, 2006).

Implications for Oncology Advanced Practice Nurses

Many patients want to be directly involved in the diagnosis, planning, and delivery of their own health care, and they are seeking information from various sources and investing significant out-of-pocket dollars in health and wellness. While in essence self-motivated health behavior is beneficial for individuals and society, patients sometimes are seeking interventions without consultation with oncology APNs. Engaging in open dialogue and offering positive direction in acquiring reliable information can assist patients in being fully informed to make critical healthcare decisions. APNs can direct patients to safe and reliable sources of information to facilitate decision making. It also is imperative that oncology APNs use evidence-based CAM resources to assess patient situations affected by or likely to be affected by integrative therapies. Such resources contribute to accurate assessments and preventive approaches.

Conclusion

Complementary and integrative therapies are common in the oncology population, where they are used for cancer prevention, cancer treatment, and management of symptoms caused by treatment. Knowledge of specific characteristics of people who use CAM can assist oncology APNs in detection of CAM users who may not disclose that information readily. Access to and proper interpretation of evidence-based resources are crucial to people with cancer and oncology APNs. Many current resources are available, such as Natural Standard. CAM is becoming a specialized area of nursing with opportunities for additional education for oncology APNs. But many issues are left to be resolved with respect to curriculum development for certification, reimbursement for services, and improvement of patient communication with oncology APNs about use of CAM.

Case Study

Date of visit: October 2006

History of Present Illness

L.L. is a 32-year-old white male with progressive Ewing sarcoma who was diagnosed in January 2003. He is now one-year post–nonmyeloablative stem cell transplant and graft-versus-host disease. Recently, he was treated with levofloxacin 500 mg daily for two weeks for pneumonia followed by diarrhea, which was positive for *Clostridium difficile* and treated with metronidazole 250 mg every eight hours for two weeks with resolution. He returned to the clinic for a scheduled chest computed tomography (CT) on October 2, 2006, which showed disease progression. He and his wife recently returned from a one-week cruise, which he enjoyed and tolerated well. Because of disease progression, he began radiation therapy to the chest wall for five days starting the same day as the CT documenting progression, per radiation oncology. He is seen today in the clinic following an aerosolized pentamidine treatment and is found to be febrile and tachypneic, with an oxygen saturation of 91%. He complains of auditory wheezing and intermittent nonproductive cough. His right lateral chest wall pain is controlled with oral opioids.

> **Past Medical History:**
> - Ewing sarcoma diagnosed, January 2003
> - Pneumonia, September 2006
> - Pulmonary emboli, October 2004—currently on enoxaparin
>
> **Medications:**
> - Oxycodone controlled release (CR) 10 mg every 12 hours
> - Oxycodone 5 mg every 4 hours prn
> - Enoxaparin (Lovenox®, Sanofi-Aventis) 80 mg every 12 hours
> - Pentamidine (Pentam®, American Pharmaceutical Partners) monthly
> - Valacyclovir (Valtrex®, GlaxoSmithKline) 500 mg every day
> - Clotrimazole troches 10 mg every 6 hours
> - Docusate sodium (Colace®, Purdue Pharma) 100 mg every 12 hours
> - Penicillin V potassium (VK) 500 mg every 12 hours
> - Diazepam (Valium®, Hoffmann-LaRoche) 5 mg every 6 hours prn

He has no known drug allergies. He is married, does not use tobacco or alcohol, operates a part-time business, and lives in a rural area. His family history is noncontributory.

Temperature is 102°F (38.9°C), pulse is 120, and respirations are 24. He is a well-developed, alert male in no acute distress. Pupils are equal and react to light and accommodation; extraocular muscles are intact; no nystagmus is present. No oral ulcers or candidiasis is present, nor is any lymphadenopathy. He has expiratory wheezes bilaterally in all lobes and decreased breath sounds in the right posterior lobes. The apical pulse is 130, regular rate and rhythm, no murmur, rub, or gallop, S3 or S4; no jugular vein distention or carotid bruits found. The abdomen is soft and nontender with positive bowel sounds. No hepatosplenomegaly or costovertebral angle tenderness is present. Pedal pulses are 2+; no edema. Skin is warm and dry. Healing bruises are present on the abdomen from subcutaneous injections; the right lateral chest wall has radiation therapy markings; and the patient has a healing anterior right chest wall chest tube site.

The patient is alert and oriented times three. The cranial nerves 2–12 are intact. Deep tendon reflexes are 1+ upper and lower extremities. Strength is 5/5. Gait is normal. Patient has full range of motion in the neck and all extremities.

- White blood cells = 24.8/ul
- Red blood cells (RBCs) = $3.12 \times 10^6/mm^3$
- Hemoglobin = 10.2 g/dl
- Hematocrit = 32.4%
- Mean corpuscular volume = 100.4 fl
- RBC distribution width = 18.7
- Platelets = $283 \times 10^3/ul$
- Neutrophils = 79.0%
- Lymphocytes = 50.0%
- Monocytes = 15%
- Eosinophils = 1.0%
- Basophils = 1.0%
- Blood cultures and sputum cultures are pending.

This is a 32-year-old male with stage IV progressive Ewing sarcoma who presents with fever, recurrent dyspnea, and desaturation. No obvious source of infection is noted on exam. Chest x-ray demonstrates an obstructive component. Recommendations include levofloxacin (Levaquin®, Ortho-McNeil), metronidazole (Flagyl®, Pfizer Inc.) 750 mg once a day for four weeks, then Flagyl 250 mg every eight hours for four weeks. Additional recommendations were for the patient to continue radiation therapy per radiation oncology and return to the clinic in one week for follow-up.

Treatment Planning

The goals of therapy are to (1) treat obstructive pneumonia, (2) complete radiation therapy (two days remaining), and (3) promote comfort and quality of life. L.L. and his wife are aware of the grave prognosis and completed a home hospice referral prior to the cruise. They are interested in combining complementary approaches for pain management, intermittent nausea, occasional constipation (and possible diarrhea while on an extended course of antibiotics), and dyspnea.

Proposed Integrative Treatment Plan

L.L. reports that his spirits are good and that he and his wife are adjusting to his prognosis. He would like to spend as much of his time at home helping his wife with the business, maximize his energy, and minimize his symptoms. His nutritional status is good, and he is able to eat a variety of foods and maintain his weight. For the management of any of the symptoms L.L. reports, you explain that no modality has been tested sufficiently yet to determine whether strong evidence of efficacy exists. Good evidence exists for the use of imagery and music therapy for pain management (see Table 8-3). They ask about acupuncture and whether it would be contraindicated because he is taking enoxaparin. You explain that there may be some concern about using acupuncture needles for the pain because he is on a low-molecular-weight heparin, but acupuncture-related interventions such as acupressure and acustimulation wrist bands are noninvasive and may be helpful for the nausea. For occasional constipation (and now possible diarrhea while on an extended course of antibiotics), you explain that for both conditions, good evidence exists that psyllium is effective (but can be abrasive to the intestines) and available over the counter. For dyspnea, the evidence is conflicting, but many patients enjoy the benefits of yoga and find it eases breathing. L.L. and his wife decide that they would like to see an acupuncturist, and you provide a referral for a licensed provider in addition to the name of the yoga instructor in the cancer center. You discuss that you cannot assure them that these services would be covered under their current insurance, and they verbalize understanding. You provide an opportunity for questions, document your discussion in the progress note, and schedule a follow-up appointment for two weeks.

Summary

As an APN, you have suggested a conservative integrated treatment plan that has no known interactions with L.L.'s current medications. You provided the opportunity for questions and open discussion. Following the visit, you initiate a phone consultation with the acupuncturist, discuss the referral, and request a summary letter for the patient's file after the first and subsequent visits for other HCPs on L.L.'s team to review.

1. Has a comprehensive medication assessment been conducted?
   - A complete medication assessment includes prescription and over-the-counter medications along with those products that may not come to mind as quickly such as aerosols, topical creams, dietary supplements, enhanced sports drinks, or suppositories.
2. Is there a history of previous and current CAM therapies? (If so, what kind? Duration? Reason? Did it help? Who provided it? Was it costly?)
   - Symptom management in cancer care may involve CAM modalities such as guided imagery, progressive relaxation, cognitive-behavioral therapy, yoga, exercise, aromatherapy, massage, reflexology, and acupuncture, to name a few. Documenting the patient's experience with any modality, its impact on the patient's symptoms, and cost/benefit analysis is advantageous when creating an integrative plan of care.
3. How is L.L.'s overall well-being and endurance? Nutritional status? Stress level and management? View toward the status of his illness?
   - Knowing the overall well-being of the patient physically, emotionally, and spiritually is important for the APN, as it assists in effective treatment planning. For example, if a patient is not able to eat solids, is he or she receiving adequate caloric intake to provide energy for daily activities? Or is he experiencing hopelessness that may affect his outlook and his relationships with family members?

4. Does the treatment plan include any additional chemotherapy or surgery? Is continuing the radiation desirable to the patient? Are there safe and effective CAM therapies available for his symptoms? What are your thoughts as a provider about L.L. integrating CAM therapies at this time? Do he and his wife have some therapies in mind? Do they anticipate a cost, and can they pay if insurance does not cover it? Does L.L. need to be monitored for particular side effects or interactions? Is there a plan for consistent follow-up?

Participation in healthcare decision making is desirable for many patients, and treatment planning should reflect their input along with a method of evaluation. The benefits and drawbacks of any intervention should be explained well. Many patients would like to try CAM therapies outside of conventional interventions. This patient is experiencing pain, nausea, constipation, and dyspnea. He may be interested in meeting with an acupuncturist to discuss the benefits, risks, and cost of a series of treatments for his pain. For the nausea, you may suggest drinking a cup of ginger tea. Psyllium often is used in conventional approaches for the relief of constipation but also is considered to be CAM. Some patients with dyspnea benefit from progressive relaxation and special breathing techniques taught in yoga classes. The patient or family member can keep a log of what works and what does not and how the intervention was tolerated. As a provider, the APN can review the possible interventions, check for potential interactions, and make a plan for follow-up evaluation in several weeks.

Key Points

- Many patients want to be directly involved in the diagnosis, planning, and delivery of their care.
- Patients are seeking information from various sources and are investing and spending significant out-of-pocket dollars in health and wellness.
- Many patients with cancer use CAM without the knowledge of APNs.
- Safe and effective CAM therapies exist for some conditions.
- CAM research must urgently fill the gaps between what is used by patients daily and what is proved to be safe and reliable in well-controlled studies.
- APNs must know how to access safe and reliable sources of CAM information, maintain knowledge about CAM, and assess for CAM use among patients.
- CAM licensure and credentialing is governed by state bodies, and requirements vary by state.
- Informed consent is suggested for patients utilizing CAM services within an inpatient or outpatient setting.
- APNs can serve as facilitators in maintaining an open dialogue between patients and the oncology care team.

Recommended Resources for Oncology Advanced Practice Nurses

- Alternative Link Systems, Inc. (2001). *The state legal guide to complementary and alternative medicine and nursing.* Albany, NY: Delmar Thomson Learning.

- Bridevaux, I.P. (2004). A survey of patients' out-of-pocket payments for complementary and alternative medicine therapies. *Complementary Therapies in Medicine, 12,* 48–50.
- Cassileth, B.R., & Lucarelli, C.D. (2003). *Herb-drug interactions in oncology.* Hamilton, Ontario, Canada: BC Decker.
- Centers for Medicare and Medicaid Services coverage: www.medicare.gov/coverage /home.asp
- Cohen, M.H., Ruggie, M., & Micozzi, M.S. (2007). *The practice of integrative medicine: A legal and operational guide.* New York: Springer.
- Decker, G.M. (Ed.). (1999). *An introduction to complementary and alternative therapies.* Pittsburgh, PA: Oncology Nursing Society.
- Decker, G.M. (2003). Commonly used vitamin supplements: Implications for clinical practice. *Clinical Journal of Oncology Nursing, 7*(Suppl. 2), 1–28.
- Lee, C.O. (2005). Herbs and cytotoxic drugs: Recognizing and communicating potentially relevant interactions. *Clinical Journal of Oncology Nursing, 9,* 481–487.
- National Cancer Institute. (2005). *Thinking about complementary and alternative medicine: A guide for people with cancer* [NIH Publication No. 04-5541]. Bethesda, MD: Author.
- NIH Office of Dietary Supplements: http://dietary-supplements.info.nih.gov
- ONS Complementary and Alternative Therapies Clinical Resource Area (Bibliography): www.ons.org/clinical/treatment/complementary/bibliography.shtml
- *Physicians desk reference for nonprescription drugs and dietary supplements* (26th ed.). (2005). Montvale, NJ: Thomson PDR.

References

AARP & National Center for Complementary and Alternative Medicine. (2007). *Complementary and alternative medicine: What people 50 and older are using and discussing with their physicians.* Retrieved January 23, 2007, from http://assets.aarp.org/rgcenter/health/cam_2007.pdf

Alternative Link. (2007). *ABC coding solutions. Alternative link.* Retrieved January 15, 2007, from http://www.alternativelink.com/ali/home/

American Botanical Council. (2007). *The ABC herbal information course.* Retrieved January 23, 2007, from http://abc.herbalgram.org/site/DocServer/HIC.pdf?docID=401

American Holistic Nurses Association. (n.d.-a). *Position on the role of nurses in the practice of complementary and alternative therapies.* Retrieved January 22, 2007, from http://www.ahna.org/about/statements .html#role

American Holistic Nurses Association. (n.d.-b). *The school endorsement program.* Retrieved January 23, 2007, from http://www.ahncc.org/pages/1/index.htm

Ashikaga, T., Bosompra, K., O'Brien, P., & Nelson, L. (2002). Use of complimentary and alternative medicine by breast cancer patients: Prevalence, patterns and communication with physicians. *Supportive Care in Cancer, 10,* 542–548.

Astin, J.A. (1998). Why patients use alternative medicine: Results of a national study. *JAMA, 279,* 1548–1553.

Barnes, P.M., Powell-Griner, E., McFann, K., & Nahin, R.L. (2004). *Complementary and alternative medicine use among adults: United States, 2002. Advance data from vital and health statistics; no 343* [DHHS Publication No. PHS 2004-1250 04-0342]. Hyattsville, MD: National Center for Health Statistics.

Bernstein, B.J., & Grasso, T. (2001). Prevalence of complementary and alternative medicine use in cancer patients. *Oncology (Huntington), 15,* 1267–1272.

Burman, M.E. (2003). Complementary and alternative medicine: Core competencies for family nurse practitioners. *Journal of Nursing Education, 42,* 28–34.

Center for Mind-Body Medicine. (2007). *Science. Training. Community. Outreach.* Retrieved January 23, 2007, from http://www.cmbm.org

Chong, O.T. (2006). An integrative approach to addressing clinical issues in complementary and alternative medicine in an outpatient oncology center. *Clinical Journal of Oncology Nursing, 10,* 83–88.

Cochrane Library. (n.d.). *Welcome to the Cochrane library*. Retrieved January 23, 2007, from http://www3 .interscience.wiley.com/cgi-bin/mrwhome/106568753/home

Cohen, M. (2001). Legal and ethical issues in complementary and alternative medicine. In E. Ernst (Ed.), *The desktop guide to complementary and alternative medicine: An evidence-based approach* (pp. 404–411). London: Mosby.

Committee on the Use of Complementary and Alternative Medicine by the American Public, Institute of Medicine of the National Academies. (2005). *Complementary and alternative medicine in the United States*. Washington, DC: National Academies Press.

Consortium of Academic Health Centers for Integrative Medicine. (2006). *Consortium of Academic Health Centers for Integrative Medicine*. Retrieved January 23, 2007, from http://www.imconsortium .org/cahcim/members/home.html

Decker, G., & Lee, C. (2005). Complementary and alternative medicine (CAM) therapies. In C.H. Yarbro, M.H. Frogge, & M. Goodman (Eds.), *Cancer nursing: Principles and practice* (6th ed., pp. 590–620). Sudbury, MA: Jones and Bartlett.

Decker, G.M., Lee, C.O., & Krebs, L. (Eds.). (in press). *Complementary and alternative therapies: A symptom approach*. Pittsburgh, PA: Oncology Nursing Society.

Eisenberg, D.M., Cohen, M.H., Hrbek, A., Grayzel, J., Van Rompay, M.I., & Cooper, R.A. (2002). Credentialing complementary and alternative medical providers. *Annals of Internal Medicine, 137,* 965–973.

Eisenberg, D.M., Davis, R.B., Ettner, S.L., Appel, S., Wilkey, S., Van Rompay, M., et al. (1998). Trends in alternative medicine use in the United States, 1990–1997: Results of a follow-up national survey. *JAMA, 280,* 1569–1575.

Fouladbakhsh, J.M., Stommel, M., Given, B.A., & Given, C.W. (2005). Predictors of use of complementary and alternative therapies among patients with cancer. *Oncology Nursing Forum, 32,* 1115–1122.

Goldstein, M.S., Brown, E.R., Ballard-Barbash, R., Morgenstern, H., Bastani, R., Lee, J., et al. (2005). The use of complementary and alternative medicine among California adults with and without cancer. *Evidence-Based Complementary and Alternative Medicine, 2,* 557–565.

Halcon, L.L., Chlan, L.L., Kreitzer, M.J., & Leonard, B.J. (2003). Complementary therapies and healing practices: Faculty/student beliefs and attitudes and the implications for nursing education. *Journal of Professional Nursing, 19,* 387–397.

Jonas, W.B., Linde, K., & Walach, H. (1999). How to practice evidence-based complementary and alternative medicine. In W.B. Jonas & J.S. Levin (Eds.), *Essentials of complementary and alternative medicine* (pp. 72–87). Philadelphia: Lippincott Williams & Wilkins.

Karnofsky, D.A. (1959). Cancer quackery: Its causes, recognition and prevention. *American Journal of Nursing, 59,* 496–500.

Kenner, D. (2002). Putting it all together: Practicing oriental medicine. In C.M. Cassidy (Ed.), *Contemporary Chinese medicine and acupuncture* (pp. 125–135). Philadelphia: Churchill Livingstone.

Kessler, R.C., Davis, R.B., Foster, D.F., Van Rompay, M.I., Walters, E.E., Wilkey, S.A., et al. (2001). Long-term trends in the use of complementary and alternative medical therapies in the United States. *Annals of Internal Medicine, 135,* 262–268.

Kinsel, J.F., & Straus, S.E. (2003). Complementary and alternative therapeutics: Rigorous research is needed to support claims. *Annual Review of Pharmacology and Toxicology, 43,* 463–484.

Kozachik, S.L., Wyatt, G., Given, C.W., & Given, B.A. (2006). Patterns of use of complementary therapies among cancer patients and their family caregivers. *Cancer Nursing, 29,* 84–94.

Lafferty, W.E., Downey, L., McCarty, R.L., Standish, L.J., & Patrick, D.L. (2006). Evaluating CAM treatment at the end of life: A review of clinical trials for massage and meditation. *Complementary Therapies in Medicine, 14,* 100–112.

Lee, C.O. (2005a). Communicating facts and knowledge in cancer complementary and alternative medicine. *Seminars in Oncology Nursing, 21,* 201–214.

Lee, C.O. (2005b). Herbs and cytotoxic drugs: Recognizing and communicating potentially relevant interactions. *Clinical Journal of Oncology Nursing, 9,* 481–487.

Lengacher, C.A., Bennett, M.P., Kip, K.E., Gonzalez, L., Jacobsen, P., & Cox, C.E. (2006). Relief of symptoms, side effects, and psychological distress through use of complementary and alternative medicine in women with breast cancer. *Oncology Nursing Forum, 33,* 97–104.

Maizes, V., Koffler, K., & Fleishman, S. (2002). Revisiting the health history: An integrative medicine approach. *Advances in Mind-Body Medicine, 18*(2), 31–34.

Maskarinec, G., Shumay, D.M., Kakai, H., & Gotay, C.C. (2000). Ethnic differences in complementary and alternative medicine use among cancer patients. *Journal of Alternative and Complementary Medicine, 6,* 531–538.

Mumber, M.P. (2006a). Clinical decision analysis. In M.P. Mumber (Ed.), *Integrative oncology principles and practice* (pp. 145–164). New York: Taylor and Francis.

Mumber, M.P. (2006b). Principles of integrative oncology. In M.P. Mumber (Ed.), *Integrative oncology principles and practice* (pp. 3–15). New York: Taylor and Francis.

National Cancer Institute. (2006). *NCI's cancer CAM research portfolio.* Retrieved January 24, 2007, from http://www.cancer.gov/cam/research_portfolio.html

National Cancer Institute. (n.d.). *Search for clinical trials.* Retrieved January 23, 2007, from http://www.cancer.gov/clinicaltrials/search

National Cancer Institute Office of Cancer Complementary and Alternative Medicine. (2007). *Understanding CAM.* Retrieved January 22, 2007, from http://www.cancer.gov/cam/health_understanding.html

National Institutes of Health National Center for Complementary and Alternative Medicine. (2007a). *Complementary and alternative medicine funding by NIH institute/center.* Retrieved January 22, 2007, from http://nccam.nih.gov/about/budget/institute-center.htm

National Institutes of Health National Center for Complementary and Alternative Medicine. (2007b). *Complementary and alternative medicine online continuing education series.* Retrieved January 24, 2007, from http://nccam.nih.gov/videolectures/

National Institutes of Health National Center for Complementary and Alternative Medicine. (2007c). *What is CAM?* Retrieved January 22, 2007, from http://nccam.nih.gov/health/whatiscam/

National Institutes of Health Office of Dietary Supplements. (n.d.). *About the Office of Dietary Supplements (ODS).* Retrieved January 23, 2007, from http://dietary-supplements.info.nih.gov/About/about_ods.aspx

Offit, K., & Siddiqui, R. (2004). Genetic factors: Hereditary cancer predisposition syndromes. In M.D. Abeloff, J.O. Armitage, M.B. Kastan, & W.G. McKenna (Eds.), *Clinical oncology* (3rd ed., pp. 227–251). Philadelphia: Elsevier Churchill Livingstone.

Oncology Nursing Society. (2006). *The use of complementary, alternative, and integrative therapies in cancer care* [Position statement]. Retrieved January 22, 2007, from http://www.ons.org/publications/positions/complementarytherapies.shtml

Oncology Nursing Society. (n.d.). *Outcomes resource area: Putting evidence into practice.* Retrieved September 4, 2007, from http://www.ons.org/outcomes/index.shtml

Richardson, M.A., Masse, L.C., Nanny, K., & Sanders, C. (2004). Discrepant views of oncologists and cancer patients on complementary/alternative medicine. *Supportive Care in Cancer, 12,* 797–804.

Richardson, M.A., Sanders, T., Palmer, J.L., Greisinger, A., & Singletary, S.E. (2000). Complementary/alternative medicine use in a comprehensive cancer center and the implications for oncology. *Journal of Clinical Oncology, 18,* 2505–2514.

Rizzo, J.A., & Xie, Y. (2006). Managed care, consumerism, preventative medicine: Does a causal connection exist? *Managed Care Interface, 19*(7), 46–50.

Ropka, M.E., & Spencer-Cisek, P. (2001). PRISM: Priority symptom management project phase I: Assessment. *Oncology Nursing Forum, 28,* 1585–1594.

Silverman, H., & Schneider, T. (2006). Spirituality. In M.P. Mumber (Ed.), *Integrative oncology principles and practice* (pp. 221–241). New York: Taylor and Francis.

Sofhauser, C.D. (2002). Development of a minor in complementary health. *Nurse Educator, 27,* 118–122.

Sparber, A., Bauer, L., Curt, G., Eisenberg, D., Levin, T., Parks, S., et al. (2000). Use of complementary medicine by adult patients participating in cancer clinical trials. *Oncology Nursing Forum, 27,* 623–630.

Strickland, P.T., & Kensler, W. (2004). Environmental factors. In M.D. Abeloff, J.O. Armitage, M.B. Kastan, & W.G. McKenna (Eds.), *Clinical oncology* (3rd ed., pp. 173–189). Philadelphia: Elsevier Churchill Livingstone.

Swisher, E.M., Cohn, D.E., Goff, B.A., Parham, J., Herzog, T.J., Rader, J.S., et al. (2002). Use of complementary and alternative medicine among women with gynecologic cancers. *Gynecology Oncology, 84,* 363–367.

University of Maryland Complementary Medicine Program. (n.d.). *Integrative medicine: Cochrane CAM field.* Retrieved January 23, 2007, from http://www.compmed.umm.edu/cochrane.asp

U.S. Department of Health and Human Services. (2002). *White House Commission on Complementary and Alternative Medicine Policy* [NIH Publication No. 03-5411]. Washington, DC: U.S. Government Printing Office.

U.S. Food and Drug Administration. (n.d.). *Dietary supplement health and education act of 1994.* Retrieved January 23, 2007, from http://www.fda.gov/opacom/laws/dshea.html

Verhoef, M.J., & White, M.A. (2002). Factors in making the decision to forgo conventional cancer treatment. *Cancer Practice, 10,* 201–207.

Winnick, T.A. (2005). From quackery to "complementary" medicine: The American medical profession confronts alternative therapies. *Social Problems, 52,* 38–61.

Yates, J.S., Mustian, K.M., Morrow, G.R., Gillies, L.J., Padmanaban, D., Atkins, J.N., et al. (2005). Prevalence of complementary and alternative medicine use in cancer patients during treatment. *Supportive Care in Cancer, 13,* 806–811.

CHAPTER 9

Clinical Research

Barbara A. Biedrzycki, RN, MSN, CRNP, AOCNP®

Introduction

Clinical research is the systematic investigation of human biology, health, or illness that contributes to generalizable knowledge (Grady, 2007). In clinical research, a hypothesis is tested through specific activities outlined in a protocol. Conclusions obtained through the scientific process advance health care for society, not individuals. Although participants may benefit from clinical research, the intent is to benefit the common good.

The National Cancer Institute (NCI) provides the same definition for clinical trial and clinical study: research that tests new methods of screening for, preventing, diagnosing, or treating a disease (NCI, 2007). The World Health Organization (WHO) provides the following definition.

> A clinical trial is any research study that prospectively assigns human participants or groups of humans to one or more health-related interventions to evaluate the effects on health outcomes. Interventions include but are not restricted to drugs, cells and other biological products, surgical procedures, radiologic procedures, devices, behavioral treatments, process-of-care changes, preventive care, etc. (WHO, n.d.)

Common names for clinical research include *study, trial, investigation, experiment,* and *nursing research.* Throughout the chapter, these terms will be used interchangeably, reflective of user preferences. For researchers and healthcare providers, the many terms used to describe clinical research may be interchangeable; however, to the public and potential research participants, the terms may have different meanings. Sugarman et al. (1998) found that lay people respond differently to the many terms in use. For example, the term *investigation* may imply that something was in error, and the term *study* often is preferred, as patients believed that the researchers were providing an in-depth exploration of the patient's case.

Advanced practice nurses (APNs) are essential in the recruitment, conduct, evaluation, and dissemination of clinical research. This chapter will review the foundations for clinical research and its relevance to oncology APNs. The processes and outcomes of research influence the clinical decisions of oncology APNs in their daily practice.

Historical Development of Clinical Research

While most of the historical references to clinical research were descriptive in nature, following the natural course of diseases, there is documentation of an early reference to a comparison study found in an unlikely source, the book of Daniel in the Bible. The experiment tested the effects of a rich food diet compared to a vegetarian diet.

> Then Daniel said to the steward . . .
> 'Test your servants for ten days; let us be given vegetables to eat and water to drink. Then let your appearance and the appearance of the youths who eat the king's rich food be observed by you, and according to what you see deal with your servants:
> So he harkened them in this matter, and tested them for ten days. At the end of ten days it was seen that they were better in appearance and fatter in flesh than all of the youths who ate the king's rich food. So the steward took away their rich food and the wine they were to drink and gave them vegetables.' Daniel 1:11–16 (English Standard Version)

The 20th century brought significant advances in health care through research fueled by academia, as well as investments by the government and pharmaceutical industries (Gallin, 2007). Prior to this time, few, if any, differences existed between clinical research and practice, as not much was known about medicine. Therefore, most of the care provided was experimental (Grady, 2007).

Although a number of significant historical advances have occurred in health care and clinical research, only a few will be discussed in this chapter. With the discovery of penicillin by Alexander Fleming of Scotland in 1932 and the discovery of insulin by Frederick G. Banting and Charles H. Best of Canada in 1921, the amount of interest in pharmaceutical research became tremendous. Clinical research began in earnest to discover more antibiotics, hormonal agents, vaccines, and antiviral agents (Gallin, 2007).

Advances flourished in the science of clinical research. In his agricultural work with plant fertility, Ronald A. Fisher applied experimental design and statistics when he introduced the concepts of randomization and analysis of variance in his work from the 1920s to the 1930s (Efron, 1998). Although as far back as 1784, Benjamin Franklin ensured that his subjects did not know whether they were receiving the research product or placebo, the concept of "blinding" was not well integrated into science until the 1930s, when Torald Sollman demonstrated the importance of controlled experiments (Beecher, 1966). Essential elements of clinical research design are based in history and refined through time. Table 9-1 defines some of the most common design components. Familiarity with these terms will assist oncology APNs in interpretation and application of clinical trial findings to oncology practice.

Very serious ethical concerns accompanied these clinical research advances. Concerns regarding unethical practices in clinical research led to the regulations that mandate clinical research standards today. The Nazi experiments with prisoners that took place in Germany during World War II, the syphilis experiments with poor African American men that occurred in Tuskegee, Alabama, from 1930 to 1972, and the hepatitis experiments performed on children with Down syndrome at Willowbrook State School in New York during the 1950s are all examples of experiments that are considered highly unethical. One of the chief ethical concerns in these studies is that participants were forced to participate. Their inalienable rights as human beings were violated.

Not only do all subjects need to know that they are participating in an experiment, but they also must voluntarily participate. Participants such as children, prisoners, the

Table 9-1. Clinical Research Design Components

Component	Definition
Bias	Bias is a measurement error that affects the validity of the data. May be related to how participants are recruited, data are analyzed, or conclusions are determined.
Blinding	Research participants are not aware of their investigational product assignment (single blinding), or researchers are not aware of the participants' investigation assignments (double blinded). Also known as masking.
Clinical significance	Clinical research outcome is important to patient outcomes. Also known as meaningful significance.
Data analysis	Method of data analysis is dependent on the research questions, design of the study, and the type and number of variables.
Placebo	Placebo is an inactive substance used in comparison against the investigational product to determine efficacy.
Randomization	Research participants are assigned to investigational cohort (or arm) based on chance. Assignments may be generated by computer programs or other methods.
Sample size	Sample size is the number of research participants in a clinical research study. Sample size goal needs to be predetermined based on anticipated research effect and power needed to answer the research question.
Statistical significance	If the null hypothesis was true, the results would be very unusual. Usually referred to as $p < .5$.
Survival curves	This is the output of statistical method to evaluate survival using censored data. Actuarial (life table) and Kaplan-Meier methods commonly are used.

Note. Based on information from Friedman et al., 1998; Munro, 2005; Stone, 2006.

cognitively impaired, and people with life-threatening illnesses need additional protection when participating in clinical research. In an attempt to diminish ethical complications and protect research participants, the medical community developed guidelines to protect all subjects, including those with a diminished capacity for voluntary decision making. Legal actions and guidelines from governmental agencies, as well as international organizations such as the World Medical Assembly, have significantly improved human subject protection in clinical research. Table 9-2 provides an overview of some of these protecting guidelines, laws, and codes published over the past 60 years. With an understanding of these, oncology APNs can effectively reassure patients about safety concerns when they are considering entry into a clinical trial.

Phases of Clinical Research

Clinical research is a costly and time-consuming endeavor. Time, finances, and the recruitment of research participants are carefully considered in planning the advancement of a product from the original concept to commercial availability (after the U.S. Food and Drug Administration's [FDA's] approval). Only about 1 out of 10,000 com-

Table 9-2. Documents for Protection of Human Subjects

Originally Published	Title	Purpose
1949	Nuremberg Code www.hhs.gov/ohrp/references/nurcode.htm	Established voluntary consent and justification for the research
1953	*Guidelines for the Conduct of Research Involving Human Subjects at the National Institutes of Health* http://ohsr.od.nih.gov/guidelines/graybooklet82404.pdf	Required medical review of research at the newly opened NIH Clinical Center
1962	Kefauver-Harris amendments to the Food and Drug Administration Act www.fda.gov/cder/about/history/Page32.htm	Mandated consent for drug testing
1964	Declaration of Helsinki http://www.wma.net/e/policy/b3.htm	Declared that potential benefits must outweigh potential risks
1979	Belmont Report http://ohsr.od.nih.gov/guidelines/belmont.html	Defined principles of respect for persons, beneficence, and justice
1991	*Code of Federal Regulations,* Title 45, Part 46: Protection of Human Subjects; also known as the "Common Rule" www.hhs.gov/ohrp/humansubjects/guidance/45cfr46.htm	Established role of the institutional review board (IRB) to protect human subjects

Note. Based on information from Gallin, 2007.

pounds discovered will eventually receive an FDA indication for use in oncology. Figure 9-1 illustrates the lengthy process through which a pharmacologic agent must proceed prior to earning an FDA review (Pharmaceutical Research and Manufacturers of America [PhRMA], 2007b). This process includes preclinical and clinical testing of many potential agents that are discarded during the process. Figure 9-2 demonstrates the time commitment from the FDA and sponsor in developing new investigational products. The time for the research and development of a pharmacologic agent averages approximately 9 years but could take as long as 15 years.

Once preclinical testing is complete, oncology clinical research for new drug development usually consists of three phases of research. Each phase has specific goals that must be achieved prior to progression to a higher phase. Subsequent phases build upon the data obtained in previous phases. The sample size of different phases of research is dependent upon the purpose of the research. A small sample usually is needed for the initial phase of research, whereas a larger sample is required in order to reach statistical significance for the stated outcomes in a higher phase.

Preclinical Testing

Originating from test tube or computer-based discoveries, research products often are tested in animals prior to being tested in humans. Mice and rats commonly are the first recipients of new medical discoveries. Based on small animal data, medium- and larger-sized animals such as dogs or apes may be tested before the research is translat-

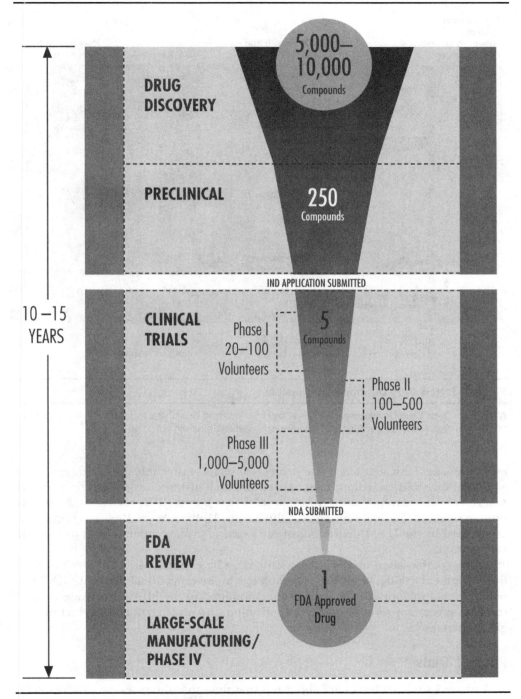

Figure 9-1. The Research and Development Process: Long, Complex, and Costly

Note. From "Pharmaceutical Industry Profile 2007" (p. 6), by Pharmaceutical Research and Manufacturers of America, March 2007, Washington, DC: Author. Copyright 2007 by the Pharmaceutical Research and Manufacturers of America. Reprinted with permission.

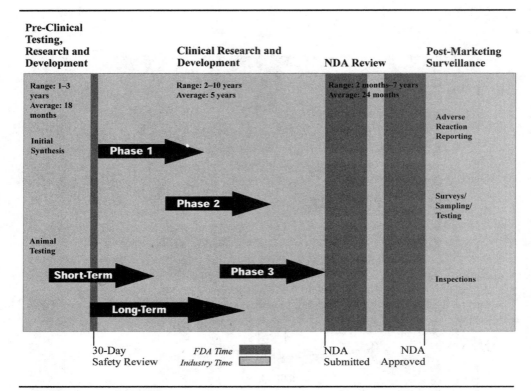

Figure 9-2. New Drug Development Timeline

Note. From "New Drug Development Timeline," by U.S. Food and Drug Administration. Retrieved April 9, 2008, from http://www.fda.gov/fdac/graphics/newdrugspecial/drugchart.pdf

ed to humans. Ethical practice also protects animals in preclinical testing. Institutional animal care and use committees at each research institute review and regulate animal research as carefully as an institutional review board (IRB) reviews and regulates human research. Federal laws, such as the Animal Welfare Act of 1966 and regulations established by the U.S. Department of Agriculture, protect animals used in biomedical research.

An acceptable safety and efficacy profile must be established in the preclinical setting via animal testing. Once this is completed, an investigational new drug (IND) application that includes this information is submitted to the FDA for consideration. If the FDA grants approval of the IND application, the investigational product may begin human testing.

Phase I Trials

A phase I study collects data about the first time that the research product is given to humans. One goal of this phase of research is to determine whether the product is safe in humans. Phase I studies examine the pharmacokinetics of the product. Data are collected on various doses of the agent to determine what constitutes the optimal dose. Based on all the knowledge gained from the study, recommendations are made by the researchers to the FDA as to whether additional research on this product should proceed.

Most often, researchers do not know the optimal dose or schedule for the new investigational product. Phase I studies also are known as dose-finding studies. The phase I study of an allogeneic granulocyte macrophage–colony-stimulating factor (GM-CSF) secreting tumor vaccine for pancreatic cancer is an example of a traditional dose-escalating scale (Jaffee et al., 2001). During phase I study, three research participants received the lowest dose level believed to be efficacious in humans. After determining that the lowest dose level was safe, the next group of three participants received a higher second dose level. This sequence proceeded to a third and then fourth dose level—the dose that ultimately demonstrated safety as well as evidence of a dose-dependent antitumor immunity through an increased postvaccination delayed type hypersensitivity response against autologous tumor injections (Jaffee et al.).

Challenges arise when more than one investigational product is tested simultaneously. Determining the offending agent for a particular toxicity may be difficult and deter the discovery of the optimal dose. An excellent example of an efficient statistical strategy used to find optimal doses of multiple products can be found in the phase I research of an allogeneic GM-CSF secreting breast cancer vaccine given in a specifically timed sequence with immunomodulating doses of cyclophosphamide and doxorubicin (Emens et al., 2004).

Phase II Trials

Phase II clinical trials are designed to further define the safety and efficacy of the research product. Efficacy may be examined in various types of cancer or disease states. Phase II enrollment often is limited to fewer than a hundred participants with a specific cancer diagnosis. Phase I and II clinical trial participants often participate for altruistic purposes, as the chance of direct personal benefit is little.

Although this is the second step for new investigational products, drugs previously approved by the FDA for a particular indication also may be examined in phase II research to determine safety and efficacy in a new combination of therapy or for a new indication. Such is the case in the phase II research testing of a combination of bevacizumab, a monoclonal antibody designed to bind to and inhibit the human antivascular endothelial growth factor, and erlotinib, a tyrosine kinase inhibitor that targets the epidermal growth factor receptor. Bevacizumab was first approved by the FDA for use in colon cancer and later approved for use in non-small cell lung cancer. In this phase II, multiarm study, research participants received either bevacizumab and erlotinib, bevacizumab and chemotherapy with either docetaxel or pemetrexed, or chemotherapy alone. The research participants had nonsquamous, non-small cell lung cancer and had progressed during or after one platinum-based regimen. The outcome data indicated an acceptable safety profile with no unexpected toxicities. Furthermore, favorable progression-free survival and overall survival occurred in the groups receiving bevacizumab in combination with erlotinib or chemotherapy when compared to the chemotherapy-only group (Herbst et al., 2007).

Bevacizumab, in combination with carboplatin and paclitaxel, is FDA approved as first-line therapy for advanced nonsquamous non-small cell lung cancer (the same pathology as the previously described phase II research participants). Erlotinib also is FDA approved as monotherapy in this group of patients. The results of such a clinical trial combining bevacizumab and erlotinib provide data that could lead to a new FDA recommendation for therapy in non-small cell lung cancer.

Phase III Trials

In phase III clinical trials, the research product may be compared to the current standard of care, and participants may be randomized to the standard or experimental treatment group. Larger numbers of participants usually are required to demonstrate statistical significance of the efficacy of the product over the control. These often are the most expensive, time-consuming, and complex trials to design and complete. Compilation of toxicities and safety issues continues through phase III trials as well. Data from phase III research on the safety and effectiveness of the research product over time will be presented for the FDA's consideration.

The value of quality cancer research is clearly demonstrated in the Cancer and Leukemia Group B 89803 study (Saltz et al., 2007). As a result of randomized research studies demonstrating a survival benefit, irinotecan, a topoisomerase 1 inhibitor, received FDA approval as first-line therapy for advanced colorectal cancer in combination with fluorouracil (FU) and leucovorin (LV) and as second-line therapy as a single agent. Although the drug was approved only for advanced colorectal cancer, patients were also receiving it as adjuvant therapy. Saltz et al. conducted a study of 1,264 research participants with completely resected stage III adenocarcinoma of the colon who had no evidence of disease. They were randomized to receive either the standard of care adjuvant therapy of FU plus LV or irinotecan with FU plus LV. Surprisingly, the data indicated that no significant disease-free survival or overall survival advantage resulted from adding the irinotecan to the standard adjuvant therapy of FU plus LV for people with stage III colon cancer. The researchers acknowledged that before and during their research, patients were being treated off-label in the adjuvant setting based on the promising results from the metastatic study with the combination of irinotecan and FU plus LV. The unfounded belief that an agent effective in the metastatic setting also will be beneficial in the adjuvant setting exposed many patients to the toxicities of this combination without evidence-based benefit. This study demonstrates the benefit of clinical research and the potential hazards of off-label use (Saltz et al.).

Optional Phase IV (Postmarketing) Research

After FDA approval is granted, occasionally the FDA may request or mandate or the product manufacturer may desire that additional research be conducted to identify long-term positive and negative effects of the approved product. Phase IV research may target a special population, such as older adults or people with compromised renal function. Data collected from a phase IV clinical trial may clarify unanswered questions from previous research and may affect the continuing approval and indications for the product (NCI, n.d.-a; PhRMA, 2007a).

The Ethics of Phase IV Clinical Trials

Grady (2007) defined ethics as "a systematic method of inquiry that helps us to answer questions about how we ought to live and behave and why" (p. 15). Grady explained that clinical research poses two fundamental ethical questions: Should we, and how should we, do clinical research? Although ideally all clinical trials have the same high standards and scientific integrity, phase IV research studies, also known as therapeutic use studies, are more challenging to monitor for this standard of ethics (Bickerstaff et al., 2006). Some clinicians and patients may be misdirected by clever marketing strategies used in phase IV clinical trials. Instead of focusing on long-term surveillance of efficacy and safety, motivations for phase IV research may be the realization of long-term profits. Bickerstaffe et al. suggested that if clinicians have any ethical concerns about a phase IV clinical trial, they may report their concerns to the sponsor of the clinical trial. If the concern continues, they should contact their ethics committee.

Although minimal literature exists on the topic, perhaps because of the sparsity of unethical phase IV issues, one research study explored physician remuneration for the enrollment of phase IV research participants. La Puma et al. (1995) found that 36% of doctors surveyed indicated that they were asked to participate in phase IV clinical research. Almost half (43%) reported that they received between $5 and $5,000 for each phase IV research participant enrolled, with a median of $80. Discordance occurred in the data between patients and physicians on acceptability of the doctor to accept a "finder's fee." Patients most frequently thought $10 would be a reasonable fee for a physician to accept, whereas most frequently physicians thought $100 was reasonable (La Puma et al.).

Clinical Research Review

Before enrolling the first research participant on a clinical research study, certain approvals must be received. All clinical research must be reviewed by the IRB. The IRB is the regulatory body authorized to review, approve, and regulate research. An IRB may be part of an academic or healthcare institution or an independent entity. The IRB's purpose includes (a) to protect the rights and welfare of research participants, (b) to determine that potential benefits are greater than the risks, (c) to ensure that research participant recruitment is equitable, and (d) to ensure that consent is obtained and documented, when appropriate (FDA, 2007b). The IRB also reviews and approves the informed consent form for the clinical research study. The IRB will "stamp" its mark on the approved informed consent form. Originally, a traditional inked stamp was used; now a logo or another electronic mark along with the date of approval and expiration date of the approval is used to identify the approved informed consent form.

According to the FDA (2007b), only two categories of new clinical research are exempt from IRB review. The first is an emergency use of an investigational product (also known as a test product) as long as it is reported to the IRB within five working days. The second exemption from review is for certain taste and food quality evaluations and consumer acceptance studies. However, qualifications are built into the second exemption related to the safety of the food product (FDA, 2007b). The U.S. Department of Health and Human Services (DHHS) has different qualifications for exemption from review (DHHS, 2004). Regardless, in all cases, the IRB determines whether a study is exempt from review, not the researchers.

Clinical research may need to have an expedited or convened meeting review. If the research does not involve more than minimum risk to the research participant, it may qualify for an expedited review and may fit into one of the expedited categories (DHHS, 1998). Examples of research that may qualify for expedited review include surveys, chart reviews, noninvasive testing, and some blood sampling research. The IRB renders the final ruling regarding expedited review status.

Depending on the investigational product, approval by another regulatory body in addition to the IRB may be required. This regulatory body may be either internal or external to the institution. For example, if the investigational product involves a toxin, an infectious agent, a pathogen, recombinant DNA or RNA, or gene transfer, an approval from the institutional biosafety committee (IBC) also will be required before research can commence. If the research involves collecting human research samples, a human tissue registration may also need to be filed with the IBC. The IBC ensures that investigational products, procedures, and settings comply with federal, state, and local biosafety regulations and institutional biosafety policies.

Additional reviews may be mandated by particular institutions before research information can be presented to the IRB. An internal scientific review committee reviews the research application for its scientific merit. A nursing research review committee evaluates the science of the proposed research and subsequent nursing implications. An administrative review evaluates presence of required documents needed for the IRB application. Specific institutional policies must be consulted regarding the requirements for initiating a new clinical research study.

Components of Clinical Research

Many components are essential to clinical research. The sponsor of a clinical trial is the developer of the research product and holds the IND application. The sponsor may be an individual or an entity that selects and trains the investigators and decides where the research will be conducted. Financial support for the study may come from the sponsor or from other sources. The sponsor is responsible to the FDA for all research conducted on the investigational product. The principal investigator, who is usually the lead clinician on the study, is responsible for the research conduct at the practice setting. Principal investigators do not directly interact with the FDA; that is the responsibility of the sponsor. Table 9-3 describes other critical components. These must be considered during the conception of the clinical research, the review process, the implementation phase, and the evaluation.

Informed Consent

Informed consent is a legal process whereby a person gives permission for some action based on thorough understanding of the implications of that action. Informed consent begins with the introduction of clinical research to the potential participant and leads to the participant's signature on the informed consent document. The signature is a legal formalization or documentation that the informational process has been sufficient for the person to make a decision about participation in the clinical research. Some suggest that the informed consent process should continue even when the research participant is off study if new developments might arise that may affect the research participant's safety. However, in most clinical research, the obligation ends after a protocol-specified time.

Mandates from the FDA and DHHS provide the essential ingredients for an informed consent (see Table 9-4). The IRB reviews informed consent documents to ensure the required elements of the informed consent document are present. IRBs may provide informed consent templates to facilitate compliance with the federal mandates.

On occasion, the FDA issues letters to sponsors and investigators mandating sharing new information about adverse drug effects long after the research has ended and/or extending the follow-up period. For example, a "Dear Gene Therapy IND Sponsor/

Table 9-3. Components of Clinical Research

Element	Description
Protocol	Guide to conduct of clinical research that includes • Background and significance • Primary and secondary aims • Design • Methods • Statistical analysis • Adverse reactions • Dissemination plan
Informed consent	Formal documentation in which the research participant acknowledges information about the study (see Table 9-4)
Investigator's brochure	The investigator's source of information about the research and development of the investigational product • Written and maintained by holder of the investigational new drug (IND) application • Contains preclinical, clinical, and manufacturing details • Defines the sponsor (person or organization responsible to the U.S. Food and Drug Administration [FDA]) • Details side effects that have occurred in animals and humans • Defines indications for and proper usage of the investigational product • Is updated whenever significant changes occur during the course of the research
Standard operation procedure (SOP) manual	Guidelines that facilitate consistent methods in conducting the research and may include • SOPs already in practice as well as those specific to the research (such as storage, accountability, preparation, and administration of the investigational product) • Information regarding specimen procurement and processing • Guidance on communicating with the sponsor and the internal regulatory bodies • Reporting of serious drug reactions
Curricula vitae, professional licenses, financial disclosures	Required for all principal and subinvestigators (coinvestigators) who are responsible for the conduct of the study • Document the qualifications needed to perform the clinical research responsibilities • Disclose financial involvement that may provide a real or perceived conflict of interest • Require dated signature of each investigator

Regulatory documents	Institutional review board (IRB) correspondence that may include
	• IRB approval letters for the initial submission and amendments
	• Continuing review reports; frequency and content depend on each IRB's policies (frequency is at least annually)
	• Unexpected problem/event reports (such as a death)
	• IND safety reports received from the sponsor
	• Acknowledgment of the IRB's receipt of IND safety
	• IRB-approved consent forms
	• IRB-approved advertisement
	• Form FDA 1572 (the Statement of the Investigator)
	  – Documents investigators' responsibility
	  – Names subinvestigators, sites of research, laboratory facilities, and IRB
	• Research participant log
	• Sponsor correspondence, including conference calls, meeting summaries, and reports
	• IRB membership list
	• Product inventory and shipping logs
	• Laboratory certifications and reference ranges for lab values
	• Monitoring visit logs
	• Blank set of case report forms

Note. Based on information from Guralnik & Manolio, 2007; Kvochak, 2007; Stone, 2006; Zoon & Yetter, 2007.

Table 9-4. Required Elements of Informed Consent

Factor	Details
General requirements	• Consent must be obtained from the participant or participant's legal representative. • Process must allow sufficient opportunity for the patient to consider whether to participate. • Process must minimize the possibility of coercion or undue influence. • Language of consent must be understandable to the participant or representative. • Agreement must not release or appear to release the investigator, sponsor, institution, or its agents from liability for negligence.

Basic elements	• States that the study involves research
	• Describes purpose, expected duration, and procedures
	• Describes foreseeable risks
	• Describes benefits
	• Discloses alternatives
	• Describes how confidentiality will be maintained
	• Explains what compensation or treatments are available if injury occurs
	• Defines whom to contact for questions about
	  – The research
	  – The participant's rights
	  – Research-related injury that occurs
	• Includes statements such as
	  – Participation is voluntary.
	  – Refusal to participate will not result in any penalty or loss of benefits.
	  – Participant may withdraw at any time without penalty or loss of benefits.

Additional elements that could possibly be included	• Reasons participation may be stopped by the investigator without the participant's consent • Additional costs for participation • Consequences of participant's withdrawal and procedures for orderly termination • Notice that if significant new findings occur that relate to the study product, this information will be provided to the participant • The approximate number of participants to be enrolled

Note. Based on information from U.S. Department of Health and Human Services, 2000; U.S. Food and Drug Administration, 2007a.

Principal Investigator Letter" was issued to ensure the continued safety of research participants who received a genetically modified investigational product. The letter informed the sponsor and investigator of a need for prolonged monitoring and the necessity of reporting adverse events to the National Institutes of Health/Office of Recombinant DNA Activities and the Center for Biologics Evaluation and Research (FDA, 1999).

Recruiting Clinical Trial Participants

An ever-present challenge facing researchers and the research team is the recruitment of research participants. Only an estimated 3%–5% of people with cancer participate in a cancer clinical trial (Elting et al., 2006; Lara et al., 2005). The suspected reasons vary for this disparaging low enrollment rate, but participation in cancer clinical research cannot increase without effective recruitment. Oncology APNs, because of their in-depth knowledge of the science that supports clinical research endeavors and oncology care, as well as their educational and communication skills, are the ideal practitioners to recruit research participants.

Several methods are commonly used to recruit individuals, including screening for and offering appropriate clinical trials to patients, referrals from other healthcare providers, community activities, databases, and advertisements about the clinical trial (Dunn & Chadwick, 2004). When research is conducted at multiple clinical sites, effective communication and a designated point person may enhance clinical trial participation (Berger, Neumark, & Chamberlain, 2007). IRB approval of recruitment strategies usually is required in advance of approving a protocol.

Accrual data timelines are an important topic for IRB review. If the clinical research is not meeting accrual goals, revised recruitment strategies may need to be submitted to the IRB with the continuing review application. Great variability exists in the financial and time requirements of recruitment strategies. Consideration of successful recruitment strategies used to target similar sample populations and to establish community commitment may be beneficial. Consulting with clinical research colleagues, healthcare providers, and patients within the targeted community may lead to valuable recruitment initiatives.

A common method of recruiting research participants is to deliver a message directly to the targeted sample. Direct advertisement may take many forms, including traditional or electronic mail to patients, flyers, Web postings, phone calls, magazine and newspaper postings, and radio or television announcements. Most advertisements for clinical research require IRB approval prior to their posting or implementation because advertisement for clinical research is considered part of the informed consent process. The first information that people receive about the research needs to be clear, concise, and free of misleading text.

The IRB's policy may mandate that the IRB approval stamp, along with the date of approval, be physically present on all direct advertisements. When reviewing a prospective advertisement, the IRB ensures that it contains no potential for misinterpretation, coercion, bias, or discrimination. Information about payments, benefits, and safety should not be overly emphasized. Some elements of marketing are required whenever marketing to professionals or the public (Dunn & Chadwick, 2004; Stone, 2006). They include
- Name and contact information for the principal investigator and coordinator
- Description of rationale, eligibility criteria, risks, and commitment
- Note that a drug is experimental, if the clinical trial involves the use of a drug and it is not FDA approved
- Conservative description of benefit and payment
- IRB's approval stamp and date.

An exception exists to obtaining preapproval for advertisement from the IRB. If the advertisement is aimed directly to healthcare providers, then messages sent by the principal investigator, sponsor, or institution can be in the form of direct mailings such as "dear doctor" letters and news reports without IRB approval (Stone, 2006).

Traditionally, clinical research teams have relied on research nurses for the recruitment of participants (Barrett, 2002). However, every healthcare provider must understand basic clinical research principles and how to access information about the availability of trials for any particular cancer. Oncology APNs may be involved in developing and reviewing clinical research advertisements. Knowledge of recruitment materials available to consumers regarding clinical research options is required for oncology APNs to interpret the relevance of this information for patients.

Interpreting Clinical Trials

On review of a clinical research abstract or article, clinicians may quickly scan to find the survival data and the significance level. Although these components are very important outcomes, the safety profile may not be given the acknowledgment it deserves. The safety profile includes adverse events, side effects, and toxicities. All of these terms have the same general meaning of reflecting a change from baseline for any sign, symptom, or abnormal assessment, such as a vital sign, lab result, or test result, that has a temporal association with the investigational product. Other logistical and psychosocial factors associated with the investigational product, such as the scheduling, insurance coverage, out-of-pocket expenses, and administration, also must be considered when interpreting clinical trial results.

In order to conduct survival analysis of any research study, only two data time points are needed for each research participant, a start and end date. Individual researchers define these two time points differently, thus causing a lack of uniformity across all research studies. The concern in having varying meaning for data points is that comparison across studies is compromised and may be impossible. For example, to define the start date for research participants in a resectable pancreatic cancer clinical trial, various dates could be used, such as when the first computed tomography scan visualized the mass, when the tumor was biopsied, when the tumor was removed via a pancreaticoduodenectomy, when the person signed consent, when eligibility to participate in the study was confirmed, or when the first investigational product was administered. Depending on which of these definitions is used, the start date may vary by months. In an aggressive disease like pancreatic cancer, the definition of the start date is carefully considered when evaluating survival data.

For the end time point, variability may be more restricted. For example, when using overall survival, no variations exist in the definition of date of death. However, for some participants, the date of death may be unknown. The research participant may be lost to follow-up or may withdraw from the study, or the study may end while research participants are still alive. In those cases, the data would be censored. The last date of contact typically is the censored date for overall survival analysis.

Johnson and Shih (2007) pointed out that "although the term *survival* is used, the event of interest is not limited to death or failure" (p. 273). Herein lies another area where caution is required in interpreting data. Perhaps the most common survival end point after overall survival is progression-free survival. Each clinical researcher defines the meaning of progression-free survival. It could be the date the research participant had a study visit, the date of the imaging studies that indicated progression, or another measure. Consideration must be given to how progression was determined and if that determination is typical of general clinical practices. To standardize when imaging studies provide significant results, many oncology researchers working with patients who have solid tumors use the Response Evaluation Criteria in Solid Tumors (RECIST). It provides concrete guidelines for evaluation of target, nontarget, and new lesions to determine the overall response (Therasse et al., 2000). Hematologic malignancies have similar guidelines to determine what constitutes progression.

Progression-free survival data also may be censored. Options include censoring research participants when they complete all or part of the investigational product regimen, or not censoring subjects at all, wherein the researchers continue to track the research participants' status (Allegra et al., 2007).

Survival data may be analyzed using the actuarial or Kaplan-Meier methods. The outputs are different in that the actuarial method divides time into sections and provides survival data for each time interval. An example using the actuarial methods would be survival data calculated at every three months of the research study. The Kaplan-Meier method calculates survival every time a research participant dies.

Allegra et al. (2007) have coined a new term: *time to failure of strategy* (TFS). They distinguished this new end point from time to treatment failure (TTF), which could be either the date of death, date of last treatment, or date of disease progression. It appears obvious that this definition could confuse efficacy with the toxicities of clinical research. Also, the researchers clarified that TTF is not the same as progression-free survival, which they preferred to label as *duration of disease control,* perhaps a more acceptable terminology. Research participants would reach the new clinical research end point (TFS) when "they require the addition of a non-protocol-specified new agent for further management, have disease progression while on all planned agents, experience progression and receive no further therapy within one month, or die" (Allegra et al., p. 3574). A strong feature of this new end point is that it allows consideration for maintenance therapies, breaks for holidays or toxicities, and the reintroduction of therapy if disease progresses.

Another type of clinical research end point uses a composite of variables to determine a clinical benefit response. Several subjective and objective measures relative to the condition being studied may be analyzed. For example, the FDA approved gemcitabine for treatment of advanced pancreatic cancer based on dates that included survival, time to progression, and clinical benefit response. The clinical benefit response was determined through an algorithm that analyzed the variables of weight change, pain scores, analgesic consumption, and performance status (Burris et al., 1997).

Sample size and power are determined during the design phase of the clinical research development. An inadequate sample size will affect the outcomes. Some researchers claim it is unethical to conduct clinical research without adequate sample sizes, as participants face the risks of research without making contributions to science (Halpern, Karlawish, & Berlin, 2005).

Recently, 423 randomized clinical trials reported at the American Society of Clinical Oncology's annual meeting as having negative results were analyzed post hoc. Bedard, Krzyzanowska, Pintilie, and Tannock (2007) determined that more than half of these negative studies had a sample size that could not detect a medium effect. Aware of the challenges in recruiting to cancer clinical trials, one may assume that this was a factor influencing these small sample sizes. However, only 35 (7.1%) of the studies reviewed indicated their reasons for a small sample size. Of these 35 studies, 13 (37%) indicated "slower than anticipated accrual" and 9 (26%) indicated "an interim analysis suggested lack of efficacy of the experimental treatment" as the reasons for the early termination (Bedard et al., p. 3484).

Another area of caution in interpreting research results is to not infer research conclusions to other conditions. As previously mentioned in Herbst et al.'s (2007) adjuvant colon cancer research, both clinicians and patients may misinterpret the conclusions of research and incorrectly infer that research findings apply to other conditions where research has not been completed. Oncology APNs' interpretations of clinical research findings are integral to informed decision making, whether the decision is for standard of care treatment or for cancer clinical research.

Clinical Trials Resources

As of August 3, 2007, 14,637 cancer clinical trials were posted to the NCI Web site database, also known as Physician Data Query (PDQ®) (available at www.cancer.gov/ search/searchclinicaltrialsadvanced.aspx) (NCI, n.d.-b). However, less than half of those listed (6,642) were actively recruiting subjects (National Institutes of Health National Library of Medicine, n.d.). Although it initially may seem odd that the database includes clinical trials that are closed, there is a good rationale. The WHO fueled the momentum that prompted the current clinical trial registry mandate. Registering all clinical trials prior to knowing the success of the research and providing a summary of its results promotes the public's trust in the way research is conducted and removes some of the mystery surrounding research. It also allows standardization of findings and avoids unnecessary duplication of research. Scientific and ethical integrity of clinical research is enhanced by the use of a universal system to register clinical trials.

The International Committee of Medical Journal Editors (ICMJE) mandated that only manuscripts originating from clinical trials registered before enrolling the first human subject would be considered for publication in peer-reviewed journals. Although the WHO recognizes clinical trial transparency and public trust as global issues and the subsequent rationale for their recommendation of a universal research registry, the ICMJE had a slightly different goal. The rationale for the ICMJE's stand regarding clinical trial registry was "to promote the public good by ensuring that everyone can find information about every clinical trial whose principal aim is to help shape medical decision making" (Deangelis et al., 2005, p. 2928). This policy applies to all clinical trials, not just cancer clinical trials, that began enrollment on or after July 1, 2005. Clinical trials that started before July 1, 2005, had another 10 weeks to complete the registration process. The ICMJE defines a clinical trial as a prospective intervention research project with a concurrent control or comparison group designed to affect a health outcome. The intervention may include a drug, surgical procedure, device, behavioral treatment, and process-of-care changes. Because the ICMJE feels that the public needs to know about clinical trials that may affect clinical practice, trial registration also is required for all phase III clinical trials regardless of the study design. The ICMJE does not currently mandate that all clinical trials, such as those exploring safety of the research product or pharmacokinetics, be registered; however, individual journals may have more strict guidelines mandating the registration of all clinical trials (Deangelis et al.).

The WHO established the essential elements for clinical trial registration at its 2004 meeting. Table 9-5 lists the WHO's criteria as well as comments adapted from the ICMJE.

Oncology APNs have options when choosing a clinical trial registry for their clinical research as well as searching for cancer research for their patients. All reputable clinical trial registries must be electronically searchable and free for the public's access (Deangelis et al., 2005). APNs may prefer NCI's database (PDQ) for finding cancer clinical trials. NCI's database is easy to navigate with both basic and advanced search options; it is the gold standard for locating a cancer clinical trial. NCI's Web site (www.cancer.gov/clinicaltrials) also is a valuable resource for finding results of recently completed cancer clinical trials and for accessing general educational materials on clinical research and specific information about conducting clinical research.

Although research has been ongoing since Biblical times, the phenomenon of reviewing research for purposes of strengthening health care is relatively new. Professor Archie Cochrane, author of *Effectiveness and Efficiency: Random Reflections of Health Ser-*

Table 9-5. World Health Organization Clinical Research Minimal Registration Data Set

World Health Organization Criteria Item	Comments by International Committee of Medical Journal Editors
1. Unique trial number	Assigned by registry
2. Trial registration date	Established by registry
3. Secondary identification (optional)	May be assigned by sponsor, institution, cooperative group, or other party
4. Funding source(s)	Organization that is supporting the trial
5. Primary sponsor	Main entity responsible for performing the research
6. Secondary sponsor(s)	Secondary entities, if any, responsible for performing the research
7. Responsible contact person	Public contact person for people interested in participating
8. Research contact person	Person to contact regarding scientific inquiries
9. Title of the study	Brief title
10. Official scientific title of the study	The title must include the name of the intervention, the condition being studied, and the outcome.
11. Research ethics review	Has the study at the time of registration received appropriate ethics committee approval?
12. Condition	The medical condition being studied
13. Intervention	A description of the study and comparison/control intervention(s). The duration of the intervention must be specified.
14. Key inclusion and exclusion criteria	Characteristics that determine if a person is eligible for the clinical trial
15. Study type	Randomized or nonrandomized, type of masking, type of controls, and group assignment
16. Anticipated trial start date	Estimated enrollment date for the first participant
17. Target sample size	Total number of participants that investigators plan to enroll
18. Recruitment status	Is this information available? If yes, provide the electronic link.
19. Primary outcome	Primary outcome that the study was designed to evaluate
20. Key secondary outcomes	As specified in the protocol

Note. Based on information from Deangelis et al., 2005; World Health Organization, n.d.

vices (1972), may have conceptualized the evidence-based practice movement, and the term *evidence-based medicine* was first coined by Gordon Guyatt, David Sayatt, and their colleagues in 1992 (Evidence-Based Medicine Working Group). From 1992 to 1996, the Agency for Health Care Policy and Research (AHCPR) released 19 clinical practice guidelines. Many oncology APNs will recall the clinical practice guideline No. 9, *Management of Cancer Pain* (Jacox et al., 1994). Although this specific guideline is no longer recommended for practice because the content is dated, it is available for historical review at www.ncbi.nlm.nih.gov/books/bv.fcgi?rid=hstat6.chapter.18803.

Jacox et al. (1994) and their Cancer Pain Management Panel introduced many to the value of evidence-based practice. Figure 9-3 displays the levels and strength of evidence provided in this first clinical practice guideline focused on cancer. The guideline was published in four versions: clinicians' guidelines, quick version, and an English and Spanish version of the consumers' guidelines. The impact of this guideline revolutionized cancer pain management.

Type of evidence
  I. Meta-analysis of multiple, well-designed controlled studies.
     A. Studies of patients with cancer.
     B. Studies of other clinical populations.
  II. At least one well-designed experimental study.
     A. Studies of patients with cancer.
     B. Studies of other clinical populations.
  III. Well-designed, quasiexperimental studies such as nonrandomized controlled, single group pre-post, cohort, time series, or matched case-controlled studies.
     A. Studies of patients with cancer.
     B. Studies of other clinical populations.
  IV. Well-designed nonexperimental studies, such as comparative and correlational descriptive and case studies.
     A. Studies of patients with cancer.
     B. Studies of other clinical populations.
  V. Case reports and clinical examples.
     A. Studies of patients with cancer.
     B. Studies of other clinical populations.

Strength and consistency of evidence
  A. There is evidence of type I or consistent findings from multiple studies of types II, III, or IV.
  B. There is evidence of types II, III, or IV, and findings are generally consistent.
  C. There is evidence of types II, III, or IV, but findings are inconsistent.
  D. There is little or no evidence, or there is type V evidence only.

Panel Consensus—Practice recommended on the basis of opinion of experts in pain management

---

Figure 9-3. Type, Strength, and Consistency of Evidence

Note. From *Clinical Practice Guideline No. 9: Management of Cancer Pain,* by A. Jacox, D.B. Carr, R. Payne, C.B. Berde, W. Breitbart, J.M. Cain, et al., March 1994, Rockville, MD: Agency for Health Care Policy and Research, U.S. Department of Health and Human Services, Public Health Service.

In 1997, the AHCPR evolved to the Agency for Healthcare Research and Quality (AHRQ) along with a different approach of bringing evidence-based practice to those who make healthcare decisions. The AHRQ now works with 12 Evidence-Based Practice Centers that also may include input from outside organizations to develop evidence reports and technology assessments. Rigorous syntheses and analyses of the scientific literature are the foundations for these reports designed to facilitate decisions made on many levels. Decisions made on the basis of evidence-based reports may be related to health policy, insurance benefits, clinical practice guidelines, or individual patients (Havighurst, Hutt, McNeil, & Miller, 2001). To date, 18 cancer-related evidence reports exist. The first cancer-related report was released in 2000, titled *The Efficacy of Interventions to Modify Di-*

etary Behavior Related to Cancer Risk, and the most recently released report is *Hereditary Nonpolyposis Colorectal Cancer: Diagnostic Strategies and Their Implications.* Many additional topics, although not specific to oncology, may be of interest to oncology APNs, such as meditation practices for health; preventive care, economic incentives; nurse staffing and the quality of patient care; and systematic reviews, criteria for distinguishing effectiveness from efficacy trials (AHRQ, 2007). All of these reports can be reviewed at www.ahrq.gov/clinic/epcindex.htm#hematology.

In addition to the AHRQ reports to facilitate evidence-based practice, many other resources also are available. The increased prevalence of practice guidelines and the recognition of their value are not surprising. The purpose of clinical practice guidelines is to determine the best care for patients without increasing healthcare costs (Goode et al., 2000). The National Guideline Clearinghouse (www.guidelines.gov) is a comprehensive electronic database of evidence-based clinical guidelines. The National Comprehensive Cancer Network (www.nccn.org) offers a collection of oncology clinical practice guidelines on treatments, detection, prevention, risk reduction, and supportive care. The main product of the Cochrane Collection (www.cochrane.org), named after Professor Archie Cochrane, is a comprehensive database of systematic reviews on a variety of oncology and non-oncology health topics.

The Oncology Nursing Society (ONS) is taking the lead among nursing organizations to facilitate the incorporation of evidence-based practice into daily oncology nursing practice. The ONS Putting Evidence Into Practice® (PEP) resource cards are designed to be carried into the practice setting. These pocket-sized cards provide a concise summary of analyses and recommendations from oncology nurse experts. Currently, PEP cards are available on a variety of oncology nursing sensitive outcomes: fatigue; chemotherapy-induced nausea and vomiting; prevention of infection; sleep-wake disturbances; caregiver strain and burden; constipation; depression; dyspnea; mucositis; peripheral neuropathy; prevention of bleeding; pain; anorexia; anxiety; diarrhea; and lymphedema. More information about the PEP resource cards can be found at www.ons.org/outcomes/measures.

Measuring Quality of Life in Clinical Trials

Research interest in the quality of life of people with cancer became evident in the 1980s (Buchanan et al., 2007). As in clinical research for drug development, challenges and controversies exist within quality-of-life research. Efficace and Bottomley (2002) proposed several reasons why quality-of-life studies cannot improve patient care. They claim that quality-of-life studies often are of weak methodologic character, are inadequately reported, and lack agreed-upon standards for conducting and reporting quality of life (Efficace & Bottomley).

Although challenges exist in quality-of-life studies partly because of the multitude of measurement tools available to evaluate this important construct, many recognize the value of quality-of-life research and its relation to evidence-based clinical practice guidelines (Griffin, Koch, Nelson, & Cooley, 2007; Guyatt et al., 2000; Guyatt & Schunemann, 2007). Buchanan et al. (2007) published a report based on their NCI-sponsored workshop titled "Quality of Life Assessment in Cancer Symptom Management Trials." Although many recommendations were made as a result of the workshop, the first major recommendation was that "researchers should always consider the possibility that HRQOL [health-related quality of life] assessment has potential research value" (Buchanan et al., p. 1623). This clearly differentiates HRQOL from quality of life that could include all components of a person's life: employment, education, environment, and so on. Recommendations were made that clearly defining HRQOL and using a conceptual model enhances the research value. During the two-day workshop, experts discussed how variations within the four components of a global quality-of-life measure (functional status, disease symptoms, psychological functioning, and social functioning) could be masked in one global score. The workshop participants concluded that agreement on a single definition and measurement tool for HRQOL was unlikely to occur in the near future (Buchanan et al.).

Oncology Nursing Research

Historical milestones in the interest of oncology nursing research paralleled or closely followed that of the general nursing community (see Table 9-6). During the 1940s and 1950s, the focus was on the nursing profession, education, and administrative issues. In the 1960s, the focus was redirected to patient care (McGee, 1989). Now, research priorities are multicentered on the many facets of nursing (see Table 9-6). Research involving nursing-sensitive patient outcomes will validate oncology nursing's value to the healthcare enterprise. In clinical research, translational research takes preclinical discoveries to the clinic, whereas in nursing, translational research explores system and clinician factors that affect healthcare outcomes when evidence-based clinical guidelines are implemented.

Oncology nursing's rich legacy in research is well-documented within the ONS publication *It Took Courage, Compassion, and Curiosity—Recollections and Writings of Leaders in Cancer Nursing: 1890–1970*. Although many are identified as oncology nurse researchers, Jeanne Quint Benoliel has been labeled by her peers as a leader in cancer nursing and research (Johnson, Baird, & Hilderley, 2001). As early as 1959, she knew the value of advanced oncology nursing research when she enrolled in an experimental research post-master's program at the University of California, Los Angeles. Benoliel was known as a nurse researcher/scientist pioneer at a time when most nurses were direct caregivers or teachers (Johnson et al.). She is also known for her research work in the landmark mastectomy study of 1961 funded by the National Institute of Mental Health.

Throughout the years, oncology nursing research has continued to be a formidable force within quality cancer care. Oncology APNs lead and participate in clinical research studies that affect not only how services can be provided most efficiently but also patient outcomes. Even when not directly working within cancer research, oncology APNs are essential to identifying research questions, evaluating research, and implementing evidence-based practice—all vital components of quality cancer research.

Funding Sources

Limited research funding sources are available. The government remains the largest supporter of cancer clinical research, but the pharmaceutical industry and various organizations also provide substantial support. The ONS Foundation is one of the largest supporters of oncology nursing research, providing more than $8 million since the foundation began in 1981 (ONS Foundation, n.d.). ONS's position is that increased research funding is essential for the continuum of cancer research, from cancer prevention to survivorship issues (ONS, 2006).

Table 9-6. Historical Nursing Research Milestones With Empahsis on Oncology Nursing

Year	Event
1859	Florence Nightingale's *Notes on Nursing* published.
1900	First nursing journal, *American Journal of Nursing,* published.
1952	First nursing research journal, *Nursing Research,* published.
1955	Inception of American Nurses' Foundation, a source for research funding.
1963	Seminal research article published by oncology nurse scientist Jeanne Quint Benoliel.
1965	American Nurses Association begins funding nursing research.
1973	"American Cancer Society Proceedings of the National Conference on Cancer Nursing" published.
1974	*Cancer Nursing Newsletter* (forerunner to the *Oncology Nursing Newsletter,* and then the *Oncology Nursing Forum*) published.
1977	First oncology nursing journal, *Oncology Nursing Forum,* published.
1981	Inception of Oncology Nursing Foundation, source for research funding, later renamed to ONS Foundation.
1986	National Center for Nursing Research (NCNR), source for research funding, established within National Institutes of Health.
1993	NCNR becomes the National Institute of Nursing Research.
2001	First Oncology Nursing Society (ONS) Research Agenda published.
2005	First ONS Putting Evidence Into Practice® (PEP) cards released.

Note. Based on information from Oncology Nursing Society, n.d.; Polit & Beck, 2006.

Many organizations have application information available on their Web sites (see Table 9-7) along with their research priorities or goals in funding clinical research. These funding priorities may be based on the mission of the organization or determined by their members.

ONS conducted a descriptive, cross-sectional survey in which more than 2,800 randomly selected ONS members were invited to participate. Although the overall response rate was only 15%, sufficient data were collected to establish the top research priorities for 2005–2007 (Berger et al., 2005). Based on the most recent membership survey, the revised 2005–2009 ONS Research Agenda lists six priority areas and topics that are equally important (see Figure 9-4). Additional details on these priority headings can be found at the ONS Foundation Web site (www.onsfoundation.org).

Conclusion

Opportunities for oncology APNs to become involved with clinical research are diverse. APNs may (a) refer patients for research, (b) design the protocol, (c) consent, screen, examine, and evaluate research participants, (d) manage regulatory affairs, (e) be a co- or subinvestigator, (f) be a principal investigator, (g) analyze the data, (h) disseminate research findings, (i) serve as a consultant to clinical researchers to identify and manage complications, and (j) serve on a committee or board that provides scientific, regulatory, or ethical review. Many APNs are active in more than one of these clinical research roles. In fact, as a principal investigator, the APN has an active role in participating in all of the aforementioned listed opportunities or providing direct oversight for assigned colleagues.

APNs have several options for strengthening their knowledge on clinical research. One resource is the NIH complimentary three-hour online training on the principles, policies, and regulations that guide ethical human research (http://phrp .nihtraining.com). Although this training was designed for researchers seeking federal funding for their research, it is available for all interested APNs. Another comprehensive resource is the research section of the ONS Web site (www.ons.org /research). Up-to-date information can be found specific to ONS such as the ONS research agenda and priorities, available awards, opportunities for funding, research expert profiles, and the research consultation program, as well as links to a variety of research resources.

Table 9-7. Sources for Clinical Nursing Research Funding

Organization	Web Site
American Cancer Society	www.cancer.org/docroot/RES/RES_0.asp
American Nurses Foundation	www.anfonline.org/anf/nrggrant.htm
Komen Foundation	http://cms.komen.org/komen/GrantsProgram/index.htm
National Institute of Nursing Research	www.ninr.nih.gov
ONS Foundation	www.onsfoundation.org
Sigma Theta Tau International	www.nursingsociety.org/research/main.html

Note. Based on information from Berry et al., 2007.

- Research in cancer symptoms and side effects
- Individual and family-focused psychosocial and behavioral research
- Research in health promotion: Primary and secondary prevention
- Research that considers the late effects of cancer treatment and long-term survivorship issues for patients and families
- Research in nursing-sensitive patient outcomes
- Translational research to develop, test, and evaluate strategies designed to determine which system- and clinician-related factors affect the clinical application of already created evidence-based guidelines

Figure 9-4. 2005–2009 Oncology Nursing Society Research Agenda: Content Areas

Note. Based on information from Berry et al., 2007.

Case Study

C.S. is a 54-year-old female patient with advanced pancreatic cancer who wants to participate in a phase I clinical trial that was featured on the news two weeks ago. When the oncology APN first meets C.S., she tells her that since hearing the news that "a cure for pancreatic cancer has been found," she could hardly wait to get started. The APN notes that her handshake is weak and she appears frail. Her family reports that she did not eat any breakfast that morning because she is so nervous. C.S. shares that her appetite has not been good for the past few days because of the anxiety of waiting for this first consultation visit. She has been traveling with her family since before dawn to arrive for this early afternoon appointment. Her partner, her two adult children, and her father accompany her and appear very distressed over C.S.'s current condition. C.S. is extremely fatigued and was transported from the car to the office via a wheelchair. Her family indicates that she usually is more energetic and is "sleepy" now only because they all needed to wake up so early to arrive in time for this appointment. Her family believes that her fatigue and anorexia are related to this visit.

The plan of care was to obtain an informed consent at this visit for the cancer clinical trial and to initiate screening to determine eligibility.

1. After introductions are made and comfort measures are provided for the patient and her family, how should the oncology APN begin the consenting process?
   - During the initial greeting, C.S. shared information about how she learned about the cancer clinical trial. Earlier this week on the local evening news, a report indicated that the phase I study for a new investigational product that rid some mice of advanced pancreatic cancer was going to start. The oncology APN could begin the consenting process by discussing the research history of the new investigational product. The oncology APN could briefly explain the phases of research, including the preclinical phase, in which mice are treated with the investigational product. The APN would note that the successful results seen in mice do not always happen in humans. C.S. and her family need to know that the purpose of the phase I research study is to find out if the new investigational product can be given safely to humans and to determine the best dose. All phase I research studies are not designed to offer a therapeutic benefit.
   - C.S. and the family are puzzled now. They thought they heard reliable news that reported the existence of a cure for pancreatic cancer. C.S.'s partner said, "You are just saying that to keep the publicity and malpractice claims under control. We know that you have the cure. Your lawyers are probably telling you to say that, right?" The oncology APN assures C.S. and her family that because this is the first time the investigational product will be given to humans, the effects are unknown. The drug may help, but it also may be harmful. The APN explains that this is a phase I, dose-escalating study and that even if the investigational product is found to be helpful, neither C.S. nor the healthcare providers will know if she will be receiving the optimal dose.
2. After the oncology APN provides an overview of the essential elements of the informed consent, C.S. asks, "Can I sign the papers now?" Her partner asks, "She's ready to sign up. Just tell her where to sign and let's be on with it." How should the oncology APN respond?

- The oncology APN knows that ensuring an adequate informed consent benefits the research participant and the cancer clinical trial. By knowing as much as possible about the cancer clinical trial, the research participant can be a partner in research. Having research participants understand their essential role in the cancer clinical trial can affect retention. The APN anticipated that C.S. would bring family and friends with her and provided extra copies of the informed consent document. Each person receives a copy of the consent and is asked to read the document thoroughly. The APN could encourage them to mark the areas of the consent that they find to be unclear or have questions about. After they have read the consent, the oncology APN will return to answer their questions.
- Twenty minutes later, the family indicates that they have read the consent, and the nurse finds C.S. in a deep sleep. She arouses but is having difficulty staying awake. The family suggests that they allow C.S. to sleep, as she already signed the informed consent document. They ask if she needs to be awake to receive the treatment.

3. What about this situation would cause concern to the APN?
- A few events could cause the oncology APN to become concerned. The oncology APN knows that the informed consent form needs to be signed in her presence. She tells the family that she needs to review the consent with C.S. to determine her understanding of the content of the informed consent document. The oncology APN explains to the family that part of the routine consenting process includes validation from the research participant about what information is contained in the document that is being signed. This includes that the purpose and process of the cancer clinical trial be explained in the patient's own words. The oncology APN also needs to assess her understanding of the time commitment required to be a research participant. Because C.S. is not mentally alert enough to continue with the consenting process, the oncology APN suggests they return another day to continue. The family indicates that they were planning to drive back home today and that these long drives are taking a toll on C.S. They ask if their local APN can sign the consents with C.S. tomorrow.

4. Can the oncology APN arrange this for C.S.'s convenience?
- No, this is not an option. The oncology APN explains why C.S. will need to return to the clinical site to continue the consenting process. The oncology APN knows that only certain investigators who have received training about the study and have adequate education and experience are allowed to obtain informed consent. Also, for each study, investigators are selected by the principal investigator and approved by the IRB. Within the cancer clinical trial's regulatory binders, the oncology APN's signed and dated curriculum vita, APN license, and financial disclosure form are on file. Another healthcare provider would not have approval by the IRB nor have the training to perform this function.

The oncology APN is sensitive to the family's desire to help their loved one. She shares information about the signs and symptoms of advanced pancreatic cancer. She acknowledges that while the long drive and the excitement of today's visit probably affected C.S.'s energy level, the decreasing performance status actually may reflect advancing disease. C.S.'s inability to eat also may be reflective of the anorexia that accompanies advanced pancreatic cancer. The APN encourages the family to call the clinic tomorrow when C.S. is more alert. They do have a speaker phone at home, and all who are present today plan to talk tomorrow on the call. The oncology APN provides the family with several educational materials. The topics include dealing with advanced cancer, pancreatic cancer, hospice care, clinical trial information, and Internet resources. She also plans to discuss with C.S.'s oncology healthcare provider that C.S. may not be a good candidate for the cancer clinical trial.

Key Points

- Clinical research is the systematic investigation of human biology, health, or illness that contributes to generalizable knowledge.
- General requirements of informed consent include
  - Consent must be obtained from the participant or the participant's legal representative.
  - Process must allow sufficient opportunity to consider whether to participate.
  - Process must minimize the possibility of coercion or undue influence.
  - Language of consent must be understandable to the participant or representative.
  - Consent must not release or appear to release the investigator, sponsor, institution, or its agents from liability for negligence.
- Only about 1 out of 10,000 compounds discovered will eventually receive an FDA indication for use in oncology. The time for the research and development of a pharmacologic agent averages approximately 9 years but could take as long as 15 years.
- Only an estimated 3%–5% of people with cancer participate in a cancer clinical trial; thus, recruitment of participants to oncology trials must be a priority for oncology APNs.
- Oncology APNs have diverse roles in clinical research and may
  - Refer patients for research
  - Design the protocol
  - Consent, screen, examine, and evaluate research participants
  - Manage regulatory affairs
  - Be a co- or subinvestigator
  - Be a principal investigator
  - Analyze the data
  - Disseminate research findings
  - Serve as a consultant to clinical researchers to identify and manage complications
  - Serve on a committee or board that provides scientific, regulatory, or ethical review.

Recommended Resources for Oncology Advanced Practice Nurses

- CenterWatch Clinical Trials Listing Service™: www.centerwatch.com/index.html

- National Comprehensive Cancer Network oncology clinical trial information for patients: www.nccn.org/clinical_trials/patients.asp
- NCI Clinical Trials Web page: www.cancer.gov/clinicaltrials

References

Agency for Healthcare Research and Quality. (2007). *EPC evidence reports.* Retrieved August 3, 2007, from http://www.ahrq.gov/clinic/epcindex.htm#hematology

Allegra, C., Blanke, C., Buyse, M., Goldberg, R., Grothey, A., Meropol, N.J., et al. (2007). End points in advanced colon cancer clinical trials: A review and proposal. *Journal of Clinical Oncology, 25,* 3572–3575.

Barrett, R. (2002). A nurse's primer on recruiting participants for clinical trials. *Oncology Nursing Forum, 29,* 1091–1095.

Bedard, P.L., Krzyzanowska, M.K., Pintilie, M., & Tannock, I.F. (2007). Statistical power of negative randomized controlled trials presented at American Society of Clinical Oncology annual meetings. *Journal of Clinical Oncology, 25,* 3482–3487.

Beecher, H.K. (1966). Ethics and clinical research. *New England Journal of Medicine, 94,* 1280–1300.

Berger, A.M., Berry, D., Christopher, K.A., Greene, A.L., Maliski, S., Swenson, K.K., et al. (2005). Oncology Nursing Society's 2004 nursing research priorities survey. *Oncology Nursing Forum, 32,* 281–290.

Berger, A.M., Neumark, D.E., & Chamberlain, J. (2007). Enhancing recruitment and retention in randomized clinical trials of cancer symptom management [Online exclusive]. *Oncology Nursing Forum, 34,* E17–E22.

Berry, D.L., Champion, V., Dodd, M., Given, B., Haase, J.E., Jacobs, L.A., et al. (2007). *Oncology Nursing Society 2005–2009 research agenda.* Retrieved October 5, 2007, from http://www.ons.org/research/information/documents/pdfs/executive05.pdf

Bickerstaffe, R., Brock, P., Husson, J.-M., Rubin, I., Bragman, K., Paterson, K., et al. (2006). Ethics and pharmaceutical medicine—the full report of the Ethical Issues Committee of the Faculty of Pharmaceutical Medicine of the Royal Colleges of Physicians of the UK. *International Journal of Clinical Practice, 60,* 242–252.

Buchanan, D.R., O'Mara, A.M., Kelaghan, J.W., Sgambati, M., McCaskill-Stevens, W., & Minasian, L. (2007). Challenges and recommendations for advancing the state-of-the-science of quality of life assessment in symptom management trials. *Cancer, 110,* 1621–1628.

Burris, H.A., Moore, M.J., Andersen, J., Green, M.R., Rothenberg, M.L., Modiano, M.R., et al. (1997). Improvements in survival and clinical benefit with gemcitabine as first-line therapy for patients with advanced pancreas cancer: A randomized trial. *Journal of Clinical Oncology, 15,* 2403–2413.

Cochrane, A.L. (1972). *Effectiveness and efficiency: Random reflections of health services.* London: Nuffield Provincial Hospitals Trust.

Deangelis, C.D., Drazen, J.M., Frizelle, F.A., Haug, C., Hoey, J., Horton, R., et al. (2005). Is this clinical trial fully registered? A statement from the International Committee of Medical Journal Editors. *JAMA, 293,* 2927–2929.

Dunn, C.M., & Chadwick, G.L. (2004). *Protecting study volunteers in research: A manual for investigative sites* (2nd ed.). Boston: CenterWatch.

Efficace, F., & Bottomley, A. (2002). Do quality-of-life randomized clinical trials support clinicians in their decision-making? *Journal of Clinical Oncology, 20,* 4126–1427.

Efron, B. (1998). R.A. Fisher in the 21st century. Invited paper presented at the 1996 R. A. Fisher lecture (with comments). *Statistical Science, 13,* 95–122.

Elting, L.S., Cooksley, C., Bekele, B.N., Frumovitz, M., Avritscher, E.B., Sun, C., et al. (2006). Generalizability of cancer clinical trial results: Prognostic differences between participants and nonparticipants. *Cancer, 106,* 2452–2458.

Emens, L.A., Armstrong, D., Biedrzycki, B., Davidson, N., Davis-Sproul, J., Fetting, J., et al. (2004). A phase I vaccine safety and chemotherapy dose-finding trial of an allogeneic GM-CSF-secreting breast cancer vaccine given in a specifically timed sequence with immunomodulatory doses of cyclophosphamide and doxorubicin. *Human Gene Therapy, 15,* 313–337.

Evidence-Based Medicine Working Group. (1992). Evidence-based medicine: A new approach to teaching the practice of medicine. *JAMA, 268,* 2420–2425.

Friedman, L.M., Furberg, C.D., & DeMets, D.L. (1998). *Fundamentals of clinical trials* (3rd ed.). New York: Springer.

Gallin, J.I. (2007). A historical perspective on clinical research. In J.I. Gallin & F.P. Ognibene (Eds.), *Principles and practice of clinical research* (2nd ed., pp. 1–13). Burlington, MA: Academic Press.

Goode, C.J., Tanaka, D.J., Krugman, M., O'Connor, P.A., Bailey, C., Deutchman, M., et al. (2000). Outcomes from use of an evidence-based practice guideline. *Nursing Economic$, 18,* 202–207.

Grady, C. (2007). Ethical principles on clinical research. In J.I. Gallin & F.P. Ognibene (Eds.), *Principles and practice of clinical research* (2nd ed., pp. 15–26). Burlington, MA: Academic Press.

Griffin, J.P., Koch, K.A., Nelson, J.E., & Cooley, M.E. (2007). Palliative care consultation, quality-of-life measurements, and bereavement for end-of-life care in patients with lung cancer: ACCP evidence-based clinical practice guideline (2nd edition). *Chest, 132*(Suppl. 3), 404S–422S.

Guralnik, J.M., & Manolio, T.A. (2007). Design and conduct of observational studies and clinical trials. In J.I. Gallin & F.P. Ognibene (Eds.), *Principles and practice of clinical research* (2nd ed., pp. 197–217). Burlington, MA: Academic Press.

Guyatt, G., & Schunemann, H. (2007). How can quality of life researchers make their work more useful to health workers and their patients? *Quality of Life Research, 16,* 1097–1105.

Guyatt, G.H., Haynes, R.B., Jaeschke, R.Z., Cook, D.J., Green, L., Naylor, C.D., et al. (2000). Users' guides to the medical literature. XXV. Evidence-based medicine: Principles for applying the users' guides to patient care. *JAMA, 284,* 1290–1296.

Halpern, S.D., Karlawish, J.H., & Berlin, J.A. (2005). Ethics and sample size. *American Journal of Epidemiology, 161,* 105–110.

Havighurst, C.C., Hutt, P.B., McNeil, B.J., & Miller, W. (2001). Evidence: Its meaning in health care and in law. *Journal of Health Politics, Policy and Law, 26,* 195–216.

Herbst, R.S., O'Neill, V.J., Fehrenbacher, L., Belani, C.P., Bonomi, P.D., Hart, L., et al. (2007). Phase II study of efficacy and safety of bevacizumab in combination with chemotherapy or erlotinib compared with chemotherapy alone for treatment of recurrent or refractory non–small-cell lung cancer. *Journal of Clinical Oncology, 25,* 4743–4750.

Jacox, A., Carr, D.B., Payne, R., Berde, C.B., Breitbart, W., Cain, J.M., et al. (1994). *Clinical practice guideline No. 9: Management of cancer pain* [AHCPR Publication No. 94-0592]. Rockville, MD: Agency for Health Care Policy and Research, U.S. Department of Health and Human Services, Public Health Service.

Jaffee, E.M., Hruban, R.H., Biedrzycki, B., Laheru, D., Schepers, K., Sauter, P.R., et al. (2001). Novel allogeneic granulocyte-macrophage colony-stimulating factor-secreting tumor vaccine for pancreatic cancer: A phase I trial of safety and immune activation. *Journal of Clinical Oncology, 19,* 145–156.

Johnson, J.B., Baird, S.B., & Hilderley, L.J. (2001). *It took courage, compassion, and curiosity—recollections and writings of leaders in cancer nursing: 1890–1970.* Pittsburgh, PA: Oncology Nursing Society.

Johnson, L.L., & Shih, J.H. (2007). An introduction to survival analysis. In J.I. Gallin & F.P. Ognibene (Eds.), *Principles and practice of clinical research* (2nd ed., pp. 273–282). Burlington, MA: Academic Press.

Kvochak, P.A. (2007). Legal issues. In J.I. Gallin & F.P. Ognibene (Eds.), *Principles and practice of clinical research* (2nd ed., pp. 109–123). Burlington, MA: Academic Press.

La Puma, J., Stocking, C.B., Rhoades, W.D., Darling, C.M., Ferner, R.E., Neuberger, J., et al. (1995). Financial ties as part of informed consent to postmarketing research—attitudes of American doctors and patients. *BMJ, 310,* 1660–1663.

Lara, P.N., Paterniti, D.A., Chiechi, C., Turrell, C., Morain, C., Horan, N., et al. (2005). Evaluation of factors affecting awareness of and willingness to participate in cancer clinical trials. *Journal of Clinical Oncology, 23,* 9282–9289.

McGee, R. (1989). Oncology nursing: Five decades of growth. *Journal of Cancer Education, 4,* 167–173.

Munro, B.H. (2005). *Statistical methods for health care research* (5th ed.). Philadelphia: Lippincott Williams & Wilkins.

National Cancer Institute. (2007). *Dictionary of cancer terms: Clinical study.* Retrieved August 3, 2007, from http://www.cancer.gov/templates/db_alpha.aspx?cdrid=44195

National Cancer Institute. (n.d.-a). *Clinical trials: Questions and answers.* Retrieved August 3, 2007, from http://www.cancer.gov/cancertopics/factsheet/Information/clinical-trials

National Cancer Institute. (n.d.-b). *Search for clinical trials: Advanced search.* Retrieved August 3, 2007, from http://www.cancer.gov/search/searchclinicaltrialsadvanced.aspx

National Institutes of Health. (n.d.). *Protecting human research participants.* Retrieved March 15, 2008, from http://phrp.nihtraining.com

National Institutes of Health National Library of Medicine. (n.d.). *ClinicalTrials.gov: Linking patients to medical research.* Retrieved August 3, 2007, from http://clinicaltrials.gov

Oncology Nursing Society. (2006). *Cancer research and cancer clinical trials* [Position statement]. Retrieved August 3, 2007, from http://www.ons.org/publications/positions/CancerResearch.shtml

Oncology Nursing Society. (n.d.). *Outcomes measures.* Retrieved August 3, 2007, from http://www.ons.org/outcomes/measures

Oncology Nursing Society Foundation. (n.d.). *Donations at work.* Retrieved April 9, 2008, from http://www.onsfoundation.org/donations.shtml

Pharmaceutical Research and Manufacturers of America. (2007a, February). *Drug, discovery and development: Understanding the R & D process.* Washington, DC: Author.

Pharmaceutical Research and Manufacturers of America. (2007b, March). *Pharmaceutical industry profile 2007.* Washington, DC: Author.

Polit, D.F., & Beck, C.T. (2006). *Essentials of nursing research: Methods, appraisal, and utilization* (6th ed.). Philadelphia: Lippincott Williams & Wilkins.

Saltz, L.B., Niedzwiecki, D., Hollis, D., Goldberg, R.M., Hantel, A., Thomas, J.P., et al. (2007). Irinotecan fluorouracil plus leucovorin is not superior to fluorouracil plus leucovorin alone as adjuvant treatment for stage III colon cancer: Results of CALGB 89803. *Journal of Clinical Oncology, 25,* 3456–3461.

Stone, J. (2006). *Conducting clinical research: A practical guide for physicians, nurses, study coordinators, and investigators.* Cumberland, MD: Mountainside MD Press.

Sugarman, J., Kass, N.E., Goodman, S.N., Perentesis, P., Fernandes, P., & Faden, R.R. (1998). What patients say about medical research. *IRB: A Review of Human Subject Research, 20*(4), 1–7.

Therasse, P., Arbuck, S.G., Eisenhauer, R.A., Wanders, J., Kaplan, R.S., Runinstein, L., et al. (2000). New guidelines to evaluate the response to treatment in solid tumors. *Journal of the National Cancer Institute, 92,* 205–216.

U.S. Department of Health and Human Services. (1998). *Categories of research that may be reviewed by the institutional review board (IRB) through an expedited review process.* Retrieved October 5, 2007, from http://www.hhs.gov/ohrp/humansubjects/guidance/expedited98.htm

U.S. Department of Health and Human Services. (2000). *Informed consent checklist: Basic and additional elements.* Retrieved March 15, 2008, from http://www.hhs.gov/ohrp/humansubjects/assurance/consentckls.htm

U.S. Department of Health and Human Services. (2004). *Office for Human Research Protections policy guidance: Human subject regulation decision charts.* Retrieved March 15, 2008, from http://www.hhs.gov/ohrp/humansubjects/guidance/decisioncharts.htm

U.S. Food and Drug Administration. (1999, November 5). *Dear gene therapy IND sponsor/principal investigator letter.* Retrieved October 5, 2007, from http://www.fda.gov/cber/ltr/gt110599.htm

U.S. Food and Drug Administration. (2007a). *Title 21—Food and Drugs—Chapter I—Food and Drug Administration Department of Health and Human Services: Subchapter A—General—Part 50. Protection of human subjects.* Retrieved March 15, 2008, from http://www.accessdata.fda.gov/scripts/cdrh/cfdocs/cfcfr/CFRSearch.cfm?CFRPart=50

U.S. Food and Drug Administration. (2007b). *Title 21—Food and Drugs—Chapter I—Food and Drug Administration Department of Health and Human Services: Subchapter A—General—Part 56. Institutional review boards.* Retrieved October 5, 2007, from http://www.accessdata.fda.gov/scripts/cdrh/cfdocs/cfcfr/CFRSearch.cfm?CFRPart=56

World Health Organization. (n.d.). *Welcome to the WHO international clinical trials registry platform.* Retrieved August 3, 2007, from http://www.who.int/ictrp/en/

Zoon, K., & Yetter, R.A. (2007). The regulation of drugs and biological products by the Food and Drug Administration. In J.I. Gallin & F.P. Ognibene (Eds.), *Principles and practice of clinical research* (2nd ed., pp. 97–108). Burlington, MA: Academic Press.

CHAPTER 10

Pain, Fatigue, and Cognitive Dysfunction

Wendy H. Vogel, MSN, FNP, AOCNP®, and
Jean M. Rosiak, RN, MSN, ANP-BC, AOCNP®

Introduction

Pain, fatigue, and cognitive dysfunction are common problems encountered by advanced practice nurses (APNs) in oncology practice. Each of these may have a profound effect on patient quality of life and daily function. Assessment, diagnosis, and management of each will be addressed in this chapter.

Cancer Pain

Introduction

Pain is one of the most common concerns and most feared symptoms associated with cancer and cancer treatments. Pain can severely affect the quality of life of patients with cancer. The Agency for Healthcare Research and Quality (AHRQ) evidence report/technology assessment on management of cancer symptoms noted that most patients with cancer encounter pain at some time during their cancer experience (Carr et al., 2002). The World Health Organization (WHO) estimates that about one-third of patients receiving cancer treatments and 60%–90% of patients with metastatic disease experience moderate to severe pain (WHO, 1996). Actual pain incidence rates vary depending on the extent of the disease, the study setting, the type of cancer, the definition of pain, and measurement methods (Wool & Mor, 2005). Because of the increasing number of cancer survivors, the incidence of chronic pain following successful cancer treatment also is increasing (Burton, Fanciullo, Beasley, & Fisch, 2007). Post-treatment pain syndromes (such as postmastectomy or post-thoracotomy pain and peripheral neuropathies) account for many cases of chronic pain.

Several professional societies have position statements about the treatment of cancer pain, including the Oncology Nursing Society (ONS, 2006), the American Society for Pain Management Nursing (ASPMN, 2003a), the Alliance of State Pain Initiatives (1998), the American Pain Society (APS) (Miaskowski et al., 2005), and the American Academy of Pain Medicine (AAPM, 1998), among others. Several organizations have practice guidelines or standards of care for cancer pain treatment, such as the National Comprehensive Cancer Network (NCCN, 2007a), the Joint Commission on the Accreditation of Healthcare Organizations (Phillips, 2000), APS (Miaskowski et al., 2005), the American Society of Anesthesiologists (1996), and AHRQ (Goudas et al., 2001). Patient advocacy groups, along with several professional organizations, have made pain the "fifth vital sign." However, despite the many position statements, practice guidelines, and patient advocacy group petitions, cancer pain often is underrecognized and undertreated (AAPM; Miaskowski, 2005). The most common error in the treatment of cancer pain is inadequate assessment and failure to act upon that assessment by treating adequately or underdosing (AAPM; APS, 2003; Cleeland et al., 1994; Cohen et al., 2003). The optimal management of cancer pain is one of the most important tasks of the oncology APN and is accomplished through a multidisciplinary approach: blending various skills, knowledge, tools, therapies, policies, and beliefs of each member of the healthcare team, including the patient.

Definitions and Incidence

The concept of *pain* is complex, varying by individual and culture. The International Association for the Study of Pain (Merskey, 1986) created a definition for pain that is used by multiple disciplines, defining pain as an unpleasant sensory and emotional experience related to actual or potential tissue damage. Pain generally is described as one of two types: acute or chronic. Acute pain is of shorter, limited duration, has an identifiable cause, and functions to warn and protect from tissue damage. Chronic pain continues well past the expected recovery time following injury to the body. In general, chronic pain continues for longer than one to six months or recurs at various intervals. The pain may have no identifiable cause or association with the usual physical and psychological changes occurring with acute pain. Cancer pain may be acute or chronic, or both may occur simultaneously depending upon the disease state, diagnostic procedure, or treatment. Three mechanisms of cancer pain exist: somatic, visceral, and neuropathic pain (Coyne, Watson, McGuire, & Yeager, 2005). Each mechanism of pain can be acute or chronic and has differing characteristics and responses to treatments. Patients with cancer may have one or a combination of the three mechanisms of pain.

Breakthrough pain is defined as transitory pain that "breaks through" a well-controlled pain plan (Portenoy & Hagen, 1990; Portenoy, Payne, & Jacobsen, 1999). Breakthrough pain may be somatic, visceral, neuropathic, or a combination of these. It can occur without stimulus or as a result of certain activities or biologic events and is associated with decreased quality of life and increased cost and hospitalizations (Fortner, Okon, & Portenoy, 2002). The incidence of breakthrough pain is difficult to quantify. A prospective study of 63 patients by Portenoy and Hagen of patients with cancer pain reported that 64% had breakthrough pain of severe or excruciating intensity. Twenty-nine percent of the cases of breakthrough pain in this study were related to fixed opioid dosing, occurring at the end of the dosing interval. Fifty-five percent of the cases of breakthrough pain were precipitated by some activity. Less than one-third were considered idiopathic and not under voluntary control (such as pain occurring with flatulence or coughing). Other studies report similar findings with the prevalence of breakthrough pain ranging from 24%–95% (Svendsen et al., 2005). A task force of the International Association for the Study of Pain performed a prospective, cross-sectional survey of cancer pain and found that almost 65% of patients had breakthrough pain (Caraceni et al., 2004).

Confusion exists about the issue of addiction, even among healthcare providers, and this confusion often leads to suboptimal cancer pain management. Optimal pain management requires understanding of tolerance, addiction, and physical dependence. *Addiction* is a disease that has genetic, psychosocial, and environmental influences causing a state of dependence upon some substance and is caused by habitual use of this substance for nonmedical reasons. Addiction is associated with deviant behavior, such as inadequate self-control over drug use, continued use despite harm, drug craving, and drug-seeking behaviors (Colleau & Joranson, 1998). Opioid addiction is rare among patients with cancer (American Cancer Society [ACS], 2007). Pseudoaddiction occurs because of inadequate pain management (Colleau & Joranson). Pseudoaddictive behaviors are pain-relief–seeking behaviors that occur when a patient's pain is unrelieved and healthcare clinicians view the patient's request for more pain medication as addictive behavior. This is more likely to occur when the clinician is inadequately trained in pain management and opioid administration.

Conversely, *physical dependence* is a physiologic consequence of opioid use when needed for pain control and rarely is associated with deviant behavior (Colleau & Joranson, 1998). It is a normal response to ongoing opioid therapy and does not mean that the patient is addicted. Physical dependence may occur within a few days; however, it varies among patients. Physical dependence may be seen as a withdrawal syndrome if the drug is abruptly stopped, if a rapid dose reduction occurs, or if an antagonist is administered. Withdrawal symptoms can be avoided if the narcotic is tapered over a period of time (ACS, 2007).

Tolerance is the need to increase the dosage of drug or the frequency of use in order to achieve the same level of pain relief and results from chronic administration (Colleau & Joranson, 1998). This does not occur in every patient with cancer and pain, but if it does, the frequency of dosing may be increased or another opiate could be tried.

Etiology and Pathology

Nociceptors are specialized receptors (sensory neurons) located throughout the body (skin, viscera, and musculoskeletal tissues) that respond to painful stimuli. When nociceptors are activated by either mechanical or chemical stimuli, nociceptive information is sent along A-delta and C fibers to the brain, and the individual then experiences somatic and/or visceral pain. Non-nociceptive information (caused by damage to the nervous system) is conveyed by A-beta fibers, and when the brain receives them, neuropathic pain results (Coyne et al., 2005; Foley, 2005). A-delta fibers are small, thinly myelinated fibers that are activated by stimuli such as pinpricks. C fibers are thin and unmyelinated and are activated by tissue damage. Tissue damage causes C fibers to release chemical metabolites called transducers, such as epinephrine, prostaglandins, leukotrienes, serotonin, bradykinin, and substance P, that sensitize the area of damage (causing inflammation) and activate nociceptors, thus causing pain. A-beta axons are larger and more heavily myelinated and are activated by light touch, therefore transmitting information much more rapidly than the A-delta or C fibers. Pain information enters the spinal cord via the dorsal root synapse, and transmission is mediated by excitatory amino acids, mainly glutamate but also aspartate, substance P, and calcitonin gene-related peptide. The pain information then crosses to the spinothalamic tracts and is transmitted to the thalamus and cortex. From there, the sensory cortex, frontal lobe, and reticular formation process the information, resulting in the perception of pain (Coyne et al.; Foley; Hickey & Brown, 2003). Opioid receptors are located on ascending and descending pain pathways and will produce the analgesic effects of opioid pharmaceuticals. More opioid receptors are located in certain parts of the brain and spinal cord.

Understanding of the neurotransmitters involved in pain transmission has led researchers to explore targeted strategies for cancer pain management (Grossman, Dunbar, & Nesbit, 2006). Strategies include blocking pain at the periphery (as with nonsteroidal anti-inflammatory drugs [NSAIDs] and anesthetics), activation of inhibitory processes in the spinal cord and brain (as with opioid treatments), and interference with the perception of pain (as with relaxation therapy).

Somatic pain originates from skin, bone, muscle, blood vessels, subcutaneous tissue, and connective tissue. It is well localized when cutaneous but more diffuse when originating deeper. Patients may describe somatic pain as dull, constant, or aching. An example of somatic pain in oncology is bone metastases or postsurgical incision pain. Approximately one-third of all cancer pain is somatic (Chang, Janjan, Jain, & Chau, 2006).

Visceral pain comes from organs and linings of body cavities when a tumor infiltrates, compresses, or stretches an area. It usually is poorly localized in nature and may be described as deep, squeezing, cramping, splitting, or pressure-like. Visceral pain can occur with metastases to an organ or intraperitoneal metastases and often is referred to areas away from the actual site of disease. Causes include the tumor itself or injury resulting from chemotherapy, radiation therapy, or surgery.

Neuropathic pain is poorly localized and may be described as sharp, strange, shooting, hot or burning, electric shock–like, vise-like, or "painfully numb." If localized, it usually occurs at the site of injury, and this area may be hypersensitive to other stimuli. Neuropathic pain may be delayed in onset, occurring days to years after the nerve-damaging event. Approximately 9% of patients with cancer have only neuropathic pain; mixed types of pain syndromes occur more commonly (Chang et al., 2006). Postmastectomy syndrome, plexopathies, chemotherapy-induced peripheral neuropathy, and post-thoracotomy pain are examples of neuropathic pain.

Several pain syndromes commonly appear in patients with cancer (see Table 10-1). Many of these are post-treatment pain syndromes (Burton et al., 2007), such as chemotherapy-induced peripheral neuropathy caused by an agent or combination of agents such as vincristine, thalidomide, bortezomib, platinum compounds, and the taxanes. Even years after radiation therapy, patients may experience the onset of pain from neural damage, compromising correct diagnosis.

The etiology of breakthrough pain in patients with cancer is not always clear (Svendsen et al., 2005). It can occur spontaneously or be precipitated by an activity such as walking, turning, or standing (volitional pain). Breakthrough pain may be nonvolitional, such as with abdominal distention or coughing, or incidental, as related to a procedure or a therapeutic intervention. Breakthrough pain also may result from "end-of-dose failure" caused by declining analgesic levels, that is, pain occurring before the next scheduled dose of pain medication. Breakthrough pain is estimated to be caused by cancer in 68%–80% of cases (Gutgsell, Walsh, Zhukovsky, Gonzales, & Lagman, 2003; Portenoy & Hagen, 1990) but may be caused by cancer treatment in 10%–20% of cases (Portenoy & Hagen). The pathophysiology of breakthrough pain is believed to be con-

Table 10-1. Common Oncologic Pain Syndromes

Pain Syndrome	Description
Bone metastasis pain	• Form of nociceptive pain • Sensitive to nonsteroidal anti-inflammatory drugs • Localized, sharp, aching, deep pain that may worsen with activity
Brachial plexopathy	• Often occurs following radiation for breast cancer • Incidence up to 9% • Onset varies from 6 months to 20 years after cancer treatment • Dysesthesia, pain, weakness, flaccid arm, loss of hand function
Herpetic neuralgia	• Painful paresthesia and dysesthesia, burning, aching, shock-like • Risk factors: Increasing age, immunosuppression
Inflammatory pain	• Results from tissue damage that leads to inflammation (migration of white blood cells to site that release cytokines, prostaglandins, and bradykinin, thus activating nociceptors) • Common causes: Tumor mass effect, treatment-induced gout, abscesses
Osteonecrosis (avascular necrosis)	• Often caused by corticosteroid use, usually within 3 years, most often in the femoral head • Focal necrosis from radiation or chemotherapy could occur. • Decreased range of motion, pain with activity, arthritis
Peripheral neuropathy	• Painful paresthesias and dysesthesias, hyporeflexia • Could lead to motor and sensory loss, including autonomic dysfunction • May be chemotherapy-induced • Preexisting nerve damage may increase incidence and severity.
Postamputation "phantom" pain	• Prevalence rates vary (7%–72%). • Phantom sensations, phantom pain, stump pain, burning dysesthesias • Pain may be exacerbated by movement. • Risk factors: Preamputation pain, female sex, severe postoperative pain, poorly fitted prosthesis, more proximal amputation, chemotherapy treatment
Postmastectomy pain syndrome	• Tight, burning pain in mastectomy site, axilla, and back of arm; paresthesia, dysesthesia, allodynia, hyperalgesia, or loss of shoulder function; neuroma pain (scar pain); phantom breast pain • Caused by intercostobrachial neuralgia and/or other nerve injuries • Worse with arm movement • Prevalence rates are approximately 50%. • Risk factors: Postoperative radiation therapy, extent of axillary dissection, negative psychological states
Postnephrectomy pain syndrome	• Dysesthesias, fullness and heaviness in flank, abdomen, groin
Postradiation pain syndrome (radiation-induced plexopathy)	• Radiation-induced neural damage • May have late onset (even up to 20 years) after treatment
Postradiation pelvic pain syndromes	• Etiology: Pelvic insufficiency fracture, enteritis, visceral dysfunction, neural damage, prostate brachytherapy • Often underreported

(Continued on next page)

Table 10-1. Common Oncologic Pain Syndromes *(Continued)*

Pain Syndrome	Description
Post–radical neck dissection	• Tight, burning pain in surgical site • Dysesthesias, shock-like pains • Incidence of neck pain is around 33%; shoulder pain is around 37%; myofascial pain, 47%; loss of sensation, 65% • Radiation-induced neural damage may cause pain years after treatment.
Post-thoracotomy pain syndrome	• Aching, sharp pain in incision site, more intense at medial and apical points of incision • Prevalence rates are around 50%, with half of these reporting moderate to severe pain. • Etiology: Intercostal nerve injury
Radiation myelopathy	• Injury to spinal cord by radiation • Paresthesia, thermesthesia, algesthesia, muscle weakness, gait disturbance, hemiplegia • Pain or dysesthesia at or below level of injury
Skeletal fractures	• Pain that increases in severity; severe pain; reports of a "cracking" sound • May exacerbate with activity
Tumor infiltration of peripheral nerve	• Dysesthesia; localized, constant burning pain • Pain may radiate.
Visceral pain	• Most often found in abdominal cancers • Associated with distention • Dull, cramping pain, difficult to localize

Note. Based on information from American Pain Society, 2003; Burton et al., 2007; Chang et al., 2006.

sistent with the mechanisms outlined previously. However, hyperexcitability in the central nervous system or periphery may play a role as well (Svendsen et al.). Mechanical stimuli, nerve injuries, changes in the chemical environment of nociceptors, and the release of tumor growth factors may cause sensitization, and thus breakthrough pain may be evoked by stimuli that normally are minimally painful (i.e., hyperalgesia) or by stimuli that are not normally painful (i.e., allodynia).

Risk Factors

Certain factors increase the risk of cancer pain. Advanced disease increases the risk of pain. Additionally, the type of metastases may increase risk; for example, patients with bone metastasis report more pain than those whose tumors do not commonly metastasize to the bone (Foley, 2005). The location of the cancer influences the risk of pain. Studies show that psychosocial factors, such as depression, anxiety, and feelings of isolation, influence pain reports (Marazzita, Mungai, Vivarelli, Presta, & Dell'Osso, 2006; Wool & Mor, 2005). Patients with inadequate pain management during treatment are more likely to have subsequent chronic pain (Burton et al., 2007). Patients who catastrophize (ruminate or exaggerate) report greater intensity of pain and have greater risk for the development of chronic pain (Marazzita et al.).

Factors also exist that increase the risk of inadequate pain management. These factors include increasing age (> 70), young age (< 3), female sex, cognitive impairment, a history of substance abuse, and minority races (ACS, 2007; Im, 2006; ONS, 2006; Vallerand, Hasenau, Templin, & Collins-Bohler, 2005). A cross-sectional, descriptive study of 281 ambulatory patients with cancer concluded that African American patients had significantly higher pain intensity, more pain-related distress, and more pain-related interference with function than Caucasian patients (Vallerand et al., 2005). However, when controlling for perceptions of control over pain, the disparities in these populations diminished to an insignificant level (but did not alleviate pain), revealing the importance of a patient's perception of control over pain (Vallerand, Saunders, & Anthony, 2007).

Signs and Symptoms

Acute, chronic, and neuropathic pain will have varying clinical signs and symptoms (see Figure 10-1). Autonomic signs are present in acute pain but may be absent in chronic pain. The absence of autonomic signs does not necessarily indicate absence of pain. Neuropathic pain presents unique symptoms. Nonverbal or cognitively impaired patients may be more difficult to assess because of absence of a self-report. In such patients, clinicians should rely on observation of the patient's behavior (Herr et al., 2006). However, these behaviors do not necessarily reflect pain intensity.

Acute
- Autonomic signs*
  - Tachycardia
  - Pallor
  - Diaphoresis
  - Elevated blood pressure

Chronic
- Autonomic signs absent
- Insomnia
- Fatigue
- Depression
- Decreased appetite
- Decreased libido
- Constipation
- Social withdrawal

Neuropathic
- Dysesthesias
- Hyperesthesia
- Allodynia
- Hyperalgesia
- Hyperpathia
- May follow neural pathway

Figure 10-1. Clinical Signs and Symptoms of Pain

* Autonomic signs are not sensitive in differentiating pain from other sources of distress (Herr et al., 2006). Absence of autonomic signs does not indicate absence of pain.

Note. Based on information from Miaskowski et al., 2005; National Comprehensive Cancer Network, 2007a.

Assessment of Pain

Assessment of cancer pain quantifies and qualifies pain but also considers the impact on physical and emotional functioning, previous interventions, success of interventions, and effects of symptoms or adverse events produced by the treatment (Chang et al., 2006; Gordon et al., 2005). A comprehensive pain assessment is completed following any pain report. Failure to perform an adequate pain assessment is one of the most common causes of inadequate pain management (NCCN, 2007a). Maladaptive behaviors related to ongoing pain, such as reduced socialization and altered sleep patterns, are assessed (Burton et al., 2007). An essential part of the assessment is the patient's self-report (Miaskowski et al., 2005). Description, pain characteristics, and quantity are elicited from patients (NCCN, 2007a). Pain descriptions, thresholds, expressions, and perceptions may differ not only because of physiologic differences but also because of sex, culture, and ethnicity (Im, 2006). Remembering the acronym PQRST (see Table 10-2) assists clinicians in obtaining a complete assessment of pain or other symptoms.

Breakthrough pain assessment also must consider the location, intensity, and timing. Temporal patterns, precipitating or exacerbating factors, relieving factors, and response to interventions are part of a thorough assessment. The number of episodes per day should be documented. The relationship of breakthrough pain to the overall clinical status requires examination as well (Portenoy & Hagen, 1990).

Table 10-2. Pain Assessment Using PQRST Mnemonic Device

Letter	Definition	Illustration
P	Provocative or palliative	What causes pain? What relieves pain? What have you tried to relieve pain? How are you currently taking your pain medications?
Q	Quality	Describe pain characteristics. Has the pain changed in any way? Have you had this pain in the past? Was the onset of pain gradual or sudden?
R	Radiation (associated symptoms)	Where is the pain located? Does the pain radiate to another location? Are there any associated symptoms? How is pain affecting you emotionally? Spiritually? How are you sleeping? Are any other medical conditions affecting or contributing to your pain?
S	Severity	Rate pain intensity • At rest • With activity. Rate pain intensity after intervention. How is pain affecting daily activities? Has the intensity varied over time?
T	Timing	When did the pain start? How often does it occur? How long does it last? Does pain vary as to time of day or night? Is the pain constant or episodic? How long does intervention give relief?

Because pain data are difficult to quantify and some patients are poor historians, a number of pain assessment tools are available to assist patients and clinicians (Patrick et al., 2003). Assessment tools also assist in standardizing pain assessments for comparisons in clinical trials. Pain is assessed at regular intervals and whenever a change occurs in the patient's pain or when the patient has a new pain (Miaskowski et al., 2005). Many assessment tools exist, with various strengths and weaknesses. The choice of tool depends upon the dimension of pain that the clinician decides is most relevant for that particular situation (Coyne et al., 2005). In general, the baseline assessment is more comprehensive, whereas ongoing reassessment tools are more succinct. Table 10-3 lists common cancer pain assessment tools. No universally accepted tool exists for the assess-

Table 10-3. Pain Assessment Tools

Tool	Description	Advantages/Disadvantages
Numerical Rating Scale (McCaffery & Pasero, 1999)	0–10 scale where 0 = no pain and 10 = worst pain imaginable	Rapid, good for assessment of intervention efficacy
Breakthrough Pain Questionnaire (Portenoy et al., 1999)	Structured interview	Designed to characterize breakthrough pain
Checklist of Nonverbal Pain Indicators (Feldt, 2000)	Six-item checklist rated by observer with 0 = behavior not observed and 1 = behavior observed	For patients who are cognitively impaired or otherwise unable to verbally rate pain presence or intensity
Edmonton Symptom Assessment Scale (Bruera et al., 1995)	Nine-item visual analog scale for symptoms of patients receiving palliative care	Gives a numerical score; higher scores reflect greater severity of patient condition; easy to perform
Memorial Symptom Assessment Scale (Fishman et al., 1987)	Assesses 32 symptoms in three dimensions: intensity, frequency, and distress	Broader range of information, more time-consuming; two abbreviated forms available that assess 32 or 14 symptoms in one dimension; valid in patients with or without cancer
Wong-Baker FACES (Wong et al., 2001)	Six faces that vary from smiling (0 and no pain) to crying (10 and worst pain)	Recommended for people age 3 years or older; useful in patients with language barriers
McGill Pain Questionnaire (MPQ) (Melzack, 1975, 1987)	Three major classes of word descriptors: sensory, affective, and evaluative, used by patients to describe subjective pain experience; also has intensity scale	Qualitative and quantitative information; originally developed for nonmalignant pain, but valid in cancer populations as well; short form has been developed with 15 descriptors
Multidimensional Affect and Pain Scale (Knotkova et al., 2006)	101 descriptors rated by patient as to closeness to his or her own feelings, emotions, and experiences	Similar to MPQ; no more than 15 minutes to complete; assesses somatosensory and emotional experiences and feelings of well-being
Brief Pain Inventory (Cleeland & Ryan, 1994; Tittle et al., 2003)	Measures pain by severity and interference with function	Developed for use in patients with cancer; established validity across cultures and various languages; validated in surgical patients with cancer and chronic nonmalignant pain; time-intensive

ment of pain in patients with cancer. It is recommended that every cancer care setting have a standard for the assessment and documentation of pain (Gordon et al., 2005). Documentation must be very visible to each member of the healthcare team to facilitate regular review at each interface.

Reassessment is performed following any intervention and uses the patient's self-report and the initial assessment tools. Reassessment includes assessment of intervention side effects, adverse events, and effects on quality of life (Gordon et al., 2005). A pain management diary may be helpful to better assess the efficacy of treatment strategies. This may give patients an enhanced awareness of pain and its contributing factors as well as an increased sense of control over pain.

The patient report will guide the physical examination. Areas claimed to be painful are examined for any physical changes, such as redness, bruising, edema, or tenderness. Activities, movements, or positions that reproduce the pain are evaluated. Diagnostic studies are ordered based on findings from the physical examination and patient report as well as the medical history. Chapter 3 gives more information on diagnostic studies that may be appropriate for patients with cancer who are experiencing pain.

Differential Diagnosis

The differential diagnosis of pain may be related to its etiology and pathophysiology and may be further defined as acute or chronic. Potential specific cancer pain syndromes (see Table 10-1) and potential oncologic emergencies should be considered in the differential (see Chapters 14 and 15 on oncologic emergencies). The pain is determined to be continuous or intermittent (breakthrough). Cancer pain and chronic nonmalignant pain should be differentiated, although the distinction often is unclear (Burton et al., 2007).

Treatment of Cancer Pain

An individualized, multidisciplinary, and multimodal pain management approach that considers physical, mental, psychological, cultural, and social factors will provide an optimal outcome for patients with cancer (Cahill, 2005; ONS, 2006; Wool & Mor, 2005). The pain management plan begins with treatment of the underlying pathology (Cahill) to remove, control, or palliate the tumor burden. Clinicians should initiate pain treatment promptly while awaiting work-up for specific etiology of the pain (Miaskowski, 2005). Interventions may include pharmacologic analgesia; pharmacologic treatment of contributing factors such as mood disorders; invasive interventions; and nonpharmacologic interventions, including alternative interventions and behavioral approaches.

Pharmacologic treatment: Initial pharmacologic intervention is based on the patient's report of pain severity (Miaskowski et al., 2005). Morphine continues to be the opioid of choice for moderate to severe cancer pain management. Although no controlled trials demonstrate its superiority over other agents, it is easily available, is relatively inexpensive, and has multiple routes of administration (Grossman et al., 2006). Morphine is not generally associated with organ toxicity and has expected and manageable side effects, such as nausea and drowsiness, that usually improve within a few days of regular intake.

Opioids are used for moderate to severe pain based on the WHO analgesic ladder (WHO, 1996). The only absolute contraindication to opioid use is hypersensitivity (Coyle & Layman-Goldstein, 2007). Opioids' mechanism of action is binding to mu and kappa receptors in the central and peripheral nervous systems (APS, 2003). Opioid analgesics often are compounded with a nonopioid such as acetaminophen, which confers a ceiling dose because of the nonopioid component. Opioid classifications and effects are listed in Table 10-4. Opioid use has the potential for addiction, but this potential must not compromise appropriate pain management. The most common error in using opioids for cancer pain management is underdosing. Pure opioid agonists (e.g., morphine, hydromorphone) are the most common opioids used in cancer pain management. Partial agonists (e.g., buprenorphine) have little use in cancer pain because of their ceiling effects and ability to precipitate withdrawal syndrome in patients on pure agonist agents (Coyle & Layman-Goldstein). Patients receiving mixed agonist-antagonist agents (e.g., butorphanol, nalbuphine, pentazocine) may have more side effects, such as agitation, dysphoria, and confusion, than with pure opioid agonists. These agents are not recommended for cancer pain treatment.

Table 10-4. Opioid Pharmacology

Opioid Class	Class Effects	Agents	Comments
Pure opioid agonists	Increasing dose increases effectiveness but with no ceiling effect. Will not reverse or decrease effects of other pure opioid agonists if given together Caution with impaired breathing, bronchial asthma, increased intracranial pressure, or liver failure	Morphine	Opioid of choice for cancer pain; standard of comparison for opioids
		Hydromorphone	Synthetic short half-life opioid Useful in those intolerant of morphine More potent than morphine Peak effect slightly more rapid than morphine, but with slightly shorter duration of action May cause less nausea and hallucinations than morphine
		Oxycodone	Synthetic opioid, better oral absorption than with morphine May cause less nausea and hallucinations than morphine but more constipation No parenteral route May cause more nausea and constipation

(Continued on next page)

Table 10-4. Opioid Pharmacology *(Continued)*

Opioid Class	Class Effects	Agents	Comments
		Fentanyl	Short half-life opioid use Much more rapid onset of action, but effect of shorter duration Transdermal and transmucosal routes May be less constipating than morphine When given transdermally, the drug is stored in subcutaneous fat, and serum concentration may take several hours to decline.
		Methadone	Unique characteristics such as excellent oral and rectal absorption, long duration of action, low cost, and no known active metabolites Severe pain situations such as neuropathic pain Accumulates with repetitive dosing After a few days, the interval of administration can be increased, while maintaining analgesic effects. For use by experienced prescribers Careful titration and follow-up required
		Codeine	Many combination preparations with aspirin or acetaminophen 10% of population cannot metabolize this agent. May cause nausea and constipation
		Hydrocodone	Considered a weaker opioid than oxycodone agents Often used in antitussive agents
		Propoxyphene	Weak opioid Not often used in treating cancer pain
Partial agonists	Less effects than full agonists at the opioid receptor	Buprenorphine	This class of opioids is not recommended for the treatment of cancer pain. Ceiling effects May precipitate withdrawal in patients on pure opioid
Mixed agonist-antagonists	Block or are neutral at one receptor, but activate another; contraindicated in patients receiving an opioid agonist	Butorphanol Nalbuphine Pentazocine	This class of opioids is not recommended for the treatment of cancer pain. Ceiling effects Risk of psychotomimetic effects such as dysphoria, delusions, and hallucinations

Note. Based on information from American Pain Society, 2003; Coyle & Layman-Goldstein, 2007.

NCCN (2007a) and APS (Miaskowski et al., 2005) have established clinical practice guidelines for cancer pain management based on the WHO (1996) three-step analgesic ladder. Clinical practice guidelines provide evidence-based information to reduce variation in the clinical management of cancer pain and improve patient outcomes. Figure 10-2 defines some of the key concepts of cancer pain management based on these guidelines and current literature. A crucial concept is that pain is what the patient says it is, and treatment is based on pain intensity.

Following a comprehensive pain assessment, if the patient has a pain intensity of 1 to 3, a nonopioid analgesic agent such as an NSAID or acetaminophen may be administered, or a short-acting opioid can be considered. Any NSAID, including one that the patient has used successfully in the past, can be considered (NCCN, 2007a). Figure 10-3 lists common NSAIDs used in the management of cancer pain. NSAIDs often are combined with opioids and are particularly effective in treating metastatic bone pain. NSAIDs have a ceiling effect and do not produce tolerance, dependence, or addiction. Acetaminophen appears to have fewer side effects than NSAIDs; however, hepatic toxicity can occur and is more likely in alcoholic individuals and those with liver disease (Coyle & Layman-Goldstein, 2007). NSAIDs are used cautiously in patients at risk for gastrointestinal or renal toxicities. If two different NSAIDs are tried without successful control of pain, another strategy should be considered.

If the patient's pain intensity is rated 4 or greater, a short-acting opioid is ordered and titrated to adequate analgesic effect (NCCN, 2007a). Adjuvant analgesics are given as indicated by assessment and response to initial opioid treatment. A pain reassessment is completed within 24 hours of initiating treatment. Upon reassessment, if the patient's pain is rated 1–3, then conversion to a sustained-release agent is recommend-

---

Pain is what the patient says it is.
Use the oral route whenever possible; avoid intramuscular route.
Scheduled dosing is preferable to episodic dosing.
Opioid prescribing
• Pain intensity 1–3: Increase dose by 25%.
• Pain intensity 4–6: Increase dose by 25%–50%.
• Pain intensity 7–10: Increase dose by 50%–100%.
• Pain intensity < 4 and unmanageable side effects: Consider dose reduction of 25% and reassess.
• Rescue doses of the short-acting form of the sustained-release medication at 10%–20% of the 24-hour dose should be given every hour as needed.
• Patients on pure agonists should not be switched to either mixed agonist-antagonists or partial agonists, as the antagonistic element may precipitate withdrawal.
• When acetaminophen dose of fixed combination opioid is > 4 g/day, switch to single-entity opioid.
• Convert from short-acting to long-acting opioid when total 24-hour opioid dose is achieving adequate pain control.
• Adjuvant pharmacologic agents (non-narcotic) may be required.
• Consider opioid rotation (switching) if more than two side effects (not including constipation) are present and/or if pain is not managed with increasing doses.
• Opioid-induced side effects must be monitored and managed (e.g., a bowel regimen should begin whenever the patient begins an opioid intervention).
• Meperidine, mixed agonist-antagonists, partial agonists, placebos, and propoxyphene are not recommended for treatment of adult cancer pain.

Figure 10-2. Key Concepts of Cancer Pain Management

Note. Based on information from Coyle & Layman-Goldstein, 2007; Grossman et al., 2006; Miaskowski et al., 2005; National Comprehensive Cancer Network, 2007a; World Health Organization, 1996.

- Aspirin
- Etodolac
- Salsalate
- Ibuprofen
- Diflunisal
- Ketoprofen
- Acetaminophen
- Meclofenamate
- Fenoprofen calcium
- Nonacetylated salicylate
- Naproxen and naproxen sodium
- Ketorolac (also has parenteral route)
- Selective cyclooxygenase-2 inhibitors
- Choline and magnesium salicylate combinations

Figure 10-3. Common Nonsteroidal Anti-Inflammatory Drugs Used for Mild Cancer Pain or Adjunctive Treatment

Note. Based on information from American Pain Society, 2003; National Comprehensive Cancer Network, 2007a.

ed (see example in Figure 10-4). If pain continues to be rated 1–3, then the patient may be assessed weekly until comfortable, and then at each healthcare visit. However, if upon reassessment, the patient's pain intensity is 4 or greater, opioid titration should continue, and a specialty consultation might be considered.

Short-acting opioids have a peak effect of 60 minutes if given orally and 15 minutes if given intravenously. Generally, when prescribing opioids, the dose is increased by 25% for pain intensity of 1–3; 25%–50% for pain intensity of 4–6; and 50%–100% for pain intensity of 7–10 (NCCN, 2007a). For the example in Figure 10-4, a patient is currently taking opioids but now reports pain rated at 8, and the total 24-hour dose (including the breakthrough doses) is calculated. The new scheduled dose is determined by the previous total 24-hour dose and increased by 50%. The new breakthrough dose is calculated at 10%–20% of this new 24-hour dose and is given every one hour as needed. The most appropriate dose for any patient with cancer pain is whatever dose it takes to relieve the individual's pain.

Patient-controlled analgesia (PCA) is useful when a patient has uncontrolled pain or requires quick relief, or when the clinician is trying to determine the required opioid dose for adequate pain relief. This method allows the patient to self-administer a preset dose of an analgesic within a prescribed time period (usually every 15–30 minutes), enabling timely and highly individualized management. A maximum safe usage dose is set as well (usually prescribed in 1–4-hour dose limits). An effective safeguard of the PCA is that excessively sedated patients will not be able to activate the dosing button, thereby preventing delivery of further opioid (APS, 2003). A continuous infusion may be prescribed along with patient-administered bolus doses. Once pain is controlled, the IV pharmacologic agent can be converted to an equianalgesic oral dose. PCA management is a poor choice of pain management for a cognitively impaired patient. Caution is vital in prescribing and managing opioid-naïve patients with PCA (APS). PCA by proxy (i.e., someone other than the patient activates the bolus dose delivery) is considered unsafe, and ASPMN (2006) issued a position statement against this practice.

APNs must be familiar with concepts of narcotic equianalgesia and dosage conversions from drug to drug and also from one route to another. Conversions to a dif-

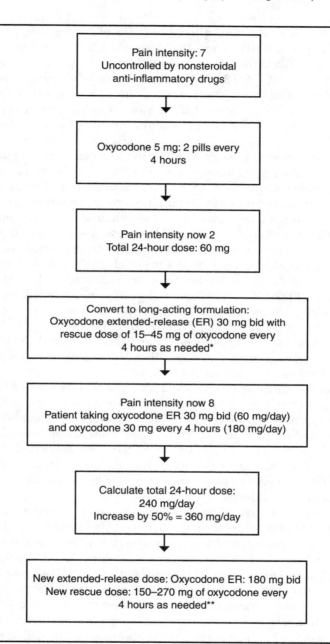

Figure 10-4. Opioid Titration Example

* Rescue dose calculated by multiplying total 24-hour dose by 10%–20% to be given every hour (60 mg × 10%–20% = 6–12 mg every hour). Given in 4-hour intervals: 24–48 mg every 4 hours prn. Oxycodone tablets come in 5, 15, and 30 mg tablets; therefore 15–45 mg every 4 hours is appropriate for break-through dose.

** Rescue dose calculated by multiplying 24-hour dose by 10%–20% as above (360 × 10%–20% = 36–72 mg every hour). Given in 4-hour intervals: 144–288 mg every 4 hours prn; therefore, using oxy-codone 30 mg tablets, dose is 5–9 pills (150–270 mg).

Note. Based on information from National Comprehensive Cancer Network, 2007a.

ferent opioid or route may be required because of inadequate analgesia, intolerable side effects, inability to use the oral route, insurance coverage, or formulary coverage. This information is found in many pain management references, including the NCCN (2007a) guidelines on adult cancer pain. Doses of various opioid analgesics are compared to the equivalent of 10 mg of parenteral morphine (and 30 mg of oral morphine). Conversion of regularly scheduled parenteral to regularly scheduled oral morphine is calculated by a 1:3 ratio (APS, 2003). It is critical to note that the parenteral route is always more potent than the oral route. Oncology APNs maintain a consistent method of conversion to promote safety, using the same equianalgesic chart or program. In most cases, the equianalgesic dose is reduced by 25% to account for incomplete cross-tolerance and patient variations in metabolism. When rounding a dose, rounding downward is preferred. An adequate breakthrough dose of the new medication also must be prescribed, and analgesia should be assessed within 24 hours.

Breakthrough pain can, at times, be anticipated and prevented. When managing breakthrough pain, it is critical to consider the etiology. Patients with metastatic bone pain located in the back or pelvis may be at risk for resistant breakthrough pain (Hwang, Chang, & Kasimis, 2003). If the breakthrough pain is of neuropathic etiology, it may be beneficial to add an antidepressant, anticonvulsant, or other neuropathic agent. If the etiology is bone-related, then an NSAID or corticosteroid might be beneficial. Pretreatment for events expected to cause pain should be considered (NCCN, 2007a). For breakthrough pain caused by end-of-dose failure, increasing the dosage or frequency of the regular analgesic can improve pain control.

Treatment for breakthrough pain should have a rapid onset and short half-life. Adjustments in regularly scheduled analgesic dosing are considered if frequent episodes of breakthrough pain are reported (Portenoy & Hagen, 1990). The rescue dose should reflect the amount of the regularly scheduled medication. Usually this dose is 10%–20% of the total daily opioid dose and may be given every hour as needed (NCCN, 2007a); however, this can vary greatly among patients (Hagen, Fisher, Victorino, & Farrar, 2007). Titration of the dose to patient response is necessary to adequately manage pain and to balance untoward side effects.

Neuropathic pain may be treated with an antidepressant, anticonvulsant, or topical agents such as capsaicin or local anesthetics. Figure 10-5 lists common agents used in the treatment of neuropathic pain. If neuropathic pain is not controlled within two to three weeks, referral to a pain specialty service or anesthesia is recommended (NCCN, 2007a).

Treatment of metastatic bone pain requires not only NSAIDs and opioids but also bisphosphonate therapy, which currently is accepted to provide moderate analgesic effects (Fulfaro, Casuccio, Ticozzi, & Ripamonti, 1998; Saad et al., 2002). Local treatments such as external beam radiotherapy, radiofrequency ablation, and surgical interventions (e.g., bone stabilization procedures) also may be utilized. Strontium-89 and samarium-153 may be employed for widespread bone metastases. Chapter 6 provides more information on radiologic interventions.

Interventional strategies: Interventional strategies may be considered if adequate oral pain management has produced intolerable side effects or if pain is more likely to be controlled with a nerve block, as in the case of a celiac plexus block for uncontrolled pancreatic pain. Interventional approaches may include nerve blocks (temporary or permanent), neurostimulation, neuraxial analgesic infusion, neuroablation, and surgical intervention (Hickey & Brown, 2003; NCCN, 2007a). Common procedures for neuraxial infusions include an epidural or intrathecal infusion of opioids, local anesthetic, or

Antidepressants
- Doxepin
- Duloxetine
- Venlafaxine
- Desipramine
- Nortriptyline

Anticonvulsants
- Pregabalin
- Gabapentin
- Clonazepam

Topical agents
- Capsaicin
- Lidocaine

Opioid
- Methadone

Figure 10-5. Common Agents Used for Neuropathic Pain Management

Note. Based on information from Coyle & Layman-Goldstein, 2007; Grossman et al., 2006; Miaskowski et al., 2005; National Comprehensive Cancer Network, 2007a.

other analgesics to diffuse into the dorsal laminae and affect nociception (Chang et al., 2006). Neuroablative procedures such as brachial plexus neurolysis or cordotomy may be considered for well-localized pain syndromes. Neurostimulation procedures such as transcutaneous electrical nerve stimulation (TENS) modulate the pain stimulus transmission, thereby relieving pain (Hickey & Brown). Surgical interventions such as a vertebroplasty or kyphoplasty may also be considered. Vertebroplasty involves injection of orthopedic cement into fractured vertebrae. Kyphoplasty includes the insertion and then inflation of a "balloon" tamp to restore the height of the vertebrae before injecting orthopedic cement. Other surgeries for pain management might include amputation, tumor debulking, organ excision, or skeletal fixation (Cahill, 2005; Chang et al.).

Management of treatment side effects: Pharmacologic intervention for pain, particularly opioids, may produce a variety of side effects, many occurring as a result of the effects on the gastrointestinal system. The most common side effects of opioids are constipation, cognitive impairment, sedation, somnolence, nausea and vomiting, reduced libido, and delirium. Constipation, the one side effect that does not improve with routine opioid use, is best treated prophylactically. Initiation of a bowel regimen including a stimulant laxative and a stool softener and titrated to effect is critical when patients are started on opioid therapy (NCCN, 2007a). Caffeine, methylphenidate, dextroamphetamine, or donepezil may be appropriate for the treatment of persistent opioid-induced sedation (Reissig & Rybarczyk, 2005; Slatkin & Rhiner, 2003; Westberg & Gobel, 2004). Research shows that psychomotor and cognitive functioning usually is not affected after stable doses of opioids are attained (Gaertner et al., 2006). Gaertner et al. found that the use of long-term (at least four weeks) controlled-release oxycodone did not prohibit driving, but they emphasized that individual assessment is vital. Treatment of many common pain management side effects is discussed in other chapters of this book.

Nonpharmacologic treatment: Nonpharmacologic approaches to cancer-related pain have a role in pain management strategies. Rehabilitative interventions, such as physical therapy, may improve range of motion, strength and endurance, and neuromuscular control, thus improving cancer pain (Menefee & Monti, 2005). Massage, TENS, ultrasonic stimulation, and other modalities also may be appropriate to manage pain (Chang et al., 2006; Hickey & Brown, 2003). Applications of heat or cold may be beneficial in certain types of pain, particularly postsurgical pain (Menefee & Monti). Patients must be warned about the potential for burns, especially if neuropathy or other disorders are present that would disrupt the individual's perception of pain or temperature.

Many other symptoms may occur during the disease trajectory that contribute to the distress associated with cancer pain (Mystakidou et al., 2006). These symptoms must be controlled for optimal pain management (Foley, 2005). Psychiatric symptoms, including anxiety and depression, of patients with cancer pain should first be considered to be a result of uncontrolled pain and then reassessed after pain is controlled. Patients with pain that interferes with their daily activities express more anxiety, which compounds intolerance of daily activities (Mystakidou et al.). Psychosocial support is vital, and patients and families should understand that emotional reactions to pain are normal and should be treated as part of the pain management plan (NCCN, 2007a). Reinforcing positive coping skills, enhancing personal control, and focusing on optimal quality of life are all part of psychosocial support to the patient and family or support systems.

Treatment of patients with substance abuse: Treatment of cancer pain in people with a history of substance abuse is an issue that oncology APNs should be prepared to encounter. While maintaining a healthy respect for the potential for abuse of controlled substances such as opioid analgesics, one must understand that these medications are the most effective way to treat cancer pain. Twenty-one health organizations (including ONS and ACS) and the Drug Enforcement Administration have issued a joint statement titled *Promoting Pain Relief and Preventing Abuse of Pain Medications: A Critical Balancing Act* (ASPMN, 2003b). This statement reinforces the need to prevent abuse of prescription pain medications while still ensuring availability for those who need them. Patients with addictive disease and pain have the right to be treated with dignity, respect, and the same quality of pain management (ASPMN, 2002). Figure 10-6 lists some recommendations for management of pain in patients with addictive disease. Higher doses may be required because the patient may have developed a tolerance to some medications or increased sensitivity to pain because of drug use. A pain contract that includes clear, written patient expectations and responsibilities with non-negotiable limits will help to deter aberrant behavior. Careful documentation protects the clinician while providing rationale for proper management.

Patient and family education: A vital part of the pain management plan is patient and family education. Lack of knowledge and incorrect beliefs about pain are barriers to optimal pain relief (Cohen et al., 2003). Research shows improvements in cancer pain management when patients and families are taught about their pain and its management (Aubin et al., 2006; Miaskowski et al., 2004; Vallerand, Collins-Bohler, Templin, & Hasenau, 2007). Individualized education may reduce the disparity in cancer pain management among minorities (Kalauokalani, Franks, Oliver, Meyers, & Kravitz, 2007). Both professional position statements and management guidelines emphasize the patient's right to education about the pain process and its treatment (Cohen et al.).

Complementary and alternative treatments: The treatment of pain with complementary or alternative medicine (CAM) is a science now developing an evidence base. The National Cancer Institute (NCI) has a panel of experts to further CAM cancer research (Smith, 2004). A wide variety of CAM pain interventions exists, including yoga, Qi gong, Reiki, Shiatsu, hypnosis, imagery, massage, nutrition, meditation, acupuncture,

- Use a nonjudgmental approach, and assume self-report of pain is true.
- Involve patient and family in pain management plan and goal setting.
- Use a pain contract or medication agreement that outlines patient and clinician responsibilities, patient expectations, and consequences of aberrant behavior, setting clear, non-negotiable limits.
- Designate a single pharmacy and prescriber, and refill prescriptions only during face-to-face contacts.
- Prescribe the appropriate amount of pain medication, understanding that higher doses may be required, as the patient may have tolerance to some medications or increased sensitivity to pain because of drug use.
- Consider methadone for pain control, as it is effective, inexpensive, and less likely to be diverted.
- Monitor patient with periodic pill counts and drug screens (include this in the pain contract).
- Document the etiology of pain, assessment, education, prescription, management, and follow-up carefully.

Figure 10-6. Management of Cancer Pain in Patients With Addictive Disease

---

Note. Based on information from American Society for Pain Management Nursing, 2002; Grant et al., 2007; Penson et al., 2003; Weaver & Schnoll, 2002.

acupressure, aromatherapy, magnet therapy, mind-body medicine, reflexology, spiritual cures, therapeutic touch, and traditional Chinese medicine (Chang et al., 2006; Hickey & Brown, 2002; Menefee & Monti, 2005). Patients with cancer use CAM for many reasons, but a common reason is unrelieved pain (Berenson, 2007). Chapter 8 provides more detailed information about CAM. Cognitive-behavioral interventions, such as keeping a pain diary or a journal about thoughts and emotions surrounding the pain experience, may promote feelings of control over the pain (Menefee & Monti; NCCN, 2007a). Perceived control over pain is an influential aspect of pain response (Vallerand, Saunders, et al., 2007). Behavioral interventions examine behaviors that influence the pain experience. Biofeedback, hypnosis, music and art therapy, distraction training, systematic desensitization, and relaxation therapy are examples of behavioral interventions. Some evidence demonstrates that cognitive-behavioral interventions are effective in immediate pain relief but not long term (Anderson et al., 2006). Randomized, controlled clinical trials are needed to evaluate CAM interventions in the management of cancer pain.

Evaluation of Outcomes

Following reassessment of cancer pain after therapeutic intervention, if pain control appears to be inadequate, the oncology APN should assess the patient for factors that impede pain relief. Numerous studies have identified a range of barriers to optimal cancer pain management. Figure 10-7 is a nonexhaustive list of barriers to adequate pain management. Successful outcomes of pain interventions include not only a decrease in pain intensity but also an increase in functional abilities and quality of life. Reassessment should include the patient's continued ability to obtain and afford medications or treatment (Coyne et al., 2005). Documentation of outcomes is essential for continuity of care and for legal obligations. Compliance with the therapeutic regimen and follow-up also must be documented.

Continuous quality improvement is vital to increase the quality of cancer pain management (Gordon et al., 2005; Patrick et al., 2003). Continuing education of physicians, nurses, and ancillary staff improves the quality of pain management (Stevenson, Dahl, Berry, Beck, & Griffie, 2006). Ideally, all practice settings should have a formal process for evaluation and improvement of cancer pain management (Miaskowski et al., 2005).

- Stoicism
- Fear of addiction
- Language barriers
- Healthcare staff turnover
- Desire to be a "good patient"
- Poor access to pain specialists
- Cost of medications/procedures
- Patients' lack of support people
- Misconceptions about cancer pain
- Lack of national policies on pain relief
- Healthcare provider's resistance to change
- Lack of consistent use of assessment tools
- Low expectations that pain can be relieved
- Inadequate dosing of pharmacologic agents
- Fear of side effects of pharmacologic agents
- Legal concerns on part of healthcare provider
- Inadequate time on part of healthcare provider
- Incomplete effectiveness of some interventions
- Inadequate reimbursement for healthcare providers
- Inadequate knowledge about cancer pain etiology and control
- Organizational factors (increasing paperwork, documentation, etc.)
- Varying rules and regulations on controlled substances state to state
- Nurses' or support people's reluctance to administer opioids
- Inadequate knowledge about cultural variations regarding pain responses
- Unmanaged negative psychosocial factors (such as depression and anxiety)
- Reluctance to report pain because of fear that pain stems from progressive or recurrent disease
- Shortages of healthcare providers, particularly those specializing in cancer pain management
- Poor recognition of importance of pain control or low priority of pain control in optimal cancer treatment and care
- Disagreement between patient and support system or patient and provider on presence and severity of pain
- Fear of tolerance (i.e., that cancer pain will worsen toward death and interventions will then be ineffective)
- Poor communication (between healthcare provider and patient; provider and provider; provider and support systems; patient and support systems; etc.)

Figure 10-7. Barriers to Optimal Cancer Pain Management

Note. Based on information from American Cancer Society, 2007; Cohen et al., 2003; Coyne et al., 2005; Gordon et al., 2005; Im, 2006; Patrick et al., 2003; Wool & Mor, 2005; World Health Organization, 1996.

The whole healthcare team must follow evidence-based standards of care. When the patient transitions from one healthcare setting to another (such as from the hospital to home), care is taken to ensure that optimal pain management is maintained. Sharing performance data with the team can assist in setting goals for improved outcomes, and collaboration between disciplines is essential (Gordon et al.).

Fatigue

Introduction

One of the most frequently recurring symptoms oncology APNs confront in practice is fatigue. It is a nearly universal side effect of cancer and cancer treatment, affecting physical, psychological, and social functioning and causing significant distress for patients and caregivers (NCCN, 2007b; Portenoy & Itri, 1999). It often is underrecognized and undertreated and has a strong relationship with quality of life (Lawrence, Kupelnick, Miller, Devine, & Lau, 2004; Tchen et al., 2003). Fatigue is subjective and multidimensional and often is reported as the most distressing symptom associated with cancer and its treatment, causing the most interference with daily life (Lawrence et al.; NCCN, 2007b).

Definitions and Incidence

NCI (n.d.-b) defines fatigue as a condition of extreme tiredness and inability to function because of lack of energy. NCCN (2007b) defines cancer-related fatigue as "a distressing persistent, subjective sense of tiredness or exhaustion related to cancer or cancer treatment that is not proportional to recent activity and interferes with usual functioning" (p. FT-1). Vogel, Wilson, and Melvin (2004) defined it as "an overwhelming, unremitting sense of exhaustion resulting in decreased capacity for physical and mental work" (p. 339). Fatigue may be acute or chronic. Acute fatigue occurs because of excessive exertion and is relieved by rest. Chronic fatigue continues over a prolonged period of time and is not responsive to rest (NCI, n.d.-b; Portenoy & Itri, 1999; Vogel et al.). Disruptive symptoms of chronic fatigue are reported to persist for months to years after completion of cancer therapy (NCCN, 2007b).

Research studies have reported the occurrence of fatigue to be anywhere from 4%–91% depending on the population studied and the method of assessment (Lawrence et al., 2004). However, subjective reports of fatigue in patients with cancer approach 100% in patients receiving cytotoxic chemotherapy, radiation therapy, stem cell transplant, or biologic therapy. Radiation therapy is associated with a 65%–80% incidence of fatigue (Hickok, Morrow, McDonald, & Bellg, 1996; Irvine, Vincent, Graydon, & Bubela, 1998; Jereczek-Fossa, Marsiglia, & Orecchia, 2002). Nearly 99% of patients with breast and lung cancer report fatigue, and 61% of patients receiving chemotherapy or radiation therapy state that fatigue persists after treatment has stopped (NCI, 2005). Incidence and prevalence rates of fatigue in long-term cancer survivors range from 17%–53% depending on the criteria used for evaluation (NCCN, 2007b). Women are more likely than men to report experiencing daily fatigue (Fu, McDaniel, & Rhodes, 2005).

Etiology and Pathophysiology

Because of the various causative factors and multiple confounding factors, the biologic processes causing the development of fatigue are unknown. Fatigue most likely occurs as a side effect of treatment as well as a biologic effect of the disease itself (see Figure 10-8) (Lawrence et al., 2004; NCCN, 2007b). Proposed mechanisms include abnormal accumulation of metabolites, proinflammatory cytokine effects, changes in neuromuscular function, abnormalities in adenosine triphosphate synthesis, serotonin dysregulation, and vagal afferent activation (Collado-Hidalgo, Bower, Ganz, Cole, & Irwin, 2006; NCCN, 2007b). Abnormalities in energy metabolism related to increased requirements because of tumor growth, infection, fever, or surgery also may cause fatigue (Portenoy & Itri, 1999).

Aberrant cytokine production (of cytokines such as interleukin-1, interleukin-6, and tumor necrosis factor-alpha), as noted in post-treatment breast cancer survivors, may

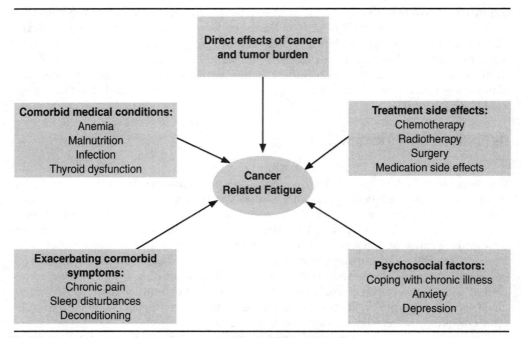

Figure 10-8. Factors Contributing to Cancer-Related Fatigue

Note. From "Fatigue and Cancer: Causes, Prevalence and Treatment Approaches," by L.I. Wagner and D. Cella, 2004, *British Journal of Cancer, 91,* p. 823. Copyright 2004 by Cancer Research UK. Reprinted with permission.

be associated with persistent fatigue (Collado-Hidalgo et al., 2006). Some cytokines may be produced by tumors and directly cause fatigue. Alterations in cytokine production also are linked to cancer treatments (Collado-Hidalgo et al.). They may contribute indirectly to fatigue by promoting cachexia and muscle wasting (Gullatte, Kaplow, & Heidrich, 2005).

Persistent activation of the immune system or late effects of treatment on major organ systems may account for long-term fatigue in patients with cancer (NCCN, 2007b). Endocrine abnormalities, such as a blunted cortisol response to stressors suggesting hypothalamic-pituitary-adrenal dysregulation, may result from cancer treatment (Bower, Ganz, & Aziz, 2005).

Chemotherapy and radiation therapy may have direct effects causing fatigue. Accumulation of end products of cell destruction and increased energy requirements needed to repair cell damage may be factors (Fu et al., 2005; Tchen et al., 2003). Treatments with chemotherapy or radiation therapy depress the bone marrow and disrupt erythrocyte production, resulting in a normocytic, normochromic anemia with a low reticulocyte count. With decreased circulating red blood cells, it is not surprising for the patient to feel fatigued during treatments because of loss of oxygen-carrying capacity to the muscles and brain. Nail (1997) described a depletion hypothesis to explain the fatigue of anemia. In addition to decreasing the oxygen-carrying capacity of the blood, anemia also inhibits the delivery of essential nutrients to the cells while at the same time decreasing the energy available to the organism.

Risk Factors

NCCN (2007b) identified seven causative factors of cancer-related fatigue: pain, emotional distress (i.e., depression, anxiety), sleep disturbance, anemia, alteration in nutrition, deconditioning resulting from decreased activity level, and comorbidities. Fatigue may occur alone but more frequently occurs in combination with other symptoms or symptom clusters (Gullatte et al., 2005; NCCN, 2007b). For example, anxiety, depression, and stress contribute to fatigue and often occur concurrently with fatigue.

People with certain preexisting conditions may be at increased risk for development of or increased level of fatigue. Tchen et al. (2003) identified a strong association among profound fatigue, menopausal symptoms, and quality of life. Individuals who have had a stroke or congestive heart failure have decreased reserves and may develop fatigue more easily (Gullatte et al., 2005). Concurrent endocrine, pulmonary, cardiac, or other conditions affecting major organ systems also intensify fatigue. Sleep disturbances, including hypersomnia, insomnia, or sleep apnea, contribute to fatigue. Physiologic stress may be a contributing factor. Pain, infection, dehydration, hypoxia, anemia, and malnutrition can intensify fatigue. Paraneoplastic syndromes, such as syndrome of inappropriate antidiuretic hormone and hypercalcemia, cause fatigue (Gullatte et al.). Tissue injury and stress response attributable to surgery may result in fatigue that lasts six months or longer (Fu et al., 2005). People taking medications such as opioids, hypnotics, anxiolytics, antihistamines, antiemetics, anticonvulsants, or antihypertensives may experience fatigue as a result of these agents' sedative effects (Gullatte et al.; Vogel et al., 2004). Immobility can result in deconditioning and muscle wasting, thereby causing fatigue (Gullatte et al.).

Signs and Symptoms

Fatigue is multidimensional, including mental, physical, and emotional components (Nail, 2002). Alterations in behavioral patterns of sleep quality, stamina, cognition, and emotional reactivity are early indicators of impending fatigue. Eventually, body processes and social interactions are affected if the person is unable to adapt. Patients may complain of generalized weakness, tiredness, negative or unpleasant emotions, mental exhaustion, and impaired concentration and memory. Mental and physical fatigue may prevent the individual from participating in relationships, thus resulting in isolation and loneliness (Gullatte et al., 2005).

Patients may complain of physical symptoms and frequently describe feeling weary, sluggish, or dragged-out, having heavy limbs, or feeling slow, irritable, and tired (Johnston & Coward, 2001). Fatigue is a physical symptom, but mental fatigue also occurs. Difficulty concentrating and processing information may be experienced. Patients with fatigue may have difficulty understanding simple instructions or trying to complete a to-do list. Individuals may complain of forgetfulness resulting in missed appointments, omitted medications, or difficulty in communications with healthcare providers.

Activity often is the first area affected and usually presents as limited energy to complete routine tasks such as housecleaning. It also can affect recreational pastimes such as golfing or gardening. Even routine activities, such as getting dressed, require more effort than customary. Patients may find their ability to fulfill various roles has decreased. Interactions with others may change because of the inability to carry out usual responsibilities, and family dynamics may change. Patients may cease volunteerism in their community, school, or social groups.

Assessment

Assessment of fatigue is a routine part of clinical evaluation of individuals with cancer (Lawrence et al., 2004). Patient self-reports and information from family members may be solicited (NCCN, 2007b). Questions are posed about day-to-day functioning, such as the ability to work and engage in routine activities. PQRST assessment provides information regarding the onset, pattern, and duration of fatigue, changes over time, and associated or alleviating factors. Disease status, type and length of treatment, and the patients' response to treatment are documented. Comorbidities and contributing factors, such as pain, anemia, depression, altered nutritional status, medications, and sleep disturbance, are identified (NCCN, 2007b; Portenoy & Itri, 1999).

NCCN (2007b) guidelines recommend that every patient be screened for fatigue as a vital sign at regular intervals. Following a thorough history and physical examination, certain diagnostic tools may be necessary to form the diagnosis of cancer-related fatigue. However, consideration is given to the time required to complete the testing: It should not take so long that it causes fatigue (Nail, 2002).

The use of a severity scale will facilitate assessment and provide continuity over time. Fatigue over the previous seven days may be rated on a scale of 0 to 10 (0 = no fatigue, and 10 = worst fatigue imaginable) or using terms such as mild, moderate, or severe. Complaints of moderate (4–6) or severe (7–10) fatigue lead to a focused history, physical examination, and management of treatable contributing or causative factors. Multiple other instruments are available to evaluate fatigue. ONS has compiled a list of tools and references for evaluation of cancer-related fatigue, which is available at www.ons.org /research/outcomes/pdf/fatigue7.pdf. Three commonly referenced tools specific to cancer-related fatigue are the Piper Fatigue Scale (Piper et al., 1998), the Brief Fatigue Inventory (University of Texas M.D. Anderson Cancer Center, 1997), and the Functional Assessment of Chronic Illness Therapy–Fatigue (FACIT-F) (www.facit.org/qview/qlist.aspx) assessment tool (Yellen, Cella, Webster, Blendowski, & Kaplan, 1997).

Physical examination: Physical examination may provide clues to causes of fatigue and identification of contributing factors (NCCN, 2007b; Vogel et al., 2004). For example, constitutional signs might identify nutritional deficiencies, and vital signs might indicate the presence of infection. Assessment of general appearance, mood, and manner may reveal anxiety or depression. Assessing the musculoskeletal system might reveal focal or generalized weakness, muscle mass loss, joint pain, warm or edematous joints, muscle pain, muscle twitching, limitations in range of motion, or bone pain. Abnormal skin turgor could indicate that dehydration might be contributing to fatigue. Decreased or adventitious lung sounds might indicate pulmonary edema, chronic obstructive pulmonary disease, or pneumonia that is affecting activity tolerance. Abnormal heart sounds and jugular venous distention might indicate that congestive heart failure is causing fatigue.

Diagnostic testing: Diagnostic testing for evaluation of fatigue may be problematic. No identified diagnostic tests exist for fatigue specifically. However, tests are available that assist in determining the cause or causes of fatigue or ruling out other potential diagnoses. Table 10-5 gives a nonexhaustive list of diagnostic tests to consider in the work-up of patients with fatigue.

Differential diagnosis: The differential diagnoses for cancer-related fatigue are vast and may include causes or contributing factors. These may potentially be treatable or reversible, such as pain, emotional distress, sleep disturbance, anemia, and hypothyroidism (Lawrence et al., 2004). Comorbidities such as infection or cardiac, pulmonary,

Table 10-5. Diagnostic Tests* to Consider in the Work-Up of Fatigue	
Test	**Rationale**
Complete blood count and differential	Rule out anemia and infection.
Thyroid-stimulating hormone and T4 level	Evaluate thyroid function.
Electrolyte levels	Evaluate nutritional status, and rule out electrolyte imbalance.
Blood urea nitrogen and creatinine	Evaluate renal function as a potential factor in fatigue.
Liver function tests (aspartate aminotransferase, alanine aminotransferase, alkaline phosphatase, and bilirubin)	Rule out liver dysfunction or metastatic disease as a potential cause of fatigue.
Bone scan, computed tomography scans, or other diagnostic imaging tests	Rule out metastatic disease causing pain that in turn causes fatigue.

* Nonexhaustive listing

renal, hepatic, neurologic, or endocrine dysfunction also may be part of the differential. Cancer-related fatigue is now accepted as a diagnosis by the International Classification of Diseases in its 10th revision.

Treatment of Cancer-Related Fatigue

Prevention: The optimal intervention for cancer-related fatigue is prevention. APNs will assess for and treat any potential causes, such as nutritional deficiencies, anemia, pain, emotional distress, and sleep disturbances, thus avoiding the concomitant impacts of these (Fu et al., 2005). Encouraging activity and establishing a regular exercise program may prevent as well as treat fatigue (Lawrence et al., 2004). Educating patients regarding fatigue before its onset can promote early reporting of this symptom and prompt early intervention before it becomes debilitating.

Management: The management of fatigue positively affects physical, psychological, social, and vocational functioning and improves overall quality of life. However, as causes of cancer-related fatigue are poorly understood and are affected by concomitant diseases and their various treatments, few specific and effective treatments exist (Fu et al., 2005; Lawrence et al., 2004). According to Olson (2007), the goal of fatigue intervention is to focus on eliminating stressors and increase the resistance of the patient to stressors. Therapy may include modification of drug regimens and correction of metabolic abnormalities, as well as symptomatic interventions such as exercise, activity and rest modification, cognitive therapies, and nutritional support (Portenoy & Itri, 1999).

Whenever possible, the underlying cause should be eliminated or treated. Managing pain, depression, infection, dehydration, hypoxia, insomnia, anemia, nutritional deficiencies, and electrolyte imbalances may improve fatigue and eliminate other symptoms as well (Gullatte et al., 2005). Table 10-6 lists potential interventions and levels of evidence to support them (Mitchell, Beck, Hood, Moore, & Tanner, 2007).

Pharmacologic: Although no medications currently are FDA approved specifically for fatigue, certain drugs are approved to treat possible concomitant, contributing disease states that affect fatigue. Dexmethylphenidate (Focalin®, Novartis Pharmaceuticals

Table 10-6. Interventions for Preventing and Treating Fatigue During and Following Cancer and Cancer Treatment

Level of Evidence	Intervention
Recommended for practice	Exercise
Likely to be effective	Massage Relaxation Healing touch Education/information provision Measures to optimize sleep quality Energy conservation and activity management Screening for potential etiologic factors and management as appropriate
Benefits balanced with harms	Correction of anemia
Effectiveness not established	Yoga Modafinil Paroxetine Donepezil Acupuncture Methylphenidate Expressive writing Bupropion sustained-release Levocarnitine supplementation Individual and group psychotherapy Adenosine 5'-triphosphate infusion Omega-3 fatty acid supplementation Distraction—virtual reality immersion Combination therapy: Aromatherapy, foot soak, and reflexology Combination therapy: Medroxyprogesterone, celecoxib, and enteral food supplementation Combination therapy: Soy protein supplementation and nutrition counseling following discharge from hospital

Note. From "Putting Evidence Into Practice: Evidence-Based Interventions for Fatigue During and Following Cancer and Its Treatment," by S.A. Mitchell, S.L. Beck, L.E. Hood, K. Moore, and E.R. Tanner, 2007, *Clinical Journal of Oncology Nursing, 11,* p. 102. Copyright 2007 by Oncology Nursing Society. Adapted with permission.

Corp.), a central nervous system stimulant used in the treatment of attention-deficit/hyperactivity disorder, is being studied in chemotherapy-related fatigue. Doses up to 50 mg/day are well tolerated, with common mild to moderate side effects of headache and nausea (NCI, 2005). Other psychostimulants, such as methylphenidate (Ritalin®, Novartis Pharmaceuticals Corp.) and modafinil (Provigil®, Cephalon, Inc.), appear to be effective in decreasing fatigue and depression; however, the evidence is not yet sufficient to support a recommendation for routine use (Gullatte et al., 2005; Mitchell et al., 2007). Adverse effects associated with psychostimulants include anorexia, insomnia, tremulousness, anxiety, delirium, and tachycardia (Portenoy & Itri, 1999).

Treatment of anemia may ameliorate fatigue and significantly improve quality of life. Transfusion may be necessary to treat acute blood loss (NCCN, 2008). The use of epoetin alfa for the correction of anemia has been shown to decrease fatigue (Lawrence et al., 2004). Correction of hemoglobin to a target level of 11–12 g/dl seems to produce the greatest benefit in reducing fatigue and improving quality of life. Side effects include a slight increased risk of thrombotic events, hypertension, and theoretical concerns of increased tumor growth in certain disease sites (Steensma & Loprinzi, 2005).

Use of antidepressants, such as selective serotonin-reuptake inhibitors (SSRIs), tricyclics, or bupropion, occasionally is associated with the experience of increased energy, even in nondepressed patients. An empiric trial may be considered in severe or refractory cases of fatigue (Portenoy & Itri, 1999). The rationale for use of these agents is that a neurotransmitter mechanism induced by cancer treatment may contribute to fatigue (Nail, 2002).

Nonpharmacologic: Exercise and rest are the most frequently recommended and used strategies to relieve fatigue (Fu et al., 2005). Exercise is the only intervention supported by a body of evidence in controlling fatigue during and following cancer treatment (Mitchell et al., 2007) and is associated with lower levels of emotional distress and improved sleep patterns (NCCN, 2007b). Physical exercise training programs can decrease the loss in physical performance associated with toxic treatment, increase functional capacity, and improve cardiopulmonary function. Referral to physical therapy or physical medicine and rehabilitation for assessment and exercise prescription may be indicated. Comorbidities such as bone metastasis, neutropenia, thrombocytopenia, or other treatment complications may limit prescribed activity. If appropriate, a progressive program of 20–30-minute sessions, three to five days per week, at an intensity of 60%–80% of maximum heart rate is recommended.

Strategies for energy conservation may be helpful (Lawrence et al., 2004). NCCN (2007b) defines energy conservation as "deliberately planned management of one's personal energy resources to prevent their depletion" (pp. MS-13–14). The goal of energy conservation is to maintain a balance between rest and activity, so that valued activities may be completed. Patients may envision the concept of an "energy checkbook" in which "withdrawals" in the form of participating in activities need to be offset with "deposits" of rest. "Withdrawals" for some activities can be anticipated and planned for appropriately by prioritizing important activities, delegating tasks to others, pacing oneself, taking extra rest periods, or altering the environment to decrease the amount of energy required (Gullatte et al., 2005; NCCN, 2007b).

Attention-restoring therapy may improve the capacity to concentrate or direct attention during times of stress. Enjoyment of natural environments improves cognitive ability and decreases attentional fatigue (NCCN, 2007b). Keeping the mind active, even when the body is fatigued, improves the ability to concentrate (Gullatte et al., 2005). Psychosocial interventions also have a strong evidence base for treating fatigue and include education, support groups, individual counseling, stress management training, and tailored behavioral interventions to decrease anxiety, depression, and fatigue (NCCN, 2007b).

Nutritional consultation may be helpful in managing deficiencies resulting from anorexia, diarrhea, nausea, and vomiting. Proper nutrition is thought to provide adequate fuel for the body to function (Nail, 2002). Hydration and replacement of deficient electrolytes, such as iron and folic acid, may prevent or treat fatigue (NCCN, 2007b).

Treatment of sleep disorders through stimulus control, sleep restriction, and sleep hygiene decreases fatigue by optimizing sleep quality. Stimulus control includes going to bed when sleepy, going to bed at the same time each night, and rising at approximately the same time each morning. *Sleep restriction* refers to avoiding long naps during the day, avoiding late afternoon naps, and limiting time spent in bed to the hours designated for nighttime sleep. *Sleep hygiene* includes techniques to promote a good night's sleep, such as avoiding caffeine after noon, exercising at least six hours before bedtime, and establishing an environment conducive to sleep (i.e., quiet, dark, comfortable) (NCCN, 2007b; Portenoy & Itri, 1999).

Keeping a journal, log, or diary of activities, feelings, and evaluation of self-care actions is useful in determining triggers that worsen fatigue and interventions that lessen its impact (Fu et al., 2005). These can assist in planning essential activities for times when energy levels are higher or modifying activities based on individual reserves. Time for rest and restorative activities is easier to plan if prior patterns and interventions are evaluated.

Education about fatigue and its usual pattern, duration, and natural history ideally is offered to all patients and families at the start of treatment, before fatigue onset (NCCN, 2007b). The goal of fatigue education is to teach self-care strategies (Fu et al., 2005).

Consultation with multidisciplinary team members is an essential part of fatigue management. Referral to other expert practitioners, such as physical therapists, social services, or nutritionists, may be necessary (NCCN, 2007b). APNs are instrumental in coordinating these referrals.

Complementary and alternative therapies: Preliminary studies have noted massage therapy, acupuncture, expressive writing, yoga, muscle relaxation, healing touch, and mindfulness-based stress reduction to be effective in reducing fatigue in patients with cancer; however, further study is warranted (Mitchell et al., 2007; NCCN, 2007b). Chapter 8 gives more information about alternative therapies.

Evaluation of Outcomes

Assessment and evaluation of fatigue are essential at each clinic visit. Effectiveness of interventions is evaluated, and if ineffective, alternative strategies are considered. Assessment for the presence of seven known treatable factors (pain, emotional distress, sleep disturbance, anemia, alteration in nutrition, deconditioning, and comorbidities) is ongoing. Fatigue occurs in the context of multiple symptoms, and these symptoms may act synergistically to worsen the overall symptom experience (NCCN, 2007b). Multiple concurrent interventions may be required. Cause-specific interventions are indicated, but if no cause is identified, nonpharmacologic and pharmacologic treatments still are considered (NCCN, 2007b).

Chemotherapy-Related Cognitive Dysfunction

Introduction

As the diagnosis and treatment of cancer become more sophisticated and successful, more individuals will live longer as survivors, and the long-term sequelae of systemic treatments will become more apparent. A long-term effect of cancer and cancer treatments increasingly being recognized by healthcare professionals is referred to in the popular press as *chemo brain*. This term refers to changes in cognitive function, including short- and long-term memory, attention span, concentration, language, and motor skills, attributed to the effects of drugs or other treatments for cancer (Olin, 2001; Schagen et al., 1999).

Definition and Incidence

Cognition is "the mental process of thinking, learning, remembering, being aware of surroundings, and using judgment" (NCI, n.d.-a). Cognitive function is defined as "an intellectual process by which one becomes aware of, perceives, or comprehends ideas. It involves all aspects of perception, thinking, reasoning, and remembering" (Myers, 2006, p. 412). The multidimensional concept of cognitive function includes the domains of attention and concentration, executive function (including planning and problem solving), information processing speed, language, visuospatial skill, psychomotor ability, learning, and memory (Jansen, Miaskowski, Dodd, & Dowling, 2005; Nail, 2006).

Following chemotherapy, patients have reported difficulty in their ability to remember, think, and concentrate (Brezden, Phillips, Abdolell, Bunston, & Tannock, 2000). Some describe the sensation of being in a mental fog (LaTour, 2002). The reported incidence of cognitive dysfunction associated with cancer treatment ranges from 16%–87% (Ahles et al., 2002, 2003; Anderson-Hanley, Sherman, Riggs, Agocha, & Compas, 2003; Brezden et al., 2000; Castellon et al., 2004; Cull et al., 1996; Heflin et al., 2005; Schagen, Muller, Boogerd, Mellenbergh, & van Dam, 2006; Schagen et al., 1999; Schultz, Klein, Beck, Stava, & Sellin, 2005; Shilling, Jenkins, & Trapala, 2006; Tchen et al., 2003; van Dam et al., 1998; Wefel, Lenzi, Theriault, Buzdar, et al., 2004; Wefel, Lenzi, Theriault, Davis, & Meyers, 2004). Determining actual incidence is difficult, as existing studies measure varying domains of cognitive function, use varying control groups for comparison, examine different points in time relative to administration of treatment, do not account for confounding factors, lack pretreatment assessment for comparison, and lack consistency in many aspects of methodology. The method used for analyzing data also may account for variations in study findings. Because of these variations in available studies, caution is advised when interpreting results of trials evaluating cognitive function and when making decisions about practice changes.

Virtually no patients complain that their cognitive impairment existed prior to their diagnosis of cancer (van Dam et al., 1998). However, several studies have reported subtle declines in cognitive function in approximately one-third of patients before the start of chemotherapy treatment (Wefel, Lenzi, Theriault, Buzdar, et al., 2004; Wefel, Lenzi, Theriault, Davis, et al., 2004). Although no definite cause has been identified, it is hypothesized that this may be the result of patient factors such as nutritional, hormonal, genetic, or immune factors; disease characteristics such as cytokines produced by the tumor; or the influence of the psychological impact of a cancer diagnosis (Wefel, Lenzi, Theriault, Davis, et al.).

Etiology and Pathophysiology

Several mechanisms are hypothesized to contribute to the development of cognitive impairment. Cognitive dysfunction has been reported in patients receiving various cancer treatments, including chemotherapy (Wefel, Lenzi, Theriault, Davis, et al., 2004), radiation therapy (Omuro et al., 2005), hormonal treatments (Castellon et al., 2004), and transplantation (Syrjala, Dikmen, Langer, Roth-Roemer, & Abrams, 2004). It also has been reported following the diagnosis of cancer, prior to treatment (Wefel, Lenzi, Theriault, Davis, et al.). To detail all the possible theories of etiology is beyond the scope of this chapter. Chemotherapy-associated cognitive dysfunction is most likely multifactorial. Figure 10-9 illustrates the relationship between cancer treatment effects and cognitive functioning. Physiologic effects, such as clotting in small blood vessels, may cause cognitive dysfunction, as may psychological factors such as depression or anxiety.

Several potential mechanisms are hypothesized to account for cognitive dysfunction associated with chemotherapy (Barton & Loprinzi, 2002; Saykin, Ahles, & McDonald, 2003; Tannock, Ahles, Ganz, & van Dam, 2004; Wefel, Lenzi, Theriault, Davis, et al.,

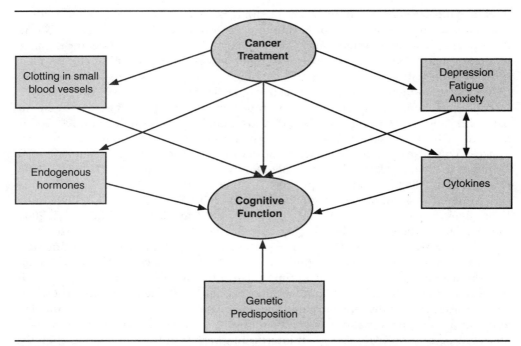

Figure 10-9. A Conceptual Framework Including Factors That Might Influence Cognitive Function in Women With Breast Cancer

Note. Figure courtesy of Patricia Ganz, MD. Used with permission.

2004). Most chemotherapy drugs are not able to cross the blood-brain barrier and thus do not directly affect the brain. However, it is possible that cytokines, produced as a result of chemotherapy's effect on cells, are able to cross this natural barrier and cause direct injury to cerebral gray and white matter, producing demyelination or altered water content in the central nervous system. Secondary injury may occur as a result of immune-mediated inflammatory responses. Cytokines released in response to inflammation, stress, or direct injury to neurons may affect cognition. Altered neurotransmitter levels and metabolites may have neurotoxic effects. Microvascular injury, such as that associated with leukoencephalopathy, may lead to obstruction of small and medium-sized blood vessels, spontaneous thrombosis, ischemia or infarction, and parenchymal necrosis.

Drugs given along with chemotherapy, such as antiemetics, steroids, sedatives, and antihistamines, also may have a short-term effect on cognitive ability. For example, steroids can have adverse effects on mental and emotional functioning, intensifying anxiety, depression, restlessness, and insomnia. Antiepileptic medications can cause sedation, distractibility, somnolence, dizziness, and impairment of attention and memory (Kayl, Wefel, & Meyers, 2006).

Effects of hormonal changes associated with menopause, whether naturally occurring or induced by chemotherapy treatment, are hypothesized to influence cognitive function. Estrogen receptors are present in areas of the brain associated with attention, memory, and learning. Estrogen may have a neuroprotective effect and support the maintenance of cognitive function (Saykin et al., 2003). However, in spite of subjective reports, research has not proved a difference in cognitive function that is attributable to menopause or hormonal changes (Schagen et al., 1999; van Dam et al., 1998; Wefel, Lenzi, Theriault, Buzdar, et al., 2004). Studies vary on the influence of additional psychological factors, such as anxiety, depression, and fatigue, on cognitive function. Heflin et al. (2005) concluded that cancer and chemotherapy treatment decrease cognitive reserve, and over time, survivors have a higher risk of reaching the threshold for measurable cognitive dysfunction.

Risk Factors

Not all patients receiving chemotherapy develop cognitive changes. Several studies have reported that cognitive impairment appears to affect a subset of patients, with the underlying risk or causative factors unknown (Brezden et al., 2000; Tchen et al., 2003; Wefel, Lenzi, Theriault, Davis, et al., 2004) and the severity of impairment varying among individuals. No significant differences have been identified in sociodemographic characteristics, such as age, sex, employment status, IQ level, or education, or clinical characteristics, such as diagnosis. Studies controlling for confounding or associated factors show that age, education level, menopausal status, mood, fatigue, anxiety, and depression have not had a significant impact on results (Brezden et al.; Schagen et al., 1999; Tchen et al.; van Dam et al., 1998).

Patients receiving high-dose regimens of chemotherapy have a higher risk of developing cognitive impairment than those receiving standard-dose regimens. van Dam et al. (1998) compared patients with early-stage breast cancer who received high-dose chemotherapy with those treated with standard-dose chemotherapy and with patients not treated with chemotherapy. At an average of two years after treatment, patients receiving high-dose chemotherapy had 8.2-times higher risk of cognitive impairment than those not treated with chemotherapy and 3.5-times higher risk than those receiving standard-dose treatment. These results did not appear to be influenced by anxiety, depression, or fatigue.

The specific chemotherapy agents received also may affect a person's risk for cognitive dysfunction. The effect is seen as deterioration over time occurring in a subset of patients and is not consistently seen with a particular agent or combination of agents (Schagen et al., 2006).

Certain psychological complaints may increase the risk of developing cognitive dysfunction. Cull et al. (1996) found that those reporting difficulty with memory and concentration had significantly higher scores on measures of anxiety, depression, and fatigue. Wefel, Lenzi, Theriault, Buzdar, et al. (2004) found that 26% of patients complaining of cognitive dysfunction also reported symptoms of anxiety and depression and significant affective distress. Tchen et al. (2003) noted a correlation but did not find a significant association between cognitive impairment and fatigue. Schagen et al. (1999) showed no significant difference on objective testing; however, self-reports of cognitive dysfunction were associated with anxiety and depression.

It is hypothesized that carrying certain genetic alleles, such as the ε4 allele of the *apolipoprotein E (APOE)* gene, might increase the risk of developing cognitive dysfunction when diagnosed with cancer or undergoing cancer treatment (Ahles et al., 2003). In this study, individuals who carried this allele scored significantly lower in the domains of visual memory, spatial ability, and psychomotor functioning than those who did not carry the allele. However, despite significant differences between carriers and noncarriers, all fell within the normal range for the neuropsychological tests administered, therefore reinforcing previous findings that cognitive impairment is usually mild.

Anemia may contribute to cognitive impairment, thereby increasing risk. It can occur as a result of the treatment effect on stem cells, secretion of anemia-inducing factors by some types of tumor, or other conditions such as blood loss, B_{12} or folate deficiency, or renal disease. Symptoms of decreased mental alertness, poor concentration, and memory problems are associated with decreased hemoglobin concentration (Cunningham, 2003).

Signs and Symptoms of Cognitive Dysfunction

Patients frequently report mild cognitive impairment, including having mildly affected thinking ability but still being able to maintain adequate functioning. Difficulty with memory is reported, such as trouble remembering names, trouble remembering the flow of a conversation, and a tendency to misplace things. Mild cognitive impairment differs from dementia. In dementia, memory loss has progressed to such a point that normal independent function is impossible, and individuals can no longer successfully manage their finances or provide for their own basic needs.

Subtle changes in memory, concentration, language, visual-motor, and executive function are observed and negatively affect quality of life (Ahles et al., 2002; Brezden et al., 2000; Schultz et al., 2005; van Dam et al., 1998; Wefel, Lenzi, Theriault, Davis, et al., 2004). Some individuals have difficulty maintaining ability to work, continuing education, or fulfilling social responsibilities (Saykin et al., 2003; Staat & Segatore, 2005). Symptoms of cognitive impairment may persist for years following the completion of treatment. Patients usually will report these symptoms when their activities of daily living are adversely affected.

Assessment of Cancer-Related Cognitive Impairment

Patients complaining of subjective symptoms of cognitive impairment may not show impairment on neuropsychological testing. Changes in cognitive function are often mild, and while assessment may show decline from baseline after initiation of treatment, results of neuropsychological testing frequently remain within the normal range (Cull et al., 1996; Grunfeld, Dhesy-Thind, & Levine, 2005; Wefel, Lenzi, Theriault, Davis, et al., 2004). This discrepancy may occur because tests are not measuring the correct construct or may be insufficiently sensitive to detect mild deficits (Brezden et al., 2000; Morse, Rodgers, Verrill, & Kendell, 2003).

Diagnostic tests and tools: Multiple measures are available to test various aspects of identified cognitive domains, but no valid and reliable clinical tool exists to evaluate the frequently subtle changes associated with cancer treatment (Jansen et al., 2005). Formal neuropsychological testing to evaluate various aspects of cognitive function is a lengthy process that takes several hours to administer and complete (Schagen et al., 1999) and is not practical for routine clinical practice. Referral of patients for specific neuropsychological evaluation may be indicated if symptoms are severe. Administration and interpretation of these tests by a healthcare professional with training in neuropsychology is recommended (Wefel, Lenzi, Theriault, Buzdar, et al., 2004).

Various forms of imaging may detect changes in gray and white matter, inflammatory and autoimmune responses, damage to the capillary microvasculature, and permeability of the blood-brain barrier leading to water space changes (Castellon, Silverman, & Ganz, 2005; Saykin et al., 2003), although further study is warranted. No specific imaging currently is indicated for the evaluation of chemotherapy-related cognitive dysfunction.

Physical examination: Clinical observation is the most useful way to assess for cognitive changes (O'Shaughnessy, 2003). Individuals are assessed for changes in attention or concentration and their ability to perform routine tasks and are questioned regarding subjective signs of impairment (Jansen et al., 2005). Asking directed questions may initiate discussion regarding problems with role function or quality-of-life issues. A physical examination is useful to rule out other causes of cognitive impairment, such as metastatic disease, electrolyte imbalance, or side effects of medications. Assessment may require laboratory tests, such as a complete blood count, metabolic panel, liver function tests, or imaging scans, as indicated.

Symptom rating scale: A relationship appears to exist between subjective cognitive problems and psychological distress (Cull et al., 1996; van Dam et al., 1998; Wefel, Lenzi, Theriault, Buzdar, et al., 2004). NCCN (2007c) has developed guidelines for distress management. Clinicians assess the level and nature of the distress by asking patients to quantify cognitive dysfunction's impact on their life by rating their level of distress on a scale of 0 to 10 (0 indicating no distress, and 10 indicating extreme distress). A rating of 4 or higher indicates moderate to severe distress, and intervention should be planned. Patients are reevaluated on an ongoing basis to determine the effectiveness of interventions.

Differential Diagnosis

Mild cognitive changes may be attributed to fatigue, anxiety, depression, mood imbalances, or hormonal changes; therefore, the differential diagnosis may include psychological disorders. Potentially reversible causes, such as endocrine or metabolic dysfunction, must be ruled out (Kayl et al., 2006). Infection, fever, nutritional deficits, sleep disorders, and advancing age may be indirect factors accounting for mild cognitive impairment and are included in the differential (O'Shaughnessy, 2003). Figure 10-10 is a nonexhaustive list of the differential diagnoses of cognitive dysfunction. Potential diagnoses could be psychological, physiologic, or pharmacologic in nature.

Psychological
- Fatigue
- Anxiety
- Depression
- Mood imbalance
- Insomnia/sleep disorder

Physiologic
- Fever
- Anemia
- Infection
- Hormonal changes
- Nutritional deficits

Pharmacologic
- Steroids
- Sedatives
- Antiemetics
- Antiepileptics
- Antidepressants

Figure 10-10. Differential Diagnoses for Cognitive Dysfunction

Treatment of Cancer-Related Cognitive Impairment

No treatment is currently approved to prevent or decrease any of the cognitive symptoms associated with chemotherapy (Barton & Loprinzi, 2002). Various treatments are proposed based on potential etiologies and are under study (see Figure 10-11). The passage of time may relieve cognitive dysfunction. Wefel, Lenzi, Theriault, Davis, et al. (2004) found that half of cognitively impaired patients noted improvement within one to two years of completion of treatment without specific intervention. Informing patients of this may be reassuring. It is important to first treat concomitant problems, such as anxiety, depression, pain, and fatigue, and maintain good nutrition, as well as to expertly manage comorbid diseases.

Pharmacologic: Hormonal strategies, antioxidants, monoamine oxidase inhibitors (MAOIs), growth factors, dopamine agonists, cholinesterase inhibitors, anti-inflammatory agents, thiamine, and steroids all have been noted to improve cognition, but studies proving effectiveness and safety in patients with cancer are lacking (Barton & Loprinzi, 2002; Saykin et al., 2003; Wefel, Lenzi, Theriault, Davis, et al., 2004).

The central nervous system stimulants methylphenidate (Ritalin) and dexmethylphenidate (Focalin) improve concentration, psychomotor slowing, fatigue, and attention.

Pharmacologic (Not yet supported by research study, and use may be limited by side effects)
- Methylphenidate (Ritalin®, Novartis Pharmaceuticals Corp.)
- Dexmethylphenidate (Focalin®, Novartis Pharmaceuticals Corp.)
- Modafinil (Provigil®, Cephalon, Inc.)
- Cholinesterase inhibitors (Aricept® [Eisai Co., Ltd.], Exelon® [Novartis Pharmaceuticals Corp.], Razadyne® [Ortho-McNeil Neurologics, Inc.])
- Erythropoietin

Nonpharmacologic
- Simplification
  - Limit/eliminate distraction.
    * Reduce background noise.
    * Clear clutter.
- Memory aids
  - Calendars/lists
  - Establish routines
- Cognitive behavioral therapy
- Restorative natural environment
- Physical/mental exercise

Complementary and Alternative Interventions
- Herbs
  - Thiamine
  - Vitamins C and E
  - Ginkgo biloba
- Body awareness and movement
  - Yoga
  - Tai Chi
- Aromatherapy
- Meditation

Figure 10-11. Treatment for Mild Cognitive Dysfunction

Note. Based on information from Barton & Loprinzi, 2002; Cimprich & Ronis, 2003; Galantino et al., 2005; McDougall, 2001; Nail, 2006; Saykin et al., 2003; Sherwood et al., 2005; Staat & Segatore, 2005; Wefel, Lenzi, Theriault, Davis, et al., 2004.

They also increase tissue perfusion, vascular dilation, and cerebral blood flow. Side effects usually are mild and easily reversed with drug discontinuation. Adverse effects include headache, nausea, nervousness, insomnia, and cardiovascular symptoms (Meyers, Weitzner, Valentine, & Levin, 1998). Contraindications include prior sensitivity to stimulants, glaucoma, symptomatic cardiovascular disease, and hyperthyroidism (Staat & Segatore, 2005).

Cholinesterase inhibitors, used for the treatment of Alzheimer disease and vascular dementia, may stabilize memory capacity and improve cognitive function by selectively inhibiting acetylcholinesterase (Barton & Loprinzi, 2002; Staat & Segatore, 2005). Drugs in this class include donepezil (Aricept®, Eisai Co., Ltd.), rivastigmine (Exelon®, Novartis Pharmaceuticals Corp.), and galantamine (Razadyne®, Ortho-McNeil Neurologics, Inc.). Side effects include nausea, diarrhea, weight loss, asthenia, arthralgias, and in rare cases, syncope and mild pancreatitis (Barton & Loprinzi).

MAOIs, such as phenelzine, or drugs with selective MAOI effects, such as selegiline and procarbazine, may act as antioxidants to decrease oxidative stress and provide some neuroprotection. However, the side effect profile and interactions with common medications and foods limit their use (Barton & Loprinzi, 2002). NSAIDs, such as aspirin and indomethacin, under study in patients with Alzheimer disease, may slow the decline of cognitive function. Autoimmune vasculitis or an allergic hypersensitivity response that damages neurons and affects cognition may be decreased or prevented by suppressing autoimmune processes with these agents (Barton & Loprinzi). Currently, no studies of NSAIDs to prevent cognitive dysfunction are under way in patients with cancer, and gastrointestinal side effects may limit their use.

In several studies, treating anemia with erythropoietin improved cognitive functioning (Leyland-Jones & O'Shaughnessy, 2003). Epoetin alfa may interfere with a hypoxia-induced cascade of events that, if not modulated, results in cognitive decline. NCCN (2008) has developed guidelines for the treatment of cancer- and treatment-related anemia.

Nonpharmacologic: Cognitive rehabilitation approaches may significantly improve functioning (Barton & Loprinzi, 2002; Saykin et al., 2003). Memorization exercises and memory aids such as the use of lists, alphabetical searching, and mental retracing (Cull et al., 1996) may be helpful. Cognitive behavioral interventions help individuals to recognize and remedy dysfunctional thoughts and behaviors (McDougall, 2001; Sherwood et al., 2005). McDougall found significant subjective and objective improvement in older adult survivors of cancer utilizing a cognitive behavioral model of everyday memory with emphasis on health promotion. This strategy incorporated skill building through modeling techniques, observing performance, developing awareness, handling mental challenges, and reducing anxiety about cognitive impairment.

Ferguson et al. (2007) developed a brief cognitive-behavioral program, referred to as Memory and Attention Adaptation Training. Instruction in memory and attention compensatory strategies is provided with application to daily life. Participants identify "at risk" situations where memory failures arise and then learn and rehearse compensatory strategies to deal with these. Ferguson et al. found significant improvements that persisted in areas of attention and concentration, spatial memory, verbal memory, and language.

Cimprich and Ronis (2003) used a natural restorative environmental intervention to counteract cognitive and attentional fatigue. Regular exposure to the natural environment, such as with gardening, walking in a scenic area, observing wildlife, listening to sounds of nature, or watching a sunset, improve the ability to focus and concentrate. This intervention must involve getting away from one's normal environment and routines and include the element of "fascination," meaning the activity must be effortless and involve no mental effort or directed attention. The individual must not find the activity boring, and it must be something the person is comfortable with and finds relaxing.

Simplifying tasks, commitments, and the environment reduces the stress caused by changes in memory, concentration, and the ability to multitask. Reducing work or dividing projects into manageable small steps, establishing a routine, decreasing work hours or academic credits, and avoiding performance of concurrent tasks may help to reduce stress. Limiting or eliminating distractions, such as background noise and clutter, makes the environment less stressful (Nail, 2006; Staat & Segatore, 2005). Keeping lists of tasks or important items to remember and using a calendar to keep track of important dates and appointments will provide prompts rather than relying on memory. Use of electronic devices such as an electronic calendar with an alarm is helpful if short-term memory is affected, and a word-based direction finder or global positioning system can assist patients if their visuospatial memory is decreased (Nail, 2006). Asking people to repeat information may aid patients in remembering the information. Mental exercise can improve cognition and slow mental decline. This could include working on crossword or math puzzles, participating in a book club, or taking a class. Use of mnemonic devices, such as a formula or rhyme, may aid patients in remembering information.

Complementary and alternative therapies: Herbs used to enhance mental alertness and memory include blessed thistle, blue cohosh, and ginkgo biloba (*Nursing Herbal Medicine Handbook,* 2006). Ginkgo biloba may have antioxidant, membrane-stabilizing, and neuroprotective effects. It may inhibit loss of cholinergic receptors. Studies in healthy volunteers and older adults with Alzheimer disease show promising results, but studies in individuals with cancer are lacking (Barton & Loprinzi, 2002). Because of an antiplatelet effect, ginkgo may potentiate anticoagulants and antiplatelet drugs and should not be used in conjunction with these agents (Barton & Loprinzi; *Nursing Herbal Medicine Handbook*; Staat & Segatore, 2005).

Nutritional products with antioxidant properties are proposed to decrease free radical formation and increase blood flow, thereby playing a role in decreasing vascular injury and preventing cognitive decline (Barton & Loprinzi, 2002). Fruits and vegetables high in vitamins C and E are thought to mediate the effects of oxidative stress. Thiamine (vitamin B_1) may improve mental attitude and maintain a healthy nervous system (*Nursing Herbal Medicine Handbook,* 2006). However, evidence-based and epidemiologic studies do not support these presumptions, and further study is required.

Body awareness and movement, artwork, spiritual exploration, psychotherapy groups, supportive-expressive groups, yoga, and Tai Chi are interventions that can improve psychological outcomes (Galantino, Henderson, & Michaels, 2005). Rigorous study of these techniques, however, is lacking. Interventions such as aromatherapy and meditation also may prove to be helpful.

Evaluation of Outcomes

Approximately 50% of patients who complain of cognitive impairment during chemotherapy demonstrate improvement 12–18 months after completion of treatment, and patients report improvement in ability to perform work-related activities one to two years following chemotherapy (Wefel, Lenzi, Theriault, Davis, et al., 2004). The expectation is that most cancer survivors return to normal activity and function once treatment is completed unless overt physical limitations exist. Most survivors "look normal"; therefore, subtle changes affecting their function and quality of life may persist without others appreciating the concerns of patients. Reinforcing, strengthening, or reestablishing previously effective mechanisms or patterns of cognitive activity that compensate for impaired processes is helpful. Quantifying changes over time to determine the benefit of various strategies used is an important aspect of rehabilitation (Galantino et al., 2005).

Implications for Oncology Advanced Practice Nurses

Oncology nurses play an important role in the assessment, diagnosis, and treatment of cancer pain, fatigue, and chemotherapy-related cognitive dysfunction. These symptoms often are seen in the cancer treatment setting and have a huge impact on the quality of life of patients with cancer. Understanding the pathophysiology of these toxicities and the elements of comprehensive assessment will enable APNs to successfully create an individualized, evidence-based management plan for each patient and adjust the plan as needed. Education about these toxicities is an essential part of initial training and ongoing continuing education programs for all cancer care providers.

Oncology APNs should be alert to vulnerable populations at risk for undertreatment of cancer pain and the barriers that exist to optimal pain management. Familiarity with myths surrounding cancer pain and its management will help APNs to disabuse patients, caregivers, and other healthcare professionals of these beliefs. Knowledge regarding the differences among addiction, tolerance, physical dependence, and pseudoaddiction will lead to optimal pain management, even in patients with a history of substance abuse.

Oncology APNs can reassure patients with cancer that fatigue is a common effect of cancer and its treatment and that fatigue does not necessarily indicate progressive disease (Lawrence et al., 2004). Management of fatigue is an integral part of the care of patients with cancer (NCCN, 2007b). Comorbidities or contributing factors are assessed and treated as part of the fatigue management plan.

Long-term cognitive impairment, even when relatively subtle, can have a profound influence on the daily lives of individuals with cancer (van Dam et al., 1998). Concerns regarding subjective symptoms of cognitive dysfunction must not be minimized or ignored. When educating patients, clinicians ideally should support verbal information with written material for reference to compensate for memory and processing problems (Nail, 2006). Patients receive information on coping methods and how to compensate for changes in cognition and are reassured that symptoms may decline over time. When considering chemotherapy-related cognitive dysfunction, implications exist for informed consent and identification of treatment-related toxicities (Brezden et al., 2000; Jansen et al., 2005). In order to make informed decisions regarding risks and benefits of proposed treatments, patients require accurate information regarding cognitive dysfunction as a potential side effect (Morse et al., 2003).

Oncology APNs can play an important role in the improvement of system barriers to adequate cancer care at a national or a regional level. There is a continued need to raise awareness and priority of cancer treatments (Patrick et al., 2003). Increased funding for research and education of healthcare providers and the public about the issues related to cancer are needed. Oncology APNs not only identify and address system barriers but also play a role in research. Understanding how to effectively assess and manage these toxicities will require ongoing research to support effective, evidence-based intervention strategies. A particular need exists for continued research in cancer pain management (Patrick et al.). Oncology APNs may conduct or participate in research on these toxicities, targeted treatment strategies, pharmacologic and nonpharmacologic treatments, and management of side effects or toxicities of treatments. Recruitment of patients, especially older adults, women, and minorities, to clinical trials is critical. According to NCCN guidelines (2007b), toxicities, such as cancer-related fatigue, are a vital part of studies of clinical health outcomes in patients with cancer.

Oncology APNs have a multifaceted role in the management of patients with cancer- or cancer treatment–related toxicities. They serve patients through assessment, diagnosis, treatment, and follow-up care. Patient and staff education is vital to bringing about improvements in patient compliance and adherence to the management plan and oncology team growth and development. Nursing research in the areas of cancer pain management, cancer fatigue, and cognitive dysfunction will improve patient outcomes and quality of life. Patient advocacy through legislative activities will broaden public understanding and awareness of cancer and increase funding for oncology research.

Conclusion

Patients who are experiencing pain, fatigue, or cognitive dysfunction are frequently seen in oncology practices. These toxicities may be related to the cancer or its treatment. Astute and timely assessment enables oncology APNs to accurately diagnose these toxicities. Advanced nursing knowledge allows oncology APNs to expertly manage pain, fatigue, and cognitive dysfunction, thus enhancing the quality of life and outcomes of patients with cancer.

Case Study

M.H. is a 43-year-old male diagnosed with non-Hodgkin lymphoma. He has received aggressive chemotherapy followed by stem cell transplant. Now he returns to the ambulatory treatment unit for weekly follow-up appointments and blood work. He volunteers to the APN that he had to stop twice on the way in from the parking lot to rest, and earlier today he had to stop and rest while just walking to the refrigerator to get milk. He states that he feels exhausted but is unable to sleep soundly. He has difficulty concentrating and almost got lost coming to the clinic, although he has been coming by the same route every week. He admits that his relationship with his wife is suffering because of his fatigue, as he does not have the energy to do things socially with her, and he feels emotionally numb.

1. What interventions would the oncology APN recommend for M.H.?
   • Although exercise is the only intervention proved to be effective, M.H. is too exhausted to begin with an activity intervention initially. The APN suggests that he keep a journal of activities with exacerbating and alleviating factors of his exhaustion. Methods to conserve energy were recommended, and concrete ways he could pace essential activities throughout the day, alternating with periods of rest, were planned. Sleep hygiene recommendations also were discussed.

- Later in M.H.'s disease trajectory, he experiences recurrence of his disease. He relates to the oncology APN that his back and lower abdominal pain are no longer controlled by his current analgesic regimen of extended-release morphine sulfate 15 mg twice a day and short-acting morphine sulfate 15 mg every four hours. He rates his pain as 5 on a scale of 1–10. He feels that this pain is affecting his ability to go to his son's ballgames and also is waking him from sleep at night.

2. How should the APN adjust M.H.'s pain medication to improve his pain relief?
   - The total previous 24-hour dose of morphine should first be calculated. He has been taking 30 mg of extended-release morphine plus 90 mg of short-acting morphine for a total of 120 mg of morphine in 24 hours. The APN decides to increase the scheduling dose by 50% of his previous 24-hour dose per the NCCN guidelines (2007a). She multiplies 150% by the total 24-hour dose of 120 mg and notes that this is 180 mg. Extended-release morphine is dosed in 30 mg and 60 mg release capsules. The APN writes a new prescription for extended-release morphine sulfate 60 mg tid. She calculates a new breakthrough dose by multiplying the total new 24-hour dose by 10% (180 mg × 10% = 18 mg) and knows 10%–20% of the total 24-hour dose may be given every hour as needed for breakthrough pain (18–36 mg). She writes a prescription for breakthrough pain as morphine sulfate 30 mg two to four tablets every four hours as needed for breakthrough pain. She advises him to expect an increase in constipation whenever pain medication is increased and instructs him in a bowel regimen to prevent this.
   - M.H.'s pain is now under control. He is receiving chemotherapy and biotherapy, and his last diagnostic scans show improvement. He reports experiencing memory changes over the past couple of months, which he has noticed since his initial diagnosis but now seem worse with the resumption of chemotherapy. He relates having difficulty in following television shows and has given up reading, one of his favorite pastimes, because of difficulty concentrating. He also has forgotten to take his oral medications several times and missed one healthcare appointment. He asks the APN if he might have "chemo brain" and what can be done about it. After ruling out other etiologies of cognitive dysfunction, such as metastatic disease, depression, and uncontrolled symptoms such as pain or sleep disorders, the oncology APN diagnoses cognitive dysfunction secondary to chemotherapy.

3. What interventions might the oncology APN suggest?
   - No medications are FDA approved for cognitive dysfunction. The APN realizes that depression can cause or contribute to cognitive dysfunction, but the patient is currently on an antidepressant (an SSRI), and his depression is well controlled. She discusses recent literature about central nervous system stimulants, such as dexmethylphenidate, that currently are undergoing study in patients with cancer with cognitive dysfunction; however, M.H. is not interested in taking another medication. Therefore, the APN recommends some behavioral interventions, such as list-making and using an alarm for medication and appointment reminders. She encourages him to try some relaxation techniques, such as meditation and progressive muscle relaxation, at least once a day. The APN also assures him that the passage of time often relieves cognitive dysfunction.

Key Points

Pain

- Many barriers exist to optimal pain management that must be assessed.
- The pathophysiology of pain drives treatment management.
- Common oncologic pain syndromes exist that have specific treatments.
- A comprehensive pain assessment includes past and present physical, emotional, mental, and educational history.
- Certain populations are at risk for inadequate pain management, including young, older adult, cognitively impaired, and minority patients.

Fatigue

- Cancer-related fatigue, one of the most common symptoms experienced by patients with cancer, is a distressing, persistent, subjective sense of tiredness or exhaustion related to cancer or cancer treatment that is not proportional to recent activity and interferes with usual functioning.
- Although cancer-related fatigue is widely prevalent, exact mechanisms of its pathophysiology are largely unknown.
- Seven treatable factors are known to contribute to fatigue: pain, emotional distress, sleep disturbance, anemia, alteration in nutrition, deconditioning, and comorbidities.
- As the mechanisms causing fatigue are poorly understood, few effective treatments are available. Exercise is the only intervention proved by evidence-based research to effectively reduce fatigue.

Cognitive Dysfunction

- A subset of individuals treated for cancer will have difficulty with memory, concentration, executive function, and/or motor function.
- The subjective complaint of cognitive dysfunction associated with chemotherapy does not necessarily correlate with objective performance on neuropsychological testing.
- Chemotherapy-related cognitive dysfunction is multifactorial and possibly related to direct effects of drugs or cytokines on the brain, genetic predisposition, and factors such as anxiety, depression, and fatigue.
- No current pharmacologic therapy is approved for the treatment of mild cognitive dysfunction associated with chemotherapy, although behavioral interventions and cognitive therapy show some benefit in improving cognitive function.

Recommended Resources for Oncology Advanced Practice Nurses

Pain

- City of Hope Pain and Palliative Care Resource Center Web site (www.cityofhope.org /prc): Extensive and comprehensive information on pain and pain management, in-

cluding clinical guidelines, information, assessment tools, resources, continuing education, patient education (including slide presentations, handouts, and outlines), staff education, and research tools
- Equianalgesic Pocket Reference Card (downloadable or orderable at http://sccpi .coh.org): Laminated pocket card including equianalgesic table and pain management principles; produced by the Southern California Cancer Pain Initiative
- National Institutes of Health National Institute on Drug Abuse (www.drugabuse .gov/medstaff.html): Web site with professional information on drug abuse and addiction
- StopPain.org (www.stoppain.org): Web site produced by Beth Israel Medical Center's Department of Pain Medicine and Palliative Care that provides continuing online education on pain management

Fatigue

- NCI Physician Data Query (www.cancer.gov/cancertopics/pdq/supportivecare/fatigue /healthprofessional): Information on fatigue for health professionals
- ONS's CancerSymptoms.org (www.cancersymptoms.org/fatigue/key.shtml): Information for patients about the symptoms, assessment, and treatment of cancer-related fatigue
- ONS (www.ons.org/research/outcomes/pdf/Fatigue7.pdf): List of tools and references for evaluation of cancer-related fatigue

Cognitive Dysfunction

- Lance Armstrong Foundation (www.livestrong.org): Resource for patients about cognitive changes (under the "Cancer Support" section of the page)
- ONS's CancerSymptoms.org (www.cancersymptoms.org/cognitivedysfunction/index .shtml): Resource for patients about the risk factors, causes, symptoms, and interventions for cognitive dysfunction

References

Ahles, T.A., Saykin, A.J., Furstenberg, C.T., Cole, B., Mott, L.A., Skalla, K., et al. (2002). Neuropsychologic impact of standard-dose systemic chemotherapy in long-term survivors of breast cancer and lymphoma. *Journal of Clinical Oncology, 20*, 485–493.

Ahles, T.A., Saykin, A.J., Noll, W.W., Furstenberg, C.T., Guerin, S., Cole, B., et al. (2003). The relationship of APOE genotype to neuropsychological performance in long-term cancer survivors treated with standard dose chemotherapy. *Psycho-Oncology, 12*, 612–619.

Alliance of State Pain Initiatives. (1998). *Bill of rights for people with cancer.* Madison, WI: Author.

American Academy of Pain Medicine. (1998). *Acute pain and cancer pain.* Glenview, IL: Author.

American Cancer Society. (2007). *Cancer facts and figures, 2007.* Atlanta, GA: Author.

American Pain Society. (2003). *Principles of analgesic use in the treatment of acute pain and cancer pain* (5th ed.). Glenview, IL: Author.

American Society for Pain Management Nursing. (2002). *Pain management in patients with addictive disease* [Position statement]. Lenexa, KS: Author.

American Society for Pain Management Nursing. (2003a). *Pain management at the end of life* [Position statement]. Lenexa, KS: Author.

American Society for Pain Management Nursing. (2003b). *Promoting pain relief and preventing abuse of pain medications: A critical balancing act* [Position statement]. Lenexa, KS: Author.

American Society for Pain Management Nursing. (2006). *ASPMN position statement: Authorized and unauthorized ("PCA by proxy") dosing of analgesic infusion pumps.* Lenexa, KS: Author.

American Society of Anesthesiologists. (1996). *Practice guidelines for cancer pain management.* Park Ridge, IL: Author.

Anderson, K., Cohen, M., Mendoza, T., Guo, H., Harle, M., & Cleeland, C. (2006). Brief cognitive-behavioral audiotape interventions for cancer-related pain. *Cancer, 107,* 207–214.

Anderson-Hanley, C., Sherman, M.L., Riggs, R., Agocha, V.B., & Compas, B.E. (2003). Neuropsychological effects of treatments for adults with cancer: A meta-analysis and review of the literature. *Journal of the International Neuropsychological Society, 9,* 967–982.

Aubin, M., Vezina, L., Parent, R., Fillion, L., Allard, P., Bergeron, R., et al. (2006). Impact of an educational program on pain management in patients with cancer living at home. *Oncology Nursing Forum, 33,* 1183–1188.

Barton, D., & Loprinzi, C. (2002). Novel approaches to preventing chemotherapy-induced cognitive dysfunction in breast cancer: The art of the possible. *Clinical Breast Cancer, 3*(Suppl. 3), S121–S127.

Berenson, S. (2007). Management of cancer pain with complementary therapies. *Oncology (Williston Park), 21*(Suppl. 4), 10–22.

Bower, J.E., Ganz, P.A., & Aziz, N. (2005). Altered cortisol response to psychologic stress in breast cancer survivors with persistent fatigue. *Psychosomatic Medicine, 67,* 277–280.

Brezden, C.B., Phillips, K.A., Abdolell, M., Bunston, T., & Tannock, I.F. (2000). Cognitive function in breast cancer patients receiving adjuvant chemotherapy. *Journal of Clinical Oncology, 18,* 2695–2701.

Bruera, E., Schoeller, T., Wenk, R., MacEachern, T., Marcelino, S., Hanson, J., et al. (1995). A prospective multicenter assessment of the Edmonton staging system for cancer pain. *Journal of Pain and Symptom Management, 10,* 348–355.

Burton, A., Fanciullo, G., Beasley, R., & Fisch, M. (2007). Chronic pain in the cancer survivor: A new frontier. *Pain Medicine, 8,* 189–198.

Cahill, B. (2005). Management of cancer pain. In C.H. Yarbro, M.H. Frogge, & M. Goodman (Eds.), *Cancer nursing: Principles and practice* (6th ed., pp. 662–697). Sudbury, MA: Jones and Bartlett.

Caraceni, A., Martini, C., Zecca, E., Portenoy, R., Ashby, M., Hawson, G., et al. (2004). Breakthrough pain characteristics and syndromes in patients with cancer pain: An international survey. *Palliative Medicine, 18,* 177–183.

Carr, D., Goudas, L., Lawrence, D., Pirl, W., Lau, J., DeVine, D., et al. (2002, July). *Management of cancer symptoms: Pain, depression, and fatigue* [Evidence report/technology assessment No. 61, AHRQ Publication No. 02-E032]. Rockville, MD: Agency for Healthcare Research and Quality.

Castellon, S.A., Ganz, P.A., Bower, J.E., Petersen, L., Abraham, L., & Greendale, G.A. (2004). Neurocognitive performance in breast cancer survivors exposed to adjuvant chemotherapy and tamoxifen. *Journal of Clinical and Experimental Neuropsychology, 24,* 955–969.

Castellon, S.A., Silverman, D.H.S., & Ganz, P.A. (2005). Breast cancer treatment and cognitive functioning: Current status and future challenges in assessment. *Breast Cancer Research and Treatment, 92,* 199–206.

Chang, V., Janjan, N., Jain, S., & Chau, C. (2006). Update in cancer pain syndromes. *Journal of Palliative Medicine, 9,* 1414–1434.

Cimprich, B., & Ronis, D.L. (2003). An environmental intervention to restore attention in women with newly diagnosed breast cancer. *Cancer Nursing, 26,* 284–292.

Cleeland, C., Gonin, R., Hatfield, A., Edmonson, J., Blum, R., Stewart, J., et al. (1994). Pain and its treatment in outpatients with metastatic cancer. *New England Journal of Medicine, 330,* 592–596.

Cleeland, C., & Ryan, K. (1994). Pain assessment: Global use of the brief pain inventory. *Annals of the Academy of Medicine, Singapore, 23,* 129–138.

Cohen, M.Z., Easley, M.K., Ellis, C., Hughes, B., Ownby, K., Rashad, B.G., et al. (2003). Cancer pain management and the JCAHO's pain standards: An institutional challenge. *Journal of Pain and Symptom Management, 25,* 519–527.

Collado-Hidalgo, A., Bower, J.E., Ganz, P.A., Cole, S.W., & Irwin, M.R. (2006). Inflammatory biomarkers for persistent fatigue in breast cancer survivors. *Clinical Cancer Research, 12,* 2759–2766.

Colleau, S., & Joranson, D. (1998). Tolerance, physical dependence and addiction: Definitions, clinical relevance and misconceptions. *Cancer Pain Release, 11*(3). Retrieved July 1, 2007, from http://www.whocancerpain.wisc.edu/contents/11_3/index.html

Coyle, N., & Layman-Goldstein, M. (2007). Pharmacologic management of adult cancer pain. *Oncology (Williston Park), 21*(2, Suppl. Nurse Ed.), 10–26.

Coyne, P., Watson, A., McGuire, D., & Yeager, K. (2005). Assessment of cancer pain. In C.H. Yarbro, M.H. Frogge, & M. Goodman (Eds.), *Cancer nursing: Principles and practice* (6th ed., pp. 639–661). Sudbury, MA: Jones and Bartlett.

Cull, A., Hay, C., Love, S.B., Mackie, M., Smets, E., & Stewart, M. (1996). What do cancer patients mean when they complain of concentration and memory problems? *British Journal of Cancer, 74,* 1674–1679.

Cunningham, R.S. (2003). Anemia in the oncology patient: Cognitive function and cancer. *Cancer Nursing, 26*(Suppl. 6), 38S–42S.

Feldt, K. (2000). The checklist of nonverbal pain indicators (CNPI). *Pain Management Nursing, 1,* 13–21.

Ferguson, R.J., Ahles, T.A., Saykin, A.J., McDonald, B.C., Furstenberg, C.T., Cole, B.F., et al. (2007). Cognitive-behavioral management of chemotherapy-related cognitive change. *Psycho-Oncology, 16,* 772–777.

Fishman, B., Pasternak, S., Wallenstein, S., Houde, R., Holland, J., & Foley, K. (1987). The Memorial Pain Assessment card: A valid instrument for the evaluation of cancer pain. *Cancer, 60,* 1151–1158.

Foley, K. (2005). Supportive care and quality of life. In V.T. DeVita, Jr., S. Hellman, & S.A. Rosenberg (Eds.), *Cancer: Principles and practice of oncology* (7th ed., pp. 2615–2649). Philadelphia: Lippincott Williams & Wilkins.

Fortner, B.V., Okon, T.A., & Portenoy, R.K. (2002). A survey of pain-related hospitalizations, emergency department visits, and physician office visits reported by cancer patients with and without history of breakthrough pain. *Journal of Pain, 3,* 38–44.

Fu, M.R., McDaniel, R.W., & Rhodes, V.A. (2005). Fatigue. In C.H. Yarbro, M.H. Frogge, & M. Goodman (Eds.), *Cancer nursing: Principles and practice* (6th ed., pp. 741–760). Sudbury, MA: Jones and Bartlett.

Fulfaro, F., Casuccio, A., Ticozzi, C., & Ripamonti, C. (1998). The role of bisphosphonates in the treatment of painful metastatic bone disease: A review of phase III trials. *Pain, 78,* 157–169.

Gaertner, J., Radbruch, L., Giesecke, T., Gerbershagen, H., Petzke, F., Ostgathe, C., et al. (2006). Assessing cognition and psychomotor function under long-term treatment with controlled release oxycodone in non-cancer pain patients. *Acta Anaesthesiologica Scandinavica, 50,* 664–672.

Galantino, M.L., Henderson, A., & Michaels, J. (2005). Cognitive challenges for women undergoing adjuvant chemotherapy for treatment for breast cancer: The role of rehabilitation oncology. *Rehabilitation Oncology, 23*(1), 7–10.

Gordon, D., Dahl, J., Miaskowski, C., McCarberg, B., Todd, K., Paice, J., et al. (2005). American Pain Society recommendations for improving the quality of acute and cancer pain management. *Archives of Internal Medicine, 165,* 1574–1580.

Goudas, L., Carr, D.B., Bloch, R., Balk, E., Ioannidis, J., Terrin, N., et al. (2001, October). *Management of cancer pain* [Evidence report/technology assessment No. 35, AHRQ publication No. 02-E002]. Rockville, MD: Agency for Healthcare Research and Quality.

Grant, M., Cordts, G., & Doberman, D. (2007). Acute pain management in hospitalized patients with current opioid abuse. *Topics in Advanced Practice Nursing eJournal, 7*(1). Retrieved July 1, 2007, from http://www.medscape.com/viewarticle/557043

Grossman, S., Dunbar, E., & Nesbit, S. (2006). Cancer pain management in the 21st century. *Oncology, 20,* 1333–1340.

Grunfeld, E., Dhesy-Thind, S., & Levine, M. (2005). Clinical practice guidelines for the care and treatment of breast cancer: Follow-up after treatment for breast cancer (summary of the 2005 update). *Canadian Medical Association Journal, 172,* 1319–1320.

Gullatte, M.M., Kaplow, R., & Heidrich, D.E. (2005). Oncology: Fatigue/asthenia. In K.K. Kuebler, M.P. Davis, & C.D. Moore (Eds.), *Palliative practices: An interdisciplinary approach* (pp. 227–229). St. Louis, MO: Elsevier Mosby.

Gutgsell, T., Walsh, D., Zhukovsky, D.S., Gonzales, F., & Lagman, R. (2003). A prospective study of the pathophysiology and clinical characteristics of pain in a palliative medicine population. *American Journal of Hospice and Palliative Care, 20,* 140–148.

Hagen, N., Fisher, K., Victorino, C., & Farrar, J. (2007). A titration strategy is needed to manage breakthrough pain effectively: Observations from data pooled from three clinical trials. *Journal of Palliative Medicine, 10,* 47–55.

Heflin, L.H., Meyerowitz, B.E., Hall, P., Lichtenstein, P., Johansson, B., Pedersen, N.L., et al. (2005). Cancer as a risk factor for long-term cognitive deficits and dementia. *Journal of the National Cancer Institute, 97,* 854–856.

Herr, K., Coyne, P., Key, T., Manworren, R., McCaffery, M., Merkel, S., et al. (2006). Pain assessment in the nonverbal patient: Position statement with clinical practice recommendations. *Pain Management Nursing, 7,* 44–52.

Hickey, J.V., & Brown, R.P. (2002). Management of chronic pain: A neuroscience perspective. In J.V. Hickey (Ed.), *The clinical practice of neurological and neurosurgical nursing* (5th ed., pp. 591–602). Philadelphia: Lippincott Williams & Wilkins.

Hickok, J.T., Morrow, G.R., McDonald, S., & Bellg, A.J. (1996). Frequency and correlates of fatigue in lung cancer patients receiving radiation therapy: Implications for management. *Journal of Pain and Symptom Management, 11,* 370–377.

Hwang, S., Chang, V., & Kasimis, B. (2003). Cancer breakthrough pain characteristics and responses to treatment at a VA medical center. *Pain, 101,* 55–64.

Im, E.-O. (2006). White cancer patients' perception of gender and ethnic differences in pain experience. *Cancer Nursing, 29,* 441–450.

Irvine, D.M., Vincent, L., Graydon, J.E., & Bubela, N. (1998). Fatigue in women with breast cancer receiving radiation therapy. *Cancer Nursing, 21,* 127–135.

Jansen, C.E., Miaskowski, C., Dodd, M., & Dowling, G. (2005). Chemotherapy-induced cognitive impairment in women with breast cancer: A critique of the literature. *Oncology Nursing Forum, 32,* 329–342.

Jereczek-Fossa, B.A., Marsiglia, H.R., & Orecchia, R. (2002). Radiotherapy-related fatigue. *Critical Reviews in Oncology/Hematology, 41,* 317–325.

Johnston, M.P., & Coward, D.D. (2001, April). Cancer-related fatigue: Nursing assessment and management: Increasing awareness of the effect of cancer-related fatigue. *American Journal of Nursing, 101*(Suppl.), 19–22.

Kalauokalani, D., Franks, P., Oliver, J., Meyers, F., & Kravitz, R. (2007). Can patient coaching reduce racial/ethnic disparities in cancer pain control? Secondary analysis of a randomized controlled trial. *Pain Medicine, 8,* 17–24.

Kayl, A.E., Wefel, J.S., & Meyers, C.A. (2006). Chemotherapy and cognition: Effects, potential mechanisms, and management. *American Journal of Therapeutics, 13,* 362–369.

Knotkova, H., Clark, W., Keohan, M., Kuhl, J., Winer, R., & Wharton, R. (2006). Validation of the multidimensional affect and pain survey. *Journal of Pain, 7,* 161–169.

LaTour, K. (2002). Lost in the fog: Breast cancer and chemobrain. *Cure, 1*(1). Retrieved March 11, 2007, from http://www.curetoday.com/backissues/v1n1/features/chemobrain/

Lawrence, D.P., Kupelnick, B., Miller, K., Devine, D., & Lau, J. (2004). Evidence report on the occurrence, assessment, and treatment of fatigue in cancer patients. *Journal of the National Cancer Institute Monographs, 32,* 40–50.

Leyland-Jones, B., & O'Shaughnessy, J.A. (2003). Erythropoietin as a critical component of breast cancer therapy: Survival, synergistic, and cognitive applications. *Seminars in Oncology, 30*(5, Suppl. 16), 174–184.

Marazzita, D., Mungai, F., Vivarelli, L., Presta, S., & Dell'Osso, B. (2006). Pain and psychiatry: A critical analysis and pharmacological review. *Clinical Practice and Epidemiology in Mental Health, 2,* 31.

McCaffery, M., & Pasero, C. (1999). *Pain: Clinical manual* (2nd ed.). St. Louis, MO: Mosby.

McDougall, G.J. (2001). Memory improvement program for elderly cancer survivors. *Geriatric Nursing, 22,* 185–190.

Melzack, R. (1975). The McGill questionnaire: Major properties and scoring methods. *Pain, 1,* 277–299.

Melzack, R. (1987). The short-form McGill pain questionnaire. *Pain, 30,* 191–197.

Menefee, L., & Monti, D. (2005). Nonpharmacologic and complementary approaches to cancer pain management. *Journal of the American Osteopathic Association, 105,* 515–520.

Merskey, H. (Ed.). (1986). *Classification of chronic pain: Descriptions of chronic pain syndromes and definitions of pain terms. Prepared by the International Association for the Study of Pain, Subcommittee on Taxonomy.* Amsterdam: Elsevier.

Meyers, C.A., Weitzner, M.A., Valentine, A.D., & Levin, V.A. (1998). Methylphenidate therapy improves cognition, mood, and function of brain tumor patients. *Journal of Clinical Oncology, 16,* 2522–2527.

Miaskowski, C. (2005). The next step to pain management. *Pain Management Nursing, 6,* 1–2.

Miaskowski, C., Cleary, J., Burney, R., Coyne, P., Finley, R., Foster, R., et al. (2005). *Guideline for the management of cancer pain in adults and children.* Glenview, IL: American Pain Society.

Miaskowski, C., Dodd, M., West, C., Schumacher, K., Paul, S., Tripathy, D., et al. (2004). Randomized clinical trial of the effectiveness of a self-care intervention to improve cancer pain management. *Journal of Clinical Oncology, 22,* 1713–1720.

Mitchell, S.A., Beck, S.L., Hood, L.E., Moore, K., & Tanner, E.R. (2007). Putting evidence into practice: Evidence-based interventions for fatigue during and following cancer and its treatment. *Clinical Journal of Oncology Nursing, 11,* 99–113.

Morse, R., Rodgers, J., Verrill, M., & Kendell, K. (2003). Neuropsychological functioning following systemic treatment in women treated for breast cancer: A review. *European Journal of Cancer, 39,* 2288–2297.

Myers, T. (Ed.). (2006). Cognitive function. In *Mosby's dictionary of medicine, nursing and health professions* (7th ed., p. 412). St. Louis, MO: Elsevier Mosby.

Mystakidou, K., Tsilika, E., Parpa, E., Katsouda, E., Galanos, A., & Vlahos, L. (2006). Psychological distress of patients with advanced cancer. *Cancer Nursing, 29,* 400–405.

Nail, L.M. (1997). Fatigue. In S.L. Groenwald, M.H. Frogge, M. Goodman, & C.H. Yarbro (Eds.), *Cancer nursing: Principles and practice* (4th ed., pp. 640–654). Sudbury, MA: Jones and Bartlett.

Nail, L.M. (2002). Fatigue in patients with cancer. *Oncology Nursing Forum, 29,* 537–546.

Nail, L.M. (2006). Cognitive changes in cancer survivors. *American Journal of Nursing, 106*(Suppl. 3), 48–54.

National Cancer Institute. (2005). *Dexmethylphenidate reduces some symptoms of chemobrain.* Retrieved April 11, 2007, from http://www.cancer.gov/clinicaltrials/results/chemobrain0605

National Cancer Institute. (n.d.-a). *Dictionary of cancer terms: Cognition.* Retrieved March 14, 2007, from http://www.cancer.gov/dictionary/?searchTxt=cognition&sgroup=Starts+with

National Cancer Institute. (n.d.-b). *Dictionary of cancer terms: Fatigue.* Retrieved April 11, 2007, from http://www.cancer.gov/Templates/db_alpha.aspx?CdrID=321374

National Comprehensive Cancer Network. (2007a). *NCCN clinical practice guidelines in oncology: Adult cancer pain, version 1.2007.* Retrieved June 10, 2007, from http://www.nccn.org/professionals/physician_gls/PDF/pain.pdf

National Comprehensive Cancer Network. (2007b). *NCCN clinical practice guidelines in oncology: Cancer-related fatigue, version 4.2007.* Retrieved June 27, 2007, from http://www.nccn.org/professionals/physician_gls/PDF/fatigue.pdf

National Comprehensive Cancer Network. (2007c). *NCCN clinical practice guidelines in oncology: Distress management, version 1.2008.* Retrieved March 11, 2007, from http://www.nccn.org/professionals/physician_gls/PDF/distress.pdf

National Comprehensive Cancer Network. (2008). *NCCN clinical practice guidelines in oncology: Cancer- and treatment-related anemia, version 1.2008.* Retrieved May 28, 2007, from http://www.nccn.org/professionals/physician_gls/PDF/anemia.pdf

Nursing herbal medicine handbook (3rd ed.). (2006). Philadelphia: Lippincott Williams & Wilkins.

Olin, J.J. (2001). Cognitive function after systemic therapy for breast cancer. *Oncology, 15,* 613–618.

Olson, K. (2007). A new way of thinking about fatigue: A reconceptualization. *Oncology Nursing Forum, 34,* 93–99.

Omuro, A., Ben-Porat, L., Panageas, K., Kim, A., Correa, D., Yahalom, J., et al. (2005). Delayed neurotoxicity in primary central nervous system lymphoma. *Archives of Neurology, 62,* 1595–1600.

Oncology Nursing Society. (2006). *Cancer pain management* [Position statement]. Pittsburgh, PA: Author.

O'Shaughnessy, J. (2003). Chemotherapy-related cognitive dysfunction in breast cancer. *Seminars in Oncology Nursing, 19*(4, Suppl. 2), 17–24.

Patrick, D.L., Ferketich, S.L., Frame, P.S., Harris, J.J., Hendricks, C.B., Levin, B., et al. (2003). National Institutes of Health state-of-the-science conference statement: Symptom management in cancer: Pain, depression, and fatigue, July 15–17, 2002. *Journal of the National Cancer Institute, 95,* 1110–1117.

Penson, R., Nunn, C., Younger, J., Schaeffer, N., Chabner, B., Fricchoine, G., et al. (2003). Trust violated: Analgesics for addicts. *Oncologist, 8,* 199–209.

Phillips, D. (2000). JCAHO pain management standards are unveiled. *JAMA, 284,* 428–429.

Piper, B.F., Dibble, S.L., Dodd, M.J., Weiss, M.C., Slaughter, R.E., & Paul, S.M. (1998). The revised Piper fatigue scale: Psychometric evaluation in women with breast cancer. *Oncology Nursing Forum, 25,* 677–684.

Portenoy, R., & Hagen, N. (1990). Breakthrough pain: Definition, prevalence, and characteristics. *Pain, 41,* 273–281.

Portenoy, R., Payne, D., & Jacobsen, P. (1999). Breakthrough pain: Characteristics and impact in patients with cancer pain. *Pain, 81,* 129–134.

Portenoy, R.K., & Itri, L.M. (1999). Cancer-related fatigue: Guidelines for evaluation and management. *Oncologist, 4,* 1–10.

Reissig, J., & Rybarczyk, A. (2005). Pharmacologic treatment of opioid sedation in chronic pain. *Annals of Pharmacotherapy, 39,* 727–731.

Saad, R., Gleason, D., Murray, R., Tchekmedyian, S., Venner, P., Lacombe, L., et al. (2002). A randomized, placebo-controlled trial of zoledronic acid in patients with hormone-refractory metastatic prostate carcinomas. *Journal of the National Cancer Institute, 94,* 1458–1468.

Saykin, A.J., Ahles, T.A., & McDonald, B.C. (2003). Mechanisms of chemotherapy-induced cognitive disorders: Neuropsychological, pathophysiological, and neuroimaging perspectives. *Seminars in Clinical Neuropsychiatry, 8,* 201–216.

Schagen, S.B., Muller, M.J., Boogerd, W., Mellenbergh, G.J., & van Dam, F.S. (2006). Change in cognitive function after chemotherapy: A prospective longitudinal study in breast cancer patients. *Journal of the National Cancer Institute, 98,* 1742–1745.

Schagen, S.B., van Dam, F.S., Muller, M.J., Boogerd, W., Lindeboom, J., & Bruning, P.F. (1999). Cognitive deficits after postoperative adjuvant chemotherapy for breast carcinoma. *Cancer, 85,* 640–650.

Schultz, P.N., Klein, M.J., Beck, M.L., Stava, C., & Sellin, R.V. (2005). Breast cancer: Relationship between menopausal symptoms, physiologic health effects of cancer treatment and physical constraints on quality of life in long-term survivors. *Journal of Clinical Nursing, 14,* 204–211.

Sherwood, P., Given, B.A., Given, C.W., Champion, V.L., Doorenbos, A.Z., Azzouz, F., et al. (2005). A cognitive behavioral intervention for symptom management in patients with advanced cancer. *Oncology Nursing Forum, 32,* 1190–1198.

Shilling, V., Jenkins, V., & Trapala, I.S. (2006). The (mis)classification of chemo-fog—methodological inconsistencies in the investigation of cognitive impairment after chemotherapy. *Breast Cancer Research and Treatment, 95,* 125–129.

Slatkin, N., & Rhiner, M. (2003). Treatment of opiate-related sedation: Utility of the cholinesterase inhibitors. *Journal of Supportive Oncology, 1,* 53–63.

Smith, W. (2004). Research methodology: Implications for CAM pain research. *Clinical Journal of Pain, 20,* 3–7.

Staat, K., & Segatore, M. (2005). The phenomenon of chemo brain. *Clinical Journal of Oncology Nursing, 9,* 713–721.

Steensma, D.P., & Loprinzi, C.L. (2005). Erythropoietin use in cancer patients: A matter of life and death? *Journal of Clinical Oncology, 23,* 5865–5868.

Stevenson, K., Dahl, J., Berry, P., Beck, S., & Griffie, J. (2006). Institutionalizing effective pain management practices: Practice change programs to improve the quality of pain management in small health care organizations. *Journal of Pain and Symptom Management, 31,* 248–261.

Svendsen, K.B., Andersen, S., Arnason, S., Arner, S., Breivik, H., Heiskanen, T., et al. (2005). Breakthrough pain in malignant and nonmalignant diseases: A review of prevalence, characteristics, and mechanisms. *European Journal of Pain, 9,* 195–206.

Syrjala, K., Dikmen, S., Langer, S., Roth-Roemer, S., & Abrams, J. (2004). Neuropsychologic changes from before transplantation to 1 year in patients receiving myeloablative allogeneic hematopoietic cell transplant. *Blood, 104,* 3386–3392.

Tannock, I.F., Ahles, T.A., Ganz, P.A., & van Dam, F.S. (2004). Cognitive impairment associated with chemotherapy for cancer: Report of a workshop. *Journal of Clinical Oncology, 22,* 2233–2239.

Tchen, N., Juffs, H.G., Downie, F.P., Yi, Q.-L., Hu, H., Chemerynsky, I., et al. (2003). Cognitive function, fatigue, and menopausal symptoms in women receiving adjuvant chemotherapy for breast cancer. *Journal of Clinical Oncology, 21,* 4175–4183.

Tittle, M., McMillian, S., & Hagan, S. (2003). Validating the brief pain inventory for use with surgical patients with cancer. *Oncology Nursing Forum, 30,* 325–330.

University of Texas M.D. Anderson Cancer Center. (1997). *Brief fatigue inventory.* Retrieved April 11, 2007, from http://www.mdanderson.org/pdf/bfi.pdf

Vallerand, A., Collins-Bohler, D., Templin, T., & Hasenau, S. (2007). Knowledge of and barriers to pain management in caregivers of cancer patients receiving homecare. *Cancer Nursing, 30,* 31–37.

Vallerand, A., Hasenau, S., Templin, T., & Collins-Bohler, D. (2005). Disparities between black and white patients with cancer pain: The effect of perception of control over pain. *Pain Medicine, 6,* 242–250.

Vallerand, A., Saunders, M., & Anthony, M. (2007). Perceptions of control over pain by patients with cancer and their caregivers. *Pain Management Nursing, 8,* 55–63.

van Dam, F.S., Schagen, S.B., Muller, M.J., Boogerd, W., Wall, E.V.D., Fortuyn, M.E., et al. (1998). Impairment of cognitive function in women receiving adjuvant treatment for high-risk breast cancer: High-dose versus standard-dose chemotherapy. *Journal of the National Cancer Institute, 90,* 210–218.

Vogel, W.H., Wilson, M.A., & Melvin, M.S. (2004). *Advanced practice oncology and palliative care guidelines.* Philadelphia: Lippincott Williams & Wilkins.

Weaver, M., & Schnoll, S. (2002). Opioid treatment of chronic pain in patients with addiction. *Journal of Pain and Palliative Care Pharmacotherapy, 16,* 5–26.

Wefel, J.S., Lenzi, R., Theriault, R., Buzdar, A.U., Cruickshank, S., & Meyers, C.A. (2004). "Chemobrain" in breast carcinoma? A prologue. *Cancer, 101,* 466–475.

Wefel, J.S., Lenzi, R., Theriault, R.L., Davis, R.N., & Meyers, C.A. (2004). The cognitive sequelae of standard-dose adjuvant chemotherapy in women with breast carcinoma: Results of a prospective, randomized, longitudinal trial. *Cancer, 100,* 2292–2299.

Westberg, J., & Gobel, B.H. (2004). Methylphenidate use for the management of opioid-induced sedation. *Clinical Journal of Oncology Nursing, 8,* 203–205.

Wong, D., Hockenberry-Eaton, M., Wilson, D., Winkelstein, M., & Schwartz, P. (2001). *Wong's essentials of pediatric nursing* (6th ed.). St. Louis, MO: Mosby.

Wool, M., & Mor, V. (2005). A multidimensional model for understanding cancer pain. *Cancer Investigation, 23,* 727–734.

World Health Organization. (1996). *Cancer pain relief with a guide to opioid availability* (2nd ed.). Albany, NY: Author.

Yellen, S.B., Cella, D.F., Webster, K.A., Blendowski, C., & Kaplan, E. (1997). Measuring fatigue and other anemia-related symptoms with the Functional Assessment of Cancer Therapy (FACT) measurement system. *Journal of Pain and Symptom Management, 13,* 63–74.

CHAPTER 11

Myelosuppression

Brenda K. Shelton, MS, RN, CCRN, AOCN®

Introduction

Bone marrow suppression is defined as a reduction in production and maturation of all blood cell lines resulting in leukopenia, thrombocytopenia, and anemia in peripheral blood (Camp-Sorrell, 2005). It is one of the most common and potentially life-threatening clinical complications experienced by patients with cancer (Shane & Shelton, 2004). It often has been coined "the silent complication" because of the absence of clinical findings with initial cell depletion until the lack of hematopoietic cells results in clinical disorders, such as infection and bleeding. *Myelosuppression* is a term used interchangeably with *aplasia* (without cells), although it may loosely correlate to suppression of only the myelocytic cell line when used in direct care practice. The depth of aplasia (also termed *nadir*) is associated with its severity score (usually grades 0–4) and the length of time the blood counts remain suppressed.

Certified oncology advanced practice nurses (APNs) possess expert knowledge of the risk factors, timing, clinical features, assessment scales, prevention strategies, and multidisciplinary management of myelosuppression. Within this text, general concepts of bone marrow suppression are addressed first, followed by specific findings and management associated with suppression of each cell line, and then general principles of patient management for all disorders as a group.

Etiology of Bone Marrow Suppression

More than 50% of patients with cancer will experience bone marrow suppression during the course of their disease (Daniel & Crawford, 2006; Hayes, 2001; National Comprehensive Cancer Network [NCCN], 2008a, 2008b, 2008c; Shelton, 2003b). Bone marrow suppression often is the result of (a) systemic cancer, (b) cancer treatment, (c) comorbid health conditions, or (d) a combination of these factors. Nutraceuticals and herbal agents (such as winter cherry, kava kava, St. John's wort, evening primrose, and ivy leaf) also may contribute to myelosuppression and even interfere with the therapeutic effects of antineoplastic chemotherapy or radiotherapy (de Lemos, John, Nakashima, O'Brien, & Taylor, 2004).

Specific health factors are documented to enhance the risk for significant bone marrow suppression when concomitant with cancer or its therapy. These risks include advanced age (older than 65 years); poor nutritional status; preexisting autoimmune disease, diabetes mellitus, gastrointestinal disorders, liver disease, and hematopoietic diseases; and substance abuse (Lyman, 2006; Lyman, Lyman, & Agboola, 2005; NCCN, 2008b; Zinner, 1998). The contribution of myelosuppression to increased morbidity and reduced quality of life is well defined in the literature (Lyman; Nirenberg et al., 2006a, 2006b; Safdar & Armstrong, 2001; Shelton, 2003a). Because of this, knowledge and skills regarding management of myelosuppression are essential for certified oncology APNs.

Cancer-Induced Bone Marrow Suppression

Cancer-induced bone marrow suppression occurs from three major mechanisms: (1) dysfunctional hematopoietic cells within the bone marrow, (2) bone marrow infiltration with tumor, and (3) general exhaustion of bone marrow reserves (Daniel & Crawford, 2006). Hematologic malignancies, such as leukemias and multiple myeloma, involve a defect of a specific blood cell type. The cancer manifests as overproduction of immature or poorly functioning cells in a specific cell line, resulting in overcrowding of the marrow compartment with suppression of other cell production. Lymphomas often present as extramedullary disease but can infiltrate the bone marrow, leading to decreased function of the cell lines. Solid tumor malignancies with the highest propensity to infiltrate the bone marrow in the course of metastasis include melanoma and cancers of the breast, lung, kidney, and prostate (Shane & Shelton, 2004). Nonspecific cancer-induced myelosuppression can occur with prolonged chronic illness, malnutrition, chronic infection, liver metastases, or gastrointestinal involvement (NCCN, 2008b).

Chemotherapy-Induced Bone Marrow Suppression

As the most rapidly dividing cells of the body, the bone marrow is most frequently and consistently affected by cancer chemotherapeutic agents. Each antineoplastic agent has predictable specific cell-line–suppressing effects, timing of its effects, and severity of suppression. The degree of bone marrow suppression is a guide for selection of an agent or combination of agents to use in a treatment plan, the dosage to be delivered, and the frequency of administration. A few chemotherapeutic agents (most notably the nitrosoureas) affect the pluripotent stem cells, thereby affecting all cell lines. A summary of common antineoplastic agents and their common myelosuppressive properties is included in Table 11-1. Oncology APNs consider this information when prescribing chemotherapy regimens, performing patient monitoring, ascertaining the need for hematopoietic growth factors, and providing staff nurse consultation for management of myelosuppression.

Cell cycle–nonspecific agents, such as nitrosoureas, have the most potent and longest effect on myelosuppression. Agents such as anthracyclines and alkylating agents are cell cycle active, phase nonspecific, and result in moderate myelosuppression. Phase-specific agents, such as antimetabolites and vinca alkaloids, have the shortest degree of

Table 11-1. Common Myelosuppressive Chemotherapy Agents

Drug Class	Degree of Myelosuppression	Nadir (Days)	Duration of Myelosuppression (Days)
Alkylating agents (e.g., cyclophosphamide, melphalan)	Moderate	10–21	18–40
Anthracyclines (e.g., doxorubicin)	Severe	6–13	21–24
Antifolates (e.g., methotrexate)	Severe	7–14	14–21
Antipyrimidines (e.g., 5-fluoropyrimidine/ 5-fluorouracil)	Severe	7–14	21–24
Antipurines (e.g., fludarabine)	Moderate	7–14	14–21
Antitumor antibiotics (nonanthracycline) (e.g., bleomycin)	Moderate	10–21	17–28
Camptothecins (e.g., topotecan)	Moderate	4–7	6–12
Epipodophyllotoxins (e.g., etoposide)	Moderate	5–15	22–28
Nitrosoureas (e.g., carmustine)	Severe	26–60	35–85
Plant alkaloids (e.g., vincristine)	Mild–moderate	4–9	7–21
Proteasome inhibitors (e.g., bortezomib)	Mild–moderate	Unknown	Unknown
Taxanes (e.g., paclitaxel)	Moderate	8–12	15–21
Tyrosine kinase inhibitors (e.g., imatinib)	Neutropenia only	Unknown	Unknown
Agents with unique myelosuppressive features (timing, depth of aplasia)			
• Alemtuzumab (Campath®, Genzyme Corp.)	Moderate–severe	Unknown	Unknown
• Arsenic trioxide	Mild–moderate	Unknown	Unknown
• Asparaginase	Moderate	10–20	10–20
• Busulfan	Severe	11–30	24–54
• Carboplatin	Severe	16	21–25
• Dacarbazine	Severe	21–28	28–35
• Denileukin diftitox (Ontak®, Ligand Pharmaceuticals)	Severe	4–15	Unknown
• Gemtuzumab (Mylotarg®, Wyeth Pharmaceuticals)	Moderate	8–15	15–20
• Hydroxyurea	Moderate	7	14–21
• Mitomycin	Moderate	28–42	42–56
• Mithramycin	Mild	5–10	10–18
• Nitrogen mustard	Severe	7–14	28
• Procarbazine	Moderate	25–36	35–50
• Tositumomab + iodine (Bexxar®, GlaxoSmithKline)	Moderate	8–15	Length of therapy
• Yttrium-90 ibritumomab tiuxetan	Moderate	8–20	Length of therapy

Note. Based on information from Polovich et al., 2005; Shane & Shelton, 2004; Zitella et al., 2006.

suppression. The only chemotherapeutic agents that are completely nontoxic to bone marrow are steroidal hormones (Polovich, White, & Kelleher, 2005).

The normal proliferation rate of erythrocytes, platelets, or leukocytes determines the severity and timing of suppression following exposure to a toxin. Granulocytes typically live only six to eight hours; platelets survive an average of 5–7 days; and erythrocytes live approximately 120 days. Depletion of the cell line is directly related to the normal turnover rate of the cell line after the antineoplastic agent destroys normal regrowth mechanisms. Leukopenia usually is the earliest indicator of bone marrow suppression, occurring about 7–15 days after treatment, but is the quickest to recover in most circumstances. When affected, platelets have the longest nadir, persisting for more than 20 days in many patients (Polovich et al., 2005). Red cells, with their long life span, only present serious problems in patients receiving highly suppressing erythrocytic agents such as anthracyclines or platinols, unless a bleeding problem also exists (Polovich et al.). The onset of anemia often is delayed, occurring in the second or third cycle of therapy. Response to stimulating therapies may require four to eight weeks (NCCN, 2008a).

Radiation-Induced Bone Marrow Suppression

Radiation therapy less frequently causes bone marrow suppression. However, myelosuppression occurs following radiation therapy when the treatment field involves marrow-producing tissue or with doses greater than 1,500 rads (Esco et al., 2005; Harrison, Shasha, White, & Ramdeen, 2000). Myelosuppression peaks in the third week of radiation therapy and often manifests as aplasia occurring simultaneously in all cell lines rather than sequentially as seen with chemotherapy. The recovery period is less predictable because radiation treatments may be required for several additional weeks after the onset of marrow suppression (Esco et al.). Today, marrow suppression usually is considered to be a dose-limiting toxicity of therapy and warrants a break from radiation until blood counts recover. Use of traditional preventive and supportive measures, such as hematopoietic growth factors, has not been well defined for use in radiation-induced myelosuppression.

Pathophysiology of Hematopoiesis

Hematopoiesis usually is confined to the proximal ends of long or flat bones of the body where the red bone marrow is found. These areas include the sternum, vertebrae, ribs, ileum, and skull. Extramedullary hematopoiesis is characterized by cell production that is reexpanded back into the long bones, spleen, or liver. This occurs with chronic hematopoietic disorders and hematologic malignancies. Adults have one to two liters of bone marrow consisting primarily of reticular tissues and hemopoietic progenitor cells. The reticular tissue and hemocytoblasts form a framework of sinusoids, which feed into the marrow drainage system and venous system of the body. The reticular tissue provides support and nutrition for developing blood cells and secretes several colony-stimulating factors. The hemocytoblast, or colony-forming unit, is the pluripotent stem cell. Pluripotent stem cells express the CD34+ surface protein or antigen that has receptors for stem cell growth factors promoting proliferation (Shelton, Rome, & Lewis, 2007). Once "committed," the hemocytoblast becomes a progenitor cell for a specific hemopoietic cell line. These cell lines are erythroid (red cells), granulocytic (defined phagocytic white blood cells [WBCs]), monocytic, lymphoid (specific immunity white cells), and megakaryocytic (platelets). Commitment, or differentiation and maturation, occurs as a result of the acquisition or loss of specific growth factor receptors and the action of cytokines (Weinreich et al., 2006).

Hematopoietic growth factors are glycoprotein hormones that regulate the proliferation, differentiation, maturation, and activation of progenitor and mature blood cells to optimally meet the body's hematopoietic needs. Each growth factor has a specific receptor, and their presence on the cell surface varies with cell lineage and stage of differentiation. Existing identified hematopoietic growth factors include interleukins 1, 3, 5, and 6, granulocyte macrophage–colony-stimulating factor, granulocyte–colony-stimulating factor, macrophage–colony-stimulating factor, stem cell factor, thrombopoietin, and erythropoietin (Weinreich et al., 2006). Normally, mature blood cells, except for platelets, enter the bloodstream by migrating through the epithelial lining of the sinusoids. Platelets are directly launched into the bloodstream via their maturation site in the sinusoid wall.

Assessment

Patients with bone marrow suppression are likely to present with an array of symptoms related to the specific hematopoietic cell line or lines affected. These cell-specific findings are addressed under the headings of leukopenia, thrombocytopenia, and anemia. Patients with myelosuppression often reveal nonspecific symptoms that are present and noticeable even before low blood counts are noted. General constitutional symptoms reported by patients with myelosuppression include anorexia, fatigue, myalgias, and cognitive dysfunction (Camp-Sorrell, 2005; Cella, 1997; Shane & Shelton, 2004). Because these symptoms are vague and nonspecific, they may not be immediately recognized as indicative of myelosuppression unless the astute clinician recognizes the timing associated with the predicted nadir.

Focused physical examination for evidence of infection and bleeding is performed routinely in patients at risk for myelosuppression. Anemia does not usually produce symptoms unique only to anemia. Fever is the most common symptom of infection. Common inflammatory symptoms, such as swelling and purulent exudate, may not be present with neutropenia. Localized pain, open and unhealing wounds, and organ dysfunction such as hypoxia are more common manifestations of infections in myelosuppressed patients. Skin, mucous membrane, and soft tissue bleeding usually is present with significant thrombocytopenia. Petechiae and ecchymoses of soft tissues, mucosal bleeding, or occult blood in emesis, urine, or stool warrants assessment of the platelet count. Anemia is most likely to present as fatigue or weakness, but cardiovascular compromise may occur.

Suspected myelosuppression is always first confirmed with a laboratory test, the complete blood count (CBC) (Shelton et al., 2007; Uthman, 2007). Components of the CBC include hematocrit, hemoglobin, total red blood cell (RBC) and WBC counts, RBC indices, WBC differential, platelet count, and blood cell morphologies. The specific components are addressed in the specific lineage disorders in the following sections. Table 11-2 defines the toxicity grading scores from the National Cancer Institute (NCI) for these hematologic parameters (NCI Cancer Therapy Evaluation Program [CTEP], 2006). An abnormal CBC may necessitate further diagnostic tests. When all cells are diminished, results are inconclusive for a specific disorder, thus necessitating

Table 11-2. National Cancer Institute Common Terminology Criteria for Adverse Events, Version 3.0

Adverse Event	Short Name	1	2	3	4	5
Bone marrow cellularity	Bone marrow cellularity	Mildly hypocellular or ≤ 25% reduction from normal cellularity for age	Moderately hypocellular or > 25–≤ 50% reduction from normal cellularity for age	Severely hypocellular or > 50–≤ 75% reduction cellularity from normal for age	–	Death
CD4 count	CD4 count	< LLN – 500/mm³ < LLN – 0.5 × 10⁹/L	< 500–200/mm³ < 0.5–0.2 × 10⁹/L	< 200–50/mm³ < 0.2–0.05 × 10⁹/L	< 50/mm³ < 0.05 × 10⁹/L	Death
Haptoglobin	Haptoglobin	< LLN	–	Absent	–	Death
Hemoglobin	Hemoglobin	< LLN – 10.0 g/dl < LLN – 6.2 mmol/L < LLN – 100 g/L	< 10.0–8.0 g/dl < 6.2–4.9 mmol/L < 100–80 g/L	< 8.0–6.5 g/dl < 4.9–4.0 mmol/L < 80–65 g/L	< 6.5 g/dl < 4.0 mmol/L < 65 g/L	Death
Hemolysis (e.g., immune hemolytic anemia, drug-related hemolysis) Also consider haptoglobin, hemoglobin.	Hemolysis	Laboratory evidence of hemolysis only (e.g., direct antiglobulin test [DAT, Coomb's], schistocytes)	Evidence of red cell destruction and ≥ 2 gm decrease in hemoglobin, no transfusion	Transfusion or medial intervention (e.g., steroids) indicated	Catastrophic consequences of hemolysis (e.g., renal failure, hypotension, bronchospasm, emergency splenectomy)	Death
Iron overload	Iron overload	–	Asymptomatic iron overload, intervention not indicated	Iron overload, intervention indicated	Organ impairment (e.g., endocrinopathy, cardiopathy)	Death
Leukocytes (total WBC)	Leukocytes	< LLN – 3000/mm³ < LLN – 3.0 × 10⁹/L	< 3000–2000/mm³ < 3.0–2.0 × 10⁹/L	< 2000–1000/mm³ < 2.0–1.0 × 10⁹/L	< 1000/mm³ < 1.0 × 10⁹/L	Death
Lymphopenia	Lymphopenia	< LLN – 800/mm³ < LLN – 0.8 × 10⁹/L	< 800–500/mm³ < 0.8–0.5 × 10⁹/L	< 500–200/mm³ < 0.5–0.2 × 10⁹/L	< 200/mm³ < 0.2 × 10⁹/L	Death

(Continued on next page)

Table 11-2. National Cancer Institute Common Terminology Criteria for Adverse Events, Version 3.0 (Continued)

Adverse Event	Short Name	1	2	3	4	5
Myelodysplasia	Myelodysplasia	—	—	Abnormal marrow cytogenetics (marrow blasts ≤ 5%)	RAEB or RAEB-T (marrow blasts > 5%)	Death
Neutrophils/granulocytes (ANC/AGC)	Neutrophils	< LLN – 1500/mm^3 < LLN – 1.5 × 10^9/L	< 1500–1000/mm^3 < 1.5–1.0 × 10^9/L	< 1000–500/mm^3 < 1.0–0.5 × 10^9/L	< 500/mm^3 < 0.5 × 10^9/L	Death
Platelets	Platelets	< LLN – 75,000/mm^3 < LLN – 75.0 × 10^9/L	< 75,000–50,000/mm^3 < 75.0–50.0 × 10^9/L	< 50,000–25,000/mm^3 < 50.0–25.0 × 10^9/L	< 25,000/mm^3 < 25.0 × 10^9/L	Death
Splenic function	Splenic function	Incidental findings (e.g., Howell-Jolly bodies)	Prophylactic antibiotics indicated	—	Life-threatening consequences	Death
Blood/bone marrow – Other (Specify, ___)	Blood – Other (Specify)	Mild	Moderate	Severe	Life-threatening; disabling	Death

LLN—lower limit of normal

Note. From *Common Terminology Criteria for Adverse Events, Version 3.0* (p. 4), by National Cancer Institute Cancer Therapy Evaluation Program, 2006. Retrieved May 4, 2007, from http://ctep.cancer.gov/forms/CTCAEv3.pdf

a search for the etiology. If an error in cell production is suspected, a bone marrow aspiration and biopsy will be performed. In many settings, oncology APNs perform this diagnostic test. If abnormal destruction is likely, cell survival (e.g., RBC survival studies performed with nuclear tagged RBCs infused and followed by body scans) and hemolysis studies (e.g., direct bilirubin, schistocytes by smear) are indicated (Shelton et al., 2007; Tas et al., 2002; Uthman, 2007).

Leukopenia

Definition and Etiology

Leukopenia is a reduced number of circulating leukocytes (WBCs). The two major types of WBCs are granulocytes and agranulocytes. Granulocytes include neutrophils, eosinophils, and basophils. Agranulocytes include lymphocytes and monocytes. The functions of these cells vary, and the specific cell deficiency may predict the nature of immune defect and potential infectious complications. For example, neutrophils are the primary phagocytic responder and the only leukocyte that can be released in an immature form (band). As such, the granulocytes (especially the neutrophil) are responsible for the body's response against bacterial invaders. Monocytes spend little time in the circulating serum before they differentiate into tissue macrophages, and hence, serum deficiencies are not well defined in clinical practice. Lymphocytes respond to specific immune threats and are important for recognition of foreign proteins, such as transplanted tissue or atypical antigens such as viruses. APNs identify which cells are deficient or dysfunctional and translate this knowledge to predict and possibly prevent specific infectious complications. Table 11-3 demonstrates specific leukopenias and immune cell defects with expected infectious complications.

Neutropenia is a decrease in the number of circulating neutrophils. Disagreement exists as to what level of deficiency constitutes definitive neutropenia, but it may be easiest viewed as a continuum of severity based upon the depth of the deficiency. The condition becomes definable when the absolute neutrophil count (ANC) is less than 1,500 cells/mm³ (NCI CTEP, 2006). An ANC less than 1,000 cells/mm³ is used to describe a threshold of moderate severity with increased risk for infection (NCI CTEP; Shane & Shelton, 2004). Neutropenia warranting infection prevention precautions or implementation of preventive bone marrow growth factors occurs when the ANC is less than 500/mm³ (NCI CTEP; Nirenberg et al., 2006a; Shelton, 2003b). Neutropenia occurs in diseases involving bone marrow production, as a result of excess destruction by autoimmune mechanisms, with certain marrow toxic treatments or with increased consumption during chronic illness. A diminished number of neutrophils alter the body's defenses against bacterial invaders. Disorders such as diabetes mellitus impair neutrophil function without necessarily reducing circulating numbers, causing similar clinical effects.

Lymphocytopenia is a reduction in the number of lymphocytes in the blood. The suppression of T-lymphocyte function results in reduced ability to recognize foreign tissue, malignant cells, atypical microbes, and viruses. Lymphocytopenia is seen most commonly in AIDS and organ transplant immunosuppression. The CD4 molecular surface antigen is the target for HIV retroviral incorporation that leads to cell destruction of all cells with this marker. This marker is found on T4 lymphocytes and some macrophages. Cell destruction most often is detected by the absolute number of T4 helper lympho-

Table 11-3. Specific White Blood Cell (WBC) Defects and Common Infectious Complications

WBC Defect	Patient Risk Groups	Common Infectious Complications
Granulocytopenia	Chronic infection/inflammation Diabetes mellitus Malnutrition Post chemotherapy Medications (allopurinol, chloramphenicol, flucytosine, trimethoprim-sulfamethoxazole, antiretrovirals, antineoplastic agents)	Bacterial for 3–7 days and throughout period of neutropenia Atypical bacteria after 7–10 days Fungal infections after 10–14 days Risk rises exponentially after 10 days; by day 21, almost all are infected.
Lymphopenia	Blood transfusions HIV disease IV drug use Medications (allopurinol, anesthetic agents, antipsychotic agents [clozapine], beta-lactam antibiotics, carbamazepine, chlorpromazine, corticosteroids, ganciclovir, immunosuppressive agents, propylthiouracil, ticlopidine, trimethoprim-sulfamethoxazole) Viral infection	Atypical and opportunistic infections Reactivation of dormant colonizations (e.g., *Pneumocystis carinii,* herpes simplex) Fungal infection
Immunoglobulin deficiency	Chronic illness Immunosuppressive therapy Severe malnutrition Recent transplant (solid organ or hematopoietic stem cell)	Sinus and pulmonary infection from a variety of sources
Splenectomy	Patient with spleen removed	Infection with encapsulated organisms normally cleared by the spleen (e.g., pneumococcus, streptococcus)

Note. Based on information from Centers for Disease Control and Prevention et al., 2000; Hughes et al., 2002; Lyman, 2006; Machado, 2005; National Comprehensive Cancer Network, 2008b; Nirenberg et al., 2006a, 2006b; Safdar & Armstrong, 2001; Shane & Shelton, 2004; Shelton, 2005.

cytes (also called T4 count or absolute lymphocyte count). AIDS is classified by the CD4 count and the presence of other defining clinical syndromes, such as opportunistic infections, immunologic cancers, and neurologic disease. Other etiologies of lymphocytopenia include therapeutic suppression to reduce rejection of a transplanted organ, chronic use of corticosteroids, recent history of viral infection, or an unexplained phenomenon that occurs with IV drug use or malnutrition. Lymphocyte dysfunction has been associated with genetic abnormalities (e.g., congenital T-lymphocyte suppression, combined immunodeficiency syndrome) and Hodgkin disease (Rome, 2007).

Leukopenia Assessment

Clinical assessment for neutropenia without concomitant infection may prove daunting because of the absence of specific symptoms. For this reason, researchers attempt to identify specific variables that predict the risk for neutropenia-related infection, better known as neutropenic fever. If patients at high or low risk for severe infection with neutropenia can be predicted, then proactive measures to minimize neutropenia and prevent infection can be implemented. Alternatively, patients with low risk for serious infection during neutropenia may have febrile episodes managed by less resource-intensive care. Figure 11-1 outlines variables known to increase the risk of a neutropenic event leading to serious infection and sepsis. Specific disease-related variables for higher risk of infection also have been identified in therapy for breast cancer and lymphoma, where neutropenic infections causing decreased dose density (delays in therapy

---

General—Patient factors
- Age > 65 years
- Poor performance status
- Poor nutritional status
- History of severe neutropenia with similar treatment regimen
- Extensive previous chemotherapy
- Previous radiotherapy to marrow containing bone
- Open wounds
- Active tissue infection
- Advanced or uncontrolled cancer
- Body surface area < 2/m²

General—Diagnostic test findings
- Preexisting neutropenia or lymphocytopenia
- Low albumin level
- Elevated lactate dehydrogenase (LDH) or serum albumin level < 3.5 mg/dl
- Elevated alkaline phosphatase
- Hyperglycemia
- Elevated bilirubin
- Low pretreatment neutrophil or lymphocyte count
- Bone marrow involvement with tumor

Early-stage breast cancer
- Myelosuppression present after first cycle of therapy
- Doxorubicin and taxane combination
- Concurrent radiotherapy
- Preexisting bone marrow involvement

Non-Hodgkin lymphoma
- Albumin < 3.5 mg/dl
- Bone marrow involvement
- Elevated LDH
- Advanced age (> 65 years)
OR
- International Prognostic Index > 2 (count one point for each variable present)
- Advanced age (> 65 years)
- Poor performance status (Karnofsky scale score < 50%)
- LDH elevated > 300
- Extranodal sites of disease (any = 1)
- Stage of disease > 2

Figure 11-1. Factors Influencing Risk of Serious Infection With Neutropenia

---

Note. Based on information from Blay et al., 1998; Blot et al., 2001; Chang, 2000; Hayes, 2001; Intraguntornchai et al., 2000; Lyman et al., 2005; Madsen et al., 2002; National Comprehensive Cancer Network, 2008b; Rosenman et al., 2002; Silber et al., 1998.

cycles or reductions of chemotherapy dose) can affect long-term remission rates and survival outcomes (Barrett-Lee et al., 2006; Blay et al., 1998; Chang, 2000; Intragumtornchai, Sutheesophon, Sutcharitchan, & Swasdikul, 2000; Madsen, Rosenman, Hui, & Breitfeld, 2002; Marangolo et al., 2006; Silber et al., 1998). These are defined within Figure 11-1.

Fever is the cardinal symptom of infection, although the degree of immune suppression also may blunt the patient's ability to mount a fever response. NCCN defines fever as a single oral temperature (or equivalent) of 38.0°C (100.4°F) twice within two hours or a single oral temperature (or equivalent) of 38.3°C (101°F) (NCCN, 2008b). Subnormal body temperature also may be a significant indicator of leukopenia-related infection; however, the specific clinical implications are not well described (Shelton, 2005). It is proposed that subnormal body temperature is reflective of more severe sepsis or the presence of gram-negative organisms, but these speculations are not yet supported by research findings (NCCN, 2008b). Neutropenic patients need temperature assessment at least four times per day and with any onset of symptoms of infection.

Inflammatory symptoms, such as erythema-enhanced capillary permeability, swelling, or pus formation, may not always be present in patients with leukopenia because of the absence of WBCs to produce inflammation. Fatigue is common even without infectious complications. Leukopenia beyond 7 days is thought to significantly increase the risk of infection, and virtually all who are leukopenic beyond 21 days become infected (Centers for Disease Control and Prevention [CDC], Infectious Diseases Society of America, & American Society of Blood and Marrow Transplantation, 2000; Ozer et al., 2000). As a result of many antimicrobial and growth factor advances, mortality from neutropenia-induced infections has decreased from 21% to 7% in the past two decades (NCCN, 2008b; Viscoli, 2002).

When WBC responses are adequate, inflammatory symptoms can occur within the affected organ or body part. Organ-specific signs and symptoms of infection may be predicted by considering the clinical effects of introducing fluid extravasation and large numbers of WBCs into that organ or body space (Shane & Shelton, 2004). Possible organ-specific inflammatory symptoms include the presence of WBCs, causing increased intracranial pressure or nuchal rigidity, cloudy urine, purulent sputum or hypoxia, wound drainage or dehiscence, and development of effusions. Recognition of these symptoms even with a single fever may provide a targeted and focused intervention. Oncology APNs ensure that patients, family, and staff understand the importance of assessing every open orifice, uncovering wounds to assess drainage, and looking for any abnormal organ function.

Diagnostic Testing for Leukopenia

Serum tests are the primary diagnostic tests used to detect leukopenia. The total WBC count and differential determines whether the number of WBCs is adequate to combat infection and mount inflammatory responses to injury. A low WBC count signals the probability of reduced neutrophil efficacy. Normally, the total WBC count is 5,000–10,000 cells/mm^3, composed mostly of neutrophils, although the percentage of each cell line may assist in defining the specific immune deficit and predicting the type of infection the patient is most likely to develop. The ANC is indicative of the number of neutrophils available to combat infection. It is calculated by using the WBC differential with the formula included in Figure 11-2. The frequency of monitoring the ANC will vary depending on the individual patient. Oncology APNs have the expertise

---

Total number of white blood cells × % neutrophils = absolute neutrophil count

Example: 3,800 x 0.52 = 1,976 cells/mm³

Calculation of the absolute neutrophil count provides the clinician with valuable information on the severity of leukopenia. The total number of white blood cells is multiplied by the percentage of neutrophils detected. This provides an absolute neutrophil count that can be applied to the toxicity scale in Table 11-2.

Figure 11-2. Calculation of the Absolute Neutrophil Count

---

to consider the therapeutic regimen and patient-based variables to identify a plan for monitoring the complete WBC and differential based on expected values and planned interventions.

The CD4 count reflects the absolute number of CD4 molecule-containing cells, which primarily are helper T-lymphocyte cells but also include monocytes (Rome, 2007). CD4 counts lower than 500/mm³ are considered a significant risk factor for opportunistic infection. CD4 counts are used for diagnosis, treatment planning, and evaluation of therapeutic response to treatment for AIDS. Despite abnormal values, monitoring these numbers has not proved helpful in the management of patients on corticosteroids or receiving organ transplant rejection inhibitors (NCCN, 2008b).

In patients with leukopenia without a clear etiology, hematologic malignancies or marrow infiltration by other cancers is suspected. A bone marrow aspiration with or without bone marrow biopsy may reveal specific pathogenic disorders, such as myelofibrosis, myelodysplasia, leukemia, or aplastic anemia. The bone marrow aspirate is obtained from the posterior iliac crest or sternum. Most patients require pain medication or sedation to tolerate the discomfort of this procedure (Giannoutsos, Grech, Maboreke, & Morganstern, 2004). Normal bone marrow is easily aspirated without being extremely painful, but for most patients with hematologic disorders, the dry aspirate is difficult to tolerate. The pain associated with a dry aspirate is thought to be related to the degree of suction imposed in an attempt to obtain a specimen (Giannoutsos et al.). Once 30–150 ml of red bone marrow is aspirated, it is smeared on pathology slides and sent to specialty hematology laboratories for genetic testing, flow cytometry, and cytopathology (Riley et al., 2004). Results usually are reported in two to three days and may direct the plan of care. The bone marrow aspirate site is covered with a sterile dressing, and pain medication may be administered for a few days. If the patient has thrombocytopenia or bleeding, this site may require additional pressure, ice, or topical hemostatics.

The discussion of leukopenia assessment would be incomplete without techniques for assessment of potential infection. Infection, severe infection, sepsis, and septic shock are potential complications of leukopenia. Chapter 14 discusses septic shock in greater detail.

Prevention and Management of Leukopenia

Leukopenia is best treated by reversing the underlying cause. Most cancer-related leukopenia is an anticipated and unavoidable effect of cancer therapy and therefore not preventable. APNs review the patient's medication profile and discuss any medications or alternative therapies that might enhance or prolong bone marrow suppression of WBCs. In some circumstances, other therapies with fewer marrow-suppressing effects may be available. Common offending prescriptive agents include allopurinol, antipsychotic agents (clozapine), beta-lactam antibiotics, carbamazepine, chlorpromazine, ganciclovir, phenytoin, propylthiouracil, ticlopidine, trimethoprim-sulfamethoxazole, and valproic acid (Schwartzberg, 2006). Vitamin E and echinacea are complementary and alternative therapies implicated in development or worsening of leukopenia (de Lemos et al., 2004).

The best strategy for overall management of cancer- or treatment-induced leukopenia is prevention of infection. Patients who are at risk or are predicted to develop any level of leukopenia are taught methods of preventing infection and how to recognize the early symptoms of possible infection to ensure prompt aggressive management of any infection that may occur. Common infection prevention practices are described in Table 11-4. Because many interventions are based upon scientific principles of infectious disease but do not have a high level of scientific evidence, interventions are labeled with the level of research-based evidence to support implementation.

Prophylactic antimicrobial agents are administered in specific circumstances in which the risk of infection and benefit of therapy outweigh the risk of developing antimicro-

Table 11-4. Infection Prevention Strategies

Objective	Strategy	Evidence Base
Avoid exposure to infection risks.	Avoid exposures (as in crowds, limiting contact with small children or pets, screening visitors).	High evidence
	Keep windows closed.	Moderate evidence
	Bathe and change linens daily; perform oral care 3–4 times daily and perineal care twice daily.	High evidence
	If moderate to high risk of respiratory infection transmission is possible, wear masks, changing every 30 minutes during contacts.	Moderate evidence
	Wear a high-particulate filter mask for exposure to construction.	High evidence
	Avoid close contact with fresh flowers in standing water or soil. Avoid gardening unless wearing gloves and high-particulate filter mask.	High evidence
	Cook or clean foods thoroughly before consumption. Store freshly made (preservative-free) foods no longer than 2–3 days under refrigeration. Avoid purchased foods with possible contamination (i.e., seafood, eggs, mayonnaise) unless circumstances of preparation are known.	High evidence (except neutropenic diet)
	Follow a neutropenic diet (i.e., cooked foods only).	Low evidence
	Consume bottled water or processed drinks only.	Low evidence
	Control blood glucose levels.	Moderate evidence
	Change IV tubing daily if blood or parenteral nutrition is infused via that line. Avoid use of stopcocks in IV lines.	High evidence

(Continued on next page)

Table 11-4. Infection Prevention Strategies *(Continued)*

Objective	Strategy	Evidence Base
	Prescribe prophylactic and therapeutic antimicrobial agents. Assess variables influencing absorption or blood levels. Perform peak or trough levels as ordered.	High evidence
	Use HEPA-filtered/negative-pressure rooms to reduce risk of acquiring airborne fungal pathogens.	High evidence
Control environmental risks of microbial invasion.	Follow strict hand washing and hand hygiene between patient contacts or procedures. Provide hand hygiene products in the hospital setting for patients and families.	High evidence
	Maintain clean living environment (e.g., no food waste on table and countertops).	Moderate evidence
	Ensure sterile management of vascular access devices in the hospital. Follow institutional protocols for clean versus sterile home management of vascular access devices.	Moderate evidence
	Cohort patients with leukopenia, or provide a private room.	High evidence
	Clean all multipurpose equipment (e.g., oximeter probes, infusion pumps, electronic thermometers) between patient uses. Use single-use equipment and supplies whenever possible.	High evidence
	Perform incentive spirometry, and encourage deep breathing and coughing and ambulation as much as tolerated to prevent atelectasis.	Moderate evidence
	Cover open lesions with sterile dressing. Change daily if drainage is present.	Moderate evidence
	Apply prophylactic antimicrobial powders or ointments in areas at high risk for infection (e.g., skin folds, perineal area).	Low evidence
	Consider immunizations required because of lymphocyte suppression. Do not use nasal inoculation for influenza immunization. Pneumococcal and meningitis vaccines may be indicated in some cases. Vaccinate healthcare professionals against influenza.	High evidence
	Change oxygen therapy equipment if it is visibly contaminated or if obvious breaks in integrity exist.	Low evidence
Avoid invasive procedures.	Avoid rectal procedures (e.g., rectal temperature).	Moderate evidence
	Use sterile procedure for an invasive procedure.	–
	Use in-line endotracheal/tracheal tube suction systems with a flush port to clean the catheter after each use.	Moderate evidence
	Consider enteral feeding rather than parenteral feeding. Even minimal use of gastrointestinal tract helps to maintain mucosal integrity, eliminating the need for high dextrose via IV line.	Moderate evidence

(Continued on next page)

Table 11-4. Infection Prevention Strategies (Continued)

Objective	Strategy	Evidence Base
Implement measures to lessen severity or longevity of leukopenia.	Give hematopoietic growth factors between 24–72 hours post-chemotherapy in individuals > 65 years of age or those with chemotherapy regimens likely to produce neutropenia in > 20% of patients.	High evidence
	Maintain good general health measures regarding nutrition, rest, and sleep.	Moderate evidence
	Administer IV immunoglobulin as indicated (IgG levels < 300 mcg/dl).	Low evidence

Note. Based on information from Bartley, 2000; Bolyard et al., 1998; Boyce & Pettit, 2002; Centers for Disease Control and Prevention et al., 2000; Daniel & Crawford, 2006; Freifeld et al., 1999; Gilliam, 2002; Guinan et al., 2003; Hahn et al., 2002; Hughes et al., 2002; Machado, 2005; Moran & Camp-Sorrell, 2002; National Comprehensive Cancer Network, 2008b; O'Grady et al., 2002; Sehulster & Chinn, 2003; Shane & Shelton, 2004; Smith & Besser, 2000; Wilson, 2002; Zitella et al., 2006.

bial resistance. The clinical indications for prophylactic antimicrobial therapy are defined by national standards (CDC et al., 2000; NCCN, 2008b), although some additional high-risk patients may also benefit from this practice (Cullen et al., 2005; Tjan-Heijnen et al., 2001). Patients with prolonged neutropenia receive prophylaxis against gastrointestinal gram-negative organisms and *Candida,* and patients with prolonged lymphopenia may receive prophylaxis against *Pneumocystis carinii* and cytomegalovirus (CDC et al.; NCCN, 2008b). Oncology APNs often are responsible for assessing and implementing these specific interventions.

Specific abrogation of the clinical severity of leukopenia can be managed by administration of growth factors (NCCN, 2008b; Ozer et al., 2000) or immune globulin (Bodey, 2005; Safdar, 2006). Specific doses and administration procedures are located in current medication resources.

In patients who become infected while neutropenic, immediate administration of broad-spectrum antimicrobials remains the most essential therapy (Hughes et al., 2002; NCCN, 2008b; Nucci, Landau, Silveira, Spector, & Pulcheri, 2001; Viscoli, 2002). Patients with a lower risk of sepsis may have febrile episodes treated with outpatient antimicrobials and include febrile neutropenia in children without respiratory symptoms, patients with suspected community-acquired infection, patients with nonhematologic malignancies or absence of active malignant disease, patients with expected neutropenia nadir less than seven days or nadir not expected to drop below $500/mm^3$, and patients with no comorbid health conditions (Intragumtornchai et al., 2000; Kern et al., 1999; Koh & Pizzo, 2002; Madsen et al., 2002; NCCN, 2008b).

Thrombocytopenia

Definition and Etiology

Thrombocytopenia is defined as inadequate numbers of circulating platelets available to participate in the initial phase of clotting. Clotting itself requires the integration of platelets, coagulation proteins made in the liver, calcium, and cytokine or inflammatory stimulators. The absence of platelets alone can result in life-threatening hemorrhage, as platelets are the first responders to a break in tissue integrity, and platelet aggregation is the triggering event for formation of a final fibrin clot. The degree of depletion is reflective of the severity of deficit (see Table 11-2). Many general medicine clinicians use the threshold of a platelet count less than $100,000/mm^3$, although this is considered to be too conservative for cancer therapy–related toxicity. Thrombocytopenia is not usually considered to be clinically significant until platelet counts drop to less than $50,000/mm^3$ (NCI toxicity grade 3) (NCI CTEP, 2006). Patients receiving therapeutic anticoagulation or undergoing surgical procedures are maintained with counts at or above $50,000/mm^3$, although most patients receiving oncologic/hematologic care require platelet transfusions when their level is less than $10,000/mm^3$ (Benjamin & Anderson, 2002) or at higher levels if they are symptomatic. Thrombocytopenia is the most common cause of bleeding in patients with cancer, although this risk only increases significantly as the counts decrease below $25,000/mm^3$ (Benjamin & Anderson). Oncology APNs assess the risk for and presence of thrombocytopenia.

Thrombocytopenia may occur because of decreased production or function, consumption, or blood loss (see Table 11-5). The most common etiologies of abnormal production of platelets are chemotherapy and radiotherapy. The chemotherapeutic agents most likely to produce significant thrombocytopenia are the platinols (Polovich et al., 2005). Medications such as histamine blockers or antiviral agents are well known for their effects upon platelet production and are used cautiously in patients with cancer. Some nutraceuticals and herbal agents are known to increase the risk of bleeding, although bleeding is more often related to interference with hepatic coagulation protein production or activity than to interference with platelets. Agents to avoid in patients with thrombocytopenia include vitamin E, garlic, ginkgo biloba, and ginger (de Lemos et al., 2004; National Center for Complementary and Alternative Medicine, 2008).

Blood loss–related or consumption thrombocytopenia occurs when platelets are lost with overt bleeding or are consumed in a microvascular bleeding process, such as disseminated intravascular coagulation (DIC). Blood losses less than 500 ml appear to be the threshold in which clotting factors also are depleted (Despotis, Zhang, & Lublin, 2007). In patients with large blood losses, significant thrombocytopenia occurs.

Thrombocytopenia Assessment

Because platelets are the first responders to breaks in vascular integrity (usually occurring first in skin and soft tissues), symptoms such as petechiae (tiny purplish-red dots) and ecchymoses (bruises) occur. Petechiae and ecchymoses can occur with minor injury, dependent pressure (e.g., from lying on one area), or gravitational pressure (e.g., an arm hanging alongside the bedrail) in fragile vessels with inadequate coagulation factors. Overt bleeding from wounds or body orifices or around existing tubes occurs immediately after injury to the vasculature if platelets are inadequate, as the platelet plug is the first step of the clotting cascade. Clinical bleeding events delayed 20 minutes to two hours indicates coagulation protein deficit, not necessarily thrombocytopenia. When large vessels are opened for any reason, spontaneous, severe, and continuous bleeding can occur. Organ-specific bleeding is most common in sites with a large mucosal or epithelial surface area, such as the gastrointestinal tract (oral, oropharynx, nasopharynx, gastric, rectal), urinary tract, and lungs. Assessment for occult and overt blood in all excrement and exudates may reveal sources of bleeding. All sources of se-

Table 11-5. Causes of Thrombocytopenia

Pathophysiologic Mechanism	Etiologic Factors
Abnormal production of platelets in the bone marrow	Alcohol Allopurinol Antineoplastic chemotherapy Aplastic anemia Burns Catecholamines Chloramphenicol Flucytosine Histamine 2 blockers Histoplasmosis Hormones Nutritional deficits Radiation (ionizing and nonionizing) exposure Thiazide diuretics
Interference with platelet function	Aminoglycosides Catecholamines Dextran Diabetes mellitus Hepatic cirrhosis Hyperthermia Hypothermia Loop diuretics Malignant lymphomas Nonsteroidal anti-inflammatory agents Phenothiazines Salicylates Sarcoidosis Scleroderma Systemic lupus erythematosis Thyrotoxicosis Tricyclic antidepressants Uremia Vitamin E
Blood loss	Epistaxis Gastrointestinal bleed Hematuria Hemoptysis Retroperitoneal bleed (spontaneous or from blunt trauma) Vascular injury
Consumptive process	Disseminated intravascular coagulation Heart valves Heat stroke Large-bore IV catheters (e.g., balloon pump, dialysis catheters) Large tumor masses Sepsis-induced consumption Sulfonamides Transfusions Trimethoprim-sulfamethoxazole
Immunologic destruction of platelets	Heparin Immune thrombocytopenic purpura or thrombotic thrombocytopenic purpura Mononucleosis Vaccinations Viral illness

Note. Based on information from Cagan et al., 2002; Polovich et al., 2005; Rome, 2007; Safdar & Armstrong, 2001; Salacz et al., 2007; Shane & Shelton, 2004; Shelton et al., 2007.

cretions and excrement (e.g., nasogastric secretions, urine, stool, sputum, nasal drainage, vaginal discharge) are examined for evidence of blood. Mucous membranes, such as in the oral cavity or gastrointestinal tract, particularly are prone to spontaneous bleeding with thrombocytopenia because vessels are so close to the membrane surface. Additionally, bleeding may be evidenced by organ dysfunction, such as pulmonary crackles with hypoxemia or enlarged and tender liver with hepatic enzyme elevation.

Under some circumstances, circulating platelet levels are reduced because of abnormal sequestration rather than decreased production or loss. The liver and spleen, which normally remove abnormal or senescent platelets, may inappropriately filter them from circulation. An enlarged and tender liver or spleen is an indication that abnormal or fragmented cells are being captured by these organs. Excessive removal can be a normal compensatory mechanism when cell fragments are present, such as with massive thromboses. This usually is accompanied by jaundice as a manifestation of abnormal hemolysis (Shelton et al., 2007).

Although thrombocytopenia is a clear myelosuppressive toxicity, many medications and disease states alter platelet function, cause similar complications, or exacerbate symptoms associated with thrombocytopenia. In patients with mild to moderate thrombocytopenia who have excess bleeding, these factors are considered and treated. Common causes of platelet dysfunction include acetaminophen, alcohol, aminoglycosides, beta-blockers, dextran, diuretics (loop, thiazide), hypothermia, nonsteroidal anti-inflammatory agents, penicillin, phenothiazines, rifampin, salicylates, tricyclic antidepressants, unfractionated heparin, uremia, and valproic acid (Shane & Shelton, 2004; Shelton et al., 2007).

The defining feature of thrombocytopenia is a low platelet count, although other diagnostic tests may help to differentiate the specific etiology of platelet depletion or clarify an etiology for symptoms present with thrombocytopenia. If thrombocytopenia is related to blood loss, commensurate decreases in hemoglobin and hematocrit usually are present (Shelton et al., 2007). Platelet production disorders usually are not independent of other hematopoietic cells; therefore, anemia and leukopenia usually accompany it (Rome, 2007). When hepatosplenic sequestration occurs, serum bilirubin levels are increased, and blood cell smears show schistocytes (fragmented RBCs) (Shane & Shelton, 2004; Shelton et al.). Coagulation factor tests such as fibrinogen level, prothrombin time, partial thromboplastin time, fibrin degradation products, or antithrombin III levels will reveal coagulation abnormalities that may contribute to bleeding diatheses (Shelton et al.).

Prevention and Management of Thrombocytopenia

When possible, serious thrombocytopenia is prevented with chemotherapy or radiotherapy dose adjustment. When this compromises possible response, platelet growth factor may be administered. The bone marrow growth factor currently approved by the U.S. Food and Drug Administration to stimulate bone marrow production of platelets is oprelvekin (Neumega®, Wyeth Pharmaceuticals) (interleukin 11). This agent is administered 24–72 hours after the last chemotherapy dose. The most common adverse effect is fluid retention, although thrombosis also is a potential complication (Bhatia, Davenport, & Cairo, 2007; Shane & Shelton, 2004). It is important to evaluate the thrombotic risk prior to prescription of this agent.

Other factors are known to deplete platelet levels and can be avoided or minimized with proactive interventions. Avoidance of temperature extremes, rigors or seizures, and large-bore invasive lines can reduce platelet consumption (Salacz, Lankiewicz, & Weissman, 2007). Preventing bleeding from other causes also is an important supportive intervention. Hepatic coagulation factors may be supported with administration of vitamin K (phytonadione) or plasma transfusions. Prevention of severe bleeding complications with general care measures is equally important, particularly when patients may be transfusion refractory as a result of antibody alloimmunization. Patients with low platelet counts require elevation of the head of their bed (to reduce the risk of increased intracranial pressure–induced capillary hemorrhage), reduction of invasive procedures, and a safe, clutter-free environment. Patients are advised to protect their hands and feet from injury, to use only electric razors, and to avoid physical activities that increase risk of injury.

Optimal management of thrombocytopenia involves determining the minimal tolerable and safe platelet count for each patient. Each patient has an individualized platelet threshold for transfusion based upon his or her clinical needs and complications (Benjamin & Anderson, 2002). For example, patients with existing uremia that alters platelet quality may require a high platelet count, as would individuals who are receiving therapeutic heparin for a recent pulmonary embolism. Patients with open wounds or erosive malignant masses also might require higher platelet counts to prevent bleeding.

Thrombocytopenia-induced bleeding often involves skin, mucous membranes, and soft tissues. Local procoagulant interventions or agents may be effective in preventing serious or persistent bleeding and often are initiated by an APN who is familiar with broader treatment options for bleeding. The most common and inexpensive measure is application of ice or pressure to the site of bleeding. This causes vasoconstriction and reduces blood loss but does not prevent bleeding from recurring. Other supportive local measures to decrease bleeding from specific sites include topical agents, such as Gelfoam® (Pfizer Inc.), topical thrombin, oxidized cellulose (Surgicel™, Johnson & Johnson), or microfibrillar collagen hemostat (Avitene®, C.R. Bard, Inc.).

Systemic treatments for bleeding involve stimulation of the body's normal processes to produce factors or agents known to decrease the bleeding tendency. Their specific indications, dosing, administration procedures, and evaluation of responses are directed by the APN. Epsilon aminocaproic acid (Amicar®, Xanodyne Pharmaceuticals, Inc.) blocks plasminogen breakdown of plasmin (Shane & Shelton, 2004). Somatostatin (octreotide) enhances activity of a normally occurring gastrointestinal enzyme with a procoagulant effect (Shane & Shelton). It may be used for management of gastrointestinal bleeding. High-dose estrogen also has been used to enhance normal clotting mechanisms, but its efficacy for use in bleeding patients is not established (Shane & Shelton). Because few effective therapies exist for platelet-induced bleeding, systemic therapies are targeted to enhance clotting via a mechanism other than the platelet arm.

Nursing management of bleeding risk or actual bleeding is supportive. No directed activities are used only with thrombocytopenia other than platelet transfusions or platelet growth factor (interleukin 11/oprelvekin) (Bhatia, Davenport, et al., 2007). Clinical studies with thrombopoietin were not as promising as anticipated (Tijssen, van der Schoot, Voermans, & Zwaginga, 2006). Table 11-6 describes bleeding precautions and patient education strategies. Platelet transfusions often are administered to patients with cancer and thrombocytopenia. Whenever possible, single-donor platelet products are administered to reduce exposure to foreign antigens and development of platelet antibodies that cause transfusion refractoriness. Platelets produce more reactions than RBCs because of the potential presence of WBCs within the product (Shelton et al., 2007). Febrile and allergic reactions are common; however, a specific antigen rarely can be

Table 11-6. Management of Thrombocytopenia

Objective	Strategy	Evidence Base
Prevent overt bleeding.	Limit invasive procedures.	High evidence
	Avoid medications that affect coagulation factors and increase bleeding risks.	High evidence
	Discourage strenuous activity, contact sports, or situations placing patient at high risk for injury (e.g., motorcycle riding).	Moderate evidence
Prevent occult bleeding.	Keep the head of the bed elevated at all times. Do not use Trendelenburg positioning for hypotension; weigh risks and benefits of its use for central line insertion.	Moderate evidence
	Allow patient out of bed only with assistance until physical therapy evaluation. Pad bedrails if patient is in danger of injuring himself on the bedrails.	Low evidence
	Avoid rectal procedures.	Low evidence
	Avoid intramuscular injections.	Low evidence
	Maintain oral hygiene, preventing gingivitis.	Moderate evidence
	Maintain hydration of mucous membranes (nares, mouth, lips) with saline nose spray, fluid intake, humidified oxygen, and frequent oral care.	Low evidence
	Avoid unnecessary venipunctures.	Moderate evidence
	Use paper tape, or tape to barrier (e.g., DuoDerm® [ConvaTec]) to prevent skin tears.	Low evidence
	Use alternate site for automatic blood pressure cuff. Reset maximum inflation pressure when possible.	Moderate evidence
	Use electric razors for shaving.	High evidence
	Help to avoid constipation and straining for bowel movement.	Low evidence
	Use red rubber catheters, lubricant with endotracheal/tracheal/nasotracheal suctioning. Do not insert catheter beyond the end of the airway, and avoid insertion until resistance (indicates that catheter is potentially injuring the carina).	Low evidence
	Monitor and aggressively treat hypertension.	Moderate evidence
Manage bleeding episodes.	Utilize local hemostatic agents (e.g., Gelfoam® [Pfizer Inc.], Surgicel™ [Johnson & Johnson], topical thrombin) to achieve skin and soft tissue hemostasis.	Moderate evidence
	Apply ice or pressure to site of bleeding.	Moderate evidence
	Administer blood components as ordered; monitor for transfusion reactions.	High evidence
	Assess fluid lost in bleeding episodes by monitoring intake and output, central venous pressure, weight, and orthostatic vital signs. Weigh bloody dressings to estimate actual blood lost.	Moderate evidence
	Hemorrhagic cystitis may require IV hydration, continuous bladder irrigations, and intrabladder hemostatic agents.	Moderate evidence

Note. Based on information from Polovich et al., 2005; Rome, 2007; Safdar & Armstrong, 2001; Salacz et al., 2007; Shane & Shelton, 2004; Shelton et al., 2007.

identified (Despotis et al., 2007; Khan et al., 2007). Patients with a history of reactions are likely to receive premedications of acetaminophen and diphenhydramine prior to platelet transfusion. Single-donor platelets usually have 6–10 units per transfusion. Each transfusion packet is estimated to provide a 20%–50% increase in platelet count (Benjamin & Anderson, 2002). Platelet transfusions do not require the same ABO/Rh compatibility as RBC products, unless the patient weighs less than 40 kilograms or platelet transfusion volume exceeds 600 ml of unmatched platelets or plasma in a 24-hour period (Khan et al.). ABO/Rh compatibility of platelets, plasma, and RBC products is core knowledge for oncology APNs (see Table 11-7).

Table 11-7. Blood Product Compatibility

Recipient's Blood Group	RBC Antigen	Serum Antibody	Compatible Donors: RBC Transfusions	Compatible Donors: Platelet or Plasma Transfusions
A	A	Anti-B	A and O	A and AB
B	B	Anti-A	B and O	B and AB
AB (universal recipient)	A and B	Neither anti-A nor anti-B	A, B, AB, O	AB
O	Neither	Anti-A and anti-B	O (universal donor)	O, A, B, AB

RBC—red blood cell

Note. Based on information from American Association of Blood Banks, 2006.

Anemia

Definition and Etiology

Anemia is most often defined by the serum levels of circulating RBCs (hematocrit) or their oxygen-carrying capacity (hemoglobin). National standards define anemia as a reduction of hemoglobin or hematocrit by one-third or more of normal (initial screening in patients with hemoglobin levels < 11 g/dl) (NCCN, 2008a). This definition is exclusively dependent on laboratory values and may not be a true reflection of this clinical syndrome without evidence of symptoms related to reduced oxygen-carrying capacity (Knight, Wade, & Balducci, 2004). Anemia is reported in 30%–90% of patients with cancer, but the wide variance of incidence is attributed to the variable definition (Knight et al.). Actual values and patient tolerance vary, and many patients with cancer slowly develop anemia tolerating much lower values without cardiopulmonary compromise. Because the life span of an RBC is up to 120 days, this hematopoietic element usually is depleted last when the source of dysfunction is within the bone marrow. Anemia in cancer or cancer therapy is common and is definitively linked to compromised quality of life and reduced survival (Caro, Salas, Ward, & Goss, 2001; Cella, 1997; NCCN, 2008a; Tas et al., 2002). Defining the optimal hemoglobin level, rate of correction, and method of correction continues to be debated (Esco et al., 2005; NCCN, 2008a).

Anemia in patients with cancer usually is categorized by the physiologic/etiologic mechanism, although it often is multifactorial. Common etiologic mechanisms include deficient or abnormal production, blood-loss anemia, hemolytic anemia, or cancer-associated anemia (King, 2005). RBC production is dependent upon a number of nutritional factors and precursor components. Nutritional anemias (iron deficiency, folate deficiency, vitamin B_{12} deficiency, inadequate transferrin) are common even among patients without cancer and should be considered when patients initially present with anemia (Campbell, 2003). Nutritional deficits occur in patients with cancer because of nausea and vomiting, fatigue and malaise, dysphagia, malabsorption syndromes, and gastric or bowel resection (King). Patients often receive gastric acid inhibition (e.g., proton pump inhibitors), placing them at risk for vitamin B_{12} deficiency (Shane & Shelton, 2004). Inadequate production of RBCs also may be the result of bone marrow infiltration with tumor, although leukopenia and thrombocytopenia are likely to precede anemia when this is the etiologic mechanism.

The RBCs of the body normally are sensitized and removed by the spleen when they are senescent, deformed, or dysfunctional. The spleen can become oversensitized by the development of RBC autoantibodies that detect normal RBCs as foreign tissue and then signal splenic macrophages to remove and destroy them (Shane & Shelton, 2004). In addition, RBC autoantibodies may be circulating in the serum and initiate extrasplenic hemolysis. Abnormal sequestration in the spleen or intravascular hemolysis results in hemolytic anemia. Hemolytic anemia is commonly a secondary disorder, arising as a complication of liver and splenic disease, autoimmune disorders, viral infections, malignancy, bone marrow transplantation, or drug toxicity (Rome, 2007; Shane & Shelton). Additionally, transfusion reactions can cause hemolysis, although a persistent hemolytic anemia is unusual in these situations. One indication of recent blood loss or hemolysis is the presence of excessive reticulocytes (Campbell, 2005; Rempher & Little, 2004). Reticulocytes are the immediate precursor cell for mature RBCs and are released early into circulation when the supply is inadequate. The reticulocyte count reflects the degree of bone marrow reserve and amount of replacement RBCs needed. The normal reticulocyte volume is less than 2% of the total RBC count, but in blood loss or hemolysis, the percentage may be as high as 4%–8% of the total RBC count (Campbell, 2005).

Cancer-associated anemia is a syndrome of chronic anemia that persists beyond the time reasonable for cancer therapy–induced anemia and occurs in the absence of bone marrow disease. It is speculated to be partly attributable to an escalated metabolic rate and tumor-related hemolysis (Spivak, 2005; Stasi et al., 2005; Varlotto & Stevenson, 2005; Vaupel & Mayer, 2007). In one study, blunted responses to normal human erythropoietin were noted in patients with persistent anemia, suggesting that anemia is not always the result of erythropoietin deficiency and amenable to erythropoietin replacement therapy (Ozuroglu et al., 2000). Recent recognition of complications of erythropoietin replacement therapy also has resulted in limitations in its use with cancer-related rather than therapy-related anemia (Rogers et al., 2007).

Anemia Assessment

Patients with anemia are first assessed for a past medical-surgical history that suggests other correctable etiologic factors. A dietary history may reveal areas for nutritional interventions. The most important nutrients for production of RBCs are iron, folate, vitamin B_{12}, and protein (Rogers et al., 2007). However, even with immediate nutritional replacement therapy, new RBC production may require two to four weeks (Shelton et al., 2007). Assessing patients' surgical history may identify individuals with lower gastric or duodenal surgeries having hydrochloric acid and intrinsic factor depletion leading to vitamin B_{12} deficiency (pernicious anemia). Because hemoglobin levels are partly dependent upon muscle mass, anemia can be noted when muscle atrophy and disuse syndrome occur (Rome, 2007). Hypermetabolism, such as with chronic infection, breaks down proteins for energy and may cause anemia (Rogers et al.). Hormones serve to regulate RBC production. When androgen or estrogen levels are manipulated in reproductive organ malignancies (e.g., ovarian, uterine, breast, testicular, or prostate cancer), RBC abnormalities can occur. Anemia is most often associated with increased estrogen or decreased androgen (Shelton, 2006).

A thorough medication history can reveal the potential etiology of marrow suppression, nutritional deficits, or hemolysis. Most antimetabolite, alkylating, and antibiotic antineoplastic agents given for more than one monthly cycle will induce anemia (Polovich et al., 2005). Other medications known to induce anemia that may be administered to patients with cancer include allopurinol, amphotericin-B, antidysrhythmics (procainamide, quinidine), anticonvulsants (phenytoin, carbamazepine), antihypertensives (methyldopa), chloramphenicol, flucytosine, isoniazid, reverse transcriptase inhibitors, and trimethoprim-sulfamethoxazole (Shane & Shelton, 2004; Shelton, 2006b; Shelton et al., 2007). Independent risk factors for development of anemia in patients with cancer include female gender; older age; lower initial hemoglobin in females; breast, lung, and gynecologic malignancies; and treatment with platinol agents (Barrett-Lee et al., 2006; Penninx, Cohen, & Woodman, 2007).

The physical signs of anemia are manifested as symptoms of inadequate oxygen delivery, compensatory symptoms to counteract hypoxia, and other symptoms of reduced RBC function (see Table 11-8). Diagnostic evaluation always begins with examination of the CBC with particular attention to the hematocrit and hemoglobin, as these are the most direct measurements of RBC depletion. In addition to the hematocrit and hemoglobin, the RBC indices reported with the CBC may provide helpful diagnostic information. The mean corpuscular volume (MCV) detects the size or mass of the RBC. Young or immature cells are larger in size and cause increased MCV. More macrocytic cells (folate and B_{12} deficiency) indicate more immature cells, also causing elevated MCV. The mean corpuscular hemoglobin (MCH) and mean corpuscular hemoglobin concentration (MCHC) detect the relative amount of iron and oxygen saturation of the hemoglobin molecule. The MCH and MCHC are decreased in iron deficiency, or hemoglobinopathies. Suspected iron deficiency from a low MCH is followed by assessment for decreased serum iron levels and high total iron binding capacity in combination with low transferrin saturation or increased soluble transferrin receptor (Coyne, 2006). When hemolysis is suspected, in addition to lower hemoglobin levels and elevated bilirubin, an increased percentage of reticulocytes and decreased transferrin and haptoglobin are present. In patients with cancer, the assumption that anemia is related entirely to cancer or its treatment may lead to weeks of ineffective therapy. To ensure that precursor proteins are adequate for production of the heme molecule and RBC, baseline ferritin levels are assessed at the onset of therapy or beginning of erythropoietin treatment. Erythropoietin levels have not been proved to be accurate for monitoring efficacy of RBC stimulation therapies (Campbell, 2005; Coyne; Rogers et al., 2007). On occasion, the mystery of anemia can be solved by administration of indium-tagged RBCs with a follow-up nuclear scan to determine whether those cells are lost via a damaged vessel or taken up by a spleen that is inappropriately hemolyzing. This most commonly is used for patients presumed to have a vascular bleed without a diagnosable source. RBC morphologic abnormalities also may be helpful in providing diagnostic clues and triggering more extensive testing. For example, Howell-Jolly bodies are highly indicative

Table 11-8. Signs and Symptoms of Anemia

Pathophysiologic Mechanism	Sign/Symptom
Inadequate oxygen delivery	Hypoxemia (decreased arterial oxygen level, decreased oxygen saturation) Dyspnea/air hunger Angina/ischemic changes on 12-lead electrocardiogram Neurologic symptoms—cognitive dysfunction, dizziness, blurred vision Oliguria Decreased bowel sounds, decreased motility, paralytic ileus, constipation Hypotension (systolic) Central cyanosis notable under eyelids, inside lips Capillary refill < 3 seconds
Compensatory mechanism for tissue hypoxia	Tachypnea, use of accessory muscles in increased ventilation Tachycardia Full bounding pulses Cool or diaphoretic extremities Cardiac murmurs
Inadequate blood viscosity/insulation	Orthostasis (heart rate increase > 20 beats/minute or blood pressure decrease > 40 mm Hg, or blood pressure systolic < 90 mm) when moving from lying to sitting or sitting to standing Hypotension Hypothermia
Indicators of hemolysis	Enlarged and tender liver or spleen Jaundice

Note. Based on information from Campbell, 2003; Cella, 1997; Harrison et al., 2000; King, 2005; Littlewood & Mandelli, 2002; Ludwig, 2004; Ludwig & Strasser, 2001; National Comprehensive Cancer Network, 2008a; Rome, 2007; Shane & Shelton, 2004; Shelton, 2006; Spivak, 2005; Tas et al., 2002.

of hepatic disease, and schistocytes may be present with DIC (Shelton et al., 2007). Unique types of anemia (e.g., sickle-cell anemia, paroxysmal nocturnal hemoglobinuria, thalassemia) can be detected through other specialized serum and urine laboratory tests. Oncology APNs are familiar with the medical-surgical and cancer-related causes and clinical signs of anemia and are able to differentiate key diagnostic test results and treatments for each type of anemia. An overview of these findings is outlined in Table 11-9.

Prevention and Management of Anemia

Anemia is a common and often unavoidable complication associated with cancer and cancer therapies. However, when first evaluating a patient with cancer, a thorough assessment of nutritional status and comorbid disease conditions can reveal the presence of preexisting anemia or risk factors for its development. Early nutritional assessment can permit iron or folate replacement therapy at the onset, preventing lengthy unsuccessful treatment with erythrocyte-stimulating factors. Patients who begin therapy with depleted iron precursors (transferrin, ferritin) or iron stores (iron binding capacity/iron saturation) also may demonstrate inadequate responses to erythropoietin-stimulating agents (Auerbach et al., 2004; Beguin, 2002). Oral iron replacement therapy is frequently ineffective because of iron's poor oral absorption; therefore, IV iron may be administered to high-risk patients (Auerbach et al.). Nutritional supplementa-

Table 11-9. Abnormal Clinical Findings of Specific Types of Anemia

Type of Anemia	Clinical Findings	Diagnostic Test Results
Suppressed bone marrow production of red blood cells (RBCs)	Infection, bleeding, and fatigue. Degree/severity and marrow suppression will predict symptoms.	• Bone marrow aspiration/biopsy shows low level of erythroblasts and other RBC precursors. • Serum leukopenia, thrombocytopenia, and anemia
Folate-deficiency anemia	Fatigue, paresthesias, headache, difficulty concentrating/cognitive impairment	• Decreased serum folate level (< 4 mg/dl) • Decreased hemoglobin • Increased mean corpuscular volume (MCV)
Iron-deficiency anemia	Fatigue, headache, smooth red tongue (painful), cracks in corners of the mouth, pica	• Decreased hemoglobin • Decreased MCV, decreased mean corpuscular hemoglobin/mean corpuscular hemoglobin concentration • Decreased ferritin • Decreased or normal serum iron • Increased total iron binding capacity • Decreased transferrin saturation
Hemolytic anemia	Enlarged and tender liver and/or spleen, jaundice, pruritus	• Decreased transferrin • Deceased haptoglobin • Increased urine urobilinogen levels • Increased schistocytes • RBC survival studies—indium-tagged RBCs administered and scanned for abnormal hepatic or splenic uptake

Note. Based on information from Cagan et al., 2002; Campbell, 2005; George-Gay & Parker, 2003; King, 2005; National Comprehensive Cancer Network, 2008a; Rempher & Little, 2004; Shane & Shelton, 2004; Shelton, 2006; Shelton et al., 2007; Uthman, 2007.

tion with foods high in iron, such as organ meats, beans, nuts, and green vegetables, or those high in B vitamins, such as green vegetables and enriched cereals and grains, may enhance restoration of nutrition.

Although chemotherapy and radiotherapy are known etiologies of anemia, the contribution of other medications to this complication often is overlooked. Anemia can potentially be prevented or reduced in severity by elimination of medications such as allopurinol or trimethoprim-sulfamethoxazole (Beguin, 2002; Campbell, 2003). Although not useful if the patient is not concomitantly hypoxic, oxygen administration is used frequently to supplement other therapies for anemia and will optimize the delivery of oxygen to tissues that may be compromised because of anemia's effects.

When anemia cannot be avoided with passive measures, recombinant erythropoietin, a stimulating growth factor for RBCs, may be administered. Given as an IV infusion or subcutaneous injection, it supports RBC regrowth and hemoglobin maintenance in two to four weeks (Campbell, 2003). The most up-to-date prescribing information is provided in medications resources. Baseline iron, ferritin, transferrin, and iron binding proteins provide information regarding variables that may interfere with erythropoietin replacement therapy efficacy. Although erythropoietin is given to stimulate bone marrow production and commitment of RBCs, no clear benefit results from monitoring erythropoietin levels during treatment. Recent studies attempting to increase hemoglobin levels to 14–15 mg/ dl for the purposes of increased quality of life or increased tumor oxygenation to improve responses to therapy have shown no clear benefit with increased incidence of thrombotic cardiovascular events (Bohlius et al., 2006; NCCN, 2008a; Rosenzweig, Bender, Lucke, Yasko, & Brufsky, 2004). Current recommendations are to first determine if the patient requires immediate correction of anemia by transfusion. The goals of cancer therapy must be weighed against potential risks when considering erythropoietic therapy (Bohlius et al.; NCCN, 2008a; Rosenzweig et al.).

Blood transfusion remains a common management strategy for anemia from all causes. The risk of transfusion-transmitted infection (hepatitis, cytomegalovirus, Epstein-Barr virus), immunosuppression (lymphocyte dysfunction), and complications of banked and preserved blood (hypothermia, hypocalcemia, hyperammonemia, hyperkalemia, acidosis) must be weighed against potential benefit (Despotis et al., 2007; Khan et al., 2007; Salacz et al., 2007; Shane & Shelton, 2004). Concentrated RBC products are used more often than whole blood because of the higher risk for reactions from blood products not filtered for WBCs and platelets. Blood compatibility is ensured by the bedside nurse prior to hanging a blood product (see Table 11-7), and the patient is closely monitored for febrile, allergic, or hemolytic reactions. Blood alternatives such as fluosol or stroma-free hemoglobin may be administered if contraindications for blood derivatives are present (Alayash, D'Agnillo, & Buehler, 2007; van Schalkwyk, 2007).

Patients with concomitant neurologic, cardiovascular, or pulmonary compromise are likely to be provided oxygen therapy in an attempt to alleviate symptoms. Excess oxygen therapy can cause absorption atelectasis and hypoventilation. Mild to moderate aerobic exercise has shown promise as a supportive therapy for patients with anemia-related fatigue (Evans, 2002). The suggested regimen involves 15–30 minutes of aerobic exercise three times a week.

Evaluation of Outcomes

Patients with myelosuppression related to cancer or its therapies present with variable complex symptoms. Although they adversely affect quality of life, these toxicities today account for less than 4% of cancer-related deaths (NCCN, 2008b). In some cases, the highest-risk patients are identified early in their treatment, and adjustment of dose or schedule and supportive therapies allow for amelioration of myelotoxicity. For most, the bone marrow suppression is temporary, and deficits return to normal upon completion of therapy. This knowledge is used to plan assessment, management, and follow-up care. As in all therapy toxicities, a few documented situations exist in which blood counts do not return to their pretreatment values. This is more common with high-dose therapies for hematologic malignancies where the targeted malignant cell line is within the bone marrow. Acute leukemia induction therapy and hematopoietic stem cell transplantation are the highest risk for prolonged marrow suppression affecting one of the identified cell lines (Shane & Shelton, 2004).

Implications for Oncology Advanced Practice Nurses

APNs are key resources for staff nurses and patients in developing an understanding of their clinical experiences with myelosuppression and the unique individual variables of management. The APN's broad knowledge base assists others to translate risk factors and the timing of myelosuppression to develop patient-specific plans of care. Implementation of preventive and treatment strategies is a key role of APNs in the management of myelosuppression. Finally, APNs play a pivotal role in developing facility-wide policies, procedures, staff education, and patient education that integrates evidence-based interventions for management of this vulnerable patient population.

Secondary Malignancies

Definition

A malignancy is considered "secondary" when arising from mutations produced by prior exposure to a carcinogen. As an adverse effect of therapy, this eliminates inclusion of those cancers related to common risk factors or genetic changes alone (see Chapters 1 and 2). The rate of occurrence of second malignancies is higher in children (approximately 4%), approximately 2%–3% in solid organ transplant recipients, and approximately 1.5%–3% in patients who have received radiation therapy (Dantal & Pohanka, 2007; Henderson et al., 2007; Jazbec, Todorovski, & Jereb, 2007; Vajdic et al., 2006). People at greatest risk for development of secondary malignancies are females treated for Hodgkin disease between 10–15 years of age and males with acute lymphoblastic leukemia treated between 4.6–6.6 years of age, although second malignancies occur in almost all childhood cancer survivors (Jazbec et al.). The risk for secondary malignancies increases steadily with time after exposure, particularly for childhood survivors of cancer (Hijiya et al., 2007; Witherby, Butnor, & Grunberg, 2007).

Most conventional antineoplastic therapies are successful because of their ability to destroy specific cells. The more nonspecific the action, the greater the number of normal cells that are damaged. In more targeted therapies, fewer normal cells are damaged, and latent carcinogenicity is less frequent. Secondary malignancies occur as a consequence of chemotherapy, radiotherapy, or T-cell suppression. Most secondary malignancies are myeloid, lymphoid, or soft tissue in origin, although a few highly aggressive forms of glioma, cervical cancer, rectal cancer, mesothelioma, and non-small cell lung cancer are associated with specific exposures (Carret et al., 2006; Chaturvedi et al., 2007; Jimenez et al., 2007; Witherby et al., 2007). Sarcomas are the most common malignancy related to radiation exposure (Henderson et al., 2007). Secondary malignancies are associated with more rapid and uncontrolled growth, higher number of genetic mutations, resistance to treatment, and poor prognosis, although the latter is less clear (Chang et al., 2007; Larson, 2007; Shali et al., 2006).

Etiology

The three main causes of secondary malignancies are chemotherapy, radiation therapy, and T-lymphocyte suppression (Inman, Frigola, Dong, & Kwon, 2007). The greater the therapy's nonspecific destruction, the higher the potential for secondary malignancy. This late effect also is related to dosage, length of exposure, and the level of growth and development of the individual patients (Dantal & Pohanka, 2007). Children have the highest incidence of secondary malignancies, although it is unclear whether this is related to a higher mutation rate, longevity of survival, or iatrogenic growth hormones enhancing mutagenesis (Dantal & Pohanka; Ergun-Longmire et al., 2006). Clearly, immunosuppressive drugs targeting T lymphocytes are more carcinogenic than those affecting cytokines such as tumor necrosis factor (Dantal & Pohanka). Additionally, a dose relationship exists, seen more commonly in patients who received prolonged immunosuppressive therapy as with mismatched renal transplant or those receiving multiple high-dose agents as with heart-lung transplant (Bakker, van Imhoff, Verschuuren, & van Son, 2007; Chang et al., 2007). Another higher-risk group of patients are individuals who received long-term corticosteroids, such as those with autoimmune disease. A summary of secondary malignancies according to their etiologic factors is listed in Table 11-10.

Pathophysiology

Secondary malignancies arise from damaged DNA that is unable to provide a normal RNA replication chain for normal cell division and maturation (Inman et al., 2007; Situm, Buljan, Bulic, & Simic, 2007). Despite clear chromosomal changes indicative of high risk for secondary malignancies, some individuals do not develop this complication. This suggests that DNA damage without impaired immune surveillance systems may not result in malignancy (Bakker et al., 2007; Situm et al.). This is supported by the evidence that the highest-risk medications for development of secondary malignancies are those that are nonspecific in their action and likely to suppress lymphocyte activity. The chemotherapeutic agents that are used extensively in management of autoimmune disease (e.g., cyclophosphamide, methotrexate) are well-known carcinogens. Common chromosomal abnormalities associated with development of secondary malignancy include chromosome 5, 7, 22, and 23 deletions and translocation, trisomy 8, and complex karyotypes (Chang et al., 2007; Larson, 2007). Sarcoma, as a secondary malignancy, occurs more frequently in a previous radiation portal (Henderson et al., 2007). Mesothelioma has been found to have a higher incidence in patients receiving radiation to the pleura (Witherby et al., 2007).

The average time from carcinogenic exposure to development of secondary malignancy varies dramatically from 13–36 months in patients receiving breast cancer treatment (Linassier et al., 2000), or 10–15 years in survivors of childhood cancers (Caglar et al., 2006; Haddy et al., 2006; Hijiya et al., 2007). Variables such as dose and exposure as well as individual factors cause variations between 2–20 years (Caglar et al.; Chaturvedi et al., 2007; Hijiya et al.; Linassier et al.).

Assessment

Because myeloproliferative, lymphoid, or soft tissue malignancies are most common, assessment of higher-risk patients includes periodic, thorough physical examinations and evaluation of any new and unexplained masses or enlarged lymph nodes. In many cases, the first symptoms of a secondary malignancy involve dysfunction of the hematopoietic cells with one of the cytopenias. Bone marrow or lymph node evaluation reveals malignant cells, and flow cytometry yields chromosomal abnormalities.

Prevention and Management

Reduced use of cell-cycle nonspecific chemotherapeutic agents, use of a more precise radiation delivery method, and decreased use of potent T-lymphocytic suppressive agents can reduce secondary malignancy after cancer treatment (Haddy et al.,

Table 11-10. Secondary Malignancies

Secondary Malignancy	Potential Etiologic Factors
Acute leukemia	Alkylating agents Antitumor antibiotics Antimetabolites Corticosteroids Epipodophyllotoxins
Brain tumors	Therapeutic radiation for other cancer
Cervical cancer, invasive	HIV infection
Kaposi sarcoma	HIV infection Transplant immunosuppression
Lung cancer	HIV infection Therapeutic radiation for other cancers
Lymphoproliferative disorder (premalignant condition)	Corticosteroids Post-transplantation
Mesothelioma	Thoracic radiation for lung neoplasms (primary and secondary)
Neuroectodermal tumors	Growth hormone replacement after childhood cancers Therapeutic radiation for other cancers
Non-Hodgkin lymphoma	Alkylating agents Antitumor antibiotics Antimetabolites Cyclosporine Tacrolimus
Rectal cancer	HIV infection
Sarcoma (soft tissue)	Therapeutic radiation for other cancers
Sebaceous tumors	Tacrolimus
Skin cancer (basal cell, squamous cell, melanoma)	Azathioprine Sun/tanning bed exposure Brachytherapy
Thyroid cancer	Therapeutic radiation

Note. Based on information from Bakker et al., 2007; Belson et al., 2007; Bhatia, Krailo, et al., 2007; Buyukpamukcu et al., 2006; Haddy et al., 2006; Heard et al., 2006; Henderson et al., 2007; Jimenez et al., 2007; Lear et al., 2007; Levi et al., 2007; Linassier et al., 2000; Situm et al., 2007; Vajdic et al., 2006; Witherby et al., 2007.

2006; Jimenez et al., 2007). However, this strategy may be impractical in cases of life-threatening malignancy, but it is an option in solid organ transplant or autoimmune disease where other therapy options exist.

When a patient presents with a secondary malignancy, the cytogenetics of the malignancy must be evaluated. This permits a choice of therapy based upon knowledge of these resistant malignancies. The most potent available therapy often is implemented to ensure a rapid and comprehensive response.

Evaluation of Outcomes

An optimal outcome for patients with secondary malignancies is usually cancer control. Few of these resistant malignancies can be cured because of the extensiveness of cytogenetic abnormalities (Larson, 2007; Linassier et al., 2000). After definitive therapy, follow-up computed tomography scans and bone marrow biopsies assess response. At times, follow-up tissue samples to validate eradication of a chromosome abnormality or viral antigen may be helpful but difficult to obtain in every clinical situation.

Implications for Oncology Advanced Practice Nurses

APNs are aware of therapies that predispose patients to develop a secondary malignancy and may direct patients for more frequent follow-up. It may be impractical at the onset of cancer or autoimmune therapy to discuss the possibility of future malignancy, although this often is included in informed consent documents. A time when the patient is stable and anxiety is less acute would be ideal to discuss this risk and potential implications for the patient.

Case Study

M.C. is a 67-year-old woman who presents with abdominal distention and palpable groin lymphadenopathy. She has a past medical history of smoking, hypertension, and a four-year history of immune thrombocytopenic purpura without known risk factors. Lymph node biopsy revealed follicular large cell lymphoma, stage IVB. The APN notes that despite an enlarged abdomen, the patient reports unintentional weight loss of 20 pounds over two months, profound fatigue, back pain, and night sweats. On physical examination, the APN notes a palpable liver and spleen. The APN realizes that M.H. has several risk factors for bone marrow suppression even before cancer treatment begins.

1. What are these risk factors?
   - In light of her advanced disease, she may have bone marrow involvement, and her age, malnourished state, and chronic diseases also may contribute to myelosuppression. Upon further assessment, the APN discovers M.H. has a history of ongoing thrombocytopenia without hemorrhagic episodes. Physical assessment reveals pale oral mucosal membranes with two small aphthous ulcers inside the lower lip, cool extremities, slow capillary refill, weak and thready pedal pulses, and truncal petechiae. The microscopic urine shows RBCs and WBCs.
   - M.H.'s initial complete blood count results

Blood Counts	Patient's Values	Normal
RBCs	2.9 cells/mm³	$3.5–5.0 \times 10^6/mm^3$
MCV	100 mcg/mm³	80–96 mcg/mm³
MCH	27 pg/cell	26–34 pg/cell
MCHC	31 g/dl	31–37 g/dl
Hematocrit	29 mg%	35%–45%

Blood Counts	Patient's Values	Normal
Hemoglobin	10.2 mg/dl	12–15 mg/dl
WBCs	3,800	5,000–10,000/mm³
Neutrophils	52%	33%–75%
Basophils	1%	2%–6%
Eosinophils	1%	1%–5%
Bands	3%	< 20%
Monocytes	6%	1%–10%
Lymphocytes	42%	12%–44%
Platelet count	34,000/mm³	150,000–250,000/mm³
Morphology/atypical cells	Hypochromia, megaloblasts	–

- After examination of this blood work, the APN realizes that M.H. has a pre-existing anemia.
2. Name the most likely type of anemia revealed in this CBC.
   - The type of anemia revealed by this CBC is megaloblastic (large immature cells) anemia as indicated by the MCV, and morphology indicates either folate or B_{12} deficiency. Her baseline anemia with increased MCV and hypochromic, macrocytic cells prompted a pretreatment assessment of ferritin and folate levels. Ferritin levels were low normal, and the folate level was 2 mg/dl, a value lower than normal. M.H. is prescribed a daily multivitamin with iron.
3. What is M.H.'s ANC based on this lab work?
   - To calculate, multiply the total number of WBCs by the percent of neutrophils = ANC ($3,800 \times 0.52 = 1,976$). M.H.'s ANC is slightly abnormal. It is concerning that she is older, has chronic illnesses, and has a starting baseline leukopenia and neutropenia prior to initiating therapy, therefore placing her at considerable risk for protracted chemotherapy-induced neutropenia and its complications. M.H. is prescribed rituximab with CHOP (cyclophosphamide, doxorubicin, Oncovin® [Eli Lilly and Co.], and prednisone) chemotherapy.
4. Based upon these WBC and neutrophil counts, what prophylactic measures will be implemented with the first cycle of chemotherapy to minimize the effects of myelosuppression?
   - Because of her baseline WBC suppression, pegfilgrastim was administered with her first cycle of chemotherapy. She and her family received extensive education on prevention of infection at home. After her second cycle of chemotherapy, she reported profound fatigue, altered cognition, and an inability to perform normal self-care activities. At that time, her hemoglobin was 9.9 mg/dl, and an erythrocyte-stimulating factor was prescribed. After four weeks and a modest increase in hemoglobin, M.H. begins IV iron supplementation with her erythrocyte-stimulating factor, with successful normalization of RBC counts.
5. Would the APN transfuse M.H. with RBCs while waiting for the erythropoietin to begin marrow stimulation?
   - This hemoglobin level of 9.9 mg/dl does not require RBC transfusions unless clinical evidence exists of tissue ischemia or cardiovascular compromise (e.g., abdominal pain with bowel ischemia and elevated lactate dehydrogenase, cardiac ischemia on electrocardiogram, chest pain, and intractable tachycardia associated with hypotension).

> • Between the second and third cycle, M.H. develops a fever of 38.3°C (100.5°F) with accompanying epistaxis. Her platelet count is stable at 26,000/mm³, but occult blood in the stool and urine prompts the clinicians to consider platelet transfusion. She is admitted to the hospital for fluids and IV antibiotics. She receives platelet transfusions, but the platelet count does not rise. After resolution of her infectious episode, the bleeding resolves spontaneously, causing the clinicians to suspect that bleeding was related to altered platelet quality from fever and infection.

Key Points

Myelosuppression

- Oncology APNs consider the following when prescribing chemotherapy regimens: patient monitoring, need for hematopoietic growth factors, and staff nurse consultation for management of myelosuppression.
- Patients at high risk for development of severe myelosuppression (and may be candidates for preventive measures) include those with advanced age (> 65 years); poor nutritional status; preexisting autoimmune disease, diabetes mellitus, gastrointestinal disorders, liver disease, or hematopoietic diseases; and substance abuse.
- Independent risk factors for development of anemia in patients with cancer include female gender; older age; lower initial hemoglobin in females; breast, lung, and gynecologic malignancies; and treatment with platinol agents.
- The normal proliferation rate of erythrocytes, platelets, or leukocytes determines the severity and timing of suppression following exposure to a toxin such as chemotherapy. Depletion of the cell line is directly related to the normal turnover rate of the cell line after the antineoplastic agent destroys normal regrowth mechanisms.
- Granulocytes live about six to eight hours, with leukopenia occurring about 7–15 days after treatment.
- Platelets live about 5–7 days; platelets have the longest nadir and may persist for more than 20 days.
- Erythrocytes live about 120 days; onset of anemia usually occurs following the second or third cycle of therapy.
- The ANC is indicative of the number of neutrophils available to combat infection. It is calculated by multiplying the total number of WBCs by the percentage of neutrophils detected.
- Radiation therapy may cause bone marrow suppression, but less frequently than chemotherapy. Myelosuppression can occur following radiation therapy when the treatment field involves marrow-producing tissue or with doses greater than 1,500 cGy. Myelosuppression peaks in the third week of radiation therapy and often manifests as aplasia occurring simultaneously in all cell lines rather than sequentially as seen with chemotherapy.

Secondary Malignancies

- Most secondary malignancies are myeloid, lymphoid, or soft tissue in origin; more rare are highly aggressive forms of glioma, cervical cancer, rectal cancer, mesothelioma, and non-small cell lung cancer. Sarcomas are the most common malignancy related to radiation exposure.

- The incidence of secondary malignancies is highest in children (approximately 4%), approximately 2%–3% in solid organ transplant recipients, and approximately 1.5%–3% in patients receiving radiation therapy. People at greatest risk are females treated for Hodgkin disease between ages 10–15 and males with acute lymphoblastic leukemia treated between ages 4.6–6.6. The risk for secondary malignancies increases steadily with time after exposure, particularly for survivors of childhood cancer.
- Evidence exists that medications with highest risk for causing the development of secondary malignancies are nonspecific in their action and are likely to suppress lymphocyte activity, such as agents used in the management of autoimmune disease (e.g., cyclophosphamide, methotrexate).
- The average time from carcinogenic exposure to development of secondary malignancy varies from 13 months to 20 years, dependent upon treatment modality, dose, and exposure as well as individual factors.

Recommended Resources for Oncology Advanced Practice Nurses

- AABB (formerly the American Association of Blood Banks) Services and Standards: www.aabb.org/content
- CDC: www.cdc.gov
- Leukemia and Lymphoma Society: www.leukemia-lymphoma.org
- National Center for Complementary and Alternative Medicine (NCCAM): http://nccam.nih.gov
- National Institutes of Health, NCI CTEP: www.ctep.cancer.gov

References

Alayash, A.I., D'Agnillo, F., & Buehler, P.W. (2007). First-generation blood substitutes: What have we learned? Biochemical and physiological perspectives. *Expert Opinion on Biological Therapy, 7,* 665–675.

American Association of Blood Banks. (2006). *Standards for blood banks and transfusion services* (24th ed.). Bethesda, MD: Author.

Auerbach, M., Ballard, H., Trout, J.R., McIlwain, M., Ackerman, A., Bahrain, H., et al. (2004). Intravenous iron optimizes the response to recombinant human erythropoietin in cancer patients with chemotherapy-related anemia: A multicenter, open-label, randomized trial. *Journal of Clinical Oncology, 22,* 1301–1307.

Bakker, N.A., van Imhoff, G.W., Verschuuren, E.A., & van Son, W.J. (2007). Presentation and early detection of post-transplant lymphoproliferative disorder after solid organ transplantation. *Transplant International, 20,* 207–218.

Barrett-Lee, P.J., Ludwig, H., Birgegard, G., Bokemeyer, C., Gascon, P., Kosmidis, P.A., et al. (2006). Independent risk factors for anemia in cancer patients receiving chemotherapy: Results from the European Cancer Anemia Survey. *Oncology, 70,* 34–48.

Bartley, J.M. (2000). APIC state-of-the-art report: The role of infection control during construction in health care facilities. *American Journal of Infection Control, 28,* 156–169.

Beguin, Y. (2002). Prediction of response and other improvements on the limitations of recombinant human erythropoietin therapy in anemic cancer patients. *Hematologica, 87,* 1209–1221.

Belson, M., Kingsley, B., & Holmes, A. (2007). Risk factors for acute leukemia in children: A review. *Environmental Health Perspectives, 115,* 138–145.

Benjamin, R.J., & Anderson, K.C. (2002). What is the proper threshold for platelet transfusion in patients with chemotherapy-induced thrombocytopenia? *Critical Reviews in Oncology/Hematology, 42,* 163–171.

Bhatia, M., Davenport, V., & Cairo, S.E. (2007). The role of interleukin-11 to prevent chemotherapy-induced thrombocytopenia in patients with solid tumors, lymphoma, acute myeloid leukemia and bone marrow failure syndromes. *Leukemia and Lymphoma, 48,* 9–15.

Bhatia, S., Krailo, M.D., Chen, Z., Burden, L., Askin, F.B., Dickman, P.S., et al. (2007). Therapy-related myelodysplasia and acute myeloid leukemia after Ewing sarcoma and primitive neuroectodermal tumor of bone: A report from the Children's Oncology Group. *Blood, 109,* 46–51.

Blay, J., Gomez, F., Sebban, C., Bachelot, T., Biron, P., Gugliemi, C., et al. (1998). The international prognostic index correlates to survival in patients with aggressive lymphoma in relapse: Analysis of the PARMA trial. *Blood, 92,* 3562–3568.

Blot, F., Cordonnier, C., Buzin, A., Nitenberg, G., Schlemmer, B., & Bastuji-Garin, S. (2001). Severity of illness scores: Are they useful in febrile neutropenic adult patients in hematology wards? A prospective multicenter study. *Critical Care Medicine, 29,* 2125–2131.

Bodey, G.P. (2005). Managing infections in the immunocompromised patient. *Clinical Infectious Diseases, 40*(Suppl. 4), S239.

Bohlius, J., Wilson, J., Seidenfeld, J., Piper, M., Schwarzer, G., Sandercock, J., et al. (2006). Recombinant human erythropoietins and cancer patients: Updated meta-analysis of 57 studies including 9353 patients. *Journal of the National Cancer Institute, 98,* 708–714.

Bolyard, E.A., Tablan, O.C., Williams, W.W., Pearson, M.L., Shapiro, C.N., & Deitchman, S.D. (1998). Guideline for infection control in healthcare personnel, 1998. Hospital Infection Control Practices Advisory Committee. *Infection Control and Hospital Epidemiology, 19,* 407–463.

Boyce, J.M., & Pittet, D. (2002). Guideline for hand hygiene in health-care settings: Recommendations of the Healthcare Infection Control Practices Advisory Committee and the HICPAC/SHEA/APIC/IDSA Hand Hygiene Task Force. Society for Healthcare Epidemiology of America/Association for Professionals in Infection Control/Infectious Diseases Society of America. *Morbidity and Mortality Weekly Report: Recommendations and Reports, 51*(RR-16), 1–45.

Buyukpamukcu, M., Varan, A., Yazici, N., Akalan, N., Soylemezoglu, F., Zorlu, F., et al. (2006). Second malignant neoplasms following the treatment of brain tumors in children. *Journal of Child Neurology, 21,* 433–436.

Cagan, D., Franco, M., & Vasquez, D. (2002). The ABCs of low blood count. *Clinical Journal of Oncology Nursing, 6,* 34–37.

Caglar, K., Varan, A., Akyuz, C., Selek, U., Kutluk, T., Yalcin, B., et al. (2006). Second neoplasms in pediatric patients treated for cancer: A center's 30-year experience. *Journal of Pediatric Hematology/Oncology, 28,* 374–378.

Campbell, K. (2003). Anaemia: Causes and treatment. *Nursing Times, 99*(43), 30–33.

Campbell, K. (2005). Laboratory diagnosis and investigation of anaemia. *Nursing Times, 101*(22), 36–39.

Camp-Sorrell, D. (2005). Chemotherapy: Toxicity management. In C.H. Yarbro, M.H. Frogge, & M. Goodman (Eds.), *Cancer nursing: Principles and practice* (6th ed., pp. 412–457). Sudbury, MA: Jones and Bartlett.

Caro, J.J., Salas, M., Ward, A., & Goss, G. (2001). Anemia as an independent prognostic factor for survival in patients with cancer: A systematic, quantitative review. *Cancer, 91,* 2214–2221.

Carret, A.S., Tabori, U., Crooks, B., Hukin, J., Odame, I., Johnston, D.L., et al. (2006). Outcome of secondary high-grade glioma in children previously treated for a malignant condition: A study of the Canadian Pediatric Brain Tumour Consortium. *Radiotherapy and Oncology, 81,* 33–38.

Cella, D. (1997). The Functional Assessment of Cancer Therapy-Anemia (FACT-An) Scale: A new tool for the assessment of outcomes in cancer anemia and fatigue. *Seminars in Hematology, 34*(3, Suppl. 2), 13–19.

Centers for Disease Control and Prevention, Infectious Diseases Society of America, & American Society of Blood and Marrow Transplantation. (2000). Guidelines for preventing opportunistic infections among hematopoietic stem cell recipients [Erratum in MMWR Recomm Rep. 2004 May 14;53(18):396]. *Morbidity and Mortality Weekly Reports: Recommendations and Reports, 49*(RR-10), 1–128.

Chang, C., Storer, B.E., Scott, B.L., Bryant, E.M., Shulman, H.M., Flowers, M.E., et al. (2007). Hematopoietic cell transplantation in patients with myelodysplastic syndrome or acute myeloid leukemia arising from myelodysplastic syndrome: Similar outcomes in patients with de novo disease and disease following prior therapy or antecedent hematologic disorders. *Blood, 110,* 1379–1387.

Chang, J. (2000). Chemotherapy dose reduction and delay in clinical practice. Evaluating the risk to patient outcome in adjuvant chemotherapy for breast cancer. *European Journal of Cancer, 36*(Suppl. 1), S11–S14.

Chaturvedi, A.K., Pfeiffer, R.M., Chang, L., Goedert, J.J., Biggar, R.J., & Engels, E.A. (2007). Elevated risk of lung cancer among people with AIDS. *AIDS, 21,* 207–213.

Coyne, D. (2006). Iron indices: What do they really mean? *Kidney International Supplement, 101,* S4–S8.

Cullen, M., Steven, N., Billingham, I., Gaunt, C., Hastings, M., Simmonds, P., et al. (2005). Antibacterial prophylaxis after chemotherapy for solid tumors and lymphomas. *New England Journal of Medicine, 353,* 988–998.

Daniel, D., & Crawford, J. (2006). Myelotoxicity from chemotherapy. *Seminars in Oncology, 33,* 74–85.

Dantal, J., & Pohanka, E. (2007). Malignancies in renal transplantation: An unmet medical need. *Nephrology, Dialysis and Transplant, 22*(Suppl. 1), 4–10.

de Lemos, M.L., John, L., Nakashima, L., O'Brien, R.K., & Taylor, S.C. (2004). Advising cancer patients on natural health products—a structured approach. *Annals of Pharmacotherapy, 38,* 1406–1411.

Despotis, G.J., Zhang, L., & Lublin, D.M. (2007). Transfusion risks and transfusion-related pro-inflammatory response. *Hematology/Oncology Clinics of North America, 21,* 147–161.

Ergun-Longmire, B., Mertens, A.C., Mitby, P., Qin, J., Heller, G., Shi, W., et al. (2006). Growth hormone treatment and risk of second neoplasms in the childhood cancer survivor. *Journal of Clinical Endocrinology and Metabolism, 91,* 3494–3498.

Esco, B.R., Valencia, J.J., Polo, J.S., Bascon, S.N., Velilla, M.C., & Lopez, M.M. (2005). Hemoglobin levels and acute radiotherapy-induced toxicity. *Tumori, 91,* 40–45.

Evans, W.J. (2002). Physical functioning of men and women with cancer. Effects of anemia and conditioning. *Oncology, 16*(9, Suppl. 10), 109–115.

Freifeld, A., Marchigiani, D., Walsh, T., Chanock, S., Lewis, L., Hiemenz, J., et al. (1999). A double-blind comparison of empirical oral and intravenous antibiotic therapy for low-risk febrile patients with neutropenia during cancer chemotherapy. *New England Journal of Medicine, 341,* 305–311.

George-Gay, B., & Parker, K. (2003). Understanding the complete blood count with differential. *Journal of Perianesthesia Nursing, 18,* 96–117.

Giannoutsos, I., Grech, H., Maboreke, T., & Morganstern, G. (2004). Performing bone marrow biopsies with or without sedation: A comparison. *Clinical and Laboratory Haematology, 26,* 201–204.

Gilliam, K. (2002). Oral care for patients undergoing cancer therapy. *Dentistry Today, 21,* 50–55.

Guinan, J.L., McGuckin, M., & Nowell, P.C. (2003). Management of health-care-associated infections in the oncology patient. *Oncology (Huntington), 17,* 415–420.

Haddy, N., Le Deley, M.C., Samand, A., Diallo, I., Guerin, S., Guibout, C., et al. (2006). Role of radiotherapy and chemotherapy in the risk of secondary leukaemia after a solid tumour in childhood. *European Journal of Cancer, 42,* 2757–2764.

Hahn, T., Cummings, K.M., & Michale, K. (2002). Efficacy of high-efficiency particulate air filtration in preventing aspergillosis in immunocompromised patients with hematologic malignancies. *Infection Control and Hospital Epidemiology, 23,* 525–531.

Harrison, L.B., Shasha, D., White, C., & Ramdeen, B. (2000). Radiotherapy-associated anemia: The scope of the problem. *Oncologist, 5*(Suppl. 2), 1–7.

Hayes, N.A. (2001). Analyzing current practice patterns: Lessons from Amgen's Project ChemoInsight. *Oncology Nursing Forum, 28*(Suppl. 2), 11–16.

Heard, I., Potard, V., & Costagliola, D. (2006). Limited impact of immunosuppression and HAART on the incidence of cervical squamous intraepithelial lesions in HIV-positive women. *Antiviral Therapy, 11,* 1091–1096.

Henderson, T.O., Whitton, J., Stovall, M., Mertens, A.C., Mitby, P., Friedman, D., et al. (2007). Secondary sarcomas in childhood cancer survivors: A report from the Childhood Cancer Survivor Study. *Journal of the National Cancer Institute, 99,* 300–308.

Hijiya, N., Hudson, M.M., Lensing, S., Zacher, M., Onciu, M., Behm, F.G., et al. (2007). Cumulative incidence of secondary neoplasms as a first even after childhood acute lymphoblastic leukemia. *JAMA, 297,* 1207–1215.

Hughes, W.T., Armstrong, D., Bodey, G.P., Bow, E.J., Brown, A.E., Calandra, T., et al. (2002). 2002 guidelines for the use of antimicrobial agents in neutropenic patients with cancer. *Clinical Infectious Diseases, 34,* 730–751.

Inman, B.A., Frigola, X., Dong, H., & Kwon, E.D. (2007). Costimulation, coinhibition and cancer. *Current Cancer Drug Targets, 7,* 15–30.

Intragumtornchai, T., Sutheesophon, J., Sutcharitchan, P., & Swasdikul, D. (2000). A predictive model for life-threatening neutropenia after the first course of CHOP chemotherapy in patients with aggressive non-Hodgkin's lymphoma. *Leukemia and Lymphoma, 37,* 351–360.

Jazbec, J., Todorovski, L., & Jereb, B. (2007). Classification tree analysis of second neoplasms in survivors of childhood cancer. *BMC Cancer, 7,* 27.

Jimenez, C., Manrique, A., Marques, E., Ortega, P., Loinaz, C., Gomez, R., et al. (2007). Incidence and risk factors for the development of lung tumors after liver transplantation. *Transplant International, 20,* 57–63.

Kern, W.V., Cometta, A., De Bock, R., Langenaeken, J., Paesmans, M., & Gaya, H. (1999). Oral versus intravenous empirical antimicrobial therapy for fever in patients with granulocytopenia who are receiving cancer chemotherapy. International Antimicrobial Therapy Cooperative Group of the European Organization for Research and Treatment of Cancer. *New England Journal of Medicine, 341,* 312–318.

Khan, H., Belsher, J., Yilmaz, M., Afessa, B., Moore, S.B., Hubmayr, R.D., et al. (2007). Fresh frozen plasma and platelet transfusions are associated with development of acute lung injury in critically ill medical patients. *Chest, 131,* 1308–1314.

King, M. (2005). Helping to understand the pathophysiology of anaemia. *Nursing Times, 101*(9), 42.

Knight, K., Wade, S., & Balducci, L. (2004). Prevalence and outcomes of anemia in cancer: A systematic review of the literature. *American Journal of Medicine, 116*(Suppl. 7A), 11S–26S.

Koh, A., & Pizzo, P.A. (2002). Empirical antibiotic therapy for low risk febrile cancer patients with neutropenia. *Cancer Investigation, 20,* 420–433.

Larson, R.A. (2007). Is secondary leukemia an independent poor prognostic factor in acute myeloid leukemia? *Best Practice and Research: Clinical Haematology, 20,* 29–37.

Lear, W., Dahlke, E., & Murray, C.A. (2007). Basal cell carcinoma: Review of epidemiology, pathogenesis, and associated risk factors. *Journal of Cutaneous Medicine and Surgery, 11,* 19–30.

Levi, Z., Hazazi, R., Kedar-Barnes, I., Hodak, E., Gal, E., & Mor, E. (2007). Switching from tacrolimus to sirolimus halts the appearance of new sebaceous neoplasms in Muir-Torre Syndrome. *American Journal of Transplantation, 7,* 476–479.

Linassier, C., Barin, C., Calais, G., Letortorec, S., Bremond, J.L., Delain, M., et al. (2000). Early secondary acute myelogenous leukemia in breast cancer patients after treatment with mitoxantrone, cyclophosphamide, fluorouracil and radiation therapy. *Annals of Oncology, 11,* 1289–1294.

Littlewood, T., & Mandelli, F. (2002). The effects of anemia in hematologic malignancy: More than a symptom. *Seminars in Oncology, 29*(3, Suppl. 8), 40–44.

Ludwig, H. (2004). rHuEPO and treatment outcomes: The preclinical experience. *Oncologist, 9*(Suppl. 5), 48–54.

Ludwig, H., & Strasser, K. (2001). Symptomatology of anemia. *Seminars in Oncology, 28*(2, Suppl. 8), 7–14.

Lyman, G.H. (2006). Risks and consequences of chemotherapy-induced neutropenia. *Clinical Cornerstone, 8*(Suppl. 5), S12–S18.

Lyman, G.H., Lyman, C.H., & Agboola, O. (2005). Risk models for predicting chemotherapy-induced neutropenia. *Oncologist, 10,* 427–437.

Machado, C.M. (2005). Reimmunization after hematopoietic stem cell transplantation. *Expert Review of Vaccines, 4,* 219–228.

Madsen, K., Rosenman, M., Hui, S., & Breitfeld, P. (2002). Value of electronic data for model validation and refinement: Bacteremia risk in children with fever and neutropenia. *Journal of Pediatric Hematology/Oncology, 24,* 256–262.

Marangolo, M., Bengala, C., Conte, P.E., Danova, M., Pronzato, P., Rosti, G., et al. (2006). Dose and outcome: The hurdle of neutropenia. *Oncology Reports, 16,* 233–248.

Moran, A.B., & Camp-Sorrell, D. (2002). Maintenance of venous access devices in patients with neutropenia. *Clinical Journal of Oncology Nursing, 6,* 126–130.

National Cancer Institute Cancer Therapy Evaluation Program. (2006). *Common terminology criteria for adverse events, version 3.0.* Retrieved May 4, 2007, from http://ctep.cancer.gov/forms/CTCAEv3.pdf

National Center for Complementary and Alternative Medicine. (2008, February). *Health information.* Retrieved April 28, 2008, from http://nccam.nih.gov/health

National Comprehensive Cancer Network. (2008a). *NCCN clinical practice guidelines in oncology: Cancer- and chemotherapy-induced anemia, version 1.2009.* Retrieved August 8, 2008, from http://www.nccn.org/professionals/physician_gls/PDF/anemia.pdf

National Comprehensive Cancer Network. (2008b). *NCCN clinical practice guidelines in oncology: Myeloid growth factors, version 1.2008.* Retrieved July 12, 2007, from http://www.nccn.org/professionals/physician_gls/PDF/myeloid_growth.pdf

National Comprehensive Cancer Network. (2008c). *NCCN clinical practice guidelines in oncology: Prevention and treatment of cancer-related infections, version 1.2008.* Retrieved July 12, 2007, from http://www.nccn.org/professionals/physician_gls/PDF/infections.pdf

Nirenberg, A., Bush, A.P., Davis, A., Friese, C., Gillespie, T.W., & Rice, R.D. (2006a). Neutropenia: State of the knowledge part I. *Oncology Nursing Forum, 33*, 1193–1201.

Nirenberg, A., Bush, A.P., Davis, A., Friese, C., Gillespie, T.W., & Rice, R.D. (2006b). Neutropenia: State of the knowledge part II. *Oncology Nursing Forum, 33*, 1202–1208.

Nucci, M., Landau, M., Silveira, F., Spector, N., & Pulcheri, W. (2001). Application of the IDSA guidelines for the use of antimicrobial agents in neutropenic patients: Impact on reducing the use of glycopeptides. *Infection Control and Hospital Epidemiology, 22*, 651–653.

O'Grady, N.P., Alexander, M., Dellinger, E.P., Gerberding, J.L., Heard, S.O., Maki, D.G., et al. (2002). Guidelines for the prevention of intravascular catheter-related infections. Centers for Disease Control and Prevention. *Morbidity and Mortality Weekly Report: Recommendations and Reports, 51*(RR-10), 1–29.

Ozer, H., Armitage, J., Bennett, C., Crawford, J., Demetri, G., Pizzo, P., et al. (2000). Update of recommendations for the use of hematopoietic colony-stimulating factors: Evidence-based, clinical practice guidelines. *Journal of Clinical Oncology, 18*, 3558–3585.

Ozuroglu, M., Arun, B., Demir, G., Demirelli, F., Mandel, N.M., Buyukunal, E., et al. (2000). Serum erythropoietin level in anemic cancer patients. *Medical Oncology, 17*, 29–34.

Penninx, B.W., Cohen, H.J., & Woodman, R.C. (2007). Anemia and cancer in older persons. *Journal of Supportive Oncology, 5*, 107–113.

Polovich, M., White, J.M., & Kelleher, L.O. (Eds.). (2005). *Chemotherapy and biotherapy guidelines and recommendations for practice* (2nd ed.). Pittsburgh, PA: Oncology Nursing Society.

Rempher, K.J., & Little, J. (2004). Assessment of red blood cell and coagulation laboratory data. *AACN Clinical Issues, 15*, 622–637.

Riley, R.S., Hogan, T.F., Pavot, D.R., Forysthe, R., Massey, D., Smith, E., et al. (2004). A pathologist's perspective on bone marrow aspiration and biopsy: Performing a bone marrow examination. *Journal of Clinical Laboratory Analysis, 18*, 70–90.

Rome, S.I. (2007). Nursing management: Hematologic problems. In S.L. Lewis, M.M. Heitkemper, S.R. Dirkson, P.G. O'Brien, & L. Bucher (Eds.), *Medical-surgical nursing: Assessment and management of clinical problems* (7th ed., pp. 684–737). Philadelphia: Elsevier Mosby.

Rosenman, M., Madsen, K., Hui, S., & Breitfeld, P. (2002). Modeling administrative outcomes in fever and neutropenia: Clinical variables significantly influence length of stay and hospital charges. *Journal of Pediatric Hematology/Oncology, 24*, 263–268.

Rosenzweig, M.Q., Bender, C., Lucke, J.P., Yasko, J.M., & Brufsky, A.M. (2004). The decision to prematurely terminate a trial of R-HuEPO due to thrombotic events. *Journal of Pain and Symptom Management, 27*, 185–190.

Safdar, A. (2006). Strategies to enhance immune function in hematopoietic transplantation recipients who have fungal infections. *Bone Marrow Transplantation, 38*, 327–337.

Safdar, A., & Armstrong, D. (2001). Infectious mortality in critically ill patients with cancer. *Critical Care Clinics, 17*, 531–570.

Salacz, M.E., Lankiewicz, M.W., & Weissman, D.E. (2007). Management of thrombocytopenia in bone marrow failure: A review. *Journal of Palliative Medicine, 10*, 236–244.

Schwartzberg, L.S. (2006). Neutropenia etiology and pathogenesis. *Clinical Cornerstone, 8*(Suppl. 5), S5–S11.

Sehulster, L.M., & Chinn, R.Y. (2003). Guidelines for environmental infection control in health-care facilities. Recommendations of CDC and the Healthcare Infection Control Practices Advisory Committee (HICPAC). *Morbidity and Mortality Weekly Report: Recommendations and Reports, 52*(RR-10), 1–42.

Shali, W., Helias, C., Fohrer, C., Struski, S., Gervais, C., Falkenrodt, A., et al. (2006). Cytogenetic studies of a series of 43 consecutive secondary myelodysplastic syndromes/acute myeloid leukemias: Conventional cytogenetics, FISH, and multiplex FISH. *Cancer Genetics and Cytogenetics, 168*, 133–145.

Shane, K., & Shelton, B.K. (2004). Myelosuppression. In B.K. Shelton, C.R. Ziegfeld, & M.M. Olsen (Eds.), *Manual of cancer nursing* (pp. 309–352). Philadelphia: Lippincott Williams & Wilkins.

Shelton, B.K. (2003a). The effects of neutropenia upon quality of life for patients with cancer. *Oncology Supportive Care Quarterly, 1*(4), 6–17.

Shelton, B.K. (2003b). Evidence-based care for the neutropenic patient with leukemia. *Seminars in Oncology Nursing, 19*, 133–141.

Shelton, B.K. (2005). Infections. In C.H. Yarbro, M.H. Frogge, & M. Goodman (Eds.), *Cancer nursing: Principles and practice* (6th ed., pp. 698–722). Sudbury, MA: Jones and Bartlett.

Shelton, B.K. (2006). Therapeutic options for patients with cancer and treatment-related anemia. *Johns Hopkins Advanced Studies in Nursing, 4*(5), 109–114.

Shelton, B.K., Rome, S.I., & Lewis, S.L. (2007). Nursing assessment: Hematologic system. In S.L. Lewis, M.M. Heitkemper, S.R. Dirkson, P.G. O'Brien, & L. Bucher (Eds.), *Medical-surgical nursing: Assessment and management of clinical problems* (7th ed., pp. 665–683). Philadelphia: Elsevier.

Silber, J.H., Fridman, M., DiPaolo, R.S., Erder, M.H., Pauly, M.V., & Fox, K.R. (1998). First-cycle blood counts and subsequent neutropenia, dose reduction, or delay in early-stage breast cancer therapy. *Journal of Clinical Oncology, 16,* 2392–2400.

Situm, M., Buljan, M., Bulic, S.O., & Simic, D. (2007). The mechanisms of UV radiation in the development of malignant melanoma. *Collegium Antropologicum, 31*(Suppl. 1), 13–16.

Smith, L.H., & Besser, S.G. (2000). Dietary restrictions for patients with neutropenia: A survey of institutional practices. *Oncology Nursing Forum, 27,* 515–520.

Spivak, J.L. (2005). The anaemia of cancer: Death by a thousand cuts. *Nature Reviews Cancer, 5,* 543–555.

Stasi, R., Amadori, S., Littlewood, T.J., Terzoli, E., Newland, A.C., & Provan, D. (2005). Management of cancer-related anemia with erythropoietic agents: Doubts, certainties, and concerns. *Oncologist, 10,* 539–554.

Tas, F., Eralp, Y., Basaran, M., Sakar, B., Argon, A., Bulutlar, G., et al. (2002). Anemia in oncology practice: Relation to diseases and their therapies. *American Journal of Clinical Oncology, 25,* 371–379.

Tijssen, M.R., van der Schoot, C.E., Voermans, C., & Zwaginga, J.J. (2006). Clinical approaches involving thrombopoietin to shorten the period of thrombocytopenia after high-dose chemotherapy. *Transfusion Medicine Reviews, 20,* 283–293.

Tjan-Heijnen, V.C., Postmus, P.E., Ardizzoni, A., Manegold, C.H., Burghouts, J., van Meerbeeck, J., et al. (2001). Reduction of chemotherapy-induced febrile leucopenia by prophylactic use of ciprofloxacin and roxithromycin in small-cell lung cancer patients: An EORTC double-blind placebo-controlled phase III study. *Annals of Oncology, 12,* 1359–1368.

Uthman, E. (2007). *Blood cells and the CBC.* Retrieved March 21, 2007, from http://web2.airmail.net/uthman/blood_cells.html

Vajdic, C.M., McDonald, S.P., McCredie, M.R., van Leeuwen, M.T., Stewart, J.H., Law, M., et al. (2006). Cancer incidence before and after kidney transplantation. *JAMA, 296,* 2823–2831.

van Schalkwyk, L. (2007). *Blood substitutes.* Retrieved February 28, 2007, from http://anesthetist.com/anaes/drugs/bloodsubs.htm

Varlotto, J., & Stevenson, M.A. (2005). Anemia, tumor hypoxemia, and the cancer patient. *International Journal of Radiation Oncology, Biology, Physics, 63,* 25–36.

Vaupel, P., & Mayer, A. (2007). Hypoxia in cancer: Significance and impact on clinical outcome. *Cancer Metastasis Reviews, 26,* 225–239.

Viscoli, C. (2002). Management of infection in cancer patients: Studies of the EORTC International Antimicrobial Therapy Group (IATG). *European Journal of Cancer, 38*(Suppl. 4), S82–S87.

Weinreich, M.A., Lintmaer, I., Wang, L., Liggitt, H.D., Harkey, M.A., & Blau, C.A. (2006). Growth factor receptors as regulators of hematopoiesis. *Blood, 108,* 3713–3721.

Wilson, B.J. (2002). Dietary recommendations for neutropenic patients. *Seminars in Oncology Nursing, 18,* 44–49.

Witherby, S.M., Butnor, K.J., & Grunberg, S.M. (2007). Malignant mesothelioma following thoracic radiotherapy for lung cancer. *Lung Cancer, 57,* 410–413.

Zinner, S.H. (1998). Relevant aspects in the Infectious Diseases Society of America (ISDA) guidelines for the use of antimicrobial agents in neutropenic patients with unexplained fever. *International Journal of Hematology, 68*(Suppl. 1), S31–S34.

Zitella, L.J., Friese, C.R., Hauser, J., Gobel, B.H., Woolery, M., O'Leary, C., et al. (2006). Putting evidence into practice: Prevention of infection. *Clinical Journal of Oncology Nursing, 10,* 739–750.

CHAPTER 12

Cardiac, Gastrointestinal, Neurologic, and Ocular Toxicities

Jeanne Held-Warmkessel, MSN, RN, AOCN®, ACNS-BC

Introduction

Oncology advanced practice nurses (APNs) play a major role in the management of patients with cancer, cancer treatment, and toxicities. Common toxicities of the gastrointestinal (GI) tract are encountered daily and are much more common than other toxicities addressed in this chapter. Most GI toxicities affect patients' quality of life, but others, such as diarrhea, are potentially life threatening. Cardiotoxicity and ocular side effects are serious, potentially dose-limiting toxicities of commonly used and important antineoplastic agents. Cardiac toxicities have the potential to be life threatening, as do several of the central nervous system toxicities. This chapter will review the role of the APN in the assessment and management of these important side effects.

Cardiac Toxicities

Introduction

Cardiac toxicities are a common side effect and toxicity of cancer care. Multiple cardiac symptoms are associated with cancer and its treatment. Symptoms also may be related to preexisting cardiac dysfunction. Radiation therapy to the heart may produce cardiac dysfunction or toxicity, as can certain antineoplastic and targeted therapy agents. Cancer may metastasize to the heart, grow directly into the cardiac structures, or rarely, present as a cardiac primary tumor. Toxicity presents as either acute or delayed, which is considered chronic. Acute toxicity includes electrocardiogram (EKG) changes (arrhythmias) or the development of coronary artery spasms or blood pressure changes during drug administration. Delayed toxicities include chronic conditions, such as cardiomyopathy and congestive heart failure (CHF). Structural changes to the heart may occur, such as pericardial effusion and cardiac tamponade (see Chapter 15).

Definition, Incidence, Risk Factors, and Etiology

Medications used for cancer therapy are a major risk factor for the development of cardiac toxicity, both acute and chronic (see Table 12-1). Agents associated with cardiotoxicity include chemotherapy such as arsenic trioxide (Trisenox®, Cell Therapeutics, Inc.),

Table 12-1. Cardiac Toxicities Associated With Chemotherapy, Targeted Therapy, and Biotherapy

Drug	Toxicities	Nursing Implications
All-trans-retinoic acid	Pericardial effusion Myocardial infarction	–
Alemtuzumab	Heart failure Arrhythmias	–
Androgen deprivation therapy	Increased fasting lipid and glucose levels Prolonged QT interval Coronary heart disease Acute myocardial infarction Sudden cardiac death	Long-term therapy may not increase the risk of cardiovascular side effects over those associated with short-term therapy. Patients need to be monitored for the development of comorbidities, such as diabetes and obesity, which increase the risk of cardiac disease. Preventive measures, such as a low-fat diet and exercise, are needed.
Anthracyclines, including doxorubicin, daunorubicin, epirubicin, and idarubicin	Arrhythmias Pericarditis Electrocardiogram (EKG) changes Congestive heart failure Cardiomyopathy that is cumulative and dose-dependent. Each of the agents has a different lifetime cumulative dose. Doxorubicin: 500–550 mg/m² (toxicity is reported to develop at doses lower than this); 450 mg/m² in patients who are receiving radiation therapy to the chest or other cardiotoxic agents such as cyclophosphamide Daunorubicin: 550 mg/m²; 450 mg/m² in patients who are receiving radiation therapy to the chest or other cardiotoxic agents such as cyclophosphamide Epirubicin: 900 mg/m² Idarubicin: Toxicity similar to daunorubicin; cumulative dose not identified.	Doxorubicin is a commonly used agent with a wide range of anticancer activity. Obtain baseline cardiac ejection fraction via multigated acquisition scan or echocardiogram prior to starting therapy and periodically thereafter. Avoid exceeding the lifetime cumulative doses. Assess patients for cardiac signs and symptoms at baseline, prior to each treatment, and then throughout remaining life span. Cardiac toxicity may develop anytime after completion of therapy. Pediatric patients may develop cardiac toxicity over a period of 15–20 years. Cardiomyopathy is an important late-term effect of these agents. Consider use of cardioprotectant agent, dexrazoxane, in patients where the benefits of ongoing doxorubicin therapy are present. **DO NOT administer with trastuzumab.**

(Continued on next page)

Table 12-1. Cardiac Toxicities Associated With Chemotherapy, Targeted Therapy, and Biotherapy *(Continued)*

Drug	Toxicities	Nursing Implications
Arsenic trioxide	Torsades de pointes Sudden death Prolonged QT interval T wave inversion Heart block	Perform assessment for cardiac toxicity at baseline and throughout treatment. Weekly EKGs are done along with twice-weekly electrolytes, ions, complete blood count, and coagulation studies. All studies are performed more often if abnormalities develop. Maintain electrolyte values with electrolyte replacements. Keep potassium level > 4 mmol/L and magnesium level > 1.8 mg/ml but not above normal levels. Monitor renal function. Obtain baseline and weekly EKGs to assess QT interval. Stop drugs that prolong the QT interval prior to starting therapy. Correct QT interval that is higher than 500 msec prior to starting therapy. Hold therapy for QT interval that exceeds 500 msec until the interval falls below 460 msec. Hospitalize patient, and check and correct electrolyte imbalances.
Bevacizumab	Hypertension Congestive heart failure Angina Myocardial infarction Arterial thromboembolic events	Monitor blood pressure (BP) at baseline and throughout therapy at least prior to each dose administered. Continue to monitor BP after therapy has been completed, as hypertension may develop after therapy is over. Patients with a history of hypertension may need to be taught to take their BP daily at home and report BP elevation to the advanced practice nurse. Initiate antihypertensive therapy at the first sign of hypertension. Patients with preexisting hypertension require more aggressive monitoring and escalation of antihypertensive therapy, including dose increments and the addition of additional antihypertensive medications. Follow American Heart Association guidelines for the management of hypertension for medication recommendations. In some patients, it may be necessary to interrupt or stop bevacizumab therapy. Additional risk factors for cardiac toxicity include anthracycline use, age older than 65, and prior arterial thromboembolic events.
Bleomycin	Chest pain Pericarditis Myocardial ischemia Myocardial infarction Coronary artery disease	Uncommon

(Continued on next page)

Table 12-1. Cardiac Toxicities Associated With Chemotherapy, Targeted Therapy, and Biotherapy *(Continued)*

Drug	Toxicities	Nursing Implications
Capecitabine	Chest discomfort Substernal chest pain Angina-like symptoms Arrhythmias are rare.	Incidence is approximately 9%. Interrupt patient dosing. Obtain cardiac enzyme, troponin and creatine kinase (CK)–MB, ion and electrolyte levels, EKG, chest x-ray and pulse oximetry. May be possible to rechallenge patients at lower doses.
Cisplatin	Ischemia Bradycardia Hypertension Cardiomyopathy ST-T wave changes Myocardial infarction Left bundle branch block Supraventricular tachycardia	Replete electrolytes as needed.
Cyclophos-phamide	Cardiomyopathy (high-dose therapy)	Risk factors include lymphoma diagnosis, older age, and possibly a history of prior higher doses of anthracyclines and abnormal ejection fraction. May be fatal.
	Pericardial effusion, tamponade	Steroids and analgesics are useful in treatment.
Cytarabine	Pericarditis with pericardial effusion and tamponade	Rare Corticosteroids may be useful.
Denileukin diftitox	Arrhythmias Myocardial infarction Congestive heart failure	–
Dasatinib	Chest pain Pericardial effusion Congestive heart failure	–
Docetaxel	Angina Cardiovascular collapse Abnormal heart conduction	Toxicity increases when given with doxorubicin.
Estramustine	Coronary ischemia Myocardial infarction	Estramustine contains an estrogen-like compound that promotes clotting.
Etoposide	Angina Hypotension Myocardial infarction	–
Fludarabine	Low BP Chest pain	In combination with melphalan, severe cardiotoxicity may develop.

(Continued on next page)

Table 12-1. Cardiac Toxicities Associated With Chemotherapy, Targeted Therapy, and Biotherapy *(Continued)*

Drug	Toxicities	Nursing Implications
5-fluorouracil Capecitabine	Low BP Pericarditis Arrhythmias Cardiac arrest EKG changes Myocardial infarction Angina-like chest pain Acute pulmonary edema Arterial vasocontractions Left ventricular dysfunction	Most cardiac symptoms occur during first 72 hours of cycle 1; however, it also can occur 3–18 hours after administration. Stop the infusion in any patients with complaints of cardiac signs and symptoms and obtain EKG, pulse oximetry, and chest x-ray. Lab work such as electrolytes, ions, and troponin and CK-MB levels should be done.
Ifosfamide	Arrhythmias EKG changes Cardiogenic shock Congestive heart failure	Toxicities are dose-related and may be reversible with medical care and medications.
Imatinib	Heart failure	Related to blocking of c-*Abl* Determine left ventricular ejection fraction (LVEF) function at baseline and periodically during therapy. Reduced LVEF may develop as early as one month into therapy or may be delayed and develop more than a year into therapy.
Interferon	Cardiomyopathy Myocardial infarction Myocardial ischemia Arrhythmias	Preexisting heart disease increases the risk of infarctions and ischemia. Anthracyclines may increase the risk of developing cardiac toxicity. Arrhythmias are common. Additional risk factors include age, prior cardiac history, and dose of interferon.
Interleukin-2	Death Ischemia Infarction Tachycardia Arrhythmias Hypotension Reduced vascular resistance	Side effects are probably a result of capillary leak syndrome. Patients with preexisting heart disease are at greater risk. Toxicities are not uncommon.
Liposomal daunorubicin	Similar side effect profile to standard daunorubicin but at lower incidence. Dose should be limited to 600 mg/m².	Avoid exceeding lifetime cumulative mg/m² dose. Perform baseline cardiac and LVEF assessment prior to starting therapy and monitoring during (at 320 mg/m², 480 mg/m², and then every additional 160 mg/m²) and after therapy for cardiac toxicities.
Liposomal doxorubicin	Similar side effect profile to standard doxorubicin but at a lower incidence. Dose should be limited to 550 mg/m² and to 400 mg/m² when used with cyclophosphamide or with radiation therapy to the chest.	Avoid exceeding lifetime cumulative mg/m² dose. Perform baseline cardiac and LVEF assessment prior to starting therapy and monitoring during and after therapy for cardiac toxicities.

(Continued on next page)

Table 12-1. Cardiac Toxicities Associated With Chemotherapy,
Targeted Therapy, and Biotherapy *(Continued)*

Drug	Toxicities	Nursing Implications
Methotrexate	Syncope Chest pain Arrhythmias Myocardial infarction	Rare
Mitomycin C	Heart failure	Dose-dependent cardiotoxicity developing at doses greater than 30 mg/m² and may be exacerbated by coadministration of doxorubicin at dose of 150 mg/m². Risk is < 10%.
Mitoxantrone	Myocarditis Arrhythmias Congestive heart failure	Limit lifetime cumulative dose to 140 mg/m². Cumulative dose is lower in patients with prior anthracycline therapy. Perform baseline cardiac and LVEF assessment prior to starting therapy and monitoring during and after therapy for cardiac toxicities.
Paclitaxel Nanoparticle albumin-bound paclitaxel	Chest pain Heart block EKG changes Cardiac arrest Low heart rate Supraventricular tachycardia	Rare Toxicity increases when given with doxorubicin.
Rituximab	Arrhythmias	Uncommon
Sorafenib	Hypertension Myocardial ischemia Myocardial infarction	Monitor BP at baseline and at least weekly during first 6 weeks of therapy. Monitor BP throughout ongoing drug therapy. Hypertension may develop at any point during therapy. Patients may need to be taught to monitor BP at home and report BP elevations. It may be necessary to hold therapy for systolic BP (SBP) > 200 mmHg or diastolic BP (DBP) > 100 mmHg. Initiate antihypertensive medications immediately at onset of hypertension.
Sunitinib	Heart failure Hypertension Myocardial ischemia Myocardial infarction Reduced ejection fraction	Monitor BP at baseline and at least weekly during first cycle of therapy. Continue to monitor BP during the two weeks off therapy, and continue to monitor BP throughout ongoing drug therapy. BP elevations begin during the first week of therapy and continue to increase throughout the 4 weeks of therapy. Hypertension may develop at any point during therapy. Patients need to be taught to monitor BP at home and report BP elevations. It may be necessary to hold therapy for SBP > 200 mmHg or DBP > 100 mmHg. Initiate antihypertensive medications immediately at onset of hypertension. Patients with preexisting hypertension will need dosage increases. Perform cardiac assessment at baseline and then throughout therapy. Assess LVEF function at baseline and periodically throughout therapy.

(Continued on next page)

Table 12-1. Cardiac Toxicities Associated With Chemotherapy, Targeted Therapy, and Biotherapy (Continued)

Drug	Toxicities	Nursing Implications
Trastuzumab	Heart failure Arrhythmias Cardiomyopathy	Discontinue therapy. Provide medical management and supportive care for cardiomyopathy and heart failure. Adhere to schedule of multigated acquisition scan monitoring recommended by manufacturer. Do not administer with doxorubicin and cyclophosphamide.

Note. Based on information from Azizi et al., 2008; Brockstein et al., 2000; Doyle et al., 2005; Elliott, 2006; Genentech BioOncology, 2006b; Keating et al., 2006; Martino et al., 1987; Ng et al., 2006; Perez-Verdia et al., 2005; Quezado et al., 1993; Ryberg et al., 1998; Schimmel et al., 2004; Sonnenblick & Rosin, 1991; Sudhoff et al., 2004; Swain et al., 2003; Unnikrishnan et al., 2001; Verweij et al., 1988; Wilkes & Barton-Burke, 2007; Yannucci et al., 2006; Yeh et al., 2004; Zimmerman et al., 1994.

fluorouracil (Adrucil®, Sicor Pharmaceuticals, Inc.), paclitaxel (Taxol®, Bristol-Myers Squibb Co.), trastuzumab (Herceptin®, Genentech, Inc.), and the anthracycline antibiotics, such as doxorubicin (Floyd, Morgan, & Perry, 2007a). Some antiemetics, such as the serotonin antagonists, may cause cardiac toxicity in the form of prolonged QTc intervals. Toxicities may develop after acute exposure or chronic administration.

Acute toxicities include EKG changes such as arrhythmias, sudden onset of coronary artery vasoconstriction, acute myocardial infarction, and sudden cardiac death. Arrhythmias may develop acutely from IV-push doxorubicin therapy but are not common, are usually not life-threatening (Wilkes & Barton-Burke, 2007), and last approximately one week (Nakamae et al., 2005).

The two most common drugs associated with symptoms similar to angina pectoris are the pyrimidine antimetabolites fluorouracil and capecitabine. Patients complain of chest pain that may radiate to the left arm or the left neck (Jensen & Sorensen, 2006). The incidence of cardiac events associated with fluorouracil is 1.2%–19% (Tsibiribi et al., 2006; Wacker, Lersch, Scherpinski, Reindl, & Seyfarth, 2003). Capecitabine, a fluorouracil prodrug, appears to be associated with a cardiotoxicity rate of 3% (Van Cutsem, Hoff, Blum, Abt, & Osterwalder, 2002). Cardiac toxicity from these agents may result in patient mortality (Jensen & Sorensen, 2006; Ng, Cunningham, & Norman, 2005). The etiology of fluorouracil and capecitabine induced-cardiotoxicity is unknown; however, fluorouracil is known to produce arterial vasocontractions, which could produce chest pain (Sudhoff et al., 2004). In addition, risk factors for the development of cardiotoxicity identified in a group of 668 patients receiving fluorouracil or capecitabine included preexisting cardiac and renal disease (Jensen & Sorensen). When cardiotoxicity from fluorouracil occurs, it most frequently is associated with the continuous infusion of the drug (Schimmel, Richel, van den Brink, & Guchelaar, 2004).

In addition to these antineoplastics, supportive antiemetics used as premedications may cause acute cardiotoxicity. Commonly used antiemetics in the serotonin antagonist group, such as palonosetron (Aloxi®, MGI Pharma), may prolong the QTc interval (Wilkes & Barton-Burke, 2007).

Serious chronic toxicities include cardiomyopathy, CHF, and the development of coronary artery disease. A major treatment modality for men with advanced or metastatic prostate cancer is the use of medications that reduce the testosterone level. Androgen deprivation therapy (ADT) reduces the testosterone levels to castration levels and results in altered lipid profiles, such as increased cholesterol, thereby increasing the incidence of cardiac disease. With ADT, the incidence of myocardial infarction increases to 5.4%, sudden cardiac death to 4.5%, and coronary heart disease to 25.3% (Keating, O'Malley, & Smith, 2006). Although ADTs, such as luteinizing hormone-releasing hormone agonists, increase the risk of cardiovascular disease, myocardial infarction, and sudden cardiac death, the same risk is not present with orchiectomy (Keating et al., 2006). ADTs alter fasting serum lipid and glucose levels and may increase the risk of cardiac disease in patients undergoing these therapies within one to four months (Keating et al.).

Anthracyclines produce a variety of acute and chronic side effects, but cardiomyopathy and CHF are the most serious. CHF may develop in up to 26% of patients treated with doxorubicin and at doses lower than 550 mg/m² (Swain, Whaley, & Ewer, 2003). Anthracyclines such as doxorubicin, daunorubicin (Cerubidine®, Bedford Laboratories), epirubicin (Ellence®, Pfizer Inc.), and idarubicin (Idamycin PFS®, Pfizer Inc.) and the anthraquinone mitoxantrone (Novantrone®, Serono, Inc.) are known cardiotoxic agents when doses exceed the drugs' lifetime recommended cumulative dose (Floyd, Morgan, & Perry, 2007b). Factors identified that increase the risk of anthracycline-induced cardiomyopathy, in a study of 1,273 patients treated with doxorubicin, included total dose, concomitant use of vincristine, bleomycin (Blenoxane®, Bristol-Myers Squibb Co.) administration prior to the anthracycline, and use of concurrent mediastinal radiation therapy (Praga et al., 1979). Additional predisposing factors for cardiac events include rate and schedule of administration, prior anthracycline therapy, concurrent use of other cardiotoxic agents, age of 65 years or older at the time of treatment after cumulative doses of 400 mg/m², preexisting heart disease, and abnormal electrolyte levels (Pai & Nahata, 2000; Swain et al.). In addition, because anthracyclines are widely used, they have the potential to produce cardiomyopathy in a large number of cancer survivors (Jensen, 2006; Johnson, 2006; Lipshultz, 2006).

A drug-drug interaction between paclitaxel (Taxol) and doxorubicin increases the cardiotoxic effects of doxorubicin (Gehl et al., 1996; Gianni et al., 1995). Studies on the pharmacokinetic interactions between paclitaxel and doxorubicin demonstrate that when paclitaxel is given before doxorubicin, either as a 24-hour continuous infusion or as a 3-hour infusion, increased cardiac toxicity occurs (Holmes et al., 1996; Moreira et al., 2001). It is thought that the interaction is caused by the liver, as both agents are hepatically eliminated (Gianni et al., 1997). When used together, the dose of doxorubicin should be capped at 360 mg/m² (Gianni & Capri, 1997). If both agents are administered as continuous infusions, the doxorubicin is to be administered before the paclitaxel (Holmes et al.). Even at low doses, anthracyclines produce some degree of cardiotoxicity (Elliott, 2006). Anthracyclines produce free radicals that interfere with myocyte function, induce cardiac muscle apoptosis, and reduce the ability of the myocytes to prevent damage from free radicals by reducing protective antioxidants that occur at naturally low levels, increase the amount of ferritin, and bind with ferritin in the myocyte, thus reducing antioxidant protection (Elliott).

Trastuzumab is a monoclonal antibody specific for human epidermal growth factor receptor 2 (HER2/neu) in patients with HER2/neu-positive breast cancer. Trastuzumab produces cardiac dysfunction as a single agent and when given in combination with other cardiotoxic agents. In a retrospective analysis of 202 patients' charts, the reported incidence of cardiac dysfunction was 3%–7% with single-agent trastuzumab; 27% when in combination with an anthracycline and cyclophosphamide (Cytoxan®, Bristol-Myers Squibb Co.); and 13% when administered with paclitaxel (Seidman et al., 2002). Most of these patients had been previously treated with anthracyclines (Feldman, Lorell, & Reis, 2000; Seidman et al., 2002). Severe CHF developed in 0.5% of patients treated with trastuzumab (Piccart-Gebhart et al., 2005). Patients who receive concurrent anthracyclines and trastuzumab have the greatest incidence of cardiac dysfunction (Seidman et al., 2002), and these drugs must never be given together (except perhaps in the setting of a clinical trial with frequent monitoring of cardiac function). Trastuzumab produces cardiotoxicity in the form of reduced left ventricular ejection fraction (LVEF) and CHF, possibly by interfering with HER2/neu expression in cardiac tissue, which appears to have a cardioprotective effect (Feldman et al.).

Multiple other antineoplastics are associated with some cardiotoxicity (see Table 12-1). As expected, combining drugs with known cardiotoxicity increases the risk of cardiac toxicity. In addition, other methods of cancer therapy, such as radiation therapy, may be cardiotoxic.

Radiation therapy to the mediastinum, chest, or breast that includes the heart in the radiation portal increases the risk of cardiac toxicity despite safeguards to shield the heart from radiation therapy when feasible. Cardiac toxicity from radiation therapy to the heart includes pericarditis, cardiomyopathy, coronary artery disease, and myocardial infarctions (Schultz-Hector & Trott, 2007). For patients who have left-sided breast cancer and receive radiation therapy as part of their treatment, the comorbidity of hypertension increases their risk of the subsequent development of coronary artery disease (Harris et al., 2006). Schultz-Hector and Trott concluded that radiation therapy–induced coronary artery disease probably is caused by damage to the lining of the endothelial cells in blood vessels supplying the heart, causing injury to those blood vessels. Even 20 years after treatment, the risk of heart disease appears to be greater in women who received radiation to the left breast as compared to the right breast (Harris et al.); hence, these patients require life-long assessment and monitoring for the development of cardiac toxicity. Doxorubicin often is used in the management of breast cancer, and its use combined with radiation therapy may increase cardiotoxic effects (Basavaraju & Easterly, 2002). Cardiomyopathy is seen in patients who also receive an anthracycline. Other toxicities, such as radiation pericarditis, are rare. See Chapter 6 for additional information.

Presenting Signs and Symptoms

Acute cardiac toxicity produces an abrupt onset of signs and symptoms, such as acute onset of chest pain, pain that radiates to the neck and arm, shortness of breath, reduced cognition, changes in vital signs, arrhythmias, irregular heart rate, and impaired oxygen exchange.

Chronic toxicity, in the form of CHF, produces signs and symptoms such as dyspnea, exercise intolerance, shortness of breath, dyspnea at rest, peripheral and pulmonary edema, fatigue, changes in vital signs, jugular vein distention, pulmonary rales, tachycardia, and other symptoms of fluid overload and inadequate tissue oxygenation (Maisel et al., 2002; Onwuanyi & Taylor, 2007).

Prevention Strategies

Oncology APNs monitor the lifetime cumulative dose of prescribed cardiotoxic agents, such as the anthracycline antibiotics. This is done so that signs and symptoms of heart disease and cardiac toxicity are identified and diagnostic tests are scheduled in a timely manner. Diagnostic studies performed to monitor for cardiac toxicity include LVEF function using echocardiogram or multigated acquisition (MUGA) scan and blood tests. An LVEF result of ≥ 50% is considered normal (Schwartz et al., 1987). Testing is performed at baseline and periodically during therapy to monitor for decreases in cardiac function using ejection fraction. In patients receiving trastuzumab, LVEF assessment follows the manufacturer's recommended schedule: before starting doxorubicin and cyclophosphamide (AC) therapy, after AC and prior to starting trastuzumab, and then 3, 5, and 15 months after initiation of trastuzumab therapy (Genentech BioOncology, 2006b). Patients receiving anthracyclines are monitored at baseline and periodically during therapy (Nousiainen, Jantunen, Vanninen, & Hartikainen, 2002; Schwartz et al.). After the baseline study is performed, studies are done three weeks after cumulative doses of 250–300 mg/m^2 and 450 mg/m^2, and then before each subsequent dose (Schwartz et al.). For patients receiving cyclophosphamide with doxorubicin or with a history of heart disease, radiation therapy to the chest, or an abnormal EKG, tests should be done when cumulative doses reach 400 mg/m^2 of doxorubicin (Schwartz et al.). For patients with an LVEF of less than 50% but more than 30%, testing should be performed before each dose of doxorubicin and should be discontinued for an LVEF less than or equal to 30% or in the presence of a 10% or higher reduction in LVEF (Schwartz et al.). Long-term monitoring after completion is crucial, as cardiotoxicity caused by anthracycline therapy may develop years after the completion of therapy (Jensen, Skovsgaard, & Nielsen, 2002). Patients who develop a reduction in LVEF after 200 mg/m^2 are especially at risk for the development of doxorubicin-induced cardiotoxicity (Nousiainen et al.). Additional results from the echocardiogram or MUGA scan that should be reviewed include regional wall motion and diastolic function (Ng, Better, & Green, 2006).

Additional test results that may be useful include troponin and B-type natriuretic peptide (BNP). Both are blood tests used in patient monitoring for cardiotoxicity. Troponin is a protein found in heart muscle. Levels increase when a patient experiences a cardiac event, such as unstable angina, myocardial injury, or infarction (Galvani et al., 1997; Gerhardt, Ljungdahl, & Herbert, 1993; Lipshultz et al., 1997). Troponin also may be used to monitor patients who receive cardiotoxic chemotherapy, such as doxorubicin (Herman et al., 1999) or high-dose chemotherapy with cardiotoxic side effects, such as cyclophosphamide (Cardinale et al., 2002). Troponin levels increase in the presence of heart muscle damage from doxorubicin (Herman et al.). In healthy individuals, troponin is undetectable using modern assays (Jaffe, 2006).

BNP levels are elevated (more than 400 pg/ml) in the presence of CHF (Prahash & Lynch, 2004). Patients with levels below 100 pg/ml most likely do not have CHF, and patients with levels of 100–400 pg/ml should be evaluated for other causes of cardiac disease (Prahash & Lynch). For patients who present with dyspnea, BNP testing helps to diagnose or rule out CHF (Maisel et al., 2002).

Use of a cardioprotective agent should be considered in patients who will benefit from ongoing therapy with an anthracycline such as doxorubicin. Dexrazoxane (Zinecard®, Pfizer Inc.) is an intravenously administered ethylenediaminetetraacetic acid–like chelator that binds free iron and reduces the risk of doxorubicin-induced cardiac toxicity in both adults and children when administered prior to doxorubicin therapy (Lipshultz et al., 2004). Treatment often is started when a cumulative dose of 300 mg/m^2 of doxorubicin is reached (Floyd, Morgan, & Perry, 2007a; van Dalen, Caron, Dickinson, & Kremer, 2005). However, it may be started in doxorubicin-naïve children with leukemia without negatively affecting their therapy (Lipshultz et al., 2004).

Eighteen patients treated for pediatric cancers were studied after receiving enalapril to reduce left ventricular end-systolic wall dysfunction caused by doxorubicin-based therapy. These patients had all been treated with a regimen that included doxorubicin. It improved left ventricular function, especially in patients with a higher than normal diastolic blood pressure, and the effect was sustained for 6–10 years, after which cardiac dysfunction worsened (Lipshultz et al., 2002). Side effects include fatigue, dizziness, and low blood pressure (Silber et al., 2004). Research using enalapril (20 mg/day) in patients who have increased troponin levels after high-dose chemotherapy showed that the early use of enalapril may reduce the risk of late cardiotoxicity (Cardinale et al., 2006). Oncology APNs should monitor the literature for ongoing research and developments in this promising area of cardiac treatment for chemotherapy-induced cardiotoxicity.

5-fluorouracil (5-FU) is an extremely important antimetabolite used in the management of several common GI cancers, such as colon cancer and esophageal cancer. When patients develop chest pain during 5-FU therapy, the infusion must be stopped. Diagnostic studies such as EKGs, a chest x-ray, pulse oximetry, and blood work to evaluate troponin levels are needed, and a cardiology consult may be required prior to resuming therapy if this is an option for the patient. To determine if a commonly used coronary artery vasodilator, nitroglycerine, would be effective in reducing bolus 5-FU–induced arterial vasocontractions, a study of 30 patients receiving 5-FU–based chemotherapy and 30 patients receiving non-5-FU–based chemotherapy was performed (Sudhoff et al., 2004). The study showed that nitroglycerine 0.8 mg sublingual may be useful in preventing cardiac arterial vasoconstriction in patients receiving bolus fluorouracil therapy (Sudhoff et al.).

Diagnosis and Assessment

Patient assessment and monitoring for early signs and symptoms of cardiac toxicity is crucial in the care of patients receiving cardiotoxic agents. A thorough cardiac evaluation includes assessment of heart sounds, jugular veins, blood pressure, breath sounds, weight, edema (abdomen for ascites, legs for peripheral edema, and lungs for pulmonary edema), temperature of extremities, and patient complaints. Complaints of new-onset acute chest pain are evaluated using troponin level assessments every eight hours to diagnose an acute myocardial infarction or other ischemic events. An EKG is always performed to assess for dysrhythmias, and a pulse oximetry is obtained to assess for hypoxia. Blood gases also may add valuable information to the assessment along with troponin and creatine kinase–MB (CK-MB) levels. MUGA scans or echocardiograms are used serially to assess and monitor cardiac toxicity. MUGA scan is the method used to accurately determine LVEF (Elliott, 2006), which is reduced in patients with cardiac dysfunction caused by cardiotoxic drugs. Cardiac dysfunction may develop within three months after epirubicin treatment and can increase in severity for up to five years; therefore, patients require ongoing monitoring of LVEF function (Jensen et al., 2002). In patients who receive doxorubicin, reduced LVEF does not predict the development of CHF in a reliable manner, and CHF may develop at doses less than 300 mg/m^2 (Swain et al., 2003). Cardiac troponin levels may be elevated after only one dose of doxorubicin (Lipshultz et al., 1997). Troponin levels (released from damaged myocytes) should be measured to assess for myocyte damage in patients who have received high-dose anthracycline therapy (Cardinale et al., 2002; Elliott, 2006; Ng et al., 2006). In a study by Cardinale et al. (2002), troponin levels were checked at baseline, after completion of the high-dose chemotherapy, and again at 12, 24, 36, and 72 hours after each cycle of therapy. Studies have evaluated the use of troponin levels to monitor for anthracycline cardiotoxicity, but its regular use as a monitoring method requires more research (Ng et al., 2006). In patients at risk for cardiotoxicity, APNs may want to monitor serial levels of troponin after the completion of cardiotoxic therapy. The frequency of assessments is unclear. Natriuretic peptides maintain blood volume and blood vessel diameter. Levels are increased in patients with left ventricular dysfunction (Elliott). Levels should be drawn in patients with dyspnea to assess for CHF as the etiology. Complete blood count is used to assess for the presence of anemia or infection, both of which may exacerbate symptoms. Liver function tests are performed to assess hepatic function (Fadol, 2006). A 12-lead EKG is done to assess arrhythmias, complaints of chest pain, and other abnormalities. Cardiac toxicity assessment should follow a standardized classification system, such as the one developed by the American Heart Association for chronic heart failure (Hunt et al., 2005).

Evidence-Based Treatment Strategies

Angiotensin-converting enzyme (ACE) inhibitors administered on a chronic basis are useful in improving cardiac function in patients who develop anthracycline-induced CHF. Ongoing administration is required to prevent ACE inhibitor withdrawal reduction in cardiac function that develops with ACE inhibitor use (Jensen et al., 2002). Standard therapies used to treat acute and chronic CHF include ACE inhibitors, angiotensin receptor blockers, beta-blockers, vasodilators, diuretics, and other agents (Colucci, 2007a, 2007b; Fadol, 2006). Consultation with a cardiologist is appropriate in all patients with cardiac toxicities related to chemotherapy. Drug discontinuation is required during patient work-up of the cardiotoxic event (Floyd, Morgan, & Perry, 2007b). EKG, pulse oximetry, and chest x-ray should be performed.

Evaluation of Outcomes

Patient education is crucial to the safe management of patients receiving cardiotoxic therapy. Initial education and consent includes the acute and chronic cardiac toxicities and their signs and symptoms and the need for and importance of periodic cardiac testing. Therefore, patients need to understand and promptly report any signs and symptoms of cardiac toxicity, such as edema, shortness of breath, palpitations, exercise fatigue, or tachycardia. APNs promptly assess and evaluate cardiac function with a physical examination, history of symptoms and their exacerbation, vital signs, and prescribing cardiac tests such as EKG, MUGA scan, or echocardiogram along with blood tests.

Dosages of medications with known cardiotoxicity are monitored and should not exceed the lifetime cumulative dose. If the patient will benefit from ongoing treatment when the lifetime cumulative dose is reached, a cardiac protectant can be used. Earlier usage of cardiac protectants at lower lifetime cumulative doses should be considered if the patient is experiencing a decrease in LVEF.

The patient must have a cardiac history, physical assessment, and LVEF evaluation at baseline, prior to each dose of cardiotoxic drug, after therapy is completed, and at each appointment. All patients are assessed for preexisting cardiac disease. At the first sign of cardiac toxicity, prompt assessment and appropriate interventions should be undertaken to prevent further cardiac decompensation. This may require interruption or discontinuation of potentially useful anticancer therapy. The benefits of ongoing therapy must be weighed against the risk of worsening cardiac status or the development of life-threatening toxicity or death.

Implications for Advanced Nursing Practice

APNs must be knowledgeable about the risk of cardiac toxicity with all the anthracyclines, taxanes, monoclonal antibodies, and multiple other antineoplastic agents. Cardiac toxicities are cumulative for many of the agents. When used in combination with other cardiotoxic agents or radiation therapy to the chest, the toxicity is additive. Oncology APNs must perform a thorough baseline cardiac history and physical examination and continually assess patients for cardiac toxicity during therapy and long after, as toxicity can develop at any time during therapy or after its completion. Long-term survivors of testicular cancer therapy with cardiotoxic drugs are at an increased risk of developing cardiac events at younger ages than their healthy counterparts who did not receive cardiotoxic agents (van den Belt-Dusebout et al., 2006). Testicular cancer was treated with regimens containing dactinomycin (actinomycin D, Cosmegen®, Merck and Co., Inc.), vinblastine, bleomycin, or etoposide (VP-16, Etopophos®, Bristol-Myers Squibb Co.). Patients experienced cardiovascular disease as early as five years after treatment. Smoking increased the risk of myocardial infarction in the patients who received chemotherapy (van den Belt-Dusebout et al.).

Gastrointestinal Toxicities

Introduction

GI side effects and toxicities are extremely common in patients with cancer for a variety of reasons, including aggressive treatment regimens, the disease process, non-oncology-related medications, non-oncology-related medical or surgical comorbidities, anxiety or other psychosocial issues, and a variety of other etiologies (see Table 12-2).

Diagnosis and Assessment

The most common diagnostic test used to monitor GI side effects is the flat plate of the abdomen or kidneys-ureters-bladder x-rays to assess for bowel obstruction or other mechanical problems in the GI tract. An upper GI fluoroscopy with small bowel follow-through will assist in the diagnosis of bowel obstruction or other mechanical or physiologic problems in the GI tract. A computed tomography (CT) or magnetic resonance imaging (MRI) scan is used to evaluate the abdomen for pathology. A colonoscopy or upper endoscopy is used to examine the GI tract for causes of GI bleeding or to evaluate the patient for tumor. *Clostridium difficile* (*C. difficile*) in patients with diarrhea can be confirmed with a series of three stool specimens, although it often is diagnosed with the first specimen. In patients receiving fluorouracil with unexpected severe diarrhea, a test for dihydropyrimidine dehydrogenase deficiency is indicated. A deficit of this enzyme may interfere with the patient's ability to receive future therapy with fluorouracil. Suspicious oral lesions should be cultured for viruses, fungi, or both. APNs monitor the patient's renal function and fluid and electrolyte balance with daily lab work (basic metabolic panel with electrolytes and ions) to determine hydration and renal status and correct electrolyte imbalance. Vomiting and diarrhea often contribute to the fluid and electrolyte losses (Held-Warmkessel, 2006).

Table 12-2. Common Gastrointestinal Toxicities From Chemotherapy, Biotherapy, and Targeted Therapies

Characteristic	Anorexia	Taste Changes	Nausea and Vomiting	Stomatitis and Mucositis	Constipation	Diarrhea
Incidence	50%–70% of patients are affected	36%–71% of patients treated with chemotherapy	Common and variable	Common	40%–60%	Based on drug therapy but is common
Signs and symptoms	Loss of appetite Early satiety	Complaints about altered food tastes (too sweet, too bitter, has no taste, tastes like cardboard or metal)	Anticipatory, acute, delayed, and chronic nausea and emesis	May affect any area of the gastrointestinal (GI) tract from the mouth to the anus and any other mucous membranes in the body Patients develop pain or discomfort in the affected areas.	Straining Small, round stools Feeling that rectum still has stool Feeling of rectal blockage Less than 3 stools each week	Increase in frequency of stools Increase in liquid nature of stools
Risk factors	Psychosocial issues Head and neck cancer Gastric cancer Chronic nausea Gastroparesis Medications Comorbidities Other GI side effects or toxicities related to treatment or disease process Abdominal disease processes	Cancer diagnosis, especially head and neck cancer Chemotherapy (often related to cisplatin-based therapy or therapy with doxorubicin) Radiation therapy Transplantation Poor oral care Infections	Dependent on many variables, including drugs and use of combination therapy, dose intensity, other medications, other medical conditions, age, gender, anxiety and other psychosocial issues, use of alcohol, and aggressiveness of antiemetic regimen prior to therapy	Concurrent radiation therapy and chemotherapy Transplantation, especially with total body irradiation Prior poor oral hygiene Diagnosis of head and neck cancer, cancer of the esophagus or GI tract, or gynecologic malignancy Combination chemotherapy, especially regimens that include antimetabolites, such as 5-fluorouracil, or irinotecan	Opioid therapy Other medications Vinca alkaloids, especially vincristine Thalidomide Low-fiber diet Low fluid intake Lack of activity Diabetes Depression Autonomic nervous system toxicity Dehydration Abnormal electrolyte levels Irritable bowel syndrome	5-fluorouracil—dihydropyrimidine dehydrogenase deficiency increases the risk of 5-fluorouracil-induced toxicity. Irinotecan Topotecan Methotrexate Cisplatin Capecitabine Docetaxel Oxaliplatin Cytarabine Infection with C. difficile and other intestinal infections

(Continued on next page)

Table 12-2. Common Gastrointestinal Toxicities From Chemotherapy, Biotherapy, and Targeted Therapies (Continued)

Characteristic	Anorexia	Taste Changes	Nausea and Vomiting	Stomatitis and Mucositis	Constipation	Diarrhea
Risk factors (cont.)	Shortness of breath				Social problems such as inability to toilet in a timely manner	Diet, tube feedings Radiation therapy that includes the intestines in the portal Medical problems such as inflammatory bowel disease may worsen problem.
Etiology and pathophysiology	Multifactorial problem related to interleukin, tumor necrosis factor, cytokine and interferon production, resulting in altered GI function caused by dysfunction of the autonomic, peripheral, and central nervous system and alterations in hormone production that helps control	Related to multiple causes including treatment-induced damage to taste buds, taste receptors, and nerves that transmit taste and smell. May be related to presence of drugs in saliva.	Several neurotransmitters and their receptors are involved in the process of nausea and vomiting. Neurotransmitters include serotonin released from the GI tract and sending signals via the peripheral afferent pathway to the 5-hydroxytryptamine (5-HT) receptor. The chemoreceptor trigger zone (CTZ) in the brain is stimulated. Stimulation of the CTZ results in signals	A multistep process involving oxidative stress and the production of reactive oxygen species by radiation or chemotherapy, production of signaling factors, damage to DNA, cell death at the basal layer followed by proinflammatory cytokines, ulceration, and then healing.	Multifactorial problem related to prolongation of GI transit time, absorption of water, reduced fiber consumption, medications, reduced mobility, and comorbidities	Chemotherapy and radiation therapy damage the mucosal lining of the GI tract, reducing its absorptive capacity and resulting in short GI transit times for food and fluids, reduced nutrient and fluid absorption, and increased bowel output. Several types of diarrhea may develop, including acute, cholinergic, secretory, and chronic.

(Continued on next page)

Table 12-2. Common Gastrointestinal Toxicities From Chemotherapy, Biotherapy, and Targeted Therapies *(Continued)*

Characteristic	Anorexia	Taste Changes	Nausea and Vomiting	Stomatitis and Mucositis	Constipation	Diarrhea
Etiology and pathophysiology *(cont.)*	food consumption and energy use.		being sent to the vomiting center (VC) in the brain that precipitates vomiting. Other neurotransmitters include dopamine, histamine, and substance P, which play a role in delayed emesis.			
Prevention strategies	Dietary education and counseling by advanced practice nurses (APNs) and registered dietitians at diagnosis and as needed throughout cancer trajectory Dietary caloric and nutritional supplements Small, frequent meals. Avoid odors.	Patient education related to dietary manipulations, trying new foods and flavors, adding spices and herbs, and experimenting with new and familiar food choices Trying cool and cold foods and avoiding aversive odors	See American Society of Clinical Oncology guidelines (http://jop.stateaffiliates-asco.org/July06Issue/193.pdf).	See the 2005 MASCC/ISOO mucositis guidelines (www.mascc.org/media/Resource_centers/Guidelines_table_12_Oct_05.pdf). Oral care needs to be a routine part of patient care. Cryotherapy may be used with edatrexate or 5-fluorouracil based—therapy that does not contain oxaliplatin. Dental care, routine tooth cleansing and flossing, patient education, and bland rinses, such as saline and baking soda, are needed.	Patient education related to use of laxatives and stool softeners administered on a regular basis, dietary manipulations to increase fiber and fluid intake, and necessity of avoiding more than two days without having a stool	Patient education on use of loperamide for all patients starting irinotecan therapy Patient education for all patients at risk for diarrhea needs to include dietary manipulations to reduce fiber, information on maintenance of fluid and electrolyte balance, and signs and symptoms to report to healthcare provider.

(Continued on next page)

Table 12-2. Common Gastrointestinal Toxicities From Chemotherapy, Biotherapy, and Targeted Therapies (Continued)

Characteristic	Anorexia	Taste Changes	Nausea and Vomiting	Stomatitis and Mucositis	Constipation	Diarrhea
Prevention strategies (cont.)	Baseline nutritional assessments on all patients			All patients who will receive head and neck radiation therapy need pretreatment dental evaluation. Amifostine may be used with head and neck radiation therapy for reducing xerostomia. Palifermin is available for patients undergoing transplantation for a hematologic malignancy.		
Resources for APNs	Cochrane reviews (see Berenstein & Ortiz, 2005)		National Comprehensive Cancer Network guidelines (www.nccn.org) Oncology Nursing Society (ONS) Putting Evidence Into Practice® (PEP) card on nausea and vomiting (www.ons.org /outcomes/volume1/ nausea/pdf /nauseaPEPCard .pdf)	National Cancer Institute Physician Data Query (PDQ®) (www.cancer .gov/cancertopics/pdq /supportivecare /oralcomplications /healthprofessional /page5) ONS PEP card on mucositis (www.ons.org /outcomes/volume2 /mucositis/pdf /pepcardshort _mucositis.pdf)	Cochrane Collaboration (www .thecochranelibrary .com) ONS PEP card on constipation (www.ons .org/outcomes /volume2 /constipation/pdf /pepcardshort _constipation.pdf)	Cochrane Collaboration (www .thecochrane library.com)

Note. Based on information from Benson et al., 2004; Boccia, 2002; Comeau et al., 2001; Davis et al., 2004, 2006; Esper & Heidrich, 2005; Halmos & Eder, 2007; Hensley et al., 1999; Hesketh, 2007; Larsson et al., 2005; Mitchell, 2006; Poutanen & Simor, 2004; Rubenstein et al., 2004; Solomon & Cherny, 2006; Sonis et al., 2004; Spielberger et al., 2004; Stepp & Pakiz, 2001; Stern & Ippoliti, 2003; Tonini et al., 2005; Trotti et al., 2003; van Kuilenburg, 2004; Viele, 2003; Wickham et al., 1999; Yavuzsen et al., 2005.

Oncology APNs complete a thorough abdominal physical examination, including a rectal examination, on all patients with GI complaints. The history includes the onset, duration, precipitating factors, current medications, and any other methods patients have tried to manage the symptom at home. Patients should describe the volume, consistency, frequency, odor, and color of the stool or emesis. APNs also assess the patients' psychosocial situation and how it pertains to the GI problems. A symptom rating scale, such as the Common Terminology Criteria for Adverse Events (http://ctep.cancer.gov/forms/CTCAEv3.pdf) by the National Cancer Institute Cancer Therapy Evaluation Program (NCI CTEP, 2006), is used to rate the severity of the side effect and guide care based on severity. Differential diagnoses in patients with GI side effects include bowel obstruction or other bowel pathology in patients with nausea, vomiting, and constipation.

Evidence-Based Treatment Strategies

Pharmacologic measures are useful in patients with GI side effects. Anorexia may be treated with appetite stimulants, such as megestrol acetate 800 mg/day in liquid form (if tablets are used, usually four 80 mg tablets are prescribed) (Berenstein & Ortiz, 2005). Corticosteroids also are effective when used for two weeks or less, as their effectiveness decreases when used for longer periods of time and the side effects may outweigh the therapeutic benefits (Yavuzen, Davis, Walsh, LeGrand, & Lagman, 2005).

Nausea and vomiting are treated with antiemetics such as ondansetron (Zofran®, GlaxoSmithKline) or granisetron (Kyril®, Roche Laboratories). Additional rescue antiemetics should be available to patients. Dietary manipulations may be useful, such as allowing patients nothing by mouth, introducing clear liquids slowly after nausea resolves, avoiding malodorous foods and odors in the environment, and using a bland diet of room temperature or cold foods once solids are tolerated.

APNs treat therapy-induced diarrhea with standard doses of over-the-counter loperamide as per package instructions (4 mg after first diarrhea, 2 mg after each diarrhea episode, up to 16 mg/day) (Wilkes & Barton-Burke, 2007). Two types of diarrhea are associated with irinotecan. Acute diarrhea occurs within 24 hours of the infusion and is cholinergic in origin. It responds to atropine (Lomotil®, Pfizer Inc.) 0.25–1 mg IV or subcutaneous and may be prevented if atropine is given as a premedication in patients with prior early diarrhea (Wilkes & Barton-Burke). Late diarrhea (occurring 24 hours or more after irinotecan) is treated with aggressive loperamide therapy (4 mg after first evidence of diarrhea, followed by 2 mg every 2 hours until diarrhea-free for 12 hours; 4 mg can be used every 4 hours during the night) (Wilkes & Barton-Burke). Patients receiving a fluorouracil- or irinotecan-based regimen who develop diarrhea require oral loperamide therapy. Those with diarrhea for longer than 24 hours or those who are neutropenic also require an oral antibiotic, such as a fluoroquinolone for seven days (Rothenberg, Meropol, Poplin, Van Cutsem, & Wadler, 2001; Van Cutsem et al., 1999). Other antidiarrheal agents include octreotide (Sandostatin®, Novartis Pharmaceuticals Corp.) (100–150 mcg subcutaneously every eight hours or 25–50 mcg/hour as an IV infusion, dose titrated to response) or paregoric (5–10 ml orally, up to four times per day, titrated to patient response) (Benson et al., 2004). Loperamide is stopped when starting other agents, such as octreotide or paregoric. In addition to medication, dietary manipulations are necessary to manage diarrhea with medication because dietary manipulations alone are not effective for irinotecan-induced and other chemotherapy-induced diarrhea.

Sugar-free foods contain sugars that act like osmotic laxatives, worsen diarrhea, and should be avoided (Stern & Ippoliti, 2003). Modifying the diet to eliminate food items that worsen diarrhea, such as fiber, most dairy products (especially milk), caffeine, and fatty foods, which may increase intestinal motility, can help to control diarrhea (Osterlund et al., 2004).

In addition to chemotherapy-induced diarrhea, infectious diarrhea may occur in patients with cancer. The most common etiology is *C. difficile*, with an incidence of 7% in a group of neutropenic patients undergoing treatment for hematologic malignancies (Gorschluter et al., 2001). *C. difficile* is treated with oral metronidazole therapy for 10–14 days dosed at 250 mg four times a day or 500 mg twice a day, or vancomycin 125 mg four times a day (Fekety, 1997). Metronidazole is the drug of choice in patient treatment, with vancomycin used as second-line therapy for recurrent disease to reduce the risk of bacteria developing resistance to vancomycin (Gerding, Johnson, Peterson, Mulligan, & Silva, 1995; Surawicz et al., 2000). Investigation of a number of probiotic microorganisms has produced conflicting outcomes for their use in managing *C. difficile* infections. Oncology APNs should monitor the literature for a systematic review of currently available data to evaluate whether probiotics are appropriate in certain patients with cancer and *C. difficile* infections (Olmos, Berenstein, & Ortiz, 2006). For patients with diarrhea and vomiting and resultant dehydration, replacement of fluids and electrolytes should occur as needed (Stern & Ippoliti, 2003). All laxative therapy is stopped in patients with diarrhea. Patients also might benefit from dietary manipulations used in patients with chemotherapy-induced diarrhea, such as consuming a low-fiber, low-lactose diet.

Constipation is treated with laxatives, stool softeners, suppositories, and enemas (Solomon & Cherny, 2006). For patients on opioid therapy or vincristine, laxatives and stool softeners are required on an ongoing basis. Increasing the fiber and fluid consumed in the diet may assist with managing constipation, but most patients with cancer require laxatives. An effective laxative is polyethylene glycol, which has better tolerability and efficacy than lactulose (Attar et al., 1999). Other laxatives have been studied, but limited evidence exists to support recommending specific laxatives or laxative combinations (Miles, Fellowes, Goodman, & Wilkinson, 2007). Additional interventions include increasing fluid consumption, ambulation, and other activities to promote bowel function (Cope, 2001).

Early-stage mucositis is treated with aggressive oral care, including saline rinses, flossing the teeth, and frequent brushing. In addition, pain is controlled with opioids, as needed, and application of mucosal protective agents, such as Gelclair® (Helsinn Healthcare SA), before meals or as often as four times a day (Buchsel, 2003; Rubenstein et al., 2004).

Evaluation of Outcomes

APNs monitor patients to minimize and prevent GI side effects and toxicities and to minimize their effects if they occur. The prevention or treatment of side effect recurrence with additional and ongoing therapy needs to be considered.

Implications for Advanced Nursing Practice

GI toxicities and side effects are common reactions to treatment. APNs need to manage GI side effects aggressively to achieve a positive outcome in the patient's quality of life. Consultation with a gastroenterologist may be appropriate for patients who do not respond to treatment as expected.

Neurotoxicities

Introduction

Neuropathies are a common, often expected, and dose-limiting side effect of several commonly used antineoplastics. Several types of neuropathies and neurotoxicities are well described in the literature and are summarized in Table 12-3. Baseline neurologic assessments and ongoing patient monitoring for the early onset of signs and symptoms of neurotoxicity should be performed prior to each dose of potentially neurotoxic therapy to provide for safe patient care.

Education for patients and families promotes self-care, which allows patients to take control of the side effects by avoiding precipitating events whenever possible. In addition, education allows patients to manage and report uncommon but potentially frightening toxicities. Many neurotoxicities, such as peripheral neuropathy, may be annoying but are reversible; however, others, such as leukoencephalopathy, are potentially life threatening.

Definition

Peripheral neuropathy occurs in several forms (see Table 12-3). Sensory neuropathy is the most common form (Hausheer, Schilsky, Bain, Berghorn, & Lieberman, 2006). It usually is bilateral and manifests as numbness and tingling in the feet and then the hands in a stocking-glove distribution with an ascending pattern. Sensation and vibration sense are altered, and pain may be present. The loss of deep tendon reflexes indicates greater toxicity (Hausheer et al.). Motor neuropathy is less common and causes motor weakness (Wickham, 2007). Acute neuropathy has an abrupt onset and may resolve between treatments. Chronic and cumulative toxicity has a more gradual onset and takes longer to resolve. The incidence of peripheral neuropathies varies widely depending on the drugs administered. Certain agents, such as oxaliplatin (Eloxatin®, Sanofi-Aventis), are associated with peripheral neuropathy, which is a dose-limiting toxicity. Other drugs commonly associated with peripheral neuropathy are cisplatin (Platinol®, Bristol-Myers Squibb Co.), the vinca alkaloids, especially vincristine, and the taxanes. Risk factors for developing peripheral neuropathies include receiving vinca alkaloids, platinum compounds, taxanes, high cumulative doses, and short intervals between drug doses (Hildebrand, 2006). Gregg et al. (1992) studied cisplatin-induced peripheral neurotoxicity. Cisplatin may cause sensory peripheral neuropathy by entering into and accumulating in the dorsal root ganglia, where it interferes with cell functioning, promotes apoptosis, and produces sensory neuropathy. Grolleau et al. (2001) discovered that oxaliplatin binds to calcium and affects nerve sodium currents resulting in peripheral neuropathy (Krishnan, Goldstein, Friedlander, & Kiernan, 2005). Vincristine-induced peripheral neuropathy is thought to develop from the disruption of tubulin, causing axonal degeneration (Peltier & Russell, 2002; Silva, Wang, Wang, Ravula, & Glass, 2006).

Central nervous system neurotoxicities are serious but occur less frequently than peripheral neurotoxicities. Metabolic encephalopathy, meningitis, leukoencephalopathy, seizures, and other toxicities have been reported (see Table 12-3). Drugs associat-

Table 12-3. Types of Neurotoxicities Associated With Chemotherapy, Biotherapy, and Targeted Therapies

Type of Neurotoxicity	Area Affected	Signs and Symptoms
Cerebellar	Cerebellum	Ataxia Diplopia Dysarthria Confusion Paresthesias Memory loss Unsteady gait Problems speaking Changes in reflexes Change in mental status
Peripheral	Peripheral, cranial, and spinal nerves	Paralysis Altered motor function Altered sensory function, such as loss of heat and cold sensation, vibration, and pain Loss of reflexes, such as deep tendon reflexes Neuropathies may be progressive with drug interruption or discontinuation. Patients may have feeling of "pins and needles" in the stocking-glove distribution of the hands and feet, weakness, loss of muscle function, or loss of sensation or vibration. Often starts distally and ascends up extremity. Pain, such as myalgia, may occur. May range in severity from mild to severe Large-fiber toxicity causes altered proprioception and altered sense of vibration. Small-fiber neurotoxicity causes pain and altered temperature sensation.
Autonomic	Autonomic nervous system	Altered cardiac, vascular, gastrointestinal, respiratory, or endocrine function. Patients may experience constipation, ileus, erectile dysfunction, urinary retention, and postural hypotension.
Central	Metabolic encephalopathy	Coma Seizures Lethargy Paranoia Delusions Sleepiness Confusion Nightmares Restlessness Hallucinations Urinary incontinence Sedation, drowsiness Altered vision (blurred) Altered motor function Altered thought processes Altered cranial nerve function

(Continued on next page)

Table 12-3. Types of Neurotoxicities Associated With Chemotherapy, Biotherapy, and Targeted Therapies *(Continued)*

Type of Neurotoxicity	Area Affected	Signs and Symptoms
Central	Leukoencephalopathy	Stupor Nausea Aphasia Seizures Vomiting Lethargy Agitation Headache Confusion Proteinuria Altered speech Neurologic deficits Vision loss/blindness Altered mental status Sudden increase in blood pressure
Central	Meningitis	Fever Nausea Vomiting Headache Change in level of consciousness

Note. Based on information from Allen et al., 2006; Camp-Sorrell, 2005; Donegan, 2001; Garg, 2001; Hildebrand, 2006; Hinchey et al., 1996; Sul & DeAngelis, 2006; Videnovic et al., 2005.

ed with central toxicities are cytarabine, methotrexate, ifosfamide (Ifex®, Bristol-Myers Squibb Co.), and interferon (Roferon-A®, Roche Laboratories) (see Table 12-4). The drug or its metabolites crossing the blood-brain barrier cause central neurotoxicities. Ifosfamide metabolites include chloracetaldehyde, which causes confusion, lethargy, and other changes in mental status (Brade, Herdrich, & Varini, 1985). Intracarotid drug administration also causes a higher incidence of central neurotoxicities.

Presenting Signs and Symptoms

The common signs and symptoms are discussed previously and in Table 12-3. Patients may present with complaints such as numbness, tingling, burning, and loss of or reduced sensations of touch or vibration (Hausheer et al., 2006; Visovsky, 2006). Some patients describe the sensation as being similar to that of one's hands or feet "falling asleep." Patients may shake their hands, thinking that the symptoms are related to impaired blood flow. Symptoms typically begin distally and ascend proximally, appearing in the feet first. Accompanying reductions in reflexes, such as deep tendon reflexes, reflect more toxicity (Hausheer et al.).

Risk Factors

Preexisting diseases and combination therapy with known neurotoxic side effects may precipitate and exacerbate peripheral neuropathy. Older patients (those older than 65)

Table 12-4. Neurotoxicities Associated With Chemotherapy, Biotherapy, and Targeted Therapies

Drug	Side Effect/Toxicity	Nursing Implications
Asparaginase	Encephalopathy Cerebellar dysfunction	Both are common.
Bevacizumab	Leukoencephalopathy (headache, seizure, lethargy, changes in mental status such as confusion, blindness, other vision abnormalities)	Discontinue agent. Monitor patient for improvement in symptoms and treat hypertension if present. With symptom resolution, evidence is lacking to support restarting therapy.
Bortezomib	Peripheral neuropathy	Incidence is greater at doses of 1.3 mg/m². Severity usually is mild to moderate but may be moderately severe. Dose reductions or treatment discontinuation may be needed to reduce severity. Severity may be increased in patients with baseline peripheral neuropathy.
Capecitabine	Leukoencephalopathy	Toxicity differs from 5-fluorouracil neurotoxicity. Discontinue agent. Improvement is seen in several days.
Carboplatin	Sensory neuropathy	Resulting neuropathy is similar to cisplatin neuropathy.
Cisplatin	Large peripheral nerve fibers affected, causing peripheral neuropathy. Loss of sensation with stocking-glove distribution. Loss of proprioception and ataxia High-frequency hearing loss Lhermitte symptom Vestibulopathy (vertigo, ataxia, seeing objects move), neuritis, and other neurotoxicities have been rarely reported. Encephalopathy with intracarotid administration	Neuropathy seen at cumulative doses of 300–500 mg/m². Risk factors include dose, length of therapy, and administration schedule. Usual pattern of presentation is gradual. May worsen after therapy is stopped and usually improves with time.
Cytarabine, high-dose	Cerebellar toxicity (common) Seizures Altered mental status Peripheral neuropathy	Assess cerebellar toxicity at baseline and prior to each dose. Hold doses for changes in cerebellar function until able to perform neurologic assessment. Toxicity usually resolves with stopping therapy. Reduce dose in older adults or those with hepatic or renal dysfunction.

(Continued on next page)

Table 12-4. Neurotoxicities Associated With Chemotherapy, Biotherapy, and Targeted Therapies *(Continued)*

Drug	Side Effect/Toxicity	Nursing Implications
Liposome for intrathecal use (DepoCyt®, Enzon Pharmaceuticals, Inc.) formulation	Encephalopathy with intrathecal administration Sustained-release formulation for intrathecal administration causes aseptic meningitis, chemical arachnoiditis.	Administer with dexamethasone 4 mg bid (IV or oral) starting on day of administration, and continue for a total of 5 days, unless contraindicated.
Etoposide	Seizures Confusion Peripheral neuropathy	Uncommon, usually mild. Assess for altered sensory and motor function prior to each cycle of therapy.
5-fluorouracil	Seizures Encephalopathy Cerebellar toxicity Other rare side effects	Stop therapy. Steroids may be useful. Toxicity may be related to dihydropyrimidine dehydrogenase deficiency and may respond to high dose of IV thymidine.
Ifosfamide	Encephalopathy, especially with higher doses Change in mental status Wide range of alterations in mentation may be seen, from mild confusion to profound obtundation. Variable onset from hours to weeks after dosing. Usually reversible 2–3 days after drug discontinuation. Incidence of toxicity is 10%–50%. May occur with any cycle of therapy but more frequent with early cycles Toxicity results from drug metabolites crossing the blood-brain barrier.	Hold doses for changes in mental status until able to perform neurologic assessment. Ensure adequate hydration and the presence of normal renal function, both of which are needed to enhance excretion of drug metabolite (chloracetaldehyde and thialysine ketamine) that is responsible for altered mentation prior to prescribing ifosfamide. Other risk factors for encephalopathy are length of administration, rate of infusion (increased with bolus infusion), route of administration (higher with oral route), presence of acidosis, impaired liver function, prior cisplatin therapy, bulky abdominal disease, medications, poor performance status, and low serum albumin. With the development of neurotoxicity, maintain hydration, hold ifosfamide, provide supportive care, and monitor neurologic status. Methylene blue IV at a dose of 1 mg/kg in a dextrose solution for high-risk patients with grade III–IV neurotoxicity or patients with recurrent neurotoxicity who need ifosfamide therapy may reduce the signs and symptoms. Administer concurrently with oral glucose supplements or IV dextrose solution. Retreat as needed. Exact frequency of dosing or how long to continue therapy is not known. Available as an oral preparation also; administer with glucose. In patients who would benefit from ongoing ifosfamide therapy, consider prophylactic administration of methylene blue.
	Peripheral neuropathy	–

(Continued on next page)

Table 12-4. Neurotoxicities Associated With Chemotherapy, Biotherapy, and Targeted Therapies *(Continued)*

Drug	Side Effect/Toxicity	Nursing Implications
Interferon	Seizures Lethargy Dementia Depression Headaches Multiple neuropsychiatric side effects are reported.	Patient education and assessment are crucial in the management of neuropsychiatric side effects. Patients need to understand that they are related to therapy and need to be assessed for depression and other neuropsychiatric problems at baseline and throughout therapy. Referral to social services or psychiatry is appropriate at the first sign of depression or if present at baseline. Neuropsychiatric toxicity requires stopping therapy. If restarted, toxicity may recur. Risk is greater in patients with prior neurologic or psychiatric diagnosis.
Interleukin	Neuropsychiatric	Side effects are expected, especially with higher doses. Effects are reversible.
Methotrexate	Seizures Myelopathy Nerve palsy Leukoencephalopathy Lumbosacral radiculopathy Encephalopathy from high-dose IV therapy Meningitis (aseptic) or arachnoiditis from intrathecal therapy	Consider steroid premedications. Several types of neurotoxicity occur, including acute, subacute, and delayed.
Oxaliplatin	Peripheral neuropathy, especially sensory, is expected. Occurs **acutely** and often suddenly after treatment, is precipitated by exposure to cold, and is common and expected. Resolves to some extent between cycles of therapy. Affects hands, feet, digits, lips, mouth, and throat. May develop during infusion or up to 2 weeks after. Severity usually is mild to moderate. Cumulative **chronic and persistent** sensory neuropathy also occurs at doses ≥ 540 mg/m². Fine motor movement may be affected. Reversible 6–8 months after therapy is completed. Neuropathy may be dose limiting. It may develop or worsen after treatment is completed.	Patient education is crucial for self-care, avoidance of precipitating factors, and management at home, as neuropathy is an **expected** side effect. Patients need to avoid cold air, cold foods, and cold liquids. Patients should keep hands and feet warm and avoid exposure to cold air.

(Continued on next page)

Table 12-4. Neurotoxicities Associated With Chemotherapy, Biotherapy, and Targeted Therapies *(Continued)*

Drug	Side Effect/Toxicity	Nursing Implications
	Acute laryngopharyngeal dysesthesias occur with exposure to cold. Patients may feel like they cannot breathe, but can, and may feel tightening of the throat or have trouble speaking or swallowing. Myotonia (inability to let go of an object) also is precipitated by the cold.	Patients can breathe on hands to feel movement of air to reduce anxiety induced by feeling of not being able to breathe. Increase infusion length to 6 hours to prevent laryngopharyngeal dysesthesia. Incidence is lower.
Procarbazine	Confusion Hallucinations Peripheral neuropathy	—
Rituximab	Leukoencephalopathy	—
Steroids	Mania Psychoses Myopathy Depression Encephalopathy	—
Tamoxifen	Headache Ischemic stroke	—
Taxanes (docetaxel, all formulations of paclitaxel)	Seizures Transient encephalopathy Peripheral sensory neuropathy Large-fiber sensory neuropathy develops at paclitaxel doses of ≥ 250 mg/m². Tends to be cumulative but may be reversible when mild. Higher doses may cause autonomic neurotoxicity. Affects legs more than upper extremities Occasionally affects motor function and autonomic function	Amitriptyline may be useful for sensory neuropathy. Paclitaxel causes more peripheral neuropathy than docetaxel. No effective treatment is known. Usually resolves with time. Greater risk of paclitaxel toxicity with higher cumulative doses, high doses over short infusion times, weekly dosing, preexisting neuropathies or cisplatin exposure, either prior or concurrent.
Thalidomide	Peripheral neuropathy (often begins after 1 year of therapy but may develop more acutely) Neuronopathy (early presentation)	May not be reversible. Dose-limiting toxicity. May develop after therapy is stopped. Treatment may need to be stopped at onset of peripheral neuropathy to prevent additional damage to nerves. Benefit of continuing therapy needs to be weighed against toxicity.

(Continued on next page)

Table 12-4. Neurotoxicities Associated With Chemotherapy, Biotherapy, and Targeted Therapies *(Continued)*

Drug	Side Effect/Toxicity	Nursing Implications
	Lethargy Sleepiness	Dose at bedtime.
Vinblastine	Peripheral neuropathy Affects legs more than upper extremities	–
Vincristine	Peripheral neuropathy (common), including cranial nerve involvement (rare) Affects legs more than upper extremities, with loss of deep tendon reflexes Progresses if therapy not stopped	Dose per week is capped at 2 mg. Do not prescribe doses of more than 2 mg/week, and question any dose of more than 2 mg/week. Older patients are less tolerant. May worsen after therapy is stopped. Usually is reversible. Peripheral neuropathy usually is seen after dose 3–4 of therapy (each a 2 mg dose or 6–8 mg cumulative dosing), worsens with cumulative doses of 15–20 mg, and produces paralysis at cumulative doses of > 30 mg.
	Autonomic neuropathy (constipation, abdominal pain, syncope, orthostatic hypotension)	Include bowel regimen, including a laxative and stool softener, in patients' therapy, as constipation is an expected side effect.
	Encephalopathy Ataxia Other neurotoxicities are reported.	
Vinorelbine	Peripheral neuropathy Affects legs more than upper extremities	–

Note. Based on information from Allen et al., 2006; Berg, 2003; Cain & Bender, 1995; Camp-Sorrell, 2005; Cavaliere & Schiff, 2006; Cersosimo, 2005; Craig, 2000; Denicoff et al., 1987; Diaz et al., 1998; Donegan, 2001; Extra et al., 1998; Furlong, 1993; Gamelin et al., 2004; Genentech BioOncology, 2006a; Glantz et al., 1999; Hausheer et al., 2006; Hensley et al., 2000; Hildebrand, 2006; Klastersky, 2003; Meanwell et al., 1986; Patel, 2006; Plotkin & Wen, 2003; Raymond et al., 1998; Richardson et al., 2006; Sul & DeAngelis, 2006; Trobaugh-Lotrario et al., 2003; Videnovic et al., 2005; Wilkes & Barton-Burke, 2007.

experience a decline in nerve function as a result of the aging process (Visovsky, 2006). Peripheral neuropathy develops in patients when cumulative doses of neurotoxic agents are reached. Cumulative doses leading to neurotoxicities vary with each agent, but in some patients, peripheral neuropathy may develop prior to reaching the cumulative dose. Risk factors that have been identified are included in Table 12-4.

Etiology and Pathophysiology

The exact etiology of peripheral neuropathy is not well understood. Hausheer et al. (2006) hypothesized that because the nerve cell bodies of the peripheral motor axons are within the blood-brain barrier, they are protected from antineoplastic agent injury, unlike the efferent portions of the peripheral motor axons, which lie outside the blood-brain barrier. The motor nerves also are less affected because they have more myelin protection than the smaller-diameter sensory nerves. Cisplatin probably causes peripheral neuropathy by inducing sensory nerve apoptosis (Gill & Windebank, 1998).

Prevention

Prompt interruption or discontinuation of therapy, dose reductions, or dose delays may be necessary to manage certain toxicities. This must always be weighed against the benefits of ongoing therapy. No agents are approved by the U.S. Food and Drug Administration (FDA) for the prevention of neurotoxicities, but the following agents have been studied in the prevention of peripheral neuropathy: glutamine (Vahdat et al., 2001); calcium and magnesium supplements administered intravenously prior to and after oxaliplatin (Gamelin et al., 2004); glutathione (Cascinu et al., 2002); and amifostine (Ethyol®, MedImmune Oncology, Inc.) (Hilpert et al., 2005). Studies were either retrospective (Gamelin et al.), had a small number of participants and therefore were not generalizable (Cascinu et al.; Hilpert et al.), or were not randomized (Vahdat et al.). Glutathione does not appear to interfere with the antineoplastic activity of oxaliplatin (Cascinu et al.). A study using calcium and magnesium supplements administered intravenously prior to and after oxaliplatin in patients receiving oxaliplatin (as part of the FOLFOX with bevacizumab regimen) was halted because the outcomes for the patients who received the infusions were worse in terms of response rate than for the patients who did not receive the infusions (Hochster, Grothey, & Childs, 2007).

Diagnosis and Assessment

No commonly used and reliable diagnostic tests exist for peripheral neuropathy. Tests to assess central neurotoxicity include CT, MRI, electroencephalogram, and lumbar puncture. Complete and thorough neurologic examinations are needed for safe patient care when treatment plans include neurotoxic agents. Physical examination and history are performed at baseline, throughout therapy, and minimally before each dose of treatment to assess for central and peripheral neuropathy. APNs assess the severity and impact of the neurotoxicity on patients' quality of life and ability to function in daily life. The severity of the impairment is weighed against the benefits and risks of continued therapy, dose reductions, or treatment breaks. To assist in testing quality-of-life issues, the APN may ask the patient to perform common activities, such as writing his or her name, picking up small objects, buttoning buttons, and walking (Cersosimo, 2005; Visovsky, 2006). Altered walking with ataxia or an abnormal Romberg test may be present related to peripheral neuropathy (Hausheer et al., 2006). Reflexes and mental status also should be monitored. Symptom rating scales, such as the NCI CTEP (2006) Common Terminology Criteria for Adverse Events, are available to rate the toxicity. Quality-of-life assessment tools for neurotoxicity may be found at www.facit.org /about/overview_measure.aspx.

APNs also should consider differential diagnoses in patients with neurotoxicity. Diabetes-induced peripheral neuropathy requires documentation of baseline signs and symptoms because chemotherapy-induced peripheral neuropathy and diabetes-induced peripheral neuropathy produce similar symptoms (Hausheer et al., 2006). Paraneoplastic syndromes may produce central or peripheral neurotoxicities (Honnorat & Cartalat-Carel, 2006). Small cell lung cancer is associated with a number of paraneoplastic syndromes that may have signs and symptoms similar to chemotherapy-induced neurotoxicities. Examples include hyponatremia-induced altered mental status changes and Lambert-Eaton myasthenic syndrome (Ghandi & Johnson, 2006). Lambert-Eaton myasthenic syndrome produces signs and symptoms such as reduced deep tendon reflexes (Lambert, Eaton, & Rooke, 1956). Lymphomas may affect cranial nerves or nerve roots either through direct growth or paraneoplastic syndromes (Glass, 2006). Postural hypotension can occur from autonomic nervous system dysfunction (Glass). Spinal cord compression causes localized back pain, nerve root pain, and altered sensory and motor function below the area of the compression. If undiagnosed and untreated, spinal cord compression can progress to paralysis with significant morbidity, including incontinence, skin breakdown, and other hazards of immobility. Alcohol abuse and resultant malnutrition can cause peripheral neuropathies. Altered electrolyte levels, such as hypocalcemia, may produce signs and symptoms that mimic peripheral neuropathy. Hypercalcemia may cause altered mental status, seizures, and altered reflexes (Richardson, 2004).

Evidence-Based Treatment Strategies

At present, no results exist from prospective randomized trials of any agents to treat peripheral neuropathy (Hausheer et al., 2006). However, a number of studies currently are enrolling patients, so APNs should monitor the literature for new developments. Symptom management and treatment of painful sensory peripheral neuropathies is important for patients' quality of life. Agents used to manage pain include gabapentinoid anticonvulsants, opioids, and antidepressants (Shaiova, 2006).

An antidepressant, such as the tricyclic antidepressant desipramine, titrated to the patient's individual needs is effective in the relief of neuropathic pain caused by diabetes (Max et al., 1992). Based on clinical trials in patients with and without cancer who have neuropathic pain, tricyclic antidepressants often are used in cancer pain management (McDonald & Portenoy, 2006). Effective tricyclic agents other than desipramine include amitriptyline and nortriptyline. A 2005 review of antidepressants for neuropathic pain showed that tricyclic antidepressants are effective in the treatment of neuropathic pain, and amitriptyline was the most effective (Saarto & Wiffen, 2005). APNs may select the agent based on the side effect profile for the patient. If a sedative effect is desired, amitriptyline may be chosen for bedtime administration, but if a dry mouth is to be avoided, a different tricyclic antidepressant is a better choice. For patients with medical problems, nortriptyline or desipramine are better choices, and amitriptyline should be avoided because of its side effects, which include cardiotoxicity, hypotension, and altered mental status (McDonald & Portenoy; Preskorn & Irwin, 1982). The serotonin reuptake inhibitors do not have analgesic properties for the treatment of neuropathic pain (Shaiova) and have limited evidence of effectiveness in pain management (McDonald & Portenoy).

The other category of antidepressants, the norepinephrine reuptake inhibitors, such as venlafaxine and duloxetine (Cymbalta®, Eli Lilly and Co.), have shown evidence of analgesic activity (McDonald & Portenoy, 2006). One study evaluated the use of venlafaxine in patients who had breast cancer and post-treatment neuropathic pain (Tasmuth, Hartel, & Kalso, 2002). Only 13 patients were accrued to the study, and the patients' pain was not reduced, but the pain relief diary and the computer analysis of the maximum pain intensity showed reduction in pain (Tasmuth et al.). Other studies in patients with painful neuropathy showed that venlafaxine was comparable in efficacy to the tricyclic antidepressant imipramine or to gabapentin (Neurontin®, Pfizer Inc.) (Rowbotham, Goli, Kunz, & Lei, 2004; Sindrup, Bach, Madsen, Gram, & Jensen, 2003). Duloxetine is FDA approved for the treatment of neuropathic pain and has better evidence of analgesic activity (McDonald & Portenoy). The drug has been studied in a variety of patients with depression. Furthermore, an evaluation of the cardiotoxic effects on the patients in those studies showed that it has no clinically significant cardiovascular side effects (Wernicke, Lledo, Raskin, Kajdasz, & Wang, 2007). Another antidepressant that may be useful for neuropathic pain management is bupropion. It blocks the reuptake of norepinephrine. Side effects include insomnia, tremor, headache, dizziness, and GI problems, such as constipation and dry mouth (Semenchuk & Davis, 2000; Semenchuk, Sherman, & Davis, 2001). In patients with a variety of neuropathic pain problems, bupropion sustained-release (150–300 mg/day) significantly reduced pain (Semenchuk et al.).

Anticonvulsants also are used to manage painful neuropathies. Gabapentin (Neurontin) administered in doses titrated to the pain caused by cancer treatment or by the cancer itself is effective (Ross et al., 2005). Caraceni et al. (2004) administered doses ranging from 600–1,800 mg/day to patients with neuropathic cancer pain who were already receiving opioids. The patients receiving both an opioid and gabapentin had statistically significant better pain control than the patients on opioids alone.

Additionally, opioids, such as oxycodone, are useful in the management of diabetic neuropathic pain (Gimbel, Richards, & Portenoy, 2003; Watson, Moulin, Watt-Watson, Gordon, & Eisenhoffer, 2003). The combination of morphine and gabapentin was better than either drug alone in reducing pain in patients with diabetic or postherpetic neuralgia (Gilron et al., 2005). Pregabalin (Lyrica®, Pfizer Inc.) is a drug similar to gabapentin and is useful in the management of neuropathic pain (Zareba, 2005). Side effects include dizziness, peripheral edema, weight gain, and somnolence (Freynhagen, Strojek, Griesing, Whalen, & Balkenohl, 2005). Doses were titrated to patient tolerance, and efficacy with pain relief was evident by the end of the first week of treatment (Freynhagen et al.).

Evaluation of Outcomes

APNs continuously monitor patients' neurologic status for the exacerbation or remission of peripheral neuropathy related to cancer therapies. Antineoplastic therapy is tailored to the patients' specific needs and problems caused by the cancer and resultant peripheral neuropathy side effects. Options include dose reductions, therapy interruptions or breaks, discontinuation of therapy, or participation in a supportive clinical trial to address neuropathy.

Implications for Advanced Nursing Practice

As neurotoxicities are common and often expected side effects of therapy, APNs must build routine evaluation of peripheral, cranial, and spinal nerves and central nervous system function into standard assessment and patient screening for toxicity and side effects.

Patient education is crucial to self-care. As such, it must be instituted with therapy and continued throughout therapy and after completion. Moreover, APNs need to be familiar with the medications used for symptom management to enhance quality of life.

Ocular Toxicities

Introduction

Ocular signs and symptoms in patients with cancer may be related to current or prior drug therapy (cancer therapy or other medications), blood or marrow transplantation, radiation therapy that includes the eye and its structures in the radiation field, paraneoplastic syndromes, preexisting ocular or connective tissue diseases, presence of contact lenses, a primary tumor of the eye, or metastases to the eye (Edman, Larsen, Hagglund, & Gardulf, 2001; Ling & Pavesio, 2003; Maher, 2005; Rudberg, Carlsson, Nilsson, & Wikblad, 2002).

Incidence

Primary tumors and eye metastases are uncommon. The majority of metastatic tumors are from breast, lung, intestinal, or prostate primaries (Wilmer Eye Institute at Johns Hopkins, n.d.). Primary retinoblastomas occur in 500–600 children each year, and melanoma of the eye occurs in 1,500–2,000 people each year (Wilmer Eye Institute at Johns Hopkins). Contact lenses are commonly worn and should always be considered as a cause of ocular toxicity. Ocular side effects and toxicities produced by cancer therapy are anticipated from antineoplastic drugs such as methotrexate, docetaxel, cytarabine, and fluorouracil or from the newer antiepidermal growth factor receptor agents. Examples of ocular signs and symptoms and toxicities include cataract development, blurred vision, night blindness, retinopathy, retinal bleeding, retinal hemorrhage, conjunctivitis, keratoconjunctivitis, neurotoxicity producing ocular signs and symptoms, excessive tearing caused by blocked tear ducts (epiphora), dry eyes, vision loss, and abnormal eyelash growth causing ocular irritation (al-Tweigeri, Nabholtz, & Mackey, 1996).

Presenting Signs and Symptoms

Patients may have an acute, gradual, or delayed onset of signs and symptoms. Examples include the development of eye pain and irritation up to a week after treatment with high-dose cytarabine, the development of epiphora after several weekly doses of docetaxel therapy, or the development of eye problems years after treatment for testicular cancer (Burstein et al., 2000; Hopen, Mondino, Johnson, & Chervenick, 1981; Rudberg et al., 2002). Signs and symptoms can develop during or after therapy. Ocular symptoms may be so subtle that the patient ignores or does not report them. Patients may not have access to APNs, and symptoms may go unrecognized. When symptoms are identified, they may not be reversible (Schmid, Kornek, Scheithauer, & Binder, 2006). Common presenting signs and symptoms of ocular toxicity include excess tearing, changes in vision, blurred vision, loss of vision, long or abnormally curly eyelashes, eye pain, eye crusting, reduced color vision, inflamed conjunctiva, inflamed ocular mucous membranes, pupil size change, red eye, change in intraocular pressure, inability to tolerate contact lenses, and photophobia (al-Tweigeri et al., 1996; Schmid et al.). Many ocular toxicities and side effects are reversible when diagnosed early and treatment is initiated. It may be necessary to discontinue the causative agent when the side effect is identified to avoid causing additional injury to the eyes. The length of time prior to the onset of problems varies by causative agent. Risk factors include drugs that affect eye metabolism or its function, irritate the eye, or cause corneal deposits or bleeding, such as antineoplastics, anticholinergics, and hormones.

Etiology

Chemotherapy, hormonal therapy, and targeted therapies (see Table 12-5) are known to produce ocular side effects. Methotrexate and docetaxel are excreted in the patients' tears and are a likely cause of ocular toxicities seen in patients undergoing therapy with these agents (Doroshow et al., 1981; Esmaeli et al., 2002). Fluorouracil is excreted in the tears, but its relationship to tearing, itching, and burning sensations is unclear (Loprinzi, Love, Garrity, & Ames, 1990). Fluorouracil may produce canalicular obstruction by causing squamous cell metaplasia resulting in excess tearing (Agarwal, Esmaeli, & Burnstine, 2002) and also may cause altered eye motor function as a result of cerebellar toxicity (Bixenman, Nicholls, & Warwick, 1977). High-dose cytarabine produces keratitis in 40%–100% of patients treated. The cause is unclear but may be related to damage to the corneal epithelium (al-Tweigeri et al., 1996; Hopen et al., 1981) or from high drug levels in the cerebrospinal fluid achieved after IV therapy (Slevin, Piall, Aherne, Johnston, & Lister, 1983). Tamoxifen (Nolvadex®, AstraZeneca Pharmaceuticals) produced drug depositions on the cornea in 72% of patients studied (Muftuoglu, Ucakhan, & Kanpolat, 2006).

Table 12-5. Ocular Side Effects and Toxicities Associated With Chemotherapy, Hormonal Therapy, and Targeted Therapy

Drug	Toxicities and Side Effects	Additional Nursing Implications
Antiandrogens (also see nilutamide); anti–luteinizing hormone-releasing hormone agents; finasteride; androgen deficiency	Eye pain Dry eyes Blurred vision Photosensitivity	Artificial tears may be useful for dry eye. Provide patient safety education for blurred vision and other ocular side effects.
BCNU/carmustine	Blurred vision Conjunctival hyperemia Multiple additional commonly occurring side effects associated with intracarotid administration Combination chemotherapy with cisplatin and cyclophosphamide is reported to cause vision loss and microvascular changes, such as retinal hemorrhage.	Intracarotid administration is associated with additional acute and delayed side effects that can be prevented by catheter advancement beyond the ophthalmic artery.
Busulfan	Cataracts Blurred vision Keratoconjunctivitis sicca	Cataracts increase in frequency and severity with dose and length of therapy.

(Continued on next page)

Table 12-5. Ocular Side Effects and Toxicities Associated With Chemotherapy, Hormonal Therapy, and Targeted Therapy *(Continued)*

Drug	Toxicities and Side Effects	Additional Nursing Implications
Capecitabine	Irritation Case studies of reversible corneal deposits and reduced vision.	Toxicity is seen in about 10% of patients. Prior history of keratoconjunctivitis may place patients at risk.
Carboplatin	Rare and reversible side effects with IV administration may include blindness or blurred vision. Mostly associated with intracarotid administration.	Effects not reported to be dose-limiting toxicities, as they were reversible.
Cetuximab	Blepharitis Trichomegaly Conjunctivitis Squamous blepharitis (tearing, itching, photophobia, crusting, feeling of foreign body in eye)	Eyelashes may grow to the extent that they interfere with vision and require cutting. Topical antibiotics for blepharitis and a treatment break may be needed.
Chlorambucil	Keratitis Other rare side effects such as diplopia	Occur after long-term use of agent
Cisplatin	May be related to neurotoxicity. Variety of potentially reversible toxicities reported, including neuritis, blurred vision, and blindness. High-dose therapy is associated with irreversible vision changes, including changes in color vision. Ocular pigment changes are not reversible. Toxicities are associated with all routes of administration, including IV and intracarotid administration. Intracarotid administration may be associated with ocular vascular changes causing ocular toxicity and vision changes.	High-dose and intracarotid drug administrations are associated with greater risk of irreversible toxicities.
Cyclophosphamide	Blurred vision, conjunctivitis, epiphora, cataracts	–
Cytarabine	Drug can be found in tears after high-dose IV therapy and is associated with keratitis including pain, tearing, sensitivity to light, and feeling of foreign body in eye. Side effects have been reported after intrathecal administration.	Administer prophylactic glucocorticoid eye drops every six hours to reduce the incidence and severity of eye toxicity from high-dose IV therapy. Eye drops should be started prior to high-dose therapy and continued during therapy. Saline eye drops may be useful. Cool compresses may be useful. Contact lenses should not be worn during high-dose therapy. Dexamethasone and diclofenac eye drops also may be useful if used together.

(Continued on next page)

Table 12-5. Ocular Side Effects and Toxicities Associated With Chemotherapy, Hormonal Therapy, and Targeted Therapy *(Continued)*

Drug	Toxicities and Side Effects	Additional Nursing Implications
Docetaxel	Secreted in tears, causing irritation of the eye May cause canalicular inflammation and blockage of tear ducts with epiphora Weekly docetaxel is associated with incidence of 64% of patients developing epiphora and canalicular stenosis. Erosive conjunctivitis (may be reversible) Punctal stenosis (may not be reversible)	Patients on weekly docetaxel should see an ophthalmologist at baseline and then as often as every four to six weeks or more often as needed. Assess patient for excess tearing at baseline and prior to each dose. Topical antibiotics and dexamethasone may be useful. Surgery with silicone intubation of canalicular and nasolacrimal ducts may be needed to manage stenosis. Docetaxel may need to be discontinued.
Doxorubicin	Rarely reported Increased tearing Conjunctivitis	–
Fludarabine	Associated with high doses and is related to neurotoxicity of drug	Ocular toxicities have not been reported with standard-dose therapy.
5-fluorouracil	Drug can be found in tears after drug administration. Blurred vision, itching, burning, watery eyes, and other symptoms have been reported. Irreversible epiphora resulting from canalicular obstruction caused by squamous metaplasia has been reported. Neuro-ophthalmologic toxicities also are reported, including nystagmus, neuropathy, and diplopia.	Application of ice packs to eyes has been reported to reduce irritation. Steroid eye drops or methylcellulose eye drops also have been reported to be effective. Consider baseline eye examination and follow-up for patients who develop eye complaints. Canalicular obstruction requires surgery with Silastic® (Dow Corning Corp.) intubation. Neuro-ophthalmologic toxicities appear to occur prior to cerebellar toxicity.
Gefitinib	Trichomegaly	–
Ifosfamide	Blurred vision, conjunctivitis	–
Interferon	Neuropathy Retinopathy Retinal hemorrhage Other rare case reports	–
Methotrexate	Secreted in tears Therapy, especially high-dose, may cause toxicity in up to 25% of treated patients. Side effects include edema, pain, blurred vision, light sensitivity, conjunctivitis, and reduced tears. Epiphora, both reversible and irreversible, has been reported. Intrathecal administration associated with optic neurotoxicity has been reported. Intracarotid administration is associated with pigment changes in retina.	Side effects usually resolve in 10 days after therapy. Eye drops to replace tears may be useful.

(Continued on next page)

Table 12-5. Ocular Side Effects and Toxicities Associated With Chemotherapy, Hormonal Therapy, and Targeted Therapy *(Continued)*

Drug	Toxicities and Side Effects	Additional Nursing Implications
Mitomycin C	Blurred vision	–
Nilutamide	Night blindness/reduced night vision Blurred vision	Common side effect; educate patients as to signs and symptoms of night blindness/reduced night vision from medication, safety issues such as not driving, and the need to report vision changes immediately. May be reversible.
Oxaliplatin	May be related to neurotoxicity. Side effects have included pain, changes in vision, and ptosis.	–
Paclitaxel	Sensation of flashing lights during infusion; is reversible. May be associated with vascular toxicity.	Educate patients.
Retinoids	Blepharoconjunctivitis (dry eyes, blurred vision, contact lens intolerance) Opacity of cornea Night blindness	Effects may be reversible after drug discontinuation. Some side effects take longer to resolve.
Tamoxifen	Corneal deposits occur in 72% of patients treated with 20 mg/day for at least six months. Multiple toxicities have been reported, including cataracts, retinopathy, keratopathy, decreased vision, neuritis, and retinal hemorrhages. Other side effects and toxicities have been reported.	Patients starting on tamoxifen should have a baseline ophthalmologic examination and periodic regularly scheduled follow-up exams. Patients should be aware of potential ocular side effects from therapy.
Steroids	Effects are common. Infection Cataracts Glaucoma Blurred vision Retinal hemorrhage and other hemorrhages Multiple ocular side effects	Educate patients as to the potential for ocular toxicities and the need to report side effects.
Vinca alkaloids	Known to produce neurotoxicity, including cranial nerve neurotoxicity, which causes eye toxicities such as optic neuropathy, palsies, ptosis, vision loss, night blindness, and other neurologic-induced ocular side effects	Educate patients as to safety measures should neurologic-induced eye toxicities develop and the need to report side effects immediately.

Note. Based on information from Agarwal et al., 2002; al-Tweigeri et al., 1996; Bixenman et al., 1977; Bouche et al., 2005; Chun et al., 1986; Dooley & Goa, 1999; Doroshow et al., 1981; Dranko et al., 2006; Esmaeli et al., 2002, 2003, 2006; Hopen et al., 1981; Imperia et al., 1989; Johnson et al., 1999; Krenzer et al., 2000; Lass et al., 1982; Loprinzi et al., 1990; Matteucci et al., 2006; Micromedex, 2006, 2007; Muftuoglu et al., 2006; Pascual et al., 2004; Schmid et al., 2006; Seidman et al., 1994; Skolnick & Doughman, 2003; Stevens & Spooner, 2001; Tonini et al., 2005; Ulusakarya et al., 2006; Walkhom et al., 2000.

Additionally, antiandrogen ablative therapies, including antiandrogens, luteinizing hormone-releasing hormone agonist agents, and finasteride, alter the hormonal milieu of patients on therapy. The loss of androgens may alter the function of the meibomian glands in the eyelids producing signs and symptoms of dry eyes, painful eyes, blurred vision, and light sensitivity (Krenzer et al., 2000). Cetuximab produces squamous blepharitis characterized by itching, light sensitivity, feeling of foreign body in eye, tearing, skin exfoliation, crusting, and oily secretions. Blepharitis is caused by dysfunction of the meibomian glands, which are responsible for tear production. Blockage of epidermal growth factor receptor and p27 may be responsible for blepharitis and abnormal eyelash growth in patients receiving cetuximab or gefitinib (Iressa®, AstraZeneca Pharmaceuticals) (Busam et al., 2001). High-dose chemotherapy with transplantation causes numerous eye toxicities. They may be related to graft-versus-host disease or chemotherapy (al-Tweigeri et al., 1996). High-dose carmustine (BCNU®, Bristol-Myers Squibb Co.) may cause changes in the blood vessels of the retina in patients undergoing transplantation (Johnson et al., 1999). In a study of 4,948 patients receiving adjuvant chemoendocrine therapy for early-stage breast cancer, 10.9% (n = 538) of the patients developed eye toxicity. Ten percent (n = 493) developed eye toxicity during the chemotherapy portion of their treatment, and 0.9% (n = 45) of the patients had eye toxicity develop during the hormonal stage of therapy (Gianni et al., 2005). Hormonal therapy consisted of tamoxifen or toremifene (Fareston®, GTx, Inc.). Toxicities of the retina, such as detachment, occurred along with other eye complications such as cataract formation, impaired vision, irritation, neuritis, and other toxicities. The authors concluded that eye irritation from hormonal therapy occurred less often than from certain types of chemotherapy (Gianni et al., 2005). Medications such as anticholinergics and antiepileptics also may affect ocular function by producing dry eyes (Hilton, Hosking, & Betts, 2004; Moore-Higgs, 2006).

Prevention Strategies

For patients at risk for or with ocular side effects and toxicities, patient education is important. When prescribing or caring for patients receiving drugs known to cause ocular toxicity, APNs provide drug-appropriate patient education on self-care management strategies for side effects. Dependent on the type and severity of the ocular toxicity, APNs should discuss safety issues such as not driving and being careful while using hazardous objects or while walking to reduce the risk of falling. Loose objects such as throw rugs and items that obstruct pathways in the home should be removed or relocated so as to not become hazards.

For patients who will be receiving high-dose cytarabine, fluorouracil, docetaxel (especially weekly), and methotrexate, a baseline eye examination should be performed by an ophthalmologist with periodic follow-up. Patients who will be starting on tamoxifen or toremifene need to be aware of the potential for ocular toxicity (Gianni et al., 2005; Muftuoglu et al., 2006). APNs should consider sending patients, especially those with a history of eye disorders or diseases or comorbidities such as hypertension or diabetes, for a baseline ocular examination, although routine examination for all patients does not seem to be warranted at this time when starting breast cancer hormonal therapy (Gianni et al., 2005).

APNs should assess patients at baseline and prior to each treatment for ocular toxicities. Patients are taught the signs and symptoms of ocular toxicities and the need to report them immediately. Patients who wear contact lenses should avoid wearing them during therapy with high-dose cytarabine, methotrexate, fluorouracil, and other drugs that are excreted in the tears. Other patients should be informed to immediately stop wearing contact lenses should any ocular effects develop, such as dry eyes or changes in vision. Patients who report a history of eye disease should be referred to an ophthalmologist. The diagnosis, assessment, and treatment of ocular disorders require immediate consultation with an ophthalmologist to perform an examination that includes pupil reflex, retinal examination, and an assessment of eye muscle function.

APNs should examine the conjunctiva for discoloration and moisture. The eyelids are examined for ptosis and the eyelashes for excess growth. An eye chart is used to assess for loss of vision, and color vision cards are helpful in assessing for loss of color vision. In addition, APNs should be suspicious of any new vision or eye complaints by patients, because for many of the antineoplastics, ocular side effects and toxicities are uncommon or rarely reported.

Evidence-Based Treatment Strategies

High-dose cytarabine ocular toxicities, such as corneal irritation, eye pain, photophobia, and foreign body sensation, are prevented and managed with steroid eye drops. Products used include 1% prednisolone phosphate (Lass, Lazarus, Reed, & Herzig, 1982) or dexamethasone plus diclofenac eye drops (Matteucci et al., 2006). If one of the products is not helpful for a given patient, the other medication should be tried. In addition, artificial tears may be useful to dilute the cytarabine found in the patients' eyes (Higa, Gockerman, Hunt, Jones, & Horne, 1991). Ice compresses over gauze pads applied five minutes prior to IV bolus fluorouracil and for 30 minutes total helps to reduce eye irritation from fluorouracil (Loprinzi et al., 1994).

For patients who will undergo weekly docetaxel therapy, epiphora is an expected side effect and is seen at median doses of 400 mg/m^2 but has been reported to occur at earlier and later doses (Burstein et al., 2000). It may be accompanied by mild conjunctivitis or eye irritation (Burstein et al.). Management of epiphora includes a baseline ophthalmologic examination with probing and irrigation of canalicular or nasolacrimal ducts prior to the start of docetaxel. Epiphora resulting from docetaxel may respond to tobramycin 0.3% and dexamethasone 0.1% (TobraDex®, Alcon Laboratories, Inc.) eye drops administered in a combination solution, one drop four times a day for seven days followed by a tapering regimen over four weeks (Esmaeli et al., 2003, 2006). If the drops are effective, ongoing reevaluations by the ophthalmologist are needed every four to six weeks. If these medications are not effective, surgical intervention, such as probing and irrigation, may reveal narrowed canaliculi. Silicone tubes may be placed in the canaliculi to promote reabsorption of tears. Additional surgery and glass tube placement may be needed in severe cases (Esmaeli et al., 2006). Artificial tears may be useful for dry eyes associated with docetaxel administration (Burstein et al.).

Evaluation of Outcomes

The patient should be monitored for ocular toxicity prior to each treatment and at each follow-up appointment. Patients require follow-up with the ophthalmologist as recommended.

Implications for Advanced Nursing Practice

APNs need to maintain a high degree of suspicion for the development of ocular toxicities in patients with a new eye complaint and for patients receiving drugs associated with eye toxicities. Some ocular toxicities and their prevention and treatment strategies are known, but for many of the agents, ocular side effects are rare or were previously reported as single case studies (see Table 12-5). Patients should have pretreatment ophthalmologic examinations when receiving drugs with known ocular toxicities. Steroid eye drops are used before treatment with high-dose cytarabine.

Conclusion

APNs must be ever vigilant in the management of GI toxicities induced by cancer therapy, as they may not only interfere with the patient's quality of life, but in some cases, such as severe diarrhea, may be life threatening. Cardiac toxicities are potentially life threatening and require prompt assessment, management, and ongoing monitoring. Although less common, ocular and neurologic toxicities have a profound effect on the patient's quality of life, and some neurotoxicities are progressive and potentially life threatening if the patient is not assessed and the drug therapy interrupted. Oncology APNs need to follow the research and evidence-based practice findings to provide the highest quality in safe patient care.

Case Study

J.S. is a 56-year-old married woman with six adult children. She has been having fevers, sweating, and complaining of being tired all the time for the past week. She has been to her family medical doctor (FMD) twice for evaluation and treatment of a presumed infection. She has been taking oral antibiotics for seven days. Her fevers have been as high as 102.5°F (39.2°C) and have lasted as long as 24 hours. Her blood cultures, urine culture, and chest x-ray have all been negative for the source of infection. She has no cutaneous lesions. Her FMD receives an emergency call from the lab where he sent her complete blood count and differential count. Her white blood cell count was 89,000/mm³, with a 60% blast count, platelet count of 54,000/mm³, hemoglobin of 8.8 g/dl, and hematocrit of 26%. He refers her to a hematology oncologist who does a bone marrow biopsy in the outpatient department and admits her for a presumptive diagnosis of acute myeloid leukemia (AML) based on his exam of the peripheral blood smear. Lab work is sent to evaluate her renal and liver function, lactate dehydrogenase, coagulation profile, ions, and electrolytes. In addition, another set of blood cultures is obtained, and the patient starts parenteral antibiotics for a presumed systemic infection. Flow cytometry is sent for evaluation of the AML, and human leukocyte antigen testing is performed for blood products and to test for compatibility with family members to serve as allogeneic transplant donors. A MUGA scan reveals an ejection fraction of 55%. The patient has no significant past medical history, and both of her parents, all siblings, and all children are alive and well. She takes no medication and has no surgical history. She has been well her entire life and cannot understand how she could have leukemia.

The day after admission, a cuffed tunneled central venous access catheter is placed in interventional radiology. After confirming the diagnosis of AML, reviewing the patient's laboratory studies and patient education, and obtaining patient consent for treatment by the treating hematology oncologist, the patient starts induction therapy with seven days of continuous infusion of cytarabine (100 mg/m^2) and three daily doses of bolus idarubicin (25 mg/m^2). Premedication included ondansetron 32 mg each day. A laxative regimen is initiated with a mild laxative to prevent constipation. No steroids are administered because of their myelosuppressive effects. Antibiotics are continued, and the patient and her supportive family receive emotional support by the staff in collaboration with the social services department. Within 36 hours of starting induction therapy, J.S. starts to spike new fevers. She is pancultured, a urinalysis and a chest x-ray are performed, and vancomycin is added to her antibiotics. She does well for several more days on treatment, when she then begins to have uncontrollable emesis that persists for several days, severely reducing her oral intake. Two days after the completion of the cytarabine, the emesis subsides, and she begins to have mucositis and diarrhea. Laxative therapy is stopped, and three daily stool specimens are sent for *C. difficile*. The third specimen is positive, and the patient is started on oral therapy. She is thrombocytopenic, anemic, and neutropenic. Twelve days after induction therapy, a second bone marrow biopsy is performed, and the patient's bone marrow demonstrates that she had achieved a response to the induction therapy. Filgrastim is initiated to enhance bone marrow recovery. She requires frequent platelet and packed red blood cell transfusions to maintain a platelet count in the teens and a hemoglobin greater than 8 g/dl. Five weeks after admission, J.S. is discharged home to recover from her hospital stay.

Four weeks later, J.S. is admitted again for consolidation therapy for AML. She receives high-dose cytarabine (2 g/m^2) IV over one hour every 12 hours on a Monday-Wednesday-Friday schedule. Steroid eye drops were started prior to the first dose of cytarabine. Prior to each dose, she receives ondansetron 16 mg. A neurologic assessment is performed prior to each drug dose to assess cerebellar function and to monitor the patient for early signs and symptoms of drug side effects. Prior to the second dose on Wednesday, the RN notes that the patient's signature had deteriorated to the extent that it was no longer legible and that her gait was altered. She is still able to perform finger-to-thumb touches and finger-to-nose touches but has trouble with rapid repetitive hand movements. The RN holds the patient's drug dose and notifies the APN to assess the patient. The APN finds a similar neurologic assessment and notifies the medical oncologist, who decides that in spite of this toxicity, treatment should proceed. J.S. receives the remaining three doses without deterioration in her neurologic status. In the morning of the day after completing high-dose cytarabine therapy, the patient awakes and complains that her eyes feel like they have glass in them and are extremely painful. Cool ice packs are applied to the eyes for comfort, the drapes are drawn to reduce outside light, and the lights in the room are dimmed for comfort. Artificial tears are administered, and the steroid eye drops are changed to a different steroid. Pain medication is administered, but the patient said it did not reduce the ocular symptoms. The patient notes symptom improvement with the combination of artificial tears, cold compresses, and the change in steroid eye drops. The symptoms subside gradually over three more days.

Because of J.S.'s type of AML and the chromosome changes, she is felt to be at high risk for relapse. She is referred to a transplant center for allogeneic transplant with her one sister as a complete match donor. During the transplant, she develops weight gain, ankle edema, shortness of breath, dyspnea on exertion, rales, and other signs of fluid overload. Her pretransplant ejection fraction was 54%. She undergoes a bedside echocardiogram, which shows an ejection fraction of 34%. She is diuresed for fluid overload, and a cardiology consult is placed to assist with the management of new-onset CHF related to the transplant conditioning regimen. She recovers some cardiac function with medications and lifestyle alterations and dies a year later related to a sudden cardiac event.

1. What laxative regimen is recommended for a patient with AML receiving induction chemotherapy?
   • No laxative regimens are recommended. A mild laxative and stool softener should be effective along with increased ambulation and oral fluid consumption.
2. What oral antibiotic is the drug of choice for the upfront treatment of *C. difficile*?
   • Metronidazole is the drug of choice administered by the oral route for best efficacy.
3. What is the etiology of both the cerebellar neurotoxicity and the ocular toxicity?
   • At high doses, cytarabine crosses the blood-brain barrier, producing neurotoxicity, most prominently cerebellar toxicity. It also is excreted in the tears and causes a chemical conjunctivitis.
4. Using the American Heart Association guidelines, what is J.S.'s stage of heart failure?
   • Using the American Heart Association criteria, this patient is stage C. The reader is referred to the Web site for the New York Heart Association Classification for cardiac patients (www.hcoa.org/hcoacme/chf-cme/chf00070.htm).
5. What categories of cardiac medications may be useful in the management of CHF?
   • ACE inhibitors, beta-blockers, diuretics, and digoxin may be useful for management of CHF.

Key Points

Cardiotoxicities

• Anthracyclines are useful agents when used appropriately with observation of lifetime cumulative doses, baseline and ongoing patient assessment, and monitoring.
• Cardiac toxicity may develop at any time during or after therapy. Combination therapy has the potential to cause additive cardiotoxic effects. Dexrazoxane (Zinecard) is a cardioprotectant that allows for ongoing treatment with doxorubicin.
• Monitoring LVEF function with MUGA scan or echocardiogram is crucial to the successful use of anthracyclines, as well as certain laboratory tests.

Gastrointestinal Toxicities

• GI side effects are common, and APNs must be vigilant and aggressive in their management.
• GI side effects have many ways of being managed. APNs should try many of them to improve patients' quality of life. If one medication does not work, try another. Consult gastroenterology for complications such as peritonitis, bowel perforations, bowel obstruction, and other serious complications.

- APNs must be familiar with the common causes of GI complaints and be suspicious of the less common problems, such as peritonitis, bowel obstruction, infection, fistula formation, and ascites.

Neurotoxicities

- Baseline and routine neurologic assessments are performed on all patients receiving neurotoxic agents. Central, peripheral, and autonomic nervous systems are included in the assessment.
- Baseline peripheral neuropathy is documented to allow for monitoring of neurotoxicity throughout therapy.
- Therapy can be held, doses reduced, or the treatment plan altered for neurotoxicity. Many peripheral neuropathies and neurotoxicities are reversible. Holding the dose or giving a dose break may reduce the severity during therapy.
- Symptom management of peripheral neuropathy improves the quality of patients' lives.

Ocular Toxicities

- Maintain a high degree of suspicion for ocular toxicities, as they are more common than thought.
- Perform baseline eye examinations on all patients who are to initiate chemotherapy.
- Patients who are anticipated to have ocular toxicities from therapy should be assessed and evaluated by an ophthalmologist prior to starting therapy.
- Provide supportive medications and symptom management to palliate ocular symptoms.
- Refer patients with ocular complaints to an ophthalmologist promptly.

Recommended Resources for Oncology Advanced Practice Nurses

Cardiotoxicities

- New York Heart Association Classification (n.d.): www.hcoa.org/hcoacme/chf-cme/chf00070.htm

Gastrointestinal Toxicities

- General
  - Camp-Sorrell, D., & Hawkins, R.A. (Eds.). (2006). *Clinical manual for the oncology advanced practice nurse* (2nd ed.). Pittsburgh, PA: Oncology Nursing Society.
  - Itano, J.K., & Taoka, K.N. (Eds.). (2005). *Core curriculum for oncology nursing* (4th ed.). St. Louis, MO: Elsevier.
  - Kogut, V.J., & Luthringer, S.L. (Eds.). (2005). *Nutritional issues in cancer care*. Pittsburgh, PA: Oncology Nursing Society.
- Nausea and vomiting
  - Tipton, J., McDaniel, R., Barbour, L., Johnston, M.P., LeRoy, P., Kayne, M., et al. (2006). *Putting evidence into practice: Chemotherapy-induced nausea and vomiting*. Pittsburgh, PA: Oncology Nursing Society.

- Constipation
  - Bisanz, A., Woolery, M., Lyons, H.F., Gaido, L., Yenulevich, M.C., & Fulton, S. (2007). *Putting evidence into practice: Constipation.* Pittsburgh, PA: Oncology Nursing Society.
- Mucositis
  - Harris, D.J., Eilers, J.G., Cashavelly, B.J., Maxwell, C.L., & Harriman, A. (2007). *Putting evidence into practice: Mucositis.* Pittsburgh, PA: Oncology Nursing Society.

Neurotoxicity

- Visovsky, C., Collins, M.L., Hart, C., Abbott, L.I., & Aschenbrenner, J.A. (2007). *Putting evidence into practice: Peripheral neuropathy.* Pittsburgh, PA: Oncology Nursing Society.

References

Agarwal, M.R., Esmaeli, B., & Burnstine, M.A. (2002). Squamous metaplasia of the canaliculi associated with 5-fluorouracil: A clinicopathologic case report. *Ophthalmology, 109,* 2359–2361.

Allen, J.A., Adlakha, A., & Bergethon, P.R. (2006). Reversible posterior leukoencephalopathy syndrome after bevacizumab/FOLFIRI regimen for metastatic colorectal cancer. *Archives of Neurology, 63,* 1475–1478.

al-Tweigeri, T., Nabholtz, J.M., & Mackey, J.R. (1996). Ocular toxicity and cancer chemotherapy: A review. *Cancer, 78,* 1359–1373.

Attar, A., Lemann, M., Ferguson, A., Halphen, M., Boutron, M.-C., Flourie, B., et al. (1999). Comparison of a low dose polyethylene glycol electrolyte solution with lactulose for treatment of chronic constipation. *Gut, 44,* 226–230.

Azizi, M., Chedid, A., & Oudard, S. (2008). Home blood-pressure monitoring in patients receiving sunitinib. *New England Journal of Medicine, 358,* 95–97.

Basavaraju, S.R., & Easterly, C.E. (2002). Pathophysiological effects of radiation on atherosclerosis development and progression, and the incidence of cardiovascular complications. *Medical Physics, 29,* 2391–2403.

Benson, A.B., Ajani, J.A., Catalano, R.B., Engelking, C., Kornblau, S.M., Martenson, J.A., et al. (2004). Recommended guidelines for the treatment of cancer treatment-induced diarrhea. *Journal of Clinical Oncology, 14,* 2918–2926.

Berenstein, E.G., & Ortiz, Z. (2005). *Megestrol acetate for the treatment of anorexia-cachexia syndrome* [Review]. *Cochrane Database of Systematic Reviews 2005,* Issue 2. Art. No.: CD004310. DOI: 10.1002/14651858. CD004310.pub2.

Berg, D. (2003). Oxaliplatin: A novel platinum analog with activity in colorectal cancer. *Oncology Nursing Forum, 30,* 957–966.

Bixenman, W.W., Nicholls, J.V., & Warwick, O.H. (1977). Oculomotor disturbances associated with 5-fluorouracil chemotherapy. *American Journal of Ophthalmology, 83,* 789–793.

Boccia, R. (2002). Improved tolerability of amifostine with rapid infusion and optimal patient preparation. *Seminars in Oncology, 29*(6, Suppl. 19), 9–13.

Bouche, O., Brixi-Benmansour, H., Bertin, A., Perceau, G., & Lagarde, S. (2005). Trichomegaly of the eyelashes following treatment with cetuximab. *Annals of Oncology, 16,* 1711–1722.

Brade, W.P., Herdrich, K., & Varini, M. (1985). Ifosfamide pharmacology, safety, and therapeutic potential. *Cancer Treatment Reviews, 12,* 1–47.

Brockstein, B.E., Smiley, C., Al-Sadir, J., & Williams, S.F. (2000). Cardiac and pulmonary toxicity in patients undergoing high-dose chemotherapy for lymphoma and breast cancer: Prognostic factors. *Bone Marrow Transplantation, 25,* 885–894.

Buchsel, P.C. (2003). Gelclair® oral gel. *Clinical Journal of Oncology Nursing, 7,* 109–110.

Burstein, H.J., Manola, J., Younger, J., Parker, L.M., Bunnell, C.A., Scheib, R., et al. (2000). Docetaxel administered on a weekly basis for metastatic breast cancer. *Journal of Clinical Oncology, 18,* 1212–1219.

Busam, K.J., Capodieci, P., Motzer, R., Kiehn, T., Phelan, D., & Halpern, A.C. (2001). Cutaneous side-effects in cancer patients treated with the antiepidermal growth factor receptor antibody C225. *British Journal of Dermatology, 144,* 1169–1176.

Cain, J.W., & Bender, C.M. (1995). Ifosfamide-induced neurotoxicity: Associated symptoms and nursing implications. *Oncology Nursing Forum, 22,* 659–668.

Camp-Sorrell, D. (2005). Chemotherapy toxicities and management. In C.H. Yarbro, M.H. Frogge, & M. Goodman (Eds.), *Cancer nursing: Principles and practice* (6th ed., pp. 412–457). Sudbury, MA: Jones and Bartlett.

Caraceni, A., Zecca, E., Conezzi, C., Arcuri, E., Tur, R.Y., Maltoni, M., et al. (2004). Gabapentin for neuropathic cancer pain: A randomized controlled trial from the gabapentin cancer pain study group. *Journal of Clinical Oncology, 22,* 2909–2917.

Cardinale, D., Colombo, A., Sandri, M.T., Lamantia, G., Colombo, N., Civelli, M., et al. (2006). Prevention of high-dose chemotherapy-induced cardiotoxicity in high-risk patients by angiotensin-converting enzyme inhibitors. *Circulation, 114,* 2474–2481.

Cardinale, D., Sandri, M.T., Martinoni, A., Borghini, E., Civelli, M., Lamantia, G., et al. (2002). Myocardial injury revealed by plasma troponin I in breast cancer treated with high-dose chemotherapy. *Annals of Oncology, 13,* 710–715.

Cascinu, S., Catalano, V., Cordella, L., Labianca, R., Giordani, P., Baldelli, A.M., et al. (2002). Neuroprotective effect of reduced glutathione on oxaliplatin-based chemotherapy in advanced colorectal cancer: A randomized, double-blind, placebo-controlled trial. *Journal of Clinical Oncology, 16,* 3478–3483.

Cavaliere, R., & Schiff, D. (2006). Neurologic toxicities of cancer therapies. *Current Neurology and Neuroscience Reports, 6,* 218–226.

Cersosimo, R.J. (2005). Oxaliplatin-associated neuropathy: A review. *Annals of Pharmacotherapy, 39,* 128–135.

Chun, H.G., Leyland-Jones, B.R., Caryk, S.M., & Hoth, D.F. (1986). Central nervous system toxicity of fludarabine phosphate. *Cancer Treatment Reports, 70,* 1225–1228.

Colucci, W.S. (2007a). *Evaluation and management of asymptomatic left ventricular systolic function.* Retrieved March 11, 2008, from http://www.uptodateonline.com

Colucci, W.S. (2007b). *Overview of the therapy of heart failure due to systolic dysfunction.* Retrieved March 11, 2008, from http://www.uptodateonline.com

Comeau, T.B., Epstein, J.B., & Migas, C. (2001). Taste and smell dysfunction in patients receiving chemotherapy: A review of current knowledge. *Supportive Care in Cancer, 9,* 575–580.

Cope, D.G. (2001). Management of chemotherapy-induced diarrhea and constipation. *Nursing Clinics of North America, 36,* 695–707.

Craig, C. (2000). Current treatment approaches for neoplastic meningitis: Nursing management of patients receiving intrathecal DepoCyt™. *Oncology Nursing Forum, 27,* 1225–1230.

Davis, M.P., Dreicer, R., Walsh, D., Lagman, R., & LeGrand, S.B. (2004). Appetite and cancer-associated anorexia: A review. *Journal of Clinical Oncology, 22,* 1510–1517.

Davis, M.P., Walsh, D., Lagman, R., & Yavuzen, T. (2006). Early satiety in cancer patients: A common and important but underrecognized symptom. *Supportive Care in Cancer, 14,* 693–698.

Denicoff, K.D., Rubinow, D.R., Papa, M.Z., Simpson, C., Seipp, C.A., Lotze, M.T., et al. (1987). The neuropsychiatric effects of treatment with interleukin-2 and lymphokine-activated killer cells. *Annals of Internal Medicine, 107,* 293–300.

Diaz, E., Sastre, J., Zaniboni, A., Labianca, R., Cortes-Funes, H., de Braud, F., et al. (1998). Oxaliplatin as a single agent in previously untreated colorectal carcinoma patients: A phase II multicentric study. *Annals of Oncology, 9,* 105–108.

Donegan, S. (2001). Novel treatment for the management of ifosfamide neurotoxicity: Rationale for the use of methylene blue. *Journal of Oncology Pharmacy Practice, 6,* 153–165.

Dooley, M., & Goa, K.L. (1999). Capecitabine. *Drugs, 58,* 69–76.

Doroshow, J.H., Locker, G.Y., Gaasterland, D.E., Hubbard, S.P., Young, R.C., & Myers, C.E. (1981). Ocular irritation from high-dose methotrexate therapy: Pharmacokinetics of drug in the tear film. *Cancer, 48,* 2158–2162.

Doyle, J.J., Neugut, A.I., Jacobson, J.S., Grann, V.R., & Hershman, D.L. (2005). Chemotherapy and cardiotoxicity in older breast cancer patients: A population-based study. *Journal of Clinical Oncology, 23,* 8597–8605.

Dranko, S., Kinney, C., & Ramanathan, R.K. (2006). Ocular toxicity related to cetuximab monotherapy in patients with colorectal cancer. *Clinical Colorectal Cancer, 6,* 224–225.

Edman, L., Larsen, J., Hagglund, H., & Gardulf, A. (2001). Health-related quality of life, symptom distress and sense of coherence in adult survivors of allogenic stem-cell transplantation. *European Journal of Cancer Care, 10,* 124–130.

Elliott, P. (2006). Pathogenesis of cardiotoxicity induced by anthracyclines. *Seminars in Oncology, 33*(3, Suppl. 8), S2–S7.

Esmaeli, B., Ahmadi, A., Rivera, E., Valero, V., Hutto, T., Jackson, D.M., et al. (2002). Docetaxel secretion in tears: Association with lacrimal drainage obstruction. *Archives in Ophthalmology, 120,* 1180–1182.

Esmaeli, B., Amin, S., Valero, V., Adinin, R., Arbuckel, R., Banay, R., et al. (2006). Prospective study of incidence and severity of epiphora and canalicular stenosis in patients with metastatic breast cancer receiving docetaxel. *Journal of Clinical Oncology, 22,* 3619–3622.

Esmaeli, B., Hidaji, L., Adinin, R.B., Faustina, M., Coats, C., Arbuckle, R., et al. (2003). Blockage of the lacrimal drainage apparatus as a side effect of docetaxel therapy. *Cancer, 98,* 504–507.

Esper, P., & Heidrich, D. (2005). Symptom clusters in advanced illness. *Seminars in Oncology Nursing, 21,* 20–28.

Extra, J.M., Marty, M., Brienza, S., & Misset, J.L. (1998). Pharmacokinetics and safety profile of oxaliplatin. *Seminars in Oncology, 25*(2, Suppl. 5), 13–22.

Fadol, A. (2006). Management of acute decompensated heart failure in patients with cancer. *Clinical Journal of Oncology Nursing, 10,* 731–736.

Fekety, R. (1997). Guidelines for the diagnosis and management of *Clostridium difficile*-associated diarrhea and colitis. *American Journal of Gastroenterology, 92,* 739–750.

Feldman, A.M., Lorell, B.H., & Reis, S.E. (2000). Trastuzumab in the treatment of metastatic breast cancer: Anticancer therapy versus cardiotoxicity. *Circulation, 102,* 272–274.

Floyd, J., Morgan, J.P., & Perry, M.C. (2007a). *Cardiotoxicity of anthracycline-like chemotherapy agents.* Retrieved January 4, 2007, from http://www.uptodateonline.com

Floyd, J., Morgan, J.P., & Perry, M.C. (2007b). *Cardiotoxicity of nonanthracycline cancer chemotherapy agents.* Retrieved January 4, 2007, from http://www.uptodateonline.com

Freynhagen, R., Strojek, K., Griesing, T., Whalen, E., & Balkenohl, M. (2005). Efficacy of pregabalin in neuropathic pain evaluated in a 12-week, randomised, double-blind, multicentre, placebo-controlled trial of flexible- and fixed-dose regimens. *Pain, 115,* 254–263.

Furlong, T.G. (1993). Neurologic complications of immunosuppressive cancer therapy. *Oncology Nursing Forum, 20,* 1337–1354.

Galvani, M., Ottani, F., Ferrini, D., Ladenson, J.H., Destro, A., Baccos, D., et al. (1997). Prognostic influence of elevated values of cardiac troponin I in patients with unstable angina. *Circulation, 95,* 2053–2059.

Gamelin, L., Boisdron-Celle, M., Delva, R., Guerin-Meyer, V., Ifrah, N., Morel, A., et al. (2004). Prevention of oxaliplatin-related neurotoxicity by calcium and magnesium infusions: A retrospective study of 161 patients receiving oxaliplatin combined with 5-fluorouracil and leucovorin for advanced colorectal cancer. *Clinical Cancer Research, 15,* 4055–4061.

Garg, R.K. (2001). Posterior leukoencephalopathy syndrome. *Postgraduate Medical Journal, 77*(903), 24–28.

Gehl, J., Boesgaard, M., Paaske, T., Vittrup, J.B., Jensen, B., & Dombernowsky, P. (1996). Combined doxorubicin and paclitaxel in advanced breast cancer: Effective and cardiotoxic. *Annals of Oncology, 7,* 687–693.

Genentech BioOncology. (2006a). Avastin [Package insert]. South San Francisco, CA: Author.

Genentech BioOncology. (2006b). *Herceptin administration and monitoring.* South San Francisco, CA: Genentech BioOncology.

Gerding, D.N., Johnson, S., Peterson, L.R., Mulligan, M.E., & Silva, J. (1995). Clostridium difficile-associated diarrhea and colitis. *Infection Control and Hospital Epidemiology, 16,* 459–477.

Gerhardt, W., Ljungdahl, L., & Herbert, A.K. (1993). Troponin-T and CK MB (mass) in early diagnosis of ischemic myocardial injury. *Clinical Biochemistry, 26,* 231–240.

Ghandi, L., & Johnson, B.E. (2006). Paraneoplastic syndromes associated with small cell lung cancer. *Journal of the National Comprehensive Cancer Network, 4,* 631–638.

Gianni, L., Bigano, L., Locatelli, A., Capri, G., Giani, A., Tarenzi, E., et al. (1997). Human pharmacokinetic characterization and in vitro study of the interaction between doxorubicin and paclitaxel in patients with breast cancer. *Journal of Clinical Oncology, 15,* 1906–1915.

Gianni, L., & Capri, G. (1997). Experience at the Istituto Nazionale Tumori with paclitaxel in combination with doxorubicin in women with untreated breast cancer. *Seminars in Oncology, 24*(1, Suppl. 3), S1–S3.

Gianni, L., Munzone, E., Capri, G., Fulfaro, F., Tarenzi, E., Villani, F., et al. (1995). Paclitaxel by 3-hour infusion in combination with bolus doxorubicin in women with untreated metastatic breast cancer: High antitumor efficacy and cardiac effects in a dose-finding and sequence-finding study. *Journal of Clinical Oncology, 13,* 2688–2699.

Gianni, L., Panzini, I., Li, S., Gelber, R.D., Collins, J., Holmberg, S.B., et al. (2005). Ocular toxicity during adjuvant chemoendocrine therapy for early breast cancer: Results from International Breast Cancer Study Group Trials. *Cancer, 106,* 505–513.

Gill, J.S., & Windebank, A.J. (1998). Cisplatin-induced apoptosis in rat dorsal root ganglion is associated with attempted entry into the cell cycle. *Journal of Clinical Investigation, 101,* 2842–2850.

Gilron, I., Bailey, J.M., Tu, D., Holden, R.R., Weaver, D.F., & Houlden, R.L. (2005). Morphine, gabapentin, or their combination for neuropathic pain. *New England Journal of Medicine, 352,* 1324–1334.

Gimbel, J.S., Richards, P., & Portenoy, R.K. (2003). Controlled-release oxycodone for pain in diabetic neuropathy: A randomized controlled trial. *Neurology, 24,* 927–934.

Glantz, M.J., Jaeckle, K.A., Chamberlain, M.C., Phuphanich, S., Recht, L., Swinnen, L.J., et al. (1999). A randomized controlled trial comparing intrathecal sustained-release cytarabine (DepoCyt) to intrathecal methotrexate in patients with neoplastic meningitis from solid tumors. *Clinical Cancer Research, 5,* 3394–3402.

Glass, J. (2006). Neurologic complications of lymphoma and leukemia. *Seminars in Oncology, 33,* 342–347.

Gorschluter, M., Glasmacher, A., Hahn, C., Schakowski, F., Ziske, C., Molitor, E., et al. (2001). Clostridium difficile infections in patients with neutropenia. *Clinical Infectious Diseases, 33,* 786–791.

Gregg, R.W., Molepo, J.M., Monpetit, V.J., Mikael, N.Z., Redmond, D., Gadia, M., et al. (1992). Cisplatin neurotoxicity: The relationship between dosage, time, and platinum concentration in neurologic tissues, and morphologic evidence of toxicity. *Journal of Clinical Oncology, 10,* 795–803.

Grolleau, F., Gamelin, L., Boisdron-Celle, M., Lapied, B., Pelhate, M., & Gamelin, E. (2001). A possible explanation for a neurotoxic effect of the anticancer agent oxaliplatin on neuronal voltage-gated sodium channels. *Journal of Neurophysiology, 85,* 2293–2297.

Halmos, B., & Eder, J.P. (2007). *Enterotoxicity of chemotherapeutic agents.* Retrieved January 26, 2007, from http://www.uptodateonline.com

Harris, E.E., Correa, C., Hwang, W.T., Liao, J., Litt, H.I., Gerrari, V.A., et al. (2006). Late cardiac mortality and morbidity in early-stage breast cancer patients after breast-conservation treatment. *Journal of Clinical Oncology, 25,* 4100–4106.

Hausheer, F.H., Schilsky, R.L., Bain, S., Berghorn, E.J., & Lieberman, F. (2006). Diagnosis, management, and evaluation of chemotherapy-induced peripheral neuropathy. *Seminars in Oncology, 33,* 15–49.

Held-Warmkessel, J. (2006). Diarrhea. In D. Camp-Sorrell & R.A. Hawkins (Eds.), *Clinical manual for the oncology advanced practice nurse* (2nd ed., pp. 425–433). Pittsburgh, PA: Oncology Nursing Society.

Hensley, M.L., Peterson, B., Silver, R.T., Larson, R.A., Schiffer, C.A., & Szatrowski, T.P. (2000). Risk factors for severe neuropsychiatric toxicity in patients receiving interferon alfa-2b and low-dose cytarabine for chronic myelogenous leukemia: Analysis of Cancer and Leukemia Group B 9013. *Journal of Clinical Oncology, 18,* 1301–1308.

Hensley, M.L., Schuchter, L.M., Lindley, C., Meropol, N.J., Cohen, G.I., Broder, G., et al. (1999). American Society of Clinical Oncology clinical practice guidelines for the use of chemotherapy and radiotherapy protectants. *Journal of Clinical Oncology, 17,* 3333–3355.

Herman, E.H., Zhang, J., Lipshultz, S.E., Rifai, N., Chadwick, D., Takeda, K., et al. (1999). Correlation between serum levels of cardiac troponin-T and the severity of the chronic cardiomyopathy induced by doxorubicin. *Journal of Clinical Oncology, 17,* 2237–2243.

Hesketh, P.J. (2007). *Prevention and treatment of chemotherapy-induced nausea and vomiting.* Retrieved January 26, 2007, from http://www.uptodateonline.com

Higa, G.M., Gockerman, J.P., Hunt, A.L., Jones, M.R., & Horne, B.J. (1991). The use of prophylactic eye drops during high-dose cytosine arabinoside therapy. *Cancer, 68,* 1691–1693.

Hildebrand, J. (2006). Neurological complications of cancer chemotherapy. *Current Opinion in Oncology, 18,* 321–324.

Hilpert, F., Stahle, A., Tome, O., Burges, A., Rossner, D., Spathe, K., et al. (2005). Neuroprotection with amifostine in the first-line treatment of advanced ovarian cancer with carboplatin/paclitaxel-based chemotherapy—a double-blind, placebo-controlled, randomized phase II study from the Arbeitsgemeinschaft Gynäkologische Onkologie (AGO) Ovarian Cancer Study Group. *Supportive Care in Cancer, 13,* 797–805.

Hilton, E.J., Hosking, S.L., & Betts, T. (2004). The effect of antiepileptic drugs on visual performance. *Seizure, 13,* 113–128.

Hinchey, J., Chaves, C., Appignani, B., Breen, J., Pao, L., Wang, A., et al. (1996). A reversible posterior leukoencephalopathy syndrome. *New England Journal of Medicine, 334,* 494–500.

Hochster, H.S., Grothey, A., & Childs, B.H. (2007). Use of calcium and magnesium salts to reduce oxaliplatin-related neurotoxicity. *Journal of Clinical Oncology, 25,* 4028–4029.

Holmes, F.A., Madden, T., Newman, R.A., Valero, V., Theriault, R.L., Fraschini, G., et al. (1996). Sequence-dependent alteration of doxorubicin pharmacokinetics by paclitaxel in a phase I study of paclitaxel and doxorubicin inpatients with metastatic breast cancer. *Journal of Clinical Oncology, 14,* 2713–2721.

Honnorat, J., & Cartalat-Carel, S. (2004). Advances in paraneoplastic neurological syndromes. *Current Opinion in Oncology, 16,* 614–620.

Hopen, G., Mondino, B.J., Johnson, B.L., & Chervenick, P.A. (1981). Corneal toxicity with systemic cytarabine. *American Journal of Ophthalmology, 91,* 500–504.

Hunt, S.A., Abraham, W.T., Chin, M.H., Feldman, A.M., Francis, G.S., Ganiats, T.G., et al. (2005). *ACC/ AHA guideline update for the diagnosis and management of chronic heart failure in the adult: A report of the American College of Cardiology/American Heart Association Task Force on Practice Guidelines* [Writing committee to update the 2001 guidelines for the evaluation and management of heart failure]. Retrieved March 24, 2008, from http://www.guideline.gov/summary/summary.aspx?doc_id=7664

Imperia, P.S., Lazarus, H.M., & Lass, J.H. (1989). Ocular complications of systemic cancer chemotherapy. *Survey of Ophthalmology, 34,* 209–230.

Jaffe, A.S. (2006). *Troponins, creatine kinase, and CK isoforms as biomarkers of cardiac injury.* Retrieved June 8, 2007, from http://www.uptodateonline.com

Jensen, B.V. (2006). Cardiotoxic consequences of anthracycline-containing therapy in patients with breast cancer. *Seminars in Oncology, 33,* S15–S21.

Jensen, B.V., Skovsgaard, T., & Nielsen, S.L. (2002). Functional monitoring of anthracycline cardiotoxicity: A prospective, blinded, long-term observational study of outcome of 120 patients. *Annals of Oncology, 13,* 699–709.

Jensen, S.A., & Sorensen, J.B. (2006). Risk factors and prevention of cardiotoxicity induced by 5-fluorouracil or capecitabine. *Cancer Chemotherapy and Pharmacology, 58,* 487–493.

Johnson, D.W., Cagnoni, P.J., Schossau, T.M., Stemmer, S.M., Grayeb, D.E., Baron, A.E., et al. (1999). Optic disc and retinal microvasculopathy after high-dose chemotherapy and autologous hematopoietic progenitor cell support. *Bone Marrow Transplantation, 24,* 785–792.

Johnson, S.A. (2006). Anthracycline-induced cardiotoxicity in adult hematologic malignancies. *Seminars in Oncology, 33,* S22–S27.

Keating, N.L., O'Malley, J., & Smith, M.R. (2006). Diabetes and cardiovascular disease during androgen deprivation therapy for prostate cancer. *Journal of Clinical Oncology, 27,* 4448–4456.

Klastersky, J. (2003). Side effects of ifosfamide. *Oncology, 65*(Suppl. 2), 7–10.

Krenzer, K.L., Dana, M.R., Ullman, M.D., Cermak, J.M., Tolls, D.B., Evans, J.E., et al. (2000). Effect of androgen deficiency on the human meibomian gland and ocular surface. *Journal of Clinical Endocrinology and Metabolism, 85,* 4874–4882.

Krishnan, A.V., Goldstein, D., Friedlander, M., & Kiernan, M.C. (2005). Oxaliplatin-induced neurotoxicity and the development of neuropathy. *Muscle and Nerve, 32,* 51–60.

Lambert, E.H., Eaton, L.M., & Rooke, E.D. (1956). Effects of neuromuscular conduction associated with malignant neoplasms. *American Journal of Physiology, 187,* 612–613.

Larsson, M., Hedelin, B., Johansson, I., & Athlin, E. (2005). Eating problems and weight loss of patients with head and neck cancer. *Cancer Nursing, 28,* 425–435.

Lass, J.H., Lazarus, H.M., Reed, M.D., & Herzig, R.H. (1982). Topical corticosteroid therapy for corneal toxicity from systemically administered cytarabine. *American Journal of Ophthalmology, 94,* 617–621.

Ling, C.P., & Pavesio, C. (2003). Paraneoplastic syndromes associated with visual loss. *Current Opinion in Ophthalmology, 14,* 426–432.

Lipshultz, S.E. (2006). Exposure to anthracyclines during childhood causes cardiac injury. *Seminars in Oncology, 33,* S8–S14.

Lipshultz, S.E., Lipsitz, S.R., Sallan, S.E., Simbre, V.C., Shaikh, S.L., Mone, S.M., et al. (2002). Long-term enalapril therapy for left ventricular dysfunction in doxorubicin-treated survivors of childhood cancer. *Journal of Clinical Oncology, 23,* 4517–4522.

Lipshultz, S.E., Rifai, N., Dalton, V.M., Levy, D.E., Silverman, L.B., Lipsitz, S.R., et al. (2004). The effect of dexrazoxane on myocardial injury in doxorubicin-treated children with acute lymphoblastic leukemia. *New England Journal of Medicine, 351,* 145–153.

Lipshultz, S.E., Rifai, N., Sallan, S.E., Lipsitz, S.R., Dalton, V., Sacks, D.B., et al. (1997). Predictive value of cardiac troponin T in pediatric patients at risk for myocardial injury. *Circulation, 96,* 2641–2648.

Loprinzi, C.L., Love, R.R., Garrity, J.A., & Ames, M.M. (1990). Cyclophosphamide, methotrexate, and 5-fluorouracil (CMF)-induced ocular toxicity. *Cancer Investigations, 8,* 459–465.

Loprinzi, C.L., Wender, D.B., Veeder, M.H., O'Fallon, J.R., Vaught, N.L., Dose, A.M., et al. (1994). Inhibition of 5-fluorouracil-induced ocular irritation by ocular ice packs. *Cancer, 74,* 945–948.

Maher, K.E. (2005). Radiation therapy: Toxicities and management. In C.H. Yarbro, M.H. Frogge, & M. Goodman (Eds.), *Cancer nursing: Principles and practice* (6th ed., pp. 283–314). Sudbury, MA: Jones and Bartlett.

Maisel, A.S., Krishnaswamy, P., Nowak, R.M., McCord, J., Hollander, J.E., Duc, P., et al. (2002). Rapid measurement of B-type natriuretic peptide in the emergency diagnosis of heart failure. *New England Journal of Medicine, 347,* 161–167.

Martino, S., Ratanatharathorn, V., Karanes, C., Samal, B.A., Sohn, Y.H., & Rudnick, S.A. (1987). Reversible arrhythmias observed in patients treated with recombinant alpha 2 interferon. *Journal of Cancer Research and Clinical Oncology, 113,* 376–378.

Matteucci, P., Carol-Stella, C., Di Nicola, M., Magni, M., Guidetti, A., Marchesi, M., et al. (2006). Topical prophylaxis of conjunctivitis induced by high-dose cytosine arabinoside. *Haematologica, 91,* 255–257.

Max, M.B., Lynch, S.A., Muir, J., Shoaf, S.E., Smoller, B., & Dubner, R. (1992). Effects of desipramine, amitriptyline, and fluoxetine on pain in diabetic neuropathy. *New England Journal of Medicine, 326,* 1250–1260.

McDonald, A.A., & Portenoy, R.K. (2006). How to use antidepressants and anticonvulsants as adjuvant analgesics in the treatment of neuropathic cancer pain. *Journal of Supportive Oncology, 4,* 43–52.

Meanwell, C.A., Blake, A.E., Kelly, K.A., Honigsberger, L., & Blackledge, G. (1986). Prediction of ifosfamide/mesna associated encephalopathy. *European Journal of Cancer and Clinical Oncology, 22,* 815–819.

Micromedex. (2006). *Cyclophosphamide.* Retrieved November 29, 2006, from http://www.thomsonhc.com/hcs/librarian

Micromedex. (2007). *Nilutamide.* Retrieved January 3, 2007, from http://www.thomsonhc.com/hcs/librarian

Miles, C.L., Fellowes, D., Goodman, M.L., & Wilkinson, S. (2007). Laxatives for the management of constipation in palliative care patients [Review]. *Cochrane Database of Systematic Reviews 2007,* Issue 4. Art. No.: CD003448. DOI: 10.1002/14651858.CD003448.pub2.

Mitchell, E.P. (2006). Gastrointestinal toxicity of chemotherapeutic agents. *Seminars in Oncology, 33,* 106–120.

Moore-Higgs, G.J. (2006). Blurred vision. In D. Camp-Sorrell & R.A. Hawkins (Eds.), *Clinical manual for the oncology advanced practice nurse* (2nd ed., pp. 873–876). Pittsburgh, PA: Oncology Nursing Society.

Moreira, A., Lobato, R., Morais, J., Silva, S., Ribeiro, J., Figueira, A., et al. (2001). Influence of the interval between the administration of doxorubicin and paclitaxel on the pharmacokinetics of these drugs in patients with locally advanced breast cancer. *Cancer Chemotherapy and Pharmacology, 48,* 333–337.

Muftuoglu, O., Ucakhan, O.O., & Kanpolat, A. (2006). Clinical and in vivo confocal microscopy findings in patients receiving tamoxifen citrate. *Eye and Contact Lens, 32,* 228–232.

Nakamae, H., Tsumura, K., Terada, Y., Nakane, T., Nakamae, M., Ohta, K., et al. (2005). Notable effects of angiotensin II receptor blocker, valsartan, on acute cardiotoxic changes after standard chemotherapy with cyclophosphamide, doxorubicin, vincristine, and prednisolone. *Cancer, 104,* 2492–2498.

National Cancer Institute Cancer Therapy Evaluation Program. (2006). *Common terminology criteria for adverse events* (version 3.0). Retrieved July 19, 2007, from http://ctep.cancer.gov/forms/CTCAEv3.pdf

New York Heart Association Classification. (n.d.). *A functional and therapeutic classification for prescription of physical activity for cardiac patients.* Retrieved January 10, 2007, from http://www.hcoa.org/hcoacme/chf-cme/chf00070.htm

Ng, M., Cunningham, D., & Norman, A.R. (2005). The frequency and pattern of cardiotoxicity observed with capecitabine used in conjunction with oxaliplatin in patients treated for advanced colorectal cancer (CRC). *European Journal of Cancer, 41,* 1542–1546.

Ng, R., Better, N., & Green, M.D. (2006). Anticancer agents and cardiotoxicity. *Seminars in Oncology, 33,* 2–14.

Nousiainen, Y., Jantunen, E., Vanninen, E., & Hartikainen, J. (2002). Early decline in left ventricular ejection fraction predicts doxorubicin cardiotoxicity in lymphoma patients. *British Journal of Cancer, 86,* 1698–1700.

Olmos, M., Berenstein, E.G., & Ortiz, Z. (2006). Probiotics for the prevention of Clostridium difficile associated diarrhea in adults (Protocol). *Cochrane Database of Systematic Reviews 2006,* Issue 3. Art. No.: CD006095. DOI: 10.1002/14651858.CD006095.

Onwuanyi, A., & Taylor, M. (2007). Acute decompensated heart failure: Pathophysiology and treatment. *American Journal of Cardiology, 99*(6B), 25D–30D.

Osterlund, P., Ruotsalainen, T., Peuhkuri, K., Korpela, R., Ollus, A., Ikonen, M., et al. (2004). Lactose intolerance associated with adjuvant 5-fluorouracil-based chemotherapy for colorectal cancer. *Clinical Gastroenterology and Hepatology, 2,* 696–703.

Pai, V.B., & Nahata, M.C. (2000). Cardiotoxicity of chemotherapeutic agents: Incidence, treatment and prevention. *Drug Safety, 22,* 263–302.

Pascual, J.C., Banuls, J., Belinchon, I., Blanes, M., & Massuti, B. (2004). Trichomegaly following treatment with gefitinib (ZD 1839). *British Journal of Dermatology, 151,* 1111–1112.

Patel, P.N. (2006). Methylene blue for management of ifosfamide-induced encephalopathy. *Annals of Pharmacotherapy, 40,* 299–303.

Peltier, A.C., & Russell, J.W. (2002). Recent advances in drug-induced neuropathies. *Current Opinion in Neurology, 15,* 633–638.

Perez-Verdia, A., Angulo, F., Handwicke, F.L., & Nugent, K.M. (2005). Acute coronary toxicity associated with high-dose intravenous methotrexate therapy: Case report and review of the literature. *Pharmacotherapy, 25,* 1271–1276.

Piccart-Gebhart, M.J., Procter, M., Leyland-Jones, B., Goldhirsch, A., Untch, M., Smith, I., et al. (2005). Trastuzumab after adjuvant chemotherapy in HER2-positive breast cancer. *New England Journal of Medicine, 353,* 1659–1672.

Plotkin, S.R., & Wen, P.Y. (2003). Neurologic complications of cancer therapy. *Neurologic Clinics, 21,* 279–318.

Poutanen, S.M., & Simor, A.E. (2004). *Clostridium difficile*-associated diarrhea in adults. *Canadian Medical Association Journal, 171,* 51–58.

Praga, C., Beretta, G., Vigo, P.L., Lenaz, G.R., Pollini, C., Bonadonna, G., et al. (1979). Adriamycin cardiotoxicity: A survey of 1273 patients. *Cancer Treatment Reports, 63,* 827–834.

Prahash, A., & Lynch, T. (2004). B-type natriuretic peptide: A diagnostic, prognostic, and therapeutic tool in heart failure. *American Journal of Critical Care, 13,* 46–55.

Preskorn, S.H., & Irwin, H.A. (1982). Toxicity of tricyclic antidepressants-kinetics, mechanism, intervention: A review. *Journal of Clinical Psychiatry, 43,* 151–156.

Quezado, Z.M., Wilson, W.H., Cunnion, R.E., Parker, M.M., Reda, D., Bryant, G., et al. (1993). High-dose ifosfamide is associated with severe, reversible cardiac dysfunction. *Annals of Internal Medicine, 118,* 31–36.

Raymond, E., Chaney, S.G., Taamma, A., & Cvitkovic, E. (1998). Oxaliplatin: A review of preclinical and clinical studies. *Annals of Oncology, 9,* 1053–1071.

Richardson, M.T. (2004). Electrolyte imbalances. In C.H. Yarbro, M.H. Frogge, & M. Goodman (Eds.), *Cancer symptom management* (2nd ed., pp. 440–453). Sudbury, MA: Jones and Bartlett.

Richardson, P.G., Briemberg, H., Jagannath, S., Wen, P.Y., Barlogie, B., Berenson, J., et al. (2006). Frequency, characteristics, and reversibility of peripheral neuropathy during treatment of advanced multiple myeloma with bortezomib. *Journal of Clinical Oncology, 24,* 3113–3120.

Ross, J.R., Goller, K., Hardy, J., Riley, J., Broadley, K., A'hern, R., et al. (2005). Gabapentin is effective in the treatment of cancer-related neuropathic pain: A prospective, open-label study. *Journal of Palliative Medicine, 8,* 1118–1126.

Rothenberg, M.L., Meropol, N.J., Poplin, E.A., Van Cutsem, E., & Wadler, S. (2001). Mortality associated with irinotecan plus bolus fluorouracil/leucovorin: Summary findings of an independent panel. *Journal of Clinical Oncology, 19,* 3801–3807.

Rowbotham, M.C., Goli, V., Kunz, N.R., & Lei, D. (2004). Venlafaxine extended release in the treatment of painful diabetic neuropathy: A double-blind, placebo-controlled study. *Pain, 110,* 697–706.

Rubenstein, E.B., Peterson, D.E., Schubert, M., Keefe, D., McGuire, D., Epstein, J., et al. (2004). Clinical practice guidelines for the prevention and treatment of cancer therapy-induced oral and gastrointestinal mucositis. *Cancer, 100,* 2026–2046.

Rudberg, L., Carlsson, M., Nilsson, S., & Wikblad, K. (2002). Self-perceived physical, psychologic, and general symptoms in survivors of testicular cancer 3 to 13 years after treatment. *Cancer Nursing, 25,* 187–195.

Ryberg, M., Nielsen, D., Skovsgaard, T., Hansen, J., Jensen, B.V., & Dombernowsky, P. (1998). Epirubicin cardiotoxicity: An analysis of 469 patients with metastatic breast cancer. *Journal of Clinical Oncology, 16,* 3502–3508.

Saarto, T., & Wiffen, P.J. (2005). Antidepressants for neuropathic pain. *Cochrane Database of Systematic Reviews 2005,* Issue 3. Art. No.: CD005454. DOI: 10.1002/14561858.CD005454.

Schimmel, K.J., Richel, D.J., van den Brink, R.B., & Guchelaar, H.J. (2004). Cardiotoxicity of cytotoxic drugs. *Cancer Treatment Reviews, 30,* 181–191.

Schmid, K.E., Kornek, G.V., Scheithauer, W., & Binder, S. (2006). Update on ocular complications of systemic cancer chemotherapy. *Survey of Ophthalmology, 51,* 19–40.

Schultz-Hector, S., & Trott, K.R. (2007). Radiation-induced cardiovascular diseases: Is the epidemiologic evidence compatible with the radiobiologic data? *International Journal of Radiation Oncology, Biology, Physics, 67,* 10–18.

Schwartz, R.G., McKenzie, W.B., Alexander, J., Sager, P., D'Souza, A., Manatunga, A., et al. (1987). Congestive heart failure and left ventricular dysfunction complicating doxorubicin therapy. Seven-year experience using serial radionuclide angiocardiography. *American Journal of Medicine, 82,* 1109–1118.

Seidman, A., Hudis, C., Pierri, M.K., Shak, S., Paton, V., Ashby, M., et al. (2002). Cardiac dysfunction in the trastuzumab clinical trials experience. *Journal of Clinical Oncology, 20,* 1215–1221.

Seidman, A.D., Barrett, S., & Canezo, S. (1994). Photopsia during 3-hour paclitaxel administration at doses > or = 250 mg/m². *Journal of Clinical Oncology, 12,* 1741–1742.

Semenchuk, M.R., & Davis, B. (2000). Efficacy of sustained-release bupropion in neuropathic pain: An open-label study. *Clinical Journal of Pain, 16,* 6–11.

Semenchuk, M.R., Sherman, S., & Davis, B. (2001). Double-blind-randomized trial of bupropion SR for the treatment of neuropathic pain. *Neurology, 57,* 1583–1588.

Shaiova, L. (2006). Difficult pain syndromes: Bone pain, visceral pain, and neuropathic pain. *Cancer Journal, 12,* 330–340.

Silber, J.H., Cnaan, A., Clark, B.J., Paridon, S.M., Chin, A.J., Rychik, J., et al. (2004). Enalapril to prevent cardiac function decline in long-term survivors of pediatric cancer exposed to anthracyclines. *Journal of Clinical Oncology, 22,* 820–828.

Silva, A., Wang, Q., Wang, M., Ravula, S.K., & Glass, J.D. (2006). Evidence for direct axonal toxicity in vincristine neuropathy. *Journal of the Peripheral Nervous System, 11,* 211–216.

Sindrup, S.H., Bach, F.W., Madsen, C., Gram, L.F., & Jensen, T.S. (2003). Venlafaxine versus imipramine in painful polyneuropathy: A randomized, controlled trail. *Neurology, 60,* 1284–1289.

Skolnick, C.A., & Doughman, D.J. (2003). Erosive conjunctivitis and punctal stenosis secondary to docetaxel (Taxotere). *Eye and Contact Lens, 29,* 134–135.

Slevin, M.C., Piall, E.M., Aherne, G.W., Johnston, H.A., & Lister, T.A. (1983). Effect of dose and schedule on pharmacokinetics of high-dose cytosine arabinoside in plasma and cerebral spinal fluid. *Journal of Clinical Oncology, 1,* 546–551.

Solomon, R., & Cherny, N.I. (2006). Constipation and diarrhea in patients with cancer. *Cancer Journal, 12,* 355–364.

Sonis, S.T., Elting, L.S., Keefe, D., Peterson, D.E., Schubert, M., Hauer-Jensen, M., et al. (2004). Perspectives on cancer therapy-induced mucosal injury. *Cancer, 100,* 1995–2025.

Sonnenblick, M., & Rosin, A. (1991). Cardiotoxicity of interferon. A review of 44 cases. *Chest, 99,* 557–561.

Spielberger, R., Stiff, P., Bensinger, W., Gentile, T., Weisdorf, D., Kewalramani, T., et al. (2004). Palifermin for oral mucositis after intensive therapy for hematologic cancers. *New England Journal of Medicine, 351,* 2590–2598.

Stepp, L., & Pakiz, T.S. (2001). Anorexia and cachexia in advanced cancer. *Nursing Clinics of North America, 36,* 735–744.

Stern, J., & Ippoliti, C. (2003). Management of acute cancer treatment-induced diarrhea. *Seminars in Oncology Nursing, 19*(4, Suppl. 3), 11–16.

Stevens, A., & Spooner, D. (2001). Lacrimal duct stenosis and other ocular toxicity associated with adjuvant cyclophosphamide, methotrexate and 5-fluorouracil combination chemotherapy for early stage breast cancer. *Clinical Oncology (Royal College of Radiology), 13,* 438–440.

Sudhoff, T., Enderle, M.D., Pahlke, M., Petz, C., Teschendorf, C., Graeven, U., et al. (2004). 5-fluorouracil induces arterial vasocontractions. *Annals of Oncology, 15,* 661–664.

Sul, J.K., & DeAngelis, L.M. (2006). Neurologic complications of cancer chemotherapy. *Seminars in Oncology, 33,* 324–332.

Surawicz, C.M., McFarland, L.V., Greenberg, R.N., Rubin, M., Fekety, R., Mulligan, M.E., et al. (2000). The search for a better treatment for recurrent Clostridium difficile disease: Use of high-dose vancomycin combined with Saccharomyces boulardii. *Clinical Infectious Diseases, 31,* 1012–1017.

Swain, S.M., Whaley, F.S., & Ewer, M.S. (2003). Congestive heart failure in patients treated with doxorubicin: A retrospective analysis of three trials. *Cancer, 97,* 2869–2879.

Tasmuth, T., Hartel, B., & Kalso, E. (2002). Venlafaxine in neuropathic pain following treatment of breast cancer. *European Journal of Pain, 6,* 17–24.

Tonini, G., Vincenzi, B., Santini, D., Olzi, D., Lambiase, A., & Bonini, S. (2005). Ocular toxicity related to cetuximab monotherapy in an advanced colorectal cancer patient. *Journal of the National Cancer Institute, 97,* 606–607.

Trobaugh-Lotrario, A.D., Smith, A.A., & Odom, L.F. (2003). Vincristine neurotoxicity in the presence of hereditary neuropathy. *Medical Pediatric Oncology, 40,* 39–43.

Trotti, A., Bellm, L.A., Epstein, J.B., Frame, D., Fuchs, H.J., Gwede, C.K., et al. (2003). Mucositis incidence, severity and associated outcomes in patients with head and neck cancer receiving radiotherapy with or without chemotherapy: A systematic literature review. *Radiotherapy and Oncology, 66,* 253–262.

Tsibiribi, P., Descotes, J., Lombard-Bohas, C., Barel, C., Bui-Xuan, B., Belkhiria, M., et al. (2006). Cardiotoxicity of 5-fluorouracil in 1350 patients with no prior history of heart disease. *Bulletin du Cancer, 93,* E27–E30.

Ulusakarya, A., Gumus, Y., Delmas-Marsalet, B., & Machover, K. (2006). Blepharitis induced by epidermal growth factor receptor-targeting therapy. *American Journal of Clinical Oncology, 29,* 531.

Unnikrishnan, D., Dutcher, J.P., Varshneya, N., Lucariello, R., Api, M., Garl, S., et al. (2001). Torsades de pointes in 3 patients with leukemia treated with arsenic trioxide. *Blood, 97,* 1514–1516.

Vahdat, L., Papadopoulos, K., Lange, D., Leuin, S., Kaufman, E., Donovan, D., et al. (2001). Reduction of paclitaxel-induced peripheral neuropathy with glutamine. *Clinical Cancer Research, 7,* 1192–1197.

Van Cutsem, E., Hoff, P.M., Blum, J.L., Abt, M., & Osterwalder, B. (2002). Incidence of cardiotoxicity with the oral fluoropyrimidine capecitabine is typical of that reported with 5-fluorouracil. *Annals of Oncology, 13,* 484–485.

Van Cutsem, E., Cunningham, C., Ten Bokkel Huinink, W.W., Punt, C.J., Alexopoulos, C.G., Dirix, L., et al. (1999). Clinical activity and benefit of irinotecan (CPT-11) in patients with colorectal cancer truly resistant to 5-fluorouracil (5-FU). *European Journal of Cancer, 35,* 54–59.

van Dalen, E.C., Caron, H.N., Dickinson, H.O., & Kremer, L.C. (2005). Cardioprotective interventions for patients receiving anthracyclines. *Cochrane Database of Systematic Reviews 2005,* Issue 1. Art. No.: CD003917. DOI:10.1002/14651858.CD003917.pub2.

van den Belt-Dusebout, A.W., Nuver, J., de Wit, R., Gietema, J.A., ten Bokkel Huinink, W.W., Rodrigus, P.T., et al. (2006). Long-term risk of cardiovascular disease in 5-year survivors of testicular cancer. *Journal of Clinical Oncology, 24,* 467–475.

van Kuilenburg, A.B. (2004). Dihydropyrimidine dehydrogenase and the efficacy and toxicity of 5-fluorouracil. *European Journal of Cancer, 40,* 939–950.

Verweij, J., Funke-Kupper, A.J., Teule, G.J., & Pinedo, H.M. (1988). A prospective study on the dose dependency of cardiotoxicity induced by mitomycin C. *Medical Oncology and Tumor Pharmacotherapy, 5,* 159–163.

Videnovic, A., Semenov, I., Chua-Adajar, R., Baddi, L., Blumenthal, D.T., Beck, A.C., et al. (2005). Capecitabine-induced multifocal leukoencephalopathy: A report of five cases. *Neurology, 65,* 1792–1794.

Viele, C.S. (2003). Overview of chemotherapy-induced diarrhea. *Seminars in Oncology Nursing, 19*(4, Suppl. 3), 2–5.

Visovsky, C. (2006). The effects of neuromuscular alterations in elders with cancer. *Seminars in Oncology Nursing, 22,* 36–42.

Wacker, A., Lersch, C., Scherpinski, U., Reindl, L., & Seyfarth, M. (2003). High incidence of angina pectoris in patients treated with 5-fluorouracil. A planned surveillance study with 102 patients. *Oncology, 65,* 108–112.

Walkhom, B., Fraunfelder, F.T., & Henner, W.D. (2000). Severe ocular irritation and corneal deposits associated with capecitabine use. *New England Journal of Medicine, 343,* 740–741.

Watson, C.P., Moulin, D., Watt-Watson, J., Gordon, A., & Eisenhoffer, J. (2003). Controlled-release oxycodone relieves neuropathic pain: A randomized controlled trial in painful diabetic neuropathy. *Pain, 105,* 71–78.

Wernicke, J., Lledo, A., Raskin, J., Kajdasz, D.K., & Wang, F. (2007). An evaluation of the cardiovascular safety profile of duloxetine: Findings from 42 placebo-controlled studies. *Drug Safety, 30,* 437–455.

Wickham, R. (2007). Chemotherapy-induced peripheral neuropathy. *Clinical Journal of Oncology Nursing, 11,* 361–376.

Wickham, R.S., Rehwaldt, M., Kefer, C., Shott, S., Abbas, K., Glynn-Tucker, E., et al. (1999). Taste changes experienced by patients receiving chemotherapy. *Oncology Nursing Forum, 26,* 697–706.

Wilkes, G., & Barton-Burke, M. (2007). *Oncology nursing drug handbook* (7th ed.). Sudbury, MA: Jones and Bartlett.

Wilmer Eye Institute at Johns Hopkins. (n.d.). *Eye tumors.* Retrieved May 10, 2007, from http://www.hopkinsmedicine.org/wilmer/Conditions/tumors.html

Yannucci, J., Manola, J., Garnick, M.B., Bhat, G., & Bubley, G.J. (2006). The effect of androgen deprivation therapy on fasting serum lipid and glucose parameters. *Journal of Urology, 176,* 520–525.

Yavuzsen, T., Davis, M.P., Walsh, D., LeGrand, S., & Lagman, R. (2005). Systematic review of the treatment of cancer-related anorexia and weight loss. *Journal of Clinical Oncology, 23,* 8500–8511.

Yeh, E.T., Tong, A.T., Lenihan, D.J., Yusuf, W., Swafford, J., Champion, C., et al. (2004). Cardiovascular complications of cancer therapy: Diagnosis, pathogenesis, and management. *Circulation, 109,* 3122–3131.

Zareba, G. (2005). Pregabalin: A new agent for the treatment of neuropathic pain. *Drugs Today, 41,* 509–516.

Zimmerman, S., Adkins, D., Graham, M., Petruska, P., Bowers, C., Vrahnos, D., et al. (1994). Irreversible, severe congestive cardiomyopathy occurring in association with interferon alpha therapy. *Cancer Biotherapy, 9,* 291–299.

CHAPTER 13

Genitourinary, Hepatic, and Pulmonary Toxicities

Shirley Triest-Robertson, RN, PhD, AOCNS®,
Wendy H. Vogel, MSN, FNP, AOCNP®,
and Barbara Holmes Gobel, RN, MS, AOCN®

Introduction

Every body system is vulnerable to cancer and cancer treatments. Dysfunction and/or toxicity occur by direct tumor effects or by treatment of the tumor. Direct tumor effects occur secondary to mass effect created by the tumor, lymphatic invasion, or tumor invasion of adjacent body structures. Treatments for the tumor may cause local or systemic toxicities. It is beyond the scope of this chapter to encompass all of the possible tumor effects or treatment toxicities for each of these body systems; therefore, select toxicities from the genitourinary (GU), hepatic, and pulmonary systems will be addressed.

Genitourinary Toxicity

Introduction

The GU system includes the kidney, bladder, ureter, and renal pelvis; the prostate, testes, urethra, and penis in males; the urethra, cervix, vagina, vulva, uterus, fallopian tubes, and ovaries in females; and the lymphatic system in both males and females. Obstruction of a ureter by tumor is an example of direct tumor effect. An example of a direct treatment effect is the surgical removal of the ovaries. Cystitis, loss of libido, erectile dysfunction, dyspareunia, and ovarian failure are examples of toxicities caused by systemic treatments. This section will focus on sexual dysfunction, infertility, and cystitis.

Bladder cancer and its treatment may cause toxicities such as cystitis, bleeding, contracture, infection, inadequate bladder emptying, loss of fullness sensation, and urinary frequency and incontinence. Almost any bladder toxicity may be interrelated to sexual functioning and reproduction by effects caused by bladder resection, urinary diversions, or body image changes related to these. In addition, almost any cancer treatment and many other cancers, particularly those that affect the pelvis, can cause sexual and reproductive dysfunction.

The intimate nature of GU toxicities often produces reluctance for dialogue between patients and clinicians about the nature and management of the dysfunction (Stead, Fallowfield, Selby, & Brown, 2007). Oncology advanced practice nurses (APNs) possess knowledge that facilitates comprehensive, compassionate management of these toxicities and the psychosocial issues that accompany them.

Sexual Dysfunction

Sexuality is a global term that encompasses not only sexual functioning but also values, beliefs, attitudes, behaviors, intimacy, practices, body image, feelings and emotions, gender identity, societal roles, reproduction, and sexual orientation. Sexual functioning as a component of human sexuality refers to the sexual response as conceptualized by Masters and Johnson (1966) and Kaplan (1979). *Sexual dysfunction* is a broad term that includes dyspareunia, anorgasmia, loss of libido, penile atrophy, vaginal dryness, introital stenosis, vaginal stenosis, ovarian failure, erectile dysfunction, ejaculatory difficulties, menopausal symptoms, and recurrent vaginal infections. Generally, the most common type of sexual dysfunction in men is premature ejaculation. Erectile dysfunction is the most common form of sexual dysfunction in men with cancer (Ukoli, Lynch, & Adams-Campbell, 2006). The most common types of sexual dysfunction reported in women are decreased libido, vaginal dryness, and dyspareunia (Amsterdam & Krychman, 2006; Krychman, 2006; Schover, 2005). The most common type of sexual problem in both sexes is decreased libido (Schover, 2005). In patients with cancer, alterations in sexual functioning occur as a result of psychological factors, physical symptoms, pharmacologic agents, GU system structure changes, endocrine dysfunction, neurologic damage, or vascular damage. Examples of each of these are noted in Table 13-1. Comorbidities or the treatment of comorbidities also can contribute to sexual dysfunction.

Incidence

Sexual dysfunction is frequent in patients with cancer, and it interferes with quality of life. In an ongoing study conducted by the Behavioral Research Center of the American Cancer Society (ACS), 41.2% of cancer survivors indicated difficulties with sexual dysfunction and listed sexual dysfunction among their top 10 concerns (Baker, Denniston, Smith, & West, 2005). In this study, men were twice as likely as women to report being less physically able to have sexual intercourse. Sexual dysfunction rates as the number-one concern for men with prostate cancer (Baker et al.). ACS predicts that 399,640 new GU cancers will be diagnosed in the United States in 2008; approximately 69% of these cases will be of the genital system and about 31% of the urinary system (Jemal et al., 2008). Numerous studies have documented sexual dysfunction following oncologic pelvic surgery, with the incidence of sexual dysfunction varying from 15% to almost 100% (Amsterdam & Krychman, 2006; Donovan et al., 2007; Galbraith, Arechiga, Ramirez, & Pedro, 2005; Huddart et al., 2005; Salonia et al., 2006; Stead et al., 2007; Ukoli et al., 2006). In patients with prostate cancer, erectile dysfunction is the most common adverse effect (Tal & Mulhall, 2006). In patients with testicular cancer, ejaculatory

Table 13-1. Causes of Sexual Dysfunction in Patients With Cancer

Cause	Examples
Psychological factors	Stress Depression Body image changes Fears (of death, cancer return)
Physical symptoms	Pain Fatigue Sleep disorders Urinary tract symptoms Gastrointestinal symptoms
Pharmacologic agents	Opioids Chemotherapy Psychotropic agents
Genitourinary structural changes	Penectomy Urethrectomy Radical prostatectomy Retroperitoneal lymph node dissection
Endocrine dysfunction	Bilateral orchiectomy Bilateral oophorectomy Androgen deprivation therapy
Neurologic damage	Damage to neural pathways (superior hypogastric plexus, inferior hypogastric plexus, pudendal, cavernosal and pelvic splanchnic nerves) from tumor encroachment or surgical resection; spinal cord lesion
Vascular damage	Damage to vasculature from pelvic radiation or surgical injury causing arterial insufficiency; venous leak allowing blood to leak from rigid penis

Note. Based on information from Amsterdam & Krychman, 2006; Col et al., 2006; Donovan et al., 2007; Krebs, 2006; Matthew et al., 2005; Miranda-Sousa et al., 2006; Schover, 2005; Schwartz & Plawecki, 2002; Tal & Mulhall, 2006.

dysfunction was the most commonly reported adverse event (Jonker-Pool et al., 2001). Even in nonpelvic cancers, such as breast cancer, sexual dysfunction may occur (Burwell, Case, Kaelin, & Avis, 2006; Schwartz & Plawecki, 2002).

Etiology and Pathophysiology

Sexual dysfunction can occur in any patient with any cancer receiving any type of treatment, including surgery, radiation, chemotherapy, immunotherapy, and hormonal therapy. Surgical treatment for cancer (particularly of the GU systems) changes the anatomy, and permanent or temporary sexual dysfunction may occur as a result of the removal of sexual organs, altered functioning of GU systems, or damage to neurovascular structures (both sympathetic and parasympathetic fibers). Surgical resection can cause body image changes that affect sexuality. Oophorectomy causes hormonal disruption and reproductive failure. Women undergoing surgery for cervical, uterine, or vaginal cancer may experience vaginal stenosis, decreased sensation, decreased vaginal lubrication, fibrosis, or development of scar tissue (Krychman, Pereira, Carter, & Amsterdam, 2006; Pieterse et al., 2006).

Surgery in men also may cause sexual dysfunction. Patients with testicular cancer who have undergone retroperitoneal lymph node dissection (RPLND) may have anejaculation (Jonker-Pool et al., 2001; Tal & Mulhall, 2006). Surgery for urologic cancer may leave men with penile deformities, fibrosis, or atrophy. The most common sexual dysfunction in males with cancer is erectile dysfunction as result of neurogenic or vasculogenic damage. Patients also experience difficulties with ejaculation, ability to maintain an erection, and orgasm. Surgical toxicities vary according to the surgeon's experience, surgical technique, and amount of resection required (Tal & Mulhall). Dysfunction may be temporary; research suggests that some men may recover erectile function following radical prostatectomy more than two years after the surgical intervention (Matthew et al., 2005).

Radiation therapy may cause sexual dysfunction in both genders. In women, vaginal fibrosis, contractures, shortened vaginal vault, and decreased lubrication and sensitivity may occur if the pelvic area is radiated (Krychman et al., 2006; Pieterse et al., 2006). A study of sexual health in women with cervical cancer indicated that radiation therapy (with or without surgery) was a consistent predictor of sexual dysfunction (Donovan et al., 2007). In men with penile cancer, radiation may cause fibrosis, deformity, skin reactions, or decreased sensation (Tal & Mulhall, 2006). Vasculogenic erectile dysfunction often occurs following radiation to the male pelvis even months to years after therapy (Jonker-Pool et al., 2001; Tal & Mulhall). Radiation toxicities vary according to radiation type, field, and dose (Krebs, 2006; Tal & Mulhall).

Pharmacologic treatments for cancer, including chemotherapy, hormonal manipulations, and immunotherapy, may be causes of sexual dysfunction in patients with cancer. Chemotherapy can result in innumerable physical symptoms that affect sexual functioning and sexuality (Krychman et al., 2006; Tal & Mulhall, 2006). Uncontrolled nausea, vomiting, diarrhea, fatigue, mucositis, dysuria, hot flashes, sleep disorders, vaginal dryness or discharge, and constipation may influence libido, the desire for sexual intimacy, or the ability to have an orgasm. Effects of chemotherapy, such as alopecia, depression, emotional lability, body image changes, and weight changes, also negatively affect sexuality. Dysfunction varies according to the pharmacologic agent, dose, and length of treatment (Krebs, 2006). When combined with another modality of treatment, sexual dysfunction may be exacerbated. In a recent study of sexual problems in patients younger than age 50 with breast cancer, chemotherapy following surgical intervention correlated with an increase in sexual dysfunction, often because of induced menopause (Burwell et al., 2006).

Other causes of sexual dysfunction in patients with cancer exist as well. Comorbid diseases, such as diabetes or depression, may cause or contribute to changes in sexual function. Numerous medications negatively affect sexual functioning, and a nonexhaustive list is noted in Figure 13-1. Aging influences sexual dysfunction, particularly in regard to dyspareunia and vaginal lubrication (Speer et al., 2005), but does not appear to be related to overall sexual health (Burwell et al., 2006). Psychological distress, including depression, body image issues, anxiety, fear, and underlying psychiatric illnesses, may cause sexual dysfunction (Fobair et al., 2006). Relationship and role changes, marital discord, and infertility are other potential sources of sexual dysfunction (Burwell et al.; Krychman et al., 2006). A study of sexual functioning determinants in breast cancer survivors found that relationship distress was the most significant variable influencing sexual function (Speer et al.).

- Opioids
- Gabapentin
- Antihistamines
- Anabolic steroids
- Tricyclic antidepressants
- Androgen deprivation therapy
- Histamine H$_2$ receptor antagonists
- Selective serotonin reuptake inhibitors
- Antiemetics (prochlorperazine, metoclopramide, scopolamine)

Figure 13-1. Medications That May Cause or Contribute to Sexual Dysfunction

Note. Based on information from Krebs, 2005; Tal & Mulhall, 2006.

Risk Factors

Many causes of sexual dysfunction in patients with cancer exist. Some identified risk factors for sexual dysfunction are aging, female gender, postmenopausal status in women, and poor performance status. Preexisting sexual dysfunction prior to a cancer diagnosis is a risk factor for sexual dysfunction during and after a cancer diagnosis. Poor self-image and having a colostomy or stoma are associated with increased risk. Treatments such as gastrointestinal (GI) or GU surgery and radiation to the pelvis, the anatomic nature of the cancer, and advanced disease are risk factors. Certain comorbidities, including depression, increase the risk for sexual dysfunction. Psychosocial issues such as poor communication with partner, lack of social support, history of rape or sexual abuse, and a more recent diagnosis of cancer also are risk factors (Burwell et al., 2006; Col et al., 2006; Donovan et al., 2007; Krebs, 2005, 2006; Miranda-Sousa, Davila, Lockhart, Ordorica, & Carrion, 2006; Speer et al., 2005; Ukoli et al., 2006).

Presenting Symptoms

Symptoms of sexual dysfunction vary according to the patient, gender, type of cancer, and treatment. In females with cancer, complaints include decreased libido, hot flashes, difficulty becoming aroused, difficulty achieving orgasm, vaginal dryness, discharge, irritation, loss of sensation, dissatisfaction with body image, dyspareunia, less frequent intercourse, and inability to relax and enjoy sex (Amsterdam & Krychman, 2006; Burwell et al., 2006; Fobair et al., 2006; Pieterse et al., 2006). Women with mucositis secondary to chemotherapy may complain of vaginal itching, soreness, and bleeding several days after chemotherapy, and these symptoms may last for up to 10 days (Katz, 2007). Males may complain of erectile dysfunction (inability to have or maintain erection), ejaculatory difficulty (anejaculation, premature ejaculation, dry ejaculation), decreased libido, hot flashes, difficulty with arousal, difficulty achieving orgasm, loss of sensation, poor body image, less frequent intercourse, and less pleasure in sex (Galbraith et al., 2005; Huddart et al., 2005; Miranda-Sousa et al., 2006). Psychosocial complaints might include feelings of decreased femininity or masculinity, anger, worry, embarrassment about the body, anxiety about relationships, fear of rejection, depression, fear about the possibility of cancer recurrence, performance anxiety, and grief about the diagnosis and resultant life changes (Col et al., 2006; Fobair et al.; Shell, 2002).

Diagnosis and Assessment

To appropriately manage sexual dysfunction, a thorough history and physical assessment are necessary. Even in the initial interview, when focus is on the cancer diagnosis, questions regarding sexual health should be included (Shell, 2002). A nonjudgmental, interested attitude will facilitate discussion. APNs can be more effective and comfortable with sexual health assessment when using a systematic and consistent set of open-ended questions used with every patient, adapting these questions to each patient's unique situation (Katz, 2007). Respect is given to sexual orientation and cultural and religious values. Whenever possible, the patient's partner's perspective is included. During dialogue, the patient should be in a comfortable position and not unclothed for a physical examination; no physical boundaries should exist between the clinician and the patient (Ohl, 2007).

A sexual frequency baseline is established, and continuing assessment throughout the disease trajectory is required. Cancer or its treatments can exacerbate a preexisting problem; therefore, precancer sexual functioning must be assessed (Sheppard & Whiteley, 2006; Ukoli et al., 2006). Assessment includes inquiry regarding feelings of inadequacy, anxiety regarding sexual performance, depression, expectations, and partner expectations and anxieties (Matthew et al., 2005). Any history of sexual abuse or rape should be ascertained. Any report of pain in the genital regions requires careful assessment. A medication review is in order, including any over-the-counter medications or alternative treatments. Men are questioned about the presence of nocturnal erections (the absence of nocturnal erections often indicates an organic cause of erectile dysfunction).

Sexual dysfunction is difficult to quantify, and no uniform methods of measurement exist (Tal & Mulhall, 2006). Multiple factors are considered, including anatomic, hormonal, physiologic, psychological, cognitive, behavioral, relational, and cultural factors (Ganz, Litwin, & Meyerowitz, 2005). However, assessment techniques can assist clinicians in obtaining more in-depth information. The ALARM and BETTER models are tools that may be used by oncology APNs and serve as reminders about needed information to request from patients. The ALARM model is reviewed in Chapter 16. The BETTER model, reviewed in Figure 13-2, presents an acronym that assists clinicians in assessment, reminding them about informational needs and guiding them through the process, ending with documentation. These models differ from the assessment tools listed in Table 13-2. These tools may be useful in clinical trials assessing sexual health in patients with cancer.

B—**B**ring up the topic.

E—**E**xplain your concern about sexuality as a key component of quality of life.

T—**T**ell patients about appropriate resources to assist them.

T—Assess **T**iming, acknowledging that patients may ask for information as they are ready to receive it.

E—**E**ducate patients about potential sexual toxicities that could occur as a result of cancer or its treatments and management options.

R—**R**ecord (document) your assessments and interventions in the medical record.

Figure 13-2. The BETTER Model for Sexual Health Assessment

Note. Based on information from Mick et al., 2004.

Table 13-2. Assessment Tools for Sexual Health and Function

Tool	Description
Derogatis Interview for Sexual Functioning (DISF) and DISF-SR (self-report) (Derogatis, 1987)	Measures quality of sexual functioning in five domains; 26-item interview
Sexual Adjustment Questionnaire (SAQ) (Waterhouse & Metcalfe, 1986)	Assesses impact of cancer or surgery on sexual function over a period of time; male and female versions
International Index of Erectile Function (IIEF) (Rosen et al., 1997, 1999)	15-item self-report addresses five domains of function postoperatively; available in a 5-item short form
Changes in Sexual Functioning Questionnaire (Clayton et al., 1997)	35 items, assessing five domains of sexual functioning; 20-minute interview
Female Sexual Function Index (FSFI) (Rosen et al., 2000)	Brief questionnaire evaluating arousal, orgasm, satisfaction, and pain
Sexual Health Inventory for Men (SHIM) (Day et al., 2001)	For screening, diagnosis, and evaluation of severity of erectile dysfunction; widely used and easily administered

Physical Examination and Diagnostic Tests

A thorough history will guide the physical examination and choice of diagnostic tests. A complete physical examination is necessary with focus on the presence of secondary sexual characteristics. The physical examination serves to further drive the diagnostic process. In men, hair patterns (assess for poor beard, slight underarm or pubic hair), testicular volume, prostate findings, height and body proportions, and breasts (for possible gynecomastia) are appraised. The penis and testicles are examined for fibrosis, atrophy, or varicocele. In women, hair patterns (female pubic, facial, and underarm hair distribution) are assessed, and breast examination is performed. Pelvic and adnexal examination includes inspecting for any signs of infection and attempts to elicit pain with cervical manipulation or during adnexal exam. A rectal examination is necessary for both genders, assessing for rectocele, hemorrhoids, or other abnormalities. Figures 13-3 and 13-4 list diagnostic tests to consider in males and females, respectively. Hormonal tests, such as testosterone levels, and glucose and thyroid testing may indicate endocrinopathy, such as hypopituitarism, hyperthyroidism, or adrenal tumors. Gonadotropin-releasing hormone (GnRH) stimulation testing assesses pituitary reserve. A semen analysis includes semen volume; a lowered volume might indicate a partial obstruction of the ejaculatory ducts or retrograde ejaculation. The pH level of semen may indicate infection, blockage of seminal vessels, or prostate abnormalities. Postejaculate urine analysis evaluates for retrograde ejaculation, which commonly is seen in patients with diabetes or after retroperitoneal lymph node dissection.

Figure 13-4 lists diagnostic tests to consider in women. Increased prolactin levels might indicate a pituitary or hypothalamus disorder. Higher levels of prolactin are associated with decreases in libido in both sexes (Barton, Wilwerding, Carpenter, & Loprinzi, 2004). Follicle-stimulating hormone (FSH) and luteinizing hormone (LH) levels assess pituitary function, gonadal function, and menopause. Excessive testosterone

- Semen analysis
- Testicular biopsy
- Testosterone assays
- Postejaculate urinalysis
- Gonadotropin-releasing hormone stimulation testing
- Luteinizing hormone*
- Follicle-stimulating hormone*
- Human chorionic gonadotropin
- RigiScan® (TIMM Medical Technologies, Inc.) (determines the extent of erectile dysfunction)
- Cultures for infection or sexually transmitted diseases

Figure 13-3. Diagnostic Tests in the Work-Up of Sexual Dysfunction in Men

* These are ordered if serum testosterone is low, and if both are appropriately elevated, then primary testicular failure is identified.

- Prolactin
- Serum estradiol
- Testosterone assays
- Cervical Pap smear
- Luteinizing hormone
- Urinalysis and culture if indicated
- Follicle-stimulating hormone
- Photoplethysmography (quantifies sexual excitement)
- Cultures for infections and sexually transmitted diseases

Figure 13-4. Diagnostic Tests in the Work-Up of Sexual Dysfunction in Women

Note. Based on information from Lin et al., 1999; Murray, 2006; Singh et al., 2005.

production in women might indicate adrenal or ovarian tumors, polycystic ovarian disease, and virilization. The Pap (Papanicolaou) smear, while ruling out precancerous and cancerous conditions, also is used for hormonal assessment and to diagnose inflammatory diseases. Other diagnostic testing to rule out medical conditions causing sexual dysfunction may be indicated.

Differential Diagnosis

Determining whether dysfunction is biologic or psychogenic in nature often is difficult. In fact, sexual dysfunction in patients with cancer frequently is both biologic and psychogenic (Derogatis & Kourlesis, 1981). It is important to determine what effects cancer treatment has had upon the body. The differential diagnoses include a wide range of potential causes of the specific problem. For instance, erectile dysfunction may be related to surgery, medication, or an endocrine disorder such as diabetes. Symptoms of cancer or cancer treatment toxicities must be adequately controlled before assessment and treatment of sexual dysfunction can proceed.

Management

Despite the fact that sexual dysfunction has potentially effective treatments and the knowledge that patients who receive sexual counseling and education have better outcomes, recent studies confirmed limited communications about sexual health between clinicians and patients (Ekwall, Ternstedt, & Sorbe, 2003; Schwartz & Plawecki, 2002; Sheppard & Whiteley, 2006; Stead et al., 2007). Myths exist and continue to be held by both clinicians and patients that impede sexual health discussions (see Figure 13-5). Time limitations, feelings of discomfort or embarrassment, or absence of perceived need are not sufficient reasons for neglecting this aspect of health.

- Older people are uninterested in sex.
- Sex is the last thing on the mind of a patient with cancer.
- Sexual contact should be avoided because cancer is contagious.
- After cancer, one should just be "happy to be alive."
- Abstinence from sexual activity will help to cure cancer.
- Birth control is not necessary during cancer treatment.
- Engaging in sexual contact will cause cancer to progress.
- Sexual health interventions are outside the clinical realm of oncology clinicians.

Figure 13-5. Myths Regarding Sexuality in Patients With Cancer

---

Note. Based on information from Derogatis & Kourlesis, 1981; Mick et al., 2004; Schwartz & Plawecki, 2002; Sheppard & Whiteley, 2006; Stead et al., 2007.

A cancer diagnosis and any treatment require discussion of their potential impact on sexual health (Donatucci & Greenfield, 2006; Leonard, Hammelef, & Smith, 2004; Tal & Mulhall, 2006) as early in the disease course as possible. Potential sexual dysfunction should be anticipated so that toxicity can be minimized (McKee & Schover, 2001). Patients are unlikely to initiate discussion about sexual health unless the clinician addresses it first. The PLISSIT model, discussed in Chapter 16, is a model for dialogue about sexual functioning and guides the clinician's intervention (Dixon & Dixon, 2006). Proficient oncology APNs are able to practice at the PLISSIT model level of specific suggestions. This level of practice includes providing anticipatory guidance and proactively assisting patients in management of their sexual health. Interventions for sexual dysfunction must not be withheld until treatment for the cancer is complete.

Educational information includes the impact of cancer, treatment, and side effects of treatment on sexual health; fertility issues; management of sexual dysfunction; and available support services (Krebs, 2006). Clinicians proactively begin with basic, factual information at the patient's level of understanding and then proceed to more sensitive or difficult topics. Just providing information validates patient concerns. Safe sex practices should be emphasized. Listening to the patient will give the APN clues about the significance of certain issues. Reassurance, support, and hope are needed throughout the cancer trajectory.

Anticipatory guidance and education specific to the patient's treatment are necessary. For instance, patients with a risk for neutropenia or thrombocytopenia are advised to avoid intercourse during these times. A condom may prevent transmission of infection and will reduce the partner's exposure to chemotherapeutic agents found in body fluids (Katz, 2007). Any effective education or intervention requires sensitivity to cultural issues, religious beliefs, and sexual orientation.

Prevention

Treatment strategies exist that can decrease the risk of sexual dysfunction. For instance, in rectal cancer, sphincter-preserving surgery eliminates the need for colostomy.

In some GI or GU cancers, nerve-sparing procedures are possible, thus preserving the patient's ability to have sexual intercourse and achieve orgasm. Nerve-sparing RPLND often preserves sexual functioning and fertility (Mezvrishvili & Managadze, 2006). In bladder cancer, the development of a "neobladder" allows maintenance of normal voiding patterns (Kanematsu, Yamamoto, & Ogawa, 2007). The choice of treatment modality may decrease post-treatment sexual dysfunction. For example, radical prostatectomy in men with prostate cancer causes more erectile dysfunction than other therapies, such as brachytherapy (Alivizatos & Skolarikos, 2005).

Interventions in Males

Management for erectile dysfunction often includes oral medications. Sildenafil, vardenafil, and tadalafil all inhibit phosphodiesterase type 5, increasing guanosine monophosphate. This enhances the effects of nitric oxide in response to sexual stimulation and leads to smooth muscle relaxation and vasodilation in the corpus cavernosum, resulting in increased blood flow and erection. Common side effects include headache, dyspepsia, back pain, myalgia, nasal congestion, vision color changes, and flushing. However, if severe neurogenic damage has occurred, erectogenic agents are ineffective. They may be less effective in situations where libido is low, such as in patients treated with androgen-ablative therapy. A contraindication for sildenafil, vardenafil, and tadalafil is concomitant use with nitrates, such as nitroglycerin, sodium nitroprusside, and amyl nitrite.

Other interventions for erectile dysfunction include use of a penile vacuum erection device, pharmacologic vasodilator injections or suppositories, and penile prostheses. However, patients often discontinue these interventions because of their inconvenience and difficulty in use (Matthew et al., 2005; McKee & Schover, 2001). An overview of interventions and issues of concern are noted in Table 13-3.

Table 13-3. Interventions in Male Sexual Dysfunction*

Intervention	Concerns
Oral erectogenic agents (sildenafil, vardenafil, tadalafil)	Contraindicated with concomitant nitrate use; must have functioning cavernosal innervations
Bupropion (for patients on antidepressants or opioids who are experiencing erectile dysfunction)	May cause concentration difficulties, sleep disturbance, and tremor
Penile vacuum erection device	Requires patient training; is cumbersome
Vasodilators (direct intracavernosal injection or intraurethral suppository)	Risk of priapism, pain, corporal scarring with injection; suppository is less effective; dose must be individually titrated.
Penile prostheses	Surgical procedure; utilization cannot occur until 8–12 weeks postoperatively; requires patient training
Testosterone	May cause mucositis, prostatic hypertrophy, acne, prolonged erections, gynecomastia, breast pain, hyperlipidemia, and hypertension

* The level of evidence of these interventions varies significantly.

Note. Based on information from Ganz et al., 2005; Masand et al., 2001; McKee & Schover, 2001; Schover, 2005; Shell, 2002; Taylor, 2006.

Interventions in Females

The treatment of menopausal symptoms (such as hot flashes, vaginal dryness, and negative emotional and cognitive states) often improves sexual functioning. Systemic or topical estrogen therapy is the most common management strategy; however, it may be contraindicated in patients with hormonally responsive cancers. Little if any systemic absorption of estrogen is reported with the estradiol-impregnated ring, and it may be helpful in minimizing menopausal symptoms. Vaginal lubricants or moisturizers may be used for vaginal dryness but often are not as effective as estrogen therapy. Hot flashes could be treated with a combination medication of belladonna, ergotamine, and phenobarbital, vitamin E, or venlafaxine (Boekhout, Beijnen, & Schellens, 2006). In women with decreased libido, androgen replacement therapy may be considered (Ganz et al., 2005). This type of therapy, as with estrogen therapy, may be contraindicated in some patients. Table 13-4 lists possible interventions for female sexual dysfunction and potential concerns for each.

Table 13-4. Interventions in Female Sexual Dysfunction*

Dysfunction	Intervention	Concerns
Altered libido	Hormonal manipulation	May be contraindicated in some patients with cancer; risk of breast cancer and cardiovascular events; estrogen must be given with progestin if uterus is intact.
	Testosterone	Under study; little is known about minimum levels of androgens required for female sexual functioning; may increase risk of breast cancer and heart disease
	Bupropion (for patients on antidepressants or opioids)	May cause concentration difficulties, sleep disturbance, and tremors
Hot flashes	Hormonal manipulation	As previously described
	Clonidine (transdermal or oral)	May cause dry mouth, dizziness, sedation, weakness, hypotension, and constipation
	Venlafaxine	May cause sexual dysfunction; increased risk of suicide in major depressive disorders
Vaginal dryness	Estrogen therapy	May be contraindicated in some patients with cancer; risk of breast cancer and cardiovascular events; oral estrogen must be given with progestin if uterus is intact.
	Lubricants/moisturizers	Local irritation; may be messy or cumbersome; can stain clothing
Vaginal fibrosis, stenosis, scarring, shortening	Vaginal dilators	Must be used daily for 10–15 minutes with lubricant; cumbersome; low adherence

(Continued on next page)

Table 13-4. Interventions in Female Sexual Dysfunction* *(Continued)*

Dysfunction	Intervention	Concerns
Dyspareunia	Analgesia	Could contribute to sexual dysfunction; sedative effects
	Topical anesthetic agents	Potential for mucosal irritation
	Kegel exercises	Requires patient education and commitment to do exercises
	Alternate coital positions	–

* The level of evidence of these interventions varies significantly.

Note. Based on information from Ganz et al., 2005; Krychman et al., 2006; Masand et al., 2001; McKee & Schover, 2001; Schover, 2005; Shell, 2002; Taylor, 2006.

Other Interventions

Selective serotonin reuptake inhibitors often are used in the oncology population. Sexual dysfunction is a common side effect of these agents. Drug holidays, dose decreases, changing the antidepressant, the use of erectile agents such as sildenafil, and the addition of bupropion or other pharmacologic agents prior to sexual activity are potential interventions (Masand, Ashton, Gupta, & Frank, 2001; Taylor, 2006).

Behavioral interventions for sexual dysfunction are noted in Figure 13-6. Because sexual dysfunction in cancer survivors often has both biologic and psychogenic causes, an approach that involves several types of interventions may be more successful. Few evidence-based interventions (Oncology Nursing Society [ONS] levels of evidence [LOE], level I) are available for the management of sexual dysfunction in patients with cancer (Shell, 2002). The evidence source for many interventions may be case studies or opinions of expert authorities, agencies, or committees (LOE III). Although sexual dysfunction is addressed liberally throughout the literature about cancer, very little practical and site-specific information exists (Shell). Most of the interventions in oncology literature do not meet ONS LOE level I designation and as such should be used with caution. Further research is needed in patients with cancer who have sexual dysfunction.

- Aerobic exercise
- Well-balanced diet
- Alternative sexual positions
- Avoidance of tobacco and alcohol
- Scheduling sexual intimacy at times when fatigue is lower
- Creation of a sensual, sexually stimulating environment
- If intercourse is painful, development of alternative, satisfying forms of nonpenetrative sex

Figure 13-6. Behavioral Interventions for Sexual Dysfunction in Patients With Cancer*

* The level of evidence of these interventions varies significantly.

Note. Based on information from Krychman et al., 2006; Shell, 2002.

In addition to specific interventions, psychosocial support is a vital part of sexual rehabilitation (Donovan et al., 2007). Information and support from clinicians decreases the negative impact of sexual dysfunction (Amsterdam & Krychman, 2006; Stead et al., 2007). Inclusion of the patient's sexual partner during education interventions may be helpful (Ekwall et al., 2003). Patients want and need practical evidence-based information in language they understand with sensitivity to culture, race, age, religious orientation, and socioeconomic factors (Schwartz & Plawecki, 2002). At times, referral to a sexual health specialist is necessary. The role of the oncology APN in this case is to coordinate the referral and to follow up as necessary to ensure the patient's needs are being met.

For various reasons, some patients turn to complementary and alternative medicine (CAM) for sexual dysfunction. Some CAM agents include ginseng, yohimbe, and withered yang (Aung, Dey, Rand, & Yuan, 2004). Other alternative therapies include acupuncture, biofeedback, and relaxation therapy. Chapter 8 addresses CAM in greater detail.

Summary and Implications

Sexual dysfunction is a common occurrence in patients with cancer, regardless of gender, and negatively affects quality of life. It is likely to become a more common occurrence as patients live longer and treatments become more complex. It may occur at any time during the cancer trajectory. Oncology APNs possess skills that enable thorough evaluation, accurate diagnosis, and individualized, compassionate management. Although sexual function may not be the primary focus of oncologic care, acknowledgment of sexuality as an important component of quality of life and the treatment of sexual dysfunction are vital in the comprehensive and holistic care of patients with cancer. Time restraints, clinician discomfort, or ignorance may be barriers to optimal care. Knowledge regarding treatment techniques that minimize sexual toxicities and state-of-the-art interventions for the management of sexual dysfunction are required of oncology APNs.

Early identification of patients at risk for sexual dysfunction can guide treatment decisions, and prophylactic measures may be possible. Many useful tools for assessment of sexual functioning exist. Oncology APNs are ideal clinicians to proactively initiate discussion about sexual health and to provide guidance about management of sexual dysfunction. Interventions are individualized and range from simple to complex strategies. Few interventions have been validated in patients with cancer by clinical research. However, regardless of the intervention, patients require permission for discussion, reassurance, and support for optimal sexual health throughout their disease course.

Reproductive Dysfunction: Infertility

Introduction

Cancer and its treatment may threaten fertility in both male and female patients. Infertility usually is defined as the inability to conceive after one year of intercourse without contraception. However, this definition does not meet the needs of many patients facing cancer treatment–related infertility who seek access to and coverage of fertility services prior to cancer treatments (U.S. Department of Health and Human Services

[DHHS], 2006). Rates of infertility following a cancer diagnosis vary and are dependent upon the cancer, its location, extent, and treatment, as well as individual patient characteristics. The effects on fertility may be transient, permanent, or late effects. An American Society of Clinical Oncology panel of experts developing recommendations on fertility preservation in patients with cancer found that available evidence suggests fertility preservation is very important to many people with cancer (Lee et al., 2006). Partridge et al. (2004) performed a Web-based study of more than 600 young women with early-stage breast cancer and found that 57% had substantial concerns about becoming infertile at the diagnosis of cancer. The President's Cancer Panel annual report (DHHS) recognized the need of cancer survivors to access infertility information, counseling, and services. This report recognizes the responsibility of oncology health professionals to identify those patients at risk for infertility, to adequately inform patients of the risk, and to understand the fertility preservation options available. Yet, many patients report that fertility issues were never discussed with them during their cancer diagnosis and treatment (Fertile Hope, 2007). In the Partridge et al. study, 72% of women reported discussing fertility concerns with their physicians, but 51% felt their concerns were not addressed satisfactorily.

Incidence

The incidence of infertility following a cancer diagnosis is difficult to quantify. Research evaluating infertility rates generally reports incidence of azoospermia and amenorrhea, but these are inadequate to quantify and often underestimate infertility (DHHS, 2006; Lefievre et al., 2007). For example, in women, infertility may occur as a result of a decrease in ovulatory reserve, even though the woman maintains or resumes cyclic menses (Lee et al., 2006). Therefore, merely assessing amenorrhea following cancer treatment could give an inaccurate estimate of infertility.

Etiology and Pathophysiology

Fertility may be compromised by the cancer itself or by treatment of the cancer. Chemotherapy and radiation therapy effects are dose dependent. The dose, frequency, route, and duration of chemotherapy influence the risk of infertility. Radiation effects on fertility depend on the size and location of the radiation field and the total dose. The patient's age, sex, pretreatment fertility, and type of cancer also influence post–cancer diagnosis fertility (Lee et al., 2006). Women older than age 35 are more likely to develop amenorrhea after chemotherapy (Goodwin, Ennis, Pritchard, Trudeau, & Hood, 1999). Women are less likely to be referred for pretreatment reproductive counseling (Schover, Brey, Lichtin, Lipshultz, & Jeha, 2002). Cancer involving a reproductive organ often requires treatment, such as surgical resection, that results in infertility.

Female Infertility

In females, infertility may occur if the hormonal balance is disrupted or if ovarian function is disturbed. If anatomic or vascular alterations to the fallopian tubes, uterus, vagina, or cervix occur, then reproduction may be inhibited (Lee et al., 2006). Treatments that decrease the number of primordial follicles may impede fertility. Single-fraction doses of 1.7–6.4 Gy (170–640 cGy) may cause temporary sterility and permanent sterility after 3.2–10 Gy (320–1,000 cGy) (Dunn & Lew, 2007). Radiation to the pelvis, abdomen, or spine often includes the ovaries and uterus within the treatment port. Uterine damage from radiation could result in future miscarriages, premature labor, and infants with low birth weights. Even in low doses, permanent ovarian failure often occurs in women older than the age of 40.

Chemotherapy also may lead to female infertility. Many chemotherapy agents can lead to temporary amenorrhea, but not all cause permanent sterility (Murray, 2006). The effect of systemic therapy on fertility is related to the chemotherapy type, the cumulative dose, the combination of chemotherapeutic agents, and the patient's ovarian reserve. Ovarian reserve declines with age; therefore, older patients' fertility is more susceptible to chemotherapy. The risk of menopause secondary to cyclophosphamide-based chemotherapy in a 40-year-old woman is approximately 5%–40%. In a 50-year-old woman, this risk increases from approximately 20% to close to 100% (Goodwin et al., 1999). Some ovarian reserve is lost with each gonadotoxic treatment, but this may not be clinically apparent (Roberts & Oktay, 2005). Cyclophosphamide and other alkylating agents are the most toxic chemotherapy agents to the ovary. Hormonal agents also can contribute to infertility. Goodwin et al. found that tamoxifen following chemotherapy increases the risk of menopause in young women with breast cancer.

Male Infertility

Male infertility may be a direct result of mechanical insult, such as that which occurs with surgery, hormonal changes, or damage to germinal stem cells (Lee et al., 2006; Puscheck, Philip, & Jeyendran, 2004). Alteration of the hypothalamic-pituitary-gonadal axis may cause secondary hypogonadism. Direct effects on erectile functioning can occur with surgery or medications, and direct effects on libido also occur (Sigman, 2007).

Spermatogenesis is a complex process of cell differentiation from germ cell to spermatozoa. Hormonal regulation guides this process, beginning with the hypothalamus releasing GnRH. This hormone regulates LH and FSH, thereby regulating testicular hormone secretion. An imbalance of any of these hormones could impair fertility.

Sperm-forming cells are exquisitely vulnerable to the effects of radiation. Doses lower than 400 cGy may cause a temporary decrease in sperm count but also may cause permanent azoospermia. Cumulative radiation doses of 2.5 Gy to the gonads may cause permanent azoospermia (Puscheck et al., 2004). Total body irradiation of 8 Gy (800 cGy) also will cause permanent azoospermia. Radiation of the testes causes irreversible infertility. Radiation scatter also can cause damage. Resection of the testicles, prostate gland, bladder, or retroperitoneal lymph nodes may result in infertility resulting from loss of a reproductive organ or damage to the nerves in the pelvis.

Chemotherapy also impairs spermatogenesis. Irreversible impairment of spermatogenesis occurs after cumulative cisplatin doses of greater than 400 mg/m^2 (Taksey, Bissada, & Chaudhary, 2003). In lesser doses, cisplatin induces an initial azoospermia in most patients, but some level of spermatogenesis usually returns, even two to four years after chemotherapy.

Risk Factors

The greatest risk for infertility in both men and women is associated with chemotherapy treatment, particularly the alkylating agents (Lee et al., 2006). Total body irradiation associated with hematopoietic stem cell transplantation is a major risk factor for infertility. Preexisting fertility problems, advancing age (particularly in women), and treatments affecting the reproductive organs increase the risk for infertility.

Presenting Symptoms

Amenorrhea is a presenting complaint of many women with infertility. Couples who are unable to become pregnant after a year are considered to be infertile. Women may report menopausal symptoms, such as hot flashes and mood variations. Various symptoms of sexual dysfunction also may be present.

Assessment and Diagnosis

Assessment of the risk for infertility must begin at the initial cancer diagnosis and be communicated with patients prior to treatment initiation. Men are questioned about history of cryptorchidism, family history of infertility, and frequency of intercourse (Taksey et al., 2003). The male physical examination includes the same evaluation as for sexual dysfunction, with careful assessment for lesions, varicoceles, and absence of vas deferens. Laboratory assessment is similar as well, with the addition of semen analysis including semen volume, sperm concentration, motility, and morphology (Taksey et al.). FSH, LH, prolactin, and testosterone levels may be assessed.

Women should be questioned about amenorrhea and menopausal symptoms. If a woman is premenopausal, a sexual and menstrual history should be taken. The female physical examination is similar to that noted previously in this chapter for sexual dysfunction. Laboratory assessment of fertility in females includes measurements of FSH and estradiol on menstrual cycle day 3 (Murray, 2006). FSH is an indirect estimate of ovarian reserve and generally will be elevated; estradiol levels will be low in infertility (Singh, Davies, & Chatterjee, 2005). Progesterone levels taken on day 21 that are less than 5 hg/ml indicate anovulation. Prolactin levels also may be assessed. Ovarian reserve testing is established in the fertility specialty and is useful to estimate patient response to ovarian stimulation for embryo or oocyte cryopreservation. Evaluation involves measurement of FSH on day 3 of the menstrual cycle or in response to clomiphene, an estrogen antagonist. An FSH level less than 10 IU/ml on cycle day 3 predicts adequate ovarian oocyte reserve. However, in the oncology setting, little evidence-based data exists on the ideal tests for ovarian reserve (Singh et al.), and data from other settings cannot be extrapolated to oncology because of the differing pathophysiology. Referral to a specialist in infertility before treatment is recommended for patients seeking specific infertility prevention or treatment guidance following a cancer diagnosis.

Differential Diagnosis

The differential diagnosis for male infertility other than cancer and cancer treatment includes cryptorchidism, Klinefelter syndrome, Leydig cell failure, hypothalamic-pituitary axial lesions, antisperm antibodies, and anatomic abnormalities (Taksey et al., 2003). The differential diagnosis for female infertility includes ovulatory dysfunction, tubal disease (secondary to pelvic inflammatory disease), appendicitis, pelvic adhesions, tubal surgery, history of intrauterine device use, and endometriosis.

Evidence-Based Treatment Strategies

The prevention and management of cancer-related infertility begins with a discussion between clinicians and patients about the likelihood that the cancer or cancer treatment might cause infertility (Lee et al., 2006). Fertile Hope (www.fertilehope.com), a national nonprofit organization dedicated to providing reproductive information to patients with cancer, maintains a list of cancer centers, hospitals, and clinics that proactively address reproductive risks with their patients. Resources should be readily available to patients. Some female interventions are menstrual cycle dependent and thus might delay cancer treatment by several weeks. Early referral to a fertility specialist may minimize delay. Data are limited, but no increased risk of cancer recurrence appears to be associated with most fertility preservation interventions, even in hormonally sensitive cancers (Lee et al., 2006). (See Tables 13-5 and 13-6 for a review of fertility preservation interventions.)

Table 13-5. Options for Male Fertility Preservation

Intervention	Description
Sperm cryopreservation	Freezing of sperm, ideally collected prior to start of treatment; most common intervention; most insurance companies do not cover
Gonadal shielding during radiation therapy	Use of shielding to prevent radiation to testes
Conservation surgical or radiation approaches	–
Testicular tissue cryopreservation and reimplantation	Freezing of testicular or germ cells and implanting following cancer treatment
Testis xenografting	Investigational
Spermatogonial isolation	Investigational

Note. Based on information from Center for Reproductive Medicine and Infertility, 2007; Lee et al., 2006.

Prevention of ovarian morbidity includes using less-toxic agents, lowering dosages, or abstaining from radiation therapy if deemed appropriate (Leonard, 2006). Partridge et al. (2004) found that 29% of young women with breast cancer believed that fertility considerations influenced their treatment decisions. Women younger than the age of 35 with a low-risk, hormonally positive breast cancer may be offered chemotherapy or tamoxifen. If patients desire a future pregnancy, the preferred option might be chemotherapy alone, understanding that a low risk of amenorrhea exists with chemotherapy and that tamoxifen use would delay pregnancy for five years. Older women would have a higher risk of amenorrhea with chemotherapy, making this a more difficult decision (Goodwin et al., 1999). However, women in both situations must weigh the risk of infertility with the risk of breast cancer recurrence following the chosen treatment. Close follow-up for recurrence is required. Ideally, these patients should be treated in a clinical trial.

Other preventive methods include applying external lead shields during radiation therapy to the female organs that may provide protection to the ovaries. Oophoropexy is the transposition of the ovaries out of the radiation port into a protected area in the abdomen. Although still exposed to radiation scatter, the radiation dose to the ovary after oophoropexy is reduced by approximately 90%–95% (Maltaris et al., 2007). This is performed as a laparoscopic procedure. Reported rates of successful fertility preservation with oophoropexy vary from 16%–90%.

Table 13-6. Options for Female Fertility Preservation

Intervention	Description
Embryo cryopreservation	Most common and successful intervention; requires two weeks of ovarian stimulation with follicle-stimulating hormone from onset of menses; oocytes are collected by ultrasound-guided transvaginal needle aspiration under sedation, then oocytes are fertilized in vitro and cryopreserved; most insurances do not cover; sperm donor is required
Oophoropexy (transposition of ovaries)	Surgical repositioning of ovaries out of pelvic radiation field
Gonadal shielding	Use of shielding to prevent radiation to reproductive organs
Conservative surgical or radiation approaches such as sparing resections and trachelectomy	Surgical expertise required; limited selection of patients; for early-stage disease only; removal of cervix, but preservation of the uterus; increased risk for midtrimester losses and preterm birth
Oocyte cryopreservation	Investigational; freezing of unfertilized eggs; requires two weeks of ovarian stimulation with follicle-stimulating hormone from onset of menses; thawed later and fertilized in vitro; useful if patient has no partner or has religious or ethical objections to embryo freezing
Ovarian tissue cryopreservation	Investigational; advantage of no ovarian stimulation or donor required; ovarian tissue is removed, frozen, and at later date, reimplanted; potential for reintroduction of cancer cells
Ovarian suppression by gonadotropin-releasing hormone agonist or antagonist	Investigational and controversial; given during chemotherapy; potential for cancer cell stimulation

Note. Based on information from Center for Reproductive Medicine and Infertility, 2007; Lee et al., 2006.

Embryo cryopreservation is the most common and successful form of fertility preservation in females. A sperm donor is required. This procedure generally requires several weeks to complete, as women must undergo hormonal stimulation and then egg harvesting. In vitro fertilization (IVF) is performed with donor sperm, and the embryos are frozen, with implantation occurring at a later time. In women with hormonally responsive cancers, hormonal stimulation with agents such as letrozole or tamoxifen may be utilized (Oktay, Buyuk, Libertella, Akar, & Rosenwaks, 2005). The cost of a single cycle of IVF may be up to $18,000 (Copperman, 2007), and insurance coverage is rare. Success rates for IVF vary and depend on many factors, such as the woman's age and the IVF facility (Leonard, 2006). Unfertilized oocyte cryopreservation may be performed. One advantage of this procedure is that no sperm donor is required. Ovarian stimulation and the oocyte harvesting procedures are similar to that of embryo cryopreservation, but no IVF occurs prior to freezing. This is still considered experimental, and live birth rates are lower than with frozen embryos (Park, Davidson, & Fox, 2006).

Ovarian tissue cryopreservation may be an option for women with a hormonally responsive cancer (Woodruff, 2007). However, it is still considered investigational. An ovary or part of an ovary is removed. The outer surface is divided into smaller strips, cryopreserved, and stored. Following recovery from cancer treatment, the strips are transplanted back to the remaining ovary or to a more superficial area in the abdomen, thus restoring estrogen production. The cost of this procedure varies but may be as high as $10,000. No ovarian stimulation is required; however, transfer of cancer cells back into the patient is possible, particularly with leukemias and lymphomas (Leonard, 2006).

Ovarian suppression with GnRH analogs during chemotherapy is a controversial, investigational method of fertility preservation. This involves the coadministration of GnRH analogs during chemotherapy and suppression of ovarian function, thus protecting the ovary from cytotoxic effects (Maltaris et al., 2007). The optimal duration of GnRH administration is unknown, as is the success rate of pregnancy following this technique. Also, no data exist on patient survival (Park et al., 2006).

In men, sperm cryopreservation is the most commonly utilized method of fertility preservation. This ideally is done before beginning chemotherapy. Only about 24% of men choose to have their sperm cryopreserved (Fertile Hope, 2007). The most common barrier found for this procedure is the lack of information about this as an option. The cost for one sperm cryopreservation storage for five years varies from $300–$500 (Schover, 2007). Testicular tissue freezing costs between $1,000–$3,000 (Turek, 2007). Most insurance policies do not cover these costs, and laws regarding insurance coverage vary from state to state (Adamson, 2007). The success rate for artificial insemination with cryopreserved sperm samples is approximately 15% per cycle. Financial assistance may be available through Fertile Hope, the LiveStrong organization, or other resources (Jacobs, 2007).

CAM treatments are utilized in the treatment of infertility. These include herbal agents, mind-body programs, and acupuncture (Domar, 2007). Chapter 8 provides more information regarding CAM therapies.

Counseling referrals are indicated for some patients, as cancer-related infertility may be associated with psychosocial distress (Lee et al., 2006). Ethical considerations also should be addressed. Directions for future disposition of the stored embryos, oocytes, ovarian tissue, and sperm should be clear in case of death. A written document should state whether stored materials may be utilized posthumously or discarded (Robertson, 2005). Other ethical concerns include harm to future offspring (such as physical health effects or psychological health effects) and balancing cancer risks with the desire for fertility.

Implications for Advanced Nursing Practice

Infertility is a risk of cancer and its therapy. Patients must be informed of this risk. Fertility preservation may be desired by many patients undergoing cancer treatment. It is a responsibility of oncology APNs to be informed regarding these options and to provide patients with this information. APNs can provide resources to patients, and referral to an infertility specialist early in the cancer trajectory is desirable. Referral for psychological counseling may be in order. Patients require information about risks of cancer recurrence if fertility preservation is undertaken. APNs must be knowledgeable about and willing to address the potential ethical issues that could arise.

Summary

Several options are available to preserve fertility in patients with cancer. However, lack of provider and patient knowledge, patient distress because of the diagnosis of cancer, time issues, and lack of insurance coverage limit the opportunity for fertility preservation. Further research is needed to advance the options and to understand the potential risks in patients with cancer.

Toxicity of the Bladder: Cystitis

Introduction

Cystitis is defined as an irritation of the bladder lining. It can be mild to severe in nature (hemorrhagic cystitis). Hemorrhagic cystitis can be life threatening. Cystitis may occur during treatment, immediately after treatment, or months to years after treatment.

Etiology and Pathophysiology

Chemotherapy, radiation therapy, and infection are the most common causes of cystitis in patients with cancer. Cystitis secondary to chemotherapeutic agents is attributed to metabolites that damage the bladder during the excretion process. Cyclophosphamide is the most common chemotherapeutic agent causing cystitis because of its metabolite, acrolein. Up to 40% of patients treated with oral cyclophosphamide will develop cystitis (Coleman & Walther, 2005). Cystitis secondary to chemotherapy may be cumulative and is dose-related (Coleman & Walther). Higher doses of chemotherapy, such as with transplantation, increase the risk of cystitis, including hemorrhagic cystitis, and may predispose patients to cystitis caused by viruses or bacteria. When given with pelvic radiation therapy, the risk of cystitis is much greater.

Intravesical chemotherapy can cause chemical or inflammatory cystitis. Intravesical treatment with thiotepa or doxorubicin causes cystitis in up to 50% of patients. Up to 33% of patients receiving intravesical treatment with mitomycin C develop cystitis (Coleman & Walther, 2005). Cystitis is more common in patients who receive intravesical bacillus Calmette-Guérin.

Radiation to the pelvis, as in cervical, bladder, or prostate cancers, may cause cystitis. Radiation therapy may potentiate the toxic effects of chemotherapy on the bladder. Intravaginal and intracavitary radiation also is associated with cystitis, and the risk increases when given with concomitant external beam radiation (Coleman & Walther, 2005). An acute inflammatory response and irritative symptoms develop as early as 10–14 days but usually within the first four to six weeks of radiation therapy (Coleman & Walther). At times, hematuria may occur. The incidence of severe hematuria following pelvic irradiation is difficult to quantify, although the incidence appears to be less than 5%, which can increase with time since irradiation (Crew, Jephcott, & Reynard, 2001). Mild symptoms occur in up to 80% of patients and may not require treatment (Coleman & Walther). Bladder capacity may be reduced as a result of vascular damage and collagen and fibroblast deposits. Late cystitis may occur as well and is proportional to the radiation dose. In late cystitis, concomitant bladder ulceration, fibrosis, and ureteral strictures may exist (Coleman & Walther).

Intravesical phototherapy for bladder tumors may cause bladder irritation that peaks on the second or third day of treatment (Coleman & Walther, 2005). Acute and chronic inflammatory reactions occur. Fibrosis and reflux are rare effects of this treatment.

Antibiotics, particularly penicillins, used to treat infections related to chemotherapy may be another cause of cystitis (Coleman & Walther, 2005). This may occur in 4%–8% of patients. Symptoms resolve shortly after cessation of the drug therapy.

Risk Factors

The risk of cystitis is increased if higher doses of urotoxic chemotherapy or radiation are given. The risk increases with the presence of a concomitant urinary tract infection (Coleman & Walther, 2005). If bladder-toxic chemotherapy is given concomitantly with radiation therapy, the risk of cystitis greatly increases. A past history of radiation to the abdomen or pelvis may enhance the risk of cystitis.

Presenting Symptoms

Patients with cystitis commonly present with suprapubic discomfort, abdominal pain, frequency, urgency, burning pain with urination, bladder spasms, reduced bladder capacity, and incomplete emptying (Coleman & Walther, 2005). Following radiation therapy, symptoms may occur as early as 10–14 days into treatment and usually resolve within a month after treatment completion. Pain may range from mild discomfort to severe pain. Clinical signs might include microscopic or gross hematuria (occurs in up to half of patients treated with cyclophosphamide) (Coleman & Walther).

Assessment and Diagnosis

The history should include fluid intake, especially of known bladder irritants (such as caffeine, alcohol, and cigarettes) and urinary output. A voiding diary may be helpful. Any past history of infection or cystitis is carefully documented. Past treatments including pelvic and abdominal irradiation are noted. Physical examination includes a pelvic examination in women and a digital rectal examination in men. Laboratory values such as coagulation profiles and platelet counts generally are normal in patients with cystitis. A urinalysis and midstream urine culture should be obtained. Abnormal urine sediment cytology may be found in patients receiving cyclophosphamide (Coleman & Walther, 2005). Cystoscopy may reveal fibrosis, telangiectasia, increased vascularity, edema, submucosal hemorrhage, mucosal thinning, ulcerations, necrosis, or malignancy. The most common cystoscopic finding in cystitis is acute diffuse inflammation. A potassium sensitivity test is useful in ruling out interstitial cystitis. This test involves introducing separate sterile water and potassium solutions into the bladder and comparing patient discomfort while each solution remains in the bladder for a period of time after instillation. Other diagnostic tests might include a hematocrit and hemoglobin, IV urogram, or pelvic (renal) ultrasound (Strohl & Camp-Sorrell, 2006).

Differential Diagnosis

Hemorrhagic cystitis and cancer recurrence or metastases to the bladder or associated innervation should be ruled out (Coleman & Walther, 2005). Other differential diagnoses include interstitial cystitis, infection, emphysematous cystitis, benign prostatic hypertrophy, chronic prostatitis, calculous disease, trauma, glomerular disease, sickle cell anemia, or infection (including viruses such as cytomegalovirus or herpes simplex, chlamydia, or bacteria) (Strohl & Camp-Sorrell, 2006).

Evidence-Based Treatment Strategies

Prevention of cystitis may be achieved by adequate hydration and diuresis, thereby diluting the metabolites in the urine (Coleman & Walther, 2005). Patients may be advised to take oral urotoxic agents (e.g., oral cyclophosphamide) early in the day to allow adequate hydration and clearing of the agent from the bladder prior to sleep (Vogel, 2007). Hydration up to three liters per day is associated with decreased cystitis and treatment completion.

Mesna is an IV agent designed to prevent bladder toxicity caused by the metabolites of ifosfamide. It usually is given in three doses: before ifosfamide and then at four and eight hours following ifosfamide. The timing of these doses is important, as the half-life of mesna is only around 30 minutes. Mesna also inhibits the breakdown of cyclophosphamide to acrolein in the urine (Coleman & Walther, 2005). Mesna often is used as a uroprotectant with high-dose cyclophosphamide. Amifostine is a cytoprotectant agent indicated for renal toxicity associated with cisplatin and may lessen the risk of hemorrhagic cystitis. It is given IV 30 minutes prior to chemotherapy.

Mild cystitis can be managed by increased hydration or cessation of the offending agent, if deemed clinically appropriate. Alkalizing agents should not be employed, as these may enhance the release of acrolein. Any infectious cause is treated. Urinary analgesics, such as phenazopyridine hydrochloride, may bring symptomatic relief of dysuria. Antispasmodics, such as oxybutynin chloride and tolterodine, may relieve symptoms of frequency, urgency, and associated incontinence (Coleman & Walther, 2005). Acetaminophen or ibuprofen also may relieve some inflammatory symptoms. Belladonna or opium suppositories might be required to relieve pain associated with cystitis. Avoidance of caffeine, alcohol, and spicy food and drinks also might be effective. Frequent bladder emptying and emptying prior to bedtime is recommended. Bladder irrigation with saline per a three-way indwelling catheter may be necessary for some patients receiving high doses of bladder-toxic chemotherapy, as in transplantation therapy.

Hyperbaric oxygen therapy has been utilized in the treatment of radiation-induced hemorrhagic cystitis (Chong, Hampson, & Corman, 2005). Urethral dilation may be indicated for urinary outlet obstruction (Hogle, 2007). Cystoscopy could be performed to cauterize bleeding vessels if needed; cystectomy is a last resort (Strohl & Camp-Sorrell, 2006).

CAM therapy for cystitis may include cranberry products (Cimolai & Cimolai, 2007), dietary modifications, bladder training, stress reduction, and sex therapy (Whitmore, 2002). Dietary modification could include elimination of bladder irritants (e.g., caffeine), fluid regulation, and a bowel regimen. Physical therapy and acupuncture also have been utilized.

Evaluation of Outcomes

Cystitis and hemorrhagic cystitis may occur with many cancer treatments. Multimodality treatment can increase this risk. Effects may occur acutely, or within a few months or years after treatment. Long-term follow-up is recommended for patients who have received urotoxic chemotherapy, bone marrow transplant, or pelvic irradiation. Referral to a urologist or other specialist may be necessary in patients with severe and unrelieved symptoms, those with decreased bladder capacity, those requiring surgical intervention, or those needing hyperbaric oxygen treatment (Strohl & Camp-Sorrell, 2006).

Hepatotoxicity

Introduction

The etiology of liver toxicity can include drugs or their metabolites, infectious agents, and immune disorders. Drug-induced toxicity is the primary cause of liver failure in the United States, accounting for 50% of its incidence (Chang & Schiano, 2007; Kaplowitz, 2004). In a review of potentially hepatotoxic drugs among major compendia sources, 59 of the 175 drugs identified were antineoplastics (Guo, Wigle, Lammers, & Vu, 2005).

Drugs must be tested on at least two animal species for at least two weeks before advancing to human testing. This approach has not proved fail-safe in avoiding drug-induced hepatotoxicity because it does not account for the individual human variables of genetics, immunology, or other comorbidities. Several agents, such as acetaminophen and isoniazid, have been approved despite hepatotoxic effects discovered in preclinical testing (Peters, 2005).

This section highlights drug-induced causes of hepatotoxicity, particularly cancer chemotherapy, supportive medications in oncology, and herbal therapies used in cancer care.

Definition and Incidence

den Brinker et al. (2000) defined hepatotoxicity as at least a three to five times elevation in serum aminotransferases (aspartate aminotransferase or serum glutamic oxaloacetic transaminase [AST or SGOT], alanine aminotransferase or serum glutamic pyruvic transaminase [ALT or SGPT], or gamma-glutamyl transpeptidase [GGT]) whether or not clinical hepatitis is present. This definition was used for a population that received highly active antiretroviral therapy. Weiss (2001) categorized the liver injury that results in hepatocellular dysfunction into chemical hepatitis, veno-occlusive disease (VOD), and chronic fibrosis. Hepatitis is an acute or chronic inflammatory injury to the liver caused by a toxin or a virus. Cirrhosis may be defined as fibrotic and nodular tissue formation that distorts the normal anatomic structure of the liver and may be caused by toxins, bacteria, or viruses. Cholestasis is a compromised flow or complete blockage of bile flow into the duodenum. VOD or sinusoidal obstruction syndrome (SOS) is associated with hepatic venous obstruction from perisinusoidal damage with dilation and congestion leading to hepatic fibrosis.

Injury to the liver by parenteral administration of drugs can occur directly from the offending drug or indirectly from the drug's metabolite and most often results in acute hepatocellular injury (hepatitis) or cholestasis, as opposed to chronic disease (Kaplowitz, 2004). Subclinical hepatotoxicity may be evident only via changes in liver enzyme tests.

Polovich, White, and Kelleher (2005) summarized the literature for incidence of hepatotoxicity related to medications in cancer care and reported ranges of less than 1% to 90%. The wide range of variability is attributed to comorbidities, specific medications used, and dose and cumulative dose of medications. The National Institutes of Health identified that the cause of drug-induced liver injury (DILI) was related to antibiotic use 43% of the time, anticonvulsants 10% of the time, and herbals, anesthetics, and nonsteroidal anti-inflammatory drugs (NSAIDs) to a lesser degree. This report did not include acetaminophen (Watkins & Seeff, 2006). Acetaminophen is the leading cause of acute liver failure. Even therapeutic doses of acetaminophen may cause significant increases in liver enzymes, which commonly manifests as jaundice (Arundel & Lewis, 2007).

Seeff (2007) pointed out that the true incidence of DILI caused by autoimmune hepatitis (liver injury with the presence of autoantibodies) is difficult to estimate because of confounding variables such as genetic susceptibility (as in hereditary hemochromatosis or Wilson disease), factors such as hepatitis, and ingestion of unsuspected drugs or herbal preparations. Reviews have presented what appeared to be DILI, but until 1999, no internationally accepted standards existed to define DILI (Alvarez et al., 1999). The scoring system includes specific measurements for autoantibodies, age at occurrence, and human leukocyte antigen associations. Clinical observation and testing of the patient after withdrawing the drug are part of the initial work-up of autoimmune hepatitis (AIH) and differentiating AIH from a genetic manifestation or subclinical form of hepatocellular injury (Seeff). Acute liver injury is considered to be disease that resolves within six months, whereas chronic hepatic injury lasts longer than six months (National Academy of Clinical Biology [NACB], 2000).

Presenting Signs and Symptoms

Edema, pruritus, jaundice, malaise, headache, anorexia, ecchymosis, low-grade fever, muscle and joint aches, and urine and stool color changes (such as clay-colored stools in liver injury) are the most common presenting signs and symptoms of DILI. Jaundice is not typically a presenting sign, except when late-stage disease is present, in the metabolic liver diseases such as hemochromatosis (Ryder & Beckingham, 2001).

Risk Factors

Hepatotoxicity is influenced by the chemical property of the drug, individual genetics, and environmental factors. Examples of these influences might include age, gender, the use of other drugs (including illicit drug use) or alcohol, cirrhosis, and comorbidities such as HIV, diabetes, and prior or current hepatitis (DeLeve & Kaplowitz, 2000; Kaplowitz, 2004; Zimmerman, 1999). Nonalcoholic steatohepatitis (NASH) can progress to cirrhosis and is associated with obesity, diabetes, and insulin resistance. Patients have a fatty liver. It is the most common cause of hepatic injury second to viruses and alcohol and is the most common cause of cryptogenic cirrhosis or cirrhosis caused by unknown etiology. NASH can be induced by chemotherapy agents such as tamoxifen (Astegiano et al., 2004).

Cancer Treatment

Hepatocellular dysfunction most likely occurs from viral hepatitis, hepatic metastasis, antidepressants, hormonal agents, and chemotherapies such as asparaginase, cytarabine, interferons in high doses, streptozotocin, thalidomide, regular-dose interferon-beta, flutamide, 6-thioguanine, and imatinib mesylate (Arundel & Lewis, 2007; Weiss, 2001) (see Table 13-7). Other chemotherapy agents also may contribute to hepatotoxicity when administered in high doses, such as busulfan, carmustine, cyclophosphamide, cytarabine, dactinomycin (especially in frequent cycles) (Weiss, 2001), methotrexate, and mitomycin. Asparaginase has one of the highest risks for hepatotoxicity (King & Perry, 2001). Intrahepatic cholestasis, which can be fatal, has been linked to the administration of 6-mercaptopurine (Weiss).

Table 13-7. Chemotherapy Drugs Associated With Hepatotoxicity

Drug	↑ AST/ ALT	↑ Bilirubin	↑ Alkaline Phosphatase	Reversible	Type	High Potential for Hepatotoxicity	High Potential at High Dose
Asparaginase	✓	✓	✓	✓	H	✓	
Bevacizumab		✓					
Bortezomib	✓	✓		✓	VOD		
Busulfan					H, C, VOD		✓
Capecitabine	✓	✓	✓				
Carboplatin	✓	✓	✓	✓			
Carmustine	✓	✓	✓	✓	VOD		✓
Cisplatin	✓	✓		✓	H, C		✓
Cyclophosphamide	✓	✓		✓	VOD		✓
Cytarabine	✓	✓			C	✓	✓
Dacarbazine							
Dactinomycin	✓				H, VOD		
Daunorubicin		✓					
Denileukin diftitox	✓			✓			
Docetaxel	✓		✓				
Doxorubicin	✓	✓					
Etoposide	✓	✓			H	✓	✓
Floxuridine	✓	✓	✓			✓	
Fluorouracil	✓	✓	✓	✓	H	✓	
Flutamide	✓	✓		✓	H, C		
Gefitinib	✓	✓	✓				
Gemcitabine	✓	✓	✓				
Gemtuzumab ozogamicin	✓	✓	✓		VOD		
Ifosfamide	✓	✓	✓				
Imatinib	✓	✓	✓				
Interferon–α	✓		✓				✓
Interleukin-2	✓	✓	✓	✓	C		
Irinotecan	✓	✓	✓				
Lomustine	✓	✓	✓	✓	H		✓
Megestrol					C		
Melphalan	✓	✓			VOD		
Mercaptopurine	✓	✓	✓	✓	H, C		✓
Methotrexate	✓	✓		✓		✓	✓

(Continued on next page)

Table 13-7. Chemotherapy Drugs Associated With Hepatotoxicity *(Continued)*

Drug	↑ AST/ ALT	↑ Bilirubin	↑ Alkaline Phosphatase	Reversible	Type	High Potential for Hepatotoxicity	High Potential at High Dose
Mithramycin					H	✓	
Mitoxantrone	✓	✓		✓			
Oxaliplatin	✓	✓			VOD		
Paclitaxel	✓	✓	✓				
Procarbazine	✓	✓					
Streptozocin	✓					✓	
Tamoxifen	✓	✓			H		
Thioguanine	✓	✓			VOD		
Topotecan	✓	✓					
Vinblastine	✓	✓					
Vincristine	✓	✓	✓			✓	
Vinorelbine	✓	✓					

ALT—alanine aminotransferase; AST—aspartate aminotransferase; type C—cholestatic disease; type H—hepatocellular damage; type VOD—veno-occlusive disease

Note. Based on information from Chang & Schiano, 2007; DeLeve, 2003; Duong & Loh, 2006; Floyd et al., 2006; Holmes Gobel, 2003; and manufacturers' package inserts.

Chronic low-dose methotrexate has been reported to cause portal fibrosis that can progress to full-blown cirrhosis, potentially through the disruption of folate homeostasis (a B vitamin that contributes to cellular purine and thymidine synthesis) (DeLeve, 2003). Although methotrexate used for cancer treatment can cause acute and reversible liver damage, long-term and consistent use, especially for nonmalignant diseases such as rheumatoid arthritis, can lead to irreversible hepatic fibrosis. In a systematic review of studies published before May 2006 (Zorzi et al., 2007), fluorouracil was associated with hepatic steatosis (a benign mild case of nonalcoholic fatty liver disease), which often progresses to a potentially fatal outcome. NASH has been linked to the administration of irinotecan, particularly in obese patients (a body mass index exceeding 25 kg/m^2) and those with metabolic syndrome. NASH also may increase postoperative morbidity. NASH can progress to fibrosis or cirrhosis, and ultimately, liver failure (Zorzi et al.). Oxaliplatin has been implicated in the development of SOS. VOD is associated with the administration of chemotherapy agents such as cytarabine, cyclophosphamide, dacarbazine, 6-mercaptopurine, mitomycin, and 6-thioguanine, as well as high doses of busulfan, carmustine, cyclophosphamide, and mitomycin for stem cell transplant (Weiss, 2001).

Many supportive medications used in cancer care can be risk factors in the development of hepatotoxicity. Amoxicillin-clavulanic acid is one of the most frequent drugs associated with liver toxicity, but antiretrovirals also are problematic (Chang & Schiano, 2007). Acetaminophen can lead to acute hepatitis. Chlorpromazine may cause acute cholestasis. Tamoxifen, a medication commonly used in breast cancer, is linked to the development of NASH. Fibrosis and cirrhosis have been reported with the use of methotrexate. Busulfan and cyclophosphamide are occasionally associated with VOD (Kaplowitz, 2004). Seeff (2007) listed nitrofurantoin, minocycline, clometacine, alpha-methyldopa, and oxyphenisatin as drugs associated with liver injury. Drugs for which autoimmune hepatitis associations have been less compelling include atomexitine, benzarone, diclofenac, fenofibrate, 3-hydroxy-3-methyl-glutaryl coenzyme A reductase inhibitors (e.g., atorvastatin, rosuvastatin, simvastatin), pemoline, and phenprocoumon. Herbal drugs associated with hepatotoxicity include Dai-saiko-to, germander, 3,4-methylenedioxymethamphetamine (Ecstasy), *Morinda citrifolia* or Noni juice, dihydralazine, and tienilic acid.

Herbal drugs can damage hepatocytes directly through parent herbal preparation or indirectly by its metabolites that may be toxic, mutagenic, or carcinogenic. Examples include quercetin, safrole, methyleugenol, estragole, pulegone in mint group, teucrin A in *Teucrium chamaedrys* found in dietary supplements, echimidine, and jacobine (Zhou, Xue, Yu, & Wang, 2007).

Herbal drugs may be indirectly responsible for liver injury by competing for liver metabolism of concurrently used medications. Herbal drugs often are metabolized by the same cytochrome P450s (CYPs) that standard medications use, and some herbal drugs conjugate enzymes to reactive agents that are associated with drug toxicity. Many complementary and alternative substances that cause indirect hepatotoxicity include flavonoids (e.g., quercetin) and alkenylbenzenes (e.g., safrole), methyleugenol, and estragoles, which are metabolized to a genetoxic substance. Some herbals, such as capsaicin, glabridin (from licorice root), oleuropein (in olive oil), daily sulfone (in garlic), and resveratrol (in red wine), can inhibit CYPs and thus can contribute to herb-drug interactions. This interaction may also be responsible for inhibiting CYPs so that a desired response of less-toxic metabolites from standard medications is formed (Zhou et al., 2007).

Case reports exist of hepatotoxicity related to the administration of epidermal growth factor receptor inhibitors, including cases of severe hepatitis from gefitinib and erlotinib. Generally, serum transaminases returned to baseline normal after the drug was discontinued (Ramanarayanan & Scarpace, 2007).

Etiology and Pathophysiology

The liver is responsible for the metabolism of fats, proteins, and carbohydrates. The liver also converts drugs into active metabolites or nontoxic substances for excretion. Pathophysiologic changes that occur related to hepatotoxicity are of a neoplastic, inflammatory, or fibrotic nature (Bryant, 2006). Kupffer cells, macrophages of the liver, respond to toxins by releasing inflammatory substances, growth factors, reactive oxygen ions, free radicals, and peroxides. This release of substances regulates acute hepatocyte injury and other chronic responses of the liver, which includes hepatocarcinoma through a multistep process of DNA damage that alters cell growth so that mutations are allowed to continue (Roberts et al., 2007). The term *liver damage* or *injury* is preferred rather than *hepatitis* because not all liver injury includes an inflammatory component (Thapa & Walia, 2007). Hepatocytes that are damaged cannot metabolize or eliminate bilirubin, synthesize many of the coagulation factors, synthesize glucose, uptake lactate acid, or moderate intracellular lactate generation from anaerobic glycolysis (Bryant).

Damage may occur to the liver from the toxic parent drug or the metabolite because of direct chemical damage to the biochemistry of the hepatocyte or indirectly through autoimmune response damage. This will lead to hepatic injury from hepatocyte death. Sinusoidal endothelial cells and bile duct epithelium also can be damaged (Kaplowitz, 2002, 2004; Odin, Huebert, Casciola-Rosen, LaRusso, & Rosen, 2001; Zimmerman, 1999).

Disruption in bilirubin consists of either overproduction, reduction in uptake or conjugation, or decreased flow by cell mechanisms, such as intrahepatic cholestasis, or by duct obstruction, such as extrahepatic cholestasis (Bryant, 2006). Portal inflammation and biliary injury occurs from a hypersensitivity-induced autoimmune reaction probably within the canaliculi of the bile ducts (Kaplowitz, 2004). Certain drugs, such as chlorpromazine, are more likely to produce hepatotoxicity in the form of cholestasis including portal inflammation and biliary damage (Watanabe et al., 2007). Signs and symptoms of cholestasis may occur three to four weeks after the drug is discontinued. This latent onset may be a result of the slow repair and regeneration potential of cholangiocytes (Kaplowitz, 2004). VOD, commonly found in patients who have had a stem cell transplant, occurs from blockage of venous circulation in the centrilobular and sublobular hepatic blood vessels from certain chemicals such as busulfan and cyclophosphamide (Weiss, 2001). A great deal of individual variation exists in the metabolism of IV cyclophosphamide, which modifies the risk of VOD for each person. If VOD develops, it is presumed to occur from the formation of acrolein, a toxic metabolite to the sinusoidal endothelial cells in the liver (DeLeve, 2003).

Prevention Strategies

Routine monitoring of aminotransferases, specifically ALT, can be used to identify potential hepatotoxicity in high-risk individuals. Cost and adherence factors require careful consideration when using this intervention (Kaplowitz, 2004). If an immune-modulated hepatotoxicity manifests shortly after therapy is initiated with a rapid onset of symptoms, the offending agent may need to be discontinued. Assessment for and discontinuation of any other hepatotoxic drugs also is indicated. Similar reactions in the patient's history and subsequent successful treatment are verified, including discontinuation of the offending drug. Other potential causes of hepatotoxicity, such as alcohol, must be ruled out. These interventions have the goal of preventing irreversible liver damage (DeLeve, 2003). Normal-risk individuals (i.e., healthy, nonfasting, nonalcoholic adults) should avoid the ingestion of more than 4 g/day of acetaminophen (Arundel & Lewis, 2007).

The Invader® (Third Wave Technologies, Inc.) is a molecular assay on the uridine-5'diphospho-glucuronosyltransferase 1A1 (UGT1A1) enzyme that is used to determine whether genetic variations exist that will affect how drugs that use this enzyme are metabolized and excreted. To date, this test is used with patients receiving irinotecan. It is the beginning of a new age of drug personalization that may provide information about individualized, accurate therapeutic dosing for individuals while potentially avoiding harmful effects such as hepatotoxicity (Third Wave Technologies, Inc., 2005).

Diagnosis and Assessment

Once the diagnosis of liver injury has been made through a history, physical examination, and abnormal laboratory parameters, the cause of the injury must be considered. Testing now occurs using viral serology or liver imaging and by evaluating the presence of potentially offending drugs (DeLeve, 2003). A cardiovascular evaluation also is in order.

AIH or DILI usually is diagnosed because of elevated serum aminotransferases and alkaline phosphatase (ALP) (Seeff, 2007). How the liver responds when a drug is given can determine whether the injury is drug induced. Most liver test abnormalities occur 5–90 days after drug ingestion, and this time shortens with rechallenge of the drug between 1–15 days. If serum aminotransferases decrease by 50% within eight days of stopping the drug, this is diagnostic of DILI. If decreases in serum aminotransferases occur within 30 days, this is still suspicious for DILI. If the drug is continued and aminotransferases stay the same or continue to rise, this is a strong clue that the liver injury is drug-induced. But, if aminotransferases decrease or normalize, it is unlikely that the liver injury is caused by the drug. If the drug is restarted after a drug holiday and abnormal labs reoccur, DILI is almost certain (DeLeve, 2003).

Laboratory Diagnostics and Monitoring

The goals of evaluating liver function tests are to determine the presence of liver disease, the etiology, the severity, and the prognosis, and to follow the efficacy of therapy (Thapa & Walia, 2007). NACB (2000) recommended the following tests to diagnose suspected liver disease, and they currently are approved for reimbursement by Medicare: ALT, AST, albumin, total protein, total bilirubin, direct bilirubin, total protein, albumin, and ALP.

Serum aminotransferases AST and ALT are used most frequently and typically are elevated with liver damage that includes injury and necrosis. Hepatocyte or bile duct damage usually is detected using the serum aminotransferases and cholestasis if ALP is elevated. The highest values of serum ALP are associated with people who have cholestatic liver diseases. Elevations in serum bilirubin, urine bilirubin, and urobilinogen all may contribute to the diagnosis of abnormal liver transport of substances from circulation. Serum albumin and coagulation factors detect abnormalities of liver metabolism and synthesis. A decrease in serum albumin occurs in patients with cirrhosis and ascites. Serum albumin levels typically are normal in viral hepatitis, DILI, and obstructive jaundice. Immunoglobulins and serologic tests for viral hepatitis may help with the diagnosis of liver injury but do not contribute information about liver function (Astegiano et al., 2004; Thapa & Walia, 2007).

ALT is more specific for liver damage than AST because this substance is more localized in the liver than any other area of the body (Bryant, 2006). AST is a more general test for liver damage; however, it is more sensitive in alcohol-related liver damage and muscle damage (Bryant).

Mild elevations related to liver tests (AST < 2–3 upper limit of normal [ULN], ALT < 2–3 ULN, ALP < 1.5–5 ULN, GGT < 2–3 ULN) are associated with fatty liver, NASH, and chronic viral hepatitis. Moderate elevations (3–20-fold increase of ULN of AST and AST) indicate acute or chronic hepatitis, including viral hepatitis, autoimmune, drug-induced, or alcoholic liver injury (Astegiano et al., 2004; Gopal & Rosen, 2000). Severe elevations of liver tests (AST > 20, ALT > 20, ALP > 5, GGT > 10) are associated with viral hepatitis, hepatic necrosis from drugs or toxins, and ischemic hepatitis (Martin & Friedman, 1998; Moseley, 1996). The extent of aminotransferase abnormality does not correlate with the amount of necrosis in the liver or clinical outcome (Astegiano et al.; Gopal & Rosen).

ALP levels are elevated in biliary obstruction (extrahepatic). Obstruction can be caused by primary biliary cirrhosis, drug-induced cholestasis, primary sclerosing cholangitis, and certain infiltrative processes (Gopal & Rosen, 2000), as well as cholestatic problems or some type of bile duct disorder, such as primary biliary tree cancer (Astegiano et al., 2004; Bryant, 2006). ALP levels can be very high in hepatotoxicity because of prolonged cholestasis and extrahepatic and intrahepatic obstruction (Bryant). Lactate dehydrogenase, because of its lack of specificity resulting from its ubiquitous presence in many tissues of the body, is a poor predictor for liver injury (Astegiano et al.). Elevated levels of unconjugated hyperbilirubinemia (levels between 1.2–5 mg/dl) signify abnormal production (increased), impaired transport, or defective conjugation of bilirubin in the hepatocytes. This abnormal test result is seen with hemolytic anemia, congenital enzyme deficiencies, and severe chronic liver damage (Bryant). If serum bilirubin levels are more than 5 mg/dl or the serum bilirubin level is between 1.2–5 mg/dl, and other liver function tests are abnormal, a strong association exists with liver disease (Astegiano et al.). A moderately elevated bilirubin level is present with drug-induced liver damage (Thapa & Walia, 2007).

The GGT level is used as a diagnostic value in hepatobiliary disease but also can indicate renal failure, myocardial infarction, pancreatic disease, and diabetes mellitus. The result of the GGT is influenced if the patient is taking phenytoin or is drinking alcohol. In a Japanese study, the correlation of abnormally elevated GGT and alcohol intake was strongest if the daily consumed alcohol amount was less than 70 g of ethanol (Matsuka et al., 2003). It is most useful to rule out a primary bone problem, such as liver metastasis to the bone, if ALP is abnormally high but GGT is normal (Gopal & Rosen, 2000).

NACB (2000) recommendations included using an ALT level in excess of 10 times the upper reference limit and an ALP level lower than three times the normal upper reference limit to diagnose acute hepatic injury. Direct bilirubin is nondiagnostic but should be used as a differential to rule out hemolysis.

In summary, elevations in AST, ALT, and bilirubin are detectable in hepatocellular dysfunction. Prolonged prothrombin and thrombin times also may be indicators of compromised renal function resulting from injury and especially has been noted after asparaginase administration. Many of the abnormal lab tests return to normal after the drug is discontinued (Weiss, 2001). However, it may take several months. Fatty changes after asparaginase persist for months after discontinuation of the drug (Weiss).

The most consistent feature of hepatic injury is a notable increase of aminotransferases—usually more than eight times the upper reference limit—and usually is paired with an elevated bilirubin, but clinicians might appreciate some protein synthesis abnormalities, such as abnormally low albumin lab results. If liver injury is chronic, only a slight elevation of aminotransferases (less than four times the upper normal limit) and no disruption in protein synthesis or bilirubin levels may be present. The ALP level may be normal in both instances because this test will yield abnormalities if biliary drainage obstructions exist. Total protein also is affected by immunoglobulin levels and synthesis; therefore, it is not useful in evaluating liver function. If globulins are increased, an autoimmune disease as the cause of liver injury may become part of the differential work-up process (NACB, 2000). See Table 13-8 for laboratory values seen in hepatotoxicity.

Radiologic Diagnostics

Abdominal ultrasounds are useful to detect dimensions of the hepatobiliary tree and view intra- or extrahepatic lesions and gallstones. It is difficult to obtain accurate data in obese patients or if excess bowel air is present (Bryant, 2006). A computed tomography (CT) scan will delineate dilated bile ducts and soft abdominal masses, pancreatic lesions,

Table 13-8. Laboratory Values Seen in Hepatotoxicity

Hepatocellular Damage	Seen In	Comments
1. Liver Injury		
↑ ALT (SGPT)	• Mild in fatty liver, NASH, chronic viral hepatitis, DILI, chronic hepatitis C • Moderate elevations with DILI, hepatitis C virus, acute and chronic hepatitis, autoimmune disease • Highest in viral-, drug-, or toxin-induced damage	• Highest concentrations in liver; most cost effective • AST:ALT < 1 = viral hepatitis • AST:ALT > 1 = liver metastases or liver congestion from chemotherapy • ↑ ALT, normal ALP and GGT = hepatitis • ↑ ALP and GGT and normal ALP = biliary cirrhosis
↑ AST (SGOT)	• More specific for alcohol abuse, MI	• AST:ALT > 2:1 = alcoholic liver disease
Obstruction	–	• AST/ALT > 300 u/L acute biliary obstruction, rapid peak and decline in lab values over 24–72 hours
↑ ALP	• Highest levels seen in cholestatic disease	• More diagnostic when used with other findings
↑ Bili	• Biliary cirrhosis, hepatic failure, prolonged fasting, hemorrhage, hemolytic diseases, pernicious anemia	–
↑ GGT	• Cholelithiasis and other biliary tract disease, chronic alcoholism, renal disease, obesity, diabetes mellitus, COPD, MI, pancreatic disease • Persistent and significant increase in nonalcoholic liver disease, alcoholic liver disease, chronic hepatitis, and cirrhosis	• Correlates with ALP levels • If elevated with AST:ALT > 2:1 more diagnostic of alcoholic liver disease
2. Liver Transport Capacity		
Serum bilirubin	• Conjugated—elevated with hepatobiliary disease even if total bilirubin is normal • Unconjugated—elevated hemolysis and Gilbert syndrome	–
3. Ability of Liver to Metabolize Drug		
Plasma clearance of substances metabolized by liver	–	–
4. Liver Synthesis Function—extent of injury or function of liver		
↓ Albumin	• Ascites, cirrhosis, nephritic syndrome, protein losing enteropathy, burns	• Most important plasma protein made by the liver • Tells more about the severity of liver disease but is affected by protein loss in urine or gastrointestinal tract

(Continued on next page)

Table 13-8. Laboratory Values Seen in Hepatotoxicity *(Continued)*

Hepatocellular Damage	Seen In	Comments
↑ PT	• Liver failure • Indicates deficiency of 1 or > liver synthesized factor	• Frequent fluctuations in levels, so ideal monitoring tool • ↑ INR and ↑ bili = poor prognosis in nonacetaminophen acute liver failure and poor prognosis in severe alcoholic hepatitis, jaundice also adds to confirmation of prognosis
↑ INR	• More specific for vitamin K deficiency, also seen in DIC, warfarin therapy	
Coagulation factors	• Full liver failure indicated by < 20% normal of factor V = very poor prognosis	–
5. Assists With Accurate Diagnosis—does not assess liver function		
Ig level	• ↑ serum globulin level indicates nonspecific chronic liver disease • ↑ IgG = autoimmune hepatitis • ↑ IgM = primary biliary cirrhosis	–
Autoantibody levels	• Primary biliary cirrhosis, autoimmune hepatitis	–
Serologic tests for viral hepatitis	–	–

ALP—alkaline phosphatase; ALT—alanine aminotransferase or serum glutamic pyruvic transaminase (SGPT); AST—aspartate aminotransferase or serum glutamic oxaloacetic transaminase (SGOT); bili—bilirubin; COPD—chronic obstructive pulmonary disease; DIC—disseminated intravascular coagulation; DILI—drug-induced liver injury; GGT—gamma glutamyl transpeptidase; Ig—immunoglobulin; IgG—immunoglobulin G; IgM—immunoglobulin M; INR—international normalized ratio; MI—myocardial infarction; NASH—nonalcoholic steatohepatitis; PT—protime

Note. Based on information from Astegiano et al., 2004; Donnan et al., 2007; Duong & Loh, 2006; Gopal & Rosen, 2000; Kaplowitz, 2004.

or any other space-occupying lesions (Bryant). The CT scan is best to determine vertical liver span and overall size. Magnetic resonance imaging is more sensitive than a CT scan for determining metastasis, hemangioma, hepatoma, or other liver lesions (Bryant). A percutaneous transhepatic cholangiogram examines the biliary tree within and outside of the liver. It especially is useful when ultrasound and CT are positive and an obstruction is being ruled out. An endoscopic retrograde cholangiopancreatography is also used to determine if biliary tree obstruction is present. Hepatobiliary iminodiacetic acid scans assist in evaluating gallbladder and bile duct disease with nuclear imaging.

Liver biopsy can determine the etiology of the hepatotoxicity and the pathology of masses or lesions identified after imaging (Bryant, 2006). Liver biopsy can prove to be definitive, especially if clinical signs of hepatotoxicity are present but serologic, autoimmune, metabolic, and other measures fail to yield diagnostic information. Biopsy also is used to verify DILI and rule out hepatocellular carcinoma, infiltrative disorders, cirrhosis, and viral hepatitis. Cultures may be obtained on liver biopsy tissue to determine the success of therapy for metabolic or viral liver disease. Liver biopsy is contraindicated in patients who have coagulopathy abnormalities, suspected hemangioma, ascites, or pleural effusion (Gopal & Rosen, 2000).

Physical Examination

General signs and symptoms correlated with liver disease include fever, jaundice, ecchymosis, petechiae, and icteric sclera. Neurologic problems associated with liver disease include altered behavior, level of orientation, mental status, and asterixis (flapping tremor of wrist in extension). Cardiac and pulmonary changes that may indicate liver disease include congestive heart failure signs, such as peripheral edema, extra heart sounds, and rales. The abdominal examination can yield much information about liver injury. Tenderness of the abdomen may reflect inflammation of the liver. Hepatomegaly may represent liver disease, and splenomegaly may reflect cirrhosis. Other signs and symptoms in the abdominal examination that may demonstrate liver injury include ascites from cirrhosis or malignancy, abdominal vein distention with spider angiomas, portal hypertension from acute or chronic liver damage, palpable abdominal mass suggesting malignancy, palpable gallbladder indicative of common bile duct obstruction with jaundice, or Courvoisier sign and/or Charcot triad, which includes fever, chills, jaundice, and right upper quadrant pain from gallstones (Bryant, 2006).

The most common causes of an enlarged palpable liver are acute and chronic liver injury, metastatic carcinoma, fatty liver, and right heart failure (Wolf, 1990). Fever, eosinophilia, and other allergic signs are more indicative of immune-mediated damage to the liver (Liu & Kaplowitz, 2002). Cholestatic hepatitis presents with jaundice, pruritus, and high elevations of ALP with slight increases in ALT (Kaplowitz, 2004).

DILI will mimic many acute and chronic liver diseases, but the primary presentation is acute icteric hepatitis or cholestatic liver disease. Appreciable elevations occur in serum transaminase levels along with slight elevations in ALP with acute icteric hepatitis. If the liver injury is severe, then coagulopathy and encephalopathy are present. If the pathology is of a cholestatic nature, the abnormal labs may take months to normalize (Kaplowitz, 2004). These symptoms normally will abate after the drug is withdrawn (Bryant, 2006).

In VOD, acute onset occurs of painful hepatomegaly, ascites, peripheral edema, and elevated liver function tests, especially hyperbilirubinemia and hepatic encephalopathy, usually within a week of a stem cell transplant. Thrombosis also contributes to the ischemia and necrosis, as does direct chemical injury (Sinicrope, 2003). The National Cancer Institute (2006) has an extensive grading scale to classify acute and subclinical toxicities including liver function tests (see Table 13-9).

Differential Diagnosis

The differential diagnosis is used to determine if a cause other than cancer chemotherapy or supportive medications is contributing to hepatotoxicity. The clinical work-up for issues related to portal/hepatic circulation needs to include a detailed work-up for portal hypertension, Budd-Chiari syndrome (obstruction of hepatic vein), thrombosis of hepatic vein, congestive heart failure, or VOD. Hepatobiliary tract problems can be caused by primary biliary cirrhosis, sclerosing cholangitis, and malignancy. Cirrhosis can be caused by alpha-1 antitrypsin deficiency, hemochromato-

Table 13-9. Common Terminology Criteria for Hepatic Toxicity

Adverse Event	Grade				
	1	2	3	4	5
Metabolic/Laboratory					
Albumin, serum-low (hypoalbuminemia)	< LLN – 3 g/dL < LLN – 30 g/L	< 3– 2 g/dL < 30 – 20 g/L	< 2 g/dL < 20 g/L	–	Death
Alkaline phosphatase	> ULN – 2.5 x ULN	> 2.5 – 5.0 x ULN	> 5.0 – 20.0 x ULN	> 20.0 x ULN	–
ALT, SGPT (serum glutamic pyruvic transaminase)	> ULN – 2.5 x ULN	> 2.5 – 5.0 x ULN	> 5.0 – 20.0 x ULN	> 20.0 x ULN	–
AST, SGOT (serum glutamic oxaloacetic transaminase)	> ULN – 2.5 x ULN	> 2.5 – 5.0 x ULN	> 5.0 – 20.0 x ULN	> 20.0 x ULN	–
Bilirubin (hyperbilirubinemia)	> ULN – 1.5 x ULN	> 1.5 – 3.0 x ULN	> 3.0 – 10.0 x ULN	> 10.0 x ULN	–

REMARK: Jaundice is not an AE, but may be a manifestation of liver dysfunction/failure or elevated bilirubin. If jaundice is associated with elevated bilirubin, grade bilirubin.

Adverse Event	Grade				
GGT (γ-Glutamyl transpeptidase)	> ULN – 2.5 x ULN	> 2.5 – 5.0 x ULN	> 5.0 – 20.0 x ULN	> 20.0 x ULN	–
Hepatobiliary/Pancreas					
Liver dysfunction/failure (clinical)	–	Jaundice	Asterixis	Encephalopathy or coma	Death

REMARK: Jaundice is not an AE, but occurs when the liver is not working properly or when a bile duct is blocked. It is graded as a result of liver dysfunction/failure or elevated bilirubin.
ALSO CONSIDER: Bilirubin (hyperbilirubinemia).

AE—adverse event; ALT—alanine aminotransferase; AST—aspartate aminotransferase; ULN—upper limit of normal

Note. From *Common Terminology Criteria for Adverse Events* (Version 3.0), by National Cancer Institute Cancer Therapy Evaluation Program, 2006. Retrieved March 30, 2008, from http://ctep.cancer.gov/forms/CTCAEv3.pdf

sis, Wilson disease (inherited disorder of metabolism creating copper overload), Reye syndrome, or diabetes mellitus.

Evidence-Based Treatment Strategies

Treatment of hepatotoxicity includes removal of the offending agent, if known, or otherwise treating the cause to stop the liver injury from progressing and to prevent irreversible damage. Frequent monitoring of laboratory values is an important intervention to monitor treatment effectiveness. APNs need to consider referral to a gastroenterologist for a more complex and inexplicable course of hepatotoxicity.

Imatinib is approved for the treatment of chronic myelocytic leukemia. A 1%–5% incidence of severe liver injury has been associated with the use of imatinib that necessitates permanent discontinuation of the drug. In a case review of five patients, all the patients experienced grade 3–4 hepatotoxicity, as measured by increased AST and ALT values, two to eight months after initiation of imatinib (Ferrero et al., 2006). These patients were rechallenged with lower doses, and two of the patients again presented with liver toxicity. The authors used prednisone or methylprednisolone 25–40 mg/day, with resolution of the hepatotoxicity occurring within three to eight weeks. The patients subsequently were able to continue on full doses of imatinib. Steroids were tapered after three to five months. Tyrosine kinase inhibitors have been well tolerated, but a 2%–5% incidence of hepatotoxicity exists with imatinib. This case study report illustrated one intervention in which corticosteroids were used to reverse the severe hepatotoxicity. Erlotinib, an epidermal growth factor receptor inhibitor, also has been reported to cause hepatotoxicity in a patient with pancreatic cancer. The patient developed increased levels of AST, ALT, and ALP, which did not peak until two weeks after discontinuation of erlotinib (Ramanarayanan & Scarpace, 2007).

Silymarin is a commonly used herb in cancer care because of its anti-inflammatory and antifibrotic effects (Verma & Thuluvath, 2007). Extract of milk thistle (silymarin) also is known as a liver tonic. It is thought to prevent or reverse hepatotoxicity of damaging drug metabolites or other toxins. Silymarin possesses low drug interaction potential, but clinical trials are still determining its effectiveness (Kroll, Shaw, & Oberlies, 2007). Natural Standard (2007), an evidence-based Web site on CAM, uses a level-of-evidence grading scale (from A to F) to review all available literature on silymarin. Silymarin received a grade of "B," meaning it has good scientific support for treatment of cirrhosis and chronic hepatitis. Natural Standard reviewed at least one randomized trial or one meta-analysis to support the use of this herb in liver injury. Unclear or conflicting support exists for the use of milk thistle in acute viral hepatitis, cancer prevention, or drug- or toxin-induced hepatotoxicity.

A current clinical trial is looking at DILI by collecting and studying patients' serum and lymphocytes. Patients are eligible if they have experienced DILI caused by isoniazid, phenytoin, amoxicillin/clavulanic acid, or valproic acid (National Institutes of Health, 2006).

Evaluation of Outcomes

Oncology APNs have several toxicity resources (see Table 13-9) available to objectively evaluate the outcome of treating hepatotoxicity. The inadequacy of many of the methods to measure hepatotoxicity and the latency of symptom onset in many types of liver injury, especially if drug-induced, make it necessary for APNs to monitor serial liver function testing following baseline testing at the first visit and correlate it with the history and physical examination findings.

Implications for Advanced Nursing Practice

Liver injury may remain subclinical in nature or only produce subtle signs and symptoms. More than 1,000 drugs have been implicated in DILI, many of which include medications used in the treatment and support of patients with cancer. Oncology APNs have frequent contact with patients with cancer who are at high risk for hepatotoxicity because of their history, cancer diagnosis, or treatment. The opportunity exists to screen high-risk individuals for liver disease and monitor their status closely for early signs of liver injury. APNs can order appropriate diagnostic and monitoring studies and make gastroenterology consults in a timely fashion to accomplish the goals of prevention and early diagnosis. Patients and families will require assistance to understand the results of their tests.

Pulmonary Toxicity Related to Cancer Therapy

Introduction

Pulmonary toxicity in patients with cancer is associated with acute and late effects from primary or metastatic disease or treatment of disease with radiation therapy, chemotherapy, and biotherapy. The use of chemotherapy, biotherapy, and radiation therapy, alone or combined, can be associated with clinically significant pulmonary toxicity. Treatment-induced pulmonary toxicities include pneumonitis, pulmonary fibrosis, and an overall decrease in pulmonary function. Radiation pneumonitis and radiation pulmonary fibrosis are the two main dose-limiting factors when irradiating the lung. Stem cell transplantation also may be associated with pulmonary toxicity, including idiopathic pneumonia syndrome and bronchiolitis obliterans. This section will review toxicities caused by radiation therapy, chemotherapy, and biotherapy. For a review of pulmonary toxicities related to stem cell transplantation, see Chapter 7.

Definition and Incidence

Treatment-related pulmonary toxicity is the parenchymal pulmonary disease caused by radiation therapy, chemotherapy, and biotherapy used for the treatment of cancer. Radiation pneumonitis is an acute inflammatory reaction of the lung parenchyma related to thoracic radiotherapy, involving alveolar cell depletion and inflammatory cell accumulation in the interstitial space (Tsoutsou & Koukourakis, 2006). Radiation pneumonitis generally occurs within 12 weeks after thoracic radiotherapy. The threshold dose of radiotherapy to the lung is about 6 Gy (600 cGy) (Srinivas, Agarwal, & Agarwal, 2007). Acute radiation pneumonitis is reported in patients who have been treated for lung cancer, Hodgkin disease, breast cancer, and other cancers that require radiation therapy to the thorax (Carver et al., 2007). Radiation pneumonitis occurs in 5%–15% of patients receiving external beam radiation therapy for lung cancer (McDonald, Rubin, Phillips, & Marks, 1995). The incidence of radiation pneumonitis is lower in patients with Hodgkin disease and breast cancer who have received mediastinal radiation therapy than in patients with lung cancer (Carver et al.). A study reviewing 560 patients with stage IA–IIIB Hodgkin disease demonstrated a 3% risk of radiation pneumonitis with radiation therapy alone, which increased to 11% when radiation therapy was combined with chemotherapy (Tarbell, Thompson, & Mauch, 1990). A risk of less than 1% exists for patients with breast cancer who undergo radiation therapy as part of a breast-conserving approach (Harris, 2001). The incidence of radiation-induced pneumonitis increases with concurrent chemotherapy administration.

Radiation-induced pulmonary fibrosis is a late effect of thoracic radiotherapy and is chronic in nature. Radiation fibrosis occurs 6–24 months after the completion of radiation therapy (Srinivas et al., 2007). Changes seen with radiation fibrosis include fibroblast proliferation, collagen accumulation, and destruction of the normal architecture of the lung (Morgan & Breit, 1995). The result of pulmonary fibrosis is permanent scarring of the lung tissue, which leads to permanent impairment of oxygen transfer. The incidence of radiation fibrosis is significantly lower than that of radiation pneumonitis.

Many chemotherapy agents may cause pulmonary toxicity, but bleomycin is the most studied. Bleomycin-induced pneumonitis is the most common form of bleomycin-related pulmonary toxicity (Carver et al., 2007). Early-onset chemotherapy-induced pulmonary toxicity generally is referred to as inflammatory interstitial pneumonitis, also known as hypersensitivity-type reaction. Early-onset chemotherapy-induced pneumonitis can develop after the initial dose of chemotherapy or can occur several months after completion of chemotherapy (Abid, Malhotra, & Perry, 2001). Chemotherapy agents associated with chemotherapy-induced pneumonitis include bleomycin, busulfan, carmustine, cyclophosphamide, cytosine arabinoside, gemcitabine, methotrexate, mitomycin, paclitaxel, and procarbazine (see Table 13-10). A recent study reported that taxane-based adjuvant chemotherapy used for the treatment of high-risk breast cancer increases the incidence of radiation pneumonitis up to 35% (Yu et al., 2004).

Table 13-10. Chemotherapy Drugs Associated With Pulmonary Toxicity

Drug	Type of Pulmonary Toxicity	Risk Factors
Bleomycin	Pneumonitis and pulmonary fibrosis	Age older than 60, concomitant chemotherapy or radiation therapy, renal insufficiency, cumulative doses > 400–500 units, supplemental oxygen (> 35% [even years later])
Busulfan	Pneumonitis and pulmonary fibrosis	No known risk factors, no relation to dose
Carmustine	Pneumonitis and pulmonary fibrosis	Dose dependent (especially greater than 1,500 mg/m^2), concurrent radiation, preexisting pulmonary disease
Cyclophosphamide	Pneumonitis Pulmonary fibrosis (< 1% incidence)	Cumulative doses ranging from 150–250 mg
Cytosine arabinoside	Pneumonitis	No risk factors
Gemcitabine	Pneumonitis	Prolonged infusion time (> 60 minutes), no relation to dose
Methotrexate	Pneumonitis and pulmonary fibrosis	Concomitant use of other chemotherapy drugs
Mitomycin	Pneumonitis and pulmonary fibrosis	Supplemental oxygen (> 35%), concurrent radiation to the lung, concomitant use of other chemotherapy drugs (e.g., bleomycin, cisplatin, cyclophosphamide, doxorubicin, vinca alkaloids)
Paclitaxel	Pneumonitis	Concurrent radiation to the lung
Procarbazine	Pneumonitis (rare)	No risk factors

Note. Based on information from Abid et al., 2001; Matthews, 2005; Wilkes & Barton-Burke, 2007.

Another early-onset chemotherapy-induced pulmonary toxicity is that of acute, non-cardiogenic pulmonary edema. This complication most commonly is associated with cytosine arabinoside (Abid et al., 2001). Interleukin-2 (IL-2) is associated with a unique capillary leak syndrome that is strongly expressed in pulmonary tissues. Capillary leak syndrome leads to a loss of vascular tone in the lungs, which can lead to an increase of capillary permeability and pulmonary edema.

Late-onset chemotherapy-induced pulmonary toxicity is defined as toxicity presenting more than two months after therapy is completed. The most common manifestation of late-onset chemotherapy-induced pulmonary toxicity is pulmonary fibrosis. The chemotherapy agents most closely associated with pulmonary fibrosis include bleomycin, busulfan, carmustine, and mitomycin (see Table 13-10) (Abid et al., 2001; Matthews, 2005). The incidence of bleomycin-induced pulmonary fibrosis is approximately 10%, with a mortality rate of 1%–2% in the patients developing pulmonary fibrosis (Hinson & McKibben, 2001).

Presenting Signs and Symptoms of Treatment-Induced Pulmonary Toxicity

The symptoms associated with treatment-induced pneumonitis are nonspecific respiratory symptoms. These symptoms include mild cough, mild to progressive dyspnea, nonproductive cough, and low-grade fever (generally less than 38.3°C [101°F]). Patients who experience acute radiation-induced pneumonitis often have a self-limited course, with complete resolution of the condition. A minority of patients develop progressive pulmonary fibrosis with signs and symptoms that include progressive exertional dyspnea and nonproductive cough (Carver et al., 2007). Signs of late-stage pulmonary fibrosis include orthopnea, cyanosis, cor pulmonale, and respiratory failure (Tsoutsou & Koukourakis, 2006).

Capillary leak syndrome results from extravasation of plasma proteins and fluid into the extravascular space, leading to a loss of vascular tone. This loss of vascular tone, which occurs within 2–12 hours of starting IL-2, causes a decrease in mean arterial blood pressure and decreased organ perfusion, which may be severe and can result in death. Resolution of the symptoms of capillary leak syndrome generally occurs with discontinuation of IL-2.

Risk Factors

Evidence is inconclusive and inconsistent for the factors that predict the occurrence or severity of radiation pneumonitis. Factors that may increase the risk of radiation-induced pneumonitis include radiation dose, volume of lung irradiated, fractionation schedule, concomitant chemotherapy, history of smoking (Lind et al., 2002), previous irradiation to the lung, recent withdrawal of steroids, preexisting lung disease, poor pulmonary function, unknown genetic predisposition (Kasten-Pisula, Tastan, & Dikomey, 2005), and older age (Matthews, 2005; Rancati, Ceresoli, Gagliardi, Schipani, & Cattaneo, 2003). The primary risk factor related to the development of radiation-induced pulmonary fibrosis is a history of pulmonary pneumonitis. A recent evaluation of treatment-related pneumonitis in patients with advanced-stage non-small cell lung cancer treated with concurrent chemotherapy and intensity-modulated radiotherapy (IMRT) found that IMRT resulted in significantly lower levels of grade ≥ 3 pneumonitis compared with three-dimensional conformal radiation therapy (3D-CRT) (Yom et al., 2007).

Risk factors related to the development of chemotherapy-induced pneumonitis include age older than 60, smoking history, preexisting pulmonary disease, concomitant radiation therapy to the lungs, history of radiation therapy to the lungs, and oxygen therapy at high doses (Matthews, 2005). Drug-specific risk factors are listed in Table 13-10. Risk factors for capillary leak syndrome associated with IL-2 include previous chemotherapy, bolus IL-2 infusions, and pretreatment reduction in forced expiratory volume in one second (FEV_1) (Abid et al., 2001).

Etiology and Pathophysiology

Radiation produces free radicals that damage pneumocytes and endothelial cells. The damage of these cells leads to a diffuse inflammatory process within the lung. This acute reaction, or pneumonitis, triggers an immune response similar to the hypersensitivity pneumonitis that is seen with chemotherapy and inhaled antigens (Srinivas et al., 2007). The diffuse inflammation results in edema in the alveolar walls caused by vascular permeability and exudation of proteins in the alveolar space (Gross, 1980). DNA damage in all cellular components occurs with this diffuse inflammation. Intraalveolar hemorrhage also may occur as a result of possible vessel thrombosis (Tsoutsou & Koukourakis, 2006). The interplay among these activities in the lung leads to accumulation of collagen and destruction of the normal architecture of the lung (Tsoutsou & Koukourakis).

Radiation-induced pulmonary fibrosis is thought to be a distinct pathologic phenomenon. Radiation-induced pulmonary fibrosis is driven by an increase in cytokine production, presumably tumor necrosis factor-alpha and platelet-derived growth factor. The result of this process is a loss of capillaries and an increase in alveolar septal thickness (McDonald et al., 1995). Changes associated with pulmonary fibrosis also lead to destruction of the normal architecture of the lungs, which can result in permanent destruction.

The pathogenesis of chemotherapy-induced lung changes involves the release of chemotactic factors from alveolar macrophages (Hinson & McKibben, 2001). Generally, toxicity is more reliably predictable with higher cumulative doses of drugs and concomitant, previous, or subsequent radiation therapy to the lungs. Pulmonary edema seen with cytosine arabinoside and IL-2 involves endothelial inflammation and vascular leak.

Physical Examination and Diagnosis

The diagnosis of pneumonitis and pulmonary fibrosis is primarily a clinical diagnosis with the aid of pulmonary function tests (PFTs). The onset of pneumonitis is characterized by nonspecific symptoms including mild cough, mild dyspnea, and low-grade fever. Physical examination may reveal scattered fine crackles, crepitations, bronchial breathing, and possible pleural effusion. A chest x-ray or CT may demonstrate ground-glass opacification and consolidation that conforms to the portals of irradiation (even though pneumonitis is a diffuse process). Bronchoscopic lavage and biopsy are tests that can exclude the possibility of infection (Srinivas et al., 2007).

A variety of PFTs can determine the gas exchange in the lung, which may give an indication of the presence and severity of lung involvement related to treatment-induced lung pathology. PFTs demonstrate gas movement (measured by FEV_1), lung capacity (measured by forced expiratory capacity [FEC]), and diffusion of gases (measured by carbon monoxide diffusing capacity [DL_{CO}]) (Mehta, 2005). The DL_{CO} is considered to be the most essential test for estimating the severity of pneumonitis and fibrosis (McDonald et al., 1995). Outcomes of PFTs that indicate pulmonary fibrosis include a reduced DL_{CO}, an intermediate reduction in FEC, and a reduction in the FEV_1 (Srinivas et al., 2007).

Toxicity Criteria for Radiation-Induced Pneumonitis

A variety of grading scales are used to determine the degree of toxicity related to radiation-induced pneumonitis. These scales include the Common Terminology Criteria for Adverse Events, the Radiation Therapy Oncology Group/European Organisation for Research and Treatment of Cancer (Late Effects on Normal Tissues–Subjective, Objective, Management and Analytic scales), and the Southwest Oncology Group criteria (see Table 13-11). These scales are used most often for grading toxicity in patients participating in clinical trials.

Table 13-11. Toxicity Criteria for Pneumonitis

Criteria	1	2	3	4	5
Common Terminology Criteria for Adverse Events	Asymptomatic; radiographic findings only	Symptomatic; not interfering with activities of daily living (ADLs)	Symptomatic; interferes with ADLs; oxygen indicated	Life-threatening; ventilation support required	Death
Radiation Therapy Oncology Group/European Organisation for Research and Treatment of Cancer (Late Effects on Normal Tissues–Subjective, Objective, Management and Analytic scales)	Asymptomatic or mild symptoms (dry cough), with radiographic findings	Moderate symptoms (severe cough, fever)	Severe symptoms	Severe respiratory insufficiency; continuous O_2/assisted ventilation support	Death
Southwest Oncology Group	Asymptomatic or symptoms not requiring steroids, with radiographic findings	Initiation of or increase in steroids required	Oxygen required	Assisted ventilation necessary	Death

Differential Diagnosis

The diagnosis of radiation- or chemotherapy-induced pneumonitis or fibrosis generally is a clinical diagnosis based on the timing of the treatment and the physical symptoms that the patient is experiencing. A chest radiograph or CT scans and PFTs help to establish the diagnosis of treatment-induced pneumonitis or fibrosis. Differentiation from recurrent malignancy, infection, or other pulmonary disease can be difficult. A lung biopsy is necessary to help to establish a diagnosis in situations where these other causes for the symptoms are considered (Abid et al., 2001). This can be done by fiberoptic bronchoscopy with transbronchial lung biopsy (Wesselius, 1999).

Prevention of Treatment-Induced Pulmonary Toxicity

Pulmonary toxicity related to radiation therapy can be a dose-limiting toxicity. Unfortunately, research demonstrates that interrupting radiotherapy or decreasing dosage because of toxicity significantly reduces overall survival, locoregional control, and metastasis-free survival in patients with non-small cell lung cancer (Jeremic et al., 2003). The use of newer methods of delivering radiation therapy, such as 3D-CRT or IMRT, may decrease the incidence of pulmonary toxicity. These methods limit the irradiation of normal lung tissue while providing improved coverage of the tumor. This type of radiation therapy is not available in all radiation treatment centers, and it requires precise targeting of the radiation beams. A recent study of 18 patients who received high-dose 3D-CRT (one of whom received neoadjuvant chemotherapy) found that none of the patients developed radiation pneumonitis ≥ grade 2 (Narayan et al., 2004). The use of IMRT reduces the exposure of normal lung tissue to radiation by approximately 10%–20% while increasing the dose to the target lung tissue (Dirkx & Heijmen, 2000; van Sornsen de Koste, Voet, Dirkx, van Meerbeeck, & Senan, 2001).

An area of study for the prevention of radiation- and chemotherapy-induced pneumonitis is the use of cytoprotective agents given while receiving therapy. The use of broad-spectrum immunomodulating therapy has been studied in relation to its protection against radiation pneumonitis. One study reported no cases of radiation pneumonitis ≥ grade 3 when corticosteroid therapy (prednisone) was given before the radiotherapy (Wurstbauer, Deutschmann, Sedlmayer, & Kogelnik, 2001). Amifostine, an aminothiol with broad-spectrum cytoprotection, has been studied for its effects against radiation-induced pneumonitis. However, results regarding the use of amifostine to protect against radiation pneumonitis are conflicting. Early studies (Antonadou, Coliarakis, et al., 2001; Antonadou, Throuvalas, et al., 2001) demonstrated that administering amifostine daily before radiotherapy or chemoradiotherapy significantly reduced the incidence of radiation pneumonitis compared to no cytoprotective therapy. In a more recent large, randomized phase III study of patients who received chemotherapy and hyperfractionated radiotherapy, the administration of amifostine did not reduce the incidence of radiation pneumonitis (Werner-Wasik et al., 2003). Other cytoprotective agents that are being studied for their pulmonary protective effects against radiotherapy include captopril, pentoxifylline, melatonin, vitamin A, carvedilol, and manganese superoxide dismutase gene therapy (Mehta, 2005; Srinivas et al., 2007).

Management of Treatment-Induced Pulmonary Toxicity

Radiation-Induced Pulmonary Toxicity

The nonspecific symptoms of radiation-induced pulmonary toxicity, including a mild cough and low-grade fever, are treated symptomatically with cough suppressants, antipyretics, and rest. Although no controlled trials exist on the effectiveness of steroid therapy in radiation pneumonitis, it is common practice to treat patients with prednisone as soon as the diagnosis of pneumonitis is made. A commonly prescribed schedule of steroid therapy is to initiate prednisolone at 1 mg/kg for several weeks, followed by a slow and cautious tapering of the medication (Abid et al., 2001; Srinivas et al., 2007; Tsoutsou & Koukourakis, 2006). Unfortunately, only about 50% of patients treated with glucocorticoid therapy respond (Matthews, 2005). No role has been demonstrated for steroid therapy in the management of radiation-induced pulmonary fibrosis. One study reported a clinical benefit (in a cohort of 43 patients) with radiation-induced pulmonary fibrosis using combination pentoxifylline and vitamin E (Delanian, Balla-Mekias, & Lefaix, 1999).

Chemotherapy-Induced Pulmonary Toxicity

Once again, no controlled trials exist on the effectiveness of glucocorticoid therapy for the management of chemotherapy-induced pulmonary toxicity, yet the use of glucocorticoid therapy is common in treating this toxicity. Other management strategies include supportive care for the nonspecific symptoms of pulmonary toxicities, limiting the cumulative dose of bleomycin to 400 units, and minimizing the use of supplemental oxygen therapy for drugs known to cause pulmonary toxicity (e.g., bleomycin, mitomycin-c, the nitrosoureas).

Evaluation of Outcomes

No standard tests currently are used to monitor patients for radiation- or chemotherapy-induced pulmonary pneumonitis or fibrosis. Generally, decisions about continuation of therapy are based on patient symptoms.

Conclusion

Toxicity to the GU, hepatic, or pulmonary systems may occur because of the cancer or because of adverse effects of cancer treatment. People with cancer often have comorbidities that increase the risk of toxicity. Some toxicities can be prevented or lessened by astute observation with the goal to discover and treat any adverse reaction early enough to prevent irreversible damage.

Case Study

J.C. is a 39-year-old female with a diagnosis of breast cancer. She was diagnosed with a stage IIB tumor, estrogen receptor positive, progesterone receptor negative, and HER2 overexpressed. She has completed a lumpectomy and is undergoing chemotherapy treatment with doxorubicin and cyclophosphamide followed by a taxane. She will receive 52 weeks of treatment with trastuzumab beginning with the taxane. Following chemotherapy, she will receive radiation to the breast with a boost to the tumor bed.

During one of her clinic visits, J.C. relates that she is worried about her sexual relationship with her husband. She has noticed that her libido has declined since her diagnosis and that sexual intercourse has become painful. The APN realizes the need to obtain more information prior to diagnosis.

1. What information should the oncology APN obtain in the sexual history?
   • The sexual history should first establish a baseline of sexual functioning prior to J.C.'s diagnosis, as cancer and its treatment could exacerbate a previous problem. The APN would inquire about feelings of inadequacy, anxiety in regard to sexual performance, depression, expectations, partner expectations, and anxieties. Specific questions about dyspareunia and libido should be posed to J.C. The ALARM and the BETTER models are useful to assist in performance of a thorough sexual history.
   • Upon further exploration, J.C. relates that she is experiencing vaginal dryness that contributes to dyspareunia. She also states that she no longer feels attractive because of her surgery and believes that her husband no longer finds her appealing. She is experiencing fatigue from her chemotherapy treatments as well.
2. What are some specific interventions that the APN could recommend?
   • The oncology APN realizes that J.C. is experiencing sexual dysfunction caused by treatment side effects as well as an alteration in self-image. The nurse schedules a meeting with the patient and her husband. For vaginal dryness, the oncology APN might recommend a water-based lubricant. The nurse suggests that scheduling intimate times when J.C.'s fatigue level is low might be beneficial. Because J.C. has had some difficulties with mucositis after chemotherapy, the APN asks about vaginal irritation or lesions, which J.C. denies.
3. J.C. tells the APN that her friend experienced vaginal dryness following her hysterectomy and that taking estrogen relieved this. She asks the APN to prescribe this for her. What should the APN do?
   • The oncology APN discusses the benefits and risks of systemic or topical estrogen therapy for menopausal symptoms such as vaginal dryness. The nurse admits that this is the most common management strategy but that it may be contraindicated in patients with hormonally responsive cancer, noting that J.C. is estrogen receptor positive. Following this discussion, J.C. decides to try vaginal lubricants for a month and if this does not prove helpful, then a vaginal estrogen agent may be considered. J.C. and her husband determine when during the chemotherapy cycle she has more energy. They decide to plan a special romantic evening during this time.
4. About 10 weeks following her radiation therapy, J.C. notices that she has a dry, nonproductive cough. Her chest wall is sore from coughing, and she is short of breath when walking down her driveway to get the mail. She has noticed an oral temperature of around 37.9°C (100.3°F) in the early evenings. What is the most likely diagnosis?
   • The oncology APN performs a thorough history and physical examination. Physical examination reveals scattered fine crackles bilaterally, and chest x-ray demonstrates fine, diffuse infiltrate corresponding to the radiation port. PFTs are normal, and no indications of an infectious process exist. The APN notes that J.C. completed radiation involving the mediastinum about 10 weeks previously and that the timing of her symptoms is consistent with radiation pneumonitis.
5. How would the APN treat J.C.'s radiation pneumonitis?
   • The APN recommends rest for conservation of respiratory effort and prescribes prednisolone at 1 mg/kg for two to three weeks and then tapered slowly. The

nurse informs J.C. that these measures are for symptomatic relief and may not shorten the duration of the pneumonitis; however, the APN encourages her with the information that usually the acute phase of pneumonitis is short-lived and resolves spontaneously.

Key Points

Genitourinary Toxicity

- Sexual dysfunction and infertility are common side effects of cancer and cancer therapy.
- Sperm and embryo cryopreservation often are viable options for fertility preservation.
- The ALARM and BETTER models are assessment techniques that may be used to elicit in-depth information. The PLISSIT model guides the clinician's dialogue and intervention.
- Despite potentially effective preventive measures and treatments for sexual dysfunction and infertility, patients with cancer continue to report limited communications about sexual health with their clinicians.
- Chemotherapy, radiation therapy, and infection are the most common causes of cystitis in patients with cancer.
- Effective preventive and treatment measures for cystitis exist.

Hepatotoxicity

- The major types of liver disease pathology include hepatocellular, cholestatic, and a mixture of both.
- The major causes of liver injury include several major drugs, such as acetaminophen, methotrexate, asparaginase, and tamoxifen.
- The most common presenting signs and symptoms of DILI include edema, pruritus, jaundice, malaise, headache, anorexia, ecchymosis, low-grade fever, muscle and joint aches, and urine and stool color changes.
- The most frequent laboratory studies used to assist in diagnosis and monitoring of liver injury are the serum aminotransferases, AST and ALT.

Pulmonary Toxicity

- Radiation pneumonitis is an acute inflammatory reaction of the lung parenchyma related to thoracic radiotherapy, which generally occurs within 12 weeks of thoracic radiotherapy. It is reported in patients who have been treated for lung cancer, Hodgkin disease, breast cancer, and other cancers that require radiation therapy to the thorax.
- The symptoms associated with treatment-induced pneumonitis are nonspecific respiratory symptoms and include mild cough, mild to progressive dyspnea, nonproductive cough, and low-grade fever (generally less than 101°F).
- Radiation-induced pulmonary fibrosis is a late effect of thoracic radiotherapy and is chronic in nature, occurring 6–24 months after the completion of radiation therapy.
- Many chemotherapy agents may cause pulmonary toxicity, but bleomycin is the most studied. The chemotherapy agents most closely associated with pulmonary fibrosis include bleomycin, busulfan, carmustine, and mitomycin.

- Early-onset chemotherapy-induced pulmonary toxicity can develop after the initial dose of chemotherapy or several months after completion of chemotherapy.
- The most common manifestation of late-onset chemotherapy-induced pulmonary toxicity is pulmonary fibrosis, which generally starts more than two months after completion of therapy.
- The diagnosis of pneumonitis and pulmonary fibrosis primarily is a clinical diagnosis with the aid of chest radiographs, CT scans, and PFTs.
- Strategies for the management of radiation- and chemotherapy-induced pneumonitis include symptom management of the respiratory symptoms as well as a course of glucocorticoid therapy. Pulmonary fibrosis is managed primarily by supportive management of the respiratory symptoms.

Recommended Resources for Oncology Advanced Practice Nurses

Genitourinary

- Fertile Hope (www.fertilehope.com): A nonprofit organization that assists patients with cancer with infertility. Provides information, resources, and financial assistance.
- Katz, A. (2007). *Breaking the silence on cancer and sexuality: A handbook for healthcare providers.* Pittsburgh, PA: Oncology Nursing Society.
- Schover, L. (1997). *Sexuality and fertility after cancer.* New York: Wiley.
- Schover, L. (2001). *Sexuality and cancer: For the man who has cancer and his partner.* Atlanta, GA: American Cancer Society.
- Schover, L. (2001). *Sexuality and cancer: For the woman who has cancer and her partner.* Atlanta, GA: American Cancer Society.
- Turnbull, G.B. (2001). *Intimacy, sexuality, and an ostomy.* May be downloaded free of charge from www.uoaa.org/ostomy_info/pubs/uoa_sexuality_en.pdf.

Hepatic

- NACB Laboratory Medicine Practice Guidelines: www.aacc.org/AACC/Members/nacb/Archive/LMPG/hepaticinjury
- Natural Standard (www.naturalstandard.com): Resource to monitor the effect of complementary and alternative therapies on the liver

Pulmonary

- CancerSymptoms.org: Dypsnea (www.cancersymptoms.org/dyspnea/index.shtml)
- Oncology Nursing Society Evidence-Based Practice Resource Area, Putting Evidence Into Practice®: Dyspnea (www.ons.org/outcomes/volume2/dyspnea.shtml)

References

Abid, S.H., Malhotra, V., & Perry, M.C. (2001). Radiation-induced and chemotherapy-induced pulmonary injury. *Current Opinion in Oncology, 13,* 242–248.

Adamson, D. (2007). Affording fertility-preserving treatment: Insurance, treatment packages, and financing. In Center for Reproductive Medicine and Infertility (Ed.), *Cancer and fertility resource guide 2007–2008* (p. 157). New York: Center for Reproductive Medicine and Infertility.

Alivizatos, G., & Skolarikos, A. (2005). Incontinence and erectile dysfunction following radical prostatectomy: A review. *Scientific World Journal, 5,* 747–758.

Alvarez, F., Berg, P.A., Bianchi, F.B., Bianchi, L., Burroughs, A.K., Cancado, E.L., et al. (1999). International Autoimmune Hepatitis Group Report: Review of criteria for diagnosis of autoimmune hepatitis. *Journal of Hepatology, 3,* 929–938. Retrieved October 9, 2007, from http://tpis.upmc.edu/tpis/schema/aih99.html#Score

Amsterdam, A., & Krychman, M. (2006). Sexual dysfunction in patients with gynecologic neoplasms: A retrospective pilot study. *Journal of Sexual Medicine, 3,* 646–649.

Antonadou, D., Coliarakis, N., Synodinou, M., Athanassiou, H., Kouveli, A., Verigos, C., et al. (2001). Randomized phase III trial of radiation treatment ± amifostine in patients with advanced-stage lung cancer. *International Journal of Radiation Oncology, Biology, Physics, 15,* 915–922.

Antonadou, D., Throuvalas, N., Petridis, A., Bolanos, N., Sagriotis, A., & Synodinou, M. (2001). Effect of amifostine on toxicities associated with radiochemotherapy in patients with locally advanced non-small-cell lung cancer. *International Journal of Radiation Oncology, Biology, Physics, 57,* 402–408.

Arundel, C., & Lewis, J.H. (2007). Drug-induced liver disease in 2006. *Current Opinion in Gastroenterology, 23,* 244–254.

Astegiano, M., Sapone, N., Demarchi, B., Rossetti, S., Bonardi, R., & Rizzetto, M. (2004). Laboratory evaluation of the patient with liver disease. *European Review for Medical and Pharmacological Sciences, 8,* 3–9.

Aung, H., Dey, L., Rand, V., & Yuan, C. (2004). Alternative therapies for male and female sexual dysfunction. *American Journal of Chinese Medicine, 32,* 161–173.

Baker, F., Denniston, M., Smith, T., & West, M. (2005). Adult cancer survivors: How are they faring? *Cancer, 104*(Suppl. 11), 2565–2576.

Barton, D., Wilwerding, M., Carpenter, L., & Loprinzi, C. (2004). Libido as part of sexuality in female cancer survivors. *Oncology Nursing Forum, 31,* 599–609.

Boekhout, A., Beijnen, J., & Schellens, J. (2006). Symptoms and treatment in cancer therapy-induced early menopause. *Oncologist, 11,* 641–654.

Bryant, G. (2006). Hepatotoxicity. In D. Camp-Sorrell & R.A. Hawkins (Eds.), *Clinical manual for the oncology advanced practice nurse* (2nd ed., pp. 553–565). Pittsburgh, PA: Oncology Nursing Society.

Burwell, S., Case, L., Kaelin, C., & Avis, N. (2006). Sexual problems in younger women after breast cancer surgery. *Journal of Clinical Oncology, 24,* 2815–2821.

Carver, J.R., Shapiro, C.L., Ng, A., Jacobs, L., Schwartz, C., Virgo, K.S., et al. (2007). American Society of Clinical Oncology clinical evidence review on the ongoing care of adult cancer survivors: Cardiac and pulmonary late effects. *Journal of Clinical Oncology, 25,* 1–18.

Center for Reproductive Medicine and Infertility. (Ed.). (2007). *Cancer and fertility resource guide 2007–2008.* New York: Author.

Chang, C.Y., & Schiano, T.D. (2007). Review article: Drug hepatotoxicity. *Alimentary Pharmacology and Therapeutics, 25,* 1135–1151.

Chong, K., Hampson, N., & Corman, J. (2005). Early hyperbaric oxygen therapy improves outcome for radiation-induced hemorrhagic cystitis. *Urology, 65,* 649–653.

Cimolai, N., & Cimolai, T. (2007). The cranberry and the urinary tract. *European Journal of Clinical Microbiology and Infectious Diseases, 26,* 767–776.

Clayton, A., McGarvey, E., & Clavet, G. (1997). The Changes in Sexual Functioning Questionnaire (CSFQ): Development, reliability, and validity. *Psychopharmacology Bulletin, 33,* 731–745.

Col, C., Hasdemir, O., Yalcin, E., Yandakci, K., Tunc, G., & Kucukpinar, T. (2006). Sexual dysfunction after curative resection of rectal cancer in men: The role of extended systematic lymph-node dissection. *Medical Science Monitor, 12,* C70–C74.

Coleman, J., & Walther, M. (2005). Urologic emergencies. In V.T. DeVita, Jr., S. Hellman, & S. Rosenberg (Eds.), *Cancer: Principles and practice of oncology* (7th ed., pp. 2301–2308). Philadelphia: Lippincott Williams & Wilkins.

Copperman, A. (2007). Infertility and IVF for the cancer patient. In Center for Reproductive Medicine and Infertility (Ed.), *Cancer and fertility resource guide 2007–2008* (p. 31). New York: Center for Reproductive Medicine and Infertility.

Crew, J., Jephcott, C., & Reynard, J. (2001). Radiation-induced hemorrhagic cystitis. *European Urology, 40,* 111–143.

Day, D., Ambegaonker, A., Harriot, K., & McDaniel, A. (2001). A new tool for predicting erectile dysfunction. *Advances in Therapy, 18,* 131–139.

Delanian, S., Balla-Mekias, S., & Lefaix, J. (1999). Striking regression of chronic radiotherapy damage in a clinical trial of combined pentoxifylline and tocopherol. *Journal of Clinical Oncology, 17,* 3283–3290.

DeLeve, L., & Kaplowitz, N. (2000). Prevention and therapy of drug-induced hepatic injury. In M. Wolfe (Ed.), *Therapy of digestive disorders: A companion to Sleisenger and Fordtran's gastrointestinal and liver disease* (8th ed., pp. 334–348). Philadelphia: Saunders.

DeLeve, L.D. (2003). Liver function and hepatotoxicity in cancer. In D.W. Kufe, R.E. Pollock, R.R. Weichselbaum, R.C. Bast, T.S. Gansler, J.F. Holland, et al. (Eds.), *Cancer medicine.* Hamilton, Ontario, Canada: BC Decker. Retrieved October 8, 2007, from http://www.ncbi.nlm.nih.gov/books/bv.fcgi ?highlight=hepatotoxicity&rid=cmed6.section.42366#42369

den Brinker, M., Wit, F.W., Wertheim-van Dillen, P.M., Jurriaans, S., Weel, J., van Leeuwen, R., et al. (2000). Hepatitis B and C virus co-infection and the risk for hepatotoxicity of highly active antiretroviral therapy in HIV-1 infection. *AIDS, 14,* 2895–2902.

Derogatis, L. (1987). The Derogatis Stress Profile (DSP): Quantification of psychological stress. *Advances in Psychosomatic Medicine, 17,* 30–54.

Derogatis, L., & Kourlesis, S. (1981). An approach to evaluation of sexual problems in the cancer patient. *CA: A Cancer Journal for Clinicians, 31,* 46–50.

Dirkx, M.L., & Heijmen, B.J. (2000). Beam intensity modulation for penumbra enhancement and field length reduction in lung cancer treatments: A dosimetric study. *Radiotherapy and Oncology, 56,* 181–188.

Dixon, K., & Dixon, P. (2006). The PLISSIT Model: Care and management of patients' psychosexual needs following radical surgery. *Lippincott's Case Management, 11,* 101–106.

Domar, A. (2007). Complementary and alternative medicine. In Center for Reproductive Medicine and Infertility (Ed.), *Cancer and fertility resource guide 2007–2008* (p. 75). New York: Center for Reproductive Medicine and Infertility.

Donatucci, C., & Greenfield, J. (2006). Recovery of sexual function after prostate cancer treatment. *Current Opinion in Urology, 16,* 444–448.

Donnan, P.T., McLernon, D., Steinke, D., Ryder, S., Roderick, P., Sullivan, F.M., et al. (2007). Development of a decision support tool to facilitate primary care management of patients with abnormal liver function tests without clinically apparent liver disease [HTA03/38/02]. Abnormal Liver Function Investigations Evaluation (ALFIE). *BMC Health Services Research, 7,* 54–65.

Donovan, K., Taliaferro, L., Alvarez, E., Jacobsen, P., Roetzheim, R., & Wenham, R. (2007). Sexual health in women treated for cervical cancer: Characteristics and correlates. *Gynecologic Oncology, 104,* 428–434.

Dunn, J., & Lew, C. (2007). Total body irradiation and total lymphoid irradiation. In M. Haas, W. Hogle, G. Moore-Higgs, & T. Gosselin-Acomb (Eds.), *Radiation therapy: A guide to patient care* (pp. 444–487). St. Louis, MO: Elsevier Mosby.

Duong, C.D., & Loh, J.-Y. (2006). Basic review: Laboratory monitoring in oncology. *Journal of Oncology Pharmacy Practice, 12,* 223–236.

Ekwall, E., Ternestedt, B., & Sorbe, B. (2003). Important aspects of health care for women with gynecologic cancer. *Oncology Nursing Forum, 30,* 313–319.

Ferrero, D., Polgiani, E.M., Rege-Cambrin, G., Fava, C., Mattioli, G., Dellacas, C., et al. (2006). Corticosteroids can reverse severe imatinib-induced hepatotoxicity. *Haematologica, 91,* 78–80.

Fertile Hope. (2007). *Community statistics.* Retrieved August 12, 2007, from http://www.fertilehope .org/participate/community-stats.cfm

Floyd, J., Mirza, I., Sachs, B., & Perry, M.C. (2006). Hepatotoxicity of chemotherapy. *Seminars in Oncology, 33,* 50–67.

Fobair, P., Stewart, S., Chang, S., D'Onofrio, C., Banks, P., & Bloom, J. (2006). Body image and sexual problems in young women with breast cancer. *Psycho-Oncology, 15,* 579–594.

Galbraith, M., Arechiga, A., Ramirez, J., & Pedro, L.W. (2005). Prostate cancer survivors' and partners' self-reports of health-related quality of life, treatment symptoms, and marital satisfaction 2.5–5.5 years after treatment [Online exclusive]. *Oncology Nursing Forum, 32,* E30–E41.

Ganz, P., Litwin, M., & Meyerowitz, B. (2005). Sexual problems. In V.T. DeVita, Jr., S. Hellman, & S. Rosenberg (Eds.), *Cancer: Principles and practice of oncology* (7th ed., pp. 2662–2676). Philadelphia: Lippincott Williams & Wilkins.

Goodwin, P., Ennis, M., Pritchard, K., Trudeau, M., & Hood, N. (1999). Risk of menopause during the first year after breast cancer diagnosis. *Journal of Clinical Oncology, 17,* 2365–2370.

Gopal, D.V., & Rosen, H.R. (2000). Abnormal findings on liver function tests. *Postgraduate Medicine, 107,* 100–114.

Gross, N.J. (1980). Experimental radiation pneumonitis: IV leakage of circulatory proteins onto the alveolar surface. *Journal of Laboratory and Clinical Medicine, 95,* 19–31.

Guo, J.J., Wigle, P.R., Lammers, K., & Vu, O. (2005). Comparison of potentially hepatotoxic drugs among major US drug compendia. *Research in Social and Administration Pharmacy, 1,* 460–479.

Harris, S. (2001). Radiotherapy for early and advanced breast cancer. *International Journal of Clinical Practice, 55,* 609–612.

Hinson, J., & McKibben, A. (2001). Chemotherapy-associated pulmonary injury. In M.C. Perry (Ed.), *The chemotherapy source book* (3rd ed., pp. 468–476). Philadelphia: Lippincott Williams & Wilkins.

Hogle, W. (2007). Male genitourinary cancers. In M. Haas, W. Hogle, G. Moore-Higgs, & T. Gosselin-Acomb (Eds.), *Radiation therapy: A guide to patient care* (pp. 234–266). St. Louis, MO: Elsevier Mosby.

Holmes Gobel, B. (2003). Chemical hepatitis. *Clinical Journal of Oncology Nursing, 7,* 99–100.

Huddart, R., Norman, A., Moynihan, C., Horwich, A., Parker, C., Nicholls, E., et al. (2005). Fertility, gonadal and sexual function in survivors of testicular cancer. *British Journal of Cancer, 93,* 200–207.

Jacobs, J. (2007). Sharing hope financial assistance program. In Center for Reproductive Medicine and Infertility (Ed.), *Cancer and fertility resource guide 2007–2008* (pp. 161–167). New York: Center for Reproductive Medicine and Infertility.

Jemal, A., Siegel, R., Ward, E., Hao, Y., Xu, J., Murray, T., et al. (2008). Cancer statistics, 2008. *CA: A Cancer Journal for Clinicians, 58,* 71–96.

Jeremic, B., Shibamoto, Y., Milicic, B., Dagovic, A., Nikolic, N., Aleksandrovic, J., et al. (2003). Impact of treatment interruptions due to toxicity on outcome of patients with early stage (I/II) non-small-cell lung cancer (NSCLC) treated with hyperfractionated radiation therapy alone. *Lung Cancer, 40,* 317–323.

Jonker-Pool, G., Van de Wiel, H., Hoekstra, H., Sleijfer, D., Van Driel, M., Van Basten, J., et al. (2001). Sexual functioning after treatment for testicular cancer. Review and meta-analysis of 36 empirical studies between 1975–2000. *Archives of Social Behavior, 30,* 55–74.

Kanematsu, A., Yamamoto, S., & Ogawa, O. (2007). Changing concepts of bladder regeneration. *International Journal of Urology, 14,* 673–678.

Kaplan, H. (1979). *Disorders of sexual desire and other new concepts and techniques in sex therapy.* New York: Brunner/Mazel Publications.

Kaplowitz, N. (2002). Biochemical and cellular mechanisms of toxic liver injury. *Seminars in Liver Disease, 22,* 137–144.

Kaplowitz, N. (2004). Drug-induced liver injury. *Clinical Infectious Diseases, 38*(Suppl. 2), S44–S48.

Kasten-Pisula, U., Tastan, H., & Dikomey, E. (2005). Huge differences in cellular radiosensitivity due to only very small variations in double-strand break and repair capacity. *International Journal of Radiation Biology, 81,* 409–419.

Katz, A. (2007). *Breaking the silence on cancer and sexuality: A handbook for healthcare providers.* Pittsburgh, PA: Oncology Nursing Society.

King, P.D., & Perry, M.C. (2001). Hepatotoxicity of chemotherapy. *Oncologist, 6,* 162–176.

Krebs, L. (2005). Sexual and reproductive dysfunction. In C.H. Yarbro, M. Frogge, & M. Goodman (Eds.), *Cancer nursing: Principles and practice* (6th ed., pp. 841–869). Sudbury, MA: Jones and Bartlett.

Krebs, L. (2006). What should I say? Talking with patients about sexuality issues. *Clinical Journal of Oncology Nursing, 10,* 313–315.

Kroll, D.J., Shaw, H.S., & Oberlies, N.H. (2007). Milk thistle nomenclature: Why it matters in cancer research and pharmacokinetics studies. *Integrative Cancer Therapies, 6,* 110–119.

Krychman, M. (2006). Sexual rehabilitation medicine in a female oncology setting. *Gynecologic Oncology, 101,* 380–384.

Krychman, M., Pereira, L., Carter, J., & Amsterdam, A. (2006). Sexual oncology: Sexual health issues in women with cancer. *Oncology, 71,* 18–25.

Lee, S., Schover, L., Partridge, A., Patrizio, P., Wallace, W., Hagerty, K., et al. (2006). American Society of Clinical Oncology recommendations on fertility preservation in cancer patients. *Journal of Clinical Oncology, 24,* 2917–2931.

Lefievre, L., Bedu-Addo, K., Conner, S., Machado-Oliveira, G., Chen, Y., Kirkman-Brown, J., et al. (2007). Counting sperm does not add up anymore: Time for a new equation? *Reproduction, 133,* 675–684.

Leonard, M. (2006). Fertility preservation options for women with cancer. *Current Topics in Cancer Fertility, 1,* 1–2, 6.

Leonard, M., Hammelef, K., & Smith, G. (2004). Fertility considerations, counseling and semen cryopreservation for males prior to initiation of cancer therapy. *Clinical Journal of Oncology Nursing, 8,* 127–132.

Lin, E., Aikin, J., & Good, B. (1999). Premature menopause after cancer treatment. *Cancer Practice, 7,* 114–121.

Lind, P.A., Marks, L.B., Hollis, D., Fan, M., Zhou, S.M., Munley, M.T., et al. (2002). Receiver operating characteristic curves to assess predictors of radiation-induced symptomatic lung injury. *International Journal of Radiation Oncology, Biology, Physics, 54,* 340–347.

Liu, Z.X., & Kaplowitz, N. (2002). Immune-mediated drug-induced liver disease. *Clinical Liver Disease, 6,* 467–486.

Maltaris, T., Seufert, R., Fischl, F., Schaffrath, M., Pollow, K., Koelbl, H., et al. (2007). The effect of cancer treatment on female fertility and strategies for preserving fertility. *European Journal of Obstetrics, Gynecology, and Reproductive Biology, 130,* 148–155.

Martin, P., & Friedman, L.S. (1998). Assessment of liver function and diagnostic studies. In L.S. Friedman & E.B. Keeffe (Eds.), *Handbook of liver disease* (pp. 1–14). Philadelphia: Churchill Livingstone.

Masand, P., Ashton, A., Gupta, S., & Frank, B. (2001). Sustained-release bupropion for selective serotonin reuptake inhibitor-induced sexual dysfunction: A randomized double-blind, placebo-controlled, parallel-group study. *American Journal of Psychiatry, 158,* 805–807.

Masters, W., & Johnson, V. (1966). *Human sexual response.* St. Louis, MO: Little, Brown.

Matsuka, Y., Wang, D.H., Suganuma, N., Imai, K., Ikeda, S., Taketa, K., et al. (2003). Differential responses of serum gamma-glutamyltransferase to alcohol intake in Japanese males. *Acta Medica Okayama, 57,* 171–178.

Matthew, A.G., Goldman, A., Trachtenberg, J., Robinson, J., Horsburgh, S., Currie, K., et al. (2005). Sexual dysfunction after radical prostatectomy: Prevalence, treatments, restricted use of treatments and distress. *Journal of Urology, 174,* 2105–2110.

Matthews, L.V. (2005). Alterations in ventilation. In J.K. Itano & K.N. Taoka (Eds.), *Core curriculum for oncology nursing* (4th ed., pp. 347–379). St. Louis, MO: Elsevier Saunders.

McDonald, S., Rubin, P., Phillips, T.L., & Marks, L.B. (1995). Injury to the lung from cancer therapy: Clinical syndromes, measurable endpoints, and potential scoring systems. *International Journal of Radiation Oncology, Biology, Physics, 31,* 1187–1203.

McKee, A., & Schover, L. (2001). Sexuality rehabilitation. *Cancer, 92,* S1008–S1012.

Mehta, V. (2005). Radiation pneumonitis and pulmonary fibrosis in non-small-cell lung cancer: Pulmonary function, prediction, and prevention. *International Journal of Radiation Oncology, Biology, Physics, 63,* 5–24.

Mezvrishvili, Z., & Managadze, L. (2006). Complications of nerve sparing retroperitoneal lymph node dissection. *Georgian Medical News, 132,* 20–23.

Mick, J., Hughes, M., & Cohen, M. (2004). Using the BETTER model to assess sexuality. *Clinical Journal of Oncology Nursing, 8,* 84–86.

Miranda-Sousa, A., Davila, H., Lockhart, J., Ordorica, R., & Carrion, R. (2006). Sexual function after surgery for prostate or bladder cancer. *Cancer Control, 13,* 179–187.

Morgan, G.W., & Breit, S.N. (1995). Radiation and the lung: A reevaluation of the mechanisms mediating pulmonary injury. *International Journal of Radiation Oncology, Biology, Physics, 31,* 361–369.

Moseley, R.H. (1996). Evaluation of abnormal liver function tests. *Medical Clinics of North America, 80,* 887–906.

Murray, R. (2006). Fertility sparing options for breast cancer patients. *Breast Disease, 23,* 73–80.

Narayan, S., Henning, G.T., Ten Haken, R.K., Sullivan, M.A., Martel, M.K., & Hayman, J.A. (2004). Results following treatment to doses of 92.4 or 102.9 Gy on a phase I dose escalation study for non-small cell lung cancer. *Lung Cancer, 44,* 79–88.

National Academy of Clinical Biology Laboratory Medicine Practice Guidelines. (2000). *LMPG: Laboratory guidelines for screening, diagnosis and monitoring of hepatic injury.* Retrieved October 8, 2007, from http://www.aacc.org/AACC/Members/nacb/Archive/LMPG/hepaticinjury

National Cancer Institute Cancer Therapy Evaluation Program. (2006). *Common terminology criteria for adverse events* (Version 3.0). Retrieved March 30, 2008, from http://ctep.cancer.gov/forms/CTCAEv3.pdf

National Institutes of Health. (2006). *Drug-induced liver injury (DILN) retrospective.* Retrieved October 7, 2007, from http://clinicaltrials.gov/ct2/show/NCT00360646

Natural Standard. (2007). *Silymarin professional monograph.* Retrieved October 9, 2007, from http://www.naturalstandard.com

Odin, J.A., Huebert, R.C., Casciola-Rosen, L., LaRusso, N.F., & Rosen, A. (2001). Bcl-2-dependent oxidation. *Journal of Clinical Investigation, 108,* 223–232.

Ohl, L. (2007). Essentials of female sexual dysfunction from a sex therapy perspective. *Urologic Nursing, 27,* 57–63.

Oktay, K., Buyuk, E., Libertella, N., Akar, M., & Rosenwaks, Z. (2005). Fertility preservation in breast cancer patients: A prospective controlled comparison of ovarian stimulation with tamoxifen and letrozole for embryo cryopreservation. *Journal of Clinical Oncology, 23,* 4347–4353.

Park, M., Davidson, R., & Fox, K. (2006). Preservation of fertility and the impact of subsequent pregnancy in patients with premenopausal breast cancer. *Seminars in Oncology, 33,* 664–671.

Partridge, A., Gelber, S., Peppercorn, J., Sampson, E., Knudsen, K., Laufer, M., et al. (2004). Web-based survey of fertility issues in young women with breast cancer. *Journal of Clinical Oncology, 22,* 4174–4183.

Peters, T.S. (2005). Do preclinical testing strategies help predict human hepatotoxic potentials? *Toxicologic Pathology, 33,* 146–154.

Pieterse, Q., Maas, C., Kuile, M., Lowik, M., Eijkeren, M., Trimbos, J., et al. (2006). An observational longitudinal study to evaluate miction, defecation, and sexual function after radical hysterectomy with pelvic lymphadenectomy for early-stage cervical cancer. *International Journal of Gynecologic Cancer, 16,* 1119–1129.

Polovich, M., White, J.M., & Kelleher, L.O. (Eds.). (2005). *Chemotherapy and biotherapy guidelines and recommendations for practice* (2nd ed.). Pittsburgh, PA: Oncology Nursing Society.

Puscheck, E., Philip, P., & Jeyendran, R. (2004). Male fertility preservation and cancer treatment. *Cancer Treatment Reviews, 30,* 173–180.

Ramanarayanan, J., & Scarpace, S.L. (2007). Acute drug induced hepatitis due to erlotinib. *Journal of the Pancreas, 8,* 39–43.

Rancati, T., Ceresoli, G.L., Gagliardi, G., Schipani, S., & Cattaneo, G.M. (2003). Factors predicting radiation pneumonitis in lung cancer patients: A retrospective study. *Radiotherapy and Oncology, 67,* 275–283.

Roberts, J., & Oktay, K. (2005). Fertility preservation: A comprehensive approach to the young woman with cancer. *Journal of the National Cancer Institute, 34,* 57–59.

Roberts, R.A., Ganey, P.E., Ju, C., Kamendulis, L.M., Rusyn, I., & Klaunig, J.E. (2007). The role of Kupffer cell in mediating hepatic toxicity and carcinogenesis. *Toxicological Sciences, 96,* 2–15.

Robertson, J. (2005). Cancer and fertility: Ethical and legal challenges. *Journal of the National Cancer Institute Monographs, 34,* 104–106.

Rosen, R., Brown, C., Heiman, J., Leiblum, S., Meston, C., Shabsigh, R., et al. (2000). The female sexual function index (FSFI): A multidimensional self-report instrument for the assessment of female sexual function. *Journal of Sex and Marital Therapy, 26,* 191–208.

Rosen, R., Cappelleri, J., Smith, M., Lipsky, J., & Pena, B. (1999). Development and evaluation of an abridged, 5-item version of the International Index of Erectile Dysfunction (IIEF-5) as a diagnostic tool for erectile dysfunction. *International Journal of Impotence Research, 11,* 319–326.

Rosen, R., Riley, A., Wagner, G., Osterloh, I., Kirkpatrick, J., & Mishra, A. (1997). The International Index of Erectile Function (IIEF): A multidimensional scale for assessment of erectile dysfunction. *Urology, 49,* 822–830.

Ryder, S.D., & Beckingham, I.J. (2001). ABC of disease of liver, pancreas, and biliary system. *BMJ, 322,* 290–292.

Salonia, A., Briganti, A., Deho, F., Zanni, G., Rigatti, P., & Montorsi, F. (2006). Women's sexual dysfunction: A review of the "surgical landscape". *European Urology, 50,* 44–52.

Schover, L. (2005). Sexuality and fertility after cancer. *Hematology: The Education Program of the American Society of Hematology,* pp. 523–527.

Schover, L. (2007). Sperm banking: Basics for the cancer patient. In Center for Reproductive Medicine and Infertility (Ed.), *Cancer and fertility resource guide 2007–2008* (p. 243). New York: Center for Reproductive Medicine and Infertility.

Schover, L., Brey, K., Lichtin, A., Lipshultz, L., & Jeha, S. (2002). Knowledge and experience regarding cancer, infertility, and sperm banking in younger male survivors. *Journal of Clinical Oncology, 20,* 1880–1889.

Schwartz, S., & Plawecki, H. (2002). Consequences of chemotherapy on the sexuality of patients with lung cancer. *Clinical Journal of Oncology Nursing, 6,* 212–216.

Seeff, L.B. (2007). *AASLD-FDA-NIH-PhRMA-Hepatotoxicity special interest group meeting. 2007 presentations.* Retrieved October 9, 2007, from http://www.fda.gov/cder/livertox/presentations2007/seeff.htm

Shell, J. (2002). Evidence-based practice for symptom management in adults with cancer: Sexual dysfunction. *Oncology Nursing Forum, 29,* 53–66.

Sheppard, C., & Whiteley, R. (2006). Psychosexual problems after gynaecological cancer. *Journal of the British Menopause Society, 12,* 24–27.

Sigman, M. (2007). Medications that impair male fertility. *Sexuality and Reproductive Medicine, 6,* 11–16.

Singh, K., Davies, M., & Chatterjee, R. (2005). Fertility in female cancer survivors: Pathophysiology, preservation and the role of ovarian reserve testing. *Human Reproduction Update, 11,* 69–89.

Sinicrope, F.A. (2003). Gastrointestinal complications: Ascites. In D.W. Kufe, R.E. Pollock, R.R. Weichselbaum, R.C. Bast, T.S. Gansler, J.F. Holland, et al. (Eds.), *Cancer medicine* (6th ed.). Hamilton, Ontario, Canada: BC Decker. Retrieved October 8, 2007, from http://www.ncbi.nlm.nih.gov/books/bv.fcgi?highlight=ascites&rid=cmed6.section.42637

Speer, J., Hillenberg, B., Sugrue, D., Blacker, C., Kresge, C., Decker, V., et al. (2005). Study of sexual functioning determinants in breast cancer survivors. *Breast Journal, 11,* 440–447.

Srinivas, R., Agarwal, R., & Agarwal, A.N. (2007). A deferred dilemma. *American Journal of Medicine, 120,* 594–597.

Stead, M., Fallowfield, L., Selby, P., & Brown, J. (2007). Psychosexual function and impact of gynecological cancer. *Best Practice and Research: Clinical Obstetrics and Gynaecology, 21,* 309–320.

Strohl, R., & Camp-Sorrell, D. (2006). Hemorrhagic cystitis. In D. Camp-Sorrell & R.A. Hawkins (Eds.), *Clinical manual for the oncology advanced practice nurse* (2nd ed., pp. 661–663). Pittsburgh, PA: Oncology Nursing Society.

Taksey, J., Bissada, N., & Chaudhary, U. (2003). Fertility after chemotherapy for testicular cancer. *Archives of Andrology, 49,* 389–395.

Tal, R., & Mulhall, J. (2006). Sexual health issues in men with cancer. *Oncology, 20,* 294–300.

Tarbell, N.J., Thompson, L., & Mauch, P. (1990). Thoracic irradiation in Hodgkin's disease: Disease control and long-term complications. *International Journal of Radiation Oncology, Biology, Physics, 18,* 275–281.

Taylor, M. (2006). Strategies for managing antidepressant-induced sexual dysfunction: A review. *Current Psychiatry Reports, 8,* 431–436.

Thapa, B.R., & Walia, A. (2007). Liver function tests and their interpretation. *Indian Journal of Pediatrics, 74,* 663–671.

Third Wave Technologies, Inc. (2005). Invader. UGT1A1 molecular assay [Package insert]. Madison, WI: Author. Retrieved October 8, 2007, from http://www.twt.com/pdfs/UGT1A1PackInsert.pdf

Tsoutsou, P.G., & Koukourakis, M.I. (2006). Radiation pneumonitis and fibrosis: Mechanisms underlying its pathogenesis and implications for future research. *International Journal of Radiation Oncology, Biology, Physics, 66,* 1281–1293.

Turek, P. (2007). Testicular tissue freezing. In Center for Reproductive Medicine and Infertility (Ed.), *Cancer and fertility resource guide 2007–2008* (p. 299). New York: Center for Reproductive Medicine and Infertility.

Ukoli, F., Lynch, B., & Adams-Campbell, L. (2006). Radical prostatectomy and quality of life among African Americans. *Ethnicity and Disease, 16,* 988–993.

U.S. Department of Health and Human Services. (2006). *Assessing progress, advancing change: President's Cancer Panel 2006–2006 annual report.* Bethesda, MD: Author.

van Sornsen de Koste, J., Voet, P., Dirkx, M., van Meerbeeck, J., & Senan, S. (2001). An evaluation of two techniques for beam intensity modulation in patients irradiated for stage III non-small cell lung cancer. *Lung Cancer, 32,* 145–153.

Verma, S., & Thuluvath, P.J. (2007). Complementary and alternative medicine in hepatology: Review of the evidence of efficacy. *Clinical Gastroenterology and Hepatology, 5,* 408–416.

Vogel, W. (2007). Chemoradiotherapy. In M. Haas, W. Hogle, G. Moore-Higgs, & T.K. Gosselin-Acomb (Eds.), *Radiation therapy: A guide to patient care* (pp. 327–354). St. Louis, MO: Elsevier Mosby.

Watanabe, N., Takashimizu, S., Kojima, S., Kagawa, T., Nishizaki, Y., Mine, T., et al. (2007). Clinical and pathological features of a prolonged type of acute intrahepatic cholestasis. *Hepatology and Research, 37,* 598–607.

Waterhouse, J., & Metcalfe, M. (1986). Development of the sexual adjustment questionnaire. *Oncology Nursing Forum, 13,* 53–59.

Watkins, P.B., & Seeff, L.B. (2006). Drug-induced liver injury: Summary of a single topic clinical research conference. *Hepatology, 43,* 618–631.

Weiss, R.B. (2001). Miscellaneous toxicities. In V.T. DeVita, Jr., S. Hellman, & S.A. Rosenberg (Eds.), *Cancer: Principles and practice of oncology* (6th ed., pp. 2974–2976). Philadelphia: Lippincott Williams & Wilkins.

Werner-Wasik, M., Scott, C., Movsas, B., Langer, C., Sarna, L., Nicolaou, N., et al. (2003). Amifostine as mucosal protectant in patients with locally advanced non-small cell lung cancer (NSCLC) receiving intensive chemotherapy and thoracic radiotherapy (RT): Results of the radiation therapy oncology group. *International Journal of Radiation Oncology, Biology, Physics, 57*(Suppl. 1), S216.

Wesselius, L. (1999). Pulmonary complications of cancer therapy. *Comprehensive Therapy, 25,* 272–277.

Whitmore, K. (2002). Complementary and alternative therapies as treatment approaches for interstitial cystitis. *Reviews in Urology, 4*(Suppl. 1), S28–S35.

Wilkes, G.M., & Barton-Burke, M. (Eds.). (2007). *Oncology nursing drug handbook* (11th ed.). Sudbury, MA: Jones and Bartlett.

Wolf, D.C. (1990). Evaluation of the size, shape, and consistency of the liver. In H.K. Walker, W.D. Hall, & J.W. Hurst (Eds.), *Clinical methods: The history, physical, and laboratory examination* (3rd ed., pp. 478–481). Stoneham, MA: Butterworths.

Woodruff, T. (2007). Ovarian tissue freezing. In Center for Reproductive Medicine and Infertility (Ed.), *Cancer and fertility resource guide 2007–2008* (p. 201). New York: Center for Reproductive Medicine and Infertility.

Wurstbauer, K., Deutschmann, H., Sedlmayer, F., & Kogelnik, H.D. (2001). Non-small-cell lung cancer: Dose escalation by target splitting with asymmetric collimation. *Clinical Lung Cancer, 3,* 151–153.

Yom, S.S., Liao, Z., Liu, H.H., Tucker, S.L., Hu, C.S., Wei, X., et al. (2007). Initial evaluation of treatment-related pneumonitis in advanced-stage non-small-cell lung cancer patients treated with concurrent chemotherapy and intensity-modulated radiotherapy. *International Journal of Radiation Oncology, Biology, Physics, 68,* 94–102.

Yu, T.K., Whitman, G.J., Thames, H.D., Buzdar, A.U., Strom, E.A., Perkins, G.H., et al. (2004). Clinically relevant pneumonitis after sequential paclitaxel-based chemotherapy and radiotherapy in breast cancer patients. *Journal of the National Cancer Institute, 96,* 1676–1681.

Zhou, S.F., Xue, C.C., Yu, X.O., & Wang, G. (2007). Metabolic activation of herbal and dietary constituents and its clinical and toxicological implications: An update. *Current Drug Metabolism, 8,* 526–553.

Zimmerman, H. (1999). *Hepatotoxicity: The adverse effects of drugs and other chemicals on the liver* (2nd ed.). Philadelphia: Lippincott Williams & Wilkins.

Zorzi, D., Laurent, A., Pawlik, T.M., Lauwer, G.Y., Vauthey, J.N., & Abdalla, E.K. (2007). Chemotherapy-associated hepatotoxicity and surgery for colorectal liver metastasis. *British Journal of Surgery, 94,* 274–286.

CHAPTER 14

Metabolic Emergencies

Diane G. Cope, PhD, ARNP-BC, AOCNP®

Introduction

Metabolic emergencies have a lower incidence rate in patients with cancer when compared to the more common side effects of pain, nausea, vomiting, and fatigue. However, when metabolic emergencies occur, they can be associated with significant morbidity and mortality in patients with cancer. The advanced practice nurse (APN) must be knowledgeable in recognizing risk factors for metabolic oncologic emergencies and the signs and symptoms of impending crisis in order to initiate immediate treatment to ameliorate the devastating consequences and prevent mortality. This chapter will review the incidence, pathophysiology, assessment, and treatment strategies for disseminated intravascular coagulation (DIC), sepsis, tumor lysis syndrome (TLS), hypercalcemia of malignancy, syndrome of inappropriate secretion of antidiuretic hormone (SIADH), and anaphylaxis.

Disseminated Intravascular Coagulation

DIC is an oncologic emergency characterized by overstimulation of normal coagulation that causes a paradoxical disorder of diffuse clotting and profuse hemorrhage. Although DIC is associated with a wide variety of clinical conditions, including myeloproliferative disorders and certain solid tumors, the most common clinical condition associated with DIC is sepsis and frequently is present in patients with cancer who present with neutropenic fever (Levi & ten Cate, 1999). APNs should be knowledgeable about the pathophysiology, diagnostic assessment, and treatment strategies for DIC to help prevent life-threatening consequences.

Definition and Incidence

DIC is a condition involving widespread activation of the normal coagulation system that causes intravascular formation of fibrin and thrombotic occlusion, resulting in diffuse clotting. Simultaneously, the depletion of platelets and coagulation proteins induces profuse hemorrhaging (Levi & ten Cate, 1999). DIC may be acute or chronic in nature. Acute DIC is associated with more bleeding, whereas chronic DIC is more associated with thrombus formation (Ezzone, 2006a). The exact incidence of DIC in patients with cancer is difficult to determine because of the numerous etiologies that can cause DIC. However, approximately 10% of all patients with cancer are estimated to develop DIC (Maxson, 2000).

Presenting Signs and Symptoms

The most obvious sign of DIC is bleeding. Clinically, patients may have continuous oozing from body orifices, surgical wounds, and venipuncture sites. In addition, patients may have sclera and conjunctival bleeding, gingival bleeding, epistaxis, hemoptysis, ecchymoses, blood in urine and stool, heavy prolonged vaginal bleeding, and petechiae. In more severe cases, intracranial, gastrointestinal (GI), genitourinary, pleural, and pericardial bleeding will occur.

Other signs of DIC result from the simultaneous thrombosis that is occurring; however, signs of thrombosis are less clinically evident. The formation of fibrin and small clots obstruct the microvascular system and large vessels, thereby decreasing organ function, especially the cardiac, pulmonary, renal, hepatic, central nervous system (CNS), and dermatologic systems (Bick, 2003; Maxson, 2000). Skin involvement is the most obvious manifestation of thrombosis, including deep tissue bleeding and large subcutaneous hematomas that can develop into gangrene and tissue ischemia. Lung involvement may be manifested as shortness of breath, tachypnea, and diminished oxygen saturation. Renal involvement may be exhibited by hematuria and, later, anuria and oliguria. Other organ involvement may be seen with signs such as hypotension, tachycardia, weak thready pulse, and altered mental status and confusion (Bick; Ezzone, 2006b; Maxson).

Risk Factors

DIC occurs as a result of an underlying condition; therefore, risk factors are related to the underlying condition. Numerous clinical conditions are associated with the development of DIC (see Table 14-1). Tissue damage and activation of the coagulation system can result from hematologic and hepatic abnormalities, trauma, vascular disorders, obstetric complications, metabolic acidosis, immune reactions, and prosthetic devices. In patients with cancer, specific malignancies and treatment-related consequences can place individuals at a higher risk for the development of DIC. The most common cause of DIC is septicemia, which occurs in approximately 30%–50% of patients with gram-negative sepsis (Franchini, Lippi, & Manzato, 2006; Levi & ten Cate, 1999). Other microorganisms, such as fungi, viruses, and parasites, also may cause DIC (Franchini et al.). In patients with cancer, a higher risk of DIC is related to the underlying malignancy and sepsis. Leukemias, especially acute promyelocytic leukemia, and solid tumor malignancies (mucin-producing adenocarcinomas) are associated with DIC. With sepsis, release of cytokines and activation of the coagulation pathway releases bacterial endotoxins and cell membrane material that stimulates the inflammatory response, subsequently resulting in hypercoagulation and DIC (Levi, 2004). Hematologic malignancies and solid tumors are hypercoagulable states that release two tumor-derived mediators of DIC, a protease

Table 14-1. Conditions Underlying Disseminated Intravascular Coagulation

Clinical Condition	Specific Associated Dysfunction	Pathophysiologic Process
Bacterial infections	Gram-negative bacteria Meningococcus, salmonella, *Pseudomonas* species, *Enterobacteriaceae, Haemophilus* Gram-positive bacteria Pneumococcus, staphylococci, hemolytic streptococci	Initiation of coagulation by endotoxin-bacterial coat lipopolysaccharide. Endotoxin activates factor XII to factor XIIa and induces a platelet release reaction, causing endothelial sloughing, damage, and permeability and release of granulocyte procoagulant materials.
Viral infections	Varicella, hepatitis, cytomegalovirus, HIV	–
Parasitic infections	–	–
Malignancy	Hematologic • Acute promyelocytic leukemia • Acute myeloid leukemia • Acute lymphocytic leukemia • Chronic myeloid leukemia • Myeloproliferative diseases Solid tumors • Adenocarcinomas of the lung, breast, prostate, stomach, ovary, and gastrointestinal tract	Activation of coagulation with hemolysis, endothelial damage, and release of cytokines
Hematologic	Polycythemia rubra vera Heparin-induced thrombocytopenia with thrombosis	Hemolysis, hyperfibrinolysis, activation of coagulation, bleeding, and increased tendency for thrombosis and thromboembolization
Trauma	Burns Brain injury Fat embolism Massive tissue destruction	Microhemolysis with release of red cell membrane phospholipids or red cell adenosine diphosphate (ADP) with release of tissue and cellular enzymes into systemic circulation
Vascular disorders	Brain infarction, cerebrovascular accident, cerebral hemorrhage, large hemangioma, aortic aneurysm	Endothelial sloughing and activation of coagulation
Obstetric complications	Abruptio placentae, abortions, amniotic fluid embolism, hemorrhagic shock, dead fetus syndrome, preeclampsia	Release of placental enzymes, uterine tissue and thromboplastin-like materials enter maternal systemic circulation and activate coagulation system
Intravascular hemolysis	Transfusion reactions, multiple transfusions of whole blood	Triggers intravascular coagulation with release of red cell ADP or red cell phospholipoprotein that activates the procoagulant system

(Continued on next page)

Table 14-1. Conditions Underlying Disseminated Intravascular Coagulation *(Continued)*

Clinical Condition	Specific Associated Dysfunction	Pathophysiologic Process
Hepatic failure	Obstructive jaundice, acute hepatic failure	Coagulation abnormalities seen with hepatic dysfunction and intrahepatic or extrahepatic cholestasis
Metabolic acidosis	–	Endothelial sloughing with activation of XII to XIIa, activation of XI to XIa and platelet release reaction. Release of tumor necrosis factor, interleukins, and interferon activates the coagulation pathway. Decreased thrombomodulin and inhibition of thrombin-mediated activities. Antithrombosis from activation of protein C and S system with thrombus formation and end-organ damage.
Toxic and immunologic reactions	Snake or spider bites, recreational drugs, transplant rejections	Tissue and endothelial damage with circulating antigen-antibody complexes, endotoxemia, platelet damage and release, and hemolysis
Prosthetic devices	Aortic balloon-assist devices, LeVeen or Denver shunts	Thrombosis or thromboembolism with activation of the coagulation system

Note. Based on information from Bick, 2003; Ezzone, 2006a, 2006b; Gobel, 1999; Messmore & Wehrmacher, 2002.

and tumor necrosis factor, which activate the clotting cascade. Cancer treatment also can promote a hypercoagulable state from chemotherapy, surgery, and radiation with subsequent endothelial damage and activation of the coagulation pathways (Ornstein & Zacharski, 2000).

Pathophysiology

Normally, the body maintains a balanced state between clot formation or thrombosis and clot breakdown or fibrinolysis (see Figure 14-1). When vascular or tissue injury occurs, the endothelium is damaged, and the procoagulant subendothelial tissue is uncovered. Vasoconstriction and platelet attraction occur at the site, and a platelet plug is formed. The release of procoagulant substances and tissue factor activates the coagulation cascade. The coagulation cascade is a sequential activation of clotting factors that ends with the formation of a stable fibrin clot. When the coagulation cascade is initiated, the fibrinolytic pathway is activated. The fibrinolytic pathway controls for excessive clot formation and eventually dissolves the clot and repairs tissue (Ezzone, 2006b).

In DIC, the vascular endothelial injury causes overstimulation of the coagulation system and an imbalance between coagulation and fibrinolysis (see Figure 14-2). As a result of the overstimulation, excessive thrombin formation, consumption and depletion of clotting factors and platelets, and activation of the fibrinolytic pathway occur (Levi, 2004; Messmore & Wehrmacher, 2002). As a result of the excess thrombin formation, the conversion of plasminogen to plasmin is enhanced, and fibrinolysis occurs. Fibrin degradation products that possess procoagulant activity increase and result in hemorrhage into the subcutaneous tissues, skin, and mucous membranes. Simultaneously, en-

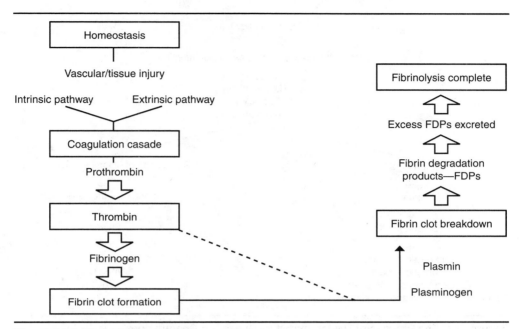

Figure 14-1. Normal Hemostasis

Note. From "Metabolic Emergencies" (p. 384), by B.H. Gobel in J.K. Itano and K.N. Taoka (Eds.), *Core Curriculum for Oncology Nursing* (4th ed.), 2005, St. Louis, MO: Elsevier. Copyright 2005 by Elsevier. Reprinted with permission.

hanced fibrin formation exists, with hypercoagulation and microvascular thrombosis resulting in end-organ damage (Franchini et al., 2006).

Prevention Strategies

For DIC, no interventional or treatment strategies are available that can prevent the process from occurring, except for strategies to treat the underlying disorder. Once DIC is suspected, APNs should facilitate the initiation of treatment immediately to prevent or reduce significant morbidity and mortality.

Diagnosis and Assessment

DIC may have an abrupt or insidious onset, may be active or chronic, and may be compensated or decompensated depending on the degree of consumption and utilization of the various procoagulant substances and platelets (Becker & Wira, 2008; Bick, 2003; Franchini et al., 2006). Therefore, a thorough history and physical examination and review of laboratory studies are critical in diagnosing DIC.

The history should include a review of any risk factors associated with an increased risk of DIC as outlined in Table 14-1. Patient evaluation also should cover any prior history of bleeding tendencies, bleeding episodes, or history of blood clots, such as deep vein thrombosis (DVT) or pulmonary embolism.

The physical examination should evaluate for any signs and symptoms that may be seen with bleeding or thrombosis. This necessitates a thorough assessment of each or-

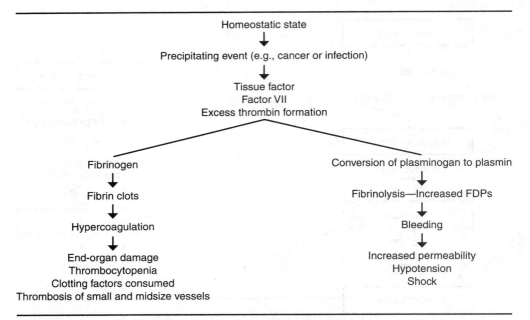

Homeostatic state
↓
Precipitating event (e.g., cancer or infection)
↓
Tissue factor
Factor VII
Excess thrombin formation

Fibrinogen
↓
Fibrin clots
↓
Hypercoagulation
↓
End-organ damage
Thrombocytopenia
Clotting factors consumed
Thrombosis of small and midsize vessels

Conversion of plasminogan to plasmin
↓
Fibrinolysis—Increased FDPs
↓
Bleeding
↓
Increased permeability
Hypotension
Shock

Figure 14-2. The Process of Disseminated Intravascular Coagulation

FDPs—fibrin degradation products

Note. From "Disseminated Intravascular Coagulation" (p. 890), by B.H. Gobel in C.H. Yarbro, M.H. Frogge, and M. Goodman (Eds.), *Cancer Nursing: Principles and Practice* (6th ed.), 2005, Sudbury, MA: Jones and Bartlett. Copyright 2005 by Jones and Bartlett. Reprinted with permission.

gan system (see Table 14-2). Bleeding from at least three unrelated sites is highly suspicious for DIC (Becker & Wira, 2008).

No single laboratory test has significant sensitivity or specificity to diagnose DIC (Franchini et al., 2006). The laboratory tests should be evaluated in correlation to the patient's clinical presentation and risk factors associated with DIC (see Table 14-3). The classic laboratory findings seen with DIC include prolonged clotting times (prothrombin time [PT], activated partial thromboplastin time [PTT], and thrombin time), increased levels of fibrin degradation products and D-dimers, low platelet count and fibrinogen levels, and low plasma levels of coagulation factors and coagulation inhibitors (such as antithrombin and protein C) (Yu, Nardella, & Pechet, 2000). The Scientific Subcommittee on DIC of the International Society on Thrombosis and Haemostasis (Taylor, Toh, Hoots, Wada, & Levi, 2001) has proposed a scoring system for the diagnosis of DIC. The system consists of a five-step algorithm that designates a score based upon the severity of abnormality of the platelet count, fibrin-related markers, PT, and fibrinogen level (see Figure 14-3). A score of 5 or greater is compatible with overt (or acute) DIC. This scoring system has recently been found to have a greater than 90% sensitivity and specificity in diagnosing DIC; however, the use of this algorithm is based upon the presence of a known underlying disorder associated with DIC (Bakhtiari, Meijers, de Jonge, & Levi, 2004; Levi, 2004). Differential diagnoses may include hemolytic uremic syndrome or idiopathic thrombocytopenic purpura in addition to the numerous underlying disorders discussed previously.

Table 14-2. Physical Assessment for Patients at Risk for Bleeding or Thrombosis

Organ	Assessment
CNS: Symptoms dependent on site and size of bleeding or clot	Headache, nausea/vomiting, retching, mental status changes (restlessness, confusion, lethargy, obtundation, coma), vertigo, seizures, changes in pupil size and reactivity; eye deviations, sensory or motor strength alterations, speech alterations, paralysis
Eyes	Visual disturbances—blurring, diplopia, absent or altered fields of vision, nystagmus, increased injections in sclera, conjunctival hemorrhage, periorbital edema; note if sclera are icteric
Nose	Petechiae, blood-tinged drainage, epistaxis
Mouth	Petechiae of oral mucosa, pain, dysphagia, hematemesis, bleeding gums/mucosa, blood-tinged secretions, ulcerations with frank bleeding
Upper gastrointestinal: Esophagus/stomach	Dysphagia, hematemesis, blood-tinged secretions, substernal burning and pain, epigastric discomfort (burning, tenderness, or cramping), coffee ground emesis, nausea, vomiting, fever, weakness, anorexia, melena, hyperactive bowel sounds
Lower gastrointestinal: Duodenum/anus	Pain (location, occurrence, duration, quality), nausea, vomiting, tarry stools, diarrhea, bowel sounds (hyper- or hypoactive), cramping, occult blood in stools, frank blood in stools (rectum or lower), blood around anus, frequency and quantity of stools, pain with bowel movements (hemorrhoids)
Lungs	Tachypnea, dyspnea, air hunger, respiration rate, depth, and exertion Crackles, rubs, wheezing, diminished breath sounds, hemoptysis (frothy BRB sputum—major airway bleeding), stridor, tickling in throat or chest with desire to cough
Cardiovascular	Tachycardia and hypotension (characteristic of anemia and acute blood loss) Changes in VS, color and temperature of extremities, peripheral pulses (present, quality), and changes in peripheral perfusion Pericardial effusions: dyspnea, cough, pain, orthopnea, venous distension, tamponade (muted heart sounds, hypotension, pulsus paradoxus, tachycardia, angina, palpitations)
Abdomen	Hepatomegaly (liver disease—possible coagulation disorder), RUQ pain, abdominal distension Splenomegaly (increased risk for bleeding): Assess for any history of trauma; if spleen ruptures, rapid hypovolemic shock ensues; left flank or left shoulder pain Retroperitoneal bleeding: vague abdominal complaints, ecchymoses over flank, occasional bulging flanks and tenderness; associated with hypovolemia
Genitourinary	Decreased urinary output due to massive bleeding is associated with hypovolemia and shock Hematuria: dysuria, burning, frequency, pain on urination, suprapubic pain and cramping, gross blood in urine, clots Menorrhagia: suprapubic pain and cramping, gross blood in urine, clots (may need to straight catheterize female patients to distinguish between urinary or vaginal bleeding) Frequency and size of clots, number of sanitary napkins used and color of urine are important in measuring bleeding

(Continued on next page)

Table 14-2. Physical Assessment for Patients at Risk for Bleeding or Thrombosis (Continued)

Organ	Assessment
Musculoskeletal	Bleeding into the joints is usually associated with alterations in coagulation; swollen, warm, sore joint with decreased mobility (active and passive ROM); usually unilateral; tapping the joint's synovial fluid is frequently required to distinguish infection from bleeding Unilateral swelling of affected extremity, with or without positive Homan's sign
Skin	Petechiae, ecchymosis, purpura, hematoma; oozing from venipuncture sites, central lines, catheters, injection sites, incisional wounds, nasogastric tubes Gangrene, alterations in skin color (e.g., pallor, cyanosis), alterations in skin temperature

BRB—bright red blood; CNS—central nervous system; ROM—range of motion; RUQ—right upper quadrant; VS—vital signs

Note. From "Bleeding and Thrombotic Complications" (p. 238), by P.H. Friend and J. Pruett in C.H. Yarbro, M.H. Frogge, and M. Goodman (Eds.), *Cancer Symptom Management* (3rd ed.), 2004, Sudbury, MA: Jones and Bartlett. Copyright 2004 by Jones and Bartlett. Reprinted with permission.

Evidence-Based Treatment Strategies

As a result of the wide variety of underlying disorders and clinical manifestations seen with DIC, treatment should be individualized to the specific patient presentation. The first priority in managing DIC is to treat the underlying disorder. Other goals of management include administration of replacement therapies aimed at reducing or ameliorating the hemorrhagic episodes, control of coagulation processes, and supportive care.

Replacement therapies are administered to replace deficiencies resulting from coagulation factors, inhibitors, and platelet consumption in an effort to reverse the hemorrhagic events associated with DIC (Franchini et al., 2006). Fresh frozen plasma (FFP) and platelet transfusions are the standard blood components used in patients with significant bleeding. FFP is preferred over specific coagulation factor concentrates because it contains all of the deficient coagulation factors and inhibitors seen in DIC. The usual dose of FFP is 15–20 ml/kg IV and is indicated in patients with significant DIC-associated bleeding and a fibrinogen level below 100 mg/dl (Franchini et al.). The administration of FFP has been controversial because FFP contains fibrinogen that can aggravate the DIC process (Bick, 2003). Platelet transfusions should be given if the patient's platelet count is less than 20,000 cells/mm³ or if the platelet count is less than 50,000 cells/mm³ and the patient is actively bleeding. Washed packed red blood cells should be given if the patient's hemoglobin is less than 8 mg/dl. Washed packed blood cells are preferred over whole blood because they limit volume and immune complications (Becker & Wira, 2008). Patients with severe hyperfibrinolysis and low fibrinogen levels may be treated with cryoprecipitate at a dosage of 1 U/10 kg (Franchini et al.).

Anticoagulant therapy is used when the patient has persistent DIC four to six hours after receiving treatment for the underlying disorder and is aimed at reversing ongoing thrombosis that can ultimately result in end-organ damage. Heparin may be used; however, clinical studies thus far have been inconclusive in regard to patient benefit and often have shown contradictory results (Feinstein, 1982; Hoyle, Swisky, Freedman,

Table 14-3. Laboratory Data in Disseminated Intravascular Coagulation (DIC)

Laboratory Test	Result	Comments
Prothrombin time varies: Compare with normal control.	Prolonged	Prolonged, shortened, or normal in DIC Coagulation deficiency of the extrinsic and common pathway May be prolonged because of several coagulation factors May be the result of liver disease, vitamin K deficiency, obstructive biliary disease, or warfarin therapy
Partial thromboplastin time varies: Compare with normal control.	Prolonged	Prolonged, shortened, or normal in DIC Deficiency of intrinsic and common pathways Decreased quantity of any coagulation factor, except VII or XIII May be caused by heparin therapy, increased fibrin degradation products, and consumption of clotting factors
International normalized ratio	Prolonged	Prolonged, shortened, or normal in DIC Evaluates overall coagulation
Fibrin degradation products	Elevated	Measures the breakdown of fibrin and fibrinogen Elevated level may occur with surgery, obstetric complication, various medical problems, and DIC.
D-dimer	Elevated	Elevated levels indicate hyperfibrinolysis. Common in DIC, pulmonary and cerebral embolism, phlebitis, thrombosis, and postoperative prothrombotic risks
Antithrombin III level	Decreased	Accelerated coagulation
Activated partial thromboplastin time	Prolonged, shortened, or normal	Nonspecific in DIC
Thrombin time	Elevated	Estimate of plasma fibrinogen Prolonged because of heparin, streptokinase, or urokinase therapy Prolonged in DIC, liver disease, or fibrinogen deficiency
Fibrinogen	Decreased	Nonspecific in DIC Plasma concentration of fibrinogen Low because of congenital or acquired hypofibrinogenemia, DIC, fibrinolysis, severe liver disease, malignant processes, or obstetrical trauma Elevated in some malignancies or inflammatory conditions
Platelet count	Decreased	Nonspecific finding in DIC
Peripheral smear	Schistocytes present	Nonspecific finding in DIC
Plasminogen levels	Decreased	Hyperfibrinolysis
Alpha-1 antiplasmin levels	Decreased	Hyperfibrinolysis
Fibrinopeptide A level	Elevated	Indicates accelerated coagulation and fibrin formation

Note. Based on information from Friend & Pruett, 2004; Gobel, 2005a, 2005b.
From "Disseminated Intravascular Coagulation" (pp. 43–44), by S.A. Ezzone in M. Kaplan (Ed.), *Understanding and Managing Oncologic Emergencies: A Resource for Nurses,* 2006, Pittsburgh, PA: Oncology Nursing Society. Copyright 2006 by the Oncology Nursing Society. Reprinted with permission.

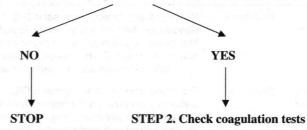

Step 1. Risk assessment

Does the patient have un underlying disorder known to be associated with DIC?

NO   YES

STOP   **STEP 2. Check coagulation tests**

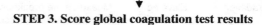

Platelet count, PT, fibrinogen, soluble fibrin monomers, FDPs

STEP 3. Score global coagulation test results

- Platelet count (x10^9/L): >100 = 0; <100 = 1; <50 = 2

- PT (sec.): <3 = 0; >3 but >6 = 1; >6 = 2

- Fibrinogen (g/L): >1 = 0; <1 = 1

- Fibrin-related markers: no increase = 0; moderate increase = 2; strong increase = 3

STEP 4. Calculate score

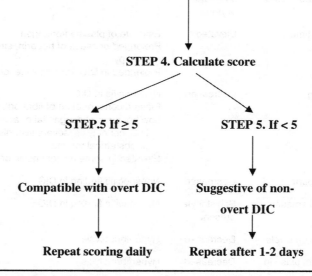

STEP.5 If ≥ 5   STEP 5. If < 5

Compatible with overt DIC   Suggestive of non-overt DIC

Repeat scoring daily   Repeat after 1-2 days

Figure 14-3. Diagnostic Algorithm and Scoring System for Disseminated Intravascular Coagulation (DIC)

FDPs—fibrin degradation products; PT—prothrombin time

Note. From "Recent Acquisitions in the Pathophysiology, Diagnosis, and Treatment of Disseminated Intravascular Coagulation," by M. Franchini, G. Lippi, and F. Manzato, February 21, 2006, *Thrombosis Journal, 4,* p. 4. Copyright 2006 by Franchini et al.; licensee BioMed Central Ltd. Reprinted from open access article that permits unrestricted use, distribution, and reproduction.

& Hayhoe, 1988; Levi & ten Cate, 1999). Heparin acts to inhibit further thrombogenesis and prevent reaccumulation of a clot after spontaneous fibrinolysis (Becker & Wira, 2008). The usual heparin dose is 80–100 U/kg subcutaneously every four to six hours or 20,000–30,000 U/day continuous IV infusion. As a result of the high risk of excessive bleeding, heparin therapy requires close monitoring and is contraindicated in patients who have CNS disorders or open wounds or who have had recent surgery (Gobel, 2005b). Antithrombin III also may be administered to increase the anticoagulation effects of heparin. Antithrombin III is indicated when significantly low levels of antithrombin III are present or in patients with severe DIC. The usual dose of antithrombin III consists of a loading dose of 100 U/kg IV over three hours followed by continuous infusion of 100 U/kg/day (Becker & Wira). Patients receiving antithrombin III should be monitored closely for localized bleeding or hematoma, hypotension, and shock. Recombinant human activated protein C, drotrecogin alfa, is indicated in patients with severe sepsis to reduce mortality (see the following discussion on sepsis). In patients with DIC, drotrecogin alfa exerts an antithrombotic effect, has indirect profibrinolytic activity, and exerts anti-inflammatory effects by inhibiting tumor necrosis factor production, blocking leukocyte adhesion, and limiting thrombin-induced inflammatory responses within microvascular endothelium (Becker & Wira; Toh & Dennis, 2003). Drotrecogin alfa is contraindicated in patients with a less than six-week history of GI bleeding, less than three-week history of thrombolytic therapy, less than seven-day history of platelet inhibitor administration, less than three-month history of ischemic stroke, or history of intracranial arteriovenous malformation or aneurysm, intracranial neoplasm, chronic severe hepatic disease, recent hemorrhagic stroke, or recent intracranial surgery (Becker & Wira). The usual dosage is 24 mcg/kg/hour continuous IV infusion over 96 hours. If clinically significant bleeding occurs, the infusion should be stopped immediately.

If all therapies have been unsuccessful in reversing the process of DIC, antifibrinolytic agents may be given. Two antifibrinolytic agents used to treat DIC are aminocaproic acid (Amicar®, Xanodyne Pharmaceuticals) and tranexamic acid (Cyklokapron®, Pfizer Inc.). Aminocaproic acid inhibits fibrinolysis by inhibiting plasminogen activator substances. The usual dosage is a loading dose of 5–10 g IV followed by 2–4 g per hour IV, not to exceed 30 g per day. Tranexamic acid inhibits fibrinolysis by displacing plasminogen from fibrin. The usual dose is 1–2 g IV every 8–12 hours (Becker & Wira, 2008). Both of the antifibrinolytic agents should be used with caution because of the inhibition of intrinsic fibrinolysis that can lead to profuse fibrin deposition and end-organ dysfunction (Maxson, 2000).

Additional medical treatment strategies include IV hydration to treat hypotension and intracellular volume depletion and specific therapies for possible complications that may include acute renal failure, cardiac tamponade, hemothorax, intracerebral hematoma, and gangrene.

Implications for Advanced Nursing Practice

The care of patients with DIC is very complex and necessitates prompt treatment and close monitoring. It is critical that APNs recognize early signs and symptoms of DIC and either initiate or support the nursing staff in the pharmacologic management and supportive care of patients immediately. Nurses should assess vital signs, noting any hypotension, tachycardia, tachypnea, or temperature change, all of which may indicate bleeding. The physical examination can give the APN the opportunity to identify any signs and symptoms of bleeding or thrombosis and to begin appropriate clinical interventions (Maxson, 2000). Hemorrhaging or oozing from gums, suture lines, and IV sites, and epistaxis, hematuria, or hemoptysis are all highly suggestive of DIC. Other less overt signs and symptoms of bleeding that may suggest DIC and should be continually monitored are guaiac-positive stools, headache, joint and abdominal pain, skin petechiae, ecchymosis, purpura, or acral cyanosis (cyanosis of peripheral structures such as extremities, digits, metatarsals, and ears). Patients should have direct pressure placed on any areas of bleeding, and skin protective measures should be initiated to prevent further injury. Venipuncture and blood draw sticks should be kept to a minimum. For gingival oozing, patients should only use soft oral swabs (such as Toothettes®, Sage Products, Inc.) and normal saline mouth rinses. Patients with epistaxis should have pressure placed on the bridge of the nose and be placed in an upright position. GI bleeding should be assessed carefully, and patients should start on stool softeners and a stool diary, recording melanous stools and estimated blood loss.

The patient's fluid status should be followed closely with monitoring of intake and output to assess for early signs of acute renal failure. With any bleeding, the patient should be well hydrated with IV fluids to maintain vascular pressure. Patients should increase fluid intake unless contraindicated.

Close assessment of signs or symptoms of thrombosis is necessary. Microvascular emboli of the skin or extremities may be evidenced by small necrotic lesions or skin-mottling. DVT may present as unilateral extremity swelling with localized erythema. To help to prevent DVT, patients should have elevation of the extremity, passive or active range of motion performed on all extremities to prevent stasis, and avoidance of any restrictive clothing or compression of the posterior popliteal knee (Gobel, 2005b; Maxson, 2000).

Pharmacologic agents, as discussed in the treatment section, should be administered promptly to make every attempt to eradicate the process of DIC. Evaluation of laboratory studies should occur every eight hours in order to monitor treatment effectiveness and the need for additional therapy (Becker & Wira, 2008).

Patients with acute DIC are critically ill and require intensive care monitoring. The overall disorder can be very frightening for both patients and the family members; therefore, significant social, spiritual, and psychological services may be required. Patients and family members should be kept informed and educated about the current clinical status, and the healthcare team should answer questions in a timely manner to reduce anxiety.

Sepsis

Sepsis is a complex interaction between an infecting microorganism and an individual's immune, inflammatory, and coagulation responses. Sepsis in patients with cancer is a life-threatening event, especially when patients are receiving chemotherapy and may be neutropenic. APNs can play a key role in prevention and also in directing immediate treatment to reverse the devastating clinical decline related to sepsis that can rapidly progress to death. Therefore, it is critical that the APN is knowledgeable about the pathophysiology and management of sepsis.

Definition and Incidence

Sepsis and *septic shock* are terms previously used to define a wide variety of inflammatory responses. In 1992, the term *systemic inflammatory response syndrome* (SIRS) was introduced (Bone et al., 1992). Infection/bacteremia is the presence of viable bacteria or fungi in the blood with positive blood cultures (Moore, 2005). SIRS is the systemic response to infection and is described as two or more of the following: temperature higher than 38°C (100.4°F) or less than 36°C (96.8°F); heart rate greater than 90 beats/minute; respiratory rate greater than 20 breaths/minute; or a white blood cell count greater than 12,000/mm^3, less than 4,000/mm^3, or greater than 10% bands (Mackenzie & Wilson, 2001; Russell, 2006; Stoll, 2001). Sepsis is the systemic inflammatory response to a variety of clinical insults to the body and is manifested by two or more of the SIRS criteria. Sepsis occurs in response to an overwhelming bacterial infection that enters the bloodstream. Severe sepsis is associated with organ dysfunction, hypotension, and organ hypoperfusion. Septic shock is sepsis with hypotension/hypoperfusion that is unresponsive to aggressive fluid resuscitation with organ dysfunction (Mackenzie & Wilson; Russell). Multiple organ dysfunction syndrome is the presence of dysfunction in more than one organ requiring aggressive treatment to maintain homeostasis (Moore).

The incidence of sepsis is approximately 750,000 per year in the United States, with approximately 210,000 fatalities (Angus et al., 2001; Martin, Mannino, Eaton, & Moss, 2003). The mortality rate associated with sepsis is approximately 40% but can surpass 50% in critically ill patients, even with aggressive treatment. Patients with neutropenia have a greater incidence of septic shock and mortality in comparison with those patients who have a normal or elevated white blood cell count (Stoll, 2001). Approximately 25%–40% of patients with cancer will develop infection at some time during their treatment (Dale, 2002).

Presenting Signs and Symptoms

The classic signs and symptoms of sepsis are fever, shaking chills and rigors, hypotension, tachycardia, tachypnea, and mental status changes. Patients who are neutropenic may present with no significant signs and symptoms with the exception of fever because of immunosuppression and depression of the normal phagocytic and inflammatory responses (Wade & Rubenstein, 2001). Additional manifestations depend on the stage of sepsis. Signs and symptoms of severe sepsis reflect the extensive vasodilation that is occurring in various organ systems, whereas the signs and symptoms of septic shock reflect the hypoperfusion and widespread alterations in circulation, tissue oxygenation, and organ dysfunction (see Figure 14-4).

Risk Factors

Risk factors associated with sepsis include infections of the pulmonary, cutaneous, renal, and GI organ systems; exposure to bacteria, fungi, and viruses; medical therapies; trauma; invasive devices; and miscellaneous risk factors, such as age, comorbidities, and frequent hospitalizations (see Figure 14-5). In patients with cancer, numerous factors may enhance an individual's susceptibility for infection. In healthy individuals, three immune defense mechanisms are present in the setting of infection (Safdar & Armstrong, 2001). The first line of defense is granulocytes that phagocytize and kill bacteria. The second line of defense is cell-mediated immunity that activates monocytes, macrophages, and T lymphocytes to eliminate pathogens, viruses, and malignant cells. The third line of defense is humoral immunity that activates the B lymphocytes to produce antibodies specific to foreign bodies or antigens. Most patients with

Severe Sepsis (Vasodilation)
- Dry, warm, flushed skin
- Anxiety, confusion, agitation
- Normal or elevated temperature
- Normal or low blood pressure
- Tachycardia
- Bounding pulse
- Tachypnea
- Diminished breath sounds, rales
- Decreased gastrointestinal (GI) motility, nausea
- Decreased urine output
- Leukopenia/leukocytosis
- Thrombocytopenia
- Elevated prothrombin time (PT)/partial thromboplastin time (PTT)
- Decreased fibrinogen
- Increased fibrin degradation products
- Lactic acidosis
- Hyperglycemia

Septic Shock (Hypoperfusion)
- Cold, clammy, pale skin
- Lethargy or coma
- Subnormal temperature
- Hypotension
- Tachycardia
- Weak, thready pulse
- Tachypnea
- Diminished breath sounds, rales with pulmonary edema
- Decreased GI motility, jaundice, elevated liver function tests
- Anuria, elevated blood urea nitrogen/creatinine, acute renal failure
- Leukopenia/leukocytosis
- Anemia
- Thrombocytopenia
- Elevated PT/PTT
- Decreased fibrinogen
- Increased fibrin degradation products
- Lactic acidosis
- Hyperglycemia
- Hyponatremia, hypokalemia, hypocalcemia
- Decreased albumin, magnesium, phosphate

Figure 14-4. Signs and Symptoms of Severe Sepsis and Septic Shock

Note. Based on information from Moore, 2005; Stoll, 2001.

cancer are affected by all three of these mechanisms because of either the cancer process or treatment. Patients with cancer undergoing treatment characteristically have granulocytopenia. Patients with hematologic cancers and patients undergoing stem cell transplant have diminished function of T lymphocytes. Patients with multiple myeloma, Waldenström macroglobulinemia, and chronic lymphocytic leukemia, and patients who are asplenic or are receiving chemotherapy can have impaired function of B lymphocytes (Moore, 2005).

Before the 1980s, the major documented pathogen in infected neutropenic patients was gram-negative organisms originating from bowel colonization (Freifeld et al., 2004). Since that time, gram-positive bacteria (associated with increasing use of ve-

System	Major Pathogens	Therapies	Invasive Devices	Other
Cutaneous	Gram-positive bacteria	Chemotherapy	Venous access devices	Age
• Trauma	• *Staphylococcus epidermidis*	Radiation therapy	Urinary catheters	• < 1 year
• Burns		Immunosuppressive agents	Gastrostomy tubes	• > 65 years
• Skin or wound infections		Antibiotics	Nasogastric tubes	Comorbidities
• Abscesses	• *Staphylococcus aureus*	Blood transfusions	Arterial catheters	• Autoimmune disease
• Cysts		Splenectomy	Ommaya reservoirs	• Diabetes mellitus
• Tumor involvement	• *Staphylococcus viridans*	Surgical procedures	Chest tubes	• Renal disease
Pulmonary	Gram-negative bacteria		Surgical drainage tubes	• Alcoholism
• Upper respiratory infections	• *Escherichia coli*			• HIV disease
• Sinus infections	• Klebsiella			• Hepatic disease
• Pneumonia	• Pseudomonas			Frequent hospitalizations
Renal	• Enterobacter			Malnutrition
• Lower urinary tract infections	Fungi			Neutropenia
• Upper urinary tract infections	• Candida			Trauma
Gastrointestinal	• Aspergillus			Exposure to gram-positive or gram-negative bacteria
• Upper	Viruses			
– Mucositis	• Herpes simplex			
– Esophagitis				
• Lower				
– Peritonitis				
– Diverticulitis				
– Cholelithiasis				
– Bowel infections				

Figure 14-5. Risk Factors Associated With Sepsis

Note. Based on information from Freifeld et al., 2004.

nous access devices) and fungi have become more common causative agents for infection in neutropenic patients with fever (Bochud & Calandra, 2005; Freifeld et al.; Martin et al., 2003).

Pathophysiology

The body's normal defense system works to recognize and destroy foreign bacteria and antigens. At the site of an injury, the endothelium secretes adherence molecules that attract leukocytes. Activation of polymorphonuclear leukocytes produces additional adhesion molecules that promote aggregation and margination to the vascular endothelium and is responsible for the cardinal signs of local inflammation, which include local vasodilation, hyperemia, and increased microvascular permeability. Lymphocytes also release cytokines, including tumor necrosis factor and interleukins, which are responsible for local vasodilation and increased vascular permeability to facilitate neutrophil saturation in the tissue and phagocytosis of bacteria (Hotchkiss & Karl, 2003; Moore, 2005; Stoll, 2001).

Without this normal inflammatory response, microbes can enter the body's circulatory system and tissue and cause an uncontrolled inflammatory response. Endotoxins, associated with gram-negative bacteria, and exotoxins, associated with gram-positive bacteria, stimulate release of inflammatory substances. The inflammatory substances, macrophages, monocytes, neutrophils, and plasma cells, activate tumor necrosis factor and cytokines that promote tissue inflammation, extensive widespread vasodilation, decreased arterial and venous tone, and activation of the clotting mechanisms. As a result, capillary leak syndrome occurs with third-spacing of fluids, hypoperfusion and decreased oxygenation of tissue and organs, ischemia, cell death, and coagulopathies seen in sepsis (Moore, 2005).

Prevention Strategies

APNs can facilitate prevention strategies through ongoing thorough assessment of patients receiving chemotherapy and initiating prophylactic treatment immediately if any patient is identified as being at high risk for infection. Patients who are at high risk for infection, including patients with hematologic malignancies, stem cell transplant recipients, or patients expected to have prolonged neutropenia, should receive treatment with quinolone therapy for seven days (Gafter-Gvili, Fraser, Paul, & Leibovici, 2005; National Comprehensive Cancer Network [NCCN], 2008; Shelton, 2003). Standard therapy for any patient receiving antineoplastic treatment that poses more than a 20% risk of febrile neutropenia should include colony-stimulating factors (NCCN; Shelton). Patient and caregiver education should include instructions to prevent infection, such as practicing good hand-washing techniques, avoiding exposure to others with known infections, and knowing the signs and symptoms to report to the healthcare provider, for example, fever, cough, purulent sputum production, urinary complaints, nausea, vomiting, diarrhea, or any skin erythema or open wounds.

Diagnosis and Assessment

Diagnosis of sepsis and septic shock is based upon the patient's history, physical examination, and diagnostic studies. The history should include a complete review of the patient's cancer, treatment, any recent immunosuppressive or antibiotic agents, recent blood product administration, comorbidities, and insertion of invasive devices. Presenting symptoms may facilitate identification of the source of infection, and therefore patients should be evaluated for any history of fever, cough with productive sputum, shortness of breath, weakness, mental status changes, syncope, burning on urination, urinary incontinence, oliguria, nausea and vomiting, or diarrhea (Russell, 2006). The physical examination should include complete vital signs with temperature, blood pressure, pulse rate, respiratory rate, and oxygen saturation. Sites of possible infection, such as the oral cavity, perianal region, skin wounds, or catheter exit sites, should be carefully evaluated. Although all systems require examination, the respiratory, cardiovascular, GI, and neurologic systems should receive special consideration, as review of these systems may provide specific data that contribute to the diagnosis and possible source of infection. On examination, patients with sepsis may present with adventitious or absent breath sounds, tachypnea, tachycardia, bounding pulse, abdominal tenderness with hypoactive or hyperactive bowel sounds, and generalized weakness with mental status changes.

Diagnostic studies include blood, urine, sputum, stool, and drainage cultures, complete blood count, complete metabolic panel, coagulation studies, pulse oximetry, chest x-ray, and electrocardiogram (EKG). The complete blood count in patients with sepsis may reflect an elevated white blood cell count (> 12,000 cells/mm³), a decreased white blood cell count (< 4,000 cells/mm³), > 10% blasts, low hemoglobin level secondary to hemorrhage, hemodilution or hemolysis, and a low platelet count secondary to platelet destruction or decreased production of platelets (Moore, 2005). With both sepsis and septic shock, hyperglycemia will occur as a result of the compensatory anti-inflammatory response with gluconeogenesis and the reduction of insulin secretion (Mackenzie & Wilson, 2001). Hypoglycemia may be seen in prolonged septic shock. In addition, elevated blood urea nitrogen (BUN) and creatinine levels will occur as a result of dehydration or renal failure in both sepsis and septic shock. In the presence of septic shock, electrolyte alterations that may occur include decreased sodium, potassium, calcium, albumin, magnesium, and phosphate (Hotchkiss & Karl, 2003). Prolonged PT and PTT frequently is seen as a result of possible liver dysfunction and alterations in the coagulation pathway. Assessment of the pulmonary system will include pulse oximetry and chest x-ray. Pulse oximetry values will reflect hypoxia and poor oxygenation, and the chest x-ray may note the presence of pneumonia, effusions, or pulmonary edema. However, in patients with neutropenia, radiographic abnormalities may not be present (Donawitz, Harman, & Pope, 1991). Arterial blood gases can provide additional information regarding a patient's oxygenation and presence of respiratory alkalosis and metabolic acidosis (Gobel & Peterson, 2006). An EKG should be performed to rule out possible cardiac causes of hypotension and to evaluate for possible arrhythmias (Mackenzie & Wilson).

Differential diagnoses may include DIC, acute myocardial infarction, acute pulmonary embolus, acute pancreatitis, acute GI hemorrhage, tumor fever, and adverse drug reactions. Other differential diagnoses may involve metabolic or volemic alterations, such as diabetic ketoacidosis, diuretic-induced hypovolemia, and adrenal insufficiency.

Evidence-Based Treatment Strategies

Treatment for sepsis involves respiratory support, fluid resuscitation, inotropic and vasopressor agents, DVT prophylaxis, insulin therapy, antibiotic and antifungal agents, activated protein C, blood transfusion support, and nutritional and electrolyte replacement (Moore, 2005; Russell, 2006) (see Table 14-4). Once the diagnosis of severe sepsis has been made, intensive therapy should begin, and the patient should be admitted to the critical care unit for aggressive fluid resuscitation and continuous monitoring of blood pressure, mean arterial pressure (MAP), central venous pressure (CVP), venous oxygen saturation (ScvO₂), arterial saturation, and arterial blood gases (Rivers et al., 2001). Initial resuscitation (within the first six hours after the diagnosis of severe sepsis) should maintain a CVP of 8–12 mm Hg, MAP greater than or equal to 65 mm Hg, urine output greater than 0.5 ml/kg/hour, and ScvO₂ greater than 70% (Gobel & Peterson, 2006).

Patients should be assessed for an adequate airway, and initiation of oxygen therapy should occur immediately with continuous pulse oximetry monitoring to decrease the risk for acute lung injury and to decrease associated mortality (Rivers et al., 2001; Russell, 2006). In patients with severe sepsis, intubation and mechanical ventilation may be required, as a majority of patients develop significant pulmonary complications secondary to pulmonary edema, poor gas exchange, encephalopathy, and altered level of consciousness (Mackenzie & Wilson, 2001; Sessler, Perry, & Varney, 2004). More than 50% of patients will develop acute respiratory distress syndrome, which is the most severe form of acute lung injury. Without correction, patients will progress and develop pulmonary fibrosis (Mackenzie & Wilson; Moore, 2005).

Table 14-4. Treatment Strategies for Severe Sepsis	
Treatment	**Goals of Therapy**
Respiratory Support	
Oxygen therapy Continuous pulse oximetry monitoring Intubation and ventilation as required	Venous oxygen saturation > 70%
Fluid Resuscitation	
May require up to 10 L in 24 hours Normal saline Lactated ringers Albumin	Central venous pressure of 8–12 mm Hg Mean arterial pressure (MAP) ≥ 65 mm Hg Urine output > 0.5 ml/kg/hour Increase in blood pressure Decrease in pulse rate Improvement in organ function
Drug Therapy—Vasopressors	
Dopamine 2–25 mcg/kg/min IV	At lower doses: Vasodilation with increased urinary output and sodium excretion At higher doses: Vasoconstriction with increased cardiac contractility, blood pressure, and pulse
Norepinephrine 1–30 mcg/min IV	Vasoconstriction, increased MAP
Drug Therapy—Inotropics	
Phenylephrine 40–180 mcg/min IV	Vasoconstriction, increased blood pressure
Epinephrine 1–20 mcg/min IV	Vasoconstriction, increased MAP
Vasopressin 0.01–0.04 unit/min IV	Vasoconstriction with decreased urine output and water retention
Dobutamine 5–15 mcg/kg/min IV	Vasoconstriction, increased cardiac contractility and heart rate
Low-Molecular-Weight Heparin	Deep vein thrombosis prophylaxis
Insulin	Maintain serum blood glucose levels between 80–110 mg/dl.
Antibiotic Agents—Monotherapy	
Cefepime 2 g IV every 12 hours Ceftazidime 2 g IV every 12 hours Imipenem/cilastatin 500 mg IV every 6 hours Meropenem 500–1,000 mg IV every 8 hours Piperacillin/tazobactam 3–4 g IV every 4–6 hours	Broad-spectrum antibacterial activity
Antibiotic Agents—Double Coverage Therapy	
Gentamicin 1 mg/kg IV every 8 hours plus antipseudomonal penicillin Piperacillin/tazobactam plus cefepime or ceftazidime Ciprofloxacin 50 mg/kg IV every 4 hours plus piperacillin/tazobactam Vancomycin 500 mg IV every 6 hours if appropriate	Broad-spectrum antibacterial activity

(Continued on next page)

Table 14-4. Treatment Strategies for Severe Sepsis (Continued)

Treatment	Goals of Therapy
Antifungal Agents	
Fluconazole 400 mg initial dose then 200 mg IV daily	Empiric antifungal for *Candida* organisms
Amphotericin B (test dose 1 mg) 1–1.5 mg/kg/day IV	Empiric antifungal for aspergillosis
Caspofungin 70 mg loading dose on first day followed by 50 mg/day IV	Empiric antifungal for aspergillosis
Activated Protein C Replacement	
Drotrecogin alfa 24 mcg/kg/hour IV for 96 hours	Promote fibrinolysis, decrease thrombin formation, decrease inflammation, and ultimately improve organ function
Metabolic and Electrolyte Replacement	
Enteral or parenteral nutrition 25–30 kcal/kg/usual body weight/day 1.3–2 g protein per kg/day 30%–70% of daily glucose caloric intake 15%–30% of daily lipid caloric intake Sodium, potassium, magnesium, calcium, phosphate, zinc: Maintain normal serum levels.	Nutritional and electrolyte support

Note. Based on information from Gobel & Peterson, 2006; Mackenzie & Wilson, 2001; Moore, 2005.

Because of the decreased vascular tone and third-spacing of fluid that occurs in sepsis, patients develop hypotension and decreased intracellular fluid. Rapidly administered fluid resuscitation is critical to replace the intracellular fluid deficits and to replenish organ perfusion. Fluid replacement may include colloids or crystalloids, such as normal saline or lactated ringers, and may necessitate large quantities of as much as 10 L within the first 24 hours. Although specific evidence-based guidelines do not exist pertaining to the type of fluid, crystalloids rapidly replace the extracellular volume; therefore, patients require larger volumes for intracellular resuscitation (Mackenzie & Wilson, 2001). In patients with preexisting cardiac disease, fluid replacement must be administered with caution, and close monitoring of patients' CVP is necessary to guide fluid resuscitation. Overall, an increase in blood pressure, decrease in pulse rate, and improvement in organ function demonstrates response to fluid replacement.

If fluid replacement does not achieve improvement in the patient's clinical status, the patient may have inadequate myocardial contractility or persistent vasodilation. If the patient appears to have persistent vasodilation, a vasopressor is appropriate to increase the blood pressure. If the patient has clinical signs of poor organ perfusion with cool extremities, an inotropic agent should be considered. Vasopressor agents, which include norepinephrine and dopamine, are adrenergic agonists and cause increased cardiac contractility and vasoconstriction in high doses. Inotropic agents (usually used as second-line drugs) include phenylephrine, epinephrine, vasopressin, or dobutamine (Dellinger et al., 2004).

Transfusional support is necessary to control active bleeding and correct severe anemia. Platelets should be administered for acute bleeding or if the platelet count is less than 5,000 cells/mm^3. Packed red blood cells should be administered for hemoglobin levels below 7 g/dl. Maintaining hemoglobin levels above 10 g/dl has not been shown to improve patients' outcome related to sepsis (Mackenzie & Wilson, 2001).

Empiric antibiotic therapy should be administered immediately after cultures have been obtained and patients have a high suspicion for sepsis. Patients with neutropenia who present with fever, or any potential signs of infection, should be immediately treated (within one hour) with a broad-spectrum antibiotic. A delay in treatment has been associated with significant mortality (Hughes et al., 2002). According to the NCCN guideline, *Prevention and Treatment of Cancer-Related Infections* (2008), initial therapy should be based on the most common potentially infecting organism, the potential sites of infection, the antimicrobial susceptibilities of locally isolated pathogens, the broad-spectrum antibacterial activity of the agent, the patient's infection risk assessment, clinical instability such as hypotension, organ dysfunction, the patient's medication allergies, and the previous antibiotic therapy history. The NCCN guidelines present two risk assessment classification systems: the Multinational Association of Supportive Care in Cancer (for identifying low-risk neutropenic patients with cancer) and the Talcott Risk Assessment (for identifying neutropenic patients at risk for sepsis). Detailed discussion regarding these risk assessment classification systems is beyond the scope of this chapter, and the reader is referred to the NCCN guidelines for further information. Both monotherapy and double coverage therapy have been found to be appropriate initial treatment for the management of febrile neutropenia (NCCN). Monotherapy may consist of cefepime, ceftazidime, imipenem and cilastatin, meropenem, or piperacillin and tazobactam. Double coverage therapy may consist of an aminoglycoside plus antipseudomonal penicillin or an extended-spectrum antipseudomonal cephalosporin, or ciprofloxacin plus antipseudomonal penicillin (NCCN). The addition of empiric vancomycin to either monotherapy or to double coverage therapy remains controversial. The use of vancomycin is indicated in some infections caused by gram-positive pathogens that can lead to rapid death; however, vancomycin is associated with an increased incidence of nephrotoxicity and hepatotoxicity, and the increased use of vancomycin has led to a recent increase in vancomycin-resistant organisms (NCCN). Vancomycin may be considered for serious catheter-related infections, for known colonization with beta-lactam–resistant pneumococci or methicillin-resistant *Staphylococcus aureus*, for patients whose blood cultures are positive for gram-positive bacteria (prior to final identification and susceptibility testing), for patients who have been previously treated prophylactically with ciprofloxacin or trimethoprim and sulfamethoxazole, or for those patients with hypotension or septic shock without an identified pathogen (NCCN).

Empiric antifungal agents also should be considered in the treatment of sepsis in patients with cancer who are unresponsive to broad-spectrum antibacterial agents, with proven or probable fungal infections. The most common fungal infections in patients with neutropenia are *Candida* and aspergillosis (Moore, 2005; NCCN, 2008). Fluconazole is indicated for patients with uncomplicated candidemia, and amphotericin B is indicated for treatment of aspergillosis. Amphotericin B is a common empiric antifungal and also is administered in patients who have been treated with broad-spectrum antibiotics and have persistent fevers.

Severe sepsis and septic shock are manifested as a significant inflammatory response with the possibility of adrenal insufficiency that occurs with major illness. Corticosteroids are commonly used for adrenal insufficiency and for inflammatory diseases. However, corticosteroids, regardless of dose and duration of treatment, have shown no significant impact on mortality associated with sepsis and are not recommended as standard treatment, but have shown at least mild effectiveness in treating the inflammatory response of sepsis (Annane et al., 2004). Use of corticosteroids may increase the risk of secondary infections.

Activated protein C, an anticoagulant and anti-inflammatory agent, has been found to decrease mortality and improve organ dysfunction in patients with severe sepsis (Bernard et al., 2001). Activated protein C acts to promote fibrinolysis, decrease thrombin formation, and decrease inflammation by reducing mast-cell degradation and platelet and neutrophil aggregation (Hinds, 2001; Moore, 2005; Russell, 2006; Tazbir, 2004). Drotrecogin alfa, a recombinant human activated protein C, is indicated for severe sepsis in adults. The major side effect of drotrecogin alfa is bleeding related to the most common sites of hemorrhage, which include skin and soft tissue sites, intracranial, GI, intra-abdominal, intrathoracic, retroperitoneal, and genitourinary sites. Drotrecogin alfa should not be administered to patients with the following: a platelet count less than 30,000 cells/mm^3, a prolonged PT with an international normalized ratio greater than 3, history of GI bleeding within six weeks, thrombolytic therapy within three days, oral anticoagulants within seven days, aspirin use or other platelet inhibitor within seven days, ischemic stroke within three months, known bleeding diathesis, or chronic severe hepatic disease (Becker & Wira, 2008).

During this critical, prolonged clinical illness, patients will require nutritional support to meet metabolic requirements and electrolyte replacement. Enteral tube feedings are preferred over IV nutrition, which often is associated with significant complications such as infection. In addition to standard electrolyte replacement, patients will require insulin to treat hyperglycemia that occurs as a result of the decreased insulin secretion seen with severe illness (Mackenzie & Wilson, 2001).

Implications for Advanced Nursing Practice

APNs act as a facilitator and coordinator of care for patients diagnosed with sepsis. APNs should be able to identify patients who are at high risk for infection and employ infection prevention strategies. All patient procedures should be performed using aseptic technique, especially those involving care of invasive devices. Recognition of signs and symptoms of impending sepsis is critical so that appropriate treatment can be started immediately. In addition to the treatment strategies outlined in Table 14-4, APNs should promote patient safety and institute preventive measures that decrease further complications during the patient's critical illness. Daily skin assessment is critical to evaluate for the presence of wounds, and patients should have skin protective devices in place, such as mechanical floatation beds as needed, sequential compression devices, and heel protectors. Patients experiencing altered mental status or agitation may require sedation to prevent patient injuries.

APNs also can facilitate the promotion of long-term care during the acute phase of illness. The long-term goal is resolution of infection and return to normal organ function; therefore, communication and environmental orientation should be maintained. Daily physical therapy can promote prevention of muscle atrophy and loss of physical function.

Family and caregiver support is critical during the patient's acute illness. Family members require ongoing information regarding the patient's status and should be educated about the rationale for procedures and treatments. Emotional support is of utmost priority, as the diagnosis of sepsis and its associated clinical manifestations can be frightening for family members. Family members also should be offered other supportive resources, such as social work and chaplain services. APNs should be prepared to discuss advance directives and appropriate palliative and hospice services, if necessary.

Tumor Lysis Syndrome

TLS is characterized by electrolyte and metabolic disturbances caused by cell lysis as a result of chemotherapy, radiation therapy, biotherapy, or surgery. The release of intracellular products from the cell lysis overloads the body's normal homeostatic mechanisms. Without treatment, these metabolic disturbances can lead to acute renal failure, multiple organ failure, cardiac arrhythmias, and death. APNs should be knowledgeable about the pathophysiology, diagnosis, assessment, and treatment of TLS; however, of utmost importance is knowledge of preventive strategies.

Definition and Incidence

TLS is a metabolic oncologic emergency characterized by rapid cell lysis caused by surgery, radiation therapy, or the administration of chemotherapy or biotherapy. Following cell lysis, intracellular contents including potassium, phosphorus, and uric acid are released into the vascular system. The characteristic metabolic disturbances associated with TLS include hyperkalemia, hyperuricemia, hyperphosphatemia, and hypocalcemia.

The exact incidence of TLS is not known, but estimated incidence rates range from 5%–25% in patients with leukemia and lymphoma (Truini-Pittman & Rossetto, 2002). Although the incidence of TLS does not vary by age or gender, older patients are more at risk for TLS and have more significant complications when diagnosed with TLS because of the possibility of having preexisting renal dysfunction (Cairo & Bishop, 2004).

Presenting Signs and Symptoms

Patients with TLS present with signs and symptoms that are dependent on the degree of metabolic abnormalities. Hyperkalemia, defined as serum potassium levels greater than 6.5 mEq/L, is often the first metabolic abnormality, occurring 6–72 hours after the initiation of therapy, and can produce symptoms that include nausea, vomiting, paresthesia, muscle weakness, paralysis, syncope, lethargy, muscle cramps, increased bowel sounds, and diarrhea. EKG changes can include bradycardia and/or tachycardia, P-wave and T-wave changes, and life-threatening arrythmias, such as ventricular fibrillation (Gobel, 2006; Kaplow, 2002; Secola, 2006).

Hyperuricemia is defined as serum uric acid levels above 10 mg/dl and can occur 24–48 hours after the initiation of therapy (Altman, 2001). Symptoms of hyperuricemia are malaise, nausea, vomiting, diarrhea, anorexia, edema, flank pain, fatigue, weakness, oliguria, and anuria (Krishnan & Hammad, 2006). Severe hyperuricemia, defined as uric acid levels above 20 mg/dl, can cause acute and chronic renal failure with extreme lethargy, extreme somnolence, seizures, paresthesias, endocarditis, azotemia, anuria, edema, and hypertension (Gobel, 2006; Kaplow, 2002).

Hyperphosphatemia is defined as serum phosphorus levels above 5 mg/dl and usually occurs 24–48 hours after the initiation of therapy (Gobel, 2006). Symptoms of hyperphosphatemia generally are the result of compromised renal function and include azotemia, oliguria, numbness, tingling, muscle cramps, muscle twitching, anuria, edema, hypertension, and acute renal failure (Kaplow, 2002).

Hypocalcemia occurs as a result of calcium-phosphorus binding that decreases ionized calcium in the systemic circulation and is defined as serum calcium levels less than 8.7 mg/dl, which usually occur 24–48 hours after initiation of therapy (Kaplow, 2002). Symptoms of hypocalcemia include diarrhea, muscle cramps, muscle spasms, tetany, positive Chvostek sign (exhibited as facial muscle spasms following a tap on one side of the face), positive Trousseau sign (exhibited as upper-arm muscular spasms following pressure to the principal vessel and nerve of the limb), seizures, syncope, laryngospasm with stridor, and anorexia. Cardiac signs of hypocalcemia include hypotension, cardiac arrythmias such as ventricular arrythmias and prolonged QT wave, heart block and sudden death, and cardiac arrest. Mental status changes may include irritability, anxiety, confusion, depression, and hallucinations (Kaplow).

Risk Factors

TLS occurs most frequently in patients with lymphoproliferative malignancies or in patients with elevated white blood cell counts, such as high-grade lymphomas or acute leukemias (Krishnan & Hammad, 2006; Secola, 2006). Although more rare, patients with various types of solid tumors can experience TLS, but these are associated to a greater degree with large bulky tumors that are chemotherapy sensitive (see Figure 14-6). Other risk factors include an elevated serum uric acid level, an elevated lactate dehydrogenase (LDH) level, preexisting renal dysfunction, and volume depletion (Lydon, 2005).

Several therapies may enhance metabolic abnormalities that contribute to the development of TLS (see Figure 14-7). Potassium and phosphorus oral supplements and enteral and parenteral nutrition can alter the normal electrolyte balance. Potassium-

---

Common or High-Risk Cancers
- Acute leukemias
- Hodgkin disease
- High-grade non-Hodgkin lymphoma (NHL)

Less Common Cancers
- Chronic leukemias
- Other NHL

Rare Cancers
- Solid tumors
  - Breast
  - Ovarian
  - Lung
- Soft tissue sarcomas
- Thymoma
- Metastatic melanoma
- Seminoma
- Neuroblastoma

Figure 14-6. Malignancies Associated With Tumor Lysis Syndrome

Note. Based on information from Del Toro et al., 2005; Gobel, 2006; Krishnan & Hammad, 2006; Secola, 2006.

- Potassium, phosphorus oral supplements
- Enteral/parenteral nutrition
- Potassium-sparing diuretics
- Concurrent nephrotoxic medications
- Angiotensin-converting enzyme inhibitors
- Clindamycin

Figure 14-7. Therapies Enhancing Tumor Lysis Syndrome

Note. Based on information from Gobel, 2005b, 2006.

sparing diuretics have the potential for elevating serum potassium and enhancing dehydration. Concurrent nephrotoxic drugs, such as aminoglycosides, amphotericin B, and nonsteroidal anti-inflammatory drugs (NSAIDs), and angiotensin-converting enzyme inhibitors also can elevate serum potassium. Clindamycin contains potassium and phosphate and should be avoided (Gobel, 2005b, 2006).

Certain chemotherapy agents and radiation therapy have been associated with TLS. However, these clinical presentations have only been described as case reports. Patients with non-small cell lung cancer have been diagnosed with TLS when treated with docetaxel (Ajzensztejn, Hegde, & Lee, 2006), with irinotecan and cisplatin (Persons, Garst, Vollmer, & Crawford, 1998), and with zoledronic acid (Kurt et al., 2005). TLS was documented in one patient with small cell lung cancer after receiving topotecan (Beriwal, Singh, & Garcia-Young, 2002) and in two patients with metastatic melanoma after receiving IV hydrocortisone (Beriwal et al.; Habib & Saliba, 2002). In patients with multiple myeloma, TLS has been associated with thalidomide (Cany, Fitoussi, Boiron, & Marit, 2002; Fuente et al., 2004) and bortezomib (Jaskiewicz, Herrington, & Wong, 2005). Patients receiving total body irradiation (Linck et al., 2003; Yamazaki et al., 2004) and palliative radiation (Fleming, Henslee-Downey, & Coffey, 1991) have experienced TLS.

Pathophysiology

TLS is characterized by electrolyte and metabolic disturbances as a result of cellular changes. Following chemotherapy administration, predominantly malignant cells undergo rapid cell lysis/death. Cell lysis releases intracellular components into the vascular circulation. These include potassium, phosphorus, and nucleic acid, all of which are believed to be in higher concentrations in cancerous cells compared to normal cells. Without prompt removal from the circulatory system, a variety of untoward effects can develop, such as fatal cardiac arrythmias. Nucleic acids, also released into the circulation, are further broken down into uric acid in the kidneys. Decreased renal function can cause an inability to adequately excrete uric acid, resulting in hyperuricemia, precipitation of urate crystals, and acute renal failure (Cervantes & Chirivella, 2004; Kaplow, 2002; Krishnan & Hammad, 2006).

Diagnosis and Assessment

The diagnosis of TLS is based on clinical symptoms and laboratory findings. The exact timing of the onset of TLS has not been defined but can range from hours to 14 days after chemotherapy administration. A complete metabolic profile can identify the key laboratory values associated with TLS, which include potassium, phosphorus, calcium, and creatinine. The other key laboratory study that should be performed is uric acid. Typically, hyperkalemia is the initial sign of TLS.

Cairo and Bishop (2004) developed a definition of laboratory values and clinical TLS symptoms that aids in rapid assessment (see Figure 14-8). These definitions have been incorporated into the Cairo-Bishop risk grading classification, which assists in determining the need for aggressive prevention and treatment of TLS (see Table 14-5) (Cairo & Bishop). The first part of the grading classification is based on laboratory values. If two or more of these values are abnormal three days before or seven days after chemotherapy administration, more caution and earlier intervention and treatment may be necessary. The second part of the grading classification is based on clinical status. Clinical TLS is defined as laboratory TLS plus one or more of the clinical TLS categories.

Laboratory Tumor Lysis Syndrome
- Potassium: > 6 mEq/L or 25% increase from baseline
- Phosphorus: > 6.5 mg/dl or 25% increase from baseline
- Calcium: < 7 mg/dl or 25% decrease from baseline
- Uric acid: 8 mg/dl or 25% increase from baseline
- Creatinine: 1.5 times the upper limit of normal

Clinical Tumor Lysis Syndrome
- Cardiac arrhythmias or sudden death
- Seizures

Figure 14-8. Cairo-Bishop Definition of Laboratory and Clinical Tumor Lysis Syndrome

---

Note. Based on information from Cairo & Bishop, 2004.

The history and physical examination should include a thorough assessment for all presenting symptoms suggestive of TLS, which may include neurologic changes, GI complaints, urinary symptoms, and neuromuscular alterations (Lydon, 2005). The most significant physical examination abnormality may involve the neurologic/neuromuscular assessment. TLS can result in lethargy and generalized weakness associated with metabolic toxicities and hyperuricemia in addition to muscle weakness, muscle spasms, paresthesias, and positive Trousseau and Chvostek signs related to hypocalcemia and hyperkalemia that can progress to paralysis (Lydon). Other neurologic changes may consist of restlessness, irritability, confusion, lethargy, weakness, and possible seizures. GI complaints may include diarrhea, nausea, vomiting, anorexia, and abdominal cramping and pain associated with hyperuricemia and hyperkalemia. Reported symptoms associated with urinary effects may include flank pain, hematuria, oliguria, and anuria related to acute renal failure. Complete vital signs should be obtained, especially noting blood pressure and pulse changes. Hyperkalemia associated with TLS may result in hypotension and bradycardia; however, decreased renal function and fluid retention may result in hypertension. In performing the physical examination, lung assessment may reveal rales or rhonchi when auscultating breath sounds secondary to acute renal failure and fluid overload. The cardiac examination may reveal bradycardia in early TLS and later tachycardia, arrhythmias, and EKG changes. Hyperactive bowel sounds may be noted on abdominal examination with generalized abdominal tenderness upon palpation secondary to hyperkalemia.

Table 14-5. Cairo-Bishop Grading Classification of Tumor Lysis Syndrome

	Grade 0*	Grade I	Grade II	Grade III	Grade IV	Grade V
LTLS	–	+	+	+	+	+
Creatinine[†,‡]	≤ 1.5 × ULN	1.5 × ULN	> 1.5–3.0 × ULN	> 3.0–6.0 × ULN	> 6.0 ULN	Death[§]
Cardiac arrhythmia[‡]	None	Intervention not indicated	Non-urgent medical intervention indicated	Symptomatic and incompletely controlled medically or controlled with device (e.g. defibrillator)	Life-threatening (e.g. arrhythmia associated with CHF, hypotension, syncope, shock)	Death[§]
Seizure[‡]	None	–	One brief generalized seizure; seizure(s) well controlled by anti-convulsants or infrequent focal motor seizures not interfering with ADL	Seizure in which consciousness is altered; poorly controlled seizure disorder; with breakthrough generalized seizures despite medical intervention	Seizure of any kind which are prolonged, repetitive or difficult to control (e.g. status epilepticus, intractable epilepsy)	Death[§]

Clinical tumour lysis syndrome (CTLS) requires one or more clinical manifestations along with criteria for laboratory tumour lysis syndrome (LTLS). Maximal CTLS manifestation (renal, cardiac, neuro) defines the grade.

* No laboratory tumour lysis syndrome (LTLS).
[†] Creatinine levels: patients will be considered to have elevated creatinine if their serum creatinine is 1.5 times greater than the institutional upper limit of normal (ULN) below age/gender defined ULN. If not specified by an institution, age/sex ULN creatinine may be defined as: > 1 < 12 years, both male and female, 61.6 µmol/l; ≥ 12 < 16 years, both male and female, 88 µmol/l; ≥ 16 years, female, 105.6 µmol/l; ≥ 16 years, male, 114.4 µmol/l.
[‡] Not directly or probably attributable to a therapeutic agent (e.g. rise in creatinine after amphotericin administration).
[§] Attributive probably or definitely to CTLS.

Note. From "Tumour Lysis Syndrome: New Therapeutic Strategies and Classification," by M.S. Cairo and M. Bishop, 2004, *British Journal of Haematology, 127*, p. 6. Copyright 2004 by Blackwell Publishing Ltd. Reprinted with permission.

Evidence-Based Treatment Strategies

The most important factors in TLS are prevention and thorough assessment for stage of disease, concomitant therapies, comorbidities, renal function, and a complete review of laboratory values prior to initiating any type of treatment. For those patients felt to be at high risk for TLS, prevention strategies traditionally have included oral allopurinol for 24–48 hours before chemotherapy, fluid loading with normal saline to maintain a urine output of greater than 2.5 L/day, and urinary alkalinization with sodium bicarbonate, administered with fluid hydration, to achieve a urine pH level in the range of 6.5–7.0 (Gobel, 2006). The use of sodium bicarbonate for urinary alkalinization is controversial. The recent guidelines of the American Society of Clinical Oncology (Coiffier, Altman, Pui, Younes, & Cairo, 2008) state that because of the potential complications associated with alkalinization, including metabolic alkalosis and calcium phosphate precipitation, the use of sodium bicarbonate for the prevention and management of TLS currently is not recommended.

Once TLS has been diagnosed, each laboratory and clinical abnormality must be addressed (see Table 14-6). Patients may need to be admitted to the intensive care unit for cardiac monitoring based upon laboratory value alterations and symptoms. Aggressive fluid hydration should be employed if cardiac status permits, in order to maintain a urine output of 100 ml/m^2 per hour or greater. Loop and osmotic diuretics also should be considered if patients are not hypovolemic (Halfdanarson, Hogan, & Moynihan, 2006). Hyperphosphatemia can be normalized by restricting phosphate intake and administering phosphate-binding, aluminum hydroxide antacids. Calcium gluconate can be administered for low calcium levels, although hypocalcemia usually is corrected following correction of phosphate levels. Calcium gluconate is usually reserved for those patients who are symptomatic related to their hypocalcemia, and it should be used with caution in patients with severe hyperphosphatemia (Halfdanarson et al.). Furthermore, aggressive treatment for hyperkalemia should be instituted, as severe hyperkalemia can lead to fatal cardiac arrythmias. Specific treatment includes the administration of calcium gluconate, sodium bicarbonate, sodium polystyrene sulfonate, insulin, and dextrose.

The two pharmacologic agents utilized in practice for hyperuricemia are allopurinol, either oral or IV, and rasburicase IV. Allopurinol is used specifically to prevent TLS and

---

Table 14-6. Standard Treatment for Tumor Lysis Syndrome

Metabolic Abnormality	Treatment
Renal insufficiency	IV fluids: Normal saline 3 L/m^2/day or enough to keep urine output > 100 ml/hour Diuresis with loop or osmotic diuretics Dialysis with renal failure
Hyperphosphatemia	Phosphate binders: Aluminum hydroxide 50–150 mg/kg/day Dialysis with renal failure
Hyperkalemia	Regular insulin 10 units IV Hypertonic glucose 50–100 ml IV Calcium gluconate or calcium chloride 100–200 mg IV Sodium bicarbonate 45 mEq IV Sodium polystyrene sulfonate (Kayexalate®, Sanofi-Aventis) 15–30 g every 6 hours po or rectal Dialysis with renal failure
Hypocalcemia	Calcium gluconate 50–200 mg IV
Hyperuricemia	IV fluids: Normal saline 3 L/m^2/day or enough to keep urine output > 100 ml/hour Rasburicase 0.05–2 mg/kg IV daily for 7 days Dialysis with renal failure

Note. Based on information from Gobel, 2002; Halfdanarson et al., 2006; Lydon, 2005.

should be initiated at least 24–48 hours prior to chemotherapy. Allopurinol acts to inhibit the conversion of the enzyme hypoxanthine, in the presence of xanthine oxidase, to xanthine to uric acid. By blocking the formation of uric acid and crystals, renal insufficiency and failure may be prevented. Allopurinol acts to reduce serum uric acid levels in two to three days. Side effects of allopurinol include rash, nausea, vomiting, hypersensitivity, and renal insufficiency and failure.

Rasburicase also may be used to lower serum uric acid levels and acts to oxidize uric acid to allantoin, a metabolite of uric acid that has a greater solubility than uric acid and therefore is easier to excrete. Rasburicase reduces serum uric acid levels within 24 hours and is used for both prevention and management of hyperuricemia. Side effects include hypersensitivity reaction, fever, nausea, vomiting, and headaches. Rasburicase is contraindicated in patients with glucose-6-phosphate dehydrogenase deficiency, as rasburicase can cause hemolytic anemia or methemoglobinemia in these patients (Holdsworth & Nguyen, 2003).

Implications for Advanced Nursing Practice

APNs can play a key role in the prevention and management of TLS. Through initial assessment and identification of risk factors, APNs can recognize patients who are in need of prophylactic treatment and vigilant monitoring once chemotherapy has been initiated. Prior to treatment, laboratory values and urine pH should be reviewed to assess pretreatment kidney function, calcium, uric acid, potassium, and lactate dehydrogenase levels to identify high-risk patients. Patients should be started on prophylactic hydration and diuresis, and medications such as allopurinol should be started at least 24–48 hours prior to therapy. After initiation of treatment, patient monitoring should include vital signs every 4 hours, electrolyte labs every 8 hours during the first 48–72 hours after chemotherapy administration, urinalysis to monitor urine pH every 6–8 hours, strict intake and output measurement, daily weight and EKG, and seizure precautions if hypocalcemia occurs. Dialysis should be considered if treatment strategies do not improve metabolic abnormalities and renal failure. Early initiation of dialysis can avoid irreversible renal failure. Patients with persistent hypocalcemia, hyperuricemia, hyperkalemia, hyperphosphatemia, volume overload, and uremia should be evaluated for dialysis (Krishnan & Hammad, 2006). Phosphate and uric acid clearance rates are greater with hemodialysis in comparison to peritoneal dialysis and therefore are the preferred treatment approach. Patient and caregiver education should include risk factors for the development of TLS, signs and symptoms, goals of treatment, and dietary restrictions, including potassium and phosphorus. Patients should receive written instructions about prophylactic strategies, including allopurinol medication administration and the importance of this medication in their treatment, the importance of good hydration, and when to notify the healthcare provider.

Hypercalcemia of Malignancy

Hypercalcemia can be induced by a variety of disorders, with the major causes being cancer and hyperparathyroidism. Hypercalcemia of malignancy may occur in patients with both solid tumors and hematologic malignancies and usually is associated with advanced disease. APNs should be knowledgeable of the risk factors, signs and symptoms, and treatment strategies for hypercalcemia in an effort to correct calcium levels, manage and treat symptoms, and provide quality-of-life care to patients.

Definition and Incidence

Hypercalcemia can be classified as mild, moderate, or severe, based on laboratory values. Mild hypercalcemia is defined as a serum calcium level of 12 mg/dl; moderate hypercalcemia is defined as a serum calcium level ranging from 12–14 mg/dl; and severe hypercalcemia is defined as a serum calcium level greater than 14 mg/dl. Hypercalcemia occurs in an estimated 10%–40% of all adults with cancer and to a lesser extent in children with cancer (estimated to occur in approximately 0.5%–1% of all pediatric cancers) (McDonnell Keenan & Wickham, 2005). Solid tumors, such as squamous cell cancers of the lung, breast tumors, and certain hematologic malignancies (e.g., multiple myeloma), are most frequently associated with hypercalcemia (see Table 14-7).

Table 14-7. Incidence of Hypercalcemia by Tumor Type

Tumor Type	Incidence of Hypercalcemia
Breast cancer with bone metastases	30%–40%
Multiple myeloma	20%–40%
Lung cancer with bone metastases	12.5%–35%
Unknown primary	7%
Lymphoma/leukemia	Up to 50%
Renal cancer	3%–17%
Gastrointestinal cancer	4%–10%
Head and neck cancer	2.9%–25%

Note. Based on information from Kaplan, 2006.

Presenting Signs and Symptoms

Patients with hypercalcemia present with a variety of symptoms that generally are nonspecific. Many symptoms may correlate to advanced disease and can be confounded by factors such as cancer treatment side effects, medications, and comorbidities. The most common symptoms are associated with calcium's action in the neuromuscular, GI, renal, and cardiovascular systems (McDonnell Keenan & Wickham, 2005). Patients may present with fatigue, weakness, anorexia, depression, vague abdominal pain, constipation, thirst, and polyuria. CNS impairment can be exhibited as delirium, disorientation, and hallucinations, which can progress to obtundation and stupor or coma as serum calcium levels increase. Cardiovascular changes associated with hypercalcemia are seen with EKG changes, including prolonged P-R interval, widened QRS complex, shortened Q-T interval, shortened or absent S-T segments, bundle branch block, and bradycardia. As calcium levels increase, widened T waves and ventricular arrhythmias may develop and progress to complete heart block, asystole, and cardiac arrest.

Risk Factors

In addition to the diagnosis of cancer, specifically squamous cell cancer of the lung, breast cancer, and multiple myeloma, several other factors place patients at increased risk for hypercalcemia. Cancer-induced hypercalcemia most often occurs as a result of increased bone breakdown or resorption, and destruction with the mobilization of calcium into the extracellular fluid and concurrent renal calcium clearance dysfunction. Patients with metastatic bone disease or renal insufficiency are at high risk for hypercalcemia (Kaplan, 2006). Immobility, often associated with metastatic bone disease, can increase calcium resorption from bone (Richerson, 2004). Dehydration, anorexia, nausea and vomiting, fever, and renal failure can reduce renal blood flow and reduce renal calcium excretion. Furthermore, certain medications, such as hormonal therapy and thiazide diuretics, may increase renal calcium reabsorption and precipitate or exacerbate hypercalcemia (Kaplan).

Pathophysiology

Calcium in the body is responsible for numerous metabolic, physiologic, and structural mechanisms. Calcium regulates cardiac, smooth, and skeletal muscle contractility, transmission of nerve impulses, cell permeability, maintenance of normal clotting mechanisms, and bone remodeling and structure. Serum calcium levels indicate both ionized and bound forms, with bound forms composing the majority (99%) of the body's calcium in the bones and teeth. Ionized calcium is the active form (1%) in the serum and is bound to albumin, bicarbonate, and phosphate. Regulation of calcium levels is maintained by the parathyroid hormone (PTH), 1,25-dihydroxyvitamin D, and calcitonin. Serum ionized calcium is regulated by PTH that is secreted by the parathyroid glands when serum ionized calcium is decreased. PTH acts on target cell receptors to increase renal tubular calcium reabsorption, enhance calcium resorption from mineralized bone and inhibit osteoblasts, and promote synthesis of 1,25-dihydroxyvitamin D that increases intestinal absorption of calcium and phosphorus, resulting in an increase in serum calcium levels (McDonnell Keenan & Wickham, 2005).

The primary causes of hypercalcemia of malignancy are humoral hypercalcemia of malignancy (HHM) or local osteolytic hypercalcemia (LOH). Patients with HHM may or may not have bone metastasis but can have tumors that secrete humoral factors consisting of hormones and cytokines that act systemically or locally to stimulate excessive calcium bone resorption and subsequent hypercalcemia (Warrell, 1992). The tumors most likely to be associated with HHM are squamous cell carcinomas of the head and neck, esophagus, cervix, or lung; renal carcinoma; ovarian carcinoma; endometrial carcinoma; and breast carcinoma (Stewart, 2005). One of the hormones that plays a key role in hypercalcemia in patients with solid tumors is parathyroid hormone-related protein (PTH-rP), which closely resembles PTH (Warrell, 2001). Similar to PTH, PTH-rP increases osteoclast bone resorption, reduces bone formation, and stimulates the renal tubules to increase calcium resorption with subsequent hypercalcemia and hypercalciuria resulting in impaired sodium and water resorption with polyuria and dehydration. The decreased fluid volume causes proximal tubular calcium and sodium resorption that further increases serum calcium concentrations. Increased calcium concentrations in the glomerular filtrate can result in nephrocalcinosis, or calcium precipitation in the renal tubules. PTH-rP secreted by tumors does not have normal negative feedback mechanisms; therefore, serum calcium levels increase without regulatory control. Other tumor-induced mediators of HHM, including interleukins 1 and 6, transforming growth factor (alpha and beta), epidermal growth factor, and tumor necrosis factor, stimulate osteoclastic bone resorption and can potentiate the effects of PTH-rP on osteoclast activity and calcium homeostasis (Mundy & Guise, 1997).

LOH is caused by increased bone resorption from direct bone destruction by primary or metastatic tumors that release calcium into the systemic circulation. LOH usually is seen in advanced disease with extensive osteolytic bone metastases (Morton & Ritch, 2002). Tumor cells produce local cytokines, osteoclast-regulating factors, and PTH-rP that induces local bone resorption, osteoclast migration to the tumor site, osteolysis, and hypercalcemia (McDonnell Keenan & Wickham, 2005).

Diagnosis and Assessment

Patients presenting with vague symptoms of weakness, fatigue, malaise, and nausea and vomiting who also have known bone metastasis should be considered to be at high risk for hypercalcemia. Complete laboratory studies should be performed, including complete blood count, complete metabolic panel, phosphorus, magnesium, and PTH-rP, if available. Laboratory results that have a direct impact on hypercalcemia and treatment are calcium and phosphorus, which have an inverse relationship; BUN and creatinine to assess renal function; magnesium, which can exacerbate neuromuscular effects of hypercalcemia with decreased levels; and albumin, which is directly related to calcium levels. Serum calcium levels reflect ionized calcium levels, except in the presence of hypoalbuminemia. Patients with cancer often have hypoalbuminemia, and therefore the total serum calcium should be corrected for the albumin level by calculating as follows: measured serum calcium + (0.8 × 4 − measured serum albumin concentration).

The patient assessment should include a thorough history and physical examination. Several areas of the patient's history may provide specific information that is directly related to hypercalcemia, such as the patient's symptoms, disease status and treatment, and medication record. Symptoms that have a rapid onset are more indicative of hypercalcemia of malignancy in comparison to a history of slower symptom onset that is associated with hyperparathyroidism or other diseases. Disease status is important to assess, as more advanced disease and the presence of metastatic bone disease are risk factors for hypercalcemia. Medication records should be reviewed to note the use of any medications known to enhance hypercalcemia, such as hormonal therapy, thiazide diuretics, calcium, or vitamin D (Kaplan, 2006).

The physical examination also may highlight specific abnormalities that are suggestive of hypercalcemia (see Table 14-8). Neurologic manifestations of hypercalcemia may be most prominent in patients presenting with lethargy and confusion that can progress to obtundation and coma as the calcium level continues to increase. Increased calcium levels cause slowing of gastric motility that may be exhibited on physical examination as abdominal distention, and hypoactive bowel sounds, which correlate with complaints of nausea, vomiting, constipation, and indigestion. Renal system dysfunction is characterized by a reduction in urine concentration and polyuria. As a result, patients can be dehydrated with dry mucous membranes, poor skin turgor, increased thirst, and

---

Table 14-8. Physical Examination Abnormalities Associated With Hypercalcemia

System	Abnormality
Neuromuscular	Decreased muscle strength and tone, decreased deep tendon reflexes
Neurologic	Fatigue, lethargy, confusion
Cardiovascular	Orthostatic hypertension, bradycardia, electrocardiogram changes such as prolonged P-R and QRS intervals, shortened Q-T and S-T intervals, sinus bradycardia, and arrythmias
Gastrointestinal	Abdominal tenderness and distention, hypoactive bowel sounds
Renal	Polyuria, polydipsia, nocturia, dehydration

Note. Based on information from Kaplan, 2006; McDonnell Keenan & Wickham, 2005.

orthostatic hypotension. Hypercalcemia also causes cardiovascular abnormalities that can include bradycardia, hypertension, and EKG changes, such as a prolonged P-R interval, a prolonged or widened QRS, a shortened Q-T interval, or widened T waves. Differential diagnosis can include TLS, hyperparathyroidism, adrenal insufficiency, hypophosphatemia, immobility, endocrine disorders, medication, dehydration, hyponatremia, and progressive disease.

Evidence-Based Treatment Strategies

Hypercalcemia usually occurs late in a patient's disease trajectory. Therefore, before any treatment is initiated, the patient and family or caregiver should receive information regarding the patient's overall prognosis and expected risks and benefits of treatment. Treatment for hypercalcemia may temporarily improve symptoms, although no ultimate effect on survival occurs (Stewart, 2005). For any possible prolonged normalization of the serum calcium levels, antitumor therapy should be initiated. The decision to consider no treatment is an option; however, proceeding with treatment also can improve quality of life.

Treatment for hypercalcemia initially focuses on fluid replacement and diuretics to improve renal calcium excretion followed by specific hypercalcemic treatment that inhibits bone resorption of calcium. The severity of hypercalcemia influences specific treatment strategies (see Table 14-9). Thiazide diuretics are not administered, as this class of diuretics increases renal tubular calcium absorption and may exacerbate hypercalcemia. Loop diuretics inhibit calcium resorption in the ascending loop of Henle and facilitate hypercalciuria. Agents that inhibit bone resorption include bisphosphonates, calcitonin, plicamycin, and gallium nitrate (see Table 14-10). Bisphosphonate therapy is the most frequently prescribed treatment because of its effectiveness in lowering serum calcium levels in comparison to calcitonin, plicamycin, and gallium nitrate. In

Table 14-9. Hypercalcemia Treatment According to Severity

Calcium Level	Treatment Strategies
Mild Serum calcium level < 12 mg/dl	Administer IV hydration followed by observation. Treat with antiemetic agents. Limit sedative medications.
Moderate Serum calcium level 12–13.5 mg/dl	Administer IV hydration: Normal saline (NS) 3,000–6,000 ml first 24 hours. After rehydration: Administer loop diuretics—furosemide 20–40 mg every 12 hours. Treat with antiemetic agents. Limit sedative medications. Implement bisphosphonate therapy (see Table 14-10).
Severe Serum calcium level > 14 mg/dl	Administer IV hydration: NS 3,000–6,000 ml first 24 hours. After rehydration: Administer loop diuretics—furosemide 20–40 mg every 12 hours. Treat with antiemetic agents. Limit sedative medications. Implement bisphosphonate therapy (see Table 14-10).

Note. Based on information from Hussein & Cullen, 2002; Kaplan, 2006.

Table 14-10. Pharmacologic Agents That Inhibit Bone Resorption

Agent	Dose	Mechanism of Action	Side Effects	Comments
Pamidronate	60–90 mg IV over 2 hours	Binds to hydroxy-apatite in calcified bone to block dissolution of minerals and prevent release of calcium from bone Reduces number of osteoclasts	Transient low-grade temperature elevations Local reactions at infusion site	Onset of action within 24 hours with maximum effect in 7–10 days
Zoledronic acid	4 mg IV over at least 15 minutes	Inhibits bone resorption and inhibits tumor-related osteoclast activity	Nausea, vomiting, fever, chills, bone pain, and/or arthralgias and myalgias, elevated creatinine	Onset of action within 24 hours, but can be up to 4–7 days
Calcitonin	4 IU/kg SC or IM every 12 hours with dose escalations after 1–2 days: 8 IU/kg every 12 hours to 8 IU/kg every 6 hours	Inhibits calcium and phosphorous resorption from bone Decreases renal calcium resorption	Mild nausea, transient cramping, abdominal pain, cutaneous flushing	Onset of action within 24–36 hours with brief effect
Plicamycin (no longer marketed in the United States)	25–30 ug/kg IV over 30 minutes	Inhibits osteoclast RNA synthesis	Nausea, vomiting, thrombocytopenia, nephrotoxicity, flulike syndrome, dermatologic reactions, and stomatitis	Onset of action within 12 hours with maximum response 48 hours after administration persisting for 3–7 days
Gallium nitrate	200 mg/m² per day IV over 24 hours for 5 days	Inhibits bone resorption and calcium release from bone	Nephrotoxicity	Given after adequate rehydration Onset of action within 24 hours lasting for 7–8 days

Note. Based on information from Novartis Pharmaceuticals Corporation, 2002a, 2002b; Wilkes & Barton-Burke, 2007.

addition, the action of calcitonin is limited, and plicamycin and gallium are no longer marketed in the United States (Wilkes & Barton-Burke, 2007).

Other antihypercalcemic therapies include corticosteroids and dialysis. Corticosteroids act to inhibit vitamin D metabolism, inhibit calcitriol-induced GI calcium absorption, and increase urinary calcium excretion. Steroid therapy is used most frequently with hematologic malignancies, although no evidence exists to support their effectiveness (Morton & Lipton, 2004). The antihypercalcemic effect of corticosteroids may not be seen for days to weeks (Kaplan, 2006), and long-term use may cause side effects such as immunosuppression, hyperglycemia, GI bleeding, and bone demineralization.

Dialysis is indicated for patients who require rapid lowering of the serum calcium level to prevent life-threatening side effects and have tumors that are chemosensitive. The effect of dialysis on lowering serum calcium is brief but can remove 200–2,000 mg of calcium in a 24–48-hour period (Kaplan, 2006).

Implications for Advanced Nursing Practice

APNs can play a key role in the management of hypercalcemia (see Figure 14-9). Prevention strategies are of utmost importance and include the identification of patients who are at risk for hypercalcemia, promotion of adequate hydration at all times, especially during chemotherapy, and education of patients and family members regarding signs and symptoms that should be reported to the healthcare provider. Patient instructions should reinforce the importance of maintaining oral fluid intake of 3 L per day, the importance of performing weight-bearing activities and, at minimum, the importance of standing at least four to six times per day. Patients who are bedridden should perform passive range-of-motion activities at least twice a day. Patients also should receive instruction about the importance of using assistive devices, such as canes, walkers, or handrails, to prevent falls and injuries. If a patient has any signs or symptoms of neurologic changes, even minor, living arrangements should be evaluated for the need of additional support. With each encounter, patients should be assessed for any signs and symptoms of hypercalcemia, and patients should have laboratory studies performed at least every two

---

Prevention strategies
- Adequate hydration
- Identification of high-risk patients
- Patient safety to prevent injury and potential fractures

Patient and family/caregiver education
- Symptoms to report to healthcare provider
  - Fatigue
  - Lethargy
  - Weakness
  - Confusion
  - Constipation
  - Nausea and vomiting

Symptom management
- Confusion
- Constipation
- Nausea and vomiting

Hypocalcemic agents
- Pamidronate 60–90 mg IV over 2 hours
- Zoledronic acid 4 mg IV over no less than 15 minutes
- Calcitonin 4 IU/kg SC or IM every 12 hours
- Plicamycin 25–30 ug/kg IV over 30 minutes
- Gallium nitrate 200 mg/m² per day IV over 24 hours for 5 days

Figure 14-9. Hypercalcemia Management and the Advanced Practice Nurse Role

to three weeks. Prompt diagnosis and treatment is critical to alleviate symptoms and enhance the patients' quality of life. Once the diagnosis has been made, APNs should begin fluid hydration, diuretics, and bisphosphonate agents as previously discussed. Patients and family members will require psychological and social support, as the patient may require other needs such as hospice and palliative care (Kaplan, 2006).

Syndrome of Inappropriate Secretion of Antidiuretic Hormone

SIADH is a fluid and electrolyte imbalance that is one of the most common underlying causes of hyponatremia in adults with cancer. Early recognition of this syndrome is critical because if untreated, patients may experience life-threatening seizures, coma, and death. APNs should be able to identify patients who are at risk for SIADH in order to initiate prompt therapy and prevent an oncologic emergency.

Definition and Incidence

SIADH is defined as an endocrine paraneoplastic syndrome that causes an increased production and secretion of antidiuretic hormone (ADH), also known as vasopressin, and results in increased reabsorption of water in the renal tubules, fluid overload, water intoxication, dilutional hyponatremia, and inappropriately concentrated urine (Mazzone & Arroliga, 2003). An endocrine paraneoplastic syndrome is the abnormal ectopic production of hormones by malignant tumors. Although hyponatremia frequently is seen in the oncology setting, the incidence of SIADH is approximately 10% in patients with small cell lung cancer (Keenan, 2005) and 1%–2% in adults with cancer (Langfeldt & Cooley, 2003).

Presenting Signs and Symptoms

The presenting signs and symptoms of SIADH are directly related to the onset and degree of hyponatremia and subsequent water intoxication of intracellular fluids. The greatest effect is on the neurologic system because of swelling of brain cells. When SIADH has a rapid onset or if the serum sodium level is less than 110 mEq/L, acute neurologic symptoms related to cerebral edema, such as delirium, hypoactive reflexes, ataxia, gait disturbances, seizures, coma, and death can occur (Flombaum, 2000; Keenan, 2005). With slower onset or if the serum sodium level is 125–134 mEq/L, patients may be asymptomatic (Flounders, 2003). Other abnormalities are exhibited with the cardiovascular, GI, renal, and musculoskeletal systems (see Table 14-11).

Risk Factors

Several factors are associated with an increased risk of SIADH, including malignancy, comorbidities, and medications (see Figure 14-10). The most common malignancy, accounting for approximately 80% of all cases of SIADH, is small cell lung cancer (Mazzone & Arroliga, 2003). Other malignancies include non-small cell lung, head and neck, pancreatic, prostate, or colon cancer, lymphomas, thymoma, and primary brain tumors. Drug-induced SIADH is relatively common and can be caused by medications such as chemotherapy, narcotics, sedatives, antidepressants, general anesthetics, thiazide diuretics, and hypoglycemic agents.

Table 14-11. Signs and Symptoms of Syndrome of Inappropriate Secretion of Antidiuretic Hormone

	Mild	Moderate	Severe
	Sodium 125–134 mEq/L	Sodium 115–124 mEq/L	Sodium < 115 mEq/L
General	May be nonspecific or none; weakness, fatigue, malaise	–	–
Neurologic	Headache	Confusion Disorientation Personality changes Hypoactive reflexes Altered mental status	Coma Ataxia Tremors Seizures Delirium Psychosis Papilledema Focal neurologic signs
Cardiovascular	–	–	No edema Normal skin turgor Usually normal pulse Usually normal blood pressure
Gastrointestinal	Thirst Nausea Diarrhea Anorexia Vomiting Abdominal cramping Moist mucous membranes	–	–
Renal	–	Oliguria (< 400 ml/24 hours) Weight gain Incontinence	–
Musculoskeletal	Muscle cramps	Myoclonus	–

Note. Based on information from Ezzone, 2006c; Flounders, 2003.

Pathophysiology

Normally, ADH that is released from the posterior pituitary gland and is secreted in response to increased serum osmolality and decreased plasma volume regulates sodium and water in the body. Fluid and electrolytes maintain a homeostasis between the intracellular and extracellular compartments. When the extracellular fluid has a high osmolality, or concentration of solutes in the solution, water moves freely out of the intracellular compartment. In the case of low osmolality, as seen with hyponatremia, water moves from the intracellular into the extracellular compartments. Arginine vasopressin, the biologic active form of ADH, is released in response to an increased serum

Diagnosis		Medications		Other
Malignancy	**Nonmalignancy**	**Chemotherapy**	**Other**	History of smoking
Bladder carcinoma	Acute intermittent	Cisplatin	Angiotensin	Idiopathic syn-
Carcinoid tumor	porphyria	Cyclophosph-	converting en-	drome of inap-
Central nervous	AIDS	amide	zyme inhibitors	propriate antidi-
system tumors	Central nervous	Ifosfamide	Acetaminophen	uretic hormone
• Primary	system disor-	Interferon—alpha	Barbiturates	secretion in the
• Metastatic	ders	or gamma	Chlorpropamide	elderly
• Ewing carci-	• Cerebral vas-	Melphalan (high	Dopaminergic	Current nicotine
noma	cular accident	dose)	drugs	use
Gastrointestinal	• Cerebral hem-	Vinca alkaloids	General anes-	Pain
cancer	orrhage		thetic	Positive pressure
• Colon	• Cerebral ab-		Isoproterenol	respirators
• Duodenum	scess		Morphine	Postoperative time
• Esophagus	• Encephalitis		Opioids	period
• Pancreas	Guillain-Barre		Oxytocin	Stress
Gynecologic can-	syndrome		Nonsteroidal anti-	Trauma
cer	Lupus erythema-		inflammatory	
• Ovary	tosus		drugs	
• Cervix	Pulmonary disor-		Somatostatin	
Head and neck	ders		Selective sero-	
cancer	• Infections		tonin reuptake	
Hematologic can-	• Status asth-		inhibitors	
cer	maticus		Thiazide diuretics	
• Acute myelog-	• Chronic		Tricyclic antide-	
enous leukemia	obstructive		pressants	
• Chronic lympho-	pulmonary			
cytic leukemia	disease			
• Lymphoma				
Lung cancer				
• Small cell				
• Non-small cell				
Mesothelioma				
Prostate cancer				
Thymoma				
Thymic neuroblas-				
toma				

Figure 14-10. Risk Factors Associated With Syndrome of Inappropriate Secretion of Antidiuretic Hormone

Note. Based on information from Akalin et al., 2001; Chan, 1997; Finley, 1998; Garrett & Simpson, 1998; Haapoja, 2000; Hirshberg & Ben-Yehuda, 1997; Keenan, 1999; Kirch et al., 1997; Langer-Nitsche et al., 2000; Miaskowski, 1997; Miller, 2001; Otto, 1997; Poe & Taylor, 1989; Robertson, 2001. From "Syndrome of Inappropriate Antidiuretic Hormone Secretion in Malignancy: Review and Implications for Nursing Management," by L.A. Langfeldt and M.E. Cooley, 2003, *Clinical Journal of Oncology Nursing, 7*, p. 427. Copyright 2003 by Oncology Nursing Society. Reprinted with permission.

osmolality. ADH acts on the V_2 receptors in the renal collecting ducts to increase water reabsorption and decrease urine output. When excess production of ADH occurs, increased water retention by the kidneys and increased body water causes expansion of the plasma volume or water intoxication (Flounders, 2003).

SIADH develops because of tumors that produce and secrete ADH or by abnormal secretion of ADH from the pituitary gland as a result of inflammation, neoplasm, vascular lesions, or drugs (Ezzone, 2006c; Flounders, 2003). The uncontrolled secretion of ADH causes increased water reabsorption, decreased urine output, hyposmolality, and hyponatremia. The normal feedback mechanism for thirst is stimulated by increased plasma concentration and decreased renal perfusion that activates the renin-angiotensin-aldosterone system, causing additional water intake. The majority of the water is in the intracellular fluid; therefore, edema is not present.

Prevention Strategies

Any patient with cancer who presents with any of the risk factors listed in Figure 14-10 should be considered to be at risk for SIADH and requires frequent evaluation for signs, symptoms, and laboratory abnormalities that may suggest the process of SIADH. Patients undergoing cancer treatment should have frequent evaluation of sodium, BUN, creatinine, uric acid, and phosphate levels (Ezzone, 2006c). Patients should report any nausea, vomiting, headaches, neurologic changes, decreased urine output, and weight gain of greater than five pounds in one day (Gobel, 2005b). Family members also must note any signs and symptoms of neurologic changes in the patient and report these immediately to the healthcare professional.

Diagnosis and Assessment

Key factors in the history and physical examination and in the laboratory studies can assist APNs in diagnosing SIADH. A thorough history should be completed that assesses onset of symptoms, disease status, comorbidities, and medications. Of significant concern are the neurologic symptoms that a patient may exhibit, because of the potential for cerebral edema. Depending on the level of hyponatremia, patients may present with confusion, lethargy, irritability, and hyporeflexia. Abdominal examination may reveal generalized tenderness and hyperactive bowel sounds. Diagnostic studies should include a complete metabolic panel, serum osmolality, urine osmolality, thyroid function tests, and computed tomography (CT) scan of the head to rule out other etiologies for neurologic changes, such as brain tumors, hemorrhage, and edema (Langfeldt & Cooley, 2003). With SIADH, serum osmolality will be decreased or < 275 mOsm/kg and urine osmolality will be increased or > 1,200 mOsm/kg water. Hyponatremia can have other etiologies in addition to SIADH. The differential diagnosis may include dehydration, fluid retention and overload, cardiac disease, drug-induced hypervolemia, Addison disease, adrenal insufficiency, hepatic and renal disorders, and thyroid disease (Ezzone, 2006c; Langfeldt & Cooley).

Evidence-Based Treatment Strategies

Treatment of SIADH is based upon the onset and severity of hyponatremia, underlying pathology, and presenting symptoms. Treatment initially is focused on correction of the underlying cause because this usually will result in significant improvement in hyponatremia (Ezzone, 2006c; Flounders, 2003; Gobel, 2005b; Keenan, 2005; Langfeldt & Cooley, 2003). For mild SIADH with sodium levels above 120 mEq/L, fluid intake should be restricted to 800–1,000 ml/day, and limited IV hydration with isotonic saline should be administered. For moderate SIADH with sodium levels between 110–120 mEq/L, fluid intake should be restricted, and IV hydration, electrolytes, and diuretics should be administered. If hyponatremia does not resolve with fluid restriction and IV hydration, demeclocycline, lithium, or urea can be administered for mild or moderate hyponatremia (Gobel, 2005b). Demeclocycline acts to interfere with the action of ADH on the renal tubules and promotes excretion of water. The usual dosage of demeclocycline is 600–1,200 mg/day orally (Rafailov & Sinert, 2007). Fluid restrictions are not required with the use of demeclocycline. Possible side effects include nausea, photosensitivity, and renal dysfunction. Demeclocycline should be used with caution in patients with hepatic or renal insufficiency. Lithium also interferes with the action of ADH on the renal tubules. The usual dosage of lithium is 900–1,200 mg/day orally (Rafailov & Sinert). Side effects may include nausea, vomiting, anorexia, weakness, and tremors. Urea acts by causing osmotic diuresis. The usual dosage of urea is 1–1.5 g/kg IV with the maximum dose of 120 g/day (Keenan, 2005). Side effects include nausea, vomiting, and anorexia (Gobel, 2005b).

For severe SIADH with sodium levels below 100 mEq/L, hypertonic (3%) saline solution should be administered to correct the sodium level by 0.5–1 mEq/L per hour with a target level of 125 mEq/L (Ezzone, 2006c). Rapid correction of hyponatremia is contraindicated and can result in brain damage and a permanent neurologic condition called central pontine myelinolysis or demyelination (Ezzone, 2006c). Patients presenting with severe SIADH should be cared for in an intensive care setting because of the need for close monitoring while correcting sodium levels.

Implications for Advanced Nursing Practice

The priority for APN practice is focused on prevention. APNs should evaluate those patients who may be at high risk for developing hyponatremia and SIADH and be able to recognize early clinical signs and symptoms. Immediate treatment is critical to prevent life-threatening side effects. Because SIADH may present with subtle changes that often are similar to other abnormalities, such as dehydration, chemotherapy side effects, and neurologic disorders, APNs need to focus on thorough assessment, history and physical examination, and close monitoring of laboratory studies that can indicate SIADH.

Patient and caregiver education also is a key component of the APN role. APNs should instruct patients to maintain adequate hydration throughout chemotherapy to prevent dehydration. They also need to instruct patients and caregivers about abnormalities to report to the healthcare provider, including weight gain, anorexia, nausea, vomiting, weakness, headaches, mental status changes, increased thirst, and decreased urine output.

APNs should initiate therapy as soon as SIADH has been diagnosed. Patients will require detailed information, both verbal and written, regarding fluid restriction. APNs can assist patients in understanding the need for fluid restrictions and in scheduling fluid intake throughout the day. Patients also should receive a list of fluids and foods that are high in sodium and protein, such as beef and chicken broth and processed meats. For patients on fluid restrictions, patient education should include information regarding frequent mouth rinses and utilization of sugar-free gum or candy for dry mucous membranes. For patients requiring drug therapy, written instructions should be given about drug administration. Patients taking demeclocycline should be instructed to take the medication two times per day, avoid taking medications with meals, avoid sun exposure and apply sunscreen and protective clothing, and monitor for nausea, vomiting, signs of infection, and urinary output alterations. Patients taking lithium should be monitored for nausea, vomiting, anorexia, and any changes in neurologic status, such as tremors or weakness. Urea administration requires monitoring patients for nausea, vomiting, and anorexia (Gobel, 2005b). For those patients who are symptomatic requiring IV hydration, APNs should monitor sodium levels at least every eight hours to ensure gradual sodium level normalization. Patient safety also is a major concern because of the mental status changes and the possibility for seizures. Institution of seizure precautions and close patient monitoring are necessary to prevent patient injury.

Anaphylaxis

Anaphylaxis is an adverse immunologic response to the exposure of an offending agent that can result in a life-threatening reaction. Anaphylactic reactions usually have a rapid onset with respiratory, cardiovascular, cutaneous, or GI manifestations. APNs should be cognizant of potential causative agents, clinical manifestations, and treatment protocols to prevent fatal allergic reactions that can occur in patients with cancer.

Definition and Incidence

Anaphylaxis and anaphylactoid reactions are allergic reactions from exposure to a causative agent. Anaphylaxis is an allergic IgE-mediated, immediate hypersensitivity reaction, whereas anaphylactoid reactions are not IgE-mediated (Joint Task Force on Practice Parameters, 2005). Both conditions are referred to as anaphylaxis because they have similar pathophysiologic processes and clinical manifestations (Tang, 2003).

The exact incidence of anaphylaxis is unknown because of variations in definition by practitioners, underdiagnosing, and underreporting of this clinical condition (Neugut, Ghatak, & Miller, 2001; Rusznak & Peebles, 2002). In the United States, approximately 1% of all emergency department visits involve anaphylaxis, with an estimated 500–1,000 fatal anaphylactic reactions per year (Neugut et al.).

Presenting Signs and Symptoms

Presenting signs and symptoms of anaphylaxis vary significantly among patients. The most common signs and symptoms are urticaria, angioedema, flushing, and pruritus. Anaphylactic manifestations can occur with the pulmonary, cardiovascular, GI, cutaneous, and neurologic systems (see Table 14-12).

Risk Factors

Several risk factors have been identified that can increase the likelihood of an anaphylactic reaction. These include a history of prior exposure to a particular agent, a history of prior anaphylactic episodes, gender, route of exposure, certain foods, certain medications and blood products, insect stings and bites, exposure to latex, and physical factors (Rusznak & Peebles, 2002; Tang, 2003).

The prior exposure history and prior anaphylactic episodes can increase the risk of anaphylaxis in an individual. The frequency and intensity of exposure and the time interval between exposures can affect anaphylactic risk. Interrupted exposure to an antigen and greater exposure to an antigen are associated with a higher risk of anaphylaxis. Individuals with a previous history of anaphylaxis to foods, antibiotics, insect bites, and radiocontrast media are at increased risk for future reactions. Short time intervals between exposure and high doses of antigen given by a rapid absorption route also are factors that can increase an individual's risk for an anaphylactic reaction. When an antigen is administered parenterally, anaphylactic reactions are more common and more severe than with oral administration.

Women in general have a higher rate of anaphylaxis than men and have a higher risk for anaphylactic reaction when exposed to aspirin, NSAIDs, latex, and neuromuscular blockers. Men have a higher risk of experiencing anaphylactic reactions to fire ants and insect stings because of occupational and recreational exposure (Tang, 2003).

Several foods are common causes of anaphylaxis, with food allergies affecting approximately 8% of children younger than three years of age and approximately 2% of adults (Sampson, 1999). Common foods that cause anaphylaxis are peanuts, tree nuts, fish, shellfish, milk, and eggs. Other foods include bananas, beets, buckwheat, chamomile tea, citrus fruits, kiwis, mustard, pinto beans, potatoes, and rice (Tang, 2003). Some food allergies, such as peanuts, tree nuts, and seafood, can be lifelong, although other food allergens can be resolved if the food is eliminated from the diet for one to two years (Sampson).

The most common medications that are related to anaphylactic reactions are aspirin, NSAIDs, and beta-lactam antibiotics, such as penicillins, cephalosporins, and sulfonamides (Tang, 2003). Other medications can include insulin, ciprofloxacin, nitrofurantoin, iron dextran, mannitol, opiates, streptokinase, thiopental, and vaccines (Tang). Certain chemotherapy agents also are more commonly associated with anaphylactic reactions. These include the taxanes, platinum compounds, methotrexate, asparaginases, rituximab, oxaliplatin, teniposide, etoposide, procarbazine, cytarabine, levamisole, topotecan, trimetrexate, melphalan, imatinib, mesylate, and pemetrexed (Camp-Sorrell, 2005). Blood products can include cryoprecipitate, immune globulin, plasma, and whole blood (Tang). Finally, radiographic contrast media, often used with diagnostic tests, can produce a wide variety of anaphylactic reactions.

Insect stings and bites are common causes of anaphylaxis and account for approximately 40–100 deaths per year (Neugut et al., 2001). Causative agents are fire ants and Hymenoptera insects, which include bees, wasps, hornets, yellow jackets, and sawflies (Rusznak & Peebles, 2002; Tang, 2003).

Latex has become a significant occupational allergen because of universal precautions and the increased use of gloves. Individuals who have a latex allergy also are at higher risk for the development of allergies to bananas, kiwis, pears, pineapples, grapes, and papayas (Tang, 2003).

Table 14-12. Signs and Symptoms of Anaphylaxis

System	Signs and Symptoms
Cutaneous	Flushing Urticaria Angioedema Lacrimation Diaphoresis Pruritus with or without rash
Pulmonary	Stridor Dyspnea Wheezing Rhinitis/rhinorrhea Nasal congestion Laryngeal edema Pulmonary arrest
Gastrointestinal	Diarrhea Abdominal pain Nausea and vomiting
Cardiovascular	Vertigo Syncope Hypotension Cardiac arrest Substernal pain Bradycardia/tachycardia
Neurologic	Seizures
Renal	Flank pain
Miscellaneous	Feelings of impending doom

Note. Based on information from Tang, 2003.

Physical factors additionally may precipitate an anaphylactic reaction. These include cold temperatures and exercise. More vigorous exertion, such as running, tennis, dancing, skiing, and bicycling, are more likely to produce anaphylaxis than less vigorous exercise, such as walking and horseback riding (Rusznak & Peebles, 2002).

Pathophysiology

Anaphylactic reactions result from activation and release of mediators from mast cells and basophils. Initially, the antigen-specific IgE (the agent causing the reaction) binds and sensitizes the mast cell to the antigen. In patients with cancer, examples of antigen-specific IgE are the chemotherapy agent, the chemotherapy agent's metabolite, or the vehicle that is used to dissolve the chemotherapy agent (Gobel, 2005b). With subsequent exposure to the antigen, degranulation of the mast cells and basophils releases histamine, tryptase, prostaglandins, and platelet-activating factor. These mediators target receptors that stimulate anaphylactic responses such as pruritus, vascular permeability, mucosal edema and mucus production, and smooth muscle constriction (Rusznak & Peebles, 2002).

Prevention Strategies

Once an antigen has been identified as causing an anaphylactic reaction, the best preventive strategy is avoidance of the antigen. If appropriate, skin testing also can be performed for diagnostic purposes. Patient education is the most important preventive strategy. Patients should receive education about the risks of future anaphylaxis and avoidance strategies. For patients receiving chemotherapy that is known to cause hypersensitivity reactions that could result in anaphylaxis, APNs should ensure administration of medications used for prophylaxis for anaphylaxis, which include corticosteroids, H_1 and H_2 blockers, and an antipyretic (Gobel, 2005b).

Diagnosis and Assessment

The diagnosis of anaphylaxis is primarily based upon clinical manifestations. Classic signs and symptoms that have an acute onset and support the diagnosis of anaphylaxis include cutaneous reactions, laryngeal edema, bronchospasm, and hypotension (Tang, 2003). Once the patient has received emergency treatment and is stabilized, a complete history and physical examination can be obtained. Any prior anaphylactic reactions should be documented in addition to any known allergies and list of foods, medications, activity, or exposure to any insects just prior to the anaphylactic event. The physical examination should assess vital signs and focus on the cutaneous, pulmonary, cardiovascular, GI, and neurologic systems (see Table 14-12). Differential diagnoses can include septic shock, vasovagal reaction, cardiogenic shock, hypovolemic shock, carcinoid syndrome, panic attack, hyperglycemia, hypoglycemia, foreign body aspiration, status asthmaticus, and pulmonary embolism.

Evidence-Based Treatment Strategies

The initial treatment for anaphylaxis is to stabilize the patient by maintaining the airway, providing oxygen administration at 8–10 L per minute unless contraindicated in patients with chronic obstructive pulmonary disease, placing the patient in a supine or Trendelenburg position, maintaining IV access and rapidly administering normal saline, and in the case of the patient with cancer, stopping the infusion of the offending agent or chemotherapy drug. Pharmacologic therapy may include the administration of epinephrine, antihistamines, bronchodilators, or corticosteroids, depending on the severity of the anaphylactic reaction (see Table 14-13) (Joint Task Force on Practice Parameters, 2005).

Implications for Advanced Nursing Practice

APNs can play a critical role in the prevention, assessment, diagnosis, and treatment of anaphylactic reactions. In the oncology setting, the potential for anaphylaxis is great with the introduction of new medications for patients with cancer. Furthermore, numerous chemotherapeutic agents and the solvents used for administration possess the potential for adverse reactions such as anaphylaxis.

APNs can identify those patients who are at high risk for anaphylaxis by performing a complete assessment that would include identification of any known allergies or prior history of allergic reactions. Although some antineoplastic agents possess greater potential for allergic reactions, all patients receiving chemotherapy or biotherapy agents should be considered to be at risk for an anaphylactic reaction. Patients who are at risk should be educated about the potential for allergic reactions

Table 14-13. Pharmacologic Treatment for Anaphylaxis		
Agent	**Dosage**	**Indication**
Epinephrine intramuscular or subcutaneous	0.3–0.5 ml in anterior or lateral thigh If no response, may repeat every 5–15 minutes	Angioedema Hypotension Laryngeal edema
Diphenhydramine	25–50 mg IV over 10–15 minutes	Mucosal edema Mucus production
Ranitidine	1 mg/kg over 10–15 minutes	Mucosal edema
Famotidine	20 mg IV	Mucus production
Albuterol	2.5–5 mg in 3 ml saline via nebulizer	Bronchospasm
Methylprednisolone Dexamethasone	125 mg IV 20 mg IV	Bronchospasm
Crystalloid solution for IV infusion (maintain blood pressure)	–	–
If inadequate response to epinephrine and saline:		
Dopamine	5–20 mcg/kg/minute	–
Norepinephrine	0.5–30 mcg/minute	–

Note. Based on information from Joint Task Force on Practice Parameters, 2005; Rusznak & Peebles, 2002; Tang, 2003.

both in the supervised treatment setting and also at home. Patients and caregivers should receive written instructions about the signs and symptoms to report to the healthcare provider.

Of paramount importance is the availability of proper equipment, including an emergency kit and medications to adequately treat patients who experience an anaphylactic reaction as a consequence of chemotherapy administration. Patient safety and stabilization once a reaction has occurred is critical, and APNs should be knowledgeable about the appropriate procedures for the treatment of anaphylaxis. Patient reassurance also must be provided to reduce anxiety and fear throughout the anaphylactic reaction.

Evaluation of Outcomes

High-quality patient care is a result of evidence-based interventions and evaluation of outcomes. APNs can play a critical role in evaluating nursing-sensitive patient outcomes because of their direct involvement in facilitating patient care. The following discussion will highlight outcomes evaluation for each of the metabolic oncologic emergencies.

Ultimately, the overall goal in the treatment of DIC is to prevent mortality and significantly reduce morbidity. Research is limited in investigating the most effective treatment for DIC because of the numerous underlying disorders and the variance in clinical presentations. Currently, some treatments remain controversial, as discussed previously; however, the standard of treatment remains directed at the individual clinical presentation and severity of the DIC process.

The overall goal of treatment for sepsis and septic shock is to eradicate the infectious organism and prevent organ failure. Results of clinical trials involving antibiotic therapy have now provided evidence to facilitate specific antibiotic guidelines for the treatment of sepsis (NCCN, 2008). Other treatment strategies are based on individual clinical presentation to provide supportive care throughout the illness trajectory.

The major priority in TLS is prevention; therefore, APNs' primary goal is to ensure that patients receive adequate oncologic therapy without complications. When TLS occurs, prompt treatment is imperative to correct metabolic abnormalities and ultimately prevent major irreversible complications, such as renal failure and cardiac arrest.

With hypercalcemia of malignancy, the major treatment goal is rapid reduction of serum calcium levels to resolve associated signs and symptoms. Outcomes evaluation should include assessment of symptom resolution and decreasing serum and urinary calcium levels. In addition to aggressive hydration and symptom management, bisphosphonate therapy has been found to be very effective in hypercalcemia prevention and treatment (Major et al., 2001; Ramaswamy & Shapiro, 2003).

The goal of treatment for SIADH is correction of hyponatremia and associated clinical manifestations. No randomized clinical trials exist to guide this therapy; however, the literature supports fluid restriction, IV hydration with hypertonic saline for severe hyponatremia, and pharmacologic agents consisting of demeclocycline, lithium, and urea.

The goal of treatment for anaphylaxis is to eradicate the allergic reaction and clinical manifestations and stabilize the patient. No randomized clinical trials exist; however, the literature supports the clinical practice of using pharmacologic agents, including epinephrine, antihistamines, vasopressors, crystalloid IV solution, bronchodilators, and antiarrhythmic medications.

Conclusion

In summary, this chapter has presented metabolic oncologic emergencies, including DIC, sepsis, TLS, SIADH, hypercalcemia of malignancy, and anaphylaxis. Metabolic oncologic emergencies can evolve rapidly. APNs have a unique role in providing direct continuous care for patients and family members as the patient experiences the cancer illness trajectory and treatment. With advanced knowledge and understanding of the metabolic emergencies that can occur in patients with cancer, APNs can facilitate prevention strategies for those patients who are thought to be at high risk for developing complications. APNs should employ treatment strategies immediately to prevent morbidity and mortality.

Case Study

L.M. is a 52-year-old female who was diagnosed in 2004 with stage IV small cell lung carcinoma with metastasis to the brain and bone. She originally received radiation therapy to the brain and received six cycles of cisplatinum and irinotecan. Follow-up CT scans, bone scan, and positron-emission tomography scan showed that L.M. was in complete remission. She did well until July 2006, when follow-up CT scan showed a right hilar mass. L.M. was enrolled in a clinical trial with vinflunine. L.M. had significant side effects with this drug and experienced constipation and overwhelming fatigue. After two cycles, L.M. described herself as "completely worn out."

Two weeks after the second cycle of vinflunine, L.M.'s husband took her to the emergency room. Her husband reported that she was incoherent and her sentences and conversation were inappropriate. He also noticed that she had twitching and tremors of her hands, but he did not witness any seizure-like activity. L.M. denied experiencing any headaches, nausea, vomiting, or paresthesias. Neurologic examination demonstrated that L.M. was disoriented to person, place, and time and was unable to answer simple questions.

A complete metabolic panel revealed a serum sodium level of 117 mEq/L and a calcium level of 11.4 mg/dl. L.M. was admitted to the intensive care unit after her stay in the emergency room.

1. Based on L.M.'s history and clinical presentation, what should be included in the list of differential diagnoses?
    • The list of differential diagnoses would include
        – Metabolic abnormalities
        – Cerebrovascular accident
        – Recurrent brain metastasis
        – Chemotherapy side effects
        – Anemia related to chemotherapy
        – Hypoxia secondary to disease progression.
2. What diagnostic tests should be performed?
    • Diagnostic tests should include both radiographic and laboratory studies. A magnetic resonance imaging study of the brain should be performed to rule out any neurologic abnormalities and possible recurrent metastasis. Laboratory tests should include a complete blood count to evaluate for anemia, and

a complete metabolic profile to evaluate for any metabolic abnormalities that may be contributing to her neurologic changes.

3. Based on this assessment data, what abnormality is most likely the cause of L.M.'s signs and symptoms?
   - L.M. presents with moderate hyponatremia with a sodium level of 117 mEq/L. Sodium levels in this range can cause symptoms of altered mental status, confusion, and myoclonus. L.M. also presents with hypercalcemia and a calcium level of 11.4 mg/dl. Hypercalcemia can cause confusion and constipation.

4. What therapies should the APN expect to be initiated for SIADH and hypercalcemia?
   - The treatment for SIADH should include fluid restriction, isotonic saline IV hydration, and diuretic therapy. If the hyponatremia does not resolve with these treatments, demeclocycline, lithium, or urea may be administered, or the saline can be changed to a hypertonic solution. The treatment for hypercalcemia should include IV hydration and bisphosphonate therapy.
   - At the time of discharge, L.M.'s sodium level was 130 mEq/L and her calcium level was 9.7 mg/dl. L.M. was discharged on demeclocycline and started on bisphosphonate therapy as an outpatient. Prior to discharge, L.M. had CT scans that showed an enlarging right hilar mass and recurrent bone metastasis. L.M.'s husband was very anxious about taking his wife home and providing her care.

5. What should the APN include in the discharge plan?
   - The APN should first address the concerns of L.M.'s husband since he is the primary caregiver and will be responsible for understanding and executing the discharge instructions. L.M.'s husband should be given education about SIADH and hypercalcemia with explanations regarding why these are frequently seen in patients with cancer. The instructions should include signs and symptoms and what to report to the healthcare provider. Discharge instructions should also include instructions to maintain a well-balanced diet and adequate fluid intake. Medication instructions should include dosage and frequency schedule for oral demeclocycline and the importance of continuing IV bisphosphonate therapy as an outpatient. The APN also should identify community resources for supportive care for L.M.'s husband, such as home health or hospice as needed.

Once discharged, L.M. continued to improve and saw her oncologist to discuss other treatment options. Her chemotherapy regimen was changed to etoposide and carboplatin. After two cycles, L.M.'s sodium level continued to improve to her current level of 132 mEq/L. A follow-up CT scan showed a decrease in the size of the hilar mass, showing a positive response to therapy. With the improvement in her disease and sodium level, her demeclocycline was discontinued. She continues on bisphosphonate therapy and has not had any further episodes of hypercalcemia.

Key Points

Disseminated Intravascular Coagulation

- Although a wide variety of clinical conditions are associated with DIC, the most common clinical condition is sepsis.

- DIC is characterized by diffuse clotting and profuse hemorrhaging.
- The classic laboratory findings in DIC are prolonged clotting times, increased levels of fibrin degradation product and D-dimers, low platelet count and fibrinogen levels, and low plasma levels of coagulation factors.
- DIC treatment strategies focus on treatment of the underlying disorder, administration of replacement therapies, and supportive care.

Sepsis

- Sepsis is a complex interaction between an infecting microorganism and the immune, inflammatory, and coagulation responses by an individual.
- Gram-positive bacteria and fungi are common causative agents for infection in neutropenic patients with fever.
- Sepsis treatment strategies involve respiratory support, fluid resuscitation, inotropic and vasopressor agents, DVT prophylaxis, insulin therapy, antibiotic and antifungal agents, activated protein C, blood transfusion support, and nutritional and electrolyte replacement.

Tumor Lysis Syndrome

- TLS is characterized by electrolyte and metabolic disturbances caused by cell lysis as a result of chemotherapy, radiation therapy, biotherapy, or surgery.
- The characteristic metabolic disturbances associated with TLS include hyperkalemia, hyperuricemia, hyperphosphatemia, and hypocalcemia.
- Prevention strategies for patients thought to be at high risk for TLS should include allopurinol, fluid loading, and urinary alkalinization.
- TLS treatment strategies are aimed at correction of the laboratory and metabolic abnormalities.

Hypercalcemia of Malignancy

- Hypercalcemia of malignancy occurs in patients with both solid tumors and hematologic malignancies and usually is associated with advanced disease.
- Patients with hypercalcemia can present with a wide variety of signs and symptoms.
- Hypercalcemia of malignancy standard treatment strategies include fluid replacement, diuretics, and bisphosphonate therapy.

Syndrome of Inappropriate Secretion of Antidiuretic Hormone

- SIADH is an endocrine paraneoplastic syndrome that causes increased ADH with fluid overload and dilutional hyponatremia.
- Signs and symptoms of SIADH are related to the onset and degree of hyponatremia.
- SIADH treatment strategies include correction of the underlying cause, oral fluid restriction, IV hydration, diuretics, and demeclocycline, lithium, or urea therapy.

Anaphylaxis

- Anaphylaxis is an adverse immunologic response to the exposure of an offending agent.

- Offending agents may include certain foods, insect bites, latex, physical exertion, and certain medications and blood products.
- Classic signs and symptoms of anaphylaxis include cutaneous reactions, laryngeal edema, bronchospasm, and hypotension.
- Anaphylactic treatment strategies include stabilization of the patient, supportive care, rapid administration of normal saline, and pharmacologic therapy with epinephrine, antihistamines, bronchodilators, or corticosteroids.

Recommended Resources for Oncology Advanced Practice Nurses

- Answers.com Web site that provides information regarding etiologies, treatment, and International Classification of Disease codes for DIC: www.answers.com/topic/disseminated-intravascular-coagulation
- UpToDate® professional-level topic review of DIC (must be a subscriber to access complete information): http://patients.uptodate.com/topic.asp?file=coagulat/9921
- Overview of sepsis regarding patient screening, risk factors, pathophysiology, and treatment with video educational materials and additional Web sites: www.sepsis.com
- International Sepsis Forum: www.sepsisforum.org
- Surviving Sepsis Campaign, a Web site for patients, healthcare professionals, and the general public regarding sepsis information: www.survivingsepsis.org
- Society of Critical Care Medicine resources for patients and family members regarding sepsis: www.myicucare.org
- Patient information regarding tumor lysis syndrome with additional Web site links: www.lymphomation.org/side-effect-tumor-lysis.htm
- UpToDate professional-level topic review of tumor lysis syndrome (must be a subscriber to access full information): http://patients.uptodate.com/topic.asp?file=chemagen/4930
- National Cancer Institute Web site with overview of hypercalcemia: www.cancer.gov/cancertopics/pdq/supportivecare/hypercalcemia/healthprofessional
- Novartis Oncology US patient Web site with information about hypercalcemia: www.us.novartisoncology.com/info/coping/hypercalcemia.jsp
- National Cancer Institute professional information the about hypercalcemia: http://cancerweb.ncl.ac.uk/cancernet/304462.html
- Answers.com patient Web site providing information about SIADH: www.answers.com/topic/syndrome-of-inappropriate-antidiuretic-hormone
- Patient information regarding anaphylactic reactions: http://adam.about.com/encyclopedia/000844.htm

References

Ajzensztejn, D., Hegde, V.S., & Lee, S.M. (2006). Tumor lysis syndrome after treatment with docetaxel for non-small-cell lung cancer. *Journal of Clinical Oncology, 24*, 2389–2391.

Akalin, E., Chandrakantan, A., Keane, J., & Hamburger, R.J. (2001). Normouricemia in the syndrome of inappropriate antidiuretic hormone secretion. *American Journal of Kidney Diseases, 37*, 1–3.

Altman, A. (2001). Acute tumor lysis syndrome. *Seminars in Oncology, 28*(2, Suppl. 5), 3–8.

Angus, D.C., Linde-Zwirble, W.T., Lidicker, J., Clermont, G., Carcillo, J., & Pinsky, M.R. (2001). Epidemiology of severe sepsis in the Unites States: Analysis of incidence, outcome, and associated costs of care. *Critical Care in Medicine, 29,* 1303–1310.

Annane, D., Bellissant, E., Bollaert, P.E., Briegel, J., Didler, K., & Kupfer, Y. (2004). Corticosteroids for severe sepsis and septic shock: A systematic review and meta-analysis. *BMJ, 329,* 480.

Bakhtiari, K., Meijers, J.C., de Jonge, E., & Levi, M. (2004). Prospective validation of the International Society of Thrombosis and Haemostasis scoring system for disseminated intravascular coagulation. *Critical Care Medicine, 32,* 2416–2421.

Becker, J.U., & Wira, C.R. (2008, March). *Disseminated intravascular coagulation.* Retrieved April 3, 2008, from http://www.emedicine.com/emerg/topic150.htm

Beriwal, S., Singh, S., & Garcia-Young, J.A. (2002). Tumor lysis syndrome in extensive-stage small-cell lung cancer. *American Journal of Clinical Oncology, 25,* 474–475.

Bernard, G.R., Vincent, J.L., Laterre, P.F., LaRosa, S.P., Dhainaut, J.F., Lopez-Rodriguez, A., et al. (2001). Efficacy and safety of recombinant human activated protein C for severe sepsis. *New England Journal of Medicine, 344,* 699–709.

Bick, R.L. (2003). Disseminated intravascular coagulation: Current concepts of etiology, pathophysiology, diagnosis, and treatment. *Hematology/Oncology Clinics of North America, 17,* 140–176.

Bochud, P., & Calandra, T. (2005). Pathogenesis of sepsis: New concepts and implications for future treatment. *BMJ, 326,* 262–264.

Bone, R.C., Balk, R.A., Cerra, F.B., Dellinger, R.P., Fein, A.M., Knaus, W.A., et al. (1992). Definitions for sepsis and organ failure and guidelines for the use of innovative therapies in sepsis. The ACCP/SCCM Consensus Conference Committee. American College of Chest Physicians/Society of Critical Care Medicine. *Chest, 101,* 1644–1655.

Cairo, M.S., & Bishop, M. (2004). Tumour lysis syndrome: New therapeutic strategies and classification. *British Journal of Haematology, 127,* 3–11.

Camp-Sorrell, D. (2005). Chemotherapy toxicities and management. In C.H. Yarbro, M.H. Frogge, & M. Goodman (Eds.), *Cancer nursing: Principles and practice* (6th ed., pp. 412–457). Sudbury, MA: Jones and Bartlett.

Cany, L., Fitoussi, O., Boiron, J.M., & Marit, G. (2002). Tumor lysis syndrome at the beginning of thalidomide therapy for multiple myeloma. *Journal of Clinical Oncology, 20,* 2212.

Cervantes, A., & Chirivella, I. (2004). Oncological emergencies. *Annals of Oncology, 15*(Suppl. 4), 299–306.

Chan, T.Y. (1997). Drug-induced syndrome of inappropriate antidiuretic hormone secretion: Causes, diagnosis and management. *Drugs and Aging, 11,* 27–44.

Coiffier, B., Altman, A., Pui, C.H., Younes, A., & Cairo, M.S. (2008). Guidelines for the management of pediatric and adult tumor lysis syndrome: An evidence-based review. *Journal of Clinical Oncology, 26,* 2767–2778.

Dale, D.C. (2002). Colony-stimulating factors for the management of neutropenia in cancer patients. *Drugs, 62*(Suppl. 1), 1–15.

Del Toro, G., Morris, E., & Cairo, M.S. (2005). Tumor lysis syndrome: Pathophysiology, definition, and alternative treatment approaches. *Clinical Advances in Hematology and Oncology, 3,* 54–61.

Dellinger, R.P., Carlet, J.M., Masur, H., Gerlach, H., Calandra, T., Cohen, J., et al. (2004). Surviving sepsis campaign guidelines for management of severe sepsis and septic shock. *Critical Care Medicine, 3,* 858–873.

Donawitz, G.R., Harman, C., & Pope, T. (1991). The role of the chest roentgenogram in febrile neutropenic patients. *Archives of Internal Medicine, 151,* 701–704.

Ezzone, S.A. (2006a). Disseminated intravascular coagulation. In D. Camp-Sorrell & R.A. Hawkins (Eds.), *Clinical manual for the oncology advanced practice nurse* (2nd ed., pp. 823–829). Pittsburgh, PA: Oncology Nursing Society.

Ezzone, S.A. (2006b). Disseminated intravascular coagulation. In M. Kaplan (Ed.), *Understanding and managing oncologic emergencies: A resource for nurses* (pp. 31–49). Pittsburgh, PA: Oncology Nursing Society.

Ezzone, S.A. (2006c). Syndrome of inappropriate antidiuretic hormone. In D. Camp-Sorrell & R. Hawkins (Eds.), *Clinical manual for the oncology advanced practice nurse* (2nd ed., pp. 685–690). Pittsburgh, PA: Oncology Nursing Society.

Feinstein, D.I. (1982). Diagnosis and management of disseminated intravascular coagulation: The role of heparin therapy. *Blood, 60,* 284–287.

Finley, J.P. (1998). Syndrome of inappropriate ADH (SIADH). In C.R. Ziegfeld, B.G. Lubejko, & B.S. Shelton (Eds.), *Manual of cancer nursing* (pp. 431–435). Philadelphia: Lippincott.

Fleming, D.R., Henslee-Downey, P.J., & Coffey, C.W. (1991). Radiation induced acute tumor lysis syndrome in the bone marrow transplant setting. *Bone Marrow Transplantation, 8,* 235–236.

Flombaum, C. (2000). Metabolic emergencies in the cancer patient. *Seminars in Oncology, 27,* 322–324.

Flounders, J.A. (2003). Syndrome of inappropriate antidiuretic hormone [Online exclusive]. *Oncology Nursing Forum, 30,* E63–E70.

Franchini, M., Lippi, G., & Manzato, F. (2006, February). Recent acquisitions in the pathophysiology, diagnosis and treatment of disseminated intravascular coagulation. *Thrombosis Journal, 4,* 4.

Freifeld, A.G., Kalil, A., & Rubenstein, E. (2004). Fever in the neutropenic cancer patient. In M. Abeloff, J.O. Armitage, J.E. Niederhuber, M.B. Kastan, & W.G. McKenna (Eds.), *Clinical oncology* (3rd ed., pp. 925–940). Philadelphia: Elsevier.

Friend, P.H., & Pruett, J. (2004). Bleeding and thrombotic complications. In C.H. Yarbro, M.H. Frogge, & M. Goodman (Eds.), *Cancer symptom management* (3rd ed., pp. 233–251). Sudbury, MA: Jones and Bartlett.

Fuente, N., Mane, J.M., Barcelo, R., Munoz, A., Perez-Hoyos, T., & Lopez-Vivanco, G. (2004). Tumor lysis syndrome in a multiple myeloma treated with thalidomide. *Annals of Oncology, 15,* 537.

Gafter-Gvili, A., Fraser, A., Paul, M., & Leibovici, L. (2005). Meta-analysis: Antibiotic prophylaxis reduces mortality in neutropenic patients. *Annals of Internal Medicine, 12,* 979–995.

Garrett, C.A., & Simpson, T.A., Jr. (1998). Syndrome of inappropriate antidiuretic hormone associated with vinorelbine therapy. *Annals of Pharmacotherapy, 32,* 1306–1309.

Gobel, B.H. (1999). Disseminated intravascular coagulation. *Seminars in Oncology Nursing, 15,* 174–182.

Gobel, B.H. (2002). Management of tumor lysis syndrome: Prevention and treatment. *Seminars in Oncology Nursing, 18*(Suppl. 3), 12–16.

Gobel, B.H. (2005a). Disseminated intravascular coagulation. In C.H. Yarbro, M.H. Frogge, & M. Goodman (Eds.), *Cancer nursing: Principles and practice* (6th ed., pp. 887–894). Sudbury, MA: Jones and Bartlett.

Gobel, B.H. (2005b). Metabolic emergencies. In J.K. Itano & K.N. Taoka (Eds.), *Core curriculum for oncology nursing* (4th ed., pp. 383–421). Philadelphia: Elsevier.

Gobel, B.H. (2006). Tumor lysis syndrome. In M. Kaplan (Ed.), *Understanding and managing oncologic emergencies: A resource for nurses* (pp. 285–306). Pittsburgh, PA: Oncology Nursing Society.

Gobel, B.H., & Peterson, G.J. (2006). Sepsis and septic shock. In M. Kaplan (Ed.), *Understanding and managing oncologic emergencies: A resource for nurses* (pp. 159–195). Pittsburgh, PA: Oncology Nursing Society.

Haapoja, I.S. (2000). Syndrome of inappropriate antidiuretic hormone. In C.H. Yarbro, M.H. Frogge, M. Goodman, & S.L. Groenwald (Eds.), *Cancer nursing: Principles and practice* (5th ed., pp. 913–919). Sudbury, MA: Jones and Bartlett.

Habib, G.S., & Saliba, W.R. (2002). Tumor lysis syndrome after hydrocortisone treatment in metastatic melanoma: A case report and review of the literature. *American Journal of the Medical Sciences, 323,* 155–157.

Halfdanarson, T.R., Hogan, W.J., & Moynihan, T.J. (2006). Oncologic emergencies: Diagnosis and treatment. *Mayo Clinic Proceedings, 11,* 835–848.

Hinds, C.J. (2001). Treatment of sepsis with activated protein C. *BMJ, 323,* 881–882.

Hirshberg, B., & Ben-Yehuda, A. (1997). The syndrome of inappropriate antidiuretic hormone secretion in the elderly. *American Journal of Medicine, 103,* 207–273.

Holdsworth, M.T., & Nguyen, P. (2003). Role of i.v. allopurinol and rasburicase in tumor lysis syndrome. *American Journal of Health-System Pharmacy, 60,* 2213–2222.

Hotchkiss, R.S., & Karl, I.W. (2003). The pathophysiology and treatment of sepsis. *New England Journal of Medicine, 348,* 138–150.

Hoyle, C.F., Swisky, D.M., Freedman, L., & Hayhoe, G.F. (1988). Beneficial effect of heparin in the management of patients with APL. *British Journal of Haematology, 68,* 187–191.

Hughes, W.T., Armstrong, D., Bodey, G.P., Bow, E.J., Brown, A.E., Calandra, T., et al. (2002). 2002 guidelines for the use of antimicrobial agents in neutropenic patients with cancer. *Clinical Infectious Diseases, 34,* 730–751.

Hussein, M., & Cullen, K. (2002). Metabolic emergencies. In P.G. Johnston & R.A. Spence (Eds.), *Oncologic emergencies* (pp. 51–73). New York: Oxford University Press.

Jaskiewicz, A.D., Herrington, J.D., & Wong, L. (2005). Tumor lysis syndrome after bortezomib therapy for plasma cell leukemia. *Pharmacotherapy, 25,* 1820–1825.

Joint Task Force on Practice Parameters. (2005). The diagnosis and management of anaphylaxis: An updated practice parameter. *Journal of Allergy and Clinical Immunology, 3*(Suppl. 2), S438–S524.

Kaplan, M. (2006). Hypercalcemia of malignancy. In M. Kaplan (Ed.), *Understanding and managing oncologic emergencies: A resource for nurses* (pp. 51–97). Pittsburgh, PA: Oncology Nursing Society.

Kaplow, R. (2002). Pathophysiology, signs, and symptoms of acute tumor lysis syndrome. *Seminars in Oncology Nursing, 18*(Suppl. 3), 6–11.

Keenan, A.M. (1999). Syndrome of inappropriate secretion of antidiuretic hormone in malignancy. *Seminars in Oncology Nursing, 15,* 160–167.

Keenan, A.M. (2005). Syndrome of inappropriate antidiuretic hormone. In C.H. Yarbro, M.H. Frogge, & M. Goodman (Eds.), *Cancer nursing: Principles and practice* (6th ed., pp. 940–945). Sudbury, MA: Jones and Bartlett.

Kirch, C., Gachot, B., Germann, N., Blot, F., & Nitenberg, G. (1997). Recurrent ifosfamide-induced hyponatraemia. *European Journal of Cancer, 33,* 2438–2439.

Krishnan, K., & Hammad, A. (2006, December). *Tumor lysis syndrome.* Retrieved December 28, 2006, from http://www.emedicine.com/med/topic2327.htm

Kurt, M., Onal, I.K., Elkiran, T., Altun, B., Altundag, K., & Gullu, I. (2005). Acute tumor lysis syndrome triggered by zoledronic acid in a patient with metastatic lung adenocarcinoma. *Medical Oncology, 22,* 203–206.

Langer-Nitsche, C., Luck, H.J., & Heilmann, M. (2000). Severe syndrome of inappropriate antidiuretic hormone secretion with docetaxel treatment in metastatic breast cancer. *Acta Oncologica, 39,* 1001.

Langfeldt, L.A., & Cooley, M.E. (2003). Syndrome of inappropriate appropriate hormone secretion in malignancy: Review and implications for nursing management. *Clinical Journal of Oncology Nursing, 4,* 425–430.

Levi, M. (2004). Current understanding of disseminated intravascular coagulation. *British Journal of Haematology, 124,* 567–576.

Levi, M., & ten Cate, H. (1999). Disseminated intravascular coagulation. *New England Journal of Medicine, 341,* 586–592.

Linck, D., Basara, N., Tran, V., Vucinic, V., Hermann, S., Hoelzer, D., et al. (2003). Peracute onset of severe tumor lysis syndrome immediately after 4 Gy fractionated TBI as part of reduced intensity preparative regimen in a patient with T-ALL with high tumor burden. *Bone Marrow Transplantation, 31,* 935–937.

Lydon, J. (2005). Tumor lysis syndrome. In C.H. Yarbro, M.H. Frogge, & M. Goodman (Eds.), *Cancer nursing: Principles and practice* (6th ed., pp. 947–958). Sudbury, MA: Jones and Bartlett.

Mackenzie, I., & Wilson, I. (2001). The management of sepsis. *Update in Anaesthesia, 13,* Article 8. Retrieved January 4, 2007, from http://www.nda.ox.ac.uk/wfsa/html/u13/u1308_01.htm

Major, P., Lortholary, J., Hon, E., Abdi, E., Mills, G., Menssen, H.D., et al. (2001). Zoledronic acid is superior to pamidronate in the treatment of hypercalcemia of malignancy: A pooled analysis of two randomized, controlled clinical trials. *Journal of Clinical Oncology, 19,* 558–567.

Martin, G.S., Mannino, D.M., Eaton, S., & Moss, M. (2003). The epidemiology of sepsis in the United States from 1979 through 2000. *New England Journal of Medicine, 348,* 1546–1554.

Maxson, J.H. (2000). Management of disseminated intravascular coagulation. *Critical Care Nursing Clinics of North America, 12,* 341–352.

Mazzone, P.J., & Arroliga, A.C. (2003). Endocrine paraneoplastic syndromes in lung cancer. *Current Opinion in Pulmonary Medicine, 9,* 313–320.

McDonnell Keenan, A.K., & Wickham, R.S. (2005). Hypercalcemia. In C.H. Yarbro, M.H. Frogge, & M. Goodman (Eds.), *Cancer nursing: Principles and practice* (6th ed., pp. 791–807). Sudbury, MA: Jones and Bartlett.

Messmore, H.L., & Wehrmacher, W.H. (2002, March). Disseminated intravascular coagulation: A primer for primary care physicians [Web exclusive]. *Postgraduate Medicine, 111*(3). Retrieved from http://www.postgradmed.com/issues/2002/03_02/messmore.shtml

Miaskowski, C. (1997). Oncologic emergencies. In *Oncology nursing: An essential guide for patient care* (pp. 225–243). Philadelphia: Saunders.

Miller, M. (2001). Syndrome of excess antidiuretic hormone release. *Critical Care Clinics, 17,* 11–23.

Moore, S. (2005). Septic shock. In C.H. Yarbro, M.H. Frogge, & M. Goodman (Eds.), *Cancer nursing: Principles and practice* (6th ed., pp. 895–909). Sudbury, MA: Jones and Bartlett.

Morton, A.R., & Lipton, A. (2004). Hypercalcemia. In M.D. Abeloff, J.O. Armitage, J.E. Niederhuber, M.B. Kasten, & W.G. McKenna (Eds.), *Clinical oncology* (3rd ed., pp. 957–972). Philadelphia: Elsevier Churchill Livingston.

Morton, A.R., & Ritch, P.S. (2002). Metabolic disorders: Hypercalcemia. In A.M. Berger, R.K. Portenoy, & D.E. Weissman (Eds.), *Principles and practice of palliative care and supportive oncology* (2nd ed., pp. 493–507). Philadelphia: Lippincott Williams & Wilkins.

Mundy, G.R., & Guise, T.A. (1997). Hypercalcemia of malignancy. *American Journal of Medicine, 103,* 134–145.

National Comprehensive Cancer Network. (2008). *NCCN clinical practice guidelines in oncology: Prevention and treatment of cancer-related infections, version 1.2008.* Retrieved April 1, 2008, from http://www.nccn.org/professionals/physician_gls/PDF/infections.pdf

Neugut, A.I., Ghatak, A.T., & Miller, R.L. (2001). Anaphylaxis in the United States: An investigation into its epidemiology. *Archives of Internal Medicine, 161,* 15–21.

Novartis Pharmaceuticals Corporation. (2002a). Aredia [Package insert]. East Hanover, NJ: Author.

Novartis Pharmaceuticals Corporation. (2002b). Zometa [Package insert]. East Hanover, NJ: Author.

Ornstein, D.L., & Zacharski, L.R. (2000). Cancer, thrombosis, and anticoagulants. *Current Opinion in Pulmonary Medicine, 4*, 301–308.

Otto, S. (1997). Syndrome of inappropriate antidiuretic hormone secretion. In *Oncology nursing* (3rd ed., pp. 463–474). St. Louis, MO: Mosby.

Persons, D.A., Garst, J., Vollmer, R., & Crawford, J. (1998). Tumor lysis syndrome and acute renal failure after treatment of non-small-cell lung carcinoma with combination irinotecan and cisplatin. *American Journal of Clinical Oncology, 21*, 426–429.

Poe, C.M., & Taylor, L.M. (1989). Syndrome of inappropriate antidiuretic hormone: Assessment and nursing implications. *Oncology Nursing Forum, 16*, 373–381.

Rafailov, A., & Sinert, R. (2007, May). *Syndrome of inappropriate antidiuretic hormone secretion.* Retrieved April 5, 2008, from http://www.emedicine.com/emerg/fulltopic/topic784.htm

Ramaswamy, B., & Shapiro, C.L. (2003). Bisphosphonates in the prevention and treatment of bone metastases. *Oncology, 17*, 1261–1270.

Richerson, M.T. (2004). Electrolyte imbalances: Hypercalcemia. In C.H. Yarbro, M.H. Frogge, & M. Goodman (Eds.), *Cancer symptom management* (3rd ed., pp. 440–453). Sudbury, MA: Jones and Bartlett.

Rivers, E., Nguyen, B., Havstad, S., Ressler, J., Muzzin, A., Knoblich, B., et al. (2001). Early goal-directed therapy in the treatment of severe sepsis and septic shock. *New England Journal of Medicine, 19*, 1368–1377.

Robertson, G.L. (2001). Antidiuretic hormone: Normal and disordered function. *Endocrinology and Metabolism Clinics of North America, 30*, 671–695.

Russell, J.A. (2006). Management of sepsis. *New England Journal of Medicine, 355*, 1699–1713.

Rusznak, C., & Peebles, S. (2002). Anaphylaxis and anaphylactoid reactions. A guide to prevention, recognition, and emergent treatment. *Postgraduate Medicine, 5*, 101–114.

Safdar, A., & Armstrong, D. (2001). Infectious morbidity in critically ill patients with cancer. *Critical Care Clinics, 17*, 531–570.

Sampson, H.A. (1999). Food allergy. Part 1: Immunopathogenesis and clinical disorders. *Journal of Allergy and Clinical Immunology, 103*, 717–728.

Secola, R. (2006). Tumor lysis syndrome: Nursing management and new therapeutic options. *Advanced Studies in Nursing, 3*, 41–48.

Sessler, C.N., Perry, J.C., & Varney, K.L. (2004). Management of severe sepsis and septic shock. *Current Opinion in Critical Care, 10*, 354–363.

Shelton, B.K. (2003). Evidence-based care for the neutropenic patient with leukemia. *Seminars in Oncology Nursing, 19*, 133–141.

Stewart, A.F. (2005). Clinical practice: Hypercalcemia associated with cancer. *New England Journal of Medicine, 352*, 373–379.

Stoll, E.H. (2001). Sepsis and septic shock. *Clinical Journal of Oncology Nursing, 5*, 71–72.

Tang, A.W. (2003). A practical guide to anaphylaxis. *American Family Physician, 68*, 1325–1332, 1339–1340.

Taylor, F.B., Jr., Toh, C.H., Hoots, W.K., Wada, H., & Levi, M. (2001). Towards definition, clinical and laboratory criteria, and a scoring system for disseminated intravascular coagulation. *Thrombosis and Haemostasis, 86*, 1327–1330.

Tazbir, J. (2004). Sepsis and the role of activated protein C. *Critical Care Nurse, 24*, 40–45.

Toh, C.H., & Dennis, M. (2003). Disseminated intravascular coagulation: Old disease, new hope. *BMJ, 327*, 974–977.

Truini-Pittman, L., & Rossetto, C. (2002). Pediatric considerations in tumor lysis syndrome. *Seminars in Oncology Nursing, 18*(3, Suppl. 3), 17–22.

Wade, J.C., & Rubenstein, E.B. (2001). NCCN: Fever and neutropenia. *Cancer Control, 8*(6, Suppl. 2), 16–21.

Warrell, R.P. (1992). Etiology and current management of cancer-related hypercalcemia. *Oncology, 6*, 37–43.

Warrell, R.P. (2001). Metabolic emergencies. In V.T. DeVita, Jr., S. Hellman, & S.A. Rosenberg (Eds.), *Cancer: Principles and practice of oncology* (6th ed., pp. 2633–2644). Philadelphia: Lippincott Williams & Wilkins.

Wilkes, G., & Barton-Burke, M. (2007). *2007 oncology nursing drug handbook.* Sudbury, MA: Jones and Bartlett.

Yamazaki, H., Hanada, M., Horiki, M., Kuyama, J., Sato, T., Nishikubo, M., et al. (2004). Acute tumor lysis syndrome caused by palliative radiotherapy in patients with diffuse large B-cell lymphoma. *Radiation Medicine, 22*, 52–55.

Yu, M., Nardella, A., & Pechet, L. (2000). Screening tests of disseminated intravascular coagulation: Guidelines for rapid and specific laboratory diagnosis. *Critical Care Medicine, 6*, 1777–1780.

CHAPTER 15

Structural Oncologic Emergencies

Heather L. Brumbaugh, RN, MSN, ANP, AOCN®

Introduction

Oncologic emergencies are complications that can occur in patients with cancer at initial diagnosis as the presenting symptom or at any time throughout the cancer journey. Oncologic emergencies can have a significant impact on quality of life; therefore, it is important that they are recognized and treated expeditiously to prevent long-term consequences. This chapter will cover the structural emergencies of superior vena cava syndrome (SVCS), cardiac tamponade, spinal cord compression (SCC), and increased intracranial pressure (ICP).

Superior Vena Cava Syndrome

The superior vena cava (SVC) is the major vein that carries blood from the head, neck, upper chest, and arms to the heart. SVCS is a collection of symptoms caused by partial blockage or compression of the SVC. This mechanical obstruction causes compromise of venous drainage from the head, neck, upper extremities, and upper thorax. The obstruction results because of intrinsic or extrinsic factors to the SVC. Intrinsic compression is the result of thrombosis or intraluminal tumor in the SVC. Extrinsic obstruction more commonly results from tumor and/or enlarged lymph nodes. The obstruction causes impairment of the venous return to the heart from the head, neck, thorax, and upper extremities and results in increases in venous pressure with decreased cardiac output. SVCS can become an emergency when it becomes severe and results in decreased cardiac filling, cerebral edema, and respiratory distress (Aurora, Milite, & Vander Els, 2000). Advanced practice nurses (APNs) need to be alert to patients who are potentially at risk for SVCS, as well as be able to recognize it early so that intervention can occur before it becomes life threatening.

Incidence

SVCS was first described in 1757 in a patient who had a syphilitic aneurysm of the ascending aorta (Hunter, 1757). Syphilitic aneurysms and tuberculosis mediastinitis caused 40% of the cases of SVCS in 1954 (Schechter, 1954). Malignant disease is now the most common cause of SVCS, occurring in 70%–80% of the cases (Yahalom, 2005). SVCS has been most closely associated with thoracic neoplasms since the late 1900s (Rice, Rodriguez, & Light, 2006). An estimated 15,000 people in the United States develop SVCS annually (Wudel & Nesbitt, 2001). Nonmalignant causes of SVCS account for as many as 22% of the cases (Parish, Marschke, Dines, & Lee, 1981; Rice et al.; Schraufnagel, Hill, Leech, & Pare, 1981), which most likely is because of the increased use of pacemakers and central venous catheters.

Signs and Symptoms

The clinical manifestations of SVCS vary depending on the rapidity of onset and are directly related to obstruction of venous drainage in the upper body (see Figure 15-1). Symptoms can be gradual and vague or have a sudden onset. SVCS is more likely to be life threatening when the onset is sudden, as collateral veins have not had time to develop. Intravascular thrombosis is more likely to have a rapid onset of symptoms (Moore, 2006; Uaje, Kahsen, & Parish, 1996). The clinical signs and symptoms associated with SVCS also are affected by the underlying cause, with dyspnea at rest, cough, and chest pain being more frequent in patients with malignancy (Rice et al., 2006). Symptoms often are worse in the morning after the patient has been supine at night sleeping. The symptoms usually will improve after the patient has been upright for several hours (Uaje et al.). Patients also may notice that symptoms are exacerbated with bending over or stooping.

Early Signs and Symptoms
- Dyspnea
- Facial swelling upon arising
- Neck and thoracic vein distention
- Redness and edema in conjunctivae
- Nonproductive cough, hoarseness
- Swelling of neck, arms, and hands (Stoke sign)

Late Signs and Symptoms
- Congestive heart failure
- Stridor
- Irritability
- Dysphasia
- Hemoptysis
- Tachycardia
- Severe headache
- Dizziness, syncope
- Horner syndrome
- Changes in mental status
- Decreased blood pressure
- Visual disturbances, blurred vision

Figure 15-1. Superior Vena Cava Syndrome: Signs and Symptoms

Note. Based on information from Flounders, 2003b; Hunter, 2005; Moore, 2006; Rice et al., 2006.

The most common signs and symptoms of SVCS are face or neck swelling (82%), upper extremity swelling (68%), dyspnea (66%), cough (50%), and dilated chest vein collaterals (38%) (Rice et al., 2006). Patients often report a sense of "fullness" in the head. Patients may have swelling in the face, neck, and arms in the morning causing their shirt collar to be tight (Stoke sign). Women may develop breast swelling and have trouble removing their rings because of swelling of the fingers. Periorbital edema, conjunctival edema, and chest pain or discomfort can also occur (Flounders, 2003b; Moore, 2006).

Late signs and symptoms of SVCS can be severe and life threatening. Respiratory symptoms can include stridor and respiratory distress. Involvement of the recurrent laryngeal nerve (cranial nerve X) by lymph nodes can result in a paralyzed true vocal cord, leading to dysphagia and hoarseness (Moore, 2006). Late signs and symptoms related to the cardiovascular system can include tachycardia, decreased blood pressure, congestive heart failure, and cyanosis. Late symptoms of SVCS in the central nervous system (CNS) include severe headache, irritability, visual disturbances (blurred vision), dizziness, and syncope (Hunter, 2005). Mental status changes occur as SVCS progresses, including confusion, decrease in consciousness, seizures, and coma, which can indicate increased ICP. Hemoptysis also may be present in patients with SVCS. Horner syndrome (unilateral ptosis, constricted pupil, and ipsilateral loss of sweating from pressure on the cervical sympathetic nerves) can occur rarely in SVCS (Moore).

Risk Factors and Etiology

The most common cause of SVCS is mediastinal malignancy causing obstruction of the upper venous return to the heart. Men ages 50–70 with primary or metastatic tumors of the mediastinum have the most frequent occurrence of SVCS (Haapoja & Blendowski, 1999). More than 75% of the cases of SVC obstruction resulting from malignancy are caused by advanced lung cancer, with small cell lung cancer being the most common histology (Flounders, 2003b; Rice et al., 2006; Yahalom, 2005). The second most common histology of lung cancer that is responsible for SVCS is squamous cell carcinoma (Yahalom). Right-sided lung cancers are more likely to cause SVCS. Non-Hodgkin lymphoma involving the mediastinum can cause SVCS, and diffuse large cell lymphoma and lymphoblastic lymphoma are the most common histologies (Yahalom). Although Hodgkin lymphoma commonly involves the mediastinum, it rarely causes SVCS (Yahalom). Breast cancer is the most common metastatic cause of SVCS (Yahalom). Other cancers that can cause SVCS include Kaposi sarcoma, thymoma, and germ cell tumors (Rice et al.).

The most common etiology of nonmalignant SVCS is an intravascular device—central venous catheters or pacemakers causing thrombosis (Rice et al., 2006). Mediastinal fibrosis is the second most common nonmalignant cause because of either previous radiation therapy to the mediastinum or infection from tuberculosis or histoplasmosis (Flounders, 2003b; Rice et al.). Other rare benign causes of SVCS are thoracic aortic aneurysm and goiter.

Pathophysiology

The SVC is a thin-walled major vessel that carries venous drainage from the head, neck, upper extremities, and upper thorax to the right atrium of the heart (see Figure 15-2). It is located in the middle mediastinum surrounded by several rigid struc-

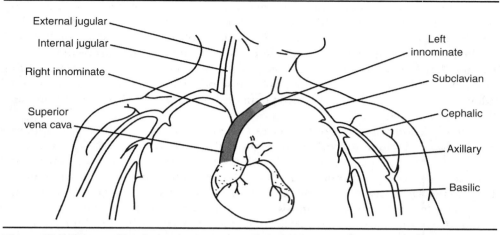

Figure 15-2. Venous Circulation Including the Superior Vena Cava

Note. From "Superior Vena Cava Syndrome," by J.A. Flounders, 2003, *Oncology Nursing Forum, 30,* p. E85. Copyright 2003 by Oncology Nursing Society. Reprinted with permission.

tures, including the sternum, trachea, right bronchus, aorta, pulmonary artery, vertebrae, and perihilar and paratracheal lymph nodes (Yahalom, 2005). The junction of the right and left brachiocephalic or innominate veins is the beginning of the SVC. It extends for 6–8 cm where it enters the pericardial sac and terminates at the right atrium. Unlike the other structures of the mediastinum, the SVC is a low-pressure vessel that is easily compressed. The SVC is completely surrounded by chains of lymph nodes that drain the structures of the right thoracic cavity and the lower part of the left thorax (Yahalom). The azygos vein empties into the SVC at the level of the main stem bronchus. The azygos venous system is an important alternative pathway if the blockage is above its entrance to the SVC.

As previously stated, SVCS is caused by extrinsic or intrinsic factors. Tumors or enlarged lymph nodes cause extrinsic compression. It can occur gradually or suddenly with complete or partial obstruction, and collateral venous drainage can develop (Flounders, 2003b). Intrinsic or intraluminal obstruction is a result of infiltration by tumor or thrombosis. Acute and complete obstruction is more common with thrombosis. Risk factors for thrombosis formation include intimal damage to the vein from central venous catheters, venous stasis from extrinsic compression, and a hypercoagulable state in patients with malignancy (Haapoja & Blendowski, 1999).

Partial or complete obstruction reduces venous blood return to the heart, increases venous congestion, and decreases cardiac output. Increased venous pressures can cause pleural and pericardial effusion, as well as edema of the face, neck, upper thorax, and extremities (Moore, 2006). Impaired venous drainage above the azygos vein causes less venous pressure, and the SVCS is less pronounced because of the distention and accommodation of the azygos system for the venous return from the upper body (Kuzin, 2006). If the SVC obstruction occurs below the azygos vein, the manifestations of SVCS are more severe because the venous return must be shunted by way of the upper abdominal veins and the inferior vena cava.

Stanford and Doty (1986) used venography patterns to classify individuals with SVCS into four categories based on the severity of obstruction and the extent of collateral venous circulation (see Table 15-1). Type I SVCS is partial SVC obstruction (with up to 90% stenosis), the azygos/right atrial pathway is not obstructed, and blood flow is in the normal direction. Type II SVCS continues to have normal blood flow and patency of the azygos/right atrial pathway, but with 90%–100% obstruction of the SVC. Patients with type III have 90%–100% SVC obstruction with reversal of the azygos flow and blood flow into the inferior vena cava. Type IV SVCS is complete obstruction of the SVC and obstruction of one or more of the major vena cava tributaries including the azygos system, along with blood flow into the inferior vena cava. Collateral development is dependent on the patency of the azygos system and the extent of the obstruction and is most pronounced in patients with type III SVC obstruction. Moderate collateral circulation is associated with types II and IV, whereas type I has minimal to no collateral development. Based on their findings, Stanford and Doty recommended that patients with type III be considered for SVC bypass as an initial therapeutic intervention because they show the most cerebral and airway compromise, will benefit most from surgery, and are better candidates, as the left brachiocephalic vein usually is open.

Prevention Strategies

Intravascular devices account for up to 14% of the cases of SVCS (Rice et al., 2006). Prophylactic low-dose anticoagulation commonly is given to patients with central vein intravascular devices to prevent clot formation and is one strategy to try to decrease thrombosis formation (Bern et al., 1990; Klerk, Smorenburg, & Buller, 2003). However, in a study by Rice et al., 18% of patients on prophylactic low-dose warfarin (Coumadin®, Bristol-Myers Squibb Co.) still developed SVCS.

Diagnosis and Assessment

The clinical history of patients is important because SVCS often is the result of malignancy, and identification of risk factors can help to develop the differential diagno-

Table 15-1. Classification of Superior Vena Cava Obstruction

Type of Obstruction	Level of Obstruction	Collateral Circulation
Type I	Partial obstruction (up to 90% stenosis) of the superior vena cava (SVC) with patency of the azygos/right atrial pathway, blood flow in normal direction	Minimal or absent collateral circulation
Type II	Near complete to complete obstruction (90%–100%) of the SVC with patency and normal blood flow in the azygos/right atrial pathway	Moderate collateral development
Type III	Near complete to complete obstruction (90%–100%) of the SVC with reversal of the azygos blood flow and blood flow into the inferior vena cava (IVC)	Significant collateral development
Type IV	Complete obstruction of the SVC and one or more of the major caval tributaries, including the azygos system, and blood flow into the IVC	Moderate collateral development

Note. Based on information from Stanford & Doty, 1986.

sis. Smoking history, previous cancer history, and presence of central venous catheters or pacemakers should be determined (Moore, 2006).

Physical Examination

Many of the physical examination findings of SVCS are specific to the syndrome (see Figure 15-1). Examination reveals edema of the face, neck, upper thorax, breast, and upper extremities along with dilated veins or prominent venous pattern. Jugular vein distention and facial plethora (ruddy complexion of the face and cheeks) along with periorbital and conjunctival edema often are present. Compensatory tachycardia often is noted.

Late signs occur more commonly in rapidly progressive, severe SVCS, which accounts for less than 2% of the cases (Kuzin, 2006). Cyanosis of the face or upper torso and engorged conjunctiva can occur. Stridor, tachypnea, tachycardia, and orthopnea are manifestations of respiratory distress. Mental status changes, visual changes, syncope, coma, seizures, and death can occur as a result of cerebral and laryngeal edema (Hunter, 2005; Kuzin).

The diagnostic evaluation has two components: imaging and tissue diagnosis, as most causes of SVCS are attributable to malignancy. Accurate, definitive histologic diagnosis is important to determine the appropriate treatment (Flounders, 2003b). A chest x-ray is positive in more than 80% of SVCS cases (Parish et al., 1981). The most common findings on chest x-ray are pleural effusion, superior mediastinal widening, and mediastinal or lung mass. A computed tomography (CT) scan of the chest provides visualization of the anatomy to determine tumor size and extent of involvement (Schwartz, Goodman, & Haskin, 1986). Magnetic resonance imaging (MRI) is another noninvasive diagnostic tool that can provide greater detail of the mediastinal structures, but it has increased cost and scan time. Once clinicians determine that the SVCS is attributable to tumor, then tissue diagnosis is needed in the least invasive way possible. Sputum cytology is diagnostic in 50% of the cases (O'Brien, 1996). Bronchoscopy can be used in most cases of small cell lung cancer for diagnosis. If a pleural effusion is present, thoracentesis can be diagnostic in 70% of patients (Schraufnagel et al., 1981). Supraclavicular node biopsy or biopsy of any palpable mass or lymph node may be performed. A bone marrow biopsy may provide diagnosis in non-Hodgkin lymphoma or small cell lung cancer, as these diseases often involve the bone marrow and assist in staging as well (Drews, 2005). Mediastinoscopy has a high success rate if less invasive measures do not result in a definitive diagnosis (Yahalom, 2005).

Differential Diagnosis

Aortic aneurysm, tuberculosis, histoplasmosis, and fungal infections would be other processes to consider in the differential diagnosis (Peralta & Guzofski, 2007). These processes can cause mediastinal changes causing symptoms associated with SVCS. A thorough history to evaluate for possible exposures and imaging studies can help to distinguish differences (Rice et al., 2006).

Evidence-Based Treatment

When SVCS develops acutely, it is an emergency and requires prompt intervention for relief of symptoms. The goals of treatment are to relieve symptoms and control the underlying disease. The etiology of the SVCS, the severity of symptoms, the patient's prognosis, the underlying malignancy, and the presence of thrombosis guide the treatment plan.

Pharmacologic therapy for the treatment of SVCS includes chemotherapy, steroids, diuretics, and thrombolytic therapy. Chemotherapy is used for malignancies that are highly chemosensitive, such as non-Hodgkin lymphoma and small cell lung cancer. Combination chemotherapy is most commonly used. For small cell lung cancer, the treatment may include cisplatin or carboplatin, etoposide, ifosfamide, cyclophosphamide, doxorubicin, vincristine, taxanes, and gemcitabine (Moore, 2006). Lymphoma regimens are based on the subtype but may include cyclophosphamide, doxorubicin, vincristine, prednisone, or fludarabine (Flounders, 2003b). Improvement in symptoms usually occurs within 7–14 days. Chemotherapy may be used in combination with radiation in some settings to provide quicker relief of symptoms. This will result in increased side effects, and patients need close monitoring (Kuzin, 2006). An important issue when using chemotherapy in patients with SVCS is the route of delivery. Because of the venous stasis in the upper thorax, chemotherapy can become concentrated if it is delivered via the upper extremities. A central line through the femoral vein may be necessary for safe drug delivery (Moore).

Other pharmacologic therapies can be used as supportive care to manage symptoms. Oxygen can be used to relieve dyspnea, and analgesics may be of benefit in patients with chest pain. Loop diuretics, such as furosemide, can be used to reduce edema, but patients need to be monitored for dehydration, which could lead to an increased risk of thrombosis (Kuzin, 2006; Yahalom, 2005). Steroids, although commonly used, have no evidence to support their use. They may decrease an inflammatory reaction to the tumor or radiation therapy, but no controlled data exist to support their use (Rowell & Gleeson, 2002; Yahalom). Steroids can be useful in SVCS caused by non-Hodgkin lymphoma because the disease is responsive to steroids, but their value in other etiologies is limited or nonexistent (Aurora et al., 2000).

Thrombolytic therapy is used to treat SVCS when the cause is catheter-induced thrombosis. The therapy should be initiated within five to seven days of onset for maximum effectiveness (Aurora et al., 2000). The thrombolytic agent is infused through the catheter to try to lyse the clot and is followed by heparin anticoagulation to prevent reembolization (Moore, 2006). Streptokinase, urokinase, and recombinant tissue plasminogen activator (rt-PA) have been used in this setting (Gray et al., 1991; Greenberg, Kosinski, & Daniels, 1991). Studies have shown urokinase to be more effective than streptokinase, but a delay beyond five days of symptom onset was associated with treatment failure (Gray et al.). Febrile reactions are more common with rt-PA, as are serious adverse effects, such as anaphylaxis and angioedema (Chodirker, 2000; Rudolf, Grond, Prince, Schmulling, & Heiss, 1999). Thrombolytics have been used to treat thrombosis in heparin-induced thrombocytopenia with success but should be used with caution (Calligaro, Kansagra, Dougherty, Savarese, & DeLaurentis, 1995; Clifton & Smith, 1986).

Nonpharmacologic therapy for the management of SVCS includes radiation, surgery, and stent placement. If the cause of SVCS is catheter-induced thrombosis, catheter removal may be necessary. Intravascular stent placement has become a treatment option for SVCS from either benign or malignant etiology. Stent placement is effective in relieving symptoms in 68%–100% of patients (Rowell & Gleeson, 2002). Results are seen within 24–72 hours with immediate relief of headache and resolution of edema within days (Rowell & Gleeson). Complication rates for stent placement range from 3%–7% and include bleeding, infection, stent migration, stent occlusion, hematoma at the insertion site, and pulmonary embolus (Hochrein, Bashore, O'Laughlin, & Harrison, 1998; Smayra et al., 2001; Uberoi, 2006). Stent placement is contraindicated if tumor invasion of the vessel exists (Uberoi). Because of the ease and safety of stent placement, it has been recommended as a first choice for palliative care of malignant SVCS until the etiology can be determined and appropriate therapy instituted (Lanciego et al., 2001; Rice et al., 2006). Balloon angioplasty can be used in combination with stent placement to allow for complete expansion of the vessel (Uberoi).

Surgical intervention is rare for malignant causes of SVCS and is reserved for patients who have failed other therapeutic options, such as chemotherapy and radiation therapy (Panneton, Andrews, & Hofer, 2001). A surgical bypass creates a circulation route around the SVC obstruction between the innominate or jugular vein on the left side to the right atrium using autologous saphenous veins, synthetic materials, or tissue from the patient's pericardium (Abner, 1993; Piccione, Faber, & Warren, 1990). If rapid progression in benign etiologies of SVCS occurs, surgical intervention for anterosternal goiter or aortic aneurysm may be used to relieve the obstruction (Kalra et al., 2003).

Radiation therapy is considered the treatment of choice for SVCS caused by non-small cell lung cancer (Armstrong, Perez, Simpson, & Hederman, 1987; Rowell & Gleason, 2002). Radiation therapy can be used for most malignant causes of SVCS and is an effective treatment if the patient's clinical status deteriorates rapidly, requiring emergent intervention (Davenport, Feree, Blake, & Raben, 1978). The radiation dose is determined by the tumor type, extent of disease, history of previous radiation in the area, and the patient's performance status. The initial two to four treatments usually are 300–400 cGy to obtain quicker symptomatic relief, followed by standard daily dose fractions of 180–200 cGy (Anderson & Coia, 2000). Patients may notice improvement in venous congestion within three to four days as a result of improved blood flow. Maximum symptom relief may occur in three weeks in 70%–95% of the patients treated with radiation therapy, with better results in lymphoma than in lung cancer (Nicholson, Ettles, & Arnold, 1997). The side effects of radiation depend on the total dose, the fraction dose, the amount of normal tissue in the radiation field, and whether concomitant chemotherapy is given. Short-term side effects include fatigue, cough, nausea, dysphagia, heartburn, and skin irritation. Long-term side effects include pneumonitis, pulmonary fibrosis, esophageal stenosis, cardiac changes, and spinal cord myelopathy (Moore, 2006).

Implications for Advanced Nursing Practice

SVCS is an obstructive complication seen in malignant and benign conditions. The most common malignancies associated with SVCS are small cell lung cancer and lymphoma. The onset typically is gradual, but it can develop rapidly. Early recognition and intervention is important to prevent progression to an emergency. Establishment of etiology is needed to determine the treatment plan. APNs can help to facilitate the recognition of early SVCS, establish a diagnosis, and implement intervention before it becomes a true emergency.

Although no formal professional guidelines exist for the management of SVCS, both the American College of Chest Physicians and the National Comprehensive Cancer Network (NCCN) recommend the consideration of radiotherapy and/or stent placement for symptomatic obstruction in lung cancer (Kvale, Simoff, & Prakash, 2003; NCCN, 2008). An area with no data to guide decision making is in recurrent obstruction of the SVC, but stent placement often is done because of the limited benefit or toxicity from further chemotherapy or radiation (Wilson, Detterbeck, & Yahalom, 2007).

Nursing management of patients with SVCS includes monitoring respiratory status and easing dyspnea with oxygen therapy, elevation of the head of the bed, and anxiety management. Cardiac monitoring and fluid balance are needed, as is neurologic assessment to monitor for any changes in mental status. Bowel management is needed to avoid performing the Valsalva maneuver, which increases venous pressure. For many patients, SVCS may be the initial presentation of their cancer, whereas for others, it indicates recurrence, so emotional care will be needed. Also important to remember is that vascular access devices are causing an increased incidence of SVCS (Moore, 2006).

Cardiac Tamponade

Cardiac tamponade is the compression of the heart caused by fluid or blood accumulation in the pericardial sac, the space between the myocardium (the muscle of the heart) and the pericardium (the outer covering sac of the heart). Cardiac tamponade can be a life-threatening oncologic emergency. The fluid causes an increase in pressure around the heart, resulting in decreased blood flow in and out of the ventricles, thus leading to compromised cardiac function and decreased cardiac output (Spodick, 2003). Pericardial effusion and cardiac tamponade are two distinct entities. Pericardial effusion is the presence of abnormal fluid that often has no hemodynamic consequences, whereas cardiac tamponade causes increased pressure with hemodynamic consequences (Reddy, Curtiss, O'Toole, & Shaver, 1978). If untreated, cardiac tamponade leads to cardiovascular collapse, shock, and death (Story, 2006).

Incidence

Cardiac tamponade is not always diagnosed in patients with pericardial effusion, as patients often are asymptomatic. The incidence of pericardial effusion in patients with malignancy has been reported to be 5%–50% but is thought to be underreported because of the vague symptoms associated with pericardial effusion (Grannis, Lily, Cullinane, & Wagman, 2005; Warren, 2000). Malignancy is the most common cause of cardiac tamponade, accounting for 16%–41% of cases (Uaje et al., 1996).

Signs and Symptoms

The signs and symptoms of cardiac tamponade (see Figure 15-3) depend on the amount of fluid and how quickly it accumulates. Initially, the symptoms can be vague and overlooked, but as the effusion becomes larger, the symptoms increase. Initial symptoms include fatigue, chest pain, apprehension/anxiety or agitation, and dyspnea at rest. Dyspnea is the most common presenting symptom of cardiac tamponade (Shepherd, 1997). Chest pain is retrosternal and may be relieved by leaning forward and worsened by lying supine, because of compression on the heart (Flounders, 2003a; Hunter, 2005). Other early symptoms are cough, hoarseness, dysphasia, and hiccups resulting from mechanical compression of the nerves of the esophagus and trachea (Uaje et al., 1996). Heart sounds are distant or muffled because of the fluid accumulation and compression of the heart (Kaplow, 2006). As the fluid continues to accumulate and the pericardium is no longer able to stretch, the signs and symptoms worsen (Uaje et al.).

Late signs and symptoms of cardiac tamponade include worsening dyspnea with the patient being unable to speak more than a word or two without becoming short of

---

Early Signs and Symptoms
- Cough
- Hiccups
- Dyspnea
- Anxiety/agitation
- Muffled heart sounds
- Retrosternal chest pain, relieved by leaning forward and intensified by lying supine

Late Signs and Symptoms
- Oliguria
- Cyanosis
- Tachypnea
- Tachycardia
- Peripheral edema
- Pulsus paradoxus
- Narrow pulse pressure
- Altered level of consciousness
- Beck triad—Classic signs of cardiac tamponade (elevated central venous pressure, hypotension, and distant heart sounds)

Figure 15-3. Cardiac Tamponade: Signs and Symptoms

Note. Based on information from Flounders, 2003a; Hunter, 2005; Shepherd, 1997; Spodick, 2003.

breath (Kaplow, 2006). Tachypnea, tachycardia, and peripheral edema begin to develop. Cardiovascular signs become more prominent with the development of pulsus paradoxus, a decrease in systolic blood pressure of greater than 10 mm Hg during inspiration. The classic signs of cardiac tamponade, the Beck triad, occur as cardiac tamponade progresses. The Beck triad includes elevated central venous pressure (CVP), hypotension, and distant heart sounds (Beck, 1935). All three signs only occur in the advanced stages of cardiac tamponade (Shabetai, 1988; Spodick, 2003). Hypotension leads to decreased perfusion of the kidneys, resulting in oliguria and decreased peripheral perfusion leading to weakness, cyanosis, and cool and clammy extremities. Mental status changes also can occur, including lethargy, restlessness, confusion, decreased level of consciousness, and seizures (Beauchamp, 1998; Shepherd, 1997).

Risk Factors and Etiology

The major cause of pericardial effusion is malignancy or its treatment, but nonmalignant causes exist as well. Although primary tumors of the pericardium are rare, they account for many of the cases of pericardial effusion leading to cardiac tamponade. Mesothelioma is the most common primary tumor of the heart; other less common tumors include malignant fibrous histiocytoma, rhabdomyosarcoma, and angiosarcoma (Warren, 2000). The tumors most commonly associated with metastatic spread or local extension to the heart include lung, breast, lymphoma, and leukemia. Other tumors that can metastasize to the heart include liver, gastric, esophageal, sarcoma, melanoma, and pancreatic malignancies (Flounders, 2003a; Knoop & Willenberg, 1999).

The treatment of malignancies can result in the development of pericardial effusion. Radiation therapy to the mediastinal area encompassing the heart can lead to pericarditis if greater than 4,000 cGy is delivered and can result in cardiac tamponade (Knoop & Willenberg, 1999). Chemotherapy and biotherapy can increase the risk of pericardial effusion. Chemotherapy agents associated with the development of pericardial effusion include anthracyclines, especially doxorubicin or daunorubicin; cytosine arabinoside; and cyclophosphamide. Biotherapy agents can increase capillary permeability, resulting in increased risk of pericardial effusion, and include interferon, interleukin-2, interleukin 11, and granulocyte macrophage–colony-stimulating factor (Story, 2006).

Nonmalignant risk factors for the development of pericardial effusion and cardiac tamponade include systemic lupus erythematosis, renal failure, rheumatoid arthritis, scleroderma, hypoalbuminemia, coexisting heart disease, and hypothyroidism (Braunwald, 2005). Infectious pericarditis caused by bacteria, viruses, fungi, or tuberculosis also can result in cardiac tamponade. Chest trauma, improper insertion of central venous catheters, aneurysm, and cardiac surgery are additional risk factors for the development of cardiac tamponade (Flounders, 2003a; Hawley, Dreher, & Vasso, 2003).

Pathophysiology

The pericardium is a double-layered, fibrous sac surrounding the heart. The outer fibrous layer is the parietal layer, which provides strength and protection for the heart. The inner layer is a serous membrane called the visceral layer and is connected to the surface of the heart. The pericardium functions to support the heart chambers, to protect the heart from friction, infection, and inflammation, and to stabilize the cardiac position against gravity (Spodick, 1983). A small amount of fluid, approximately 15–50 ml, between the two layers in the pericardial space serves to prevent friction between the layers of the heart. This fluid normally is reabsorbed and drained by the lymph channels into the mediastinum and right heart chambers (Uaje et al., 1996).

The intrapericardial pressure normally is lower than ventricular diastolic pressure and equal to pleural pressure, thereby allowing the heart chambers to fill (Kaplow, 2006). If the pressure, production of fluid, or clearance of fluid is altered, then an effusion will develop. Obstruction of the venous and lymphatic drainage of the heart is the most common cause of fluid build-up (Beauchamp, 1998). Cancer cells will stimulate the pericardium to produce excess fluid, and invasive tumors may bleed into the pericardial space. Blood accumulates more rapidly, so pericardial effusions caused by bleeding tend to progress more rapidly to cardiac tamponade (Keefe, 2000).

The amount of fluid that causes cardiac tamponade varies from 50 ml to greater than one liter depending on how rapidly the fluid develops (Hawley et al., 2003; Spodick, 2003). With slow, chronic accumulation of fluid, the pericardium has time to stretch and compensate. If the accumulation is acute and rapid, the intrapericardial pressure rises to 20 mm Hg or higher, resulting in hemodynamic instability and cardiac compromise (Uaje et al., 1996).

Increased intrapericardial pressure initially causes compression of the right atrium and right ventricle, resulting in decreased right atrial filling during diastole. Increased venous pressure occurs, causing edema, hepatomegaly, jugular vein distention, and increased diastolic pressure. Continued compression causes decreased filling of the ventricles, thus leading to decreased stroke volume and decreased cardiac output (Flounders, 2003a). Compensatory mechanisms related to increased intrapericardial pressure include cardiac stimulation by the adrenergic nervous system, causing tachycardia and peripheral vasoconstriction. This in turn activates the renin-angiotensin-aldosterone system in attempts to increase blood volume and improve stroke volume (Flounders, 2003a). These compensatory mechanisms increase the workload of the heart, and without intervention, this process leads to shock, cardiac arrest, and death (Spodick, 2003).

Diagnosis and Assessment

The clinical manifestations of cardiac tamponade will vary based on the amount of fluid accumulation, the rapidity of fluid accumulation, and the baseline cardiac function of the patient. Early symptoms are nonspecific and may be overlooked as being caused by progressive disease or pulmonary complications, as dyspnea is the most common symptom (Shepherd, 1997). A thorough and detailed history should be performed to evaluate for a history of cancer, looking for cancers that have a higher risk of causing cardiac tamponade, as well as determining previous therapies that are cardiotoxic.

Physical Examination

Early signs of cardiac tamponade on physical examination include muffled heart sounds, undetectable or weak apical pulse, or positional pericardial rub resulting from increased pericardial fluid. Mild tachycardia caused by the compensatory mechanism of the adrenergic system can be present. As venous and visceral congestion develops, peripheral edema and abdominal distention can occur (Spodick, 2003).

As cardiac tamponade progresses, pulsus paradoxus can occur. Pulsus paradoxus is measured by inflating the blood pressure cuff 20 mm Hg above the systolic pressure and slowly deflating the cuff. The first systolic pressure reading heard during exhalation is noted. The systolic pressure reading heard during both inspiration and exhalation then is noted. If the difference between the two sounds is greater than 10 mm Hg, the patient has pulsus paradoxus (Hawley et al., 2003; Shabetai, 1988). Other conditions (such as chronic obstructive pulmonary disease [COPD], pulmonary embolism, right ventricular infarction, extreme obesity, or tense ascites) can cause pulsus paradoxus; therefore, it is not specific to cardiac tamponade (Shabetai). Pulsus paradoxus may be absent or undetectable in patients with severe hypotension, atrial septal defect, left ventricular dysfunction, or aortic stenosis (Tsang, Oh, & Seward, 1999).

Hepatojugular reflux also can occur and is an elevation of the jugular venous pressure by 1 cm or more. To assess this, place the patient supine with the head of the bed elevated so that the jugular venous pulsations are visible. Exert pressure for 30–60 seconds over the right upper quadrant of the abdomen and observe for increased jugular venous pressure, which is a result of an elevated CVP (Knoop & Willenberg, 1999). As discussed previously, the Beck triad comprises elevated CVP, hypotension, and distant heart sounds, but all three signs occur only in advanced cardiac tamponade (Hawley et al., 2003; Spodick, 2003).

A routine chest x-ray is not diagnostic of cardiac tamponade but may demonstrate an enlarged cardiac silhouette as a result of increased fluid in the pericardial sac, which may raise suspicion leading to further testing (Flounders, 2003a; Uaje et al., 1996). Electrocardiogram (EKG) changes are nonspecific and include tachycardia, low-voltage QRS complex, nonspecific ST-T changes, and premature atrial or ventricular contractions (Knoop & Willenberg, 1999; Warren, 2000). Electrical alternans is a rare EKG finding that shows a variation in the height of the QRS amplitudes with alternating beats caused by the swinging of the heart in the fluid-filled pericardium (Uaje et al.).

The most precise diagnostic test in cardiac tamponade is a two-dimensional echocardiogram (Hawley et al., 2003; Spodick, 2003; van Steijn, van der Graaf, van der Sluis, & Nieboer, 2002). It is a painless and noninvasive test that assesses for the presence, location, and approximate quantity of pericardial fluid, as well as the overall cardiac function. The classic finding on echocardiogram that is suggestive of cardiac tamponade is diastolic collapse of the right atrium and ventricle because of the pressure of the increased pericardial fluid. Other findings on echocardiogram include swinging heart, left atrial and ventricular collapse, inspiratory changes in ventricle size, and inferior vena cava plethora (an excess build-up of fluid in the vena cava) (Chong & Plotnick, 1995).

Other tests used to diagnose cardiac tamponade include CT scan and MRI. CT scans can detect as little as 50 ml of pericardial fluid, and MRI scans may have superior resolution compared to echocardiogram. CT and MRI may help to distinguish between radiation fibrosis and constrictive pericarditis with effusion (Myers, 2001). Neither test is better than the echocardiogram, nor do they provide data on cardiac functioning (van Steijn et al., 2002).

Pericardial fluid evaluation can be performed to determine whether the effusion is a result of malignancy. The fluid is evaluated for cytology, lactate dehydrogenase (LDH), and total protein levels. Cytology testing has a significant false-negative rate (Hunter, 2005). The fluid is described as transudate or exudate. A transudate has a low protein level and has leaked from the blood vessels as a result of mechanical factors, such as cirrhosis. An exudate is rich in protein and has leaked as a result of increased permeability (Venes, 2005). Malignant effusions often are exudates and appear bloody, serous, or serosanguineous.

Differential Diagnosis

The differential diagnosis includes tension pneumothorax; acute right ventricle failure (acute myocardial infarction); COPD; acute pulmonary embolus; fat embolus; excessive or rapid administration of fluids; abdominal distention from ascites or ileus; increased intrathoracic pressure from pneumothorax, hemothorax, airway obstruction, or mechanical ventilation; or administration of vasopressors (Carran, 2007). A tension pneumothorax presents with a deviated trachea and unequal breath sounds to distinguish it from cardiac tamponade. A large pleural effusion can have the same signs and symptoms of cardiac tamponade, along with dyspnea and respiratory distress. An echocardiogram is needed to differentiate between the two processes (Kaplan, Epstein, Schwartz, Cao, & Pandian, 1995). Acute myocardial infarction will have characteristic EKG changes to distinguish it from cardiac tamponade. Chronic tamponade must be distinguished from congestive heart failure, and an echocardiogram can make that distinction (Shabetai & Hoit, 2006).

Evidence-Based Treatment

Cardiac tamponade is a potentially life-threatening emergency requiring removal of the pericardial fluid to restore hemodynamic stability. The patient's overall condition, presenting symptoms, diagnosis, and prognosis are taken into account in the recommended treatment plan. A surgical approach (see Table 15-2) usually is necessary initially to restore hemodynamic stability followed by medical management (Story, 2006).

Pericardiocentesis is the most common approach for the management of cardiac tamponade. It drains the fluid for initial treatment and serves as a diagnostic tool (Beauchamp, 1998; Knoop & Willenberg, 1999). Pericardiocentesis provides quick relief but has potential complications, including abscess, infection, dysrhythmias, puncture of the cardiac muscle, and introduction of air into the heart chambers (Warren, 2000). A subxiphoid approach is used to insert a needle into the pericardial sac for fluid aspiration. This usually is performed under guidance by echocardiogram or fluoroscopy, but in a truly emergent situation, it can be unguided (Maisch et al., 2004). The effusion must be drained slowly over several minutes to prevent right ventricular distention and failure. Once the fluid is

Table 15-2. Surgical Approaches to Cardiac Tamponade

Surgical Procedure	Comments
Pericardiocentesis	Removal of fluid at bedside (with surgical back-up), needle inserted via subxiphoid approach toward left shoulder, catheter can be placed for continued drainage
Pericardial sclerosis	Instillation of sclerosing agent into the pericardial sac to induce scarring and prevent recurrence of fluid accumulation
Percutaneous balloon pericardiotomy	Insertion of catheter into pericardial space, inflation of balloon to cause tear or hole in pericardium allowing fluid to drain into the mediastinum
Pericardial window	Local anesthesia with subxiphoid approach; segment of pericardium is resected, allowing fluid to drain into the mediastinum
Pericardiectomy	General anesthesia with resection of part or all of the pericardium to allow drainage and prevention of recurrence because of removal of pericardial sac

Note. Based on information from Beauchamp, 1998; Warren, 2000.

drained, a catheter can remain in place to drain over several days, and it has been theorized that the presence of the catheter may allow adhesion formation or scarring of the pericardial sac so that further intervention may not be needed (Warren).

Pericardial sclerosis often is attempted once the pericardial fluid is drained. Pericardial sclerosis is the instillation of an agent into the pericardial sac after drainage of the fluid. The agent causes inflammation and fibrosis, preventing reaccumulation of fluid. Sclerosing agents include bleomycin, doxycycline, minocycline, mitomycin C, cisplatin, fluorouracil, or radioisotopes (Knoop & Willenberg, 1999; van Steijn et al., 2002). Thiotepa has been shown to be effective in sclerosing in patients with breast cancer with a low incidence of side effects and with the added benefit of antineoplastic effect (van Steijn et al.). Radioisotope use is limited because of the expense and the need for isolation (Warren, 2000).

Several surgical options for management of cardiac tamponade exist, as pericardiocentesis is a temporary measure and reaccumulation is likely. A subxiphoid pericardiotomy or pericardial window is associated with lower morbidity and mortality than a pericardiectomy, and the procedure can be performed under local anesthesia (Warren, 2000). The pericardium is exposed, and a small incision is made with an approximate 3 cm diameter piece of pericardium removed to allow fluid to drain into surrounding tissues. Tube drainage or sclerosis may be combined with this procedure.

A subtotal pericardial resection (pericardiectomy), the partial or complete removal of the visceral pericardium, is the definitive treatment for pericardial effusion, allowing continuous fluid drainage into the pleural space (Park, Rentschler, & Wilbur, 1991). Because of the need for general anesthesia, a pericardiectomy has a longer recovery time and higher morbidity rate compared to other surgical procedures; thus, it is reserved for patients with recurrent effusions and a life expectancy of greater than one year (Beauchamp, 1998). It often is used to treat patients with radiation-induced constrictive pericarditis (Flounders, 2003a). A newer technique that is technically feasible but for which long-term results are unknown is percutaneous balloon pericardiotomy (Warren, 2000). A balloon-tipped catheter is placed across the pericardium under fluoroscopic guidance and is inflated to tear the pericardium, creating a window for drainage. No tissue is removed, so scarring and closure of the site is possible, and biopsy cannot be obtained with this technique. Complications related to this procedure include bleeding, fevers, and pneumothorax (Warren).

Systemic chemotherapy is used to treat chemotherapy-sensitive malignancies, such as lymphoma, leukemia, breast cancer, testicular cancer, and small cell lung cancer, to help to prevent recurrence of cardiac tamponade once the patient is stabilized. Chemotherapy also may be used in the setting of a slowly accumulating pericardial effusion when the patient is asymptomatic (Myers, 2001). Radiation therapy has a limited role in cardiac tamponade and pericardial effusions but can be used in patients with radiosensitive tumors who have not had prior radiation. It also can be used to prevent reaccumulation after pericardiocentesis, but it does not provide immediate relief because the patient must be stabilized first (Helms & Carlson, 1989). Response rates of 30%–100% have been seen with a dose of 1,500–4,500 cGy with best results in leukemia, lymphoma, and breast cancer and the lowest results occurring in lung cancer (Cham, Freiman, Carstens, & Chu, 1975; Vaitkus, Herrmann, & LeWinter, 1994). Other medical management involves supportive care with ongoing pharmacologic therapy to maintain blood pressure and cardiac functioning. Mild effusions initially can be treated cautiously with diuretics and corticosteroids. Steroids or nonsteroidal anti-inflammatory agents may help to reduce inflammation in constrictive pericarditis. Oxygen therapy may be needed to maintain oxygen saturation above 92% (Hawley et al., 2003). Blood products, plasma, or saline may be used to expand circulatory volume. Inotropic agents, such as dobutamine, may be used to maintain blood pressure and improve cardiac output (Beauchamp, 1998; Hawley et al.). Beta-blockers and positive pressure mechanical ventilation should be avoided, as they further decrease cardiac output (Spodick, 2003).

Implications for Advanced Nursing Practice

Cardiac tamponade is a potentially life-threatening emergency that without rapid intervention can lead to cardiac collapse and death. The symptoms can be vague and occur slowly or acutely. With intervention, rapid improvement is seen. APNs can help to facilitate the appropriate intervention, which is based on the patient's disease, prognosis, expected survival time, and clinical status (Kaplow, 2006).

Nursing management of patients with cardiac tamponade is complex, and APNs must ensure that these patients are assessed and monitored closely. Ongoing assessment of blood pressure, EKG monitoring, and oxygen therapy is critical in patients with cardiac tamponade. Patient and family education along with emotional support is needed to decrease anxiety and maintain optimal cardiac status. Preparation for procedures and monitoring after procedures for complications such as pneumothorax, bleeding, infection, or reaccumulation of pericardial fluid also are needed (Estes, 1985).

APNs always should consider pericardial effusion in patients with a history of malignancy who present with dyspnea. An echocardiogram should be obtained if pericardial effusion is suspected, because physical examination, chest x-ray, and EKG may be nonspecific (van Steijn et al., 2002).

Spinal Cord Compression

Metastatic SCC is defined as the compressive indentation, displacement, or encasement of the spinal cord's thecal sac by metastatic or locally advanced cancer (Baehring, 2005b). SCC is an oncologic emergency that affects patient function and quality of life. With early diagnosis, treatment is effective in 90% of patients (Maranzano et al., 1996). Paraplegia, quadriplegia, and loss of bowel or bladder function are potential consequences of SCC with late diagnosis. Early recognition and intervention are critical to preserve function and quality of life.

Incidence

SCC is the second most common neurologic complication of cancer, following brain metastases (Myers, 2001). SCC affects 5%–10% of the adult cancer population, more than 25,000 people per year (Schiff, 2003). Most patients with SCC have a known diagnosis of cancer, but in up to one-third of the cases, it is the first indication of malignant disease (Schiff, O'Neill, & Suman, 1997).

Signs and Symptoms

The signs and symptoms of SCC depend on the anatomic level and location of the tumor (see Figure 15-4). The thoracic spine is the most common site of spinal metastasis with SCC (70%), followed by the lumbar-sacral spine (20%), and the cervical spine (10%) (Schiff, O'Neill, Wang, & O'Fallon, 1998). Pain is the presenting symptom in up to 95% of the cases, preceding the diagnosis of SCC by days to months (Baehring, 2005b; Osowski, 2002). The pain may be localized, radicular (pain in the area of the affected dermatome), referred, or a combination. If the

---

Cervical Spine
- Breathing difficulties
- Loss of sensation in arms
- Headache, neck, shoulder, or arm pain
- Muscle weakness in neck, trunk, arms, and hands
- Paralysis involving neck, trunk, arms, and hands

Thoracic Spine
- Paralysis
- Muscle weakness
- Chest or back pain
- Positive Babinski reflex
- Bladder, bowel, and sexual dysfunction
- Loss of sensation below the tumor level
- Increased sensation above the tumor level

Lumbar-Sacral Spine
- Paralysis
- Foot drop
- Weakness in the legs and feet
- Loss of sensation in the legs and feet
- Decreased or absent reflexes in the legs
- Bladder, bowel, and sexual dysfunction
- Lower back pain that may radiate down the legs or into the perineal area

---

Figure 15-4. Signs and Symptoms of Spinal Cord Compression

Note. Based on information from Flounders & Ott, 2003; Gilbert et al., 1978; Osowski, 2002; Schiff, 2003.

pain is not recognized and evaluated, it progresses to motor weakness, sensory loss, autonomic dysfunction, and eventually paralysis (Kaplan, 2006).

Localized pain usually is the initial symptom and is dull, aching, constant, and progressive. It is the result of expansion, destruction, or fracture of the involved vertebral elements. Unlike the pain from a herniated disc, the pain from SCC is worse when patients are in a supine position. The intensity of the pain increases, and a radicular component can develop over time (Schiff, 2003). Compression of the nerve roots or cauda equina causes radicular pain, which follows the pattern of the affected dermatome. Radicular pain can be a constant, dull ache to a burning, shooting pain. Bilateral band-like pain, across the chest and abdomen, is more common with thoracic cord lesions, whereas unilateral radicular pain is characteristic of lumbar or cervical lesions (Schiff). Both localized and radicular pain is exacerbated by coughing, sneezing, movement, and the Valsalva maneuver (Baehring, 2005b; Flounders & Ott, 2003).

Weakness is the second most common symptom of SCC at presentation and is present in up to 85% of the cases (Baehring, 2005b; Greenberg, Kim, & Posner, 1980). Motor weakness typically begins in the legs regardless of the level of compression (Kaplan, 2006). Initially it is more proximal, and the patient may have difficulty getting up from a chair or the toilet and climbing steps. Patients often describe the weakness as a heaviness or stiffness, or it may present as sexual dysfunction (Wilkes, 2004b). As it progresses, the weakness leads to loss of coordination, difficulty in walking, and eventually paralysis (Schiff et al., 1997). More than two-thirds of patients are nonambulatory at diagnosis (Husband, 1998; Maranzano & Latini, 1995). Neurologic status at diagnosis is the most important predictor of post-treatment function, so it is important to diagnose and intervene early (Maranzano & Latini). Only 10% of patients who present with paraplegia will be able to ambulate after intervention (Gabriel & Schiff, 2004).

Sensory changes may develop at the same time as weakness or shortly after, and although they occur less frequently than weakness, they are present in 50% of patients (Gilbert, Kim, & Posner, 1978). Sensory loss includes numbness, paresthesia, loss of temperature sensation, loss of proprioception, and loss of vibratory sense. Sensory loss typically starts in the toes and ascends until it reaches the level of the lesion (Wilkes, 2004b). Cauda equina compression results in bilateral sensory loss and follows the dermatome path involving the perianal area, posterior thigh, and lateral leg (Flounders & Ott, 2003).

Autonomic dysfunction is a common late finding of SCC. It includes impotence and change in bladder and bowel function. Bladder dysfunction is most common, followed by bowel dysfunction (Kaplan, 2006). Bladder symptoms include hesitancy and retention followed by overflow and incontinence. Bowel dysfunction includes lack of urge to defecate and inability to bear down, leading to constipation, obstipation, and incontinence. Loss of sphincter control is a late sign and is associated with a poorer prognosis (Helweg-Larsen, Sorensen, & Kreiner, 2000). Horner syndrome (drooping eyelid, constricted pupil, and decreased sweating on the affected side of the face) can be seen with tumor involvement around the junction of the cervical and thoracic spines, causing autonomic dysfunction of the sympathetic nerves of the face (Gabriel & Schiff, 2004). Autonomic hyperreflexia may occur with injury to the spinal cord at or above the level of the sixth or seventh thoracic vertebra. Symptoms of autonomic hyperreflexia include pounding headache, bradycardia, nasal congestion, hypertension, profuse sweating, and pilomotor erection (goose bumps) above the level of the lesion (Myers, 2001).

Risk Factors and Etiology

SCC as a result of malignant neoplasm is a result of primary tumors of the spinal cord or tumors that metastasize to the spinal cord or bone (see Figure 15-5). Primary tumors of the spinal cord, such as ependymoma, astrocytoma, or glioma, are intramedullary tumors that are rare and cause a very small percentage of the cases of SCC (Myers, 2001). The most common cause is metastatic tumors, composing 85%–90% of the cases of SCC. Solid tumors that metastasize to the bone have a high incidence of SCC and include breast, lung, and prostate cancer, which account for 60% of the cases (Schiff et al., 1997). Other common tumor types associated with SCC include renal cell carcinoma, lymphoma, and myeloma. The location of the lesion correlates with the tumor type, with cervical lesions often caused by breast cancer. Thoracic lesions often are caused by breast, lung, and prostate tumors, whereas prostate malignancies commonly are the cause of lumbar lesions (Flounders & Ott, 2003).

Primary cancers of the spinal cord
- Glioma
- Astrocytoma
- Ependymoma

Cancers with a natural history of bone metastasis
- Breast
- Lung
- Renal
- Prostate
- Myeloma
- Melanoma

Cancers that metastasize to the spinal cord
- Seminoma
- Lymphoma
- Neuroblastoma

Figure 15-5. Cancer Types at Risk for Spinal Cord Compression

---

Note. Based on information from Hunter, 2005.

A study by Lu, Gonzalez, Jolesz, Wen, and Talcott (2005) identified four independent predictors of risk for development of SCC: abnormal neurologic examination, pain in the middle or upper back, known vertebral metastases, and metastatic disease at initial presentation. APNs can use these to be alert for patients who are at increased risk for the development of SCC.

Pathophysiology

The spinal column is composed of 33 vertebrae—7 cervical, 12 thoracic, 5 lumbar, 5 fused sacral (forming the sacrum), and 4 fused coccygeal (forming the coccyx). Between each disc (except the fused ones), an intervertebral disk exists that functions to absorb shocks and prevent damage to the vertebrae. This forms the spinal canal, which encloses and protects the spinal cord. The spinal cord is a long nerve cable that arises from the medulla oblongata and ends at the level of the first or second lumbar vertebra. The end of the spinal cord, the conus medullaris, is cone shaped, and the lumbar and sacral spinal nerve roots continue outward from it and are called the cauda equina because they resemble a horse's tail (Sugarman, 2006).

Three membranes or meninges cover the brain and spinal cord as a protective mechanism (see Figure 15-6). The innermost layer is the pia mater, which directly adheres to the brain and spinal cord. The subarachnoid space separates the pia mater from the middle membrane and the arachnoid membrane and contains the cerebrospinal fluid. The subdural space is between the arachnoid membrane and the outermost layer, the dura mater. The dura mater (Latin for *hard mother*) is a tough membrane to which the spinal nerves are attached. The space between the dura mater and the vertebral column is the epidural space, which contains the blood vessels and adipose tissue (Sugarman, 2006).

In the majority of cases, SCC results from metastatic disease developing outside the spinal cord (extradural) and invading the epidural space, causing direct compression on the cord. The main mechanism of tumor invasion of the epidural space is through hematogenous spread of malignant cells that have an affinity for spinal marrow (Prasad & Schiff, 2005). This results in a mass that enlarges and impinges on the thecal sac, anteriorly compressing the spinal cord and leading to collapse of the vertebral body and retropulsion of bony fragments into the epidural space. Primary tumors of the spinal cord are intramedullary and directly invade and destroy the cord. Another cause is lymph node growth from the paraspinal region through the vertebral neural foramen into the epidural space, as seen with lymphoma (Prasad & Schiff).

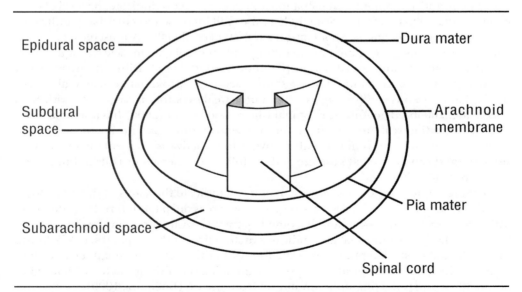

Figure 15-6. Meninges or Membranes Surrounding the Spinal Cord, With Associated Spaces

Note. From "Oncology Emergency Modules: Spinal Cord Compression," by J.A. Flounders and B.B. Ott, 2003, *Oncology Nursing Forum, 30,* p. E18. Copyright 2003 by Oncology Nursing Society. Reprinted with permission.

Neurologic defects caused by SCC are a result of direct compression on the spinal cord or cauda equina, interruption of the vascular supply to the spinal cord by tumor or bone, or compression from vertebral collapse causing bone to protrude onto the spinal cord (Flounders & Ott, 2003). Compression obstructs the normal venous blood flow in the vertebral venous plexus, resulting in vasogenic edema, swelling of the nerve axons, loss of myelin, and ischemia in the areas of compression (Byrne, 1992). Additional nerve injury results from the release of neurotoxic substances, including cytokines (interleukin-1 and interleukin-6), inflammatory mediators (prostaglandin E), and excitatory neurotransmitters (serotonin). Hypoxia of the spinal cord stimulates the production of vascular endothelial growth factor (VEGF), which increases vascular permeability and vasogenic edema. Without intervention, the vasogenic edema progresses to ischemia and cytotoxic edema, resulting in further neurologic damage that can become irreversible (Siegal, 1995).

Diagnosis and Assessment

A thorough history is important to detect early indications of SCC. Any complaint of pain in patients with cancer needs a detailed history. Back pain requires careful assessment to determine if any radicular component exists. A visual analog scale can be used to assess pain (Kaplan, 2006).

Physical Examination

The clinical manifestations of SCC correspond to the location and extent of compression. As pain is the most common presenting symptom, patients can point to the site of pain, and assessment with palpation and percussion can indicate the level of cord compression (Wilkes, 2004b). Straight leg raises will increase radicular pain, indicative of lumbar or thoracic nerve root compression (Wilkes, 2004b). A musculoskeletal examination assesses motor function, including evaluation of gait, muscle strength, involuntary movements, and coordination (Flounders & Ott, 2003). Difficulty arising from a seated position or difficulty climbing stairs is seen with proximal muscle weakness of the legs and often is the first sign of the motor weakness that is associated with SCC (Baehring, 2005b). The American Spinal Injury Association (2006) has a standardized form and grading scale to classify motor and sensory function and impairment. The grading categories are from 0 (total paralysis) to 5 (active movement against full resistance) and can be used at baseline and for follow-up assessment (Bilsky, Lis, Raizer, Lee, & Boland, 1999).

An assessment of reflexes is important and can indicate the status of the neurologic system. Normal reflexes show a brisk response, whereas deep tendon reflexes decrease with nerve root compression and become hyperactive with cord compression. A positive Babinski sign is abnormal and indicates dysfunction of the spinal tract. A Babinski sign is elicited by stroking the sole of the foot from the heel to the small toe and then arcing to the great toe. A positive response is dorsiflexion of the great toe with fanning of the other toes reflecting upper motor neuron disease (Bucholtz, 1999).

Sensory assessment should include evaluation of patients' sense of pain, temperature, touch, vibration, and position (proprioception). Careful dermatome mapping of sensory loss can indicate the level of cord damage (Bucholtz, 1999). Assessment of autonomic function also is necessary. Taking a careful history of urination is important, and a post-void residual measurement may be needed to assess for neurogenic bladder.

Change in bowel habits should be elicited, and digital rectal examination performed to assess sphincter tone. Questions about sexual function and recent onset of impotence also are important (Kaplan, 2006).

Plain films (x-rays) of the spine often are initially obtained in a patient with pain but no neurologic changes, as they are easy to obtain. Plain films can show vertebral collapse, erosion, and bone fragment dislocation, but unfortunately, they do not detect early SCC because 50% of the bone must be destroyed before it is evident on plain films (Gabriel & Schiff, 2004). Plain films also do not detect paraspinal masses that may be extending into the epidural space (Schiff, 2003). Bone scans may be useful in patients with pain alone. They are more sensitive than plain films but have limitations, as they do not provide structural detail to identify whether an epidural tumor is present (Schiff).

MRI currently is the gold standard to evaluate SCC because it is the most sensitive, specific, and accurate test for evaluating SCC. MRI allows visualization of the extent of the lesion and anatomy, detects paraspinal masses, and can image multiple levels to assess for areas of disease that are not clinically apparent (Baehring, 2005b). Myelography with or without CT scanning essentially has been replaced by MRI but is still used in patients for whom MRI is contraindicated (Baehring, 2005b).

Differential Diagnosis

Trauma, arthritis, infections, hematoma, muscle strain, epidural abscess, old vertebral injury, cauda equina syndrome, spinal cord damage from exposure to radiation, and neoplastic meningitis are other conditions to consider (Osowski, 2002). Most benign causes of SCC generally occur in the cervical or lumbar spine. Pain that worsens with lying down should be considered malignant until proved otherwise (Schiff, 2003). Radiation myelopathy occurs 9–15 months after radiation, and MRI can distinguish it from SCC (Schiff). MRI is useful to evaluate for most other conditions that may mimic SCC and can either rule in or rule out SCC.

Evidence-Based Treatment

Intervention for SCC needs to begin immediately to prevent permanent damage. Ambulatory status at the time of diagnosis is predictive of ambulation following treatment; 80%–100% of patients who are able to ambulate at diagnosis retain their ability to ambulate (Gilbert et al., 1978; Maranzano et al., 1996; Schiff, 2003). Treatment usually is considered palliative, as SCC is most commonly associated with metastatic disease (Flounders & Ott, 2003). The choice of treatment depends on several factors, including tumor type, location, rapidity of onset, radiosensitivity of the tumor, and the mechanism of cord compression (Bucholtz, 1999). The goals of treatment are to optimize quality of life with pain relief, preserve and restore neurologic function, and reduce tumor. Corticosteroids are initiated as a temporary therapy until definitive treatment with radiation or surgery, alone or in combination, can be instituted (Prasad & Schiff, 2005).

Corticosteroids decrease vasogenic edema in the spinal cord and downregulate VEGF expression, resulting in improvement in neurologic symptoms as well as pain relief. Corticosteroids also may have a direct effect on some tumors, particularly lymphoma (Schiff, 2003). Dexamethasone is the most widely used corticosteroid, usually given as a high-dose bolus initially, followed by a maintenance dose and tapered after initiation of definitive therapy. A prospective study of high-dose dexamethasone (96 mg) versus no corticosteroids showed improved outcomes in ambulation (Sorenson, Helweg-Larsen, Mouridsen, & Hansen, 1994). The recommendation in the absence of prospective randomized data is for an initial dose of 10 mg of dexamethasone IV, followed by 4 mg orally every six hours. Once the patient's condition has stabilized or improved, a slow taper is initiated every four days (Baehring, 2005b; Loblaw & Laperriere, 1998).

Radiation therapy remains the most common treatment for SCC. Indications for radiation therapy instead of surgical decompression include radiosensitive tumors, expected survival of less than three to four months, multiple levels of compression, and inability to tolerate surgery (Ferris, Bezjak, & Rosenthal, 2001; Schiff, 2003). The most frequently used dosing is 3,000 cGy in 10 daily fractions, although the optimal dose fractionation is not known (Ferris et al.; Loblaw & Laperriere, 1998; Schiff). Improvement with relief of pain usually occurs within five days of initiation of therapy (Bucholtz, 1999). Transient demyelination of spinal posterior columns and white matter necrosis can develop 12–20 weeks after therapy, causing paresthesias or Lhermitte sign, a sudden, mild, electric shock–like sensation triggered by neck flexion that radiates down the spine into the extremities (Behin & Delattre, 2004).

Indications for surgical intervention include rapidly progressing paraplegia, progression of neurologic dysfunction while receiving radiation, spinal instability, pathologic fracture with dislocation of bone fragments, biopsy for unknown tumor type, radioresistant tumors, and recurrence after previous radiation therapy (Klimo & Schmidt, 2004; Loblaw & Laperriere, 1998). A randomized clinical trial indicated an advantage for surgical intervention followed by radiation therapy, thereby increasing the chances of regaining and maintaining ambulation versus radiation alone (Patchell et al., 2005). The surgical approach depends on the tumor location, extent of tumor, type of reconstruction planned, and the general condition of the patient (Klimo & Schmidt). Anterior decompression with mechanical stabilization is the main approach for epidural metastases arising from the vertebral body because it allows for total removal of the vertebral body (Klimo & Schmidt). The anterior surgical approach allows for resection of the tumor, which then is followed by the insertion of polymethyl methacrylate (PMMA, bone cement) and instrumentation to achieve anterior stabilization (Patchell et al.). Surgery with the use of PMMA is followed by radiation therapy, with a delay of about one week. If a bone graft is used, then radiation must be delayed for six weeks to allow for fusion of the graft (Prasad & Schiff, 2005). Laminectomy has fallen out of favor, as it does not allow for complete tumor resection and increases spinal instability (Baehring, 2005b). Vertebroplasty and kyphoplasty can be used in patients who are poor surgical candidates but have pain related to their SCC (Klimo & Schmidt). Both procedures involve the percutaneous injection of PMMA into a collapsed vertebral body. In kyphoplasty, a balloon is first inflated to restore vertebral height and reduce kyphosis, and then PMMA is injected. In vertebroplasty, the vertebral body is not reexpanded, only PMMA is injected (Fourney et al., 2003). Both procedures can be performed on an outpatient basis, have rare complications, and are highly effective in reducing pain (Fourney et al.).

Chemotherapy is a treatment option for SCC in chemosensitive tumors, such as breast, lymphoma, myeloma, small cell carcinoma, or germ cell tumors. It also is useful in patients with recurrent tumors who have previously been radiated and cannot tolerate further radiation, or in nonsurgical candidates who have not responded to radiation therapy (Baehring, 2005b; Gabriel & Schiff, 2004). Chemotherapy also is used as combination therapy with radiation or as an adjunct therapy to surgery (Daw & Markman, 2000).

Implications for Advanced Nursing Practice

Timely recognition of the early signs and symptoms of SCC is critical to patients' quality of life. New onset of back or neck pain in a patient with known cancer must be evaluated as a potential cord compression. APNs must be aware of the potential for SCC and alert to any sign so that early intervention can prevent long-term complications (Osowski, 2002). No guidelines exist on the specific imaging to be done when SCC is suspected. Ruckdeschel (2005) advocated for obtaining a total spine sagittal-only view MRI with full imaging at "positive" areas in patients with new-onset back pain or change in previous symptoms within several days. Ruckdeschel showed that using the scanning MRI as the first diagnostic test was the most cost-effective and rapid means to diagnosis SCC. Based on evidence (Schiff et al., 1998) that 21% of epidural lesions are missed if thoracic and lumbar imaging is not performed, Schiff (2003) recommended thoracic and lumbar MRI at a minimum.

Other issues that APNs need to address in this patient population are pain management and prevention of constipation. As these patients are less active, deep vein thrombosis (DVT) prophylaxis is a consideration with subcutaneous heparin or sequential compression devices in moderate- to high-risk patients. Prophylaxis against DVT in patients with SCC has not been studied, nor has spinal bracing (Schiff, 2003).

Increased Intracranial Pressure

Increased ICP is an increase in normal brain pressure because of an increase in the intracranial contents from edema, hemorrhage, tumor growth, or excess cerebrospinal fluid (CSF). Increased ICP is a life-threatening complication of malignant disease that can lead to neurologic complications and death if not treated. A space-occupying lesion is the most common cause of increased ICP, either from a primary brain tumor or metastases. Early recognition and intervention are important to prevent long-term complications and death related to increased ICP (Smith & Amin-Hanjani, 2005).

Incidence

According to the American Cancer Society, an estimated 21,810 new cases of primary malignant brain tumors will be diagnosed in 2008, accounting for 1.5% of all cancers (Jemal et al., 2008). Primary brain tumors often present with symptoms of increased ICP. Brain metastases occur in approximately 24% of all patients with cancer. Brain metastases occur most frequently in lung cancer (50%), followed by breast cancer (15%–20%), unknown primary (10%–15%), melanoma (10%), and colon cancer (5%) (Lassman & DeAngelis, 2003). Other causes of ICP in patients with cancer are hemorrhage, ischemia, infection, or autoimmune inflammatory process (Baehring, 2005a).

Signs and Symptoms

The signs and symptoms of increased ICP depend on the location of the lesion and the degree of increase (see Figure 15-7). Headache is a very common presenting symptom of increased ICP. Patients often describe it as an early morning headache that subsides on rising. Bending over, coughing, or performing the Valsalva maneuver may cause or worsen the headache. It often is bilateral, located in the frontal or occipital regions, and increases in severity, frequency, and duration (Hickey, 2003).

Early Signs
- Headache—most severe in early morning
- Diplopia
- Blurred vision
- Extremity drifts
- Decreased visual fields
- Decreased visual acuity
- Change in level of consciousness (LOC)
- Lethargy, apathy, confusion, restlessness
- Gastrointestinal: Loss of appetite, nausea, occasional/unusual vomiting

Late Signs
- Abnormal posturing
- Temperature elevations
- Cardiovascular: Bradycardia, hypotension, widening pulse pressure
- Respiratory: Slow, shallow respirations, tachypnea, Cheyne-Stokes respirations
- Neurologic: Decreased ability to concentrate, decreased LOC, personality changes, hemiplegia, hemiparesis, seizures, pupil changes, papilledema (cardinal sign)
- Cushing triad (hypertension with a widening pulse pressure, bradycardia, and abnormal respirations)

Figure 15-7. Signs and Symptoms of Increased Intracranial Pressure

Note. Based on information from Arbour, 1998; Hickey, 2003.

Changes in mental status, including altered level of consciousness, confusion, short-term memory loss, and personality changes, may occur with increased ICP. Patients may note decreased attention span, drowsiness, and memory loss, whereas family members may note mood changes, irritability, poor judgment, and decreased reasoning (Arbour, 1998). Diplopia, blurred vision, decreased visual fields, and decreased visual acuity are other neurologic symptoms associated with increased ICP. Vomiting unrelated to food intake that is sudden and projectile can occur with increased ICP (Hickey, 2003). Other focal signs and symptoms of increased ICP are related to the location of the tumor and can assist APNs in localizing the affected area. These include hemiparesis, aphasia, new-onset seizures, hemisensory loss, cranial nerve deficits, and personality changes (Hickey). Involvement of the frontal lobe will affect higher-level function, personality with emotional lability or flat affect, and difficulty in concentration, problem solving, and vigilance. Speech deficits, such as word finding, and motor weakness with focal seizure activity can occur with involvement of the posterior frontal lobe. Parietal lobe tumors cause deficits in sensation, inability to recognize common objects, and neglect syndrome (a lack of awareness of the opposite side of the body) as well as seizure activity. Temporal lobe involvement results in short-term memory loss, weakness, and visual field deficits. Cerebellar signs are ataxia, incoordination, nystagmus, vertigo, and nausea (Hickey).

Papilledema is a late sign of increased ICP. It is almost always bilateral and does not affect the vision. An increase in CSF pressure around the optic nerve that impairs the outflow of venous blood, leading to edema and swelling of the optic disk, causes papilledema (Hickey, 2003). Altered vital signs typically are a late finding of increased ICP. Elevated temperature and Cheyne-Stokes respirations emerge in the decompensatory phase. Cushing triad, a combination of hypertension with a widening pulse pressure, bradycardia, and abnormal respirations, is a late finding, and the patient usually is comatose (Cushing, 1902). As increased ICP progresses, pressure on the brain stem causes loss or dysfunction of papillary, corneal, and gag reflexes, and motor dysfunction progresses to hemiplegia, decortications, or decerebration (Hickey).

Risk Factors and Etiology

Increased ICP is the result of increasing edema, hemorrhage, infection, infarction, or tumor mass. Primary or metastatic lesions can expand, taking up space, which leads to increased ICP. These lesions also can have associated edema or hemorrhage. Patients with tumors that metastasize to the brain are at risk for increased ICP. Tumors associated with brain metastases include lung, breast, colon, testicular, and melanoma (Lassman & DeAngelis, 2003). Primary brain tumors or tumors of the spinal cord can cause increased ICP. Patients with leukemia with high blast counts are at risk for increased ICP because of leukostasis that can cause diffuse cerebral edema. Increased ICP associated with leukemia also may be a result of hemorrhage because of coagulopathy or thrombocytopenia (Baehring, 2005a). Leptomeningeal metastasis or involvement can cause increased ICP resulting from obstruction of CSF flow (Graus, Rogers, & Posner, 1985). Syndrome of inappropriate antidiuretic hormone secretion can cause increased ICP, as can brain radiation because of edema (Wilkes, 2004a).

Nonmalignant causes of increased ICP include intracranial hemorrhage that can occur with traumatic brain injury, ruptured aneurysm, arteriovenous malformation, or other vascular anomalies (Smith & Amin-Hanjani, 2005). CNS infections, such as viral encephalitis, toxoplasmosis, aspergillosis, and candidiasis, or infections from an Ommaya reservoir may cause edema that can result in ICP (Hickey, 2003). Other nonmalignant causes of increased ICP are vasculitis, ischemic infarcts, hydrocephalus, and pseudotumor cerebri (Smith & Amin-Hanjani). Pseudotumor cerebri (benign intracranial hypertension) is seen most often in obese adolescent girls and young women and presents with headache, blurred vision, and papilledema (Hickey).

Pathophysiology

The intracranial cavity is a nonexpandable, closed compartment that contains three components: the brain parenchyma, CSF, and vascular tissue or blood. ICP is the pressure normally exerted by the CSF as it circulates around the brain, spinal cord, and within the ventricles. ICP is normally 5–15 mm Hg, and pathologic intracranial hypertension (commonly called increased ICP) is present at pressures greater than or equal to 20 mm Hg (Smith & Amin-Hanjani, 2005).

The first compensatory mechanism of the CNS with increasing ICP is to displace the CSF out of the cranial vault. If ICP remains high, then cerebral blood volume is altered, causing stage 1 intracranial hypertension. Vasoconstriction occurs in an attempt to decrease the ICP. If the pressure does not decrease, a state of intracranial hypertension (increased ICP) occurs. Stage 2 intracranial hypertension occurs next. Neuronal oxygenation is compromised, and systemic arterial vasoconstriction occurs, which elevates the systemic blood pressure. Hypoxia and hypercapnia begin to occur in the brain tissue. As compensatory mechanisms are exhausted, autoregulation (the ability of the brain to maintain a constant rate of cerebral blood flow regardless of variations in systemic arterial pressure and venous drainage) fails, and ICP increases. Carbon dioxide accumulates, causing vasodilation and edema and leading to increased blood volume and stage 3 intracranial hypertension (increased ICP). ICP approaches systemic blood pressure at this stage, thus resulting in cerebral pressure and perfusion decrease, causing the brain tissue to experience severe hypoxia and acidosis (Boss & Wilkerson, 2006).

If increased ICP is not reversed at this point, stage 4 intracranial hypertension (increased ICP) occurs. In stage 4 intracranial hypertension, the brain shifts or herniates because of the pressure. The herniating tissue's blood supply is further compromised, causing ischemia and hypoxia. Herniation leads to a rapid increase in ICP, and when it equals mean systolic arterial pressure, cerebral blood flow ceases (Boss & Wilkerson, 2006).

Diagnosis and Assessment

The clinical manifestations of increased ICP depend on the location of the abnormality and the degree of increased ICP. A CT scan often is performed initially to evaluate for changes in brain structure, such as hemorrhage, hydrocephalus, or mass with associated edema, as it can quickly image acute changes (Schaefer, Budzik, & Gonzalez, 1996). MRI is a superior imaging modality that provides better definition of lesions and edema (Sze, Milano, & Johnson, 1990). Magnetic resonance angiography is a useful modality to assess vascular abnormalities and has replaced angiography as an imaging tool for increased ICP (Schaefer et al.). Positron-emission tomography (PET) is used to distinguish between tumor and radiation necrosis. Single-photon emission computed tomography can differentiate between infiltrating tumor and solid tumor. A CT-guided stereotactic biopsy may be performed for tissue diagnosis (Schaefer et al.). A lumbar puncture can be useful to determine a causative infectious agent or assess for leptomeningeal metastasis but must be done with caution and after definitive imaging, because of the chance of brain herniation with pressure changes (Wilkes, 2004a).

History taking is important and should include history of cancer to assess the potential for metastatic disease. Headache is a common, nonspecific complaint. Increased ICP will cause an early morning headache that is bilateral and aggravated by coughing, bending, or performing the Valsalva maneuver. It will increase in frequency, severity, and duration as ICP increases (Hickey, 2003).

Physical Examination

Assessment of visual acuity and extraocular movements will determine cranial nerve impairment and brain stem functioning (Clancey, 2006). Cranial nerve II (the optic nerve) is evaluated by assessing visual acuity and fields. Cranial nerve III (the oculomotor nerve) is assessed with pupil size, shape, and symmetry (Wilkes, 2004a). Evaluating extraocular movements assesses cranial nerves IV (trochlear) and V (abducens), as well as cranial nerve III. Testing extraocular movement involves having the patient follow the clinician's finger through the six cardinal gazes as the clinician draws an "H" shape and evaluates for nystagmus in the upward and lateral gazes (Wilkes, 2004a). Funduscopic examination assesses for papilledema, which may be seen because of congestion of blood flow (Smith & Amin-Hanjani, 2005).

Assessment of motor defects is necessary, including coordination and balance problems as well as weakness with heel to toe walking, Romberg, finger to nose, and gait. Clinicians need to assess patients' level of consciousness, with evaluation for agitation, confusion, restlessness, or lethargy (Wilkes, 2004a). The Glasgow coma scale (see Table 15-3) can be used to assess neurologic status by evaluating eye opening response, motor response, and verbal response with a score assigned to each. A total score of 15 is best and 3 is worst, and patients with a score lower than 8 are considered to be comatose. The exam is limited in that it does not account for paraplegia or absent lower extremity function (Cho & Wang, 1997).

Changes in vital signs occur as increased ICP continues and should be assessed regularly. Cushing triad is a late and ominous finding consisting of hypertension with a widening pulse pressure, bradycardia, and abnormal respirations (Cushing, 1902).

Differential Diagnosis

The differential diagnosis for increased ICP includes ruptured aneurysm, arteriovenous malformation, ischemic infarcts, cerebral abscess, meningitis, trauma, hydrocephalus, pseudotumor cerebri, and vasculitis (Smith & Amin-Hanjani, 2005). A thorough history is helpful to begin to distinguish among these entities. As noted previously, pseudotumor cerebri is commonly seen in young women. Patients with meningitis or abscess are likely to have a fever. Patients with vasculitis usually have an elevated sedimentation rate. Imaging studies are needed to distinguish between the other diagnoses.

Table 15-3. Glasgow Coma Scale

Response	Score
Eye opening	
• Spontaneous	4
• To sound	3
• To pain	2
• Never	1
Motor response	
• Obeys commands	6
• Localized pain	5
• Normal flexion (withdrawal)	4
• Abnormal flexion	3
• Extension	1
• None	0
Verbal response	
• Oriented	5
• Confused conversation	4
• Inappropriate words	3
• Incomprehensible sounds	2
• None	1

Note. Based on information from Cho & Wang, 1997.

Evidence-Based Treatment

Early recognition and prompt intervention are needed to decrease adverse outcomes related to increased ICP. Reducing cerebral edema and controlling symptoms while determining and treating the cause of increased ICP is the goal of intervention (Smith & Amin-Hanjani, 2005). Initial intervention includes managing factors that can further increase ICP. These factors include hypercapnia, hypoxemia, respiratory procedures, vasodilating drugs, body positioning, Valsalva maneuver, coughing, emotional upset, noxious stimuli (such as invasive procedures), and clustering of nursing activities (Hickey, 2003).

Corticosteroids are effective in treating vasogenic edema caused by tumors. Corticosteroids are thought to decrease capillary permeability and promote extracellular fluid resorption, but the exact mechanism is unknown (Sitton, 1998). Steroids are initiated prior to radiation therapy or other definitive therapy and tapered to the lowest dose needed to control neurologic symptoms once definitive therapy becomes effective (Lassman & DeAngelis, 2003). Dosing is variable but generally is an IV bolus of 10–24 mg of dexamethasone followed by 2–6 mg every six hours (Lassman & DeAngelis).

Mannitol is an osmotic diuretic that draws free water out of the extracellular space in the edematous brain tissues into the circulation, where it is excreted by the kidneys, resulting in reduction of brain volume by dehydrating the brain parenchyma (Smith & Amin-Hanjani, 2005). Mannitol therapy is directed at keeping the serum osmolality at 310–315 mOsm; the maximal effect should occur within 15–30 minutes and can last for one to three hours. Dosing is 0.25–0.5 g/kg up to 1 g/kg every three to six hours as an IV bolus (Hickey, 2003). A rebound effect can occur, and furosemide, a loop diuretic, often is used to manage the resultant increase in ICP (Hickey).

Avoidance of hypotension with fluid bolus or vasopressors is important, as hypotension can lead to cerebral ischemia and secondary brain injury (Smith & Amin-Hanjani, 2005). Fever increases brain metabolism and cerebral blood flow; therefore, aggressive treatment of fever with antipyretics is important. Fluid management is needed to avoid dehydration, which causes decreased cerebral perfusion and ischemia. Using isotonic saline prevents hyponatremia, as it can further increase ICP by causing cerebral edema (Hickey, 2003). Analgesics are used to treat pain, and sedation may be necessary to decrease restlessness and anxiety, as all can increase ICP (Shapiro et al., 1995). Morphine sulfate is the preferred analgesic and can be effective in controlling pain and providing sedation, with fentanyl and hydromorphone as alternatives (Hickey). Lorazepam is the preferred drug for prolonged treatment of anxiety (Shapiro et al.).

Seizures can contribute to increased ICP as well as complicate it, so anticonvulsant therapy should be given if seizures are suspected or prophylactically in some settings. No clear guidelines exist for prophylaxis of seizures, but prophylaxis should be considered in high-risk patients who have lesions within the supratentorial cortical locations or adjacent to the cortex (subdural hematomas or subarachnoid hemorrhage) (Smith & Amin-Hanjani, 2005). Phenytoin 100 mg three to four times per day is the most common agent used with increased ICP, and carbamazepine is an alternative (Hickey, 2003).

Mechanical hyperventilation is a rapid method to decrease ICP in conjunction with osmotic therapy (Hickey, 2003). Mechanical hyperventilation lowers the $PaCO_2$ (partial pressure of arterial carbon dioxide) to 26–30 mm Hg, resulting in vasoconstriction and decreased cerebral blood volume. The effect is of short duration, lasting from 1–24 hours, so more definitive therapy is needed (Baehring, 2005a; Smith & Amin-Hanjani, 2005). Elevation of the head of the bed to 30° facilitates jugular venous drainage, thus lowering ICP (Hickey).

Surgery is indicated for life-threatening increased ICP to resect or debulk tumor or hematoma, thereby providing decompression. Ventriculoperitoneal shunt placement also can be performed to provide a pathway for CSF drainage in select patients, such as patients with gait apraxia, precipitate micturition, and cognitive decline, who are most likely to respond (Baehring, 2005a). Shunting should be avoided in patients with leptomeningeal tumor to prevent seeding of the peritoneum (Baehring, 2005a).

Radiation therapy is another intervention that is useful in treating radiosensitive tumors, either primary or metastatic. It can be used as definitive therapy of the underlying cause of increased ICP once the acute symptoms are managed (Lassman & DeAngelis, 2003). Stereotactic external beam radiation or radiosurgery is useful to treat small lesions and decrease radiation exposure to normal tissue or as an adjunct to surgical resection (Lassman & DeAngelis). Stereotactic radiosurgery uses computerized treatment planning and multiple angles to allow for delivery of higher doses to the lesion while sparing normal surrounding brain tissue. It is useful in treating one to three lesions that are less than 3.5 cm in size (Sanghavi et al., 2001).

Leptomeningeal carcinomatosis is treated with intrathecal chemotherapy (Baehring, 2005a). Agents used for intrathecal treatment are methotrexate and cytarabine. High-dose methotrexate can be used to treat CNS metastases, with dose ranges from 3.5–8 g/m² (Glantz et al., 1998; Lassman et al., 2006). Temozolomide also has shown effectiveness in treating CNS metastases (Abrey et al., 2001).

Implications for Advanced Nursing Practice

Increased ICP is an oncologic emergency that can lead to death without prompt intervention. Assessment, recognition, and treatment of early signs and symptoms are critical. Management of increased ICP requires a combined effort with oncology, neurosurgery, and radiation therapy. APNs play an important role in the recognition and coordination of care in patients with increased ICP.

Nursing management of patients with increased ICP is complex. Factors known to increase ICP include many nursing activities. Positioning is important, with the head of the bed at 30° and proper alignment when turning and positioning. Bowel management is necessary to prevent constipation, which can lead to straining. A quiet room is important with avoidance of sudden jarring of the bed or other painful stimuli to avoid increases in ICP. Clustering of nursing activities, such as assessment, turning, bathing, or suctioning, needs to be considered, as these activities can increase ICP (Hickey, 2003). Patient and family education is an essential need in this setting.

Conclusion

The importance of having an awareness of structural oncologic emergencies cannot be over emphasized. These emergencies can have a significant impact on patients' quality of life. Early assessment and intervention are critical to allow patients to maintain independence. An understanding of the presentation, etiology, pathophysiology, differential diagnosis, and treatment allows APNs to anticipate and intervene early.

Case Study

S.K. is a 23-year-old white female who presents with complaints of shortness of breath and facial swelling, particularly in the morning. She has no past medical or surgical history and works out regularly at the gym. She notes that for the past several weeks she has been fatigued and has not been to the gym. Despite not working out for several weeks, she has lost 10 pounds. She has noticed feeling warm/feverish in the evenings but has not taken her temperature. Upon questioning, she admits that she has had a dry nonproductive cough for the past few days. Initially, the shortness of breath only occurred with exertion, but now at times she is winded even at rest. She has begun to use several pillows at night in order to sleep. She also has noted swelling of her right breast.

The APN examines S.K. and notes that she has a prominent venous pattern on her chest and her right breast is larger than the left breast. She is tachycardic. She is unable to lie flat on the exam table without becoming significantly short of breath and developing flushing. S.K. has palpable lymphadenopathy in the supraclavicular areas, right greater than left, with the largest node measuring 2 cm. She also has bilateral axillary lymphadenopathy.

The APN initially obtains a chest x-ray (because she can send S.K. for it immediately). The chest x-ray shows a large anterior mediastinal mass. The APN knows that a tissue diagnosis is needed to design an appropriate treatment plan. She suspects Hodgkin or non-Hodgkin lymphoma and contacts a surgeon to arrange a biopsy. A CT of the chest, abdomen, and pelvis will be obtained, as well as an echocardiogram and bone marrow biopsy.

The echocardiogram showed an ejection fraction of greater than 55% and normal wall motion. CT scan showed edema in the right neck area; enlarged lymph nodes in both neck areas, right greater than left; bilateral axillary lymph nodes; a large mediastinal mass obstructing the SVC; and no obvious abdominal disease. Her LDH was elevated at 1,235 u/L (normal is < 600). The bone marrow biopsy showed no evidence of disease. A right supraclavicular node biopsy showed an anaplastic large cell lymphoma.

S.K. begins rituximab, cyclophosphamide, doxorubicin, vincristine, and prednisone (R-CHOP) chemotherapy given peripherally via the left arm. Allopurinol is initiated to prevent tumor lysis. Within a few days, she notes a decrease in the size of her right breast, improvement in her breathing, and a decrease in the size of the lymph nodes. At the time of her second cycle of chemotherapy, she had clear improvement, and her LDH had returned to normal. She completed six cycles of R-CHOP chemotherapy, and six weeks after completion, a PET scan was negative. She then received low-dose involved-field radiation for consolidation.

At routine follow-up three months after completing therapy, S.K. is doing well. Her chest x-ray is negative and LDH normal. She is scheduled to return in three months.

S.K. calls the office three weeks after her visit, stating she is worried that her disease had recurred. She is again experiencing shortness of breath and cough. She feels very anxious and is having chest pain when she lies down. The APN is concerned and tells her to come in immediately for evaluation.

On examination, S.K. is tachycardic, hypotensive, with jugular venous distention, and has a pulsus paradoxus of 22 mm. An EKG shows low voltage with T wave inversions. A CT scan shows a moderate to large pericardial effusion and recurrent mediastinal mass with LDH elevated at 960 u/L. An echocardiogram reveals a large pericardial effusion with respiratory flow variation and right atrial and ventricle diastolic collapse.

S.K. is taken emergently to the operating room for a subxiphoid pericardial window, where 700 ml of fluid is removed and sent for cytology. The fluid was an exudate with elevated protein level and LDH. Cytopathology demonstrates recurrent lymphoma.

S.K. begins salvage chemotherapy for recurrence of her disease with etoposide, methylprednisolone, cisplatin, and cytarabine (ESHAP). Her LDH improves after one cycle, and evaluation for autologous stem cell transplant is initiated. After completion of her second cycle, while her counts were still recovering, she notes an enlarged lymph node in the left neck. Her LDH was 1,054. She also complains of back pain. She notes it had started 7–10 days earlier while she was in the hospital for the chemotherapy, and she thought it was caused by the hospital bed. The pain has not improved and wraps around to her chest. She describes it as a burning discomfort that is worse with coughing or laughing. She also notes that it is worse if she lies down, so she has been sleeping in a recliner for the past few days.

On examination, S.K. points to the area of T10 and with palpation has pain. The APN arranges a total spine MRI. The APN elects to get an MRI because it is the gold standard and detects paraspinal masses. The MRI shows a paraspinal mass at T10.

The APN starts S.K. on corticosteroids to decrease the edema. Radiation oncology is consulted, as lymphoma is a radiosensitive tumor. S.K. clearly is in a difficult situation, because her disease has progressed on therapy. She needs to show a response to some type of therapy (further salvage therapy or experimental therapy) so that she can proceed to stem cell transplant.

1. What signs and symptoms does S.K. have that are concerning for SVCS?
    - Facial swelling in the morning, shortness of breath, prominent venous pattern on her chest, swollen right breast, tachycardia, inability to lie flat on the exam table, and flushing.
    - All of these are seen in SVCS and should make that the top diagnosis the APN needs to rule out or in. The finding of lymphadenopathy adds to the concern because it is worrisome for lymphoma, which would be a cause of SVCS in a young woman.

2. Why is the APN concerned when S.K. calls complaining of shortness of breath and cough shortly after an office visit?
    - The APN knows that oncologic emergencies can occur at any time, and the onset of shortness of breath and cough could indicate cardiac tamponade because dyspnea is the most common symptom. S.K. also had mentioned that she had chest pain when lying down and felt anxious, which increased the APN's concern.

3. Which test confirmed that S.K. had cardiac tamponade?
    A. EKG
    B. MRI
    C. CT scan
    D. Echocardiogram
    - The answer is D: Echocardiogram is the diagnostic test of choice in cardiac tamponade. The classic finding on echocardiogram that is suggestive of cardiac tamponade is diastolic collapse of the right atrium and ventricle because of the pressure of the increased pericardial fluid. Other findings on echocardiogram include swinging heart, left atrial and ventricular collapse, inspiratory changes in ventricle size, and inferior vena cava plethora (an excess build-up of fluid in the vena cava). A routine chest x-ray is not diagnostic of cardiac tamponade but may demonstrate an enlarged cardiac silhouette as a result of increased fluid in the pericardial sac and raise suspicion leading to further testing. EKG changes are nonspecific and include low-voltage QRS complex, tachycardia, nonspecific ST-T changes, and premature atrial or ventricular contractions.

4. Why does the APN order a total spine MRI on S.K. when she complains of back pain?
    - By taking a history, the APN determined that the pain is radicular (wrapping around the chest) and worsens with coughing and laughing. It also is worse with lying down, making it more likely to be caused by malignancy. The APN orders a total spine MRI because MRI allows visualization of the extent of the lesion and anatomy, detects paraspinal masses, and can image multiple levels to assess for areas of disease that are not clinically apparent.

5. How does a paraspinal mass cause cord compression?
    - Lymph nodes in the paraspinal region can grow through the vertebral neural foramen into the epidural space in lymphoma.

Key Points

Superior Vena Cava Syndrome

- The most common signs and symptoms of SVCS are cough, dyspnea, face or neck swelling, upper extremity swelling, and dilated chest veins.
- The treatment of SVCS is based on the etiology, the severity of symptoms, the underlying malignancy, the presence of thrombosis, and the patient's prognosis.

Cardiac Tamponade

- The clinical manifestations of cardiac tamponade depend on the rapidity of fluid accumulation, the amount of fluid, and the patient's baseline cardiac function.
- Echocardiogram is the most precise diagnostic test for cardiac tamponade; it is painless and noninvasive and allows for assessment of the location and quantity of fluid and overall cardiac function.

Spinal Cord Compression

- Pain is the presenting symptom in 95% of the cases of SCC; without intervention, it progresses to motor weakness, sensory loss, autonomic dysfunction, and paralysis.
- The first sign of motor weakness often is difficulty arising from a seated position or climbing stairs because of proximal muscle weakness of the legs.
- The treatment of choice for SCC depends on the tumor type, location, rapidity of onset, radiosensitivity of tumor, and mechanism of cord compression.
- The goals of treatment are preservation and restoration of neurologic function, relief of pain, optimization of quality of life, and reduction of tumor.

Increased Intracranial Pressure

- Primary or metastatic brain lesions can cause increased ICP by tumor growth, edema of surrounding tissue, or obstruction of CSF.
- Early morning headache that worsens with bending over, coughing, or performing the Valsalva maneuver and increases in severity, frequency, and duration is a common sign of increased ICP.

Study Guide—Glossary of Terms

- Babinski sign—elicited by stroking the sole of the foot from the heel to the small toe and then arcing to the great toe. A positive response is dorsiflexion of the great toe with fanning of the other toes reflecting upper motor neuron disease.
- Beck triad—consists of elevated CVP, hypotension, and distant heart sounds
- Cushing triad—a combination of hypertension with a widening pulse pressure, bradycardia, and abnormal respirations. This is a late finding, and the patient usually is comatose.
- Electrical alternans—a rare EKG finding showing a variation in the height of the QRS amplitudes with alternating beats caused by the swinging of the heart in the fluid-filled pericardium

- Hepatojugular reflux—an elevation of the jugular venous pressure by 1 cm or more. To assess, place the patient supine with the head of the bed elevated so that jugular venous pulsations are visible. Exert pressure for 30–60 seconds over the right upper quadrant of the abdomen, and observe for increased jugular venous pressure, which is a result of elevated CVP.
- Horner syndrome—consists of unilateral ptosis, constricted pupil, and ipsilateral loss of sweating from pressure on the cervical sympathetic nerves
- Pulsus paradoxus—measured by inflating the blood pressure cuff 20 mm Hg above the systolic pressure and slowly deflating the cuff. The first systolic pressure reading heard during exhalation is noted. The systolic pressure reading heard during both inspiration and exhalation then is noted. If the difference between the two sounds is greater than 10 mm Hg, the patient has pulsus paradoxus.
- Stoke sign—swelling in the face, neck, arm, and hand

Recommended Resources for Oncology Advanced Practice Nurses

- Kaplan, M. (Ed.). (2006). *Understanding and managing oncologic emergencies: A resource for nurses.* Pittsburgh, PA: Oncology Nursing Society.
- A good source for the latest treatment and research on any medical subject is www .UpToDate.com. It requires a subscription, but some institutions will have an institutional subscription for all employees to use. It is good for oncology subjects but also for primary care issues that APNs encounter in practice.
- A resource for patients is the Cancer.Net (formerly People Living With Cancer) Web site (www.cancer.net/cancer/cancer.html), which is sponsored by the American Society of Clinical Oncology. Cancer.Net covers more than 120 types of cancer or cancer-related syndromes, including information on side effects and treatment, and lists links to other reputable sites. This is helpful to guide patients to Web sites that provide accurate information.

References

Abner, A. (1993). Approach to the patient who presents with superior vena cava obstruction. *Chest, 103*(Suppl. 4), 394S–397S.

Abrey, L.E., Olson, J.D., Raizer, J.J., Mack, M., Rodavitch, A., Boutros, D.Y., et al. (2001). A phase II trial of temozolomide for patients with recurrent or progressive brain metastases. *Journal of Neuro-Oncology, 53,* 259–265.

American Spinal Injury Association. (2006). *ASIA impairment scale.* Retrieved March 30, 2008, from http://www.asia-spinalinjury.org/publications/2006_Classif_worksheet.pdf

Anderson, P.R., & Coia, L.R. (2000). Fractionation and outcomes with palliative radiation therapy. *Seminars in Radiation Oncology, 10,* 191–199.

Arbour, R. (1998). Aggressive management of intracranial dynamics. *Critical Care Nurse, 18*(3), 30–40.

Armstrong, B.A., Perez, C.A., Simpson, J.R., & Hederman, M.A. (1987). Role of irradiation in the management of superior vena cava syndrome. *International Journal of Radiation Oncology, Biology, Physics, 13,* 531–539.

Aurora, R., Milite, F., & Vander Els, N.J. (2000). Respiratory emergencies. *Seminars in Oncology, 27,* 256–269.

Baehring, J.M. (2005a). Oncologic emergencies: Increased intracranial pressure. In V.T. DeVita, Jr., S. Hellman, & S.A. Rosenberg (Eds.), *Cancer: Principles and practice of oncology* (7th ed., pp. 2281–2287). Philadelphia: Lippincott Williams & Wilkins.

Baehring, J.M. (2005b). Oncologic emergencies: Spinal cord compression. In V.T. DeVita, Jr., S. Hellman, & S.A. Rosenberg (Eds.), *Cancer: Principles and practice of oncology* (7th ed., pp. 2287–2292). Philadelphia: Lippincott Williams & Wilkins.

Beauchamp, K. (1998). Pericardial tamponade: An oncologic emergency. *Clinical Journal of Oncology Nursing, 2*, 85–95.

Beck, C.S. (1935). Two cardiac compression triads. *JAMA, 104*, 714–716.

Behin, A., & Delattre, J.Y. (2004). Complications of radiation therapy on the brain and spinal cord. *Seminars in Neurology, 24*, 405–417.

Bern, M.M., Lokich, J.J., Wallach, S.R., Bothe, A., Benotti, P.N., Arkin, C.F., et al. (1990). Very low doses of warfarin can prevent thrombosis in central venous catheters. A randomized prospective trial. *Annals of Internal Medicine, 112*, 423–428.

Bilsky, M.H., Lis, E., Raizer, J., Lee, H., & Boland, P. (1999). The diagnosis and treatment of metastatic spinal tumor. *Oncologist, 4*, 459–469.

Boss, B.J., & Wilkerson, R.R. (2006). Concepts of neurologic dysfunction. In K.L. McCance & S.E. Huether (Eds.), *Pathophysiology: The biologic basis for disease in adults and children* (5th ed., pp. 491–546). St. Louis, MO: Mosby.

Braunwald, E. (2005). Pericardial disease. In D.L. Kasper, E. Braunwald, A.S. Fauci, S.L. Hauser, D.L. Longo, & J.L. Jameson (Eds.), *Harrison's principles of internal medicine* (16th ed., pp. 1414–1420). New York: McGraw-Hill.

Bucholtz, J. (1999). Metastatic epidural spinal cord compression. *Seminars in Oncology Nursing, 15*, 150–159.

Byrne, T.N. (1992). Spinal cord compression from epidural metastases. *New England Journal of Medicine, 327*, 614–619.

Calligaro, K.D., Kansagra, A., Dougherty, M.J., Savarese, R.P., & DeLaurentis, D.A. (1995). Thrombolysis to treat arterial thrombotic complications of heparin-induced thrombocytopenia. *Annals of Vascular Surgery, 9*, 397–400.

Carran, T.S. (2007). Cardiac tamponade. In F.J. Domino (Ed.), *The 5-minute clinical consult* (pp. 212–213). Philadelphia: Lippincott Williams & Wilkins.

Cham, W.C., Freiman, A., Carstens, P.H., & Chu, F.C. (1975). Radiation therapy of cardiac and pericardial metastases. *Radiology, 114*, 701–704.

Cho, D.Y., & Wang, Y.C. (1997). Comparison of the APACHE III, APACHE II and Glasgow Coma Scale in acute head injury for prediction of mortality and functional outcome. *Intensive Care Medicine, 23*, 77–84.

Chodirker, W.B. (2000). Reactions to altepase in patients with acute thrombotic stroke [Comment]. *Canadian Medical Association Journal, 163*, 387–389.

Chong, H.H., & Plotnick, G.D. (1995). Pericardial effusion and tamponade: Evaluation, imaging modalities, and management. *Comprehensive Therapy, 21*, 378–385.

Clancey, J.K. (2006). Increased intracranial pressure. In M. Kaplan (Ed.), *Understanding and managing oncologic emergencies: A resource for nurses* (pp. 99–121). Pittsburgh, PA: Oncology Nursing Society.

Clifton, G.D., & Smith, M.D. (1986). Thrombolytic therapy in heparin-associated thrombocytopenia with thrombosis. *Clinical Pharmacology, 5*, 597–601.

Cushing, H.W. (1902). Some experimental and clinical observations concerning states of increased intracranial tension. *American Journal of the Medical Sciences, 124*, 375–400.

Davenport, D., Feree, C., Blake, D., & Raben, M. (1978). Radiation therapy in the treatment of superior vena caval obstruction. *Cancer, 42*, 2600–2604.

Daw, H.A., & Markman, M. (2000). Epidural spinal cord compression in cancer patients: Diagnosis and management. *Cleveland Clinic Journal of Medicine, 67*, 497–504.

Drews, R.E. (2005, October 18). *Superior vena cava syndrome* [UpToDate version 14.3]. Retrieved April 18, 2007, from http://www.uptodate.com

Estes, M.E. (1985). Management of the cardiac tamponade patient: A nursing framework. *Critical Care Nurse, 5*(5), 17–26.

Ferris, F.D., Bezjak, A., & Rosenthal, S.G. (2001). The palliative uses of radiation therapy in surgical oncology patients. *Surgical Oncology Clinics of North America, 10*, 185–201.

Flounders, J.A. (2003a). Cardiovascular emergencies: Pericardial effusion and cardiac tamponade [Online exclusive]. *Oncology Nursing Forum, 30*, E48–E55.

Flounders, J.A. (2003b). Superior vena cava syndrome [Online exclusive]. *Oncology Nursing Forum, 30*, E84–E88.

Flounders, J.A., & Ott, B.B. (2003). Oncology emergency modules: Spinal cord compression [Online exclusive]. *Oncology Nursing Forum, 30*, E17–E23.

Fourney, D.R., Schomer, D.F., Nader, R., Chlan-Fourney, J., Suki, D., Ahrar, K., et al. (2003). Percutaneous vertebroplasty and kyphoplasty for painful vertebral body fractures in cancer patients. *Journal of Neurosurgery, 98*(Suppl. 1), 21–30.

Gabriel, K., & Schiff, D. (2004). Metastatic spinal cord compression by solid tumors. *Seminars in Neurology, 24,* 375–383.

Gilbert, R.W., Kim, J.H., & Posner, J.B. (1978). Epidural spinal cord compression from metastatic tumor: Diagnosis and treatment. *Annals of Neurology, 3,* 40–51.

Glantz, M.J., Cole, B.F., Recht, L., Akerley, W., Mills, P., & Saris, S. (1998). High-dose intravenous methotrexate for patients with nonleukemic leptomeningeal cancer: Is intrathecal chemotherapy necessary? *Journal of Clinical Oncology, 16,* 1561–1567.

Grannis, F.W., Lily, L., Cullinane, C.A., & Wagman, L.D. (2005). Fluid complications. In R. Pazdur, L.R. Coia, W.J. Hoskins, & L.D. Wagman (Eds.), *Cancer management: A multidisciplinary approach* (9th ed., pp. 1035–1050). Melville, NY: PRR.

Graus, F., Rogers, L.R., & Posner, J.B. (1985). Cerebrovascular complications in patients with cancer. *Medicine, 64,* 16–35.

Gray, B.H., Olin, J.W., Graor, R.A., Young, J.R., Bartholomew, J.R., & Ruschhaupt, W.F. (1991). Safety and efficacy of thrombolytic therapy for superior vena cava syndrome. *Chest, 99,* 54–59.

Greenberg, H.S., Kim, J.H., & Posner, J.B. (1980). Epidural spinal cord compression from metastatic tumor: Results with a new treatment protocol. *Annals of Neurology, 8,* 361–366.

Greenberg, S., Kosinski, R., & Daniels, J. (1991). Treatment of superior vena cava thrombosis with recombinant tissue type plasminogen activator. *Chest, 99,* 1298–1301.

Haapoja, I., & Blendowski, C. (1999). Superior vena cava syndrome. *Seminars in Oncology Nursing, 15,* 183–189.

Hawley, J., Dreher, H.M., & Vasso, M. (2003). Under pressure: Treating cardiac tamponade. *Nursing Management, 34*(2), 44D–44H.

Helms, S.R., & Carlson, M.D. (1989). Cardiovascular emergencies. *Seminars in Oncology, 16,* 463–470.

Helweg-Larsen, S., Sorensen, P.S., & Kreiner, S. (2000). Prognostic factors in metastatic spinal cord compression: A prospective study using multivariate analysis of variables influencing survival and gait function in 153 patients. *Journal of Radiation Oncology, Biology, Physics, 46,* 1163–1169.

Hickey, J.V. (2003). Intracranial hypertension: Theory and management of increases in intracranial pressure. In J.V. Hickey (Ed.), *The clinical practice of neurological and neurosurgical nursing* (5th ed., pp. 286–315). Philadelphia: Lippincott Williams & Wilkins.

Hochrein, J., Bashore, T.M., O'Laughlin, M.P., & Harrison, J.K. (1998). Percutaneous stenting of superior vena cava syndrome: A case report and review of the literature. *American Journal of Medicine, 104,* 78–84.

Hunter, J.C. (2005). Structural emergencies. In J.K. Itano & K.N. Taoka (Eds.), *Core curriculum for oncology nursing* (4th ed., pp. 422–439). Philadelphia: Saunders.

Hunter, W. (1757). History of an aneurysm of the aorta, with some remarks on aneurysms in general. *Medical Observations and Inquiries, 1,* 323–357.

Husband, D.J. (1998). Malignant spinal cord compression: Prospective study of delays in referral and treatment. *BMJ, 317*(7150), 18–21.

Jemal, A., Siegel, R., Ward, E., Hao, Y., Xu, J., Murray, T., et al. (2008). Cancer statistics, 2008. *CA: A Cancer Journal for Clinicians, 58,* 71–96.

Kalra, M., Gloviczki, P., Andrews, J.C., Cherry, K.J., Bower, T.C., Panneton, J.M., et al. (2003). Open surgical and endovascular treatment of superior vena cava syndrome caused by nonmalignant disease. *Journal of Vascular Surgery, 38,* 215–223.

Kaplan, L.M., Epstein, S.K., Schwartz, S.L., Cao, Q., & Pandian, N.G. (1995). Clinical echocardiographic, and hemodynamic evidence of cardiac tamponade caused by large pleural effusions. *American Journal of Respiratory and Critical Care Medicine, 151,* 904–908.

Kaplan, M. (2006). Spinal cord compression. In M. Kaplan (Ed.), *Understanding and managing oncologic emergencies: A resource for nurses* (pp. 219–259). Pittsburgh, PA: Oncology Nursing Society.

Kaplow, R. (2006). Cardiac tamponade. In C.H. Yarbro, M.H. Frogge, & M. Goodman (Eds.), *Cancer nursing: Principles and practice* (6th ed., pp. 873–885). Sudbury, MA: Jones and Bartlett.

Keefe, D. (2000). Cardiovascular emergencies in the cancer patient. *Seminars in Oncology, 27,* 244–255.

Klerk, C.P., Smorenburg, S.M., & Buller, H.R. (2003). Thrombosis prophylaxis in patient populations with a central venous catheter. *Archives of Internal Medicine, 163,* 1913–1921.

Klimo, P., & Schmidt, M.H. (2004). Surgical management of spinal metastases. *Oncologist, 9,* 188–196.

Knoop, T., & Willenberg, K. (1999). Cardiac tamponade. *Seminars in Oncology Nursing, 15,* 168–173.

Kuzin, E. (2006). Superior vena cava syndrome. In M. Kaplan (Ed.), *Understanding and managing oncologic emergencies: A resource for nurses* (pp. 261–284). Pittsburgh, PA: Oncology Nursing Society.

Kvale, P.A., Simoff, M., & Prakash, U.S. (2003). Lung cancer: Palliative care. *Chest, 123*(Suppl. 1), 284S–311S.

Lanciego, C., Chacon, J.L., Julian, A., Andrade, J., Lopez, L., Martinez, B., et al. (2001). Stenting as first option for endovascular treatment of malignant superior vena cava syndrome. *American Journal of Roentgenology, 177,* 585–593.

Lassman, A.B., Abrey, L.E., Shah, G.G., Panageas, K.S., Begemann, M., Malkin, M.G., et al. (2006). Systemic high-dose methotrexate for central nervous system metastases. *Journal of Neuro-Oncology, 78,* 255–260.

Lassman, A.B., & DeAngelis, L.M. (2003). Brain metastases. *Neurology Clinics, 21,* 1–23.

Loblaw, D.A., & Laperriere, N.J. (1998). Emergency treatment of malignant extradural spinal cord compression: An evidence-based guideline. *Journal of Clinical Oncology, 16,* 1613–1624.

Lu, C., Gonzalez, R.G., Jolesz, F.A., Wen, P.Y., & Talcott, J. (2005). Suspected spinal cord compression in cancer patients: A multidisciplinary risk assessment. *Journal of Supportive Oncology, 3,* 305–312.

Maisch, B., Seferovic, P.M., Ristic, A.D., Erbel, R., Rienmuller, R., Adler, Y., et al. (2004). Guidelines on the management of pericardial diseases executive summary. *European Heart Journal, 25,* 587–610.

Maranzano, E., & Latini, P. (1995). Effectiveness of radiation therapy without surgery in metastatic spinal cord compression: Final results from a prospective trial. *International Journal of Radiation Oncology, Biology, Physics, 32,* 959–967.

Maranzano, E., Latini, P., Beneventi, S., Perrucci, E., Panizza, B.M., Aristei, C., et al. (1996). Radiotherapy without steroids in selected metastatic spinal cord compression patients. A phase II trial. *American Journal of Clinical Oncology, 19,* 179–183.

Moore, S. (2006). Superior vena cava syndrome. In C.H. Yarbro, M.H. Frogge, & M. Goodman (Eds.), *Cancer nursing: Principles and practice* (6th ed., pp. 925–939). Sudbury, MA: Jones and Bartlett.

Myers, J.S. (2001). Oncologic complications. In S.E. Otto (Ed.), *Oncology nursing* (4th ed., pp. 498–581). St. Louis, MO: Mosby.

National Comprehensive Cancer Network. (2008). *NCCN clinical practice guidelines in oncology: Non-small cell lung cancer, version 2.2008.* Retrieved March 30, 2008, from http://www.nccn.org/professionals/physician_gls/pdf/nscl.pdf

Nicholson, A.A., Ettles, D.F., & Arnold, A. (1997). Treatment of malignant superior vena cava obstruction: Metal stents or radiation therapy? *Journal of Vascular Interventional Radiology, 8,* 781–788.

O'Brien, J.F. (1996). The oncologic crisis part 2: Cardio respiratory and neurologic emergencies. *Emergency Medicine, 28,* 21–44.

Osowski, M. (2002, October 12). Spinal cord compression: An obstructive oncologic emergency. *Topics in Advanced Practice Nursing eJournal, 2*(4). Retrieved December 8, 2006, from http://www.medscape.com/viewarticle/442735

Panneton, J.M., Andrews, J.C., & Hofer, J.M. (2001). Superior vena cava syndrome: Relief with a modified saphenojugular bypass graft. *Journal of Vascular Surgery, 34,* 360–363.

Parish, J.M., Marschke, R.F., Jr., Dines, D.E., & Lee, R.E. (1981). Etiologic considerations in superior vena cava syndrome. *Mayo Clinic Proceedings, 56,* 407–413.

Park, J.S., Rentschler, R., & Wilbur, D. (1991). Surgical management of pericardial effusion in patients with malignancies: Comparison of subxiphoid window versus pericardiectomy. *Cancer, 67,* 76–80.

Patchell, R.A., Tibbs, P.A., Regine, W.F., Payne, R., Saris, S., Kryscio, R.J., et al. (2005). Direct decompressive surgical resection in the treatment of spinal cord compression caused by metastatic cancer: A randomised trial. *Lancet, 366,* 643–648.

Peralta, R., & Guzofski, S. (2007). Superior vena cava syndrome. In F.J. Domino (Ed.), *The 5-minute clinical consult* (pp. 1182–1183). Philadelphia: Lippincott Williams & Wilkins.

Piccione, W., Jr., Faber, L.P., & Warren, W.H. (1990). Superior vena caval reconstruction using autologous pericardium. *Annals of Thoracic Surgery, 50,* 417–419.

Prasad, D., & Schiff, D. (2005). Malignant spinal cord compression. *Lancet Oncology, 6,* 15–24.

Reddy, P.S., Curtiss, E.I., O'Toole, J.D., & Shaver, J.A. (1978). Cardiac tamponade: Hemodynamic observations in man. *Circulation, 58,* 265–272.

Rice, T.W., Rodriguez, R.M., & Light, R.W. (2006). The superior vena cava syndrome: Clinical characteristics and evolving etiology. *Medicine, 85,* 37–42.

Rowell, N.P., & Gleeson, F.V. (2002). Steroids, radiotherapy, chemotherapy and stents for superior vena caval obstruction in carcinoma of the bronchus: A systematic review. *Clinical Oncology, 14,* 338–351.

Ruckdeschel, J.C. (2005). Early detection and treatment of spinal cord compression. *Oncology, 19,* 81–92.

Rudolf, J., Grond, M., Prince, W.S., Schmulling, S., & Heiss, W.D. (1999). Evidence of anaphylaxy following alteplase infusion. *Stroke, 30,* 1142–1143.

Sanghavi, S.N., Miranpuri, S.S., Chappell, R., Buatti, J.M., Sneed, P.K., Suh, J.H., et al. (2001). Radiosurgery for patients with brain metastases: A multi-institutional analysis, stratified by the RTOG recursive partitioning analysis method. *International Journal of Radiation Oncology, Biology, Physics, 51,* 426–434.

Schaefer, P.W., Budzik, R.F., Jr., & Gonzalez, R.G. (1996). Imaging of cerebral metastases. *Neurosurgery Clinics of North America, 7,* 393–423.

Schechter, M.M. (1954). The superior vena cava syndrome. *American Journal of the Medical Sciences, 227,* 46–56.

Schiff, D. (2003). Spinal cord compression. *Neurologic Clinics of North America, 21,* 67–86.

Schiff, D., O'Neill, B.P., & Suman, V.J. (1997). Spinal epidural metastasis as the initial manifestation of malignancy: Clinical features and diagnostic approach. *Neurology, 49,* 452–456.

Schiff, D., O'Neill, B.P., Wang, C.H., & O'Fallon, J. (1998). Neuroimaging and treatment implications of patients with multiple epidural spinal metastases. *Cancer, 83,* 1593–1601.

Schraufnagel, D.E., Hill, R., Leech, J.A., & Pare, J.A. (1981). Superior vena caval obstruction. Is it a medical emergency? *American Journal of Medicine, 70,* 1169–1174.

Schwartz, E.E., Goodman, L.R., & Haskin, M.E. (1986). Role of CT scanning in the superior vena cava syndrome. *American Journal of Clinical Oncology, 9,* 71–78.

Shabetai, R. (1988). Pericardial and cardiac pressure. *Circulation, 77,* 1–5.

Shabetai, R., & Hoit, B.D. (2006, November 8). *Cardiac tamponade* [UpToDate version 15.1]. Retrieved April 18, 2007, from http://www.utdol.com

Shapiro, B.A., Warren, J., Egol, A.B., Greenbaum, D.M., Jacobi, J., Nasraway, S.A., et al. (1995). Practice parameters for intravenous analgesia and sedation for adult patients in the intensive care unit: An executive summary. *Critical Care Medicine, 23,* 1596–1600.

Shepherd, F.A. (1997). Malignant pericardial effusion. *Current Opinion in Oncology, 9,* 170–174.

Siegal, T. (1995). Spinal cord compression: From laboratory to clinic. *European Journal of Cancer, 31A,* 1748–1753.

Sitton, E. (1998). Central nervous system metastases. *Seminars in Oncology Nursing, 14,* 210–219.

Smayra, T., Otal, P., Chabbert, V., Chemla, P., Romero, M., Joffre, F., et al. (2001). Long-term results of endovascular stent placement in the superior vena caval venous system. *Cardiovascular and Interventional Radiology, 24,* 388–394.

Smith, E.R., & Amin-Hanjani, S. (2005, November 17). *Evaluation and management of elevated intracranial pressure in adults* [UpToDate version 14.3]. Retrieved January 26, 2007, from http://www.utdol.com

Sorenson, S., Helweg-Larsen, S., Mouridsen, H., & Hansen, H.H. (1994). Effect of high-dose dexamethasone in carcinomatous metastatic spinal cord compression treated with radiotherapy: A randomised trial. *European Journal of Cancer, 30A,* 22–27.

Spodick, D.H. (2003). Acute cardiac tamponade. *New England Journal of Medicine, 349,* 684–690.

Spodick, D.H. (1983). The normal and diseased pericardium: Current concepts of pericardial physiology, diagnosis, and treatment. *Journal of American College of Cardiology, 1,* 240–251.

Stanford, W., & Doty, D.B. (1986). The role of venography and surgery in the management of patients with superior vena cava obstruction. *Annals of Thoracic Surgery, 41,* 158–163.

Story, K.T. (2006). Cardiac tamponade. In M. Kaplan (Ed.), *Understanding and managing oncologic emergencies: A resource for nurses* (pp. 1–29). Pittsburgh, PA: Oncology Nursing Society.

Sugarman, R.A. (2006). Structure and function of the nervous system. In K.L. McCance & S.E. Huether (Eds.), *Pathophysiology: The biologic basis for disease in adults and children* (5th ed., pp. 411–446). St. Louis, MO: Mosby.

Sze, G., Milano, E., & Johnson, C. (1990). Detection of brain metastases: Comparison of contrast enhanced MR with unenhanced MR and contrast CT. *American Journal of Neuroradiology, 11,* 795–797.

Tsang, T.S., Oh, J.K., & Seward, J.B. (1999). Diagnosis and management of cardiac tamponade in the era of echocardiography. *Clinical Cardiology, 22,* 446–452.

Uaje, C., Kahsen, K., & Parish, L. (1996). Oncology emergencies. *Critical Care Nursing Quarterly, 18*(4), 26–34.

Uberoi, R. (2006). Quality assurance guidelines for superior vena cava stenting in malignant disease. *Cardiovascular and Interventional Radiology, 29,* 319–322.

Vaitkus, P.T., Herrmann, H.C., & LeWinter, M.M. (1994). Treatment of malignant pericardial effusion. *JAMA, 272,* 59–64.

van Steijn, J.H., Sleijfer, D.T., van der Graaf, W.T., van der Sluis, A., & Nieboer, P. (2002). How to diagnose cardiac tamponade. *Netherlands Journal of Medicine, 60,* 334–338.

Venes, D. (2005). *Taber's cyclopedic medical dictionary* (20th ed.). Philadelphia: F.A. Davis.

Warren, W.H. (2000). Malignancies involving the pericardium. *Seminars in Thoracic and Cardiovascular Surgery, 12,* 119–129.

Wilkes, G.M. (2004a). Increased intracranial pressure. In C.H. Yarbro, M.H. Frogge, & M. Goodman (Eds.), *Cancer symptom management* (3rd ed., pp. 374–385). Sudbury, MA: Jones and Bartlett.

Wilkes, G.M. (2004b). Spinal cord compression. In C.H. Yarbro, M.H. Frogge, & M. Goodman (Eds.), *Cancer symptom management* (3rd ed., pp. 359–371). Sudbury, MA: Jones and Bartlett.

Wilson, L.D., Detterbeck, F.C., & Yahalom, J. (2007). Superior vena cava syndrome with malignant causes. *New England Journal of Medicine, 356,* 1862–1869.

Wudel, L.J., & Nesbitt, J.C. (2001). Superior vena cava syndrome. *Current Treatment Options in Oncology, 2,* 77–91.

Yahalom, J. (2005). Oncologic emergencies: Superior vena cava syndrome. In V.T. DeVita, Jr., S. Hellman, & S.A. Rosenberg (Eds.), *Cancer: Principles and practice of oncology* (7th ed., pp. 2273–2280). Philadelphia: Lippincott Williams & Wilkins.

CHAPTER 16

Psychosocial Management

Nancy Jo Bush, RN, MN, MA, AOCN®

Introduction

The psychological sequelae that challenge patients with cancer and their families are interwoven within all aspects of oncologic care from diagnosis through terminal care. The definition of *psychosocial* is the association among the patient's interpersonal relationships, social conditions, and mental health (Fitch, 2006). Psychosocial issues that confront patients with cancer include but are not limited to anxiety and depression; post-traumatic stress disorder (PTSD); fear of recurrence; cognitive changes; sexual health and body image changes; family/caregiver distress; socioeconomic, occupational, and role changes; and, most profoundly, a changed life perspective.

The National Comprehensive Cancer Network (NCCN, 2008) chose the word *distress* to characterize the psychosocial nature of the cancer experience. NCCN defines distress as a multifactorial, unpleasant experience that is social, emotional, psychological, and spiritual in nature. Distress can range from normal feelings of fear, sadness, and vulnerability to disabling conditions such as clinical depression, anxiety and panic, isolation, and existential or spiritual crises (Madden, 2006; NCCN). How patients cope and adapt to cancer depends on many intervening variables, such as age, gender, lifestyle, family dynamics, culture and ethnicity, social support, socioeconomic status, religious beliefs, and spirituality.

Family systems theory provides a framework for understanding the impact of cancer not only on the patient but also on the family unit. Coping for patients and families is interdependent—the emotional and behavioral responses of one will always affect the other, positively or negatively. The family, in all its present-day permutations, is the unit of care (Bush, 1998; Jassak, 1992; Kristjanson & Ashcroft, 1994).

Definitions

Self-Esteem

Sexuality and Cancer (American Cancer Society [ACS], 2004), a mainstay of education literature for patients with cancer, shares an analogy used by Wendy Schain, EdD, a psychologist who specializes in counseling patients with cancer. She likens self-esteem to the total sum of several bank accounts that support an individual's identity. One account is the net worth of the **physical** self—this includes body health and functioning, sexuality, and body image. A second account is the **social** self—this includes personality and character, temperament and outlook on life, and interrelationships with others. The third account is the **achieving** self—this includes an individual's identity formulated through roles in work, community, and personal and family relationships. The last bank account is the **spiritual** self—this includes an individual's religious and moral beliefs and the strength found in these beliefs.

Throughout life's journey, deposits are made in each of these bank accounts. The experience and challenges of cancer draw from each account along the continuum of disease and treatment. Keeping the accounts balanced may require withdrawing from one and depositing into another. It can be analogous to effective coping—having the flexibility to adjust by not defining self-esteem or self-worth on one part of the total self. Yet a person's identity is more than the sum of its interrelated parts. Difficulty in one area of self-esteem (e.g., sexuality) will affect another part of the self (e.g., the social self). A self-image that integrates the physical and psychological changes brought about by the cancer experience is necessary for psychosocial adaptation. The ability to cope and adapt to these challenges is easier when individuals have positive self-esteem and ego-strength prior to diagnosis (Shell & Campbell-Norris, 2006), keeping their emotional accounts flexible and balanced. Individuals with high self-esteem feel personal control over their life circumstances (Barry, 2002; Grimm, 2005), but all people diagnosed with cancer may be challenged to maintain high self-esteem while confronting stressors that they may have never thought possible. Meeting these challenges with strength and endurance can lead to emotional growth and positive changes in self-esteem brought about by surviving trauma and loss (Nolen-Hoeksema, 2001).

Anxiety

Anxiety and depression are the most common emotional reactions to the cancer experience, but unfortunately, they also are the most overlooked, misunderstood, and misdiagnosed of symptoms (Schwartz, Lander, & Chochinov, 2002; Stein, 2004). Advanced practice nurses (APNs) need to understand that all mental health disorders are biologic in nature (Barry, 2002) and impart this information to patients. The diagnosis of cancer arouses fear of the unknown and the uncontrollable. Unrelenting sadness, grief, and loss often occur as a result of the physical and psychosocial losses experienced along the cancer trajectory. It is the *intensity, duration,* and *extent* to which these symptoms interfere with functioning that differentiate abnormal anxiety or a depressive disorder from the normal emotional responses that are experienced with chronic illness (Bowers & Boyle, 2003; Pasacreta, Minarik, & Nield-Anderson, 2006). Depression and anxiety consist of a cluster of psychological and physiologic symptoms that, if recognized, often are responsive to treatment, but if unrecognized, interfere with coping and quality of life. Both patients and family members may feel these emotions intensely at specific transition points: diagnosis, treatment, recurrence, and progressive illness. Even during long-term remission and survivorship, fears of recurrence and disabilities caused by cancer treatment can continue to promote feelings of uncertainty and anguish.

The most common emotional reaction to a cancer diagnosis is *fear.* At the beginning of the cancer journey, feelings of fear are related to the unknown and patients' disbelief that this is really happening to them. This response can be especially poignant for asymptomatic patients whose malignancy is discovered unexpectedly, such as during a routine mammogram (Boehmke & Dickerson, 2006). Fear is a normal affective response to the *real* threat of a cancer diagnosis, and fear involves the *cognitive appraisal* that cancer is a threat to one's well-being. Anxiety is the affective response to a *perceived* threat or danger and involves the *emotional response* to that cognitive appraisal (Beck & Emery, 1985; Bush, 2006b).

Fear and anxiety are interrelated. Fear leads to the stress response of "fight or flight," in contrast to anxiety, which can reduce a person's ability to act. Severe anxiety can cause patients with cancer to feel emotionally paralyzed. The physical symptoms of anxiety are associated with the autonomic response and include motor tension ranging from generalized aches and pains to autonomic hyperactivity, such as palpitations and shortness of breath. Patients may describe feeling restless, trembling, and dizzy, having a lump in their throat, or feeling suffocated. The physical toll of anxiety demands energy, causing patients to feel fatigue and exhaustion when facing the demands of their illness. This may be exacerbated by difficulty falling asleep or staying asleep or waking with ruminating thoughts and apprehension about what is happening to them. Patients commonly feel that they are always on "alert" and are vigilant toward any physical ache or pain that may be interpreted as cancer spread or recurrence.

The psychological symptoms of anxiety are associated with feelings of impending doom. The perceived threat of treatments may increase fear of body image changes and permanent disabilities. Fear and anxiety can range from an acute, transient distress at different stages along the continuum of disease to a major psychiatric illness, such as PTSD, or stress syndromes such as panic attacks or phobias (Bush, 2006b; Marrs, 2006). Therefore, fear and anxiety are normal responses to stressful events, such as cancer, but become pathologic if these emotions persist and interfere with patient functioning (Noyes, Holt, & Massie, 1998). Anxiety has been associated with specific illnesses (infection, hypoxia, hypoglycemia, hyperthyroidism, alcohol or drug withdrawal) and medications (steroids, antiemetics), thus demanding that a thorough health and medical history be taken for differential diagnosis (Marrs).

Kwekkeboom and Seng (2002) described the presence of trauma-related symptoms, such as avoidance behaviors, intrusive thoughts, and heightened arousal in cancer survivors. These symptoms are referred to as PTSD and resemble those observed in individuals who have experienced extreme psychological assault such as with rape, combat, or a natural disaster (Passik & Grummon, 1998). Recurrence of cancer may bring forth traumatic memories for patients who underwent intensive treatments for their cancer. Feelings of dread or doom are not unusual when recurrent disease arouses these memories. People with a history of generalized anxiety disorder also may experience a reemergence or intensification of symptoms with the diagnosis of cancer. A prior history of obsessive-compulsive disorder may be reactivated, and specific phobias (e.g., needle phobia, claustrophobia, such as with magnetic resonance imaging [MRI] scans) may interfere with cancer treatment (Gorman, Raines, & Sultan, 2002; Noyes et al., 1998) (see Table 16-1). "Conditioned" or learned responses to repetitive, aversive treatments have been found to contribute to symptoms such as anxiety, anticipatory nausea and vomiting, and other emotions, such as apprehension toward office visits and follow-up examinations (Passik & Grummon).

Gender and ethnicity may influence patterns of anxiety disorders (Stein, 2004). Research has found that depressed women are more likely to have specific phobias than depressed men, and African Americans are more likely to experience specific phobias.

Table 16-1. Classifications of Anxiety Disorders

Disorder	Defining Characteristics
Generalized anxiety disorder	Uncontrollable, unrealistic worry with accompanying physiologic symptoms, such as muscle tension, difficulty sleeping, fatigue, restlessness, irritability, and difficulty concentrating; persistent for a six-month period; interferes with functioning.
Trauma	An event that a person experiences or witnesses that involved actual or threatened death or serious injury, or a threat to the physical integrity of self or others.
Post-traumatic stress disorder	Vividly remembering a traumatic event in the form of thoughts, images, and dreams with persistent internal (physiologic) or external (behavioral) avoidance of the reminders of the trauma, detachment from others, negative emotions, a sense of a foreshortened future, and heightened sympathetic arousal.
Panic disorder	Periods of intense fear, apprehension, or discomfort that develop suddenly and reach peak intensity within 10 minutes of the initiation of symptoms, which include tachycardia, shortness of breath, fear of dying or losing control, chest pain, and feelings of suffocation.
Specific phobia	The circumscribed fear of an object or situation: animal, situational, natural environment, or blood/injection/injury. Situational phobias include acrophobia (fear of heights), agoraphobia (fear of a specific place or situation), and claustrophobia (fear of closed spaces). Common fears for patients with cancer include fear of doctors (white coat syndrome), illness and injury (needles, medications), and death (anesthesia).
Obsessive-compulsive disorder	Obsessions are intrusive, disturbing thoughts, images, or urges. Compulsions are repetitive mental or motor activities aimed to neutralize anxiety. Obsessions and compulsions intrude into a person's psychological functioning and daily life by creating distress, taking inordinate periods of time, and increasing the risk of comorbidity, such as depression.

Note. Based on information from American Psychiatric Association, 2000; Stein, 2004.

Comorbid depression also has been found to exacerbate phobic anxiety and increase the risk of suicidal behavior. More research is needed in this area to help to identify patients who are at greatest risk for comorbidities (Stein).

Depression

The diagnoses of anxiety and depression often coexist. Depression has been defined as a state of feeling hopeless, worthless, and discouraged (Grimm, 2005); a more intense and debilitating version of sadness (Bowers & Boyle, 2003); and a complex, progressive neurologic-cognitive response to loss or deprivation (Lovejoy, Tabor, Matteis, & Lillis, 2000). The normal, expected changes in thinking, feelings, and behaviors that occur in response to cancer are defined as *emotional distress* (Grimm) and can be viewed on one end of the continuum, with clinical depression, a severe form of emotional distress, on the other end of the continuum. Prolonged grief and sadness are thought to actually contribute to the neurophysiology of depression by causing an imbalance of neurotransmitters in the mood-sensitive areas of the brain—the limbic system, basal ganglia, and hypothalamus. A decrease in levels of neurotransmitters (dopamine, norepinephrine, and serotonin) negatively affects homeostasis throughout the body, causing cognitive, behavioral, and systemic symptoms (Keltner, Folks, Palmer, & Powers, 1998; Lovejoy, Tabor, & Deloney, 2000). Cognitive symptoms related to depression include feelings of guilt, sadness, and worthlessness, which negatively affect the ability to think, concentrate, and make decisions. A major behavioral symptom of depression is diminished interest or pleasure in all, or most, activities of the day, nearly every day. Systemic symptoms of depression can range from unrelenting fatigue, to changes in eating and sleeping patterns, to psychomotor agitation, such as irritable mood. The physical symptoms of depression may mimic side effects of cancer treatment; thus, a thorough assessment of the cognitive changes associated with depression should be used for definitive diagnosis (see Table 16-2). Untreated depression places patients at risk for suicide, therefore making diagnosis and treatment imperative (Albright & Valente, 2006; American Psychiatric Association [APA], 2000).

As mentioned earlier, depressive disorders are biologic in nature (Barry, 2002), and symptoms reflect a progressive derangement of underlying neurologic circuits (Lovejoy, Tabor, Matteis, et al., 2000). Individuals often find it difficult to admit to feelings or behaviors related to depression because of fear of being negatively judged as weak in character or because of personal feelings of failure. Stressful experiences can "burn out" neurologic circuits in the brain, or, as in the case of hereditary depression, neurotransmitter systems may fail, first contributing to responses of sadness and ineffective coping when faced with stressful situations such as cancer (Lovejoy, Tabor, Matteis, et al.).

Numerous diagnostic tools are available to evaluate mood disorders in the clinical and research settings. For initial diagnosis in the clinical setting, a thorough intake history, physical examination, and psychosocial assessment are appropriate and effective. A single-item screening question such as, "Do you feel low in mood or depressed?" has the benefit of being simple and efficient and begins a dialogue that is nonthreatening to both patients and nurses (Chochinov, Wilson, Enns, & Lander, 1997).

Table 16-2. Symptoms of Anxiety and Depression[a]

State	Symptoms
Anxiety	Physical symptoms: Sympathetic stimulation, including trembling, tremors, restlessness, facial tension, increased perspiration, heart palpitations, dyspnea, chest tightness, lump in throat, feelings of suffocation
	Psychological symptoms: Fear, worry, ruminating thoughts, irritability, apprehension, feelings of inadequacy, overexcitement, uncertainty, distress, fear of unspecific consequences
Depression	Physical symptoms[b]: Psychomotor agitation or retardation; weight loss while not dieting or weight gain; insomnia or hypersomnia; fatigue or loss of energy; decreased libido; sadness, crying, or despondence
	Psychological symptoms: Feelings of worthlessness or excessive or inappropriate guilt; diminished ability to think and concentrate or indecisiveness; helplessness and hopelessness; recurrent thoughts of death, suicide ideation with or without a specific plan for committing suicide

[a] States of anxiety and depression often coexist.
[b] Physical symptoms of depression are similar to side effects of cancer treatment; therefore, psychological symptoms are more indicative of depression in patients with cancer.

Note. Based on information from American Psychiatric Association, 2000; Barry, 2002; Crowley, 2005.

Cognitive Dysfunction

Cognitive dysfunction in patients with cancer can be misdiagnosed as psychological disorders such as anxiety and depression, or these psychological comorbidities can contribute to changes in cognition. *Direct/disease-related factors* causing cognitive dysfunction include primary tumors of the central nervous system (CNS) or brain metastases. Primary and metastatic brain tumors often cause diffuse cognitive dysfunction or focal deficits related to the site of the tumor (Muscari, 2006a; Walch, Ahles, & Saykin, 1998) (see Table 16-3).

Indirect/treatment-related factors contributing to cognitive dysfunction include adverse effects of treatment modalities (e.g., medications, radiation, chemotherapy, biologic response modifiers) or indirect factors, such as metabolic, endocrine, and nutritional abnormalities that commonly occur with cancer (Muscari, 2006a; O'Shaughnessy, 2003) (see Table 16-4). Radiation therapy is an effective treatment for primary CNS tumors or CNS metastases; however, treatments place patients at risk for cognitive impairment. Variables that contribute to neurotoxicity related to radiation therapy include the dose of radiation, the volume of tissue irradiated, and the total number of treatments delivered (Walch et al., 1998). Identifying the impact of radiotherapy on cognitive dysfunction may be difficult because of CNS disease progression (Muscari, 2006a). High doses of cranial irradiation concomitant with high-dose chemotherapy may place patients at even higher risk for cognitive dysfunction (Walch et al.).

Cognitive impairment caused by chemotherapeutic agents often is colloquially referred to as *chemo brain* or *chemo clutter* (Jansen, Miaskowski, Dodd, Dowling, & Kramer, 2005; Muscari, 2006a; Staat & Segatore, 2005). Reported changes include difficulties in thinking, memory, and concentrating ranging from subtle to moderate. Drawing definitive conclusions regarding the impact of chemotherapy-induced cognitive dysfunction has been difficult because of the many drug combina-

---

Table 16-3. Cognitive Dysfunction Related to Primary or Metastatic Brain Tumor

Tumor Site	Possible Effects
Frontal lobe	Emotional lability, apathy, poor judgment, impulsivity, lack of inhibition, anosognosia (lack of self-awareness of impaired neurologic or neuropsychological function), and socially inappropriate behaviors Language deficits and dysfunction of executive cognition
Temporal lobe	Auditory and perceptual changes; memory and learning impairments, and aphasia and other language disorders Mania or depressed mood, irritability or anxiety, and seizures
Parietal lobe	Somatosensory abnormalities; agraphesthesia (tactile recognition), agnosia (disorders of recognition), alexia (reading disorders), agraphia (writing disorders), and apraxias (motor abnormalities) Language comprehension impairments and homonymous visual deficits
Occipital lobe	Visual problems; hemianopia (loss of half of the visual field of both eyes), achromatopsia (impairment of color), and alexia (reading disorders) Impaired extraocular movements

Note. Based on information from Fox et al., 2006; Walch et al., 1998.

Table 16-4. Treatment-Related Cognitive Dysfunction

Treatment	Possible Results
Chemotherapy	Neurotoxicity (e.g., leukoencephalopathy), inflammatory (e.g., cytokine-induced), immunologic, and microvascular invasion Chemotherapy-induced anemia Chemotherapy-induced menopause
Radiation	Cerebral edema, demyelination, leukoencephalopathy, and radiation necrosis of brain matter
Biologics	Disorientation, psychomotor slowing, slowed speech, aphasia, and impaired concentration and memory

Note. Based on information from Jansen et al., 2005; O'Shaughnessy, 2003; Saykin et al., 2003; Staat & Segatore, 2005; Walch et al., 1998.

tions and schedules, deficiencies in estrogen and progesterone related to chemotherapy-induced menopause and estrogen-blocking medications, and chemotherapy-induced anemia (e.g., hemoglobin levels less than 12 g/dl in women and 13 g/dl in men) (Jansen et al.; Muscari, 2006a; Staat & Segatore).

Age, intelligence, and education level also contribute to the impact of disease- or treatment-related cognitive dysfunction (Muscari, 2006a). Cognitive decline is expected to occur as adults age and may be exacerbated by the decline in hearing and sight. Normal, expected cognitive changes among older adults must be differentiated from psychiatric diagnoses, such as depression, anxiety, and dementia (Muscari, 2006a; Smith & Buckwalter, 2006) and delirium (Bond, Neelon, & Belyea, 2006; Boyle, 2006a). Concurrent use of medications, such as antiemetics and antidepressants, as well as substance abuse, will adversely affect cognitive ability.

Delirium: Delirium is a medical problem that is commonly misdiagnosed as anger, anxiety, depression, or psychosis (Breitbart, Jaramillo, & Chochinov, 1998; Maynard, 2003). Delirium is defined as an acute organic brain syndrome involving a change in the level of consciousness and cognitive function (thinking, perception, and memory) that develops over a short period of time (APA, 2000). This onset of acute confusion often signifies a worsening of the primary illness or a complication of treatment. Symptoms of delirium are characterized by changes in attention and behavior that can fluctuate throughout the day (Bond et al., 2006; Caeiro, Ferro, Albuquerque, & Figueria, 2004). Delirium is estimated to occur in 18%–60% of patients with cancer (Ljubisavljevic & Kelly, 2003; Tuma & DeAngelis, 2000), with hospitalized older adult patients being at increased risk (Muscari, 2006b). As many as 90% of patients in the terminal stage of cancer exhibit delirium in the final weeks of life (Bond et al.). Variables that increase the risk of delirium in patients with cancer are comorbid illnesses and preexisting cognitive impairment, such as prior stroke or preexisting dementia. Cancer- or treatment-related factors that increase the risk of delirium include infection, use of benzodiazepines, metabolic imbalances, the use of steroids and opioids, and CNS metastases. Nurses across all settings from the hospital to ambulatory settings need to recognize delirium in patients with cancer and the impact of delirium on family caregivers who are expected to manage these complex symptoms at home (Bond et al.). Unfortunately, a paucity of research exists on delirium in older patients with cancer, contributing to misdiagnosis and a lack of early identification that could reduce symptoms (Boyle, 2006a).

Dementia: Dementia, a global loss of cognitive and intellectual functioning, is an important risk factor for delirium but is a distinctly different form of cognitive impairment (APA, 2000; Muscari, 2006b). Diagnostic criteria for dementia include impairment in memory, behavior, and personality. In contrast to delirium, dementia is a decline in cognitive functioning over a period of time. Patients experience a decline in executive functioning (e.g., problem solving) and an inability to carry out normal daily activities (e.g., dressing), and over time, their functional dependence requires care and supervision (Muscari, 2006b; Smith & Buckwalter, 2005). In patients with cancer, dementia may be the result of disease or of treatment-related involvement of the brain and spinal cord, such as with radiation therapy for brain metastases (Muscari, 2006b). The behavioral components of dementia include apathy, withdrawal, paranoia, wandering, and sleep changes (Smith & Buckwalter), in contrast to the agitation, restlessness, and fluctuating changes in cognition that are seen with delirium (Crowley, 2005). Mood states, such as depression and anxiety, also may occur in patients experiencing dementia and should be diagnosed and treated appropriately.

Differential diagnosis: Distinguishing among cognitive impairment, delirium, and dementia begins with a clear understanding of the differences in the nature of these separate but sometimes related conditions (Boyle, 2006a; Fox, Mitchell, & Booth-Jones, 2006; Maynard, 2003). Attributes commonly used to distinguish one condition from another include onset, duration, progression, memory, level of orientation, and psychomotor behavior, among others (Barry, 2002; Boyle, 2006a).

A wide variety of standardized tools are available to assess cognitive function. One of the most frequently used is the Mini-Mental State Exam (MMSE) (Folstein, Folstein, & McHugh, 1975). The MMSE assesses only gross general cognitive status (Boyle, 2006a) and "is not intended to diagnose but rather raise a flag of awareness that further testing is needed" (Muscari, 2006a, p. 196). Older adult patients suspected of having dementia should be referred for a full evaluation.

Sexuality and Altered Body Image

Sexuality is not limited to intimate relations with a partner. Sexuality encompasses self-esteem, body image, and behavioral expressions of intimacy, including hugging, kissing, touching, tenderness, and body language (Anastasia, 2006a). The definition of sexuality must be interpreted individually. What is normal for one person may be considered abnormal for another, depending on influencing factors such as cultural and religious norms, value systems, and past and present experiences (Anastasia, 2006a). The emotional responses to assaults on body image, such as with mastectomy or hysterectomy, also must be interpreted individually because of these same influencing factors. Internal as well as external body image changes can cause psychological distress related to sexual self-image.

Sexual health has been defined as an integration of the somatic, emotional, intellectual, and social aspects of a sexual being (World Health Organization, 2006). The sexual health of a patient experiencing cancer is an important component of psychosocial management, and disturbance in sexual being can negatively affect psychological health and quality of life. Sexual dysfunction related to cancer can occur as a result of disease- or treatment-induced side effects, such as fatigue and pain related to physical changes (e.g., chemotherapy-induced menopause or prostatectomy-induced erectile dysfunction), or psychological responses to the disease and treatment, such as fear, anxiety, and depression (Anastasia, 2006a; Schover, 1998). Less apparent physical and psychological factors also may negatively affect a patient's sexual health. These factors can include subtle feelings related to weight fluctuations or unspoken fears of transmitting the cancer to a partner (Nishimoto, 2005). Figure 16-1 lists characteristics that place patients at high risk for emotional distress related to sexual dysfunction.

- Younger age
- Recently married
- Pelvic irradiation
- Unmarried, single
- Hormonal therapy
- History of sexual abuse
- Treatment-related infertility
- Preexisting sexual dysfunction
- Chemotherapy-induced menopause
- Chemotherapy-induced neuropathies
- Radiation-induced erectile dysfunction
- Low self-esteem and body image changes
- Cancers involving the genitals, pelvis, or breasts
- Poor individual or couple psychological adjustment
- Psychological responses such as fear, anxiety, or depression
- Patients who have had a mastectomy/lumpectomy, hysterectomy, cystectomy, orchiectomy, radical prostatectomy, radical vulvectomy, head and neck surgery

Figure 16-1. Variables That Put Patients at High Risk for Sexual Dysfunction

Note. Based on information from Nishimoto, 2005; Schover, 1998.

APNs must ensure that patients are educated about the side effects of cancer treatment on their sexuality; for example, fertility concerns need to be addressed for young adults at the time of diagnosis and prior to treatment (Davis, 2006). Wilmoth (2006) identified four key processes that nurses must address to enable them to carry out sexual assessment: (a) achieving comfort with their own sexuality in order to talk to their patients about sexuality, (b) becoming educated about the effects of cancer and treatment on sexuality, (c) honing effective communication skills, and (d) identifying multidisciplinary team members who support incorporating sexual health care into practice. Nurses also need to take cues from the patient when they communicate sensitive issues such as sexuality. Nurses should approach the subject in a safe and nonjudgmental manner and give the patient permission to be sexually active and discuss sexual issues that may be of concern (Krebs, 2006).

Nurses can provide a screening sexual assessment as part of the general history and physical intake. Sample questions for the sexual assessment are outlined in Figure 16-2. A problem-focused sexual assessment most often is carried out when the patient has identified a specific sexual problem related to the disease and treatment. This type of sexual assessment is appropriate for the APN and includes a thorough sexual history and medication review with a more in-depth focus on the sexual dysfunction of concern (Wilmoth, 2006). If patients identify a specific problem with sexual function, a simple assessment developed by Andersen (1990) based on the acronym ALARM can be useful (see Figure 16-3).

The PLISSIT Model (Annon, 1976)—**P**ermission, **L**imited **I**nformation, **S**pecific **S**uggestions, and **I**ntensive **T**herapy—provides an intervention framework to guide nurs-

- How has cancer affected the way you feel about yourself as a woman or man?
- How has cancer affected the way your partner feels about you as a woman or man?
- How has cancer affected your role as partner?
- What aspects of your sexuality have been affected by cancer?
- How has cancer affected your ability to function sexually?

Figure 16-2. Sexual Assessment Questions

Note. Based on information from Wilmoth, 1994; Woods, 1984.
From "Life After Cancer: What *Does* Sexuality Have to Do With It?" by M.C. Wilmoth, 2006, *Oncology Nursing Forum, 33,* p. 907. Copyright 2006 by Oncology Nursing Society. Reprinted with permission.

Activity (frequency and type of sexual practice)
Libido/desire
Arousal and orgasm
Resolution, release, or relaxation
Medical information (potential influencing factors)

Figure 16-3. ALARM Assessment Model for Sexual Functioning

Note. Based on information from Andersen & Lamb, 1995.

es through sexual counseling. *Permission* encourages nurses to allow patients to express their feelings and concerns by providing an open and trusting environment. *Limited information* refers to patient education regarding the sexual side effects of medication and treatment. At this step, the nurse clarifies any fears and misconceptions that the patient verbalizes and validates specific symptoms that may interfere with sexuality (e.g., fatigue, pain). *Specific suggestions* can be provided after a thorough sexual health history that includes attitudes, patient beliefs, and a baseline sexual functioning. The nurse can provide the patient with strategies for improving sexual functioning and expression within the physical demands of the illness and treatment. In addition to assessment of treatment-related physical changes, a thorough sexual assessment must take into consideration all the psychological variables that may negatively affect sexuality, such as fear, anxiety, and depression. *Intensive therapy* by a certified sex therapist is recommended if the patient expresses prolonged or severe sexual dysfunction (Anastasia, 2006a; Annon).

Personal Control

A sense of personal control is the perception that one's behaviors and choices can bring about positive outcomes and avoid life-threatening situations—such as the diagnosis of cancer (Gorman, 2006). The perception of personal control may be emotionally shattered for individuals in good health who have made healthy lifestyle choices but find themselves confronting a diagnosis of cancer. Perception of control enables individuals to feel that they can change their life circumstances or their psychological responses to these circumstances (Barry, 2002). Feelings of control are shaped by individual and situational differences. Understanding the function of control is critical to supporting the coping process (Nail, 2001).

The biologic basis of cancer is one of the most feared aspects of the disease. Cancer is derived from a single cell that has lost control and then replicates, causing local invasion of healthy tissues. Single cells of the tumor then can break off and threaten other more distant parts of the body. Patients with cancer live in fear of these microscopic but destructive cells that threaten their well-being and survival. Even with successful treatments to control local and systemic invasion, patients may express fear that one lingering cell exists that was not destroyed. Uncertainty and fear of recurrent disease are recurring themes for long-term cancer survivors (Boyle, 2006b).

Social learning theory and the theory of learned helplessness provide the framework for research on perceived control and the concept of powerlessness (Gorman, 2006). Feelings of powerlessness are situationally determined (e.g., traumatic event such as a cancer diagnosis) but often are influenced by the individual's locus of control. Individuals who have an **internal** locus of control believe that their choices and behaviors affect outcomes, whereas individuals with an **external** locus of control believe that outcomes are dependent on the behavior of others or by fate (Gorman) (see Figure 16-4). On a continuum of personal control, feelings of powerlessness can lead to feelings of helplessness and hopelessness. The individual believes that his or her physical and psychological needs will not be met under any circumstances (e.g., "No matter what I do, I cannot beat the cancer") (Barry, 2002; Grimm, 2005). The risk of persistent anxiety and depression increases if these feelings of powerlessness endure over time (see Table 16-5).

External
- Talks of fate or luck being needed to control illness
- Has less interest in educational materials and self-monitoring programs
- Looks to family or healthcare providers to make decisions and plan treatment
- Looks to others for motivation and encouragement
- Needs to be repeatedly prodded to follow through on making appointments or to complete self-monitoring
- May respond to rewards

Internal
- Expresses belief that one can actively control the course of the illness
- Actively seeks information about the illness and takes an active part in decision making and problem solving
- Participates in self-care strategies such as exercise programs and self-help groups
- Does not need prodding or reminding to follow through with self-motivation
- Looks at how one's behavior can affect treatment
- Responds to internal rewards

Figure 16-4. Assessment of External and Internal Locus of Control

---

Note. From "Powerlessness" (p. 370), by L.M. Gorman in R.M. Carroll-Johnson, L.M. Gorman, and N.J. Bush (Eds.), *Psychosocial Nursing Care Along the Cancer Continuum* (2nd ed.), 2006, Pittsburgh, PA: Oncology Nursing Society. Copyright 2006 by Oncology Nursing Society. Adapted with permission.

Spiritual Distress

Spirituality is the belief or value system that an individual perceives to provide strength, hope, and meaning in his or her life (Grimm, 2005). Spirituality has been described as an aspect of being human that is uniquely personal yet universal and innate (Taylor, 2006). Dimensions of spirituality that have been described in the nursing literature include faith and religion, empathy and compassion, and becoming and transcendence

Table 16-5. Perceptions of Personal Control

Term	Definition
Control	The perception that one's own choices and behaviors will positively influence life circumstances. The individual has high self-esteem and a greater sense of mastery of life. Internal locus of control.
Powerlessness	The perception that one's choices and behaviors cannot effect change in life circumstances. Situationally controlled. The person has low self-esteem and an external locus of control.
Helplessness	The perception that one is helpless in effecting changes. The person feels emotionally overwhelmed and disorganized.
Hopelessness	The perception that one's needs have no chance of being met. The person feels that no choices or alternatives exist for their current life situation.
Depression	Sadness brought about by feelings of powerlessness, helplessness, and hopelessness. The individual feels worthless.

Note. Based on information from Barry, 2002; Gorman, 2006; Grimm, 2005.

(Goldberg, 1998; Kemp, 2006; Martsolf & Mickley, 1998; Taylor) (see Figure 16-5). Spirituality is based on the cherished beliefs and faith of the individual, including the presence or absence of a belief in God, the meaning of suffering and pain, or the value of living (Barry, 2002; Martsolf & Mickley). Spirituality also includes many interrelated emotional responses, such as hope, acceptance, forgiveness, guilt, and shame (Fitchett & Handzo, 1998; Kemp; Taylor) (see Table 16-6). Religion, defined as the rituals, dogma, or devotion that are a manifestation of spirituality (Kemp), is only one component of spirituality.

Finding meaning in one's life is a core component of spirituality. It is a process of introspection that motivates personal growth and development (Barry, 2002), a process of becoming the person who one is (Martsolf & Mickley, 1998). Finding meaning is analogous to feeling that one's life has a purpose or believing that one's life makes a difference for the greater good. A spiritual person feels connectedness with others and to an internal or external life force (Barry). A life-threatening disease such as cancer often challenges the basic components of spirituality. When individuals are forced to confront their own mortality, it may motivate them to question their own spiritual beliefs. Fears brought on by the disease and treatment also may cause spiritual distress in people. Painful or distressing spiritual responses to cancer include having doubts about the presence or nature of God, feeling that cancer is a punishment for wrongdoing, or never working through the anguish of finding meaning in their experience or an answer to the question, "Why me?" (Taylor, 2006).

Many patients are able to process their spiritual pain and find positive meaning to living with cancer. This has included increasing self-awareness, changing priorities to focus on meaningful activities, getting in touch with nature, and finding more joy in everyday life (Taylor, 2006). Many patients with cancer have expressed that the experience has helped them to transcend their own lives, enabling them to understand others better and give back or help others (e.g., empathy and compassion). Taking on this broader life perspective or purpose has been described as *self-transcendence* (Carroll-Johnson, 2006). The experience of self-transcendence often underlies the patients' de-

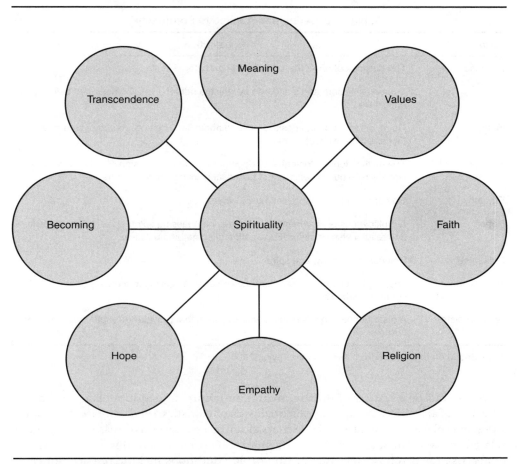

Figure 16-5. Dimensions of Spirituality

Note. Based on information from Goldberg, 1998; Kemp, 2006; Martsolf & Mickley, 1998; Taylor, 2006.

sire to volunteer to help other patients with cancer, for example, becoming a Reach to Recovery® volunteer or engaging in clinical trials to support future research.

Indications

Risk Factors for Psychosocial Disturbance

All patients diagnosed with cancer are at risk for experiencing psychosocial distress ranging from normal fear resulting from the uncertainty of disease to sadness related to the perceived loss of health and identity. Surveys of people with cancer have demonstrated that 20%–40% of patients show a significant level of distress, such as depression and anxiety, at some point along the cancer trajectory (NCCN, 2008). Patients are especially vulnerable at major transition points along the disease continuum: work-up and diagnosis, treatment cycles, at the end of treatment, at follow-up office visits, re-

Table 16-6. Definitions Applied to Spirituality

Term	Definition
Meaning	The purpose of one's life; belief in a primary force in life
Values	The belief system and standards by which a person lives. Commitment to living an ethical life.
Faith	Open, committed, and positive attitude about life. The acceptance of God or a higher power, without proof.
Religion	The myths/stories, doctrines, or dogma that is the expression of spirituality. An individual's religious beliefs are not necessarily institutional in nature.
Empathy	Compassion and understanding for others
Hope	A multidimensional, dynamic life force encompassing spiritual, cognitive, contextual, and relationship domains. Expectation of something positive.
Becoming	Unity of mind, body, and spirit
Transcendence	Looking beyond oneself and one's own suffering. Giving to the greater good. Outcome of spirituality.
Spiritual distress	A disturbance in one's belief or value system that provides strength, hope, and life purpose

Note. Based on information from Kemp, 2006; Taylor, 2006.

currence and progression of disease, treatment failure, and awareness of end of life (Bush, 2006a; NCCN). Numerous personality characteristics, such as ineffective coping styles, may place patients at an increased risk for distress, as well as disease- or treatment-related stressors, such as body image changes. Comorbid conditions also increase patients' risk for psychosocial distress. Comorbid conditions include physical illnesses, such as renal, cardiac, pulmonary, and endocrine diseases, or mental illness, such as anxiety, depression, or substance abuse.

Initial psychosocial assessment (see Table 16-7) can help to identify those patients who have had a previous psychiatric disorder, such as a history of depression or suicide attempt, or if a family member has experienced depression. Throughout the course of disease, patients with a prior history of depression should be monitored carefully. People who have experienced a major depressive episode in the past are at an increased risk for recurrent episodes, and a previous suicide attempt increases the risk for another (Albright & Valente, 2006). NCCN (2008) and others have identified those patients who require a psychological/psychiatric evaluation and referral to a mental health team (see Figure 16-6). Symptoms related to disease and treatment must be differentiated from psychological symptoms of distress. Physical side effects of treatment may mimic physical symptoms associated with distress (e.g., anorexia, weight loss, insomnia, fatigue). Signs among older adults will be more complex as a result of comorbid diseases or dementia, anxiety, alcohol or benzodiazepine use, or symptoms of psychosis (Reynolds & Kupfer, 1999). Therefore, in patients with cancer, assessment should focus on symptoms that affect appearance, behavior, or cognition and symptoms that are a change from the patients' previous level of functioning (e.g., guilt, crying, pessimism, hopelessness, flat affect, slowed speech, labile emotions; problems with concentrating and decision making).

Table 16-7. Components of a Psychosocial Assessment

Term	Description
Mental health	Personal/family history of psychiatric disorder, anxiety, depression, suicide attempt; substance abuse; cognitive impairment
Sexual health	The individual's personal meaning of sexuality and intimacy; disease- and treatment-related body image changes
Spiritual needs	Meaning or purpose of life, hope, relatedness, forgiveness, or acceptance, and transcendence
Culture and ethnicity	Limited access to medical care; communication barriers: language, literacy, and physical barriers; financial problems; inadequate social support
Phase of illness	Stage of cancer and treatment(s) along the continuum of disease/diagnosis, prognosis, active treatment, remission, recurrence, terminal progression; management of symptoms and treatment side effects (e.g., pain, fatigue)
Comorbidities	Comorbid physical illnesses such as cardiac, pulmonary, renal, and endocrine diseases; mental illness such as anxiety disorders, depressive disorders, or personality disorders
Coping style	Past history of traumatic loss or illness; internal versus external locus of control; patient-identified strengths and weaknesses, perceived social support and resources; younger age; female gender
Life stage/goals	Developmental life stage; emotional challenges, life goals, and personal dreams delayed or blocked by cancer diagnosis and treatment
Family system	Family boundaries and cohesion; family coping styles and communication skills; family/caregiver conflicts; young or dependent children
Social support	Continuity of health care, medical healthcare team, and access to health care; community support such as work environment, church, and cancer resources (e.g., American Cancer Society, Wellness Community®); inadequate social support; financial problems

Note. Based on information from Bush, 2006a; Kemp, 2006; National Comprehensive Cancer Network, 2008.

- Delirium
- Psychosis
- Dementia
- Mood disorder
- Anxiety disorder
- Manic symptoms
- Acute depression
- Severe depression
- Personality disorder
- Adjustment disorder
- Suicidal ideation or risk
- Antidepressant resistance
- Substance-related disorder/abuse

Figure 16-6. Diagnoses Warranting Psychiatric Referral

Note. Based on information from Moore, 2006; National Comprehensive Cancer Network, 2008.

Coping and Adaptation

Coping with cancer is a process—as illness demands change over time, so will patients' coping methods. Each of the stages of cancer will require different coping skills from patients. Patterns of distress are heightened at major transition points; recurrence has been found to be more disturbing than initial diagnosis because the hope for cure is gone (Bush, 2006a; Spencer, Carver, & Price, 1998). In an investigation of women's experiences with recurrent ovarian cancer, recurrence brought forth a sense of desperation to find a treatment that would control the disease (Howell, Fitch, & Deane, 2003).

Coping has been defined as a complex, ever-changing dynamic that is influenced by the situation (context), individual differences (personality traits), and previous life experiences (Nail, 2001). Important to understand is that no "right" or "wrong" way to cope exists (Nail). Coping and adaptation to illness also depend on patients' psychological makeup, cultural identity, and the social support resources available. Each person will respond to the cancer experience based on his or her own reality. Figure 16-7 summarizes the many variables that influence how an individual may cope with the challenge of cancer. Personality characteristics, such as how prone a person is to anxiety and depression, optimism versus pessimism, hardiness and ego-strength, and locus of control, will influence coping responses. Those patients who have a prior history of anxiety and depression will have the highest risk of emotional instability when challenged by cancer (Bush, 2006a).

- Nature of the illness
- Phases of illness
- Personality dimensions
- Coping styles
- Cultural, socioeconomic, and gender dimensions
- Developmental life stage
- Social networks and support
- Family coping
- Personal meaning, spirituality, and hope
- Specific coping challenges

Figure 16-7. Variables That Influence Coping

Note. From "Coping and Adaptation" (p. 69), by N.J. Bush in R.M. Carroll-Johnson, L.M. Gorman, and N.J. Bush (Eds.), *Psychosocial Nursing Care Along the Cancer Continuum* (2nd ed.), 2006, Pittsburgh, PA: Oncology Nursing Society. Copyright 2006 by Oncology Nursing Society. Reprinted with permission.

Optimism refers to people's generalized positive expectancies about future events (Aspinwall & Brunhart, 2000). Those patients who are optimists suffer fewer emotional consequences from adversity and cope more actively because they reframe stressful events related to a self-image of control and efficacy (Satterfield, 2000). Being an optimist supports finding something positive in loss (Nolen-Hoeksema, 2001). Ego-strength is a resiliency trait that engages the person to master the stress being confronted (Barry, 2002), and individuals with an internal locus of control are more likely to cope by becoming a participant in their care plan and by taking responsibility for their own health (Bush, 2006a).

Lazarus and Folkman's (1984) framework commonly is used as a basis for stress and coping research (see Figure 16-8). The theoretical principle underlying this model is

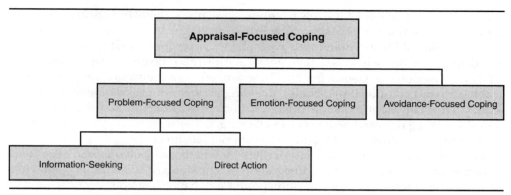

Figure 16-8. Conceptual Framework for Stress and Coping

Note. Based on information from Lazarus & Folkman, 1984.

that how people evaluate or appraise the challenge at hand determines their emotional and behavioral responses to stress. **Primary appraisal** incorporates the personal meaning of the stressful event as threatening or challenging, and **secondary appraisal** incorporates people's evaluation of their capability to reduce the threat. People with cancer experience both threat (potential for harm) and challenge (potential for mastery) appraisals at the same time (Nail, 2001). **Self-efficacy,** defined as a person's confidence in the ability to carry out the necessary behaviors and skills to overcome a threat, has been shown to positively influence the appraisal process. **Coping styles,** such as taking on a fighting spirit versus taking on a fatalistic or stoic acceptance, also influence the appraisal process (Bush, 2006a). Boehmke and Dickerson (2006) found that women with breast cancer who had positive attitudes and fighting spirits coped more effectively with the diagnosis and treatment of cancer.

Appraisal-focused coping often leads to problem-focused coping. Once the situation has been appraised, the person then focuses on solving the problem (e.g., What do I do now?). Two methods of problem solving are to gain knowledge or seek information about the challenge and to take direct action against the stressor by applying cognitive and behavioral means. Information supports effective problem solving when it is tailored to the individual's education, past experiences, and emotional needs (Bush, 2006a; Nail, 2001). Inherent in taking direct action against the stressor is the individual's need to feel empowered and in control of the situation. Because a cancer diagnosis often makes individuals feel powerless, the feeling of control will be personal and situational (Nail). It is easier for the individuals to feel empowered to fight when the disease is diagnosed at an early versus late stage.

Maintaining emotional equilibrium and safety is another function of coping. Cognitive processes, such as fears, feelings, and worries, influence the emotional responses to stress. Emotion-focused coping behaviors, such as expressing anger or crying, are effective means of regaining emotional balance (Spencer et al., 1998). Even denial in the early stages of diagnosis can help individuals from becoming overwhelmed with fear and anxiety. If the intensity and duration of emotion-focused coping causes individuals to disengage mentally or physically from the threatening situation, then this becomes *avoidance-focused coping,* and the individuals are at risk for becoming immobilized from taking direct action (Bush, 2006a). Denial has been linked to poor long-term adjustment to illness, and denial is likely to compromise one's ability to anticipate and prepare for unknown stressors (Aspinwall & Brunhart, 2000). A review of symptoms affecting the quality of life in women with gynecologic cancer found that women who used avoidance-style coping to escape their emotional distress reported a lower quality of life (Tabano, Condosta, & Coons, 2002). These women were found to have poorer physical health and emotional well-being, including greater symptoms of anxiety, depression, fatigue, and other mood disturbances. In contrast, women who used active problem-style coping reported better social well-being, better relationships with their physicians, and less confusion and mood disturbances (Tabano et al.).

Lethborg, Kissane, Burns, and Snyder (2000) found that adaptation to the experience of cancer and treatment requires integration of a new identity. The initial completion of cancer treatment is a major transition point when patients often reflect, "What shall I do with my life now?" A changed reality becomes a catalyst for adaptive adjustment. Integration of a new reality consists of dealing with the stress of uncertainty and ambiguity about the future, reintegration of a new body image and self-image, disruption of sexuality and intimacy, and self-consciousness in relationships and social situations. Returning to normalcy does not mean returning to the same place or identity (Lethborg et al.). In a qualitative study to determine the personal meanings and shared experiences of women after a diagnosis of breast cancer, women described their feelings of a changed identity as "erasure" of their former self (Boehmke & Dickerson, 2006). One woman explained, "I lost not only my hair, but my eyelashes, eyebrows, pubic hair, and nasal hairs. My best description is I felt like someone took a big eraser and erased me" (p. 1124).

The personal meaning of the cancer experience demands that assessment and interventions to support coping must be directed at those variables that strongly affect the patient's emotional and behavioral responses. This includes stage of disease and treatment, any comorbid illnesses, management of disease- and treatment-related symptoms, family and social support, gender and developmental life stage, culture and ethnicity, spirituality and hopefulness, and survivorship. Assessment also must include the phase of the disease being experienced along the illness continuum and how coping challenges change over time. Psychosocial interventions should then be both individualized and targeted to points in time when they are most needed (Nail, 2001). Adopting a focus on individual outcomes rather than on specific coping strategies and focusing interventions on modifiable stressors ensures the most effective way to support adaptation.

> Every person brings unique characteristics to dealing with illness: a
> particular personality, a way of coping, a set of beliefs and values, and
> a way of looking at the world. The goal is to take these qualities into
> consideration and make sure that they work in favor of the person at
> each point along the cancer journey. (Holland & Lewis, 2000, p. 3)

Gender and developmental life stage: Other contributing factors for psychological distress during the cancer experience include gender and developmental life stage. Rates of depression vary across the life span, and depression occurs differently among men and women. The lifetime prevalence of clinical depression is approximately twice as high in women as in men (Kornstein & McEnany, 2006). The theoretical basis for this difference may be that both biologic and social factors contribute to increased rates of depression for women. Women have differences in brain structure and function, different genetic factors, and hormonal fluctuations across the reproductive life span that increase their vulnerability to depression. Cancer treatments, such as certain chemotherapeutic agents, also may contribute to depression by placing a woman in premature, unnatural menopause. Psychosocial factors that increase women's risk for depression include gender differences in roles, socialization, coping styles, and economic and social status (Kornstein & McEnany). Men may experience similar symptoms of depression as women do, yet they are less likely to identify or report depressive moods because of fears related to stigmatization, job security, or loss of health insurance benefits (Porche, 2005). Depression in men may manifest differently because men are more apt to engage in coping efforts using drugs and alcohol, immersing themselves in work-related activities, or acting out reckless and risky behaviors. Of grave concern is that suicide can be a symptom or consequence of depression, and in the United States, men are four times more likely than women to die of suicide (Porche).

Stereotypes of men and women play a role in gender-based coping (Anastasia, 2006b). Stereotypes support the beliefs that men are rational, independent, and decisive, whereas women are emotional, dependent, sensitive, and nurturing (Geis, 1993). Therefore, emotion-focused coping is expected to be used more often by women than men. A diagnosis of cancer may bring a display of emotion from a woman, whereas a man may act stoic to remain in control. More often, men use problem-focused coping styles or even denial and avoidance to prevent relinquishing control and independence. Across the cancer continuum, women experience more personal strain because they juggle role responsibilities as wife, mother, employee, and caregiver for others. Men have demonstrated more distress related to psychosocial concerns regarding role changes in the home and workplace and financial worries (Anastasia, 2006b). APNs must be aware of and avoid using gender-based stereotypes when assessing coping styles. Assessment and interventions are most effective when based on the individual's personality and methods to cope with crisis in the past.

Age and developmental life stage also influence coping and adaptation. The risk of psychological distress increases when life tasks are interrupted at any given age (Anastasia, 2006b). Childhood survivors live with the fear of possible secondary malignancies related to their primary treatments (e.g., Hodgkin disease survivors face breast cancer risk related to mantle field radiation). Inherent developmental challenges exist that the person must resolve at each stage of psychological growth, and cancer can disrupt emotional development and the resolution of life goals (Anastasia, 2006b; Barry, 2002; Bush, 2006a). Erikson's (1963) theoretical framework of psychosocial development described the inherent tasks or challenges that a person must resolve at each stage of emotional growth (see Table 16-8). Disruption of these tasks may negatively affect patients' abilities to cope and to feel hopeful about their future. Young people experiencing cancer have reported greater adjustment problems and poorer quality of life than older people with cancer (Barsevick, Much, & Sweeney, 2000; Bush, 2006a). Older adults may be less apt to recognize and report psychological symptoms caused by cumulative physical and social losses throughout their life span (e.g., bereavement in older adults increases their risk for chronic depression). Whether young or old, the reordering of priorities and revision of life goals constitute part of the reappraisal of the event as an opportunity for growth, rather than only as a loss. This reappraisal may be a coping strategy that helps to strengthen self-esteem and coping (Nolen-Hoeksema, 2001).

Symptom management: Symptoms experienced with cancer and treatment may negatively affect patients' abilities to cope. Newly diagnosed younger patients with breast cancer have expressed emotional distress related to menopausal symptoms, such as hot flashes and insomnia, or chemotherapy-related fatigue and neuropathies that interfere with their daily functioning and activity levels (Boehmke & Dickerson, 2006). Women

Table 16-8. Erikson's Developmental Stages of Emotional Growth

Age	Psychosocial Stage	Main Developmental Tasks	Personality Outcomes
Birth–1 year	Trust versus mistrust	Establish a basic trust.	Hope, faith, and optimism
1–3 years	Autonomy versus shame	Learn to control bodies, behavior, and their environment.	Self-control and will power
3–6 years	Initiative versus guilt	Explore, imagine, and develop conscience.	Direction, purpose, and imagination
6–12 years	Industry versus inferiority	Work and produce; develop self-assurance.	Competence
12–18 years	Identity versus role confusion	Incorporate changes to the body; integrate concepts and values with society.	Devotion and fidelity
Early adulthood	Intimacy versus isolation	Develop intimate love and interpersonal relationships.	Affiliations, love, and mutuality
Young/middle adulthood	Generativity versus stagnation	Create and care for the next generation; nourish and nurture.	Care
Old age	Ego integrity versus despair	Become satisfied with life, and accept what has been.	Wisdom

Note. Based on information from Erikson, 1963.
From "Gender and Age Differences in the Psychological Response to Cancer" (p. 93), by P.J. Anastasia in R.M. Carroll-Johnson, L.M. Gorman, and N.J. Bush (Eds.), *Psychosocial Nursing Care Along the Cancer Continuum* (2nd ed.), 2006, Pittsburgh, PA: Oncology Nursing Society. Copyright 2006 by Oncology Nursing Society. Reprinted with permission.

experiencing recurrent ovarian cancer have reported difficulty coping as a result of the side effects of progressive disease and treatments (Howell et al., 2003).

As discussed, coping is affected by patients' appraisal of the disease and treatment challenges. This appraisal also may directly affect side effect and symptom experiences. Boehmke and Dickerson (2006) found that if newly diagnosed patients with breast cancer cannot move beyond the emotional reaction of shock and disbelief, the diagnosis becomes a profound loss that necessitates grieving. Grief requires both physical and emotional energy, causing women to report an increase in treatment-related symptoms, side effects, and symptom distress.

Management of disease-related and treatment-related symptoms can have a direct impact on patient coping and adaptation. Debilitating symptoms such as pain, fatigue, anxiety, and depression must be effectively managed in order to provide comprehensive psychosocial care to patients. In addition, if physical and psychological symptoms are not well controlled, cognitive impairment may result, thus interfering with the patient's ability to appraise the situation appropriately or to make necessary decisions and problem solve (Zabora, Loscalzo, & Weber, 2003). Uncontrolled physical symptoms, such as pain, accounts for high rates of suicide and requests for assisted suicide in patients with cancer (Chochinov, Wilson, Enns, & Lander, 1998).

Culture and ethnicity: Culture prescribes the beliefs, values, norms, and practices of a group of people, providing identity, meaning, and purpose to their lives. The experience of cancer cannot be understood as an event separate from the cultural context and ethnic identity of the patient (Itano, 2005). Both Western and non-Western countries are rapidly becoming multicultural. In the United States, the presence of diverse communities of Latinos, African Americans, Asian Americans, and Native Americans is increasing in demographic magnitude and cultural differentiation, including an ongoing flow of immigrants and refugees (Mezzich, Kleinman, Fabrega, & Parron, 1996). Cultural competency has become a necessity to ensure that quality health care is given to these diverse populations and communities. The components of cultural competence include assessment and interventions based on a framework that includes the cultural identity of the patient, cultural explanations of the patient's illness, cultural factors related to psychosocial functioning and the social environment, and the cultural exchange between the patient and the healthcare provider (Mezzich et al.). Guidelines for providing culturally competent care are outlined in Figure 16-9.

The expression of emotion will vary by the cultural context in which experiences are discussed (Manson, 1996). Culture also may determine different expressions of an emotion. For example, Vietnamese refugees distinguish states of sadness by the degree, duration, and frequency of their feelings (Manson). Cultural and gender norms may determine the threshold at which the expression of certain emotions is considered "normal" versus "abnormal." For example, the higher prevalence of depression reported among females compared to males may represent socially patterned expectations in the expression of emotions associated with depression and do not necessarily represent higher rates of the disorder in one gender over the other (Manson). Psychosocial assessment within a cultural framework may be most effective by considering an individual's or family's perception of a stress or problem, how they are experiencing the problem, and how they express their emotions rather than searching for distinct entities or definitions of a disorder (Tseng, 1996). How the healthcare provider relates to

---

- Accept that all people have value and are worthy of respect.
- Explore and acknowledge your own beliefs and values, biases, and prejudices.
- Respect religious and cultural norms regarding touch, eye contact, or treatment by the opposite sex.
- Acknowledge and be respectful of patient beliefs regarding alternative treatments or traditional healers.
- Learn the appropriate cultural greeting for the patients' belief system as a means of establishing rapport and trust.
- Determine the patient's preferred language prior to assessment, and arrange for a medical interpreter when appropriate.
- Regardless of education, socioeconomic status, culture, and ethnicity, all people have strengths that can be identified and built upon.
- Negotiate a treatment plan that negotiates the patient's value system and lifestyle within acceptable standards of American health care.
- Apply cross-cultural interview techniques to avoid stereotyping. Question patients about their beliefs relating to disease causation, treatment, and cure.
- Educate yourself regarding the culture, traditions, rules of interaction, family and social roles, health and illness beliefs, and practices of the populations you serve.
- If legally possible, honor the patients' and family's values regarding decision-making practices and preferences regarding the disclosure of bad news and truth-telling.
- Understand that the combined concepts of culture, perceptual world view, and health and illness beliefs are fundamental to the provision of culturally competent nursing care.

Figure 16-9. Guidelines for Cultural Competence

Note. Based on information from Salimbene, 2007.

the patient and the provider's own perception and understanding of the problem are important variables (Tseng).

Family systems: Cancer is experienced by patients and families interdependently, and thus, the family is the "unit of care" (Bush, 1998; Jassak, 1992). Family systems theory provides a framework to assess the impact of cancer on the family (Jassak; Morris, Grant, & Lynch, 2007). A family is defined as a social system with shared goals, beliefs, and history, and within the family, each member acts independently but also as part of a family unit (Morris et al.). Therefore, a life-threatening illness such as cancer will not only affect the patient but also will affect family members, particularly those who have direct caregiving responsibilities.

An assumption underlying family systems theories is that a homeostatic state or balancing of forces exists within every family—family rules, member roles, subsystems and boundaries, and expectations exist within the family to ensure internal equilibrium (Bush, 1998; Goldenberg & Goldenberg, 1996). Figure 16-10 details the aspects of family structure and organization that the experience of cancer can challenge. Family homeostasis can be disrupted at any time along the major transition points of the cancer experience, placing the family in a crisis state. The family subsystems and boundaries can be predictive of how patients and family members will cope. If the family is an open system, it will be more adaptable and open to change without losing its unity, seeking out resources and using creative and flexible problem solving (Friedman, Bowden, & Jones, 2003). Closed family units are rigid, lack flexibility for adaptation, and view change as threatening (Friedman et al.; Goldenberg & Goldenberg).

Family roles, rules, and myths are socially, culturally, and gender based. For example, Given, Given, Kozachik, and Rawl (2003) found that caregiving is more stressful for women (wives or daughters) than for men (husbands and sons). In the married couples that were studied, husbands tended to caregiving tasks while continuing their own interests and activities, whereas wife caregivers focused on the interpersonal aspects of caregiving, most often giving priority to their husbands' needs and demands. When confronting cancer, family roles and rules also will influence communication and decision making. Certain cultures have practices regarding the disclosure of bad news. For example, Hispanic beliefs maintain that family members, especially elders, should not be informed of their "real" diagnosis of cancer because truth-telling will only make them sicker (Cohen & Munet-Vilaro, 2001; Faysman & Oseguera, 2002). Additionally, a cancer diagnosis will challenge the developmental stage of the family. If cancer occurs during childbearing years, a young couple may face infertil-

---

Rules: Organized, repetitive patterns of interaction; expected member behaviors

Homeostasis: A dynamic state of balance or equilibrium; stable family function

Subsystems and boundaries: Family dyads (e.g., spouse dyad, parent-child dyad); respect of individual boundaries

Roles: Expectations of the behaviors and contributions of individual family members in order to support independence and the family unit

Myths: Beliefs that family members hold uncritically about themselves in relationship to each other and to the outside world

Developmental tasks: Stages of family growth and development with inherent tasks for individual members and for the family as a unit

---

Figure 16-10. Family Structure and Organization at Risk From a Diagnosis of Cancer

---

Note. Based on information from Bush, 1998; Friedman et al., 2003; Goldenberg & Goldenberg, 1996.

ity challenges or stressors with balancing work and parenting, in addition to other challenges (Bush, 1998).

The impact of cancer on the family will continue as changes in healthcare delivery find more patients being cared for in the home setting and with family members becoming the primary caretakers. Families must cope not only with the emotional responses to the cancer experience but also with the social, physical, and financial aspects of providing care to their loved ones. Research focused on family caregivers has shown that family members feel ill-prepared, have insufficient preparation and knowledge, and feel that they receive little support from the healthcare system (Given et al., 2003). More recent research focusing on patient-reported family distress among long-term cancer survivors identified that high levels of family distress are experienced at initial diagnosis and treatment followed by ongoing family distress related to the challenges of the disease (Morris et al., 2007). Further research is needed to identify the impact of distress on families across time (e.g., from diagnosis through transition points), to identify those families at highest risk for distress, to identify family needs based on cultural, ethnic, and socioeconomic diversity, and to identify healthcare interventions that support family coping and adaptation (Given et al.; Kitrungrote & Cohen, 2006). APNs are in a pivotal role to improve clinical outcomes for patients by identifying the physical, spiritual, and emotional needs of the family unit. Interventions should be focused on promoting adaptation and preserving normal family functioning as much as possible. Interventions also must help family caregivers to meet their own health needs and maintain quality of life (Kitrungrote & Cohen).

Social support: Social support has been shown to buffer the negative effects of cancer by providing direct intervention through physical and emotional support. According to Lazarus and Folkman's (1984) cognitive model of stress and coping, when a person is dealing with a stressful event such as cancer, social support can directly influence the person's adjustment. Family, friends, and community and religious resources, as well as the healthcare team, can positively affect the patient's coping responses by changing the person's appraisal of the event or their emotional response to it (Hudek-Knezevic, Kardum, & Pahljina, 2002). Interpersonal relationships, such as family and friends, provide emotional or **affectional** support through love, nurturance, acceptance, and intimacy. These relationships can also provide **affirmational** support or validation that the patient's feelings are accepted and understood. Community and religious resources, or **affiliational** support, provides the person with a social identity and sense of belonging. Affiliational support also may include cancer resources, such as belonging to the Wellness Community®, which prevent patients from feeling isolated in their experience. Tangible or **instrumental** support includes resources, such as a job, church, family, or the ACS, that can provide financial assistance, physical goods, or services. Healthcare providers play a major role in educational or **informational** support by providing patients with the knowledge and skills needed for effective decision making and coping (Bush, 2006a; Hudek-Knezevic et al.). **Therapeutic** support in the form of psychoeducational support has been shown to positively enhance psychological and physical well-being (Edelman, Craig, & Kidman, 2000; Neilson-Clayton & Brownlee, 2002), as well as strengthen the immune system (Fawzy, Fawzy, Arndt, & Pasnau, 1995). Participation in cancer support groups has been found to provide informational and emotional support, and sharing experiences with others may reduce fear and anxiety (Ahlberg & Nordner, 2006). Internet support has recently become an identified vehicle for meeting the psychosocial needs of patients. In a qualitative study of

Internet use for cancer care, one of the major themes that evolved was the use of the Internet to provide peer support for patients (Dickerson, Boehmke, & Brown, 2006). Internet communications minimized feelings of isolation, allowed a forum to share cancer treatment experiences, and provided hope by making the most current information available.

Social support promotes the use of positive coping strategies, but the effectiveness of social support must be evaluated as to whether it has been tailored to the patient's individual needs and situation (Fitch, 2006), in addition to what, and how strongly, the patient *perceives* his or her social support to be (Hudek-Knezevic et al., 2002). For example, hospitalized patients have reported that the most important sources of support were their family and the medical staff, whereas among nonhospitalized patients, the family was perceived as the most important social support (Hudek-Knezevic et al.). Patients may attend a cancer support group and yet not feel or perceive that their personal needs are being met, which is not an uncommon finding for minority populations (Henderson, Gore, Davis, & Condon, 2003).

When evaluating the effectiveness of social support, other intervening variables such as gender and culture must be considered. Considerable research has been done on the benefits of social support for female patients with cancer, specifically breast cancer. Men have different, although equally pressing, needs for social support, such as in the case of prostate cancer (Poole et al., 2001). APNs need to understand and respect the diversity among ethnic populations and be aware that social support will be defined within their cultural perspective. For example, family support and involvement are essential for Filipino Americans, and these patients may not comply with the instructions of healthcare providers who disregard their family's opinions. In the traditional Japanese culture, the family assumes most of the responsibility for health care; therefore, when hospitalization is necessary, family members should be encouraged to be involved to relieve the patient's anxiety and to promote emotional comfort (Lasky, Martz, & Kagawa-Singer, 2001). The psychosocial support needs must be identified in multiethnic populations in order to provide culturally sensitive interventions for these patients (Gotay & Lau, 2003).

Spirituality: Illness heightens spiritual awareness and the use of spiritual coping strategies (Taylor, 2006). In the realm of suffering and loss, and dying and death, many individuals turn to their faith, religion, and God for comfort (Kemp, 2006). Therefore, spiritual care is a vital component of quality oncology nursing care. Spiritual care focuses on meeting the spiritual needs of patients—finding meaning and purpose, hopefulness, relatedness, forgiveness or acceptance, and transcendence (Kemp). APNs can provide spiritual care through empathic listening and by helping patients to process the meaning of their illness as it relates to their beliefs, life experiences, and religious practices. Nurses need to validate patients' spiritual needs by encouraging activities of self-expression, such as meditation and prayer; storytelling (e.g., life review); journal writing; music, art, or dance therapy; and being with nature.

Taylor (2006) identified some of the reasons why oncology nurses fail to address their patients' spiritual needs. These included time restraints, ambiguity about their own spiritual beliefs, and a lack of knowledge regarding the nurse's role in spiritual care. Oncology APNs are in a prime position to educate other oncology nurses regarding spiritual assessment and the impact that spirituality has on patients' coping with their illness. APNs also are educated to include spiritual assessment as part of overall psychosocial management and refer patients to spiritual counselors, chaplains, and clergy when needed.

Supportive Cancer Care for Psychosocial Disturbance

Supportive cancer care has been defined as the necessary services for those people with or affected by cancer to meet a continuum of needs—social, practical, physical, spiritual, emotional, informational, and psychological—throughout the full continuum of living as a cancer survivor (Fitch, 2006). The goals of supportive care are to assist patients in meeting their psychosocial needs, maintaining or improving their quality of life, and optimizing their sense of well-being (Fitch). Supportive care should be directed at the expressed needs of both patients and families and continually monitored and adapted as the course of the disease and treatment unfolds. Each transition point along the cancer continuum will demand new knowledge, new skills, and different networks of support to meet the changing demands of illness, whether it is acute, chronic, or palliative (Fitch). Supportive care consists of pharmacologic, nonpharmacologic, and programmatic approaches to psychosocial support.

Pharmacologic Interventions

A thorough health history and physical examination must be initiated prior to pharmacologic interventions for psychosocial distress. If depression or anxiety, or any associated symptom, such as insomnia, is being caused by a medical condition or by a drug, the underlying problem must be identified and treated initially. After the underlying problem is treated, the patient is again assessed for mood disorder prior to initiating treatments (Massie & Popkin, 1998; NCCN, 2008).

If possible, assessment should include a family member, as many patients are not aware of changes in their affect or behavior or may minimize their feelings for fear of being stigmatized or viewed as being emotionally weak. Guidelines suggest that when generalized anxiety coexists with depressed mood, treatment should first be directed toward managing the depression (Agency for Health Care Policy and Research, 1993). A majority of antidepressants are effective in ameliorating associated anxiety. Treatment for mood or anxiety disorders should include a multimodality approach: pharmacologic management, individual or family counseling or psychotherapy, cognitive and behavioral interventions, and complementary therapies (NCCN, 2008).

In the cancer population, the medications most often used for depression and anxiety include a class of drugs called the selective serotonin reuptake inhibitors (SSRIs). General side effects of the SSRIs include agitation, gastrointestinal disturbance, and sexual dysfunction. However, because the SSRIs affect only one neurotransmitter (serotonin), they frequently are a medication of choice for depression because of their low side effect profile and their low potential for overdose. SSRIs also are the drug of choice for patients experiencing symptoms of both depression and anxiety (Bowers & Boyle, 2003; Stahl, 1998; Van Fleet, 2006).

Pharmacotherapy also may be chosen to manage some treatment-induced side effects. Venlafaxine is used to reduce chemotherapy-induced menopausal symptoms, such as mood swings, hot flashes, and insomnia. Combination therapy may be initiated to provide broader therapeutic efficacy or when patients become tolerant or resistant to one specific agent. Both serotonin and norepinephrine mediate pain pathways; therefore, a selective norepinephrine reuptake inhibitor such as bupropion may be combined with a similar drug that has serotonin properties such as venlafaxine to effectively treat patients with severe depression who also need support for pain management (Sharp, 2005). Duloxetine, a newer antidepressant, is effective against depression, generalized anxiety disorder, and neuropathic pain, which is a fairly common symptom profile in the cancer population. Bupropion, a norepinephrine and dopamine reuptake inhibitor, has proved to be effective for symptoms such as cognitive slowing or pseudodementia or in patients who are concerned about sexual dysfunction from the SSRIs. These examples point out that for therapeutic results, matching the pharmacologic profile of the drug or drug combination with the patient's clinical profile is an important criterion for successful treatment (Stahl).

Psychostimulants such as methylphenidate also may have a role in treating depression because of their rapid onset and ability to improve mood, energy levels, concentration, and attention span (Van Fleet, 2006). Psychostimulants can be effective adjuncts in pain management because they counteract opioid-induced sedation and improve mood (Pasacreta et al., 2006). Side effects of psychostimulants include insomnia, tachycardia, and agitation and therefore may exacerbate anxiety associated with depression. Psychostimulants generally are ordered to be given early in the day to avoid insomnia.

Antidepressant therapy is effective for both depressive and anxious states, but the benzodiazepines are used most often to treat isolated states of anxiety. This classification of drugs also is used for treating insomnia, chemotherapy-related nausea and vomiting, and treatment-related fears and phobias, such as claustrophobia associated with MRI, and as premedication for unpleasant procedures, such as bone marrow aspiration. Lorazepam usually is the drug of choice because its short half-life is unaffected by age, liver disease, or the concurrent use of an SSRI. The amnesic effect of lorazepam may be beneficial for patients who experience anticipatory nausea and vomiting with chemotherapy yet may be contraindicated in patients who suffer from chemotherapy-related cognitive dysfunction. Longer-acting benzodiazepines, such as clonazepam, are effective for treatment of panic disorders or generalized anxiety disorders but should be used with caution in older adults because of the risk of oversedation (Pasacreta et al., 2006). See Figure 16-11 for guidelines for ordering psychotherapeutic drugs.

- Reassess dosages regularly.
- Use caution when ordering drugs with sedative effects for patients with cognitive dysfunction.
- Drugs must be individually tailored to the age, health history, symptoms, and comorbidities of patients.
- Adjust drug and dosage for older adult patients, for patients with liver disease, and for patients with a history of seizure disorder.
- Advise patients that withdrawal symptoms may occur if medications are discontinued and that a tapering schedule should be followed.
- Know the side effect profile of each medication administered. Educate patients and families to normal and expected versus untoward side effects.
- Combination drugs also may improve clinical efficacy in severely depressed patients by their independent therapeutic actions on serotonin and norepinephrine.
- Prescribe the lowest dose, and then titrate upward after seven days in order to monitor side effects and evaluate therapeutic effectiveness. It takes approximately six to eight weeks to reach therapeutic levels.
- Antidepressants also may be chosen for their proven effectiveness against disease- or treatment-related side effects that contribute to depression and anxiety (e.g., pain, insomnia, menopausal symptoms).

Figure 16-11. Guidelines for Ordering Psychotherapeutic Drugs

Note. Based on information from Moore, 2006; Pasacreta et al., 2006; Stahl, 1998; Van Fleet, 2006.

Nonpharmacologic Interventions

An integrated and patient-centered approach to psychosocial care is required to provide comprehensive, quality cancer care (Fitch, 2006). This includes both pharmacologic and nonpharmacologic interventions tailored to meet the physical and psychological needs of patients. Initiation of medication is recommended if patients are immobilized by depression or anxiety because it is difficult for patients to engage in nonpharmacologic activities or programs until their symptoms are controlled and they have energy and focus to learn and participate. Individual counseling or psychotherapy can be very effective to support patients in the initial six to eight weeks until antidepressant therapy becomes fully effective. Individual counseling or psychotherapy should be continued as long as it meets patients' emotional needs.

Integrative oncology is the use of complementary therapies for anxiety, mood disorders, and symptom management, such as for pain (Deng & Cassileth, 2005; Kocsis, 2000; Kwekkeboom, 2003). The term *integrative* implies that standard, conventional care is combined with complementary therapies using a multidimensional and holistic approach to health and healing (Fletcher, 2006). The relationship between stress and negative mood states having a deleterious effect on immune function and health outcomes provides the basis for many of these nonpharmacologic interventions (Post-White, 2006). Interventions that modulate the immune response can be divided into two categories: sensory stimulation and cognitive-behavioral therapy. Sensory stimulation interventions involve the senses and include massage, music and art, humor or laughter therapy, prayer and spiritual healing, and aromatherapy. A number of researchers have demonstrated improvements in mood and perceived stress following massage therapy, in addition to a decrease in symptoms such as pain, and music interventions have shown a positive effect on mood, nausea, and anxiety (Post-White). The efficacy of aromatherapy has yet to be determined, but this intervention often is combined with massage, relaxation, and meditation to heighten the senses.

Cognitive-behavioral therapy is a nonpharmacologic approach to depression and anxiety that is well accepted with clinically proven outcomes. The goal underlying cognitive-behavioral therapy is to help patients to cognitively "reframe" their negative and hopeless perceptions with realistic and positive perceptions (Lovejoy, Tabor, Matteis, et al., 2000). Techniques include psychoeducation, guided imagery, and relaxation and stress management techniques, such as meditation, exercise, and expressive writing. Cognitive-behavioral techniques result in positive effects on mood, anxiety, and the overall well-being of patients with cancer (Post-White, 2006). APNs can learn, teach, and implement many of these interventions in their practice settings.

Nonpharmacologic interventions also include the use of complementary and alternative medicine (CAM), including stress-reducing techniques previously described in addition to the use of traditional and ethnic techniques and medicines (e.g., acupuncture), diet and nutritional supplements, and energy therapies (e.g., Reiki). CAM is defined as *complementary* therapy because it is used for symptom management and to improve quality of life while patients with cancer are receiving conventional medical treatment (Lengacher et al., 2006). The effective implementation of CAM therapies has been found to relieve physical symptoms and psychological distress in addition to giving patients a feeling of personal control over their illness (Lengacher). APNs need to educate patients regarding the use of CAM therapies, identify what CAM therapies the individual patient is using, monitor patient outcomes, and detect any contraindications to the use of these preparations or techniques based on the patient's conventional treatments. The National Institutes of Health has a scientific branch, the National Center for Complementary and Alternative Medicine, to investigate the role of CAM therapy in oncology care (Fletcher, 2006) and to make information available to healthcare providers and the public.

Programmatic Interventions

Cancer programs provide basic information and practical support to all patients with cancer and their families. These programs also should be able to identify those patients who need additional assistance and then refer them to the appropriate services (Fitch, 2006). Programmatic interventions range from one-to-one peer support, such as the ACS Reach to Recovery program, to individual and family support groups, such as those provided by the Wellness Community, and even support groups accessed via the Internet. Programmatic support for patients with cancer can be found on the local, state, and national levels. These programs form a network of services for social support ranging from instrumental support (e.g., equipment) to informational support (education). ACS has been a leader in providing a broad range of social services to patients with cancer. The ACS *I Can Cope* program is an excellent example of an effective programmatic approach that involves both an informational and psychosocial dimension. These types of psychoeducational approaches have been shown to provide patients with the knowledge and skills necessary for problem-focused coping and stress management, in turn increasing their sense of control and competency. Because cancer is a life-threatening diagnosis and the treatment regimens often elicit an emotional stress response of persistent anxiety along with feelings of isolation and helplessness, interventions, whether individual or group in nature, require a holistic approach and an existential perspective (Sloman, 2002). A wide variety of types of support programs are available, and all of them can be effective and help patients and families to cope (Iacovino & Reesor, 1997). The choice of the right type of support can be tailored to the individual patient based on needs and patient preferences.

Hopefulness

Hope is a multidimensional, dynamic life force. As described by Ersek (2006), the dimensions of hope are spiritual, cognitive, contextual, relationships, and behavioral. The spiritual dimension of hope is related to spiritual well-being and encompasses meaning and purpose in life, self-transcendence, and connectedness to a deity or other life force. The cognitive dimension of hope is related to the attainment of life goals and encompasses self-esteem, self-efficacy, and the sense of personal control. The contextual dimension of hope is related to life circumstances that influence hopefulness and encompasses physical and mental health, social and financial stability, and functional and cognitive abilities. Relationships form a significant dimension of hope, encompassing interconnectedness with others and social support. The behavioral dimension of hope includes those activities and thoughts that foster hope and encompass coping strategies such as problem-focused and emotion-focused coping (Ersek). Hope and maintaining hopefulness brings together all aspects of successful psychosocial coping and adaptation.

Hope can exist even in the face of a life-threatening illness such as cancer (Nail, 2001). The context of hope changes throughout the cancer trajectory, but the vital force of hope must be recognized as being present regardless of stage of disease or what the goals of care are to a person (Nail). Positive relationships have been found between hope and coping style and effectiveness, regardless of diagnosis, gender, age, marital status, or education. Hope positively influences adaptation to cancer. Hopelessness contributes to anxiety, depression, and feelings that self and life are worthless. At the extreme, hopelessness can contribute to suicide or consideration of physician-assisted suicide toward the end of life (Ersek, 2006). The impact of a patient's optimism and hope on the coping process can be fostered (Aspinwall & Brunhart, 2000). Fostering hope includes helping patients to reframe the initial appraisal of the potential stressor in a more positive light, assisting them to evaluate whether they are using the right coping mechanism and problem-solving strategy for the identified stressor, and teaching them how to use active, as opposed to avoidant, coping behaviors (Aspinwall & Brunhart). Being hopeful is not giving up in the face of challenge. Hopefulness is engagement in life (Spencer et al., 1998).

Standards of Practice

The NCCN Clinical Practice Guidelines in Oncology™ are recognized standards for clinical policy and practice in the oncology community. These comprehensive guidelines are based on scientific data and are supported by an expert panel of multidisciplinary physicians and other healthcare professionals from NCCN member institutions. The NCCN guidelines address supportive care areas, including distress management (NCCN, 2008). To guide evidence-based practice, NCCN has formulated standards of care for psychosocial management of patients with cancer and has provided algorithms outlining assessment, treatment, and management guidelines. NCCN advises that nurses and all multidisciplinary team members must be responsible for assessing patients with cancer for symptoms of distress.

Numerous other standards of care for assessment and intervention have been provided by the American Psychiatric Association (2000), the Agency for Health Care Policy and Research (1993), and the Oncology Nursing Society (2004). Standards of practice are supported by scientific research, and these guidelines support evidence-based practice for APNs.

Patient and Family Education

Patient and family education is an essential role of the APN. Education regarding psychosocial issues begins with a thorough assessment of the dynamics of patient and family structure (see Figure 16-10) and basic education regarding the impact of the disease, treatment, and side effects on patients' physical, psychological, and spiritual health. Evidence-based practice guidelines (e.g., NCCN, 2008) can provide APNs with the tools and skills to guide assessment and interventions. Psychosocial education must follow standard educational principles and respect for privacy (Agre, 2005) but must address both knowledge deficits that patients or family members may have in addition to their emotional needs and behavioral responses to the experience.

The emotional responses to the diagnosis of cancer often make patients feel as though they are "going crazy" or are out of control. Educating patients and family members regarding the expected emotional reactions to a cancer diagnosis, such as fear, shock, anxiety, and disbelief, will "normalize" their feelings and give them permission to share. When appropriate, APNs should educate patients and family members regarding the signs and symptoms of anxiety and depression, the risk factors, and the professional resources available to help them. Involve patients and family members in decision making and problem solving regarding their disease status and treatment to support their sense of control, autonomy, and self-esteem. Inform patients that emotional support and peer information are available through programs such as Reach to Recovery and CanSurmount. Patients requiring ongoing counseling or psychotherapy for emotional, spiritual, or psychosocial distress should be referred immediately. One-to-one intervention can provide patients with cognitive-behavioral techniques to reframe their experiences and decrease feelings of powerlessness. Encourage patients and family members to participate in psychoeducational programs such as the Wellness Community and *I Can Cope* to gain both educational and emotional support.

The goals of psychosocial education are to enable patients and families to integrate the experience of cancer and maintain a good quality of life. Education includes providing a safe and supportive environment for patients to talk about what personal issues are important to them. A nonjudgmental approach communicates interest and concern. APNs should take cues from patients and family members and start at a point of factual information and move from less sensitive to more sensitive areas when talking to patients about psychosocial issues (Marrs, 2006). Patients' privacy and respect must be honored to prevent them from feeling embarrassment or self-blame. Educate patients regarding ways to increase resilience to psychosocial problems, including nutrition, exercise, good sleeping habits, stress management, and the importance of open communication with healthcare providers and family members regarding their feelings and emotions.

Implications for Oncology Advanced Practice Nurses

Early psychosocial assessment can provide the healthcare team with objective information regarding the general concerns and coping skills of patients and families. Signs and symptoms of emotional or social problems may be less obvious or more difficult to identify than those of a physical nature. A concerted effort to evaluate patients and family members holistically will help to ensure that all their needs can be identified and met. If not identified and supported, emotions can occupy patients' thoughts and expend their mental energy and will not only interfere with coping effectiveness but also may increase somatic complaints and experiences (Zabora et al., 2003). Early psychosocial interventions can prevent the exacerbation of preexisting levels of distress or psychological illness (Zabora et al.). Educational programs for APNs provide the theoretical knowledge base and clinical experience to ensure that they have the expertise to carry out high-level psychosocial assessments and to plan and provide high-level interventions based on scientific data and standards of practice. APNs also can be effective role models for other nurses, healthcare professionals, and family members in addressing and dealing with patients' strong emotional reactions to a diagnosis of cancer. APNs play an integral role in the quality of life of patients with cancer and their families by intervening to ensure balance in their emotional, psychological, spiritual, and social lives as well as in their physical care. Nurses hone these skills over time with consistent application of psychosocial principles of care as well as by continuing professional education in all aspects of quality patient care. Psychosocial assessment must be a fundamental part of new patient assessments, as well as ongoing interactions. Modeling this assessment behavior and intervention techniques for colleagues and family members will support patients and help to foster a therapeutic healthcare environment.

Conclusion

With technologic advancements in prevention, diagnosis, and treatment, many patients diagnosed with cancer will be long-term survivors of this chronic illness. Biobehavioral outcomes through psychological interventions must continue to ensure that cancer survivors do not just experience longevity but that they experience a minimum of adverse long-term health effects and that their quality of life is maintained (Andersen, 2003). Psychological research must continue and expand to represent "the diversity of cancer, as the disease spares no race, gender, age, or ethnic group" (Andersen, 2003, p. 210). Future directions must focus on research and evidence-based practice, and psychosocial care must continue to be grounded in humanity.

Case Study

K.M. is a 41-year-old premenopausal attorney who presents with a diagnosis of axillary lymphadenopathy of adenocarcinoma of unknown origin. She is seeking a second medical oncology consultation regarding potential treatment options. K.M.'s mother is accompanying her for the consultation. When scheduling the appointment, the patient told the secretary that she was extremely frightened and "losing her mind" because no one could tell her what type of cancer she had, so she asked, "How can they treat me correctly?"

Prior to assessing the patient, the APN reviews K.M.'s medical record. K.M.'s breast history dated back 12 years when she underwent breast augmentation following the births and breast-feeding of her three children. Recently, she underwent revision and replacement of the implants because of a rippling effect that had occurred on the right side overlying the implant. Only 10 days previously, while shaving, the patient noticed a mobile, marble-sized mass in her left axilla that she had not appreciated when she had shaved approximately three days earlier. She immediately sought medical attention and underwent a diagnostic mammogram. No abnormalities were detected in her breast, but a 2.5 cm oval, left axillary nodule was present, consistent with lymphadenopathy, which was confirmed by ultrasound to be a 2.6 cm well-circumscribed mass. A two-week course of antibiotics was prescribed with the thought that this may represent a reactive lymphadenopathy; however, no improvement occurred. Excisional biopsy of this lymph node proved to be a $3 \times 2 \times 1$ cm poorly differentiated adenocarcinoma. A complete metastatic work-up, including PET, CT, and bone scans, was negative. At the time of her initial work-up, K.M.'s primary medical physician prescribed lorazepam and paroxetine.

When taking the patient's history, the APN observed visual signs of anxiety. K.M. appeared to be tense, worried, and somewhat tearful. She continually fidgeted, wringing her hands and darting her eyes back and forth to her mother when she answered questions. She relayed the previously discussed history at one point stating, "Can you believe this nightmare? Ten days ago my life was normal." When the APN began to ask questions regarding K.M.'s social history and support systems, she burst into tears. She expressed that her main concern was her three young children and being there for them. Through a veil of tears she asked, "Am I going to die?" The APN, sensitive to K.M.'s fears and anxious mood, intervened by communicating in a calm, caring, and supportive manner. The APN's assessment determined that K.M. worked part-time as an attorney in partnership with her husband. K.M. felt that her husband was emotionally supportive and was as frightened as she was. He had not come with her that day so that he could drive the children to school as if "everything was normal as usual." K.M. also expressed that she had a close-knit family, and she was actively involved in her church community.

Important findings from the history included that K.M. had lost several pounds as a result of the stress she had experienced over the past several weeks. K.M.'s history included the information that her father was of Ashkenazi Jewish background, and a paternal aunt died of breast cancer at age 32. The remaining review of systems and family history were unremarkable. K.M. expressed that she had been healthy and physically active her entire adult life and that she felt totally "out of control in this situation."

The medical consultation revealed important diagnostic information to support the patient's most likely diagnosis and treatment plan. The morphologic immuno-histochemical tissue staining had characteristics of breast, lung, and gastrointestinal tissue in descending order of probability. Tumor markers were negative, and the tissue was estrogen and progesterone receptor and HER2/neu negative. The thyroid transcription factor–1 also was negative, and a special mammaglobin assay was weakly positive. These findings together were supportive of breast origin as the primary site. The medical oncologist reassured K.M. that the likelihood was exceedingly high that she had a stage II breast cancer and that treatment could be planned accordingly. The oncologist recommended dose-dense chemotherapy followed by a formal axillary node dissection and that, if the nodes were pathologically clear, this would indicate a more favorable prognosis as well. A follow-up MRI of the breasts would be performed, and if it was negative, the choices would be a mastectomy, watchful waiting, or perhaps radiotherapy alone (Foroudi & Tiver, 2000).

K.M. asked numerous questions during the consultation, and the APN provided educational and social support resources to the patient and encouraged her to call with further questions if needed. The APN also discussed with K.M. the recently prescribed medications and other nonpharmacologic measures such as what and how to communicate with her children regarding her diagnosis and upcoming treatments. Referrals for psychological intervention also were provided.

1. What nursing diagnoses would the APN identify from K.M.'s assessment?
    - Diagnoses would be anxiety, powerlessness, deficient knowledge, and death anxiety. K.M.'s anxiety is apparent by both her verbal and nonverbal cues. These nonverbal cues include fidgeting, hand wringing, and darting glances. An example of her verbal expression of anxiety is the statement, "Can you believe this nightmare?" K.M.'s feelings of powerlessness are supported by her expressions that she is "losing her mind" and that she feels "out of control in this situation." Deficient knowledge is an important diagnosis in this case because of the unknown primary and rare presentation making treatment planning a challenge. K.M. asked, "How can they treat me properly?" Finally, the diagnosis of death anxiety must be considered when the patient expresses the fear "Am I going to die?"

2. What is an appropriate intervention for the APN to carry out to support the identified nursing diagnoses?
    - The APN should validate and normalize each feeling expressed by the patient. This includes providing a safe and supportive environment for the anxious patient, being calm when answering questions, and allowing the patient time to

reflect. To decrease feelings of powerlessness, the APN should encourage the patient to ask questions and encourage her to be an active member in decision making regarding treatment possibilities. Providing information about the disease and treatment is important at diagnosis and should be reinforced at each phase of treatment to prevent deficient knowledge. The diagnosis of cancer raises existential issues for the patient, and any verbal or nonverbal clues of death anxiety should be addressed directly when the patient expresses these fears.

3. What intervention is necessary when K.M. expresses concern about taking the prescribed lorazepam and paroxetine by her primary medical physician?

   • Assessment of the drug effects and education regarding the action of medication are necessary. The APN should assess K.M.'s knowledge of the purpose of the medications and their possible side effects. The APN can then educate and reinforce for K.M. the positive outcomes of pharmacologic treatment for the anxiety and depression she is feeling as a result of this sudden and frightening change in her life. Providing the patient with referrals for psychiatric follow-up and medication support if needed is another important APN intervention.

4. What nonpharmacologic interventions can the APN suggest for K.M. during her brief consultation?

   • The APN can suggest cognitive behavioral techniques. In addition to the antidepressant and anxiolytic medication prescribed, cognitive behavioral interventions will assist the patient to cope during the many stressors she is facing. The APN should encourage K.M. to attempt to eat a well-balanced diet, get adequate rest and sleep, and continue her exercise regimen if possible. The APN also can recommend that K.M. reach out to her supportive family and friends during this time for personal support and help with the children if needed. Investigating K.M.'s spiritual beliefs and religious practices and her involvement with her church community also could help the APN to guide K.M. toward utilizing social support during this crisis. In addition to referrals for psychiatric medication follow-up if needed, the APN could suggest therapeutic resources, such as the Wellness Community for both individual and family support. Lastly, the APN should provide information and resources regarding complementary therapies, such as guided imagery, relaxation techniques, massage, and hypnosis.

5. If the APN continued to care for K.M. during treatment, what behaviors displayed by the patient would be indicative of a more serious psychiatric diagnosis requiring referral?

   • Any behavior that interfered with K.M.'s ability to follow through with appropriate medical care or treatment or any behavior indicative of suicidal ideation would require referral. If K.M. were to express feelings of suicide ideation or identify a plan for suicide in order to escape the emotional pain she was experiencing, an immediate referral for a psychiatric consultation would be warranted. If K.M.'s anxiety or depression continued, unrelieved by pharmacologic and nonpharmacologic support, and if it interfered with her ability to follow medical care or the treatment plan, then psychiatric referral is necessary. Characteristics of ineffective coping include the patient's verbalization of the inability to cope or asking for help or the inappropriate use of defense mechanisms, such as denial or anger.

Key Points

- Anxiety is a normal emotional response to the cancer experience.
- Anxiety and depression often coexist.
- An individual does not choose to be anxious or depressed; these responses are situational and biologic in nature.
- Delirium is a common acute cognitive dysfunction in the cancer population and must be differentiated from depression and dementia.
- Variables that affect the emotional response to cancer include personal control, self-esteem, sexuality and altered body image, spirituality, and a history of prior anxiety or depressive disorders.
- Variables that influence coping and adaptation to the cancer experience include prior psychosocial risk factors, family systems, social support, culture and ethnicity, and spirituality.
- Both pharmacologic and nonpharmacologic interventions play an important role in the psychosocial support of patients with cancer.
- Psychosocial nursing is holistic care for the body, mind, and spirit.

Recommended Resources for Advanced Practice Nurses

- ACS (800-ACS-2345, www.cancer.org): The ACS Cancer Resource Network provides patient and family services through counseling services and educational programs.
- CURE: Cancer Updates, Research and Education (800-210-CURE, www.curetoday .com): CURE combines the science and humanity of cancer by providing education and resources to a half million survivors through its free magazine and publications.
- Cancer*Care* (800-813-HOPE, www.cancercare.org): This organization provides free support, information, and financial assistance to patients and families.
- Fertile Hope (888-994-4673, www.fertilehope.org): Fertile Hope is a nonprofit organization dedicated to educating patients about fertility issues related to cancer and treatment.
- Lance Armstrong Foundation (512-236-8820, www.livestrong.org): This organization assists patients and families through advocacy, education, research, and public education.
- National Cancer Institute (800-4-CANCER, www.cancer.gov): This comprehensive resource site provides information about cancer prevention, treatment, and clinical trials, along with providing links to cancer centers.
- NCCN (www.nccn.org): NCCN is a nonprofit alliance of 21 of the world's leading cancer centers, dedicated to the quality of care provided to patients with cancer. NCCN resources include guidelines for psychosocial care.
- National Coalition for Cancer Survivorship (877-622-7937, www.canceradvocacy.org): This organization provides advocacy and resources for cancer survivors with a focus on quality-of-life issues.
- The Wellness Community (888-793-WELL, www.thewellnesscommunity.org): Site provides free psychological help and emotional support to cancer survivors and their family members and caregivers through support groups, psychoeducational workshops, and nutritional and educational guidance.

References

Agency for Health Care Policy and Research. (1993). *Depression in primary care: Detection, diagnosis, and treatment* [AHCPR Publication No. 93-0552]. Rockville, MD: Author.

Agre, P. (2005). The education process. In J.K. Itano & K.N. Taoka (Eds.), *Core curriculum for oncology nursing* (4th ed., pp. 893–898). St. Louis, MO: Elsevier.

Ahlberg, K., & Nordner, A. (2006). The importance of participation in support groups for women with ovarian cancer [Online exclusive]. *Oncology Nursing Forum, 33,* E53–E61.

Albright, A.V., & Valente, S.M. (2006). Depression and suicide. In R.M. Carroll-Johnson, L.M. Gorman, & N.J. Bush (Eds.), *Psychosocial nursing care along the cancer continuum* (2nd ed., pp. 241–260). Pittsburgh, PA: Oncology Nursing Society.

American Cancer Society. (2004). *Sexuality and cancer.* Atlanta, GA: Author.

American Psychiatric Association. (2000). *Diagnostic and statistical manual of mental disorders* (4th ed., Text rev.). Washington, DC: Author.

Anastasia, P.J. (2006a). Altered sexuality. In R.M. Carroll-Johnson, L.M. Gorman, & N.J. Bush (Eds.), *Psychosocial nursing care along the cancer continuum* (2nd ed., pp. 327–350). Pittsburgh, PA: Oncology Nursing Society.

Anastasia, P.J. (2006b). Gender and age differences in the psychological response to cancer. In R.M. Carroll-Johnson, L.M. Gorman, & N.J. Bush (Eds.), *Psychosocial nursing care along the cancer continuum* (2nd ed., pp. 89–99). Pittsburgh, PA: Oncology Nursing Society.

Andersen, B.L. (1990). How cancer affects sexual functioning. *Oncology, 4*(6), 81–88.

Andersen, B.L. (2003). Psychological interventions for cancer patients. In C.W. Given, B. Given, V.L. Champion, S. Kozachik, & D.N. DeVoss (Eds.), *Evidence-based cancer care and prevention: Behavioral interventions* (pp. 179–217). New York: Springer.

Andersen, B.L., & Lamb, M. (1995). Sexuality and cancer. In G.P. Murphy, W. Lawrence, & R.E. Lenhard (Eds.), *American Cancer Society textbook of clinical oncology* (2nd ed., pp. 609–713). Atlanta, GA: American Cancer Society.

Annon, J. (1976). The PLISSIT model: A proposed conceptual scheme for the behavioral treatment of sexual problems. *Journal of Sex Education and Therapy, 2,* 1–15.

Aspinwall, L.G., & Brunhart, S.M. (2000). What I do know won't hurt me: Optimism, attention to negative information, coping, and health. In J.E. Gillham (Ed.), *The science of optimism and hope: Research essays in honor of Martin E.P. Seligman* (pp. 163–200). Philadelphia: Templeton Foundation Press.

Barry, P.D. (2002). *Mental health and mental illness* (7th ed.). Philadelphia: Lippincott.

Barsevick, A.M., Much, J., & Sweeney, C. (2000). Psychosocial responses to cancer. In C.H. Yarbro, M.H. Frogge, M. Goodman, & S.L. Groenwald (Eds.), *Cancer nursing: Principles and practice* (5th ed., pp. 1529–1549). Sudbury, MA: Jones and Bartlett.

Beck, A.T., & Emery, G. (1985). *Anxiety disorders and phobias: A cognitive perspective.* New York: Basic Books.

Boehmke, M.M., & Dickerson, S.S. (2006). The diagnosis of breast cancer: Transition from health to illness. *Oncology Nursing Forum, 33,* 1121–1127.

Bond, S.M., Neelon, V.J., & Belyea, M.J. (2006). Delirium in hospitalized older patients with cancer. *Oncology Nursing Forum, 33,* 1075–1083.

Bowers, L., & Boyle, D.A. (2003). Depression in patients with advanced cancer. *Clinical Journal of Oncology Nursing, 7,* 281–288.

Boyle, D.A. (2006a). Delirium in older adults with cancer: Implications for practice and research. *Oncology Nursing Forum, 33,* 61–78.

Boyle, D.A. (2006b). Survivorship. *Clinical Journal of Oncology Nursing, 10,* 407–416.

Breitbart, W., Jaramillo, J.R., & Chochinov, H.M. (1998). Palliative and terminal care. In J.C. Holland (Ed.), *Psycho-oncology* (pp. 437–449). New York: Oxford University Press.

Bush, N.J. (1998). Family systems theory: A holistic framework for oncology nursing practice. In R.M. Carroll-Johnson, L.M. Gorman, & N.J. Bush (Eds.), *Psychosocial nursing care along the cancer continuum* (pp. 329–340). Pittsburgh, PA: Oncology Nursing Society.

Bush, N.J. (2006a). Coping and adaptation. In R.M. Carroll-Johnson, L.M. Gorman, & N.J. Bush (Eds.), *Psychosocial nursing care along the cancer continuum* (2nd ed., pp. 61–88). Pittsburgh, PA: Oncology Nursing Society.

Bush, N.J. (2006b). Anxiety and the cancer experience. In R.M. Carroll-Johnson, L.M. Gorman, & N.J. Bush (Eds.), *Psychosocial nursing care along the cancer continuum* (2nd ed., pp. 205–221). Pittsburgh, PA: Oncology Nursing Society.

Caeiro, L., Ferro, J.M., Albuquerque, R., & Figueria, M.L. (2004). Delirium in the first days of acute stroke. *Journal of Neurology, 251,* 171–178.

Carroll-Johnson, R.M. (2006). Life's meaning and cancer. In R.M. Carroll-Johnson, L.M. Gorman, & N.J. Bush (Eds.), *Psychosocial nursing care along the cancer continuum* (2nd ed., pp. 55–60). Pittsburgh, PA: Oncology Nursing Society.

Chochinov, H.M., Wilson, K.G., Enns, M., & Lander, S. (1997). "Are you depressed?" Screening for depression in the terminally ill. *American Journal of Psychiatry, 154,* 674–676.

Chochinov, H.M., Wilson, K.G., Enns, M., & Lander, S. (1998). Depression, hopelessness, and suicidal ideation in the terminally ill. *Psychosomatics, 39,* 366–370.

Cohen, R., & Munet-Vilaro, F. (2001). Cancer prevention and screening among Hispanic populations. In M. Frank-Stromberg & S.J. Olsen (Eds.), *Cancer prevention in diverse populations: Cultural implications for the multidisciplinary team* (2nd ed., pp. 177–243). Pittsburgh, PA: Oncology Nursing Society.

Crowley, M.J. (2005). Supportive care: Dying and death. In J.K. Itano & K.N. Taoka (Eds.), *Core curriculum for oncology nursing* (4th ed., pp. 102–126). St. Louis, MO: Elsevier.

Davis, M. (2006). Fertility considerations for female adolescent and young adult patients following cancer therapy: A guide for counseling patients and families. *Clinical Journal of Oncology Nursing, 10,* 213–219.

Deng, G., & Cassileth, B.R. (2005). Integrative oncology: Complementary therapies for pain, anxiety, and mood disturbance. *CA: A Cancer Journal for Clinicians, 55,* 109–116.

Dickerson, S.S., Boehmke, M., & Brown, C. (2006). Seeking and managing hope: Patients' experiences using the Internet for cancer care [Online exclusive]. *Oncology Nursing Forum, 33,* E8–E17.

Edelman, S., Craig, A., & Kidman, A.D. (2000). Group interventions with cancer patients: Efficacy of psychoeducational versus supportive groups. *Journal of Psychosocial Oncology, 18*(3), 67–85.

Erikson, E.H. (1963). *Childhood and society* (2nd ed.). New York: Norton.

Ersek, M. (2006). The meaning of hope in the dying. In B.R. Ferrell & N. Coyle (Eds.), *Textbook of palliative nursing* (2nd ed., pp. 513–529). New York: Oxford University Press.

Fawzy, F.I., Fawzy, N.W., Arndt, L.A., & Pasnau, R.O. (1995). Critical review of psychosocial interventions in cancer care. *Archives of General Psychiatry, 52,* 100–113.

Faysman, K., & Oseguera, D. (2002). Cultural dimensions of anxiety and truth telling. *Oncology Nursing Forum, 29,* 757–759.

Fitch, M.I. (2006). Programmatic approaches to psychosocial support. In R.M. Carroll-Johnson, L.M. Gorman, & N.J. Bush (Eds.), *Psychosocial nursing care along the cancer continuum* (2nd ed., pp. 419–438). Pittsburgh, PA: Oncology Nursing Society.

Fitchett, G., & Handzo, G. (1998). Spiritual assessment, screening, and intervention. In J.C. Holland (Ed.), *Psycho-oncology* (pp. 790–808). New York: Oxford University Press.

Fletcher, D.M. (2006). Complementary and alternative medicine: Moving toward integrative cancer care. In R.M. Carroll-Johnson, L.M. Gorman, & N.J. Bush (Eds.), *Psychosocial nursing care along the cancer continuum* (2nd ed., pp. 531–549). Pittsburgh, PA: Oncology Nursing Society.

Folstein, M.F., Folstein, S.E., & McHugh, P.R. (1975). "Mini-mental state." A practical method for grading the cognitive state of patients for the clinician. *Journal of Psychiatric Research, 12,* 189–198.

Foroudi, F., & Tiver, K.W. (2000). Occult breast carcinoma presenting as axillary metastases. *International Journal of Radiation Oncology, Biology, Physics, 47,* 143–147.

Fox, S.W., Mitchell, S.A., & Booth-Jones, M. (2006). Cognitive impairment in patients with brain tumors: Assessment and intervention in the clinic setting. *Clinical Journal of Oncology Nursing, 10,* 169–176.

Friedman, M.M., Bowden, V.R., & Jones, E.G. (2003). *Family nursing: Research, theory, and practice* (5th ed.). Upper Saddle River, NJ: Prentice Hall.

Geis, F.L. (1993). Self-fulfilling prophecies: A social psychological view of gender. In A.E. Beall & R.J. Sternberg (Eds.), *The psychology of gender* (pp. 9–54). New York: Guilford Press.

Given, B., Given, C.W., Kozachik, S., & Rawl, S. (2003). Family caregiving interventions in cancer care. In C.W. Given, B. Given, V.L. Champion, S. Kozachik, & D.N. DeVoss (Eds.), *Evidence-based cancer care and prevention: Behavioral interventions* (pp. 332–370). New York: Springer.

Goldberg, B. (1998). Connection: An exploration of spirituality in nursing care. *Journal of Advanced Nursing, 27,* 836–842.

Goldenberg, I., & Goldenberg, H. (1996). *Family therapy: An overview* (4th ed.). Pacific Grove, CA: Brooks/Cole.

Gorman, L.M. (2006). Powerlessness. In R.M. Carroll-Johnson, L.M. Gorman, & N.J. Bush (Eds.), *Psychosocial nursing care along the cancer continuum* (2nd ed., pp. 369–381). Pittsburgh, PA: Oncology Nursing Society.

Gorman, L.M., Raines, M.L., & Sultan, D.F. (2002). *Psychosocial nursing for general patient care* (2nd ed.). Philadelphia: F.A. Davis.

Gotay, C.C., & Lau, A.K. (2003). Preferences for psychosocial interventions among newly diagnosed cancer patients from a multiethnic population. *Journal of Psychosocial Oncology, 20*(4), 23–37.

Grimm, P.A. (2005). Coping: Psychosocial issues. In J.K. Itano & K.N. Taoka (Eds.), *Core curriculum for oncology nursing* (4th ed., pp. 29–52). St. Louis, MO: Elsevier.

Henderson, P.D., Gore, S.V., Davis, B.L., & Condon, E.H. (2003). African American women coping with breast cancer: A qualitative analysis. *Oncology Nursing Forum, 30,* 641–647.

Holland, J.C., & Lewis, S. (2000). *The human side of cancer: Living with hope, coping with uncertainty.* New York: HarperCollins.

Howell, D., Fitch, M.I., & Deane, K.A. (2003). Women's experiences with recurrent ovarian cancer. *Cancer Nursing, 26,* 10–17.

Hudek-Knezevic, J., Kardum, I., & Pahljina, R. (2002). Relations among social support, coping, and negative affect in hospitalized and nonhospitalized cancer patients. *Journal of Psychosocial Oncology, 20*(2), 45–63.

Iacovino, V., & Reesor, K. (1997). Literature on interventions to address cancer patients' psychosocial needs: What does it tell us? *Journal of Psychosocial Oncology, 15*(2), 47–71.

Itano, J.K. (2005). Coping: Cultural issues. In J.K. Itano & K.N. Taoka (Eds.), *Core curriculum for oncology nursing* (4th ed., pp. 59–79). St. Louis, MO: Elsevier.

Jansen, C., Miaskowski, C., Dodd, M., Dowling, G., & Kramer, J. (2005). Potential mechanisms for chemotherapy-induced impairments in cognitive function. *Oncology Nursing Forum, 32,* 1151–1161.

Jassak, P.F. (1992). Families: An essential element in the care of the patient with cancer. *Oncology Nursing Forum, 19,* 871–876.

Keltner, N.L., Folks, D.G., Palmer, C.A., & Powers, R.E. (1998). *Psychobiological foundations of psychiatric care.* St. Louis, MO: Mosby.

Kemp, C. (2006). Spiritual care interventions. In B.R. Ferrell & N. Coyle (Eds.), *Textbook of palliative nursing* (2nd ed., pp. 595–604). New York: Oxford University Press.

Kitrungrote, L., & Cohen, M.Z. (2006). Quality of life of family caregivers of patients with cancer: A literature review. *Oncology Nursing Forum, 33,* 625–632.

Kocsis, J.H. (2000). New strategies for treating chronic depression. *Journal of Clinical Psychiatry, 61*(Suppl. 11), 42–45.

Kornstein, S.G., & McEnany, G. (2000). Enhancing pharmacologic effects in the treatment of depression in women. *Journal of Clinical Psychiatry, 61*(Suppl. 11), 18–27.

Krebs, L. (2006). What should I say? Talking with patients about sexuality issues. *Clinical Journal of Oncology Nursing, 10,* 313–315.

Kristjanson, L.J., & Ashcroft, T. (1994). The family's cancer journey: A literature review. *Cancer Nursing, 17,* 1–17.

Kwekkeboom, K.L. (2003). Music versus distraction for procedural pain and anxiety in patients with cancer. *Oncology Nursing Forum, 30,* 433–440.

Kwekkeboom, K.L., & Seng, J.S. (2002). Recognizing and responding to post-traumatic stress disorder in people with cancer. *Oncology Nursing Forum, 29,* 643–650.

Lasky, E., Martz, C.H., & Kagawa-Singer, M. (2001). The Asian American population in the United States: Cultural perspectives and their relationship to cancer prevention and early detection. In M. Frank-Stromborg & S.J. Olsen (Eds.), *Cancer prevention in diverse populations: Cultural implications for the multidisciplinary team* (2nd ed., pp. 55–99). Pittsburgh, PA: Oncology Nursing Society.

Lazarus, R.S., & Folkman, S. (1984). *Stress, appraisal, and coping.* New York: Springer.

Lengacher, C.A., Bennett, M.P., Kip, K.E., Gonzalez, L., Jacobsen, P., & Cox, C.E. (2006). Relief of symptoms, side effects, and psychosocial distress through use of complementary and alternative medicine in women with breast cancer. *Oncology Nursing Forum, 33,* 97–104.

Lethborg, C.E., Kissane, D., Burns, W.I., & Snyder, R. (2000). "Cast adrift": The experience of completing treatment among women with early stage breast cancer. *Journal of Psychosocial Oncology, 18*(4), 73–90.

Ljubisavljevic, V., & Kelly, B. (2003). Risk factors for development of delirium among oncology patients. *General Hospital Psychiatry, 25,* 345–352.

Lovejoy, N.C., Tabor, D., & Deloney, P. (2000). Cancer-related depression: Part II—Neurologic alterations and evolving approaches to psychopharmacology. *Oncology Nursing Forum, 27,* 795–808.

Lovejoy, N.C., Tabor, D., Matteis, M., & Lillis, P. (2000). Cancer-related depression: Part I—Neurologic alterations and cognitive-behavioral therapy. *Oncology Nursing Forum, 27,* 667–678.

Madden, J. (2006). The problem of distress in patients with cancer: More effective assessment. *Clinical Journal of Oncology Nursing, 10,* 615–619.

Manson, S.P. (1996). Culture and DSM-IV: Implications for the diagnosis of mood and anxiety disorders. In J.E. Mezzich, A. Kleinman, H. Fabrega, & D.L. Parron (Eds.), *Culture and psychiatric diagnosis: A DSM-IV perspective* (pp. 99–113). Washington, DC: American Psychiatric Press.

Marrs, J.A. (2006). Stress, fears, and phobias: The impact of anxiety. *Clinical Journal of Oncology Nursing, 10,* 319–322.

Martsolf, D.S., & Mickley, J.R. (1998). The concept of spirituality in nursing theories: Differing world views and extent of focus. *Journal of Advanced Nursing, 27,* 294–303.

Massie, M.J., & Popkin, M.K. (1998). Depressive disorders. In J.C. Holland (Ed.), *Psycho-oncology* (pp. 518–540). New York: Oxford University Press.

Maynard, C.K. (2003). Differentiate depression from dementia. *Nurse Practitioner, 28*(3), 18–19, 23–27.

Mezzich, J.E., Kleinman, A., Fabrega, H., & Parron, D.L. (1996). *Culture and psychiatric diagnosis: A DSM-IV perspective.* Washington, DC: American Psychiatric Press.

Moore, S. (2006). Depression management during cancer treatment. *Oncology Nursing Forum, 33,* 33–35.

Morris, M.E., Grant, M., & Lynch, J.C. (2007). Patient-reported family distress among long-term cancer survivors. *Cancer Nursing, 30,* 1–8.

Muscari, E. (2006a). Cognitive impairment in cancer. In R.M. Carroll-Johnson, L.M. Gorman, & N.J. Bush (Eds.), *Psychosocial nursing care along the cancer continuum* (2nd ed., pp. 191–201). Pittsburgh, PA: Oncology Nursing Society.

Muscari, E. (2006b). Delirium and dementia. In R.M. Carroll-Johnson, L.M. Gorman, & N.J. Bush (Eds.), *Psychosocial nursing care along the cancer continuum* (2nd ed., pp. 351–367). Pittsburgh, PA: Oncology Nursing Society.

Nail, L.M. (2001). I'm coping as fast as I can: Psychosocial adjustment to cancer and cancer treatment. *Oncology Nursing Forum, 28,* 967–970.

National Comprehensive Cancer Network. (2008). *NCCN clinical practice guidelines in oncology: Distress management, version 1.2008.* Retrieved May 16, 2008, from http://www.nccn.org/professionals/physician_gls/PDF/distress.pdf

Neilson-Clayton, H., & Brownlee, K. (2002). Solution-focused brief therapy with cancer patients and their families. *Journal of Psychosocial Oncology, 20*(1), 1–13.

Nishimoto, P.W. (2005). Sexuality. In J.K. Itano & K.N. Taoka (Eds.), *Core curriculum for oncology nursing* (4th ed., pp. 89–101). St. Louis, MO: Elsevier.

Nolen-Hoeksema, S. (2001). Growth and resilience among bereaved people. In J.E. Gillham (Ed.), *The science of optimism and hope: Research essays in honor of Martin E.P. Seligman* (pp. 107–127). Philadelphia: Templeton Foundation Press.

Noyes, R., Holt, C.S., & Massie, M.J. (1998). Anxiety disorders. In J.C. Holland (Ed.), *Psycho-oncology* (pp. 548–563). New York: Oxford University Press.

Oncology Nursing Society. (2004). *Statement on the scope and standards of oncology nursing practice.* Pittsburgh, PA: Author.

O'Shaughnessy, J. (2003). Chemotherapy-related cognitive dysfunction in breast cancer. *Seminars in Oncology Nursing, 19*(Suppl. 2), 17–24.

Pasacreta, J.V., Minarik, P.A., & Nield-Anderson, L. (2006). Anxiety and depression. In B.R. Ferrell & N. Coyle (Eds.), *Textbook of palliative nursing* (2nd ed., pp. 375–399). New York: Oxford University Press.

Passik, S.D., & Grummon, K.L. (1998). Posttraumatic stress disorder. In J.C. Holland (Ed.), *Psycho-oncology* (pp. 595–607). New York: Oxford University Press.

Poole, G., Poon, C., Achille, M., White, K., Franz, N., Jittler, S., et al. (2001). Social support for patients with prostate cancer: The effect of support groups. *Journal of Psychosocial Oncology, 19*(2), 1–16.

Porche, D.J. (2005). Depression in men. *Journal for Nurse Practitioners, 1,* 138–139.

Post-White, J.E. (2006). Psychoneuroimmunology: The mind-body connection. In R.M. Carroll-Johnson, L.M. Gorman, & N.J. Bush (Eds.), *Psychosocial nursing care along the cancer continuum* (2nd ed., pp. 465–485). Pittsburgh, PA: Oncology Nursing Society.

Reynolds, C.F., & Kupfer, D.J. (1999). Depression and aging: A look to the future. *Psychiatric Services, 50,* 1167–1172.

Salimbene, S. (2007). *Ten guidelines for culturally and linguistically appropriate care.* Retrieved April 4, 2007, from http://www.medscape.com/viewarticle/544767

Satterfield, J.M. (2000). Optimism, culture, and history: The roles of explanatory style, integrative complexity, and pessimistic rumination. In J.E. Gillham (Ed.), *The science of optimism and hope: Research essays in honor of Martin E.P. Seligman* (pp. 349–378). Philadelphia: Templeton Foundation Press.

Saykin, A.J., Ahles, T.A., & McDonald, B.C. (2003). Mechanisms of chemotherapy induced cognitive disorders: Neuropsychological, pathophysiological, and neuroimaging perspectives. *Seminars in Clinical Neuropsychiatry, 8,* 201–216.

Schover, L.R. (1998). Sexual dysfunction. In J.C. Holland (Ed.), *Psycho-oncology* (pp. 494–499). New York: Oxford University Press.

Schwartz, L., Lander, M., & Chochinov, H.M. (2002). Current management of depression in cancer patients. *Oncology (Williston Park), 16,* 1102–1110.

Sharp, K. (2005). Depression: The essentials. *Clinical Journal of Oncology Nursing, 9,* 519–525.

Shell, J.A., & Campbell-Norris, C. (2006). Body image disturbance. In R.M. Carroll-Johnson, L.M. Gorman, & N.J. Bush (Eds.), *Psychosocial nursing care along the cancer continuum* (2nd ed., pp. 191–201). Pittsburgh, PA: Oncology Nursing Society.

Sloman, R. (2002). Relaxation and imagery for anxiety and depression control in community patients with advanced cancer. *Cancer Nursing, 25,* 432–435.

Smith, M., & Buckwalter, K. (2006). Behaviors associated with dementia. *American Journal of Nursing, 105*(7), 40–52.

Spencer, S.M., Carver, C.S., & Price, A.A. (1998). Psychological and social factors in adaptation. In J.C. Holland (Ed.), *Psycho-oncology* (pp. 211–219). New York: Oxford University Press.

Staat, K., & Segatore, M. (2005). The phenomenon of chemo brain. *Clinical Journal of Oncology Nursing, 9,* 713–721.

Stahl, S.M. (1998). Selecting an antidepressant by using mechanism of action to enhance efficacy and avoid side effects. *Journal of Clinical Psychiatry, 59*(Suppl. 18), 23–29.

Stein, D.J. (Ed.). (2004). *Clinical manual of anxiety disorders.* Washington, DC: American Psychiatric Publishing.

Tabano, M., Condosta, D., & Coons, M. (2002). Symptoms affecting quality of life in women with gynecologic cancer. *Seminars in Oncology Nursing, 18,* 223–230.

Taylor, E.J. (2006). Spirituality and spiritual nurture in cancer care. In R.M. Carroll-Johnson, L.M. Gorman, & N.J. Bush (Eds.), *Psychosocial nursing care along the cancer continuum* (2nd ed., pp. 117–131). Pittsburgh, PA: Oncology Nursing Society.

Tseng, W.S. (1996). Cultural comments on mood and anxiety disorders: I. In J.E. Mezzich, A. Kleinman, H. Fabrega, & D.L. Parron (Eds.), *Culture and psychiatric diagnosis: A DSM-IV perspective* (pp. 115–121). Washington, DC: American Psychiatric Press.

Tuma, R., & DeAngelis, L.M. (2000). Altered mental states in patients with cancer. *Archives of Neurology, 57,* 1727–1731.

Van Fleet, S. (2006). Assessment and pharmacotherapy of depression. *Clinical Journal of Oncology Nursing, 10,* 158–161.

Walch, S.E., Ahles, T.A., & Saykin, A.J. (1998). Neuropsychologic impact of cancer and cancer treatments. In J.C. Holland (Ed.), *Psycho-oncology* (pp. 500–505). New York: Oxford University Press.

Wilmoth, M.C. (1994, Spring). Strategies for becoming comfortable with sexual assessment. *Oncology Nursing News,* pp. 6–7.

Wilmoth, M.C. (2006). Life after cancer: What *does* sexuality have to do with it? *Oncology Nursing Forum, 33,* 905–910.

Woods, N.F. (1984). *Human sexuality in health and illness* (3rd ed.). St. Louis, MO: Mosby.

World Health Organization. (2006). *Defining sexual health: Report of a technical consultation on sexual health 28–31 January 2002, Geneva.* Geneva, Switzerland: Author.

Zabora, J.R., Loscalzo, M.J., & Weber, J. (2003). Managing complications in cancer: Identifying and responding to the patient's perspective. *Seminars in Oncology Nursing, 19,* 1–9.

CHAPTER 17

Cancer Survivorship

Nancy G. Houlihan, RN, MA, AOCN®

Introduction

Interest in the needs of cancer survivors is growing, as people live longer after cancer treatment and require ongoing care that focuses on quality of life. As the number of people who survive cancer increases, the efforts to address their needs and provide them with adequate resources continue to develop. Many survivorship care models have evolved to meet the physical, psychological, social, and spiritual needs of survivors. Employment and insurance issues have presented some unique challenges for oncology advanced practice nurses (APNs). This chapter will address these issues from a historical to current-day perspective.

Oncology APNs are uniquely prepared to influence this care by applying their knowledge of cancer to the period of care beyond active therapy. Oncology APNs can take an active role with the physician and mental health colleagues in the effort to further education, research, and quality care initiatives that will ensure the best transition for patients to the post-treatment period and for the remainder of their lives.

Cancer Survivors in the United States

Approximately 1,437,180 Americans will be diagnosed with cancer in 2008 (Jemal et al., 2008). This number is predicted to increase along with the growing and aging population (Edwards et al., 2002). Advances in early detection and more effective treatments also have resulted in a dramatic increase in the number of cancer survivors (Hewitt, Greenfield, & Stovall, 2006). The majority of people will survive their cancer—the latest overall relative five-year survival rate from 1996–2003 is 64.9% (Ries et al., 2007), and survival rates for many cancers are even higher (Jemal et al.). In the United States, an estimated 10.8 million cancer survivors were alive as of January 1, 2004 (National Cancer Institute [NCI], Division of Cancer Control and Population Sciences, Office of Cancer Survivorship, 2007) (see Figure 17-1).

The majority of cancer survivors today are older than 65 years of age, and the average age is slightly older in women. More than half are survivors of the most common

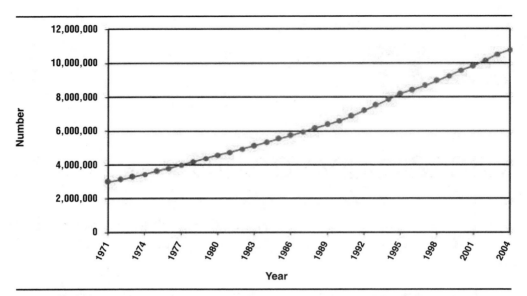

Figure 17-1. Estimated Number of Cancer Survivors in the United States From 1971 to 2003

Data source: Ries LAG, Melbert D, Krapcho M, Mariotto A, Miller BA, Feuer EJ, Clegg L, Horner MJ, Howlader N, Eisner MP, Reichman M, Edwards BK (eds). SEER Cancer Statistics Review, 1975-2004, National Cancer Institute. Bethesda, MD, http://seer.cancer.gov/csr/1975_2004/, based on November 2006 SEER data submission, posted to the SEER web site, 2007.

Note. From "Estimated U.S. Cancer Prevalence," by National Cancer Institute, Office of Cancer Survivorship, July 2007. Retrieved April 22, 2008, from http://dccps.nci.nih.gov/ocs/prevalence/prevalence.html#survivor

cancers: breast, prostate, and colorectal cancers (see Figure 17-2 and Figure 17-3). Although the data on pediatric cancer survivors are even more promising, with 78% of children surviving five years from the time of diagnosis (Ries et al., 2007), this chapter will cover only survivorship of adult-onset cancers.

These improving survival results bring new challenges for patients, caregivers, and the healthcare system. As people live longer, they will need ongoing medical care, psychosocial support, and careful monitoring of treatment complications and cancer recurrence. Cancer care providers need to develop new follow-up guidelines and systems that address the needs of this growing population so that cancer survivors can be assured the greatest quality of life (Oeffinger & McCabe, 2006).

Historical Development of a Cancer Survivorship Focus

In his essay in the *New England Journal of Medicine*, "Seasons of Survival: Reflections of a Physician With Cancer," Fitzhugh Mullan (1985) described for the first time the experience of cancer survivorship. He identified three "seasons": **acute survival,** which begins with diagnosis, is dominated by testing and therapies, and is accompanied by fear and anxiety. Next is **extended survival,** which is the period when remission occurs,

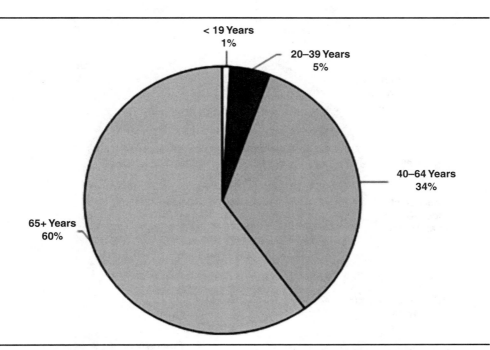

Figure 17-2. Estimated Number of Cancer Survivors in the United States on January 1, 2004, by Current Age*

* Invasive/1st primary cases only, N = 10.8M survivors.

Data source: Ries LAG, Melbert D, Krapcho M, Mariotto A, Miller BA, Feuer EJ, Clegg L, Horner MJ, Howlader N, Eisner MP, Reichman M, Edwards BK (eds). SEER Cancer Statistics Review, 1975-2004, National Cancer Institute. Bethesda, MD, http://seer.cancer.gov/csr/1975_2004/, based on November 2006 SEER data submission, posted to the SEER web site, 2007.

Note. From "Estimated U.S. Cancer Prevalence," by National Cancer Institute, Office of Cancer Survivorship, July 2007. Retrieved April 22, 2008, from http://dccps.nci.nih.gov/ocs/prevalence/prevalence.html#survivor

treatment ends, and fear of recurrence is greatest. **Permanent survival** is considered the period of "cure," when people are facing the adjustment of "normal life," dealing with the lasting impact of cancer on their ability to return to previous roles. Dr. Mullan's essay promoted recognition of the ongoing needs of individuals with cancer beyond the acute treatment period. Within a short time after this publication, a group of survivors, including Dr. Mullan, formed the National Coalition for Cancer Survivorship (NCCS) to raise awareness about quality care for survivors through advocacy.

Largely a result of the efforts in recent years of NCCS and public figures such as Lance Armstrong, increasing attention is being paid to the needs of cancer survivors. In 1996, NCI established the Office of Cancer Survivorship with the purpose of funding research that would lead to improved quality of survival for all patients with cancer and educating health professionals, survivors, and caregivers about critical issues for optimal well-being (Rowland, Aziz, Tesauro, & Feuer, 2001). Two reports, *A National Action Plan for Cancer Survivorship: Advancing Public Health Strategies* (Centers for Disease Control and Prevention, 2004) and *Living Beyond Cancer: Finding a New Balance* (Reuben,

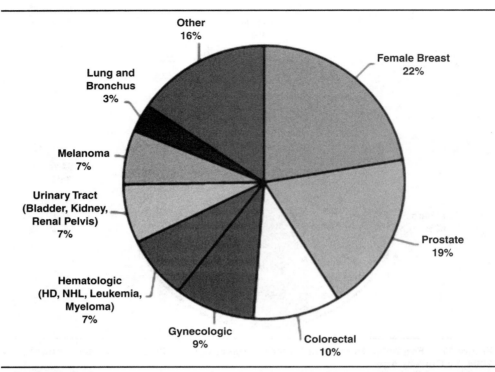

Figure 17-3. Estimated Number of Cancer Survivors in the United States on January 1, 2004, by Site*

* Invasive/1st primary cases only, N = 10.8M survivors.

Data source: Ries LAG, Melbert D, Krapcho M, Mariotto A, Miller BA, Feuer EJ, Clegg L, Horner MJ, Howlader N, Eisner MP, Reichman M, Edwards BK (eds). SEER Cancer Statistics Review, 1975-2004, National Cancer Institute. Bethesda, MD, http://seer.cancer.gov/csr/1975_2004/, based on November 2006 SEER data submission, posted to the SEER web site, 2007.

Note. From "Estimated U.S. Cancer Prevalence," by National Cancer Institute, Office of Cancer Survivorship, July 2007. Retrieved April 22, 2008, from http://dccps.nci.nih.gov/ocs/prevalence/prevalence.html#survivor

2004), outlined the issues of cancer survivorship and set specific national goals. The Institute of Medicine (IOM) of the National Academies of Science established a committee in 2005 to examine the range of medical and psychosocial issues that adult cancer survivors face and to make recommendations to improve their health care and quality of life. This resulted in the publication *From Cancer Patient to Cancer Survivor: Lost in Transition* (Hewitt et al., 2006). The IOM had produced a similar report in 2003 on pediatric cancer survivorship. Various professional organizations, such as the American Society of Clinical Oncology (ASCO), NCI, NCCS, the Lance Armstrong Foundation (LAF), and other advocacy groups are involved in efforts to promote implementation of the IOM recommendations (see Figure 17-4).

NCCS and the NCI Office of Cancer Survivorship define *cancer survivors* as the following: An individual is considered to be a cancer survivor from the time of diagnosis through the balance of his or her life. Family members, friends, and caregivers are also affected by

1. Health care providers, patient advocates, and other stakeholders should work to raise awareness of the needs of cancer survivors, establish cancer survivorship as a distinct phase of cancer care, and act to ensure the delivery of appropriate survivorship care.
2. Patients completing primary treatment should be provided with a comprehensive care summary and follow-up plan that is clearly and effectively explained. This "Survivorship Care Plan" should be written by the principal provider(s) who coordinated oncology treatment. This service should be reimbursed by third-party payors of health care.
3. Health care providers should use systematically developed evidence-based clinical practice guidelines, assessment tools, and screening instruments to help identify and manage late effects of cancer and its treatment. Existing guidelines should be refined and new evidence-based guidelines should be developed through public- and private-sector efforts.
4. Quality of survivorship care measures should be developed through public/private partnerships and quality assurance programs implemented by health systems to monitor and improve the care that all survivors receive.
5. The Centers for Medicare and Medicaid Services (CMS), National Cancer Institute (NCI), Agency for Healthcare Research and Quality (AHRQ), the Department of Veterans Affairs (VA), and other qualified organizations should support demonstration programs to test models of coordinated, interdisciplinary survivorship care in diverse communities and across systems of care.
6. Congress should support Centers for Disease Control and Prevention (CDC), other collaborating institutions, and the states in developing comprehensive cancer control plans that include consideration of survivorship care, and promoting the implementation, evaluation, and refinement of existing state cancer control plans.
7. The National Cancer Institute (NCI), professional associations, and voluntary organizations should expand and coordinate their efforts to provide educational opportunities to health care providers to equip them to address the health care and quality of life issues facing cancer survivors.
8. Employers, legal advocates, health care providers, sponsors of support services, and government agencies should act to eliminate discrimination and minimize adverse effects of cancer on employment, while supporting cancer survivors with short-term and long-term limitations in ability to work.
9. Federal and state policy makers should act to ensure that all cancer survivors have access to adequate and affordable health insurance. Insurers and payors of health care should recognize survivorship care as an essential part of cancer care and design benefits, payment policies, and reimbursement mechanisms to facilitate coverage for evidence-based aspects of care.
10. The National Cancer Institute (NCI), Centers for Disease Control and Prevention (CDC), Agency for Healthcare Research and Quality (AHRQ), Centers for Medicare and Medicaid Services (CMS), Department of Veterans Affairs (VA), private voluntary organizations such as American Cancer Society (ACS), and private health insurers and plans should increase their support of survivorship research and expand mechanisms for its conduct. New research initiatives focused on cancer patient follow-up are urgently needed to guide effective survivorship care.

Figure 17-4. Institute of Medicine Report Recommendations

Note. From *From Cancer Patient to Cancer Survivor: Lost in Transition* (pp. 3–13), by M. Hewitt, S. Greenfield, and E. Stovall (Eds.), 2006, Washington, DC: National Academies Press. Copyright 2006 by National Academy of Sciences. Reprinted with permission.

the survivorship experience and therefore are included in this definition (NCCS, n.d.). This definition has increasingly become adopted, but differing opinions exist about the definition of cancer survivors among health professionals, those with a cancer history, and the public. Some believe that survivorship begins at the completion of initial treatment or at the five-year mark from diagnosis. Some survivors reject the term completely, not wanting to be labeled as someone who is different from others (Hewitt et al., 2006).

During the past few years, the post-treatment experience has received greater emphasis. In an editorial in the *Journal of Clinical Oncology,* Ganz (2005) called for the oncology community to "turn its attention" to the period of time at which patients treated with curative intent have completed their initial therapy and require follow-up care that is currently not well studied nor well described. While recognizing the NCCS definition, IOM focused its report on the distinct period in the cancer care trajectory that begins at the end of a primary treatment provided with intention to cure (Hewitt et al., 2006). IOM defined this period as lasting until a cancer recurrence, a second cancer, or death occurs, and it may include some ongoing treatment, such as adjuvant hormonal therapy (see Figure 17-5). The NCI Office of Cancer Survivorship defines a clear focus for its research initiatives on the post-treatment phase of care (see Figure 17-6). As a result of this trend, the information contained in this chapter covers the patient experience in the post-treatment period as defined previously.

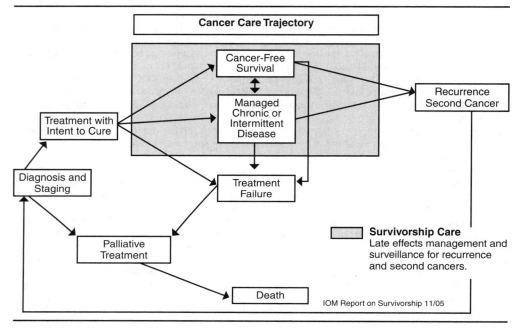

Figure 17-5. Cancer Care Trajectory

Note. From *From Cancer Patient to Cancer Survivor: Lost in Transition* (p. 190), by M. Hewitt, S. Greenfield, and E. Stovall (Eds.), 2006, Washington, DC: National Academies Press. Copyright 2006 by National Academy of Sciences. Reprinted with permission.

Cancer survivorship research encompasses the physical, psychosocial, and economic sequelae of cancer diagnosis and its treatment among both pediatric and adult survivors of cancer. It also includes within its domain, issues related to healthcare delivery, access, and follow-up care, as they relate to survivors. Survivorship research focuses on the health and life of a person with a history of cancer beyond the acute diagnosis and treatment phase. It seeks to both prevent and control adverse cancer diagnosis and treatment-related outcomes such as late effects of treatment, second cancers, and poor quality of life, to provide a knowledge base regarding optimal follow-up care and surveillance of cancers, and to optimize health after cancer treatment.

Figure 17-6. Definition of Survivorship Research

Note. From "About Cancer Survivorship Research: Survivorship Definitions," by the National Cancer Institute, 2006. Retrieved December 27, 2006, from http://dccps.nci.nih.gov/ocs/definitions.html

Quality of Life and Survivorship

Quality-of-life issues have become a vital area of concern to cancer survivors, their families, and care providers (Ferrell, Dow, Leigh, Ly, & Gulasekaram, 1995). The impact of a cancer diagnosis and treatment on health-related quality of life can be measured by assessing symptoms and functioning across an individual's physical, psychological, social, and spiritual domains. Ferrell (1996) summarized the definitions of these four domains: "Physical well-being is the control or relief of symptoms and the maintenance of function and independence" (p. 911). Psychological well-being is the attempt to maintain "a sense of control in the face of life-threatening illness characterized by emotional distress, altered life priorities, and fear of the unknown, as well as positive life changes" (p. 912). Social well-being is the effort to deal with the impact of cancer on individuals and their roles and relationships. "Spiritual well-being is the ability to maintain hope and derive meaning from the cancer experience, [which] is characterized by uncertainty" (p. 912). These patient domains represent an established focus of oncology nursing in planning care through the acute phase of treatment. As the evidence grows concerning the impact of cancer treatment on the quality of life of survivors, so too must these domains be considered through the post-treatment period. Figure 17-7 is a schematic display of a quality-of-life model developed by Ferrell and Grant that was included in the IOM report (Hewitt et al., 2006).

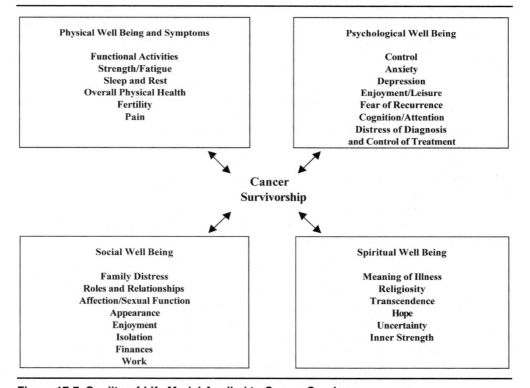

Figure 17-7. Quality-of-Life Model Applied to Cancer Survivors

Note. From *Pain and Palliative Care Resource Center: I. Quality of Life*, by Betty R. Ferrell, PhD, FAAN, and Marcia Grant, DNSc, FAAN, City of Hope City of Hope Beckman Research Institute, 2004. Retrieved April 22, 2008, from http://www.cityofhope.org/prc/pdf/cancer_survivor_QOL.pdf. Used with permission.

Physical Effects of Treatment

The physical effects of cancer and its treatment are described in terms of long-term and late effects, according to their onset. Long-term effects, also called persistent or chronic, are adverse effects that begin during treatment and continue beyond the end of treatment. Examples of long-term effects of chemotherapy and radiation therapy are cognitive problems, fatigue, amenorrhea, and peripheral neuropathies. Examples of long-term effects of cancer surgery include lymphedema, chronic pain, and structural or functional changes, such as ostomies, limb amputations, sexual dysfunction, urinary incontinence, infertility, difficulty breathing, and impaired vision, hearing, swallowing, eating, or speaking, to name a few (Ganz, 2006).

Much of the research on cancer treatment effects does not extend past the acute experience, which contributes to the challenge of designing appropriate interventions. For example, a significant body of research with corresponding management strategies for cancer treatment–related fatigue exists, yet much less is known about fatigue that can persist once treatment effects have subsided. Important considerations in planning care for survivors should include being aware of specific long-term effects that may be a problem; preventing or reducing risks during treatment when possible; and providing patients and caregivers with education about symptom management, safety, and compensatory activities (Nail, 2001).

Late effects of treatment refer to the unrecognized toxicities that are absent or subclinical at the end of treatment. They appear months to years following treatment and are related to organ injury that occurs during treatment. They manifest later as a result of the failure of repair mechanisms over time or organ senescence (Aziz & Rowland, 2003; Ganz, 2006). Survivors treated with therapy that is less intense or tissue damaging are unlikely to experience a physical late effect, whereas other patients, such as stem cell transplant recipients, have significant risk of future health problems and need careful monitoring (Oeffinger & McCabe, 2006). Late effects include risk for second cancers and a wide range of treatment-related morbidities. Table 17-1 contains possible late effects of chemotherapy, hormonal therapy, and radiation therapy by system. Note that this table also includes long-term effects, which IOM incorporates into the term *late effects* (Hewitt et al., 2006).

As cancer treatment has become more complex, late effects have become more prevalent. Risk of death from causes other than cancer recurrence is greatest among those treated with a combination of chemotherapy and radiation (Aziz, 2002). Susceptibility differs for children and younger and older adults. The increased risk of developing a second cancer, either of the same type or of a different type than the original cancer, may be the result of the cancer treatment received, genetic or other susceptibility such as health behaviors, or some interaction between the two (Hewitt et al., 2006). In particular, patients surviving Hodgkin disease are at greatest risk for developing second primary cancers, with risk associated with the age at which treatment was delivered. Solid tumors are more prevalent after treatment at a younger age, and leukemia is more frequent in those treated at an older age (Kattlove & Winn, 2003). The risk of breast cancer is higher in those treated with chest radiation before age 30 and increases with age at the end of follow-up, time since diagnosis, and radiation dose. These projections are based on older regimens associated with greater risk; more modern treatment approaches include limited-field radiation and chemotherapy with less effect on ovarian function (Travis et al., 2007). Still, the National Comprehensive Cancer Network (NCCN) guidelines recommend monitoring for breast cancer as a late effect of chest radiation beginning five to eight years after treatment (NCCN, 2008).

Table 17-1. Examples of Possible Late Effects of Radiation Therapy, Chemotherapy, and Hormonal Therapy Among Survivors of Adult Cancers

Organ System/ Tissue	Radiation Therapy Late Effects	Chemotherapy/Hormonal Therapy	
		Late Effects	Agent Responsible
All tissues	Second cancers	Second cancers	Steroids, alkylating agents, nitrosoureas, topoisomerase inhibitors, anthracyclines
Bone and soft tissue	Atrophy, deformity, fibrosis, bone death	Bone death and destruction, risk of fractures	Steroids
Cardiovascular	Scarring or inflammation of the heart, coronary artery disease; scarring of heart sac (pericardium)	Inflammation of the heart, congestive heart failure	Anthracyclines, high-dose cyclophosphamide, cisplatin, Herceptin, taxanes
Dental/oral health	Dental caries, dry mouth	–	–
Endocrine— pituitary	Various hormone deficiencies	Diabetes	Steroids
Endocrine— thyroid	Low thyroid function, thyroid nodules	–	–
Endocrine— gonadal	Men: Sterility, testosterone deficiency Women: Sterility, premature menopause	Men: Sterility, testosterone deficiency Women: Sterility, premature menopause	Alkylating agents, procarbazine hydrochloride, nitrosoureas
Gastrointestinal	Malabsorption, intestinal stricture	Motility disorders	Vinca drugs
Genitourinary	Bladder scarring, small bladder capacity	Hemorrhagic cystitis (symptoms include urinary frequency, urgency, bleeding, and pain)	Cyclophosphamide, ifosfamide, transplant therapy
Hematologic	Low blood counts, myelodysplastic syndrome and acute leukemia	Myelodysplastic syndrome and acute leukemia	Alkylating agents, nitrosoureas, topoisomerase inhibitors, purine analogs, any high-dose therapy with autologous transplantation
Hepatic	Abnormal liver function, liver failure	Abnormal liver function, cirrhosis, liver failure	Methotrexate, carmustine (BCNU)
Immune system	Impaired immune function, immune suppression	Impaired immune function, immune suppression	Steroids, anti-thymocyte globulin (ATG), methotrexate, rituximab, alemtuzumab, purine analogs, and any high-dose therapy with autologous transplantation

(Continued on next page)

Table 17-1. Examples of Possible Late Effects of Radiation Therapy, Chemotherapy, and Hormonal Therapy Among Survivors of Adult Cancers (Continued)

Organ System/ Tissue	Radiation Therapy Late Effects	Chemotherapy/Hormonal Therapy	
		Late Effects	Agent Responsible
Lymphatic	Lymphedema	–	–
Nervous system	Problems with thinking, learning, memory; structural changes in the brain; bleeding into the brain	Problems with thinking, learning, memory; structural changes in the brain: paralysis; seizure	Methotrexate, multiagent chemotherapy, bortezomib
		Numbness and tingling, hearing loss	Cisplatin
		Numbness and tingling	Vinca alkaloids, taxanes, oxaliplatin
Ophthalmologic	Cataracts, dry eyes, visual impairment	Cataracts	Steroids
Pulmonary	Lung scarring, decreased lung function	Lung scarring, inflammation	Bleomycin sulfate, carmustine (BCNU), methotrexate
		Potentiation of radiation therapy effects (gemcitabine)	Actinomycin D/doxorubicin (Adriamycin)
Renal	Hypertension, impaired kidney function	Impaired kidney function, delayed-onset renal failure	Cisplatin, methotrexate, nitrosoureas

Note. From *From Cancer Patient to Cancer Survivor: Lost in Transition* (pp. 72–73), by M. Hewitt, S. Greenfield, and E. Stovall (Eds.), 2006, Washington, DC: National Academies Press. Copyright 2006 by National Academy of Sciences. Reprinted with permission.

Psychosocial Effects

Much of the research on the psychosocial effects of cancer is devoted to early diagnosis and treatment and specific cancer sites, particularly breast cancer; few studies are devoted to the post-treatment experience (Stanton, 2006; Vachon, 2006). Psychological effects may include cancer-specific concerns and uncertainties, such as fear of recurrence, or more generalized symptoms of worry, fear of the future, insomnia, fatigue, and difficulty concentrating (Hewitt et al., 2006). NCCN used the term *psychosocial distress* in cancer in developing its guidelines for cancer distress management and defined it as "a multifactorial unpleasant emotional experience of a psychological (cognitive, behavioral, emotional), social, and/or spiritual nature that may interfere with the ability to cope effectively with cancer, its physical symptoms and its treatment" (NCCN, 2007). Distress reflects a broader set of concerns that range from common feelings of vulnerability, sadness, and fear to disabling problems of depression, anxiety, panic, social isolation, and existential and spiritual crisis (NCCN, 2007). Distress may occur as a reaction to the disease and treatment, as well as its consequential effect on social factors, such as employment, insurance, and relationships. Not all psychological effects are negative. Many cancer survivors report feelings of gratitude and good fortune and an increased sense of self-esteem and mastery (Hewitt et al., 2006; Stanton). Recent interest has emerged in how cancer survivors derive meaning from their experience. Studies have found that exploring one's spirituality is an effective way of coping, restoring sense of self, and finding purpose and meaning (Coward & Kahn, 2004; Ferrell, Smith, Juarez, & Melancon, 2003).

Overall, the majority of long-term cancer survivors do not experience serious psychological problems (Hewitt, Rowland, & Yancik, 2003). However, research has revealed subsets of survivors reporting persistent psychological sequelae. Bloom (2002) described variations according to Mullan's phases of survival, with specific issues manifesting during the acute, extended, and permanent survival. In her review article, Stanton (2006) identified risk and protective factors related to psychological adjustment outcomes. Risks factors for poor adjustment and functional limitations include treatment with chemotherapy, social isolation or conflict, expectancies for low control and negative outcomes, and concerted attempts to avoid feelings surrounding cancer. Protective factors include "having emotionally supportive relationships and using coping strategies such as problem solving, positive reappraisal, and emotional expression" (Stanton, p. 5133).

Multiple studies have focused on the psychological distress experienced by older, long-term survivors. One study investigating symptoms of general distress and post-traumatic stress disorder (PTSD) did not demonstrate clinical levels of PTSD in survivors but reported a 25% incidence of clinical depression (Deimling, Kahana, Bowman, & Schaefer, 2002). Persistent cancer-related symptoms were the strongest predictors of depression and the PTSD subdimension of hyperarousal. A survey of the cancer-related health worries and related distress of older, long-term survivors in another study revealed that one-third continued to worry about recurrence, a second cancer, and symptoms they experience as a sign of cancer (Deimling, Bowman, Sterns, Wagner, & Kahana, 2006). These worries were significant predictors of anxiety and depression and occurred least commonly among African Americans. Researchers noted that despite the prevalence of continued worries, most survivors reported little impact on overall measures of quality of life. A study of the coping styles of the same population indicated that long-term survivors used planning and acceptance most commonly and that the personal characteristic of optimism was a strong predictor of positive coping. All coping deteriorated with increasing age (Deimling, Wagner, et al., 2006). These studies indicate the need for particular attention to assessment for depression and poor coping strategies in older, long-term survivors, particularly those with comorbid or persistent cancer-related effects. Attention to this population is necessary given the current and growing numbers of older survivors.

Survivors' needs and concerns shift over time, and evidence has shown that external sources of support erode, particularly for those most distressed and of older age (Deimling, Wagner, et al., 2006; Stanton, 2006). Survivors report receiving insufficient information and support once treatment ends. The LAF (2004) surveyed more than 1,000 cancer survivors in 2004 about the impact of the cancer diagnosis and treatment on the quality of their lives. Half of the survey responders reported that their nonmedical needs were unmet. Cancer centers tend to offer many patient and family services, but surveys show that these services are inconsistent and frequently dependent on specific individuals (Tesauro, Rowland, & Lustig, 2002). Simple routine assessment of psychological well-being using tools such as the Distress Thermometer (NCCN, 2007) is an important basic intervention and can effectively identify individuals who need referral (Vachon, 2006). Information about psychological support resources, including individual, group, and Web-based groups, should be made available.

The impact of cancer treatment on people's social functioning includes family issues, such as sexual and marital relationships and adjustment of children, and work-related issues, such as concern over cancer disclosure, stigma, reentry to the workplace, changes in work priorities, discrimination, and health insurance. Although a great deal of research exists on the effects of a cancer diagnosis and treatment on family functioning, studies of family coping or core functioning in families with adult long-term survivors are limited (Lewis, 2006). Some evidence in patients with breast cancer has shown that individual and family counseling as well as support groups can be helpful (Dow, Ferrell, Leigh, Ly, & Gulasekaram, 1996). Awareness of employment and insurance laws and state and payer policy is important for patients' optimal return to career and economic stability.

Cancer Survivors and Employment

For more than 30 years, the vast majority of working-age adults who have been diagnosed with cancer want to and are able to perform their jobs and return to work (Hoffman, 2005). Most survivors work to support themselves and their families but also for the accompanying health insurance, self-esteem, and social support (Hoffman). A population-based study of cancer survivors compared to matched controls found a substantially increased burden of illness manifested in days lost from work, inability to work, general health perception, and need for help with daily activities and other concerns (Hewitt et al., 2003; Yabroff, Lawrence, Clauser, Davis, & Brown, 2004). Work limitations are dependent on many factors, including the survivor's age, stage at diagnosis, financial status, education, health insurance, transportation, the physical demands of the job, and presence of comorbid health problems (Hoffman). Most cancer survivors are able to continue working or return to work without limitations from their disease or treatment (Hoffman).

Over the past 30 years, cancer survivors have reported decreasing incidence of cancer-related employment problems, such as dismissal, failure to hire, demotion, denial of benefits, and hostility (Hoffman, 2005). Cancer survivors are protected under federal and state laws as long as they are qualified for and can perform the major responsibilities of the job. Federal laws include the Americans with Disabilities Act (ADA), the Federal Rehabilitation Act, the Family and Medical Leave Act, and the Employee Retirement and Income Security Act (Hewitt et al., 2006; Hoffman) (see Table 17-2).

Most state laws cover cancer survivors because they prohibit discrimination against people with disabilities, but the definition of "disabled" varies by state and federal law. A new focus of attention is protection of information related to genetic susceptibilities of patients. Several federal laws, including the ADA, Health Insurance Portability and Accountability Act (HIPAA), Genetic Privacy Act, and Genetic Information Nondiscrimination Act, and many state laws protect against genetic discrimination, but protection can vary widely (Hoffman, 2005).

Health Insurance Challenges

Most Americans with health insurance have coverage providing for cancer-related care (Hewitt et al., 2006). However, for those survivors who risk losing their insurance

Table 17-2. Federal Laws Protecting Cancer Survivors

Federal Law	Description of Coverage	Benefit	Restrictions
Americans with Disabilities Act (ADA)	Prohibits job discrimination by employers, employment agencies, and labor unions against people who have or had cancer and their families. Most cancer survivors are protected by the ADA from the time of diagnosis.	Prohibits discrimination for • Not hiring applicants for a job or training program • Firing a worker • Providing unequal pay, working conditions, and benefits • Punishing an employee for filing discrimination complaint • Screening out disabled employees	Disability definition may not include those without limitations of "major life activity." Does not include employers with fewer than 15 employees Does not cover the military, other than civilian members of military or people retired from the military
Federal Rehabilitation Act (FRA)	Prohibits public employers and private employers that receive public funding from discriminating based on disability Covers groups not covered by ADA: • Employees of the executive branch of the federal government • Employees of employers receiving federal contracts or federal financial assistance with fewer than 15 employees	Like the ADA, the FRA protects survivors, regardless of the extent of disability.	Does not cover the military, other than civilian members of military or people retired from the military
Family and Medical Leave Act (FMLA)	Requires employers with 50 or more employees to provide up to 12 weeks of unpaid, job-protected leave during any 12-month period for employees with a serious health condition that makes them unable to perform the functions of the position	FMLA includes leave for employees with a seriously ill child, parent, or spouse, a healthy newborn, or a newly adopted child. Benefits, including health insurance, are provided. FMLA allows intermittent or reduced work schedules or transfer to a different position with equivalent pay.	Employee must have worked at least 25 hours per week for one year. Employers may exempt highest-paid workers.
Employee Retirement and Income Security Act (ERISA)	Prohibits discrimination that prevents employees from collecting benefits under an employee benefit plan	Prohibits setting of conditions related to health status for coverage under health benefits Prohibits termination of employment for the purpose of cutting off benefits Prohibits encouraging employees to retire as a "disabled" person, which can limit benefits	Inapplicable to other forms of discrimination: • Individuals denied a new job because of medical status • Employees experiencing different treatment that does not affect benefits • Employees whose compensation does not include benefits

Note. Based on information from Hoffman, 2005.

because of employment issues, and for those who are underinsured, the expense of care after treatment can be prohibitive. Even those with good coverage can find it inadequate for the care required for surveillance or management of treatment effects. Most survivors are older than 65 and are covered by Medicare, but gaps in Medicare, particularly related to drug coverage, can create high out-of-pocket expenses. For the four million survivors younger than age 65 and not covered by Medicare, 11% are estimated to be completely uninsured, thereby creating disparity in access to needed services (Hewitt et al., 2006).

Federal laws provide some protection regarding continued insurance coverage for cancer survivors. The Consolidated Omnibus Budget Reconciliation Act (COBRA) allows survivors who lose their jobs to maintain for 18 months the insurance provided through the employer (U.S. Department of Labor Employee Benefits Security Administration, 2006). HIPAA added protection for people changing jobs by eliminating denials for preexisting conditions and denials of eligibility for benefits on the condition of health status. HIPAA provides some reassurance for survivors (and their family members who hold the insurance) who are experiencing "job lock"—the avoidance of changing jobs because of the fear of losing insurance and other health-related benefits (Hewitt et al., 2006; U.S. Department of Labor Employee Benefits Security Administration, 2004). Each state regulates health insurance polices, and laws vary significantly. Health insurers have yet to apply consistent policy on survivorship care, and costs can be high and coverage limited (Hewitt et al., 2006).

Resources include the following.

- Information on federal laws is available at the U.S. Department of Labor's Health Plans and Benefits page, which can be accessed at www.dol.gov.
- General information about employment and disability is available through the U.S. Equal Employment Opportunities Commission at www.eeoc.gov.
- Information related to health insurance can be found through NCCS (www.canceradvocacy.org) and CancerCare (www.cancercare.org/pdf/fact_sheets/fs_entitlements.pdf).
- American Cancer Society, "Medical Insurance and Financial Assistance for the Cancer Patient": www.cancer.org/docroot/MLT/content/MLT_1x_Medical_Insurance_and_Financial_Assistance_for_the_Cancer_Patient.asp?sitearea=&level=1

Components of Cancer Follow-Up Care

Care of survivors should incorporate the physical and psychosocial risks and sequelae of a cancer diagnosis and treatment. Care should be coordinated between specialists and primary care providers to ensure survivors' long-term needs are met. Follow-up care should include the following components.

Surveillance for cancer recurrence is the periodic assessment beginning at the end of treatment and extending for a period of time that is dependent on the type of cancer, stage at diagnosis, tumor characteristics, and related risk of recurrence. Surveillance includes careful review of interval history, physical examination, and appropriate diagnostic testing. The absence of evidence-based practice guidelines for adult survivors makes decision making difficult for clinicians who struggle with under- or overprescribing diagnostic tests and related follow-up. Insurance reimbursement for testing in the absence of guidelines adds to the dilemma (Hewitt et al., 2006). Discussion of clinical practice guidelines will be included later in this chapter. Follow-up visits and testing schedules tend to be frequent during the immediate post-treatment period and generally decrease in frequency over time as the more acute risks diminish. For example, most recurrences of breast cancer are detected within five years of diagnosis, with the rate of recurrence peaking in the second year (Burstein & Winer, 2000; Emens & Davidson, 2003). However, breast cancer recurrences can occur as late as 20 years after initial diagnosis, so no defined time exists for when survivors can be considered definitively cured (Hewitt et al., 2006). Thus, healthcare providers should consider a history of cancer throughout the life of the survivor. As with all survivorship care, the oncology specialist, primary care provider, or combination of both may provide surveillance for recurrence.

Monitoring for and management of disease and treatment effects, including second cancers, is essential for survivors' long-term health and quality of life. Monitoring requires knowledge of particular treatment effects and related assessments and testing. As with surveillance for recurrence, few published guidelines exist regarding the monitoring of late effects. Examples of monitoring include periodic cardiovascular evaluation for patients treated with anthracyclines, alkylating agents, or taxanes (for which no guidelines exist); breast cancer screening with annual mammography for survivors of Hodgkin disease treated with mantle field radiation eight years following therapy (NCCN, 2008); screening for hypothyroidism for patients treated with neck radiation; assessment of restoration of ovulation after treatment with alkylating or hormonal agents; and screening for anxiety and depression. Interventions for managing long-term and late treatment effects are important for the recovery and adaptation of survivors. Examples include exploring causes for persistent fatigue after lymphoma; referring patients to specialists if they have urinary incontinence and sexual dysfunction after radical prostatectomy; initiating lymphedema therapy after lymph node dissection; and referring patients to reproduction specialists for infertility. In recent years, design of initial treatment plans that can minimize the risk of late effects has had an impact on quality of life in many cancer types (Hewitt et al., 2006). New methods of tailoring treatment to individual and tumor characteristics have the potential to reduce the risk of late effects and improve outcomes for survivors.

Detection of new cancers includes ongoing screening for cancer as recommended by national guidelines. Frequently, cancer survivors and providers neglect regular cancer screening procedures because of a lack of understanding of increased risk, a feeling that surviving one cancer eliminated the need for concern about others, or fear of finding a new health problem (Hewitt et al., 2006). Routine screening for breast, colorectal, prostate, cervical, and endometrial cancers according to guidelines such as those published by the American Cancer Society (2006) should be part of ongoing healthcare recommendations.

Promotion of positive health behaviors includes counseling survivors about lifestyle changes that can reduce comorbid conditions that may be related to age, treatment, genetic susceptibility, or behaviors. Recommendations should include known risk reduction behaviors, such as initiating smoking cessation, controlling weight, moderating alcohol intake, controlling sun exposure, engaging in regular physical activity, and getting an annual influenza vaccination.

Summary of Cancer Treatment and Plan for Follow-Up Care

According to Earle (2006), quality survivor care is rooted in a plan for survivorship, and knowing what has been done, what needs to be done, and who will do it is essential for patients completing cancer treatment. The second recommendation of the IOM report states, "Patients completing primary treatment should be provided with a comprehensive care summary and a follow-up care plan that is clearly and effectively explained" (Hewitt et al., 2006, p. 151). A survivorship care plan provides patients and their current and future care providers with a source of information about the treatment they received and the related risks and recommendations. It can serve as a tool for counseling survivors about the lifetime significance of this information for their health care. The care plan should be shared with care providers throughout a cancer survivor's life as a blueprint for his or her ongoing medical needs.

The report of an IOM meeting conducted to study the implementation of formalized survivorship care calls for plans that inform patients and their providers of the long-term effects of cancer and its treatment, identify psychosocial support resources in their communities, and provide guidance on follow-up care, prevention, and health maintenance (Hewitt & Ganz, 2007). Barriers to providing these plans include the length of time required and lack of reimbursement for completion; poor access to information over time because of multiple care providers and settings; and absence of evidence- and consensus-based guidelines for follow-up care (Earle, 2006; Haylock, Mitchell, Cox, Temple, & Curtiss, 2007; Hewitt & Ganz; Hewitt et al., 2006). ASCO has established a committee to address this absence of guidelines and is developing standardized, disease-specific electronic templates for provider use. Sample templates of the ASCO treatment plan and summaries for cancer are available on the ASCO Web site (www.asco.org) on its Quality Care and Guidelines, Quality Measurement and Improvement, Chemotherapy Treatment Plan and Summary page. Figure 17-8 lists the recommended elements of a survivorship care plan.

Demographic/Contact Information
- Care providers (surgeon, medical and/or radiation oncologists)
- Treatment location (hospital, practice, etc.)
- Name, phone number, and address of institution/provider

Disease Specifics
- Diagnosis
- Pathology
- Stage of disease

Treatment Specifics
- Surgery: Date, procedure; persistent or possible late effects
- Chemotherapy/biotherapy: Dates, regimen; clinical trials; agents, doses, supportive care; persistent or possible late effects
- Hormonal therapy: Dates, agents, doses; persistent or possible late effects
- Radiation: Dates, site, type, dose; persistent or possible late effects
- Symptoms to report

Follow-Up Care Plan
- Evidence-based guidelines for surveillance, monitoring for late effects, and related interventions, as available

Cancer Screening Recommendations
- Recommendations for health promotion (nutrition, physical activity, smoking cessation)

Figure 17-8. Cancer Treatment Summary and Care Plan Elements

Note. Based on information from Earle, 2006; Haylock et al., 2007; Hewitt & Ganz, 2007; Hewitt et al., 2006.

Models of Care

The fragmented state of our healthcare system challenges the delivery of optimal survivorship care. Many barriers exist, including lack of professional education and training, lack of standards or guidelines for care, and difficulties in communication. Overcoming these barriers requires building an integrated systems approach that incorporates a team of primary care providers, oncologists, and other care providers who agree to communicate and develop streamlined transitions in care (Hewitt et al., 2006). Promising models of survivorship care have emerged, including a shared-care model and various forms of specialized follow-up clinics.

A shared-care model is described as a sharing of responsibility for health care between two or more clinicians of different specialties that involves transfer of personal communication about a patient and knowledge about the particular care requirements (Hewitt et al., 2006; Oeffinger & McCabe, 2006). Shared care has become the standard approach to managing chronic illnesses such as diabetes, where care is coordinated between an endocrinologist and a primary care physician. Analysis of data collected in the 2001 and 2002 National Ambulatory Medical Care Survey and the National Hospital Ambulatory Medical Care Survey showed that primary care physicians have a significant role in cancer care, with nearly half of cancer-related ambulatory visits characterized as shared care, although the role of each clinician during these visits is unclear (Hewitt et al., 2006). Formalizing systems, especially communication processes, for facilitating care between oncology specialists and primary care physicians could create a more comprehensive approach to meeting the long-term needs of cancer survivors.

Specialty survivorship programs are evolving in academic institutions around the United States. Initial models were developed for the care of pediatric cancer survivors, where there was early recognition of the need to monitor for late treatment effects. Most of these programs are directed by a pediatric oncologist and coordinated by an oncology nurse practitioner (NP), and about half include other providers of mental health and other specialties (Oeffinger & McCabe, 2006). Disease-specific models were the first examples of adult survivorship care programs. Oeffinger and McCabe described three distinct care models. As in the pediatric programs, NPs play a central role in care delivery. The first care model is the most basic and is described as a one-time consultative visit to a survivorship care provider, often an oncology NP. A summary of cancer treatment and a plan for monitoring late effects are developed, and needs-based counseling and risk reduction recommendations are provided. The second model is an oncology NP–led clinic that functions as an extension of the care continuum. The NP delivers ongoing care that includes a standard set of services and a follow-up plan. Contact with the primary care provider is reestablished by the oncology NP with sharing of patient information and care guidelines. This begins the transition to shared care and a potential return to community follow-up care based on the patient's risk for recurrence and late effects.

The most complex model is a specialized multidisciplinary survivor program similar to the pediatric programs. This model includes physicians with training and experience in the care of cancer survivors, NPs, and mental health and consulting specialists. The team provides risk-based care. One example of this model is a clinic that provides care for adult survivors of pediatric cancers. This resource-intense model would be challenging to adapt to groups with larger numbers of survivors.

Standards of Care

An organized set of clinical practice guidelines based on the best available evidence would assist clinical decision making and help to ensure appropriate care for survivors. The Children's Oncology Group (COG) has developed a model for these guidelines that outlines the long-term follow-up care for children, adolescent, and young adult cancer survivors. These guidelines are widely available on the Internet with a complementary set of educational materials (COG, 2006). Unfortunately, very few adult cancers have published, evidence-based clinical practice guidelines, and the guidelines available are not uniform primarily because of the absence of adequately powered, well-controlled trials of follow-up after potentially curative initial therapy (Hewitt et al., 2006). High-quality evidence on the benefits, harms, and relative cost effectiveness of follow-up strategies is needed to avoid the health and financial hazards of overuse, underuse, and misuse of resources. The IOM has called on professional organizations and public and private agencies to support the development of scientific review processes and the necessary research to address this gap in cancer care.

ASCO has published follow-up guidelines for breast (Khatcheressian et al., 2006) and colorectal (Desch et al., 2005) cancers and for fertility preservation (Lee et al., 2006). Table 17-3 is an example of the ASCO guidelines for breast cancer follow-up care. NCCN also has developed consensus-based treatment guidelines that incorporate follow-up care for some cancers.

Implications for Oncology Advanced Practice Nurses

Oncology APNs are involved in the wide spectrum of cancer care, including direct clinical practice, education of patients and other professionals, and generation of evidence-based practice standards and clinical research. APNs have much to contribute to the design, direction, and delivery of care to cancer survivors by expanding the scope of their influence beyond the end of treatment.

Oncology NPs and clinical nurse specialists need to incorporate routine approaches to designing care for survivors at key intervals, including completion of therapy, preparation for follow-up, and return for surveillance and monitoring. In all cases, the following suggestions for practice and questions to consider can serve as a guide for assessment and intervention.

1. Know patients' cancer history. Apply knowledge of treatment effects to identify the long-term risks for patients.
   - What are the cancer type, histology, and stage? What was the age of the patient during treatment? How long ago did it occur? Was there any other cancer history?
   - Did the patient have surgery? What kind and to what site? What are the functional losses and persistent effects?
   - Did the patient receive chemotherapy, biotherapy, hormonal therapy, or targeted agents? Which agents were used? What are the cumulative doses of the anthracyclines? Did the patient receive high doses and multiple cycles of any agents? Did the patient receive bisphosphonates, steroids, or multiple courses of antibiotics/antifungals? Does the patient have persistent symptoms? What are the potential late effects of agents received? Does the patient have any signs or symptoms of late effects?
   - Did the patient receive radiation? What kind, to what site, and at what dose? Does the patient have persistent symptoms? What are the potential late effects of the radiation? Does the patient have any signs or symptoms of late effects?

Table 17-3. American Society of Clinical Oncology 2006 Update of the Breast Cancer Follow-Up and Management Guidelines in the Adjuvant Setting

Mode of Surveillance	Summary of Recommendations
Recommended breast cancer surveillance	
History/physical examination	Every 3 to 6 months for the first 3 years after primary therapy; every 6 to 12 months for years 4 and 5; then annually
Patient education regarding symptoms of recurrence	Physicians should counsel patients about the symptoms of recurrence including new lumps, bone pain, chest pain, abdominal pain, dyspnea or persistent headaches; helpful websites for patient education include www.plwc.org and www.cancer.org
Referral for genetic counseling	Criteria include: Ashkenazi Jewish heritage; history of ovarian cancer at any age in the patient or any first- or second-degree relatives; any first-degree relative with a history of breast cancer diagnosed before the age of 50 years; two or more first- or second-degree relatives diagnosed with breast cancer at any age; patient or relative with diagnosis of bilateral breast cancer; and history of breast cancer in a male relative
Breast self-examination	All women should be counseled to perform monthly breast self-examination
Mammography	First post-treatment mammogram 1 year after the initial mammogram that leads to diagnosis, but no earlier than 6 months after definitive radiation therapy; subsequent mammograms should be obtained as indicated for surveillance of abnormalities
Coordination of care	Continuity of care for breast cancer patients is encouraged and should be performed by a physician experienced in the surveillance of cancer patients and in breast examination, including the examination of irradiated breasts; if follow-up is transferred to a PCP, the PCP and the patient should be informed of the long-term options regarding adjuvant hormonal therapy for the particular patient; this may necessitate rereferral for oncology assessment at an interval consistent with guidelines for adjuvant hormonal therapy
Pelvic examination	Regular gynecologic follow-up is recommended for all women; patients who receive tamoxifen should be advised to report any vaginal bleeding to their physicians
Breast cancer surveillance testing: not recommended	
Routine blood tests	CBCs and liver function tests are not recommended
Imaging studies	Chest x-ray, bone scans, liver ultrasound, computed tomography scans, FDG-PET scans, and breast MRI are not recommended
Tumor markers	CA 15-3, CA 27.29, and carcinoembryonic antigen are not recommended
FDG-PET	FDG-PET scanning is not recommended for routine breast cancer surveillance
Breast MRI	Breast MRI is not recommended for routine breast cancer surveillance

CBCs—complete blood counts; FDG-PET—fluorodeoxyglucose–positron emission tomography; MRI—magnetic resonance imaging; PCP—primary care physician

Note. From "American Society of Clinical Oncology 2006 Update of the Breast Cancer Follow-Up and Management Guidelines in the Adjuvant Setting," by J.L. Khatcheressian, A.C. Wolff, T.J. Smith, E. Grunfeld, H.B. Muss, V.G. Vogel, et al., 2006, *Journal of Clinical Oncology, 24,* p. 5092. Copyright 2006 by American Society of Clinical Oncology. Reprinted with permission.

- Did the patient have a transplant? What kind? What are the potential late effects of the transplant? Does the patient have any signs or symptoms of late effects?
2. Know the surveillance plan for the patient's cancer type. Follow guidelines as they are available.
   - How often should the person be seen and tested? What are the recommended diagnostic tests, if any? What other testing should be considered based on the systems review and examination?
3. Know what the patient's risk factors were, if any, both genetic and environmental.
   - Did the patient undergo genetic susceptibility testing? Does a related screening recommendation exist? Has the patient eliminated causal behavior, such as smoking, alcohol consumption, or occupational exposure?
4. Screen for other cancers, as indicated.
   - Has the patient been screened for other cancers? What are the particular recommendations for cancer screening for this patient?
5. Assess the patient and family for psychosocial concerns.
   - Does the patient report symptoms of anxiety or depression?
   - Has the patient experienced loss of social functioning, such as with roles, relationships, or employment?
   - Has the patient experienced discrimination, such as with employment or insurance?
   - Has the patient experienced serious economic problems?
   - How are the patient's family members or loved ones coping in this post-treatment period?
6. Know the health behaviors that increase the risk for morbidities and other cancers.
   - Does the patient smoke or use alcohol or drugs? Does the patient practice healthy behaviors, such as dietary restriction, weight control, physical exercise, and sun protection?
7. Perform a survivorship-focused history and physical examination. Review of systems includes the following (Aziz, 2002; Ganz, 2006).
   - Constitutional—weight gain/loss, fatigue, fever and night sweats, pain, changes or limitation in physical exercise ability
   - Skin and integument—skin changes, lesions; hair loss
   - Eye, ear, nose, throat, and mouth—hearing loss; dental problems, dry mouth; jaw pain; speech, sight, swallowing disturbance
   - Pulmonary—dyspnea, cough, pain
   - Cardiac and vascular—signs and symptoms of congestive heart failure; symptoms of palpitations, coronary, ischemic, and/or pleuropericardial chest pain; claudication or vascular ischemic attacks; Raynaud disease
   - Renal—hypertension
   - Gastrointestinal—chronic diarrhea or constipation; abdominal pain; ostomy function and management as well as associated sexual functioning; ascites, jaundice
   - Genitourinary—urinary incontinence, dysuria; erectile dysfunction, infertility; ostomy function and management, related urinary tract infections and sexual functioning
   - Gynecologic—premature menopause, vaginal dryness or dyspareunia; infertility
   - Endocrine—thyroid nodules or symptoms of hypothyroidism; such as unexplained weight gain, increased cholesterol; reproductive history, sexual functioning; symp-

toms of metabolic syndrome, such as increasing abdominal girth, increasing trig-
lycerides, glucose intolerance
- Hematologic—cytopenia
- Lymphatic—palpable nodules; lymphedema
- Infections—report of chronic infections
- Musculoskeletal—muscular or bone pain, osteoporosis, fracture, decreased bone density, aseptic necrosis
- Neurologic—neuropathic pain, peripheral neuropathy; hearing loss, decreased cognitive function
- Psychiatric/psychosocial—return to previous roles, symptoms of anxiety or depression, difficulty sleeping, disturbed body image; taking psychotropic medication

8. Manage symptoms.
   - Apply knowledge of symptom management of acute problems to the chronic presentation. Refer to specialists as needed.
9. Provide patients with a treatment summary and care plan.
   - Apply knowledge of the patient's cancer diagnosis and treatment history in developing a comprehensive summary and plan. Review the care plan with patients and emphasize the need to share it with their other healthcare providers. Work with colleagues to develop efficient methods to implement care plan development for all patients. Routinely communicate this plan directly to designated providers.

Professional Education

Cancer survivorship care is a new specialty, and curricula for health professionals have little, if any, content in this area (Ferrell & Winn, 2006). Few undergraduate nursing programs offer didactic training in cancer care, and the number of programs providing graduate nursing education with an oncology specialty has decreased by half in the past decade (Ferrell, Virani, Smith, & Juarez, 2003). Survivorship training is even less available. Some growth has occurred in continuing education programs offering survivorship content through specialty organizations such as the Oncology Nursing Society (ONS), but far more is needed for nurses and the other disciplines. Oncology APNs, particularly clinical nurse specialists, routinely educate and mentor other nurses and students about all aspects of cancer care in formal lectures and in the clinical arena. Incorporating survivorship content when teaching graduate or continuing education courses and mentoring other nurses and APN students can begin to build a workforce that is knowledgeable and prepared to address survivorship as part of the cancer care trajectory. APNs should seek opportunities to participate jointly with their oncology colleagues to develop survivorship practice guidelines and methods to apply them efficiently (e.g., software development). Improving the quality of care for cancer survivors is contingent on having physicians, nurses, and other professionals adequately trained in survivorship care.

Research

Oncology nurses, individually and collectively, have led many initiatives that address the needs of cancer survivors in the areas of pain, fatigue, sexuality, fertility, family coping, long-term sequelae of treatment, and psychosocial concerns (Ferrell, Virani, et al.,

2003). Much of the nursing research on cancer survivorship, supported by ONS and the ONS Foundation, the National Institute of Nursing Research, and NCI, addresses the impact of cancer treatment on quality of life (Ferrell, Virani, et al., 2003). With their intimate knowledge and understanding of the cancer treatment experience, oncology APNs can contribute to the much-needed evidence-building for the development of quality care guidelines and interventions for survivors. Through individual research studies and participation in larger initiatives addressing survivorship, such as through the ONS Putting Evidence Into Practice® project (Gobel, Beck, & O'Leary, 2006), oncology APNs have an opportunity to ensure quality care for survivors and their future.

Patient and Caregiver Education

Education of patients and their caregivers about treatment modalities, self-care, prevention and reduction of side effects, and management of symptoms to improve quality of life is a cornerstone of oncology nursing care. And yet, nurses are remiss in their preparation of patients and caregivers for the experience following treatment. Historically, celebration with patients ensued at the end of treatment, only to have patients later report feelings of abandonment, as they were unprepared to manage their ongoing needs. Quality of life commonly suffers because patients do not know what to expect (Earle, 2006). As the body of knowledge about the needs and care of cancer survivors builds, education of survivors should take on the same level of importance that is attached to active treatment.

Nurses can begin to incorporate information about survivorship during their first contact with patients. Teaching sessions on the plan of care at the start of therapy can incorporate the importance of long-term follow-up and expanding the framework of the cancer care trajectory through the post-treatment period. As patients near the end of treatment, more specific education about what to expect should be introduced and include the following categories of information.

Management Strategies for Long-Term and Late Effects

In addition to the information contained in the treatment summary and care plan, preparing patients for what to expect after treatment and teaching them symptom management strategies is important for their safety and physical and emotional well-being. Preparation can ease the transition during the period where patients see their care providers less frequently and have reduced support. Learning to adapt to these effects is important for recovery. Conversely, it is equally important that patients be made aware of symptoms that could be concerning and should be reported. Symptoms such as a new lump or onset of pain, bleeding, loss of appetite, changes in bowel habits, persistent nausea and vomiting, weight loss of 10 pounds or greater, difficulty breathing, or a cough that does not resolve could be signs of a recurrent or new malignancy or late treatment effect.

Behaviors to Promote Good Health

Cancer survivors are at increased risk for second malignancies and multiple comorbid diseases brought on by cancer treatment, genetic predisposition, or common lifestyle factors; death rates from noncancer causes are higher for cancer survivors than the general population (Demark-Wahnefried, Aziz, Rowland, & Pinto, 2005; Ganz, 2005;

Hewitt et al., 2003). As noted previously, the majority of cancer survivors today are older than 65 years of age, adding the burden of age-related comorbid conditions, which carry a poorer prognosis (Edwards et al., 2002). Comorbidities include but are not limited to obesity, cardiovascular disease, osteoporosis, diabetes, and functional decline (Demark-Wahnefried et al.). Growing evidence shows that positive changes in health behaviors by survivors, including regular exercise regimens, improved nutritional intake, smoking cessation, and sun protection, can have an impact on disease prevention (Demark-Wahnefried et al.). Much more research is needed regarding the direct impact of post-treatment behavior change on cancer-related progression, recurrence or survival, other health outcomes, and morbidity. In addition, associated interventions targeting primary and secondary prevention of morbidities and new malignancies that can reach the survivors who are most vulnerable are needed (Demark-Wahnefried et al.; Hewitt et al., 2003).

The end of primary treatment of cancer has been called a *teachable moment,* a term used to describe life transitions or health events that have the potential to motivate individuals to adopt risk-reducing or health-protective behaviors (Ganz, 2005; McBride, Emmons, & Lipkus, 2003). Transition to cancer survivorship is a teachable moment for oncology APNs to introduce healthy lifestyle behaviors. Particular attention is required for specific populations who tend to be less motivated to make health behavior changes, such as men, those with less education, older adults, and urban residents (Demark-Wahnefried et al., 2005). Oncology APNs and other providers should educate patients on existing health guidelines and encourage them to take active roles in general preventive health strategies. These strategies should include smoking cessation, alcohol abstinence, dietary modifications, exercise promotion, use of sunscreen, and cancer screening (Demark-Wahnefried et al.; Hewitt et al., 2003).

Complementary and Alternative Therapies for Cancer Survivors

Complementary and alternative medicine (CAM), as defined by the National Center for Complementary and Alternative Medicine (NCCAM, 2007), "is a group of diverse medical and health care systems, practices, and products that are not presently considered to be part of conventional medicine." CAM use among adults in the United States is widespread. When the definition of CAM includes using prayer and megavitamins specifically for health reasons, 62% of adults in the 2002 National Health Interview Survey indicated use in the previous 12 months (Barnes, Powell-Griner, McFann, & Nahin, 2004). A systematic review of prevalence studies on the use of CAM in cancer revealed a 7%–64% use with an average prevalence in adult studies of 31.4% (Ernst & Cassileth, 1998). Variability in definitions of CAM methods among researchers and patients accounts for the wide range of reports (Ernst & Cassileth; Humpel & Jones, 2006). Growing evidence supports that CAM use in cancer is becoming more prevalent (Bernstein & Grasso, 2001; Ernst, Pittler, Wider, & Boddy, 2007; Humpel & Jones). CAM use has been primarily investigated in breast cancer, revealing high use during and after treatment (Boon et al., 2000; Humpel & Jones, 2006; Lengacher et al., 2002; Matthews, Sellergren, Huo, List, & Fleming, 2007).

Studies specifically focused on survivors, although limited, also reflect common use of CAM. In a study of colorectal cancer survivors, 75% indicated use of CAM, with younger females and those with poorer perceived quality of life being more likely to participate (Lawson et al., 2007). Study of breast cancer survivors revealed high usage (69%); patients were younger and diagnosed at younger ages, and those who associated CAM use with cancer had higher trait anxiety (Matthews et al., 2007). A study of breast cancer survivors in Canada revealed that only about half of patients discuss CAM with their physicians, suggesting that care providers have a greater need to assess and counsel patients about appropriate use.

APNs need to be informed about CAM and assess patients' use of CAM methods. Many reliable resources related to CAM are available for patients and clinicians.
- NCCAM, *Cancer and CAM*: http://nccam.nih.gov/health/camcancer
- NCI, *Thinking About Complementary and Alternative Medicine*: www.cancer.gov/cancertopics /thinking-about-CAM
- American Cancer Society guide to complementary and alternative cancer methods: www.cancer.org/docroot/ETO/ETO_5.asp
- Memorial Sloan-Kettering Cancer Center, *About Herbs, Botanicals, and Other Products*: www.mskcc.org/mskcc/html/11570.cfm

Conclusion

Cancer survivorship has emerged in recent years as an important area of focus in cancer care, largely in response to the demands of cancer survivors in their pursuit of a better quality of life after treatment. Within the past decade, nurses, physicians, and mental health specialists have made significant contributions to the field of research, and NCI has organized a focus for federal sponsorship (Hewitt et al., 2006). Major publications devoted to survivorship have appeared, including the IOM report and entire issues of the *Journal of Clinical Oncology* (November 2006) and the *American Journal of Nursing* (March 2006 supplement). ASCO and ONS have incorporated content about survivorship into their annual meetings, and NCI sponsors a biannual survivorship research meeting.

Advancing survivorship care will depend on growth in research, education, and clinical practice models. IOM has called on federal agencies, private voluntary organizations, cooperative groups, and registries to urgently support initiatives related to mechanisms, prevalence, and risk of late effects; interventions to alleviate symptoms and improve function and quality of life; care models that are cost effective and address surveillance strategies and interventions; care of the underserved and supportive care and rehabilitation; insurance and employment issues; and methods to overcome barriers and challenges. The challenge lies in the availability of funding for these initiatives in a period where competing national healthcare issues and limited resources exist (Hewitt et al., 2006).

Oncology APNs coordinate care for patients throughout the cancer care trajectory. Their leadership in clinical practice, education, and research efforts for managing symptoms related to cancer treatment can be expanded beyond the acute survival period. APNs are in a position to influence quality of life in survivors by ensuring that they are prepared with the information they and their care providers need for the rest of their lives.

Case Study

Three years ago, C.R. was diagnosed at age 52 with invasive ductal carcinoma of the left breast (T1N1M0). The tumor was 1.5 cm, estrogen receptor positive, progesterone receptor negative, and HER2 negative; and 2 out of 10 lymph nodes were positive. Surgical treatment consisted of a left breast lumpectomy, sentinel lymph node biopsy, and axillary node dissection. C.R. received chemotherapy including doxorubicin (Adriamycin®, Bedford Laboratories) and cyclophosphamide (Cytoxan®, Bristol-Myers Squibb Co.) (AC) for four cycles followed by four cycles of paclitaxel (Taxol®, Bristol-Myers Squibb Co.). Her chemotherapy was followed by external beam radiation therapy with 4,500 cGy to the left breast. C.R. was postmenopausal and had stopped hormone replacement therapy at the diagnosis of her breast cancer. At completion of her chemotherapy, she started tamoxifen (Nolvadex®, AstraZeneca Pharmaceuticals).

C.R. had no prior surgical history. Her only medication for the past year was atorvastatin (Lipitor®, Pfizer Inc.) for elevated cholesterol. She has two daughters in their early 20s. Her mother was diagnosed with breast cancer at 68 years of age and died of metastatic disease four years later. Her one sister has no history of breast cancer. She and her children's father are of Italian American descent.

In the year following her treatment, C.R. experienced "terrible" hot flashes that occurred more than 12 times per day, as well as vaginal dryness and pain during sexual intercourse. She also developed a frozen right shoulder, which caused her pain and made her unable to exercise, especially to play golf. She received physical therapy for three to four months and regained some of her mobility, although she is still unable to play golf.

C.R. gained mild relief of her hot flashes from acupuncture but continued to experience a marked decrease in her quality of life. Her gynecologist prescribed megestrol acetate (Megace®, Bristol-Myers Squibb Co.) 20 mg per day to help with her symptoms. She also received treatment for a chronic yeast infection with several courses of fluconazole (Diflucan®, Pfizer Inc.). Because of her persistent vaginal complaints, C.R. was referred to a sexual medicine specialist. She was diagnosed with atrophic vaginitis associated with tamoxifen and Megace. She started vaginal estrogen (Vagifem®, Novo Nordisk Pharmaceuticals) once daily and low-dose topical estrogen and testosterone ointment. She was counseled about the potential benefits of controlling her symptoms and the breast cancer risks of hormonal therapy.

C.R.'s mammogram and clinical breast examination one year ago were normal, and her bone densitometry dual energy x-ray absorptiometry scan showed a T score of –1.5, down from a score of –1.0 the previous year. At that time, she was instructed to take calcium and vitamin D supplements.

C.R. was married just after completing her treatment. She is unable to have vaginal intercourse because of her pain and is unable to play golf with her husband, a favorite activity they shared. She also has gained 20 pounds since her treatment and complains she is unable to lose weight despite dieting. She continues to work full time as an accountant but recently avoided a promotion because she was reluctant to make any career changes for fear of jeopardizing her tenure in the corporation and losing her health insurance.

The APN in an office of a large oncology practice sees C.R. for her biannual follow-up visit. The nurse reviews her past history and plan for today's visit.

1. According to the ASCO guidelines, what testing does C.R. need for surveillance?
   - C.R. requires mammography and clinical breast examination for surveillance.
2. What late effects of treatment is C.R. experiencing?
   - C.R. is experiencing frozen shoulder as a result of radiation; loss of bone density and atrophic vaginitis from tamoxifen; and weight gain. C.R. is at risk for

continued bone loss and osteoporosis despite calcium and vitamin D replacement. She has known hypercholesterolemia, and her weight gain and diminished exercise can lead to greater risk. Although her risks for hematologic or cardiac disease from anthracycline and radiotherapy to her left breast are small, they should be considered in overall long-term assessment.

3. C.R. is concerned about her daughters' risks. Should she be referred for genetic counseling and *BRCA* testing?
   • According to the ASCO criteria, no indication for genetic testing is present. Indications include Ashkenazi Jewish heritage; history of ovarian cancer at any age in the patient or any first- or second-degree relatives; any first-degree relative with a history of breast cancer diagnosed before age 50; two or more first- or second-degree relatives diagnosed with breast cancer at any age; personal history of or relative with diagnosis of bilateral breast cancer; and history of breast cancer in a male relative.

4. C.R. is experiencing several psychosocial sequelae of her disease and treatment. What are they, and what referrals may she benefit from?
   • As a result of her illness, C.R. has experienced relationship changes in her marriage related to painful intercourse and physical limitations that prevent usual joint activities, body image disturbance related to her weight gain, and vocational changes related to anxiety over career and health insurance loss. C.R. could benefit from a session with a social worker or therapist. She might also benefit from a nutritionist and physical therapist to gain advice on diet and activity to improve her sense of control over her physical changes.

5. What laws would protect C.R. from her fears about her employment?
   • C.R. is protected against job discrimination by the ADA and by HIPAA, which guarantees her privacy and portability of health insurance.

Key Points

• Cancer survivors are increasing in numbers, and the complexity of needs is growing as the population ages and the effects of screening, early detection, and improvements in treatment are realized.

• According to NCCS, an individual is considered to be a cancer survivor from the time of diagnosis through the balance of his or her life. Family members, friends, and caregivers also are affected by the survivorship experience and therefore are included in this definition.

• Although this definition is widely embraced, increased attention is being focused on the particular needs of those in the period following curative cancer treatment.

• Cancer and its treatment can have a profound lasting effect on quality of life as measured in the assessment of all domains: physical, psychological, social, and spiritual.

• Follow-up care for cancer survivors should incorporate surveillance for signs of a cancer recurrence; monitoring and management of long-term and late treatment effects, including second malignancies; recommendations for cancer screening; counseling about health promotion behaviors; and coordination of care across providers.

• Various models of survivorship care are developing. Shared care between the oncology specialist and the primary care provider is one model that ensures continuity during the transition to long-term follow-up care. APNs are participating in the imple-

mentation of unique clinical programs with the potential to influence care of survivors across varied settings.
- All survivors should be given a written summary of their cancer treatment and a plan for follow-up care.
- APNs are in a unique position to direct and provide care to patients with cancer beyond active treatment throughout the cancer care continuum. Applying their knowledge of cancer and its treatment, APNs can contribute by incorporating the components of survivorship care into their clinical practice and research and education efforts.
- Completion of cancer treatment is a "teachable moment" and is an opportunity to guide patients to adopt behaviors that can reduce their risks of developing comorbid conditions and other cancers.
- Expansion of research and education is key to advancing the quality of life for survivors.
- Survivors treated with less intense or tissue-damaging therapy are unlikely to experience late effects, whereas others who have received more intense or multimodality therapy have significant risk of encountering future health problems and require careful monitoring and risk assessment.

Recommended Resources for Oncology Advanced Practice Nurses

Written Resources

- For patients: National Cancer Institute *Facing Forward Series*
  - *Facing Forward: Life After Cancer Treatment*
  - *Facing Forward: Ways You Can Make a Difference in Cancer*
  - *Facing Forward: When Someone You Love Has Completed Cancer Treatment*
  - To order, visit https://cissecure.nci.nih.gov/ncipubs
- Centers for Disease Control and Prevention. (2004). *A national action plan for cancer survivorship: Advancing public health strategies.* Atlanta, GA: Author. Available at www.cdc.gov/cancer/survivorship/pdf/plan.pdf.
- Hewitt, M., Greenfield, S., & Stovall, E. (Eds.). (2006). *From cancer patient to cancer survivor: Lost in transition.* Washington, DC: National Academies Press. To order, visit www.nap.edu/catalog.php?record_id=11468.
- Reuben, S.H. (2004, May). *Living beyond cancer: Finding a new balance. President's Cancer Panel 2003–2004 annual report.* Bethesda, MD: National Cancer Institute. To view report and order additional copies, visit http://deainfo.nci.nih.gov/advisory/pcp/pcp03-04rpt/Survivorship.pdf.

Groups/Internet Resources

- American Association for Cancer Research: www.aacr.org/home/survivors--advocates.aspx
- American Cancer Society Cancer Survivors Network: www.acscsn.org
- Association of Cancer Online Resources: www.acor.org
- Cancer*Care*: www.cancercare.org
- Cancer.net survivorship information: www.cancer.net/survivorship

- Cancer Survivors Project: www.cancersurvivorsproject.org
- Fertile Hope: www.fertilehope.org
- Gilda's Club Worldwide: www.gildasclub.org
- The I'm Too Young For This! Cancer Foundation (formerly Steps for Living): http://imtooyoungforthis.org
- Intercultural Cancer Council: www.iccnetwork.org
- Lance Armstrong Foundation: www.livestrong.org
- The M.D. Anderson Cancer Center complementary/integrative medicine education resources: www.mdanderson.org/departments/CIMER
- Memorial Sloan-Kettering Cancer Center survivorship information: www.mskcc.org/mskcc/html/58022.cfm
- National Cancer Institute: www.cancer.gov/cancertopics/life-after-treatment
- National Coalition for Cancer Survivorship: www.canceradvocacy.org
- OncoLink: www.oncolink.com (survivorship care plans)
- National Lymphedema Network: www.lymphnet.org
- Ulman Cancer Fund for Young Adults: www.ulmanfund.org
- The Wellness Community®: www.thewellnesscommunity.org/support

References

American Cancer Society. (2006). *American Cancer Society guidelines for the early detection of cancer.* Retrieved January 26, 2007, from http://www.cancer.org/docroot/PED/content/PED_2_3X_ACS_Cancer_Detection_Guidelines_36.asp?sitearea=PED&viewmode=print&

Aziz, N. (2002). Long-term survivorship: Late effects. In A.M. Berger, R.K. Portenoy, & D.E. Weissman (Eds.), *Principles and practice of palliative care and supportive oncology* (2nd ed., pp. 1019–1033). Philadelphia: Lippincott Williams & Wilkins.

Aziz, N., & Rowland, J.H. (2003). Trends and advances in cancer survivorship research: Challenges and opportunity. *Seminars in Radiation Oncology, 13,* 248–266.

Barnes, P.M., Powell-Griner, E., McFann, K., & Nahin, R.L. (2004). Complementary and alternative medicine use among adults: United States, 2002. *CDC Advance Data Report, 343,* 1–19.

Bernstein, B.J., & Grasso, T. (2001). Prevalence of complementary and alternative medicine use in cancer patients. *Oncology, 15,* 1267–1272.

Bloom, J.R. (2002). Surviving and thriving? *Psycho-Oncology, 11,* 89–92.

Boon, H., Stewart, M., Kennard, M.A., Gray, R., Sawka, C., Brown, J.B., et al. (2000). Use of complementary/alternative medicine by breast cancer survivors in Ontario: Prevalence and perceptions. *Journal of Clinical Oncology, 18,* 2515–2521.

Burstein, H.J., & Winer, E.P. (2000). Primary care for survivors of breast cancer. *New England Journal of Medicine, 343,* 1086–1094.

Centers for Disease Control and Prevention. (2004). *A national action plan for cancer survivorship: Advancing public health strategies.* Atlanta, GA: Author. Retrieved September 2, 2007, from http://www.cdc.gov/cancer/survivorship/what_cdc_is_doing/action_plan.htm

Children's Oncology Group. (2006). *Long-term follow-up guidelines for survivors of childhood, adolescent, and young adult cancers* [Version 2.0]. Retrieved April 11, 2008, from http://www.survivorshipguidelines.org

Coward, D.D., & Kahn, D.L. (2004). Resolution of spiritual disequilibrium by women newly diagnosed with breast cancer [Online exclusive]. *Oncology Nursing Forum, 31,* E24–E31.

Deimling, G.T., Bowman, K.F., Sterns, S., Wagner, L.J., & Kahana, B. (2006). Cancer-related health worries and psychological distress among older adult, long-term cancer survivors. *Psycho-Oncology, 15,* 306–320.

Deimling, G.T., Kahana, B., Bowman, K.F., & Schaefer, M.L. (2002). Cancer survivorship and psychological distress in later life. *Psycho-Oncology, 11,* 479–494.

Deimling, G.T., Wagner, L.J., Bowman, K.F., Sterns, S., Kercher, K., & Kahana, B. (2006). Coping among older, long-term cancer survivors. *Psycho-Oncology, 15,* 143–159.

Demark-Wahnefried, W., Aziz, N.M., Rowland, J.H., & Pinto, B.M. (2005). Riding the crest of the teachable moment: Promoting long-term health after the diagnosis of cancer. *Journal of Clinical Oncology, 23,* 5814–5830.

Desch, C.E., Benson, A.B., Somerfield, M.R., Flynn, P.J., Krause, C., Loprinzi, C.L., et al. (2005). 2005 update of ASCO practice guideline recommendations for colorectal cancer surveillance: Guideline summary. *Journal of Clinical Oncology, 23,* 8512–8521.

Dow, K.H., Ferrell, B.R., Leigh, S., Ly, J., & Gulasekaram, P. (1996). An evaluation of the quality of life among long-term survivors of breast cancer. *Breast Cancer Research and Treatment, 39,* 261–273.

Earle, C.C. (2006). Failing to plan is planning to fail: Improving the quality of care with survivorship care plans. *Journal of Clinical Oncology, 24,* 5112–5116.

Edwards, B.K., Howe, H.L., Ries, L.A., Thun, M.J., Rosenberg, H.M., Yancik, R., et al. (2002). Annual report to the nation on the status of cancer, 1973–1999. Featuring implications of age and aging on U.S. cancer burden. *Cancer, 96,* 2762–2792.

Emens, L.A., & Davidson, N.E. (2003). The follow-up of breast cancer. *Seminars in Oncology, 30,* 338–348.

Ernst, E., & Cassileth, B.R. (1998). The prevalence of complementary/alternative medicine in cancer: A systematic review. *Cancer, 83,* 777–782.

Ernst, E., Pittler, M.H., Wider, B., & Boddy, K. (2007). Complementary/alternative medicine for supportive cancer care: Development of the evidence-base. *Supportive Care in Cancer, 15,* 565–568.

Ferrell, B.R. (1996). The quality of lives: 1,525 voices of cancer. *Oncology Nursing Forum, 23,* 907–916.

Ferrell, B.R., Dow, K.H., Leigh, S., Ly, J., & Gulasekaram, P. (1995). Quality of life in long-term cancer survivors. *Oncology Nursing Forum, 22,* 915–922.

Ferrell, B.R., Smith, S.L., Juarez, G., & Melancon, C. (2003). Meaning of illness and spirituality in ovarian cancer survivors. *Oncology Nursing Forum, 30,* 249–257.

Ferrell, B.R., Virani, R., Smith, S., & Juarez, G. (2003). The role of the oncology nurse to ensure quality care for cancer survivors: A report commissioned by the National Cancer Policy Board and Institute of Medicine [Online exclusive]. *Oncology Nursing Forum, 30,* E1–E11.

Ferrell, B.R., & Winn, R. (2006). Medical and nursing education and training opportunities to improve survivorship care. *Journal of Clinical Oncology, 24,* 5142–5148.

Ganz, P.A. (2005). A teachable moment for oncologists: Cancer survivors, 10 million strong and growing! *Journal of Clinical Oncology, 23,* 5458–5460.

Ganz, P.A. (2006). Monitoring the physical health of cancer survivors: A survivorship-focused medical history. *Journal of Clinical Oncology, 24,* 5105–5111.

Gobel, B.H., Beck, S.L., & O'Leary, C. (2006). Nursing-sensitive patient outcomes: The development of Putting Evidence Into Practice resources for nursing practice. *Clinical Journal of Oncology Nursing, 10,* 621–624.

Haylock, P.J., Mitchell, S.A., Cox, T., Temple, S.V., & Curtiss, C.P. (2007). The cancer survivor's prescription for living. *American Journal of Nursing, 107*(4), 58–70.

Hewitt, M., & Ganz, P.A. (2007). *Implementing cancer survivorship care planning* [Institute of Medicine Report]. Washington, DC: National Academies Press.

Hewitt, M., Greenfield, S., & Stovall, E. (Eds.). (2006). *From cancer patient to cancer survivor: Lost in transition.* Washington, DC: National Academies Press.

Hewitt, M., Rowland, J., & Yancik, R. (2003). Cancer survivors in the United States: Age, health, and disability. *Journal of Gerontology, 58,* 82–91.

Hoffman, B. (2005). Cancer survivors at work: A generation of progress. *CA: A Cancer Journal for Clinicians, 55,* 271–280.

Humpel, N., & Jones, S.C. (2006). Gaining insight into the what, why, and where of complementary and alternative medicine use by cancer patients and survivors. *European Journal of Cancer Care, 15,* 362–368.

Jemal, A., Siegel, R., Ward, E., Hao, Y., Xu, J., Murray, T., et al. (2008). Cancer statistics, 2008. *CA: A Cancer Journal for Clinicians, 58,* 71–96.

Kattlove, H., & Winn, R.J. (2003). Ongoing care of patients after primary treatment for their cancer. *CA: A Cancer Journal for Clinicians, 53,* 172–196.

Khatcheressian, J.L., Wolff, A.C., Smith, T.J., Grunfeld, E., Muss, H.B., Vogel, V.G., et al. (2006). American Society of Clinical Oncology 2006 update of the breast cancer follow-up and management guidelines in the adjuvant setting. *Journal of Clinical Oncology, 24,* 5091–5097.

Lance Armstrong Foundation. (2004). *Livestrong poll finds nearly half of people living with cancer feel their non-medical needs are unmet by the healthcare system.* Retrieved April 10, 2008, from http://www.livestrong .org/site/apps/nl/content2.asp?c=jvKZLbMRIsG&b=738963&ct=901209

Lawson, C., DuHamel, K., Itzkowitz, S.H., Brown, K., Lim, H., Thelemaque, L., et al. (2007). Demographic, medical, and psychosocial correlates to CAM use among survivors of colorectal cancer. *Supportive Care in Cancer, 15,* 557–564.

Lee, S.J., Schover, L.R., Partridge, A.H., Patrizio, P., Wallace, W.H., Hagerty, K., et al. (2006). American Society of Clinical Oncology recommendations on fertility preservation in cancer patients. *Journal of Clinical Oncology, 24,* 2917–2931.

Lengacher, C.A., Bennett, M.P., Kip, K.E., Keller, R., LaVance, M.S., Smith, L.S., et al. (2002). Frequency of use of complementary and alternative medicine in women with breast cancer. *Oncology Nursing Forum, 29,* 1445–1452.

Lewis, F.M. (2006). The effects of cancer survivorship on families and caregivers. *American Journal of Nursing, 106*(Suppl. 2), 20S–25S.

Matthews, A.K., Sellergren, S.A., Huo, D., List, M., & Fleming, G. (2007). Complementary and alternative medicine use among breast cancer survivors. *Journal of Alternative and Complementary Medicine, 13,* 555–562.

McBride, C.M., Emmons, K.M., & Lipkus, I.M. (2003). Understanding the potential of teachable moments: The case of smoking cessation. *Health Education Research, 18,* 156–170.

Mullan, F. (1985). Seasons of survival: Reflections of a physician with cancer. *New England Journal of Medicine, 313,* 270–273.

Nail, L. (2001). Long-term persistence of symptoms. *Seminars in Oncology Nursing, 17,* 249–254.

National Cancer Institute, Department of Cancer Control and Population Sciences, Office of Cancer Survivorship. (2007). *Estimated number of cancer survivors in the United States from 1971 to 2003.* Retrieved May 5, 2007, from http://dccps.nci.nih.gov/ocs/prevalence/index.html

National Center for Complementary and Alternative Medicine. (2007, June). *Get the facts: Cancer and CAM.* Retrieved August 1, 2007, from http://nccam.nih.gov/health/camcancer

National Coalition for Cancer Survivorship. (n.d.). Retrieved December 27, 2006, from http://www .canceradvocacy.org/about/org

National Comprehensive Cancer Network. (2007). *NCCN clinical practice guidelines in oncology: Distress management, version 1.2008.* Retrieved September 2, 2007, from http://www.nccn.org/professionals /physician_gls/PDF/distress.pdf

National Comprehensive Cancer Network. (2008). *NCCN clinical practice guidelines in oncology: Hodgkin's disease/lymphoma, version 1.2008.* Retrieved March 25, 2008, from http://www.nccn.org/professionals /physician_gls/PDF/hodgkins.pdf

Oeffinger, K.C., & McCabe, M.S. (2006). Models for delivering survivorship care. *Journal of Clinical Oncology, 24,* 5117–5124.

Reuben, S.H. (2004, May). *Living beyond cancer: Finding a new balance. President's Cancer Panel 2003–2004 annual report.* Bethesda, MD: National Cancer Institute.

Ries, L.A., Melbert, D., Krapcho, M., Mariotto, A., Miller, B.A., Feuer, E.J., et al. (Eds.). (2007). *SEER cancer statistics review, 1975–2004.* Bethesda, MD: National Cancer Institute. Retrieved June 1, 2007, from http://seer.cancer.gov/csr/1975_2004

Rowland, J., Aziz, N., Tesauro, G., & Feuer, E.J. (2001). The changing face of cancer survivorship. *Seminars in Oncology Nursing, 17,* 236–240.

Stanton, A.L. (2006). Psychosocial concerns and interventions for cancer survivors *Journal of Clinical Oncology, 24,* 5132–5137.

Tesauro, G.M., Rowland, J.H., & Lustig, C. (2002). Survivorship resources for post-treatment cancer survivors. *Cancer Practice, 10,* 277–283.

Travis, L.B., Hill, D., Dores, G.M., Gospodarowicz, M., van Leeuwen, F.E., Holowaty, E., et al. (2005). Cumulative absolute breast cancer risk for young women treated for Hodgkin lymphoma. *Journal of the National Cancer Institute, 97,* 1428–1437.

U.S. Department of Labor Employee Benefits Security Administration. (2004, December). *The Health Insurance Portability and Accountability Act (HIPAA).* Retrieved May 20, 2007, from http://www.dol .gov/ebsa/newsroom/fshipaa.html

U.S. Department of Labor Employee Benefits Security Administration. (2006, September). *An employee's guide to health benefits under COBRA: The Consolidated Omnibus Budget Reconciliation Act of 1986.* Retrieved May 20, 2007, from http://www.dol.gov/ebsa/pdf/cobraemployee.pdf

Vachon, M. (2006). Psychosocial distress and coping after cancer treatment. *American Journal of Nursing, 106*(Suppl. 2), 26S–31S.

Yabroff, K.R., Lawrence, W.F., Clauser, S., Davis, W.W., & Brown, M.L. (2004). Burden of illness in cancer survivors: Findings from a population-based national sample. *Journal of the National Cancer Institute, 96,* 1322–1330.

CHAPTER 18

Palliative Care and End-of-Life Care

Deborah A. Boyle, RN, MSN, AOCN®, FAAN, and Regina M. Fink, RN, PhD, AOCN®, FAAN

Introduction

Caring for patients at the end of life has played a significant role in nursing throughout history (Murphy-Ende, 2001). The knowledge and skills required in end-of-life nursing care is a competency required within all nursing specialties (Ferrell & Coyle, 2006a; Mason, 2002). However, with the advent of the growing sophistication of drug therapies, technologic innovations, and possibilities for life extension, the denial of death has remained a challenge in clinical practice.

Rarely is end-of-life nursing an integral component of undergraduate nursing education (Coyne et al., 2007; Ferrell & Coyle, 2006b). With the exception of oncology and gerontology graduate specialty nursing education, most post-basic curricula fail to address the dying experience as a critical entity requiring nursing expertise. Rather than perceiving death as life's rightful passage, dying has increasingly become synonymous with failure (Shubha, 2007). Hence, this discordance, particularly in the United States, is largely responsible for palliative care nursing being one of the newest nursing subspecialties (Aranda, 1998).

While the genesis of formalized oncology nursing began its evolution in the early 1970s, so did end-of-life care in the form of hospice nursing. Several key health professionals are credited with increasing consciousness about the need for end-of-life care in America. This movement was largely nurse-driven in response to distinct gaps noted in the quality of patient care at that time.

Evolution of Palliative Care

In 1963, following seven years of hospice nursing practice in London, Cicely Saunders traveled to the United States to increase her knowledge about pain control by meeting with noted American researchers. Additionally, she intended to discuss the concept of hospice with healthcare leaders interested in end-of-life care. Dr. Saunders formed a longstanding friendship and collaboration with Florence Wald, then the dean of the Yale School of Nursing, who had assisted with the development of St. Christopher's Hospice in the United Kingdom in 1967. Dame Cicely Saunders assimilated modern approaches on pain relief, holistic symptom management, and bereavement counseling into the medieval monastic tradition of rendering care to pilgrims traveling to the Holy Land (Kapp & Nelson-Becker, 2007). St. Christopher's unique integration of inpatient, academic, and a research-based environment of care ultimately became the model for the first inpatient facility in the United States, the Connecticut Hospice.

In 1966, Dr. Jeanne Quint-Benoliel published her research on professional reactions to dying patients in hospital settings (Quint-Benoliel, 1966). Utilizing observational research methodology, she described nursing and physician behaviors that limited their contact with dying patients on medical-surgical units in large teaching hospitals. Quint-Benoliel postulated that the emotional distress prompted distancing behaviors utilized by staff. These were thought to emanate from several sources.

First, personal identification with dying patients occurred when similarities in age, family construct, or other characteristics elicited awareness that the health professionals themselves could be suffering or dying. Second, feelings of impotence evolved from nurses' and physicians' perception that their interventions could not change the course of the dying trajectory. Third, in the absence of communication skills training and proficiency, not knowing what to say to the dying patient evoked a sense of communication futility. Finally, distancing oneself from the dying patient was attributed to health professionals' inability to give meaning to, or rationalize, why premature death occurred in select patients.

In 1969, psychiatrist Dr. Elisabeth Kubler-Ross wrote her book *On Death and Dying*, which delineated both patients' and healthcare professionals' coping responses to the end-of-life experience. This publication marked the closure of the first decade of the American hospice movement. It set the precedent for increasing public and professional recognition of the historical neglect of a significant cohort of the medically ill—the dying.

Currently, more than 3,000 hospice and palliative care programs exist in the United States (McCarthy, Burns, Davis, & Phillips, 2003). In 2005, more than 2.4 million Americans received hospice care, and the number of Medicare recipients enrolled in hospice had risen 50% above referral statistics from 2000 (Gazelle, 2007; Wright & Katz, 2007). However, significant variability exists within established hospice programs in terms of the scope of services provided and utilization rates, based on age, sex, geography, and diagnosis (Carlson, Morrison, Holford, & Bradley, 2007; Connor, Elwert, Spence, & Christakis, 2007; Keating, Herrinton, Zaslavsky, Liu, & Ayanian, 2006). Less than 60% of American hospitals report having some degree of palliative or end-of-life care services with available experts to provide consultation (Last Acts, 2002). This is of grave concern as more than half of Americans die in acute healthcare settings (Institute of Medicine, 2001; Teno et al., 2005). Despite the growth of the hospice and palliative care movement, and Americans' well-documented preference to die at home, only about one-quarter of dying patients spend their last days of life there (Ferrell & Coyle, 2002).

The Cancer/Dying Connection

In the 1970s, the stigma associated with cancer being a "death sentence" was reality-based. The majority of patients with cancer died from their malignancy. However, these early years of oncology nursing were characterized by significant advances in drug discovery, with medical oncology becoming recognized as a new subspecialty in 1973. Cancer nursing at that time required intense collaboration with physician colleagues regarding chemotherapy administration and toxicity management (Boyle, D.A., 2006b). Decades passed while new antineoplastic drugs came to market, technologic advances offered novel drug delivery options, monitoring capabilities grew, and radiotherapy technology advanced in scope and sophistication. Concurrently, antibiotic drug development, the discovery of growth factors, and critical care as a recognized specialty evolved. It was not until these two trajectories of therapeutic and supportive care interventions matured that the ranks of cancer survivors become equivocal to those who died (Hewitt, Greenfield, & Stovall, 2006).

In the United States, as cancer care increasingly focused efforts on cure and long-term survival, end-of-life cancer care assumed a secondary focus. However, despite the evolving focus on survivorship (especially for adults), cancer remained unable to shed its distinction as a terminal diagnosis. In her highly acclaimed book, *Illness As Metaphor,* author Susan Sontag (1978) eloquently described, "Death is now an offensively meaningless event" (p. 8). Colleagues in Europe, Canada, and Australia were able to more effectively deal with this contradictory reality in cancer care. In these countries, while a pronounced attempt to eradicate cancer prevailed, so did the awareness of the need for expert end-of-life care. Hence, much of palliative and end-of-life nursing care in the United States emanates from the experiences and proficiencies of international colleagues.

Definitions and Characteristics of Palliative Care

The National Institutes of Health (NIH) State-of-the-Science in End-of-Life Care Conference in 2004 recommended efforts to improve clarity around definitions that distinguished palliative, supportive, and hospice care. Despite this clarification, a host of misperceptions exist on the nature of palliative care and palliative nursing. The confusion concerning what constitutes palliative care may be responsible in part for delayed, late, and untimely consultations (Gazelle, 2007; Pavlish & Ceronsky, 2007; Pollard, Cairns, & Rosenthal, 1999). This is of particular importance in oncology nursing, as half of all patients using palliative and hospice services are patients with cancer (Wright & Katz, 2007).

Palliative care can be characterized by what it is not, as well as what it is (Coyle, 2006). Kuebler, Lynn, and Von Rohen (2005) described it as the following.

> Palliative care is not characterized by the explanation of a specific disease status or its therapeutic interventions, but rather a distinction in the identification and management of the symptoms associated with an underlying disease for which there is no cure. In other words, palliative care may be distinguished from curative care by using interventions that predominately aim to change or improve how the patient can live with his or her illness(es). (p. 3)

A palliative philosophy of care, by the World Health Organization (n.d.), Last Acts (2002), and the National Hospice and Palliative Care Organization, have delineated eight major definitional characteristics. These include the recognition of palliative care as (Kuebler et al., 2005)

1. Identifying death as normal and natural
2. Providing relief from pain and other distressing symptoms
3. Affirming life by the provision of palliative interventions that neither hasten nor postpone death

4. Enhancing quality of life and, ideally, positively influencing the course of illness
5. Recognizing that the dying process is profoundly individualized and occurs within the dynamics of the family
6. Enhancing quality of life and integrating physical, psychological, social, and spiritual aspects of care
7. Employing the interdisciplinary team to address multidimensional needs of dying patients and their families, including bereavement counseling (if indicated)
8. Promoting the quality of life and healthy closure for patients and families via the provision of palliative interventions and the creation of a supportive environment.

The major differences between palliative, hospice, and supportive nursing care are depicted in Figure 18-1. Palliative care is the overriding construct that characterizes care provided to people with life-threatening illness not amenable to long-term survival. Hospice and supportive care are distinct entities within the broader conceptualization of palliative care.

A distinguishing characteristic of palliative care is its high functioning interdisciplinary team. The team composition usually includes nurses, physicians, social workers, chaplains, physical therapists, occupational therapists, dietitians, pharmacists, volunteers, and advanced practice nurses (APNs) (Brant, 1998). The essence of teamwork in palliative care includes collaboration differentiated by (Zollo, 1999)
• A bond among team members that demonstrates caring for one another
• Participative problem solving, goal setting, and decision making within a structure of collegiality
• Shared knowledge and mutual trust that can exist only in a balanced work culture
• A union in which participants are interdependent rather than autonomous.

Additionally, the sophistication of teamwork that is evident within a palliative care team culminates in a healthy work environment. A concerted effort exists to establish team behavioral norms that include positive attitude, accountability, and effective com-

---

Palliative care is the science that drives the practice of end-of-life care. It is an umbrella term for the provision of interdisciplinary, active, total care of patients whose disease is not responsive to curative therapy. Control of multifocal etiologies of distress is the primary goal. Palliative care's aim is to optimize living and the achievement of the best quality of life for patients and their families. This focus predominates while death is concurrently acknowledged as a normal component of life's trajectory. Family bereavement is an integral element within the continuum of palliative care.

Oncologic derivatives of **supportive care** usually relate to pharmacologic interventions that augment the patient's response to real and/or potential adverse effects associated with the disease or its treatment. Considered under the broad rubric of palliative care, supportive care interventions precede hospice care.

Hospice is one element of palliative care often used synonymously with the term "end-of-life care." It is considered the "crown jewel" of palliative care because of its historical focus and accumulated expertise. Hospice uniquely addresses patient/family care needs when the patient is dying or near death. Consultations for hospice care frequently emanate from palliative care consultative teams and services.

Figure 18-1. Nomenclature Distinctions Relative to Late-Stage Illness and Care Requirements

---

Note. Based on information from Aranda, 1998; Berger et al., 2002; Kuebler et al., 2005; World Health Organization, 2002.

munication (Parsons, Clark, Marshall, & Cornett, 2007). All of these critical characteristics coalesce to create a work culture that fosters the provision of high-quality professional care for a family dealing with affective turmoil and anticipated loss.

Indications for Palliative Care

A template for benchmarking and planning for the provision of quality palliative care was published in 2004. A joint effort of three major stakeholders (American Academy of Hospice and Palliative Medicine, Hospice and Palliative Nurses Association, and National Hospice and Palliative Care Organization) resulted in clinical practice guidelines that detailed eight domains that are imperative for the provision of comprehensive palliative care (see Figure 18-2). These domains address specific requirements related to (1) the structure and process of care; (2) the physical domain; (3) the psychological and psychiatric domain; (4) the social domain; (5) the spiritual, religious, and existential domain; (6) the cultural domain; (7) imminently dying patients; and (8) ethics and the law. Most recently, the National Quality Forum augmented these guidelines to delineate preferred

---

Domain 1: Structure and Process
- Care starts with a comprehensive interdisciplinary assessment of patients and families.
- Care addresses both identified and expressed needs of patients and families.
- Education and training are available.
- Team is committed to quality improvement.
- Emotional impact of work on team members is addressed.
- Team has a relationship with hospice.

Domain 2: Physical
- Management of pain, other symptoms, and treatment side effects uses best practice.
- Team documents and communicates treatment alternatives, permitting patients and families to make informed choices.
- Family members are educated and supported to provide safe and appropriate comfort measures to patients.

Domain 3: Psychological and Psychiatric
- Psychological and psychiatric issues are assessed and managed based on best available evidence.
- Team employs pharmacologic, nonpharmacologic, and complementary and alternative medicine as appropriate.
- A grief and bereavement program is available to patients and families.

Domain 4: Social
- Assessment includes family structure, relationships, medical decision making, finances, sexuality, caregiver availability, and access to medications and equipment.
- Individualized comprehensive care plans lessen caregiver burden and promote well-being.

Domain 5: Spiritual, Religious, and Existential
- Care assesses and addresses spiritual concerns.
- Team recognizes and respects religious beliefs and provides religious support.
- Team makes connections with community and spiritual religious groups or individuals as desired by patients and families.

Figure 18-2. Summary of the National Consensus Project Clinical Practice Guidelines for Quality Palliative Care

---

(Continued on next page)

Domain 6: Cultural
- Team assesses and aims to meet cultural-specific needs of the patient and family.
- Team respects and accommodates range of language, dietary, habitual, and religious practices of patients and families.
- Team has access to and uses translation resources.
- Recruitment and hiring practices reflect cultural diversity and community.

Domain 7: Imminently Dying Patients
- Team recognizes the imminence of death and provides appropriate care to patients and families.
- As patients decline, team introduces hospice referral option.
- Team educates family members on the signs and symptoms of approaching death in a developmentally, age, and culturally appropriate manner.

Domain 8: Ethics and Law
- Patients' goals, preferences, and choices are respected and form the basis for the plan of care.
- Team is knowledgeable about relevant federal and state statutes and regulations.

Figure 18-2. Summary of the National Consensus Project Clinical Practice Guidelines for Quality Palliative Care (Continued)

Note. Based on information from National Consensus Project for Quality Palliative Care, 2004.

practices to guide quality improvement efforts in hospice and palliative care (Ferrell et al., 2007). For the purposes of this chapter, five of these domains will be addressed.

Of important note is that these domains cannot be considered in isolation of each other, as considerable overlap exists between them. For example, issues within the social domain interface significantly with those in the realm of culture. Psychological concerns often prevail when inadequate management of physical symptoms remains problematic. This also attests to the prominence of the contagion effect associated with unrelieved symptom distress. The presence of pain, nausea, delirium, or other distressing symptoms may affect family caregivers' perceptions of poor quality of life near death or of patients having "suffered" during their last days or weeks of life (Ferrell, 1996; O'Mara, 2007; Wilson et al., 2007). Excellent evidence-based literature is available in the form of journal articles and chapters on end-of-life symptom management (Bernard & Bruera, 2000; Economou, 2006; Fink & Gates, 2006; Kedziera & Coyle, 2006; King, 2006; Knight, Espinosa, & Bruera, 2006; Kuebler, Heidrich, Vena, & English, 2006; Von Roenn & Paice, 2005; Watson, 2006; Wood, Shega, Lynch, & Von Roenn, 2007).

Physical Domain

Although the alleviation of distress in palliative care requires the same principles of symptom assessment as in other phases of the illness trajectory, symptom presentation and management in palliative care are characterized by the following unique distinctions.
- Symptoms usually evolve in clusters and rarely are isolated; their characteristics may change quickly (i.e., intensity, pattern), thus making reevaluation an ongoing necessity to optimize intervention planning.
- Sources of symptom distress are often multiple and may be related to polypharmacy or to patients' deteriorating health status (i.e., directly related to disease progression or indirectly from metabolic sequelae of advancing disease).
- Multisystem decline correlated with advanced disease complicates symptom recognition and management.

- Altered pharmacokinetics may affect the absorption, metabolism, distribution, and excretion of drugs used to relieve symptom distress.
- Prevalence of obstructive symptoms related to treatment (e.g., ileus) and extensive tumor burden (e.g., mass effects on lymphatics causing edema, blockage in the gastrointestinal system) may require that alternate routes of drug delivery be used.
- Family views regarding symptom control at the end of life may confound the choice, scheduling, and delivery of pharmacologic interventions, thereby creating barriers to optimum symptom relief.

These facets of palliative care symptom management create a complex decision-making paradigm (Gapstur, 2007).

The majority of patients treated for cancer are older than age 65 (Institute of Medicine, 2007). Thus, the issue of comorbidity may create an additional domain complicating assessment. The coexistence of symptoms often emanate from numerous etiologies (Fago, 2000). Consideration of the underlying disease state (i.e., cancer, presence of concurrent chronic illnesses), antineoplastic treatment(s), metabolic compromise, and untoward effects from polypharmacy (to manage the malignancy and comorbidities) may all interface to promote new or progressive symptom distress. Minimal information exists on drug interactions in palliative care that result from the use of prescription, over-the-counter, and oral complementary products to treat the malignancy and its clinical sequelae (Regnard & Hunter, 2005).

Evolving evidence about symptom clusters has significant relevance to palliative nursing (Barsevick, 2007; Dodd, Miaskowski, & Lee, 2004). *Symptom clusters* refers to three or more symptoms that have unique relationships with each other. The symptoms are related and occur together but are relatively independent of one another and may not share the same etiology. Identification of symptom clusters can assist with the diagnosis of symptom distress, influence the choice of drug therapy, reveal underlying pathology, and enhance syndrome recognition in palliative care (Kim, McGuire, Tulman, & Barsevick, 2005). Again, scrutiny of drug-related etiologies of symptom distress and potential adverse drug effects require vigilant assessment.

Limited research on symptom clusters exists both in cancer care and palliative care. Four symptom clusters are of particular relevance in palliative nursing. They include (Esper & Heidrich, 2005)

- Pain, constipation, and confusion
- Anxiety, agitation, and delirium
- Nausea, anorexia, and dehydration
- Cough, breathlessness, and fatigue.

These clusters require numerous assessment approaches because of their complexity (LaCasse & Beck, 2007).

Although knowledge of chemotherapy-related drug interactions has escalated, palliation-related adversity has received less attention (Bernard & Bruera, 2000). Within palliative care, adverse drug effects may diminish cognition, which in turn may influence functional status (Boyle, Abernathy, Baker, & Wall, 1998). A focus on ameliorating one priority symptom may induce a new symptom (e.g., the use of opioids for pain relief may cause acute confusion). Because of the prominence of symptom distress that evolves from disease and drug therapies (such as altered cognition, changes in sleep/wake patterns, weakness, and compromised functional status), patient safety is a major concern in end-of-life care. In particular, falls (resulting in fractures and bleeding) and medication errors (from overconsumption of medications because of memory impairment) are of critical importance in palliative care.

Drug-related adversity may stem from drug-drug, drug-disease, drug-complementary approach intervention, or drug-nutrition interactions (Bernard & Bruera, 2000). Untoward effects may stem from altered pharmacokinetics (i.e., absorption, distribution, excretion, and metabolism) (Mihelic, 2005). These pharmacokinetic alterations frequently are associated with advanced age and/or physiologic changes resulting from advanced-stage cancer. In particular, drugs that are metabolized by hepatic isoenzymes (i.e., opioids) will have delayed clearance when extensive liver metastases impair liver function. Table 18-1 summarizes potential drug interactions specific to common analgesics used in palliative care settings.

Table 18-1. Drug Interactions of Analgesics

Analgesic	Interactive Drug Class	Result
Fentanyl	Macrolides, cimetidine	Inhibition of clearance of antibiotics, cimetidine, elevated fentanyl level
Methadone	Methadone	Autoinduction, loss of effects
	Nifedipine	Inhibition of clearance of nifedipine
	Fluvoxamine	Inhibition of methadone clearance
Codeine	Theoretical for agents inhibiting CYP 2D6	Failure to activate codeine, loss of effect, large doses needed
Oxycodone	In vitro failure to convert to active agent with inhibitors of CYP 2D6	Loss of drug effect, large doses needed
Meperidine	Monoamine oxidase inhibitors	Serotonin syndrome
Morphine	Benzodiazepines, antidepressants	Antagonizes analgesic effects, increases analgesic effects

Note. Based on information from Bernard & Bruera, 2000.

Psychological and Psychiatric Domain

Evaluation of the psychological needs of patients at the end of life has emanated predominantly from quality-of-life inventories (Cohen & Mount, 1992; Cohen, Mount, Tomas, & Mount, 1996; Greisinger, Lorimor, Aday, Winn, & Baile, 1997; Teno, Byock, & Field, 1999). Early investigations focused primarily on physical distress. Most recently, greater interest has evolved in identifying parameters of psychosocial support and interventions that enhance coping with advanced disease (Chochinov, Hack, McClement, Harlos, & Kristjanson, 2002; Cohen & Mount, 2000).

In a sample of nearly 1,500 participants, which included equal representation of patients with advanced illness, families of patients with advanced illness, physicians, and other care providers, a comparison of factors considered to be important at the end of life was evaluated (Steinhauser, Christakis, et al., 2000). All four groups strongly agreed that managing pain and other symptoms, preparing for death, achieving a sense of completion, making personal decisions about treatment preferences, and being treated as a "whole person" were important. Items ranked high by patients, but not physicians, included being mentally aware, having funeral arrangements planned, not being a burden, helping others, and coming to peace with God. These priorities suggest that giving attention to cognitive clarity, diminishing burden on family members after death, maintaining functional independence, giving to others, and having a spiritual connection were prominent parameters of patients' conception of a "good death."

These researchers then interviewed focus groups of patients to further define these priorities (Steinhauser, Clipp, et al., 2000). Findings from these focus groups provided more detail about preferred states, such as

- Mental clarity fostered optimum decision making
- End-of-life planning that also entailed knowing what to expect in terms of disease progression
- Having a sense of completion, which had religious components but also involved undertaking a life review, resolving conflicts, spending time with family and friends, and having the chance to say good-bye
- Contributing to others could be actualized in many forms, such as offering the gift of time or knowledge or recognizing the impact of key personal relationships on the emotional growth and maturation of friends and family members.

These findings correlated with other investigations of patient perceptions of dying well. Cohen and Leis (2002) delineated the domains of relevance to quality of life in patients as maintaining existential well-being, feeling secure, having continuity of care, being able to deal with uncertainty, and growing close through crisis as themes that were indicative of living well while dying. Self-determination and autonomy, as manifestations of an active information-seeking style, also may foster continued choice, critical to dying well from cancer (Zanchetta & Moura, 2006).

Another theme discussed in the literature related to patient coping during advanced stages of illness has been the nature and quality of professional communication strategies in relaying bad news (Baile & Beale, 2001; Friedrichsen, Strang, & Carlsson, 2001; Fujimori et al., 2007; Hofmann et al., 1997; Rousseau, 2001; Royak-Schaler et al., 2006; Schapira, 2005). Although this historically has been the purview of oncologists, APNs are now shouldering more of this responsibility in practice. Additionally, APNs often are requested to support or console patients and families following the delivery of bad news. They also may need to mentor staff in the provision of emotional support during these times of crisis. Some distinct themes emerge from the existing literature concerning the provision of emotional support and counsel.

The first theme is the recognition that communication is a therapeutic tool. Communication can be used to clarify goals and expectations, relay information, ensure that patients' needs are being met, enhance relationships, and facilitate coping. Second, a lack of communication skill can diminish patients' disclosure, increase patient and family anxiety, thwart future exchanges, deter realistic hope, decrease satisfaction with care, and negate trust (Schapira, 2005; Sheldon, 2005). Rousseau (2001) noted that trust, communication, and truthfulness are potent deterrents to patients' sense of overwhelming fear of dying. When these features are evident in the professional-patient relationship, patients do not feel as abandoned, dependent, or susceptible. Rousseau described the following.

> Illness shrouds a patient in vulnerability, isolation and loneliness, and unless one cares for and exhibits empathy, it will be impossible to understand the patient's needs and concerns, and, consequently, to provide quality, compassionate medical care. (p. 225)

Although no guidelines exist for disclosing bad news, increasing recognition exists that individual patient preferences need to be determined prior to communication taking place. This involves ascertaining patients' preferences for information-giving early in their care. Questions that can elicit patients' communication preferences include the following.

- How much do you want to know about your cancer?
- Who are you most concerned about in your family?
- If I had to inform you of bad news, how should I do it?
- How do you usually cope when things are not going well in your life?
- Are there specific beliefs or requests related to your culture or religion that I should know about if we cannot successfully manage your cancer?

No set approach exists that works best with all patients; however, research has offered guidance as to what patients state are preferred versus contraindicated exchanges in the context of giving bad news. Figure 18-3 lists preferred components of information-giving related to the method of disclosure, the provision of emotional support, and augmentation of explanations with additional information. Evolving evidence shows that the amount of information required by both patients and family members changes as the patients' illness progresses. Patients' preferences may focus on different themes or diminish overall as their stage of illness worsens. Families, on the other hand, may need more information to prepare them for the patient's anticipated death (Parker et al., 2007).

Social Domain

The greatest degree of empiric evidence addressing coping with advanced illness and dying has concentrated on family members. The body of research on family members in palliative care primarily has targeted two themes: caregiving strain during advanced illness and family perceptions of the quality of professional interventions at the end of life.

Method of Disclosure
1. Encouraging questions
2. Breaking bad news honestly
3. Relaying the individual nature of each case
4. Explaining the progression and/or status of disease
5. Breaking bad news in a way that is easy to understand

Provision of Emotional Support
1. Saying, "Let's fight this together"
2. Saying words that soothe the patients' feelings
3. Telling in a way that is empathetic, with hope
4. Talking gently with words of realistic encouragement
5. Acknowledging the varied information needs of patients and families

Provision of Additional Information
1. Telling the proposed treatment plan
2. Explaining the process of a second opinion
3. Telling about all treatment options available
4. Telling about the latest treatment, including the risks and side effects

---

Figure 18-3. Communication Preferences in the Disclosure of Bad News

Note. Based on information from Fujimori et al., 2007; Parker et al., 2007.

Palliative care recognizes the family as the unit of care. Families generally are expected to render most of the "hands-on" care and assume the bulk of caregiving responsibility, often with minimal external professional or volunteer support in the home (Emanuel et al., 1999; Scherbring, 2002; Schumacher, Stewart, Archbold, Dodd, & Dibble, 2000). Hence, family caregiver vulnerability has become a well-acknowledged corollary of end-of-life care (Davies, 2006; Pasacreta & McCorkle, 2000).

Older women frequently are the predominant family caregivers of the terminally ill in the United States. They may experience their own symptom distress in the form of weight loss, alterations in sleep and nutrition, depression, fatigue, and memory, attention, and concentration changes. Additionally, they may have their own healthcare needs that are neglected as they focus attention on the family member with advanced cancer. Delayed new diagnoses or exacerbations of chronic illnesses may result because of the minimal time for personal interests and self-care (Aranda & Hayman-White, 2001; Cameron, Franche, Cheung, & Stewart, 2002; Grbich, Parker, & Maddocks, 2001; Kotkamp-Mothes, Slawinsky, Hindermann, & Strauss, 2005; Kristjanson, 1999; Sharpe, Butow, Smith, McConnell, & Clarke, 2005). Family members often are responsible for completing household tasks, working outside the home, being the information conduit for family and friends, providing transportation, and intervening with multiple healthcare providers (Aranda & Peerson, 2001; Bakas, Lewis, & Parsons, 2001; Hayman et al., 2001; Houldin, 2007). These demands often pose considerable challenges in an existing stress-laden situation.

The other broad family-centered research target in palliative care has focused on family caregivers' functioning as proxies in communication distress for incapacitated patients and in evaluation of the quality of end-of-life care following the death of a loved one (Lobchuk, McClement, Daeninck, Shay, & Elands, 2007; McPherson, Wilson, Lobchuk, & Brajtman, 2008). Critics argue that these studies are inherently flawed and require cautious interpretation (Hinton, 2001). Also, the studies published to date rarely have isolated families of patients with cancer in their analyses (Baker et al., 2000; Connor, Teno, Spence, & Smith, 2005; Curtis et al., 2002; Patrick, Engelberg, & Curtis, 2001; Teno et al., 2004, 2005; Tolle, Tilden, Rosenfeld, & Hickman, 2000). It remains unknown whether these findings are generalizable to patients with cancer and their families.

Lastly, a paucity of research in the United States has specifically addressed strategies to support families during palliative care. A pervasive assumption exists that families can quickly assume the multiple responsibilities of caregiving that generally are undertaken in isolation in the home setting. Nurse researcher Dr. Linda Kristjanson, the historic opinion leader and major investigator on this topic, has recommended financial support be given for further investigation to identify a sampling of intervention options for families that match individual need and circumstance (Kristjanson, Leis, Koop, Carriere, & Mueller, 1997; Kristjanson, Sloan, Dudgeon, & Adaskin, 1996; Leis, Kristjanson, Koop, & Laizner, 1997). Additionally, research that integrates perceptions of family quality of functioning and more specific indices of caregiver symptom distress would enhance the evaluation of end-of-life care that requires improvement and innovation (Hickman, Tilden, & Tolle, 2001). Instruments to evaluate the efficacy of formalized interventions that assist families with care delivery are necessary to ensure adequacy of the professional care that is provided (Bachner, O'Rourke, & Carmel, 2007; Eriksson, 2001; Kristjanson, 1993). Additional evaluation of the impact of varying modes, timing, and length of family bereavement care also warrants further investigation (Milberg, Olsson, Jakobsson, Olsson, & Friedrichsen, 2008).

Deterrents to participation in palliative care research are numerous and also require attention in research goal setting and design. Some of these considerations include (Fineberg et al., 2007; Mularski et al., 2007; Whalen et al., 2007)

- Ethical dilemmas, especially when experimental research designs may limit the use of even marginally effective interventions to ameliorate symptom distress
- Intrusiveness concerns, which involve usurping family time with the patient for purposes of research clarification, obtaining consent, and data collection
- Integration of cultural aspects of the dying experience
- Physically taxing patients who are already impaired by symptom distress and advanced cancer because of the increased demands for reading, teaching, and surveying
- Recommended and appropriate use of new technologies for data collection
- Likelihood of development of cognitive changes because of the compromising effects of palliative polypharmacy
- Lack of consensus on primary end points in determination of research outcomes.

These issues and the use of family proxies for evaluating numerous indices of end-of-life care require further investigation (Addington-Hall & McCarthy, 2001). On a positive note, intervention studies to manage caregiver strain and to evaluate the quality of services rendered to families have been topics targeted for research funding nationally and abroad (Given, Given, & Kozachik, 2001).

Spiritual, Religious, Existential, and Cultural Domains

Although generally acknowledged as important components of palliative care, little formal education about specific implications of spirituality, religious, or existential preferences and cultural norms is integrated into specialty oncology nursing education (Boyle, Sheridan, McClary, & White, 2002). In palliative care, this is of particular concern, as the process and act of dying—attitudes, behaviors, religious rituals, role of the family—are very culturally prescribed (Boyle, D.M., 1998).

Spirituality, religious beliefs, and one's cultural connection are intertwined yet interdependent phenomena. Negating any of these aspects of palliative care can deter an optimum dying experience. Braun, Pietsch, and Blanchette (2000) described: "What is seen of death is the finality of the physical body. But what is believed about the meaning of death, how it should be faced, and what happens after physical death varies by culture and its associated religion" (p. 1).

As communication technologies shrink geographical distance and historical boundaries that separated cultures disappear, the world will increasingly become more heterogeneous. In the United States, enhanced cultural awareness and sensitivity have been perceived as being most significant in large cities. Yet, even small population groups are experiencing significant shifts in their cultural mosaic.

Recent immigrants bring with them beliefs about self-care, communication, nutrition, the role of family, birthing, and dying. Even without knowing specific characteristics of cultures, oncology nurses can admit to a lack of knowledge and request help in understanding expectations for reporting and managing symptoms, the role the family will play in decision making and support, and how they should address the topic of advanced disease. Charting the results of this assessment will help professional colleagues to customize their communication and intervention planning, similar to how documentation of a pain assessment would be communicated for consistency and information sharing. Kemp (2005) suggested asking the following questions to elicit culturally prescribed meanings for alterations in a patient's health.

- What do you fear most about this illness?
- What do you think caused this to happen?
- What do you expect this treatment to do for you?
- What type of treatment do you think you should receive?
- How should your family be included in decisions and care?
- How severe is this sickness? How long do you expect to live?

Additional resources on cultural and religious aspects of cancer care are available for further reference (Boyle, D.A., 2003, 2006a).

Closely tied to culture are spiritual and religious beliefs. As with dying and sexuality, spirituality may be a difficult subject to broach. However, assessment of religious and spiritual preferences should occur, along with assessment of other aspects of the patients' profile (Halstead & Nilsson, 2006; Hermann, 2006). Asking patients about how these beliefs help in times of crisis characterizes the professional caregiver as someone open to hearing patients' stories, particularly as they attempt to assimilate a life-limiting diagnosis into their current world.

Ethical Domain

APNs' involvement in ethical dilemmas in cancer care will increase in coming years. As health care evolves into a more technologically dependent culture, characterized by dwindling fiscal resources to care for the elder majority, the humanistic view of patient and family decision making and adaptation will escalate in importance. The role of advocate will become a more formal subrole for nurses with advanced degrees.

Major areas of ethical expertise pertain to communication, shared goals between healthcare providers and patients and families, resuscitation decisions, withholding or withdrawal of treatment, the use of fluids and nutrition, definition of futility of care, and the assessment and management of symptom distress (Kinlaw, 2005). In the absence of open communication, moral distress, as studied by Elpern, Covert, and Kleinpell (2005) in nurses working in the intensive care unit, can ensue as a result of situations in which the ethically appropriate course of action is known but cannot be taken (Cohen & Erickson, 2006; Vachon, 2006).

APNs will be called on to clarify components of advance directives and surrogate decision making for patients and families (Nelson-Marten & Braaten, 2008). Interpretation of ethical principles may be needed for bedside nursing staff and interdisciplinary colleagues. Because of a variety of societal and healthcare changes, the prediction of a significantly increased role for APNs with concurrent ethics expertise is imperative. The future will be compounded by a societal duty to die as well as a right to die, as dwindling economic and social resources will preclude efforts to extend life regardless of prognosis estimates.

Standards of Hospice and Palliative Nursing Care

The most recent version of the *Scope and Standards of Hospice and Palliative Nursing* provides a comprehensive template of practice guidelines to direct specialty nursing care at the end of life (Hospice and Palliative Nurses Association & American Nurses Association, 2007). Both basic and advanced criteria are delineated within each section, along with measurement criteria. The roles of the APN in hospice and palliative care include
- Expert clinician
- Leader and facilitator of interdisciplinary teams

- Educator
- Researcher
- Consultant
- Collaborator
- Advocate
- Case manager
- Administrator.

The guidelines are divided into standards of practice (i.e., assessment, diagnosis, outcomes identification, planning, implementation, and evaluation) and standards of professional performance (i.e., quality of practice, education, evaluation of professional practice, collegiality, collaboration, ethics, research, resource utilization, and leadership). This document provides an excellent resource for benchmarking both individual and group attainment of competencies to ensure the highest level of hospice and palliative nursing care.

Patient and Family Education

Patient and family education during the trajectory of end-of-life care requires integration of several key concepts. First, clinicians must realize and address the overwhelming nature of information transmitted to patients and families. Repetition, reiteration in multiple education formats, and ongoing clarification always are required. Patients and families must understand and integrate the following categories of information into daily function.
- Medications: dosing, scheduling, titration recommendations, and assessment of response and side effects
- Physical activity: assistance with turning, out-of-bed mobilization, rest suggestions associated with the intensity of physical activity, and comfort positioning
- Nutrition: ideas for compensating for diminished appetite and compensating for taste changes and other symptoms that interfere with usual nutritional intake
- Socialization: when to have visitors, plan events, travel, and schedule appointments.

These are only some of the daily requirements for integration of information into the patients' and family members' daily experience. One attempt at explanation, reiteration of rationale, or outline of recommendations will not be enough for patients and family members to successfully comprehend what they heard. Patient and family education always needs to be repetitive and continually assessed for its understanding. Anxiety, symptom distress, cognitive changes, fatigue, and numerous other factors combine to deter optimum reception of education messages delivered by health professionals. Additionally, various mediums for information translation should be considered. Written, audio, visual, or interactive formats should never replace individual instruction. Rather, they should augment and reinforce verbal exchange. APNs should pay special attention to the development of new materials that integrate visual and audio impairments that correlate with advanced age.

Clinicians need to determine the amount of information patients and families require for optimal coping. Often these responses differ. Patients may request only limited information, whereas caregivers may need more in-depth explanation. Because each person is a vital part of the end-of-life supportive care focus, everyone's unique requirements must be individually addressed.

Lastly, a paucity of research has targeted education and support interventions that are effective with select groups of patients during palliative care. What is most efficacious is to offer a menu of options that the individual family members and patients can choose from. What is most important to remember is that teaching will not be retained, using multiple methods of information delivery works best, and the foci of teaching may change abruptly based on the evolving nature of a patient's progressive malignancy.

Implications for Oncology Advanced Practice Nurses

Oncology APNs have numerous possibilities to enhance the care of patients at the end of life. Two role options are education-focused and include role-modeling behaviors to enhance learning and the provision of formal education for colleagues. First is to role-model knowledge, behaviors, and skills that demonstrate proficiency in end-of-life care. As learning by example and emulating high-quality nursing care is increasingly viewed as highly instructive and meaningful in long-term skill acquisition, this learning opportunity should not be minimized. Role modeling that enhances skill building and the provision of formal education lay the foundation for additional opportunities to advance highly specialized and complex palliative care. These options for specialty enhancement include

- Observing the APN modeling (as a method of teaching) interview, assessment, and intervention strategies to counter popular beliefs about the lengthy and extensive nature of symptom determination and needs for emotional support (Boyle, D.A., in press-a)
- Demonstrating critical thinking by the APN, particularly in the realm of symptom assessment and management, which should integrate knowledge about polypharmacy, altered pharmacokinetics, and comorbid influences on symptom presentation (Boyle, D.A., in press-b)
- Operationalizing the translation of knowledge about symptom management approaches and opportunities from other specialties, such as reminiscence therapy from gerontologic nursing (Boyle, D.M., 2003)
- Identifying measures to counter the crisis of transition specific to palliative care as patients and families encounter new sets of professional caregivers throughout their illness trajectory (Boyle, D.A., 2002; Jenko, Gonzalez, & Seymour, 2007; Larkin, De Casterle, & Schotsmans, 2007; Lohfeld, Brazil, & Willison, 2007)
- Promoting dual certification in hospice and palliative care nursing along with oncology nursing (Esper, Lockhart, & Miller-Murphy, 2002)
- Integrating advocacy skills in individual cases and also on larger social policy scales as identified in the Oncology Nursing Society and Association of Oncology Social Work (2007) position on end-of-life care
- Educating staff nurses and colleagues about the presentation and treatment of palliative emergencies (i.e., hemorrhage, spinal cord compression, seizures, hypercalcemia, syndrome of inappropriate antidiuretic hormone secretion, superior vena cava syndrome, and pathologic bone fracture) (Heidrich & McKinnon, 2002)
- Addressing the nature and management of compassion fatigue in nurses (Aycock & Boyle, in press; Boyle, D.A., 2000, 2006b; Wilkes, 1999).

Second is the provision of formal education about the needs of dying patients and their families (Caton & Klemm, 2006; Dunn, Otten, & Stephens, 2005; Gale & Brooks, 2006). This education should be a mandate, not an option, in both undergraduate and graduate education (Coyne et al., 2007). Courses should integrate the attitudes and feelings about dying patients that could limit optimum interaction with this vulnerable cohort of patients across a variety of settings (Dunn et al.).

The American Association of Colleges of Nursing and researchers from the City of Hope National Medical Center joined forces to develop the End-of-Life Nursing Education Consortium (ELNEC) in February 2000 (Coyne et al., 2007; "ELNEC Core Curriculum," n.d.). The consortium's work, supported by the Robert Wood Johnson Foundation, included establishment of a curriculum containing nine modules that address critical aspects of end-of-life care: (1) nursing care at the end of life, (2) pain management, (3) symptom management, (4) ethical and legal issues, (5) cultural considerations, (6) communication, (7) grief, loss, and bereavement, (8) achievement of quality care at the end of life, and (9) preparation for and care at the time of death. The ELNEC core curriculum was developed to prepare qualified nurse educators to provide end-of-life education to nursing students and practicing nurses and to provide resources to facilitate that instruction. Additionally, the ELNEC curriculum provides a template for APNs' provision of quality end-of-life care. More information about the curriculum components is available at www.aacn.nche.edu/elnec/curriculum.htm.

Enhancing skill development in communication proficiency also must be integrated into formal education (Sheldon, 2005). In the absence of an existing provision to augment this competency, oncology APNs should be the lobbyists to change this paradigm. To assist with the integration of communication skills, the Joint Commission on Accreditation of Healthcare Organizations (JCAHO) mandates are available. The two new JCAHO standards in the 2004 requirements for accreditation include the following.

- To the extent possible, as appropriate to the patient's and family's needs and the hospital's services, interventions address patient and family comfort, dignity, and psychological, emotional, and spiritual needs, as appropriate, about death and grief.
- Staff are educated about the unique needs of dying patients and their families and caregivers.

Last, but certainly not least, is the benefit of APNs' counsel in quantifying the impact of palliative care. Both individual patient and program efficacy require attention (Kutner, 2008). Because much of palliative care is nurse-driven, identifying positive outcomes of such care augments the quantification of expert nursing intervention. Figure 18-4 lists a summary of quality and success factors that could be used to evaluate palliative care programs.

Future Directions

Projected changes in health and cancer care will have a significant impact on palliative services available to patients and families in the future. General issues of significance include the aging of America and the dyad of escalating technology and dwindling financial resources (Gomez, 2003; Meropol & Schulman, 2007). Cancer-specific considerations include increasing expectations on lay family members for providing care, larger patient caseloads for oncology professionals, and the need to expand the range of palliative services throughout acute care settings.

The growing number of older Americans will have a significant impact on health care and the delivery of palliative specialty services (Knickman & Snell, 2002). In 2010, the first cohort of "baby boomers" (Americans born between 1947 and 1963) will reach age 65 (Institute of Medicine, 2007). This will signal the beginning of one of the most critical epidemiologic trends to affect health care in decades (Kinsella, 2005). As age is correlated with dwindling health and limited life expectancy, increasing needs for end-of-life nursing care will prevail.

- End-of-life discussions occurred earlier, were documented
- Do-not-resuscitate orders charted prior to 48 hours before death
- Actualization of preferred place of death
- Shorter length of stay in critical care
- Overall reduction in length of stay
- Reduced number of inpatient transfers
- Decreased hospital readmissions
- Avoidance of unnecessary tests and procedures
- Cost savings
- Increased mobilization of available resources
- Lower levels of distress reported by patient
- Plan to treat emergent pain
- Use of adjuvant therapies to manage symptom distress
- Cognitive clarity
- Mood stability or improvement
- Quality of life reported by patient
- Spiritual well-being
- Perception of quality communication with team
- Responsiveness to emotional needs
- Degree of effective coordination and collaboration
- Accessibility and timeliness of interventions
- Family satisfaction with care
- Minimized primary caregiver depression
- Overall caregiver health
- Reduced sense of family isolation

Figure 18-4. Potential Outcome Measures of Effective Palliative Care

Note. Based on information from Dy et al., 2008; Lorenz et al., 2007; Rice & Betcher, 2007; Zimmermann et al., 2008.

Older adults in the future will have distinctly different defining characteristics than the current cohort of older adults (Vladeck, 2005). They will reside outside of urban areas, be predominantly more isolated from their adult children, and expect and demand collaboration and partnerships rather than be passive recipients of decisions dictated by healthcare providers. They will expect communication proficiency and sensitivity as life choices are pondered and also will request more holistic interventions that will offer them some control over their impaired health.

As previously mentioned, another consideration that will affect palliative nursing is the dyad of escalating technology and dwindling financial resources. A dichotomy will prevail in which payment for health care will influence the provision of universal health care idealized for all Americans. These projections will result from sophisticated data mining derived from historical patient samples having numerous risk factors and exposure to varied therapy modalities. Computerized programming will dictate the likelihood of survival and hence will influence decision making. This then removes the more subjective element of decision making, which is particularly relevant to end-of-life care planning. Yet, ethical dilemmas will predominate.

Ethical quandaries will require more proficient communication and interpersonal skills of health professionals around end-of-life care. Both the computerization of end-of-life projections and personal characteristics of the aged baby boomer will require physicians and APNs to have greater sophistication in end-of-life nursing and medical care. Of positive note is the opportunity for computerized monitoring of patients in the home setting (Cheek, Nikpour, & Nowlin, 2005; Viney, Batcheller, Houston, & Belcik,

2006). This, along with a broad initiative to improve the care of the dying within acute care, will optimally increase nursing proficiency in populations either remote in location or cared for within traditional settings (Billings et al., 2006; Curtis & Rubenfeld, 2005; Gale & Brooks, 2006; Meyer, Ritholz, Burns, & Truog, 2006; Mosenthal & Murphy, 2006; Puntillo & Stannard, 2006).

Finally, the individuals who will become increasingly vulnerable to competing and exaggerated demands of their time and involvement will be the end-of-life lay caregivers. Unless a major national initiative endorsing both escalated provider and financial home-based support evolves in the near future, expectations for families rendering palliative care will intensify. The ratio of young to old will dramatically change.

The current older minority (12% of Americans who consume the majority of healthcare services) have a significant cohort of adult baby boomers' children to assist with their care (Vladeck, 2005). However, the baby boomers have had fewer offspring than their parents. Hence, fewer resources will be available to provide uncompensated nursing care in the home for these future older adults. The increased mobility of Americans (both adult children and older adults) has been such that immediate family members may not be physically present or available to render care. This reversal of the old-to-young ratio will significantly burden families in their efforts to provide support to ill and infirmed family members. Therefore, the responsibility of the bulk of end-of-life care, particularly in the home, will be on the shoulders of lay caregivers, having numerous expectations to render informal care on an increasing number of older family members.

Of particular importance is the recognition of the need for palliative radiation therapy programs (Fine, 2002; Konski, Feigenberg, & Chow, 2005; McCloskey, Tao, Rose, Fink, & Amadeo, 2007). Because a significant percentage of patients receiving radiation therapy do so for the control of symptoms associated with advanced disease, the creation of a more formal service to meet the palliative needs of patients and families in radiation oncology is indicated (Konski et al.). APNs in radiation oncology can improve continuity of care by acting as an expert clinician, case manager, and educator to clarify expectations during and following a palliative course of radiation therapy.

Conclusion

This chapter began with commentary concerning the critical nursing role in palliative care, and it is fitting that it ends with comparable discourse. Noted nursing leader Florence Henderson identified that "hospice nursing is the essence of nursing" (Henderson, 1961, p. 42). In the foreword to Ferrell and Coyle's (2006b) comprehensive text on palliative nursing, Dame Cicely Saunders (2006) also eloquently described:

> Palliative care stems from the recognition of the potential at the end
> of life for discovering and for giving, a recognition that an important
> dimension of being human is the lasting dignity and growth that can
> continue through weakness and loss. No member of the interdisciplin-
> ary team is more central to making these discoveries possible than the
> nurse. (p. v)

Palliative nursing will grow in demand based solely on the evolving demographics of American society. However, the quality of palliative nursing will be enhanced only with the assimilation of evidence-based end-of-life care and formal nursing research that augments best practices. Although unique considerations in undertaking research in palliative care must be considered, this does not preclude investigative necessity.

Documentation of the efficacy of nursing interventions in reducing patient symptom distress, choice of effective holistic intervention, the creation of family-directed models for education and support, and the reduction of decisional conflict all require empiric study. A major opportunity exists to describe and evaluate care provided by APNs with this special patient population.

The choreography of patient care is at the foundation of nursing competency. Wilkes (1998) noted the fine line between therapeutic effectiveness of palliative nursing care and overcompensating based on unaddressed personal issues. She noted that nurses need to provide symptom control but not overmedication. Further parallels include the need to offer hope but not suggest the extraordinary; to try to foster acceptance but not hasten the dying trajectory; to assist with the completion of unfinished business but not force connectedness; and finally to be there for families but not impose on family privacy.

The complex and evolving nature of patient and family needs in palliative care provides a unique platform for APNs to document outcomes of care directed by nurses with advanced education and skills in prevention, early recognition, and management of sequelae that predominate when curative treatment is not an option. Additionally, the continuity of care that they can provide could minimize the relational discontinuity of professional care providers that frequently occurs and adds to patient and family uncertainty (Lohfeld et al., 2007).

Palliative nursing care experts also have extensive opportunities to enhance fellow specialty nurses with their own end-of-life competency in their chosen field. The translation of palliative nursing expertise to colleagues is of particular urgency to ensure that quality end-of-life care is enacted regardless of setting, specialization, or experience. The aversion to dying also may be countered by sharing exemplars of success emanating from palliative nursing practice and expertise. Either way, the call to arms for all nurses is a real and profound one. Ferrell and Coyle (2006a) articulated:

> The basic assumptions of palliative nursing—the principles of attention to physical pain and suffering as well as existential distress; inclusion of the family as the unit of care; extension of care into bereavement; interdisciplinary care; and many other tenets of the field—are applicable across the very diverse profession of nursing. For this reason, we believe that every nurse should be a palliative care nurse. (p. ix)

Case Study

A.C. is a 44-year-old Hispanic woman who was diagnosed with a stage II cervical cancer two years ago. She underwent a hysterectomy and was treated with radiation therapy because of an incompletely resected tumor. She later developed a pelvic recurrence and was treated with chemotherapy (cisplatin and fluorouracil) and did well for almost a year. Additionally, she has a history of morbid obesity, manic depression, and severe asthma requiring multiple hospitalizations and steroid therapy.

Recently, she developed some right buttock pain and foot drop with sensory changes in her right lower leg. A work-up revealed a new soft tissue mass in the right psoas muscle and a tumor at the L4–5 vertebral level impinging on the cauda equina nerves. A neurosurgeon debulked the tumor, and A.C. received postoperative radiation therapy to the site. She lost her appetite after radiation therapy; food did not appeal to her.

Three weeks after the completion of her radiation therapy, A.C. came to the hospital's emergency department with excruciating pain. She described her pain as "sharp, burning, radiating, electrical jolts occurring without warning." The pain started in her right hip and radiated down her leg. She also had continuous pain in her lumbar-sacral spine area, the site of the unhealed surgical wound. "The pain medication doesn't seem to be working," she said. A.C. had been taking acetaminophen with codeine prn and had none left. She could not schedule an appointment with her primary care physician for another week. Upon further evaluation, A.C. was febrile, had an elevated white blood cell count, and was clearly septic from an infected surgical wound. She was admitted for evaluation and treatment of her pain and infection.

Upon admission, A.C. started on hydrocodone with acetaminophen (Vicodin®, Abbott Laboratories) 1 tablet every four to six hours prn pain with morphine 1–2 mg IV for severe pain. She consented to extensive surgical wound debridement and aggressive antibiotic therapy. Postoperatively, A.C. was intubated for acute respiratory failure. The intensive care nurses administered opioid analgesics (morphine IV infusion at 2 mg/hour) and sedation (lorazepam 1 mg IV prn) for pain and agitation. Assessment of pain was difficult because of A.C.'s inability to speak and her trouble understanding English. Frequent repositioning by the nurses was difficult because of the patient's pain and inability to assist. Multiple attempts at weaning the patient off the ventilator over a few days were unsuccessful. A.C. was clearly uncomfortable, but the surgeons were reluctant to increase the pain medication because of concerns with respiratory depression. The nurses advocated for her relief and were able to increase her morphine to 4 mg/hour. Unfortunately, one of the senior surgeons insisted, "We are killing this patient with these doses of morphine, and she is delirious," and ordered the medication to be stopped.

A.C. did not have decisional capacity for her own care because of her decreased level of consciousness, and she had no advance directives. A.C.'s husband of 11 years cared deeply about her and understood the seriousness of her complex problems. He made it clear to the surgical team that she would not want to continue to live in this dependent and disabling circumstance with its attendant procedures, surgeries, and multiple medications. Despite his suffering over her serious illness, he was clearly capable of speaking for his wife and repeatedly related to the nurses that she would not want this treatment but would want comfort care. He talked about the experience of his wife attending her own brother's 67-day stay in a surgical intensive care unit following severe central nervous system trauma from a motor vehicle accident. She remained with her brother until he died and stated she would not wish to receive life-sustaining treatment if she were in a similar circumstance. The surgical team was reluctant to abide by his directive, particularly regarding withdrawal of hydration and nutrition.

1. True or False: Once A.C. was unable to speak for herself, it would have been inappropriate for a palliative care consultation.
   • False. Palliative care for patients can be offered for a number of reasons, including providing relief from pain and other distressing symptoms as well as enhancing the quality of life (Kuebler et al., 2005). Providing for palliative care

does not necessitate a hospice consult but is the overriding construct that characterizes care provided to people with life-threatening illness.

2. List four characteristics of palliative care.
   - Identifying death as normal and natural
   - Providing relief from pain and other distressing symptoms
   - Affirming life by the provision of palliative interventions that neither hasten nor postpone death
   - Enhancing quality of life and, ideally, positively influencing the course of illness
   - Recognizing that the dying process is profoundly individualized and occurs within the dynamics of the family
   - Enhancing quality of life and integrating physical, psychological, social, and spiritual aspects of care
   - Employing the interdisciplinary team to address multidimensional needs of dying patients and their families, including bereavement counseling (if indicated)
   - Promoting the quality of life and healthy closure for patients and families via provision of palliative interventions and creation of a supportive environment

3. List some of the barriers or factors that influenced optimal pain management for this patient.
   - Inability to communicate because of a language barrier
   - Inability to communicate because of her intubation
   - Lack of healthcare professional's knowledge about pain medications and symptom management
   - Lack of healthcare professional's knowledge about the differences between narcotic addiction and narcotic tolerance
   - The husband's fear of causing addiction
   - The nurse's concern of overmedication
   - The patient's narcotic tolerance

Key Points

- Although palliative expertise has been required of nurses historically, it is one of the newest recognized nursing specialties.
- Palliative care is the umbrella term related to the science of caring for patients and families confronted with life-threatening disease that is unresponsive to conventional evidence-based medical interventions.
- Hospice is one component of palliative care that focuses on issues proximal to the end of life.
- The genesis of a palliative care evidence base to direct individualized planning has evolved slowly, in part because of special considerations in patient consent, accrual time for clinical trials, and ethical concerns about conducting research with the dying.
- Assessment of symptom distress in palliative care is a complex process because of the presence of multiple concurrent symptoms, the use of polypharmacy, evolving metabolic compromise, and the presence of altered cognition that interferes with symptom reporting.

- Family members hesitate to request help for themselves, yet their quality of life often is impaired. The absence of formal family education concerning future expectations based on disease course and the delivery of home-based comfort care fosters increased anxiety that in turn interferes with knowledge assimilation and comprehension.
- Responses to the dying process are highly culturally prescribed.
- APN interventions should employ skills that role-model ideal communication proficiency, assist staff with critical thinking via collaborative exchanges, pose novel interventions based on evidence-based findings, offer exemplars of advocacy on behalf of patients and families, and emulate optimum self-care in the context of multiple losses.

Recommended Resources for Oncology Advanced Practice Nurses

- CD
  - Education in Palliative and End-of-Life Care for Oncology (EPEC™–O) curriculum: www.cancer.gov/aboutnci/epeco
- Journals
  - *International Journal of Palliative Nursing:* www.ijpn.co.uk
  - *Journal of Hospice and Palliative Nursing:* www.jhpn.com
  - *Journal of Pain and Symptom Management:* www.elsevier.com/locate/jpainsymman
  - *Journal of Palliative Care:* www.ircm.qc.ca/bioethique/english/publications/journal _of_palliative_care.html
- Organizations
  - American Association of Colleges of Nursing ELNEC: www.aacn.nche.edu /ELNEC
  - End-of-Life/Palliative Education Resource Center: www.eperc.mcw.edu
  - Hospice and Palliative Nursing Association: www.hpna.org
- Texts
  - Ferrell, B.R., & Coyle, N. (Eds.). (2006). *Textbook of palliative nursing* (2nd ed.). New York: Oxford University Press.
  - Kuebler, K.K., Berry, P.H., & Heidrich, D.E. (Eds.). (2002). *End-of-life care: Clinical practice guidelines*. Philadelphia: Saunders.

References

Addington-Hall, J.M., & McCarthy, M. (2001). Survey research in palliative care using bereaved relatives. In D. Field, D. Clark, J. Corner, & C. Davis (Eds.), *Facing death: Researching palliative care* (pp. 27–36). Buckingham, England: Open University Press.

Aranda, S. (1998). Palliative care principles: Masking the complexity of practice. In J. Parker & S. Aranda (Eds.), *Palliative care: Explorations and challenges* (pp. 21–31). Melbourne, Australia: Ausmed.

Aranda, S., & Peerson, A. (2001). Caregiving in advanced cancer: Lay decision making. *Journal of Palliative Care, 17,* 270–276.

Aranda, S.K., & Hayman-White, K. (2001). Home caregivers of the person with advanced cancer. *Cancer Nursing, 24,* 300–307.

Aycock, N., & Boyle, D.A. (in press). National survey reveals interventions to manage compassion fatigue in oncology nursing. *Clinical Journal of Oncology Nursing.*

Bachner, Y.G., O'Rourke, N., & Carmel, S. (2007). Psychometric properties of a modified version of the Caregiver Reaction Assessment Scale measuring caregiving and post-caregiving reactions of caregivers of cancer patients. *Journal of Palliative Care, 23,* 80–86.

Baile, W.F., & Beale, E.A. (2001). Giving bad news to cancer patients: Matching process and content. *Journal of Clinical Oncology, 19,* 2575–2577.

Bakas, T., Lewis, R.R., & Parsons, J.E. (2001). Caregiving tasks among family caregivers of patients with lung cancer. *Oncology Nursing Forum, 28,* 847–853.

Baker, R., Wu, A., Teno, J.M., Kreling, B., Damiano, A.M., Rubin, H.R., et al. (2000). Family satisfaction with end-of-life care in seriously ill hospitalized patients. *Journal of the American Geriatrics Society, 48,* 561–569.

Barsevick, A.M. (2007). The elusive concept of the symptom cluster. *Oncology Nursing Forum, 34,* 971–980.

Berger, A., Portenoy, R.K., & Weissman, D.E. (2002). Preface. In A. Berger, R.K. Portenoy, & D.E. Weissman (Eds.), *Principles and practice of palliative care and supportive oncology* (p. xix). Philadelphia: Lippincott Williams & Williams.

Bernard, S.A., & Bruera, E. (2000). Drug interactions in palliative care. *Journal of Clinical Oncology, 18,* 1780–1799.

Billings, J.A., Keeley, A., Bauman, J., Cist, A., Coakley, E., Dahlin, C., et al. (2006). Merging cultures: Palliative care specialists in the medical intensive care unit. *Critical Care Medicine, 34*(Suppl. 11), S388–S393.

Boyle, D.A. (2000). Pathos in practice: Exploring the affective domain of cancer nursing. *Oncology Nursing Forum, 27,* 915–919.

Boyle, D.A. (2002). Families facing cancer: The forgotten priority [Guest editorial]. *Clinical Journal of Oncology Nursing, 6,* 69–70.

Boyle, D.A. (2003). Culturally competent care: An annotated bibliography. *Oncology Nursing Forum, 30,* 23–24.

Boyle, D.A. (2006a). Cultural diversity considerations in oncology nursing: An updated bibliography. *Oncology Nursing Forum, 33,* 705–709.

Boyle, D.A (2006b). Desperate nursewives [Guest editorial]. *Oncology Nursing Forum, 33,* 11.

Boyle, D.A. (in press-a). Communication skill competencies required of oncology nurses. *Nursing Clinics of North America.*

Boyle, D.A. (in press-b). Recent pharmacologic recommendations in the treatment of the older adult with cancer. *Clinical Nurse Specialist.*

Boyle, D.A., Sheridan, A., McClary, J., & White, J. (2002). A multifocal education strategy to enhance hospital-based cultural competency in professional staff. *Oncology Nursing Forum, 29,* 764–768.

Boyle, D.M. (1998). The cultural context of dying from cancer. *International Journal of Palliative Nursing, 4,* 70–83.

Boyle, D.M. (2003). Establishing a nursing research agenda in gero-oncology. *Critical Reviews in Oncology/Hematology, 48,* 103–111.

Boyle, D.M., Abernathy, G., Baker, L., & Wall, A.C. (1998). End-of-life confusion in patients with cancer. *Oncology Nursing Forum, 25,* 1335–1343.

Brant, J.M. (1998). The art of palliative care: Living with hope, dying with dignity. *Oncology Nursing Forum, 25,* 995–1004.

Braun, K.L., Pietsch, J.H., & Blanchette, P.L. (2000). An introduction to culture and its influence on end-of-life decision-making. In K.L. Braun, J.H. Pietsch, & P.L. Blanchette (Eds.), *Cultural issues in end-of-life decision-making* (pp. 1–9). Thousand Oaks, CA: Sage.

Cameron, J.I., Franche, R.L., Cheung, A.M., & Stewart, D.E. (2002). Lifestyle interference and emotional distress in family caregivers of advanced cancer patients. *Cancer, 94,* 521–527.

Carlson, M.D., Morrison, R.S., Holford, T.R., & Bradley, E.H. (2007). Hospice care: What services do patients and their families receive? *HSR: Health Services Research, 42,* 1672–1690.

Caton, A.P., & Klemm, P. (2006). Introduction of novice oncology nurses to end-of-life care. *Clinical Journal of Oncology Nursing, 10,* 604–608.

Cheek, P., Nikpour, L., & Nowlin, H.D. (2005). Aging well with smart technology. *Nursing Administration Quarterly, 28,* 329–338.

Chochinov, H.M., Hack, T., McClement, S., Harlos, M., & Kristjanson, L. (2002). Dignity in the terminally ill: A developing empirical model. *Social Science in Medicine, 54,* 433–443.

Cohen, J.S., & Erickson, J.M. (2006). Ethical dilemmas and moral distress in oncology nursing practice. *Clinical Journal of Oncology Nursing, 10,* 775–780.

Cohen, S.R., & Leis, A. (2002). What determines the quality of life of terminally ill cancer patients from their own perspective? *Journal of Palliative Care, 18,* 48–58.

Cohen, S.R., & Mount, B.M. (1992). Quality of life assessment in terminal illness: Defining and measuring subjective well-being in the dying. *Journal of Palliative Care, 8,* 40–45.

Cohen, S.R., & Mount, B.M. (2000). Living with cancer: "Good" days and "bad" days—what produces them? *Cancer, 89*, 1854–1865.

Cohen, S.R., Mount, B.M., Tomas, J., & Mount, L. (1996). Existential well-being is an important determinant of quality of life: Evidence from the McGill Quality of Life questionnaire. *Cancer, 77*, 576–586.

Connor, S.R., Elwert, F., Spence, C., & Christakis, N.A. (2007). Geographic variation in hospice use in the United States in 2002. *Journal of Pain and Symptom Management, 34*, 277–285.

Connor, S.R., Teno, J., Spence, C., & Smith, N. (2005). Family evaluation of hospice care: Results from voluntary submission of data via website. *Journal of Pain and Symptom Management, 30*, 9–17.

Coyle, N. (2006). Introduction to palliative nursing care. In B. Ferrell & N. Coyle (Eds.), *Textbook of palliative nursing* (2nd ed., pp. 5–11). New York: Oxford University Press.

Coyne, P., Paice, J.A., Ferrell, B.R., Malloy, P., Virani, R., & Fennimore, L.A. (2007). Oncology end-of-life consortium training program: Improving palliative care in cancer. *Oncology Nursing Forum, 34*, 801–807.

Curtis, J.R., Patrick, D.L., Engelberg, R.A., Norris, K., Asp, C., & Byock, I. (2002). A measure of the quality of dying and death: Initial validation using after-death interviews with family members. *Journal of Pain and Symptom Management, 24*, 17–30.

Curtis, J.R., & Rubenfeld, G.D. (2005). Improving palliative care for patients in the intensive care unit. *Journal of Palliative Care, 8*, 840–854.

Davies, B. (2006). Supporting families in palliative care. In B. Ferrell & N. Coyle (Eds.), *Textbook of palliative nursing* (2nd ed., pp. 545–560). New York: Oxford University Press.

Dodd, M., Miaskowski, C., & Lee, K.A. (2004). Occurrence of symptom clusters. *Journal of the National Cancer Institute Monographs, 32*, 76–78.

Dunn, K.S., Otten, C., & Stephens, E. (2005). Nursing experience and the care of dying patients. *Oncology Nursing Forum, 32*, 97–104.

Dy, S.M., Shugarman, L.R., Lorenz, K.A., Mularski, R.A., & Lynn, J. (2008). A systematic review of satisfaction with care at the end of life. *Journal of the American Geriatrics Society, 56*, 124–129.

Economou, D.C. (2006). Bowel management: Constipation, diarrhea, obstruction and ascites. In B. Ferrell & N. Coyle (Eds.), *Textbook of palliative nursing* (2nd ed., pp. 219–238). New York: Oxford University Press.

ELNEC core curriculum. (n.d.). Retrieved August 14, 2007, from http://www.aacn.nche.edu/elnec/curriculum.htm

Elpern, E.H., Covert, B., & Kleinpell, R. (2005). Moral distress of staff nurses in a medical intensive care unit. *American Journal of Critical Care, 14*, 523–530.

Emanuel, E.J., Fairclough, D.L., Slutsman, J., Alpert, H., Baldwin, D., & Emanuel, L.L. (1999). Assistance from family members, friends, paid care givers, and volunteers in the care of terminally ill patients. *New England Journal of Medicine, 341*, 956–963.

Eriksson, E. (2001). Caring for cancer patients: Relatives' assessments of received care. *European Journal of Cancer Care, 10*, 48–55.

Esper, P., & Heidrich, D. (2005). Symptom clusters in advanced illness. *Seminars in Oncology Nursing, 21*, 20–28.

Esper, P., Lockhart, J.S., & Miller-Murphy, C.M. (2002). Strengthening end-of-life care through specialty nursing certification. *Journal of Professional Nursing, 18*, 130–139.

Fago, J.A. (2000). Physical aspects of dying. In K.L. Braun, J.H. Pietsch, & P.L. Blanchette (Eds.), *Cultural issues in end-of-life decision making* (pp. 13–22). Thousand Oaks, CA: Sage.

Ferrell, B., Connor, S.R., Cordes, A., Dahlin, C.M., Fine, P.G., Hutton, N., et al. (2007). The national agenda for quality palliative care: The National Consensus Project and the National Quality Forum. *Journal of Pain and Symptom Management, 33*, 737–744.

Ferrell, B.R. (Ed.). (1996). *Suffering*. Sudbury, MA: Jones and Bartlett.

Ferrell, B.R., & Coyle, N. (2002). An overview of palliative nursing care. *American Journal of Nursing, 102*(5), 26–30.

Ferrell, B.R., & Coyle, N. (2006a). For every nurse—a palliative care nurse [Preface]. In B. Ferrell & N. Coyle (Eds.), *Textbook of palliative nursing* (2nd ed., pp. ix–x). New York: Oxford University Press.

Ferrell, B.R., & Coyle, N. (Eds.). (2006b). *Textbook of palliative nursing* (2nd ed.). New York: Oxford University Press.

Fine, P.G. (2002). Palliative radiation therapy in end-of-life care: Evidence-based utilization. *American Journal of Hospice and Palliative Care, 19*, 166–170.

Fineberg, I.C., Grant, M., Aziz, N.M., Payne, R., Kagawa-Singer, M., Dunn, G.P., et al. (2007). Prospective integration of cultural consideration in biomedical research for patients with advanced cancer:

Recommendations from an international conference on malignant bowel obstruction in palliative care. *Journal of Pain and Symptom Management, 34*(Supp. 1), S28–S39.

Fink, R.M., & Gates, R.A. (2006). Pain assessment in the palliative care setting. In B.R. Ferrell & N. Coyle (Eds.), *Textbook of palliative nursing* (2nd ed., pp. 97–130). New York: Oxford University Press.

Friedrichsen, M.J., Strang, P.M., & Carlsson, M.E. (2001). Receiving bad news: Experiences of family members. *Journal of Palliative Care, 17,* 241–247.

Fujimori, M., Akechi, T., Morita, T., Inagaki, M., Akizuki, N., Sakano, Y., et al. (2007). Preferences of cancer patients regarding the disclosure of bad news. *Psycho-Oncology, 16,* 573–581.

Gale, G., & Brooks, A. (2006). Implementing a palliative care program in a newborn intensive care unit. *Advances in Neonatal Care, 6,* 37–53.

Gapstur, R. (2007). Symptom burden: A concept analysis and implications for oncology nurses. *Oncology Nursing Forum, 34,* 673–680.

Gazelle, G. (2007). Understanding hospice—an underutilized option for life's final chapter. *New England Journal of Medicine, 357,* 321–324.

Given, B.A., Given, C.W., & Kozachik, S. (2001). Family support in advanced cancer. *CA: A Cancer Journal for Clinicians, 51,* 213–231.

Gomez, E. (2003). Handheld technology improves the delivery of palliative care. *ONS News, 18,* 7.

Grbich, C., Parker, D., & Maddocks, I. (2001). The emotions and coping strategies of caregivers of family members with terminal cancer. *Journal of Palliative Care, 17,* 30–36.

Greisinger, A.J., Lorimor, R.J., Aday, L.A., Winn, R.J., & Baile, W.F. (1997). Terminally ill cancer patients: Their most important concerns. *Cancer Practice, 5,* 147–154.

Halstead, M.T., & Nilsson, H.C. (2006). Spiritual care of the older adult with cancer. In D.G. Cope & A. Reb (Eds.), *An evidence-based approach to the treatment and care of the older adult with cancer* (pp. 529–559). Pittsburgh, PA: Oncology Nursing Society.

Hayman, J.A., Langa, K.M., Kabeto, M.U., Katz, S.J., DeManner, S.M., Chernew, M.E., et al. (2001). Estimating the cost of informal caregiving for elderly patients with cancer. *Journal of Clinical Oncology, 19,* 3219–3225.

Heidrich, D.E., & McKinnon, S. (2002). Palliative care emergencies. In K.K. Kuebler, P.H. Berry, & D.E. Heidrich (Eds.), *End-of-life care: Clinical practice guidelines* (pp. 383–408). Philadelphia: Saunders.

Henderson, F. (1961). *Basic principles of nursing care.* London: International Council of Nurses.

Hermann, C.P. (2006). Development and testing of the spiritual needs inventory for patients near the end of life. *Oncology Nursing Forum, 33,* 737–744.

Hewitt, M., Greenfield, S., & Stovall, E. (Eds.). (2006). *From cancer patient to cancer survivor: Lost in transition.* Washington, DC: National Academies Press.

Hickman, S.E., Tilden, V.P., & Tolle, S.W. (2001). Family reports of dying patients' distress: The adaptation of a research tool to assess global symptom distress in the last week of life. *Journal of Pain and Symptom Management, 22,* 565–572.

Hinton, J. (2001). How reliable are relatives' retrospective reports of terminal illness? Patients' and relatives' accounts compared. In D. Field, D. Clark, J. Corner, & C. Davis (Eds.), *Facing death: Researching palliative care* (pp. 98–109). Buckingham, England: Open University Press.

Hofmann, J.C., Wenger, N.S., Davis, R.B., Teno, J., Connors, A.F., Desbiens, N., et al. (1997). Patient preferences for communication with physicians about end-of-life decisions. SUPPORT Investigators. Study to Understand Prognoses and Preference for Outcomes and Risks of Treatment. *Annals of Internal Medicine, 127,* 1–12.

Hospice and Palliative Nurses Association & American Nurses Association. (2007). *Hospice and palliative nursing: Scope and standards of practice* (4th ed.). Silver Spring, MD: American Nurses Association.

Houldin, A.D. (2007). A qualitative study of caregivers' experiences with newly diagnosed advanced colorectal cancer. *Oncology Nursing Forum, 34,* 323–330.

Institute of Medicine. (2001). *Improving palliative care for cancer.* Washington, DC: National Academies Press.

Institute of Medicine. (2007). *Cancer in elderly people: Workshop proceedings.* Washington, DC: National Academies Press.

Jenko, M., Gonzalez, L., & Seymour, M.J. (2007). Life review with the terminally ill. *Journal of Hospice and Palliative Nursing, 9,* 159–167.

Joint Commission on the Accreditation of Healthcare Organizations. (2004). *Hospital accreditation standards.* Oakbrook Terrace, IL: Joint Commission Resources.

Kapp, S.A., & Nelson-Becker, H.B. (2007). Evaluating hospice services for improvement: A manageable approach. *Journal of Pain and Palliative Care Pharmacotherapy, 21,* 17–26.

Keating, N.L., Herrinton, L.J., Zaslavsky, A.M., Liu, L., & Ayanian, J.Z. (2006). Variations in hospice use among cancer patients. *Journal of the National Cancer Institute, 98*, 1053–1059.

Kedziera, P., & Coyle, N. (2006). Hydration, thirst and nutrition. In B. Ferrell & N. Coyle (Eds.), *Textbook of palliative nursing* (2nd ed., pp. 239–248). New York: Oxford University Press.

Kemp, C. (2005). Cultural issues in palliative care. *Seminars in Oncology Nursing, 21*, 44–52.

Kim, H.J., McGuire, D.B., Tulman, L., & Barsevick, A.M. (2005). Symptom clusters: Concept analysis and clinical implications for cancer nursing. *Cancer Nursing, 28*, 270–282.

King, C. (2006). Nausea and vomiting. In B. Ferrell & N. Coyle (Eds.), *Textbook of palliative nursing* (2nd ed., pp. 177–194). New York: Oxford University Press.

Kinlaw, K. (2005). Ethical issues in palliative care. *Seminars in Oncology Nursing, 21*, 63–68.

Kinsella, K.G. (2005). Future longevity—demographic concerns and consequences. *Journal of the American Geriatrics Society, 53*, S299–S303.

Knickman, J.R., & Snell, E.K. (2002). The 2030 problem: Caring for aging baby boomers. *Health Services Research, 37*, 849–884.

Knight, P., Espinosa, L.A., & Bruera, E. (2006). Sedation for refractory symptoms and terminal weaning. In B. Ferrell & N. Coyle (Eds.), *Textbook of palliative nursing* (2nd ed., pp. 467–489). New York: Oxford University Press.

Konski, A., Feigenberg, S., & Chow, E. (2005). Palliative radiation therapy. *Seminars in Oncology, 32*, 156–164.

Kotkamp-Mothes, N., Slawinsky, D., Hindermann, S., & Strauss, B. (2005). Coping and psychological well being in families of elderly cancer patients. *Critical Reviews in Oncology/Hematology, 55*, 213–229.

Kristjanson, L. (1993). Validity and reliability testing of the FAMCARE scale: Measuring family satisfaction with advanced cancer care. *Social Science in Medicine, 36*, 693–701.

Kristjanson, L. (1999). Families of palliative care patients: A model for care. In S. Aranda & M. O'Connor (Eds.), *Palliative care nursing: A guide to practice* (pp. 279–293). Melbourne, Australia: Ausmed.

Kristjanson, L.J., Leis, A., Koop, P.M., Carriere, K.C., & Mueller, B. (1997). Family members' care expectations, care perceptions and satisfaction with advanced cancer care: Results of a multi-site pilot study. *Journal of Palliative Care, 13*(4), 5–13.

Kristjanson, L.J., Sloan, J.A., Dudgeon, D., & Adaskin, E. (1996). Family members' perceptions of palliative cancer care: Predictors of family functioning and family members' health. *Journal of Palliative Care, 12*(4), 10–20.

Kubler-Ross, E. (1969). *On death and dying.* New York: Macmillan.

Kuebler, K.K., Heidrich, D.E., Vena, C., & English, N. (2006). Delirium, confusion and agitation. In B. Ferrell & N. Coyle (Eds.), *Textbook of palliative nursing* (2nd ed., pp. 401–420). New York: Oxford University Press.

Kuebler, K.K., Lynn, J., & Von Rohen, J. (2005). Perspectives in palliative care. *Seminars in Oncology Nursing, 21*, 2–10.

Kutner, J.S. (2008). Assuring quality end-of-life care: Imperative to expand the evidence base in concert with growth in the field. *Journal of the American Geriatrics Society, 56*, 160–162.

LaCasse, C., & Beck, S.L. (2007). Clinical assessment of symptom clusters. *Seminars in Oncology Nursing, 23*, 106–112.

Larkin, P.J., De Casterle, B.D., & Schotsmans, P. (2007). Transition towards end of life in palliative care: An exploration of its meaning for advanced cancer patients in Europe. *Journal of Palliative Care, 23*, 69–79.

Last Acts. (2002, November). *Means to a better end: A report on dying in America today.* New York: Author.

Leis, A.M., Kristjanson, L.J., Koop, P.M., & Laizner, A. (1997). Family health and the palliative care trajectory: A cancer research agenda. *Cancer Prevention and Control, 1*, 352–360.

Lobchuk, M.M., McClement, S.E., Daeninck, P.J., Shay, C., & Elands, H. (2007). Asking the right question of informal caregivers about patient symptom experiences: Multiple proxy perspectives and reducing interrater gap. *Journal of Pain and Symptom Management, 33*, 130–145.

Lohfeld, L., Brazil, K., & Willison, K. (2007). Continuity of care for advanced cancer patients: Comparing the views of spousal caregivers in Ontario, Canada, to Dumont et al.'s theoretical model. *Journal of Palliative Care, 23*, 117–126.

Lorenz, K.A., Rosenfeld, K., & Wenger, N. (2007). Quality indicators for palliative and end-of-life care in vulnerable elders. *Journal of the American Geriatrics Society, 55*(Suppl. 2), S318–S326.

Mason, D.J. (2002). Are we specializing in neglect? *American Journal of Nursing, 102*(5), 7.

McCarthy, E.P., Burns, R.B., Davis, R.B., & Phillips, R.S. (2003). Barriers to hospice care among older patients dying with lung and colorectal cancer. *Journal of Clinical Oncology, 21*, 728–735.

McCloskey, S.A., Tao, M.L., Rose, C.M., Fink, A., & Amadeo, A.M. (2007). National survey of perspectives of palliative radiation therapy: Role, barriers and needs. *Cancer Journal, 13*, 130–137.

McPherson, C.J., Wilson, K.G., Lobchuk, M.M., & Brajtman, S. (2008). Family caregivers' assessment of symptoms in patients with advanced cancer: Concordance with patients and factors affecting accuracy. *Journal of Pain and Symptom Management, 35,* 70–82.

Meropol, N.J., & Schulman, K.A. (2007). Cost of cancer care: issues and implications. *Journal of Clinical Oncology, 25,* 180–186.

Meyer, E.C., Ritholz, M.D., Burns, J.P., & Truog, R.D. (2006). Improving the quality of end-of-life care in the pediatric intensive care unit: Parents' priorities and recommendations. *Pediatrics, 117,* 649–657.

Mihelic, R.A. (2005). Pharmacology of palliative medicine. *Seminars in Oncology Nursing, 21,* 29–35.

Milberg, A., Olsson, E.C., Jakobsson, M., Olsson, M., & Friedrichsen, M. (2008). Family members' perceived needs for bereavement follow-up. *Journal of Pain and Symptom Management, 35,* 58–69.

Mosenthal, A.C., & Murphy, P.A. (2006). Interdisciplinary model for palliative care in the trauma and surgical intensive care unit: Robert Wood Johnson Foundation demonstration project for improving palliative care in the intensive care unit. *Critical Care Medicine, 34*(Suppl. 11), S399–S403.

Mularski, R.A., Rosenfeld, K., Coons, S.J., Dueck, A., Cella, D., Feuer, D.J., et al. (2007). Measuring outcomes in randomized prospective trials in palliative care. *Journal of Pain and Symptom Management, 34*(Suppl. 1), S7–S19.

Murphy-Ende, K. (2001). Barriers to palliative and supportive care. *Nursing Clinics of North America, 36,* 843–853.

National Consensus Project for Quality Palliative Care. (2004). *Clinical practice guidelines for quality palliative care.* Retrieved September 17, 2007, from http://www.nationalconsensusproject.org

Nelson-Marten, P., & Braaten, J.S. (2008). Advance directives, end of life decisions and ethical dilemmas. In R.A. Gates & R.M. Fink (Eds.), *Oncology nursing secrets* (3rd ed., pp. 619–630). St. Louis, MO: Elsevier Mosby.

O'Mara, A.M. (2007). "Will I suffer?" *Journal of Clinical Oncology, 25,* 1645–1646.

Oncology Nursing Society & Association of Oncology Social Work. (2007). Oncology Nursing Society and Association of Oncology Social Work joint position on palliative and end-of-life care. *Oncology Nursing Forum, 34,* 1097–1098.

Parker, S.M., Clayton, J.M., Hancock, K., Walder, S., Butow, P.N., Carrick, S., et al. (2007). A systematic review of prognostic/end-of-life communication with adults in advanced stages of a life-limiting illness: Patient/caregiver preferences for the content, style, and timing of information. *Journal of Pain and Symptom Management, 34,* 81–93.

Parsons, M.L., Clark, P., Marshall, M., & Cornett, P.A. (2007). Team behavioral norms: A shared vision for a healthy patient care workplace. *Critical Care Nursing Quarterly, 30,* 213–218.

Pasacreta, J.V., & McCorkle, R. (2000). Cancer care: Impact of interventions on caregiver outcomes. *Annual Review of Nursing Research, 18,* 127–148.

Patrick, D.L., Engelberg, R.A., & Curtis, J.R. (2001). Evaluating the quality of dying and death. *Journal of Pain and Symptom Management, 22,* 717–726.

Pavlish, C., & Ceronsky, L. (2007). Oncology nurses perceptions about palliative care. *Oncology Nursing Forum, 34,* 793–800.

Pollard, A., Cairns, J., & Rosenthal, M. (1999). Transition in living and dying: Defining palliative care. In S. Aranda & M. O'Connor (Eds.), *Palliative care nursing: A guide to practice* (pp. 5–19). Melbourne, Australia: Ausmed.

Puntillo, K., & Stannard, D. (2006). The intensive care unit. In B. Ferrell & N. Coyle (Eds.), *Textbook of palliative nursing* (2nd ed., pp. 401–420). New York: Oxford University Press.

Quint-Benoliel, J. (1966). Awareness of death and the nurses' composure. *Nursing Research, 15,* 49–55.

Regnard, C., & Hunter, A. (2005). Increasing prescriber awareness of drug interactions in palliative care [Letter]. *Journal of Pain and Symptom Management, 29,* 219–221.

Rice, E.M., & Betcher, D.K. (2007). Evidence base for developing a palliative care service. *Medsurg Nursing, 16,* 143–149.

Rousseau, P. (2001). The fear of death and the physician's responsibility to care for the dying. *American Journal of Hospice and Palliative Care, 18,* 224–226.

Royak-Schaler, R., Gadalla, S.M., Lemkau, J.P., Ross, D.D., Alexander, C., & Scott, D. (2006). Family perspectives on communication with healthcare providers during end-of-life cancer care. *Oncology Nursing Forum, 33,* 753–760.

Saunders, D.C. (2006). Foreword. In B.R. Ferrell & N. Coyle (Eds.), *Textbook of palliative nursing* (2nd ed., pp. v–vi). New York: Oxford University Press.

Schapira, L. (2005). Palliative information: Doctor-patient communication. *Seminars in Oncology, 32,* 139–144.

Scherbring, M. (2002). Effect of caregiver perception of preparedness on burden in an oncology population. *Oncology Nursing Forum, 29,* 70–76.

Schumacher, K.L., Stewart, B.J., Archbold, P.G., Dodd, M.J., & Dibble, S.L. (2000). Family caregiving skill: Development of the concept. *Research in Nursing and Health, 23,* 191–203.

Sharpe, L., Butow, P., Smith, C., McConnell, D., & Clarke, S. (2005). The relationship between available support, unmet needs and caregiver burden in patients with advanced cancer and their careers. *Psycho-Oncology, 14,* 102–114.

Sheldon, L.K. (2005). Communication in oncology care: The effectiveness of skills training workshops for healthcare providers. *Clinical Journal of Oncology Nursing, 9,* 305–312.

Shubha, R. (2007). Psychosocial issues in end-of-life care. *Journal of Psychosocial Nursing and Mental Health Services, 45*(8), 24–29.

Sontag, S. (1978). *Illness as metaphor.* New York: Farrar, Straus & Giroux.

Steinhauser, K.E., Christakis, N.A., Clipp, E.C., McNeilly, M., McIntyre, L., & Tulsky, J.A. (2000). Factors considered important at the end of life by patients, family, physicians and other care providers. *JAMA, 284,* 2476–2482.

Steinhauser, K.E., Clipp, E.C., McNeilly, M., Christakis, N.A., McIntyre, L.M., & Tulsky, J.A. (2000). In search of a good death: Observations by patients, families and providers. *Annals of Internal Medicine, 132,* 825–832.

Teno, J.M., Byock, I., & Field, M.J. (1999). Research agenda for developing measures to examine quality of care and quality of life of patients diagnosed with life-limiting illness. *Journal of Pain and Symptom Management, 17,* 75–82.

Teno, J.M, Clarridge, B., Casey, V., Welch, L., Wetle, T., Shield, R., et al. (2004). Family perceptions on end-of-life care as the last place of care. *JAMA, 291,* 88–93.

Teno, J.M., Mor, V., Ward, N., Roy, J., Clarridge, B., Wennberg, J.E., et al. (2005). Bereaved family member perceptions of quality of end-of-life care in U.S. regions with high and low usage of intensive unit care. *Journal of the American Geriatrics Society, 53,* 1905–1911.

Tolle, S.W., Tilden, V.P., Rosenfeld, A.G., & Hickman, S.E. (2000). Family reports of barriers to optimal care of the dying. *Nursing Research, 49,* 310–317.

Vachon, M.L. (2006). The experience of the nurse in end-of-life care in the 21st century. In B. Ferrell & N. Coyle (Eds.), *Textbook of palliative nursing* (2nd ed., pp. 1011–1029). New York: Oxford University Press.

Viney, M., Batcheller, J., Houston, S., & Belcik, K. (2006). Transforming care at the bedside: Designing new care systems in an age of complexity. *Journal of Nursing Care Quality, 21,* 143–150.

Vladeck, B.C. (2005). Economic and policy implications of improving longevity. *Journal of the American Geriatrics Society, 53,* S304–S307.

Von Roenn, J.H., & Paice, J.A. (2005). Control of common, non-pain cancer symptoms. *Seminars in Oncology, 32,* 200–210.

Watson, A.C. (2006). Urgent syndromes at the end of life. In B. Ferrell & N. Coyle (Eds.), *Textbook of palliative nursing* (2nd ed., pp. 443–465). New York: Oxford University Press.

Whalen, G.F., Kutner, J., Byock, I., Gerard, D., Stovall, E., Sieverding, P., et al. (2007). Implementing palliative care studies. *Journal of Pain and Symptom Management, 34*(Supp. 1), S40–S48.

Wilkes, L. (1998). Reflection on the good death and the nurse in palliative care. In J. Parker & S. Aranda (Eds.), *Palliative care: Explorations and challenges* (pp. 115–125). Melbourne, Australia: Ausmed.

Wilkes, L. (1999). Occupational stress for nurses providing palliative care. In S. Aranda & M. O'Connor (Eds.), *Palliative care nursing: A guide to practice* (pp. 69–81). Melbourne, Australia: Ausmed.

Wilson, K.G., Chochinov, H.M., McPherson, C.J., LeMay, K., Allard, P., Chary, S., et al. (2007). Suffering with advanced cancer. *Journal of Clinical Oncology, 25,* 1691–1697.

Wood, G.J., Shega, J.W., Lynch, B., & Von Roenn, J.H. (2007). Management of intractable nausea and vomiting in patients at the end of life. *JAMA, 298,* 1196–1207.

World Health Organization. (2002). *National cancer control programmes: Policies and managerial guidelines* (2nd ed.). Geneva, Switzerland: World Health Organization.

World Health Organization. (n.d.). *Palliative care.* Retrieved August 4, 2007, from http://www.who.int/cancer/palliative/definition/en

Wright, A.A., & Katz, I.T. (2007). Letting go of the rope: Aggressive treatment, hospice care and open access. *New England Journal of Medicine, 357,* 324–327.

Zanchetta, M.S., & Moura, S.L. (2006). Self-determination and information seeking in end-stage cancer. *Clinical Journal of Oncology Nursing, 10,* 803–807.

Zimmermann, C., Riechelmann, R., Krzyzanowska, M., Rodin, G., & Tannock, I. (2008). Effectiveness of specialized palliative care: A systematic review. *JAMA, 299,* 1698–1709.

Zollo, J. (1999). The interdisciplinary palliative care team: Problems and possibilities. In S. Aranda & M. O'Connor (Eds.), *Palliative care nursing: A guide to practice* (pp. 21–35). Melbourne, Australia: Ausmed.

CHAPTER 19

Roles of the Oncology Advanced Practice Nurse

Sandra A. Mitchell, CRNP, PhD, AOCN®

Introduction

Today's healthcare environment is characterized by higher acuity, more complex treatments for cancer, and a shift from the delivery of cancer care in specialized inpatient settings to community hospitals and outpatient treatment facilities. The challenges presented by these trends occur at a time when demand for cancer services is expanding because of the aging of the population. Against this backdrop, the skill set of the oncology advanced practice nurse (APN) seems ideally suited to improve care quality and enhance clinical outcomes. This improvement occurs through the delivery of advanced nursing services together with program development, consultation and education, and evidence-based practice development. This chapter outlines the components of the oncology APN role, examines cross-cutting skills oncology APNs need in order to optimize role outcomes, and highlights contemporary challenges in role development.

Background

Advanced practice nursing in oncology can be characterized as the delivery of services to patients, families, care providers, and organizations based on expanded and specialized knowledge and skills concerning the care of individuals with a risk of or experiencing the diagnosis of cancer. APNs employ theory and advanced clinical skills to assemble and critically examine the evidence necessary for complex, autonomous clinical decision making that contributes to improved outcomes for patients and families (Styles, 1996).

The functions of the oncology APN encompass several differing elements, including that of clinician, consultant, educator, researcher, and case manager/coordinator. The functional emphasis depends upon the specific advanced practice role (nurse practitioner [NP] or clinical nurse specialist [CNS]), the organizational structure, the setting (in-patient, ambulatory care, office-based practice, home care, or educational institution) in which the APN role is operationalized, the needs of patients and staff, and the expectations and goals of the APN. A distinction exists between specialized nursing practice and advanced nursing practice. *Specialized* nursing practice involves concentration in a selected clinical nursing area and may be developed from clinical experience and continuing education. *Advanced* nursing practice employs advanced education and specialized practice preparation that integrates theoretical, empirical, and practice knowledge at the graduate level. Particular advanced practice roles may have additional specific competency requirements. Within states, advanced practice role titles, scopes of practice, and role responsibilities may be regulated and governed by the state board of nursing (see Chapter 20 for additional information).

Recently, the paradigm of fluid and divergent roles in advanced practice nursing has shifted, and a national consensus is developing around a new regulatory model for advanced practice nursing (APRN Joint Dialogue Group, 2008; Nelson, 2006). Debate continues about the need for APNs to be educated at the doctoral level (Chase & Pruitt, 2006; Dracup, Cronenwett, Meleis, & Benner, 2005; Eisenhauer & Bleich, 2006; McCabe, 2006), the role of the clinical nurse leader (American Association of Colleges of Nursing, 2007; National Association of Clinical Nurse Specialists [NACNS], 2005; Stanley et al., 2004), and the responsibilities of state boards of nursing and specialty organizations in the regulation and certification of APN practice (Lancaster, 2006). This evolution emerges in part from recognition that many APN roles overlap, making it difficult to logically differentiate roles as distinct and unique entities. When these varying roles are offered as the organizing framework, it is easy to conclude that because both CNSs and NPs have comparable expertise, they must have similar role emphases as APNs. Studies suggest, however, that various settings conceptualize advanced practice nursing differently and that both the CNS and the NP make a distinct contribution to improving patient outcomes (Hall, 2007; Lincoln, 2000; Mick & Ackerman, 2000).

NACNS issued a practice statement outlining the core competencies and outcomes for CNS practice. NACNS conceptualizes the CNS role as the use of clinical expertise with a specialty focus to improve clinical and economic outcomes within three spheres of influence or practice domains: patients/clients, nursing personnel, and the organization/network (NACNS, 2004). The National Organization of Nurse Practitioner Faculties (NONPF) identified core competencies of the NP, specifying additional competencies for nurse practitioners in acute care, primary care (adult, family, gerontologic, pediatric, and women's health), and psychiatric-mental health. Core NP competencies that cross-cut all subspecialties include (a) management of health and illness through assessment/diagnosis and development and implementation of a plan of care to optimize health and prevent and treat illness, (b) development of therapeutic relationships with patients and families that respect cultural differences and optimize healthy behaviors, self-management, and effective coping, (c) teaching and coaching patients and families, (d) professional leadership that incorporates critical and reflective thinking, interprofessional collaboration, ethical decision making, and the translation of new knowledge into practice and policy, (e) navigating and strengthening care delivery systems, and (f) monitoring practice and implementing change to reduce practice variation, improve access to care and patient outcomes, and strengthen the quality of care processes (NONPF, 2006). The Oncology Nursing Society (ONS) recently developed competency domains for the oncology NP role that closely parallel those identified by NONPF (ONS, 2007), and competencies for the oncology CNS are in development. Despite continued evolution in the definition and regulation of advanced practice roles, oncology APNs share the goals of promoting professional autonomy, improving outcomes for patients, and broadening access to high-quality effective care (Jacobs, 2003c).

Although APN role functions and priorities may be setting specific, the practice of APNs is characterized by several common features, including the use of advanced specialty knowledge in practice; critical thinking; autonomous clinical judgment and ethical decision making; application of evidence to improve practice; and professional leadership (Hamric & Hanson, 2003; Macdonald, Herbert, & Thibeault, 2006; Mantzoukas & Watkinson, 2006). Ackerman, Norsen, Martin, Wiedrich, and Kitzman (1996) and Gardner, Chang, and Duffield (2007) defined an operational framework for establishing and evaluating APN function. The service parameters of the APN role include direct comprehensive care, support of systems, education, research, and professional leadership. Cutting across all APN roles, spheres of influence, and functions are the essential APN skills of leadership, collaboration, management of change, scholarly practice, mentorship, negotiation, and conflict resolution. Factors that affect the implementation of advanced nursing roles are summarized in Figure 19-1.

ONS offers several documents to guide the educational preparation and role development of the oncology APN (Jacobs, 2003a, 2003b, 2003c; ONS, 2007). Current and future challenges for oncology APN role development include role definition, advanced specialty education, certification and regulation, prescriptive authority, reimbursement, relationships with other staff groups, and evaluation of different models for APN role implementation (Belcher & Shurpin, 1995; Cunningham, 2004; Jacobs, Scarpa, Lester, & Smith, 2004; Jones, 2005; Lynch, Cope, & Murphy-Ende, 2001; McCabe & Burman, 2006; Mick & Ackerman, 2000; Spross & Heaney, 2000; Vaz & Small, 2007). Before considering approaches to address these challenges, the APN role components of expert practitioner, case manager, coordinator, consultant, educator, and researcher are examined.

Expert Direct Practitioner

APNs integrate and apply specialty knowledge to improve outcomes for patients. They take a holistic or biopsychosocial orientation to clinical practice, with an emphasis on communication, counseling, conflict resolution, and coordination. ONS stated that APNs should be utilized to achieve quality in the delivery of all aspects of cancer care (ONS, 2005). Studies suggest that the expert practice of oncology APNs results in better patient education and adherence, decreased length of stay, and fewer hospital readmissions, as well as improved quality of life, patient satisfaction, and access to care (Berger et al., 1996; Cunningham, 2004; Fulton & Baldwin, 2004; Piano & Zerwic, 1998; Ritz et al., 2000; Spross & Heaney, 2000; Volker, Kahn, & Penticuff, 2004). Unique APN roles in oncology have been described in the general oncology setting (Berger et al., 1999; Blackburn, 1998; Bush & Watters, 2001; Fitch & Mings, 2003; Kinney, Hawkins, & Hudmon, 1997; Moore & Sweedman, 2004; Murphy-Ende, 2002), in nurse-led clinics (Loftus & Weston, 2001), as well as in radiation oncology (Carper & Haas, 2006; Kelvin & Moore-Higgs, 1999; Kelvin et al., 1999; Shepard & Kelvin, 1999), pediatric oncology (Callahan & De La Cruz, 2004), breast cancer care (McKenney, 2005; Vogel, 2003), gynecologic oncology (Allen, 2003; Parkinson & Pratt, 2005), head and neck cancer (Scarpa, 2004), palliative care (Kuebler, 2003; Skalla, 2006), cancer genetics (Calzone, Jenkins, & Masny, 2002), hematopoietic stem cell transplantation (Lin, 1994), and cancer survivorship (Hobbie & Hollen, 1993; Kolb Smith, 2002).

Characteristics of the Advanced Practice Nurse (APN)
- Adaptability, stamina, creativity
- Confident, assertive, patient, optimistic, proactive
- Strong decision-making and problem-solving skills
- Strong skills in negotiation, conflict resolution, and relationship building
- Accepts personal accountability for quality of relationships and achievement of outcomes

Previous Experience of the APN
- Specialty experience
- Previous experience as a staff nurse
- Previous experience as an APN

Quality of APN Relationships
- Effective working relationships with managers and supervisors, nursing staff colleagues, APN colleagues, physicians, and other key stakeholders

Professional and Educational Issues
- Sustained mentoring
- Performance measurement
- Adequate orientation to the role
- Maintaining clinical competence
- Clear regulatory framework for APN practice
- Effective role modeling during educational preparation
- Compensation package commensurate with responsibilities
- Educational preparation encompasses both generic APN skills (e.g., evidence-based practice skills, research skills, time management) and specialty skills

Organizational Issues
- Organizational positioning and status of the APN role within the organization
- Proactive and inclusive planning; transparent decision-making processes
- Clear, flexible, evolving, and responsive APN role definitions and boundaries
- Highly valued interdisciplinary teamwork, expertise, outcomes management, and evidence-based practice
- Clearly articulated goals and priorities that include employee satisfaction and individual and team productivity
- APN role expectations that encourage autonomy and are realistic, compatible with those of the APN, and well matched to the resources provided to the APN

Available Resources
- Office space
- Library access
- Full-time funding for the role
- Educational support for continuing education
- Computer, appropriate software, and technologic support
- Secretarial support, transcription services, billing management
- Seed funding and expert consultative support for research projects
- Knowledgeable, timely, and supportive guidance and advocacy from other nurse leaders

---

Figure 19-1. Factors Influencing Advanced Practice Nurse Role Development

---

Note. Based on information from Brykczynski, 2000; Cummings et al., 2003; Glen & Waddington, 1998; Irvine et al., 2000; Jones, 2005; Kleinpell & Hravnak, 2005; Lynch et al., 2001.

For APNs in the NP role, expert practice includes comprehensive assessment, diagnosis, and care management in collaboration with physicians and other healthcare team members. NPs also promote wellness and health maintenance, prevent complications, and provide acute and chronic care. Responsibilities of the NP role include conducting physical examinations and other health assessment/screening activities; diagnosing and treating acute and chronic conditions; performing, ordering, and interpreting laboratory and diagnostic studies; and prescribing pharmacologic and nonpharmacologic therapies. Delivery of these services requires that NPs enter into an explicit collaborative practice with physician colleagues, while simultaneously achieving and maintaining a high degree of autonomy in their practice. The requirements, limitations, scope, and regulation of prescriptive authority varies widely from state to state (see Chapter 20). Acquisition of advanced technical skills often is a requirement for NP practice. These procedures can include chest tube insertion, bone marrow aspiration, skin biopsy, lumbar puncture, or accessing an Ommaya reservoir for administration of intrathecal chemotherapy. It is important that these skills be gained under appropriate conditions of supervision and direction and that methods for demonstrating continuing competence to perform these procedures are in place. ONS recently developed competencies for the oncology NP role (ONS, 2007). These competencies complement and extend the core competencies for all NP practice (NONPF, 2006) and are summarized in Figure 19-2.

CNS expert practice includes the delivery of interventions to patients and their families to prevent or ameliorate symptom distress and functional limitations, provide emotional support, and enhance comfort. CNSs also intervene to reduce behaviors such as nonadherence; promote effective coping, problem solving, and self-care management;

Health Promotion, Health Protection, Disease Prevention, and Treatment
Describes the role of the ONP in assessment of patients' health status using evidence-based clinical practice guidelines to identify needs, to diagnose, and to plan interventions

Nurse Practitioner-Patient Relationship
Reflects the personal, collaborative, and therapeutic approaches ONPs apply in the delivery of patient care

Teaching-Coaching Function
Identifies the ONPs' contributions to delivering knowledge and skills necessary for self-care and advocating for, supporting, and reinforcing patient autonomy and control in treatment decision making and self-care to prevent complications, optimize adherence, and maximize well-being

Professional Role
Outlines the contributions of ONPs relative to advancing the profession, enhancing direct care and management, and sustaining and extending the role

Negotiating Healthcare Delivery Systems
Describes the ONP application of expert knowledge of reimbursement systems, case management principles, and interventions to enhance continuity of care and timely referral in achieving improved outcomes for patients and for the care delivery system

Monitoring and Ensuring the Quality of Healthcare Practice
Identifies the ONP role in ensuring quality of care through consultation, collaboration, continuing education, certification, and evaluation

Caring for Diverse Populations
Summarizes the ONP role in providing culturally competent care to populations that are diverse with respect to culture, race, ethnicity, religion, gender, or lifestyle

---

Figure 19-2. Oncology Nurse Practitioner (ONP) Competencies

Note. From *Oncology Nurse Practitioner Competencies,* by Oncology Nursing Society, 2007, Pittsburgh, PA: Author. Copyright 2007 by Oncology Nursing Society. Adapted with permission.

and enhance physical, psychological, and spiritual well-being (McKinley, 2007). The delivery of these interventions is based on a systematic assessment, including health history, physical examination, and review of relevant laboratory and diagnostic studies. Many CNSs provide direct care to high-risk, multiproblem patients and their families and patients at highest risk for adverse outcomes, whereas others improve outcomes for patients by influencing the direction and quality of staff nurses' problem solving. Even when providing direct care, CNSs may simultaneously address other role components and spheres of influence, for example, by educating staff or gathering information needed to address a system problem that is adversely affecting care delivery.

Documentation of services is a key component of the direct practice role. Clear and precise documentation of APN services is important for several reasons. First, APN documentation of the assessment, diagnosis, and interventions assists in ensuring coordination of care and achievement of desired clinical outcomes. Second, APN documentation reflects the achievement of outcomes in important areas of APN practice, including comprehensive evaluation and holistic intervention. Quality APN documentation supports an image of the APN as a knowledgeable and effective member of the care team and reinforces visibility of the APN role. Documentation of services also is necessary to meet qualifications for reimbursement of APN services. Lastly, documentation allows appropriate utilization review and quality of care evaluation, as well as collection of data useful for research and education. The elements that should be included in an APN consultation note are illustrated in Figure 19-3. An example of an APN consultation is provided by Mitchell (2001).

Barriers to reimbursement for delivery of expert clinical services may exist for APNs practicing in either the NP or CNS role. Although the federal government provides for reimbursement of all healthcare providers in its programs, individual states and private payers control which providers are eligible for reimbursement and may limit reimbursement for services not provided directly by physicians.

- Reason for consultation
- History of present illness, past medical history, current concerns, review of systems
- Limited physical examination
- Current medications
- Relevant laboratory studies
- Assessment and recommendations
- Plans for reevaluation and follow-up
- Signature

Figure 19-3. Elements of an Advanced Practice Nurse Consultation Note

---

Case Manager

Case management is recognized as an important aspect of the care continuum. Although operationalized differently in various settings, case management is a practice framework designed to integrate quality, productivity, and cost to achieve desired patient and organizational outcomes, improve access to healthcare services, and achieve enhanced care coordination between providers and continuity across settings (Cohen & Cesta, 2001). Case management requires knowledge of the disease process and treatment options together with expertise and skills that optimize quality and cost effectiveness across the whole continuum of care. At the advanced level, case management is a process frequently encompassing a broad range of activities, such as disease management or population-based case management (Stanton, Swanson, Sherrod, & Packa, 2005). Organizational goals supporting the use of an APN case manager may include reducing the length of stay, preventing readmission, optimizing resource use and costs, increasing access to services, and creating desire to become a recognized center of excellence for a particular service. Accountability of the case manager typically extends across repeated episodes of care and beyond traditional geographic boundaries.

As shown in Table 19-1, APN case management functions align closely with the traditional roles of the APN (clinical practice, consultation, education, and research) and

Table 19-1. Advanced Practice Nurse Competencies and Nurse Case Management Functions

Advanced Practice Nurse (APN) Competency	APN Case Management Functions
Direct care	• Identify and screen cases. • Conduct health assessments. • Apply critical pathways and evidence-based guidelines. • Coordinate interventions with other providers. • Link patient to appropriate resources. • Monitor patient's progress toward goals. • Evaluate effects of interventions.
Expert guidance and coaching	• Educate other providers about clinical, fiscal, and system processes. • Coach patients and families through developmental, health, and illness transitions.
Consultation	• Provide expert case consultation. • Recommend systemwide process improvements (e.g., documentation tools, referral processes, measures to improve continuity, documentation tools, comprehensiveness of care).
Critical analysis and application of research	• Collect, analyze, and synthesize data. • Review and interpret literature. • Evaluate program outcomes, such as quality, patient satisfaction, and costs of care. • Establish and facilitate quality improvement teams.
Collaboration	• Communicate, coordinate, and negotiate with other providers to improve care outcomes for patients and families. • Develop critical pathways, protocols, and other clinical guidelines.
Change agent	• Initiate systemwide change to effect improvements in comprehensiveness and continuity of care. • Plan new services and programs.
Ethical decision making	• Recognize and raise for discussion ethical dilemmas occurring in the process of care delivery. • Identify all options available to the client. • Demonstrate ethical decision making in terms of autonomy, beneficence, nonmaleficence, and justice in meeting system, fiscal, and client goals.

Note. Based on information from Connors, 1993; Hamric, 1992; Mahn & Spross, 1996.
From "The Advanced Practice Nurse Case Manager" (p. 568), by V.A. Mahn and D. Zazworsky in A.B. Hamric, J.A. Spross, and C.M. Hanson (Eds.), *Advanced Nursing Practice: An Integrative Approach* (2nd ed.), 2000, Philadelphia: Saunders. Copyright 2000 by Saunders. Adapted with permission.

incorporate APN skills in clinical leadership, collaboration, communication, and managing change. Both Mahn and Zazworsky (2000) and Hamric and Hanson (2003) defined case management as an advanced practice role that requires competency in directing expert care, provides guidance and coaching, consults with staff, interprets research, coordinates multidisciplinary collaboration, and acts as a change agent.

Although case management may be a component of the advanced practice role, at the present time, given a global shortage of nurses, it is not feasible for all nurse case managers to be APNs. At least one author suggests that basic care coordination functions be differentiated from APN case management on the basis of patient complexity (physical, emotional, or social) and the predictability of the clinical course (Mahn & Zazworsky, 2000).

Coordinator

Because cancer is often a long-term or chronic illness, patients experience an extended period of contact with an increasingly specialized and complex healthcare system. Achieving integration across settings and among members of the interdisciplinary cancer care team is of paramount importance for quality cancer care.

Although continuity of care has been variously defined in the literature (Beddar & Aikin, 1994), most definitions suggest that continuity of care is a philosophy and a quality standard of care. Continuity of care involves patients, lay caregivers, and healthcare providers working together to provide a coordinated, comprehensive continuum that meets the needs of patients, provides for transitions between settings, results in improved clinical outcomes, and promotes a cost-effective use of healthcare resources. Shortell (1976) defined continuity of care as the "extent to which services are received as a coordinated uninterrupted succession of events consistent with the needs of the patient" (p. 378). *Coordination* is a term used in many definitions of continuity of care. However, a distinction should be made between the coordination and the integration of care (Gerteis, 1993). Coordination suggests a smooth and efficient operation, whereas integration implies a more holistic, systematic, and goal-oriented concept (Beddar & Aikin; Lauria, 1991). When defining continuity of care, two different dimensions of continuity should be distinguished: (1) continuity of plan and (2) longitudinality. Continuity of plan is the means by which separate episodes of care are joined and structured, whereas longitudinality is a relationship between a patient and a regular source of care that lasts over time (Rogers, J., & Curtis, 1980; Starfield, 1980). Many clinical approaches to strengthening continuity of care, such as primary nursing and case management, emphasize longitudinality. Discharge planning models, multidisciplinary planning teams, formalized communication and referral mechanisms between providers, and integrated documentation tools and case management plans across settings are examples of models that emphasize continuity of plan.

Barriers to continuity of care include a sense of threat regarding the involvement of healthcare providers outside of one's own institution together with interagency and interprofessional competition and territoriality. Lack of knowledge regarding the services of other disciplines and resources is compounded when accompanied by hesitancy or resistance to collaborate. Suboptimal communication between providers and healthcare settings is magnified by the fact that health records are not easily shared among agencies and providers. Reimbursement issues also affect the range, intensity, duration, and location of services that are available to a patient, at the expense of both quality and continuity of care (Harris & Zwar, 2007).

Continuity of care aims to achieve and maintain a maximum level of functional health while simultaneously optimizing physical and psychospiritual comfort, facilitating transitions between settings and caregivers, and optimizing the use of healthcare resources (Buckwalter, 1985). Figure 19-4 lists seven essential elements of continuity of care. An interdisciplinary approach to care that acknowledges the whole person, including the family, and addresses the highly technical and often complex problems of cancer care is essential and should be accessible throughout the illness continuum. Although team composition and leadership may shift over time, mutual respect and recognition of each provider's unique contribution are fundamental characteristics of an interdisciplinary approach. Case conferences, shared documentation tools, and interdisciplinary care standards can be effective strategies to facilitate communication and collaboration. A comprehensive, systematic assessment of patient and family needs contributes to continuity of care. Once the needs for care are identified, three key questions should be posed to promote goal setting, teaching, and resource coordination: (1) What activities are to be performed to maintain or enhance individual and family functioning? (2) Who will perform these activities, and who is the designated alternate? and (3) What health teaching, referrals, and/or equipment and supplies are required?

- Interdisciplinary approach to care
- Comprehensive assessment of patient and family needs and strengths
- Patient and family education and involvement in decision-making
- Measurable goals and a documented plan of care
- Identification and coordination of supplemental resources
- Integration of care through each transition
- Evaluation

Figure 19-4. Essential Elements of Continuity of Care

Note. From "Continuity of Care: A Challenge for Ambulatory Oncology Nursing," by S.M Beddar and J.L. Aikin, 1994, *Seminars in Oncology Nursing, 10,* p. 259. Copyright 1994 by Elsevier. Reprinted with permission.

Because successful continuity of care requires active participation of patients and families, another required element of continuity of care is patient and family education and involvement in decision making. The identification of measurable goals, development of the plan together with patients and family members, and coordination of supplemental resources (such as home nursing care, laboratory services, medications, rehabilitation, and respite care) also are essential.

Lastly, care must be integrated through each transition in care setting or care providers. An area that can cause particular difficulties for patients with cancer is the transfer of specific medical procedures and technology into the community (McMillan et al., 2006; Winkler, Ross, Piamjariyakul, Gajewski, & Smith, 2006). It is essential to determine whether the community setting has the necessary educational, procedural, financial, and material supports to effectively transfer the technology into the community. Careful exploration of these issues, together with referral to agencies well in advance of the transition of care, provision of copies of clinic procedures and protocols, and/or an opportunity to observe the care procedure, are essential to ensure a smooth transition in care.

APN interventions to promote continuity of care also include efforts to help patients and families verbalize feelings of fear, vulnerability, and helplessness, build trust and confidence in new caregiver personnel, and develop realistic problem solving and contingency planning. Outcome indicators of continuity of care include optimal patient functioning (including physical, psychological, and social function), patient comfort, and patient and family satisfaction (McKeehan & Coulton, 1985). Continuity of care outcomes are now incorporated into existing quality measurement and accreditation programs (Fletcher, O'Malley, Fletcher, Earp, & Alexander, 1984).

A recent paper described the role of the APN in the provision of transition services (Betz & Redcay, 2005), incorporating the advanced practice dimensions of clinical expert, change agent, leader, researcher, and educator. This transition planning framework can be applied to guide the development and testing of care delivery models that are designed to improve coordination and enhance the continuity of multidisciplinary oncology care (Kennedy, Sloman, Douglass, & Sawyer, 2007).

Consultant

Although consultation is a core competency of advanced practice, the term itself may be used in different ways in various situations. Consultation refers to a two-way interaction designed to solicit, provide, and receive help. The consultant is recognized as having specialized expertise. The consultee requests the assistance of that expert in management of a problem that he or she believes to be within the expertise of the consultant. Consultants try to aid an individual, group, or organization in identifying and utilizing resources to deal with problems and manage change. Internal consultants are part of the system with which they are consulting, whereas external consultants function from outside the system. Caplan (1970) recognized four types of consultation. *Client-centered case consultation* has a primary goal of assisting the consultee to develop an effective plan of care for patients with a difficult or complex problem. *Consultee-centered case consultation* emphasizes the consultee's difficulties (whether lack of skills, knowledge, confidence, or objectivity) in handling the complex problem. In client-centered case consultation, the consultant often performs a one-time evaluation of the patient upon which to base recommendations. On the other hand, in consultee-centered case consultation, the task is to understand and address the gaps in knowledge, skill, confidence, or objectivity that hinder the consultee in ideal management of a particular case. This typically would not require an evaluation of the patient, but rather the consultant offers education, suggests actions, provides validation, or explores the consultee's perceptions about the case, strengthening professional objectivity or clarifying boundaries. The third type of consultation is *program-centered administrative consultation*. This type of consultation focuses on planning or administering clinical services. The fourth type of consultation, *consultee-centered administrative consultation,* addresses the consultee's difficulties as they interfere with the organization's objectives.

Regardless of the type of consultation, several principles are fundamental. First, the problem focus is always identified by the consultee. Furthermore, the professional responsibility for patients always remains with the consultee, and the consultant is not responsible for the consultee's work. The consultee remains free to accept or reject the ideas and recommendations of the consultant. Barron and White (2000) recommended that the consultation process address assessment, consultation focus, consensus on consultant and consultee responsibilities, and evaluation. Based on the information gathered during assessment, the consultant verifies that consultation is an appropriate strategy for this problem (versus referral, for example) and affirms that the consultant has the necessary skills to assist. The focus of the consultation must then be identified and may or may not be the problem for which help was initially sought. Reframing of the problem focus for the consultation requires discernment, skill, and tact, particularly if the problem is the consultee's lack of expertise. When reframing a consultation request, both the consultant and the consultee must agree that the reframed issue is the one on which they will work and must mutually agree to their roles and responsibilities. Once the specific issue is identified, the consultant and consultee jointly consider interventions, negotiate how the interventions will be carried out and by whom, and come to consensus on each participant's ongoing responsibilities. It is advantageous for the consultant to offer choices rather than forcing a specific kind of help onto a consultee. Using the phrase "would that be helpful?" can invite clarification and feedback about an action, plan, or advice that the consultant has offered. Resistance often means the consultant is pressing solutions onto others or that the consultee desires more control in the situation. Dialogue such as "I'm sensing that these suggestions are not fitting well for you; what would you rather be doing?" will provide feedback about resistance. Following the intervention, the consultant and consultee engage in evaluation, examining both the process of consultation and the achieved outcomes. Thoughtful negotiation of roles and responsibilities, together with strong communication and relationship development skills, will improve the consultant's effectiveness. Figure 19-5 further develops these core principles of effective APN consultation.

The Consultant Remains Self-Aware.
- The consultant remains conscious of whether, instead of consulting, he or she is operating in another role (such as avenger, rescuer, bully, nag, friend, disciplinarian, confidante, confederate, or playmate).
- The consultant regularly evaluates his or her own performances and uses that evaluation as an opportunity for learning.

Consultation Requires Developed Communication and Relationship-Building Skills.
- Consultation is always about relationship, particularly listening and valuing.
- Consultation begins when the objectives of the consultee and the type of consultation desired are clarified, and agreement about roles and responsibilities exists.
- Consultation should be deferred if the consultant or consultee is upset or frustrated.

The Consultant Helps Consultees to Develop Their Own Solutions.
- Consultation is based on the belief that people want to do a good job; communicate high expectations and trust in the consultee's abilities.
- The consultant provides options, recommends resources, and gives opinions, but ultimately, the consultee must decide upon the final solution.
- The consultant solicits ideas from the consultee using active listening and without critiquing, prior to offering his or her own ideas.
- Inviting feedback about an action plan or advice the consultant has offered allows the consultee to be in control of the process.
- Sometimes consultation provides solutions, and sometimes it provides assistance that helps consultees to find the solution themselves; consider the difficulty of the task and the experience and preferences of the consultee.
- Consider whether the consultee is essentially seeking reassurance and confirmation; use this as an opportunity to offer validation and strengthen competence.

Consultation Should Focus on Strengths and Opportunities, Not Weaknesses and Problems.
- Asking "why" may be experienced as a blaming or fault-finding question.
- The consultant should avoid giving advice, but rather should provide information the consultee can use to solve the problem.
- Acknowledge and show appreciation for each person's contribution.

The Consultant Is Always an Educator.
- The consultant should educate people as a supportive partner and coach, promoting self-sufficiency.
- The consultant should provide consultees with the tools needed to build skills for success in their goals.

Figure 19-5. Principles of Effective Consultation

Note. Based on information from Block, 1999; Lippitt & Lippitt, 1986; Yoder-Wise & Kowalski, 2006.

The process of consultation described here is formal, but consultation also may be informal. Informal consultations include brief interactions around a circumscribed problem, quick questions to the consultant, or a brief and simple request for specific information. The consultant considers whether meeting these informal requests for information fully addresses the problem or whether the request signals a broader problem requiring a more comprehensive approach. In the latter situation, the APN may still meet the informal consultation request, while at the same time suggesting that a more comprehensive and thorough investigation of the problem and potential solutions might be considered.

Barron and White (2000) distinguished consultation from clinical and administrative supervision and from comanagement, collaboration, and referral. Clarity regarding the differences among these processes is important in APN consultation, in part because the APN role includes expert practice. Although consultation and clinical and administrative supervision share the goal of developing the knowledge, skills, self-esteem, and autonomy of another (hereafter referred to as the subordinate), a hierarchical relationship exists. The supervisor is responsible for safeguarding the care of the subordinate's patients, and the supervisor is accountable for the subordinate's work. Comanagement, collaboration, and referral may result from a consultation, but they are not considered to be consultative activities. Comanagement of the patient or referral of the patient to the APN for specific services may occur during the delivery of care. For example, the APN may manage some aspects of care for a patient (such as providing complex teaching, running a family meeting, or performing a complex dressing change) while the staff nurse manages other aspects of that same patient's care. The staff nurse may refer a patient to the APN for sexual counseling, and the APN may refer a patient to the staff nurse for management of a potentially occluded central venous catheter. Given the multidimensional nature of their roles, APNs are engaged in all of these activities, but what differentiates the activities is the issue of responsibility for the outcome of care. In comanagement, collaboration, and referral, the APN and the RN each share specific responsibilities for delivering the intervention and evaluating its effects. With consultation, the staff nurse retains responsibility for delivering the intervention to the patient under his or her care, and the APN is responsible for the quality of the recommendations to the RN and for clearly managing and documenting the process of consultation.

Resistance to change, complacency or apathy, feelings of implied threat or criticism, and unfamiliarity of seeking consultation with an APN can impede development of the consultant role. As APNs enter a new organization or team as a consultant, it is important that they meet with administrators, physicians, nurses, and leaders and members of the interdisciplinary team to learn more about the needs of the team, identify key players, and describe their role and areas of expertise. Visibility is essential to be utilized as a consultant. For example, in an inpatient setting, making regular unit rounds and attending interdisciplinary team meetings, shift reports, and family conferences will help APNs to identify patients with complex clinical needs who could benefit from consultation. With each consultation request, APNs have an opportunity to demonstrate their areas of expertise and to provide informal education about the types of cases that are appropriate for future consultations.

Educator

Delivering education to patients and families, serving as an educator and preceptor for nurses in graduate nursing education, and providing specialty education to staff nurses and other members of the healthcare team are key components of the APN role. In fulfilling the role of educator with patients, families, students, and staff, APNs must apply a systematic process to the development, implementation, and evaluation of education. The educational process begins with a learning needs assessment, followed by development of learning objectives, selection of the method or methods of instruction, and design of the program, and concludes with program evaluation. Each of these steps in the educational process is guided by one or more learning theories and by adult learning principles.

Theoretical perspectives relevant to learning: Educational interventions are guided by a number of different theoretical orientations. Some interventions are drawn from the disciplines of educational, social, cognitive, behavioral, or developmental psychology, whereas others are based on stress and coping, change, or systems theories. In an educator role, APNs may apply several of these theoretical frameworks simultaneously.

Integrating new information at a time of vulnerability, crisis, anxiety, and fear presents challenges. Shortened length of inpatient hospital stays, the shifting of care to outpatient settings, the aging of the population, and the costs and complexities of technologically advanced treatment modalities compound these challenges. Increasing diversity within the U.S. population creates an imperative that educators incorporate theoretical knowledge of cultural, ethnic, and religious diversity in healthcare beliefs, lifestyle practices, and communication styles into adult learning theory (Chachkes & Christ, 1996). Table 19-2 summarizes theoretical perspectives that can be applied to explain and understand the process of teaching and motivating health behavior change in adults.

Table 19-2. Theoretical Perspectives for Teaching and Motivating Healthy Behavior

Theory	Major Concept(s)	Key Principles	Application to Teaching, Motivating, and Health Behavior Change
Operant/conditioned learning behavioral models	Stimulus-response linkages conditioned by reinforcements (rewards)	Reinforced behaviors will occur frequently. Desired behaviors can be elicited through shaping and reinforcement.	Assessment of learner includes consideration of • Factors reinforcing undesirable health behaviors • Factors for motivating and reinforcing desired health behaviors.
Cognitive/information processing	Behavior and affect result from insights, principles, concepts, relationships, generalizations, rules, or theories held by the individual, and effecting change in one or more of these dimensions mediates all behavior change.	Teaching-learning occurs by reorganizing perceptual or cognitive fields (including principles, relationships, concepts, theories, or rules) through purposive involvement, cooperative and interactive inquiry, problem solving, and problem raising.	Suggests importance of insights, memory, outlook, and thought patterns for cognitive, affective, and psychomotor learning and problem solving

---

(Continued on next page)

Table 19-2. Theoretical Perspectives for Teaching and Motivating Healthy Behavior
(Continued)

Theory	Major Concept(s)	Key Principles	Application to Teaching, Motivating, and Health Behavior Change
Mastery learning	Any behavior or task can be broken down into its component behaviors.	Breaks down complex units of instruction into the smallest component parts and then builds complex behaviors/tasks by putting the smaller units together.	Offers helpful principles when learning requires mastery of several skills
Social learning	Beliefs that one is capable of performing a certain behavior and that performance of that behavior will produce the desired outcome	Four sources of information influence the process of learning: personal mastery, vicarious experiences, verbal persuasion, and physiologic feedback.	Suggests that health education should include strategies to build self-confidence and enhance self-efficacy as a means to achieve sustained behavior change
Compliance model	The extent to which a patient's health behaviors (taking medication, following a diet) coincides with the recommendations and/or prescriptions of healthcare providers	Control of health and illness is associated directly with compliance with provider-directed regimens. An individual's noncompliance with the provider's recommendations/prescriptions may be the result of a lack of knowledge, defiance/opposition/denial, or emotional distress.	Emphasizes importance of interventions to motivate patients to accept treatment plans as valuable and provides them with knowledge, skills, and encouragement to change behavior patterns to fit the requirements of the regimen
Health belief model	Contrast of compliers and noncompliers relative to • Their perceptions of the severity of illness • Their susceptibility to illness and its consequences • The value of the benefits of treatment • The barriers to and costs of treatment • The cues that stimulate health-related actions	Identifies factors that influence compliance or noncompliance with a health professional's recommendations for care. Emphasizes an avoidance orientation related to seeking preventive care to decrease the probability of negative health and illness outcomes	Helpful in identifying barriers to and costs of prevention, early detection, and treatment as prominent factors associated with preventive health practices or maintenance of illness regimens

(Continued on next page)

Table 19-2. Theoretical Perspectives for Teaching and Motivating Healthy Behavior
(Continued)

Theory	Major Concept(s)	Key Principles	Application to Teaching, Motivating, and Health Behavior Change
Health promotion model	Individuals strive for health, well-being, enjoyment, and fulfillment, and they self-initiate behaviors directed toward attaining higher levels of health.	Cognitive-perceptual factors that determine health promotion activities include the importance of health, perceived self-efficacy, and perceived benefits and barriers. These cognitive-perceptual factors are modified by demographic variables, expectations, past experiences with health professionals and with other behavioral change, biologic variables, and situational variables, such as access. The likelihood of engaging in health promotion behaviors depends upon cues to action, including a desire for increased well-being, interaction with others interested in health promotion, advice, and information.	Identifies the essential role of the healthcare professional in assisting individuals to overcome barriers to health-promoting activities, increasing the importance of positive consequences of preferred behaviors, and reducing the frequency of negative consequences.
Transtheoretical model of the stages of change	Change is a series of stages, each with its own characteristics and each amenable to different interventions.	Stages of change are precontemplation, contemplation, preparation, action, and maintenance.	Can be used to guide assessment of stage of change and to tailor interventions
Stress and coping theory	Evaluation of a stimulus as stressful depends upon the individual's cognitive appraisal of the situation as exceeding available personal resources within one's environment. Cognitive appraisal includes two dimensions: (1) Does this situation threaten me? and (2) What can I do about it?	Coping consists of cognitive and behavioral efforts to manage specific demands that are appraised as stressful or exceeding personal resources. Coping resources include positive beliefs, problem-solving skills, and social skills. Coping styles in responding to stressful or threatening situations lie along a continuum from monitoring (a tendency to seek information, worry, and remain vigilant) to blunting (a tendency to avoid or distract oneself).	Healthcare providers can assist patients in managing stress by providing educational interventions to enhance problem-solving and social skills and strengthen positive beliefs.

(Continued on next page)

Table 19-2. Theoretical Perspectives for Teaching and Motivating Healthy Behavior
(Continued)

Theory	Major Concept(s)	Key Principles	Application to Teaching, Motivating, and Health Behavior Change
Self-regulation or common sense theory	An individual's understanding of an illness is the critical factor in his or her decisions about compliance with recommendations, self-care management, and coping response.	Illness representations are constructed from accumulated experiences over time and are an integration of knowledge gathered from the media, personal contacts, health professionals' input, symptoms and body sensations, and past experiences with illness. An illness representation has four features: identity of concrete symptoms, the cause of the problem, the timeline of the problem (how long it will last), and the consequences of the problem.	Assessment of the learner should include an evaluation of his or her illness representation and consideration of how this representation shapes behavior, self-care management, and coping responses.
Explanatory models of health and illness	In an attempt to attribute meaning to seemingly disordered events, patients and families interpret the events, symptoms, and illnesses they experience into explanatory models.	Explanatory models of health and illness are shaped by cultural factors. Explanatory models of health and illness shape individuals' understanding of what caused their health problem, why it started, what the illness is doing to their body, how long the illness will occur, and what kind of treatment they should be given.	Assists healthcare professionals to tailor educational interventions to harmonize with patients' explanatory model and/or to evolve with the patients a mutual representation of the healthcare problem that promotes healthy behaviors and progress toward improved health and well-being
Ecological systems theory	Individuals can only be understood in reciprocity with their environmental context. Environmental contexts are nested within each other and include the chronosystem (the developmental processes and life transitions experienced by the individual), the microsystem (activities, family relationships, and material environment of the home), the mesosystems (e.g., school, work, social network), exosystems (social systems, institutions, government), and macrosystems (cultures, larger society).	Individuals and their behavior can only be understood with the context of their chronosystem, microsystem, mesosystem, exosystem, and macrosystem.	Individual behavior is shaped, restricted, and reinforced by a variety of systems, and thus, much less "individual choice" may exist than other theories of learning suggest.

(Continued on next page)

Table 19-2. Theoretical Perspectives for Teaching and Motivating Healthy Behavior
(Continued)

Theory	Major Concept(s)	Key Principles	Application to Teaching, Motivating, and Health Behavior Change
Life span developmental frameworks	The interrelationships among chronologic age, normative developmental trajectories, cohort experiences, and non-normative life events	Biologic, environmental, and behavioral determinants, in conjunction with specified developmental influences, shape the life span of individuals and families.	In developing patient education, factors that should be considered include normative chronologic or age-graded factors (e.g., reading ability), historical events that influence particular birth cohorts (e.g., war, natural disasters), and life events that occur asynchronously with the life course (e.g., illness in young adults).
Motivational interviewing	Fears of, need for, and commitment to behavior change	Emphasizes resolution of ambivalence regarding change Includes respectful and individualized discussion that addresses six key elements: (1) feedback about personal risk factors, (2) personal responsibility for change, (3) advice to change, (4) suggestions or a menu of approaches by which change might be achieved, (5) empathy and listening style of counseling, and (6) messages that support self-efficacy for change	Details principles for the delivery of interventions to help patients to resolve ambivalence about changing health-related behaviors and adhering to health professional recommendations

Note. Based on information from Leventhal & Cameron, 1987; Rankin & Stallings, 1996; Rankin et al., 2005; Saarmann et al., 2000.

Patient and family education: Ensuring that patients and families are active participants in their health care requires that they possess necessary knowledge and skill. Knowledge enables patients to take necessary self-care actions to prevent the development of complications, to intervene quickly when problems develop, and to comply with needed procedures and therapies. It also assists them in interacting effectively with healthcare personnel, making decisions that are congruent with their preferences, and taking the necessary steps to maintain or regain health. From a cognitive-behavioral perspective, knowledge promotes a constructive understanding of the illness process, eliminates erroneous beliefs, enhances coping and problem solving, and mitigates anxiety, fear, uncertainty, and worry. In providing education, the entire family unit, including any people who are significant to the patient's daily life, must be included.

The process begins with an evaluation of patient and family learning needs (Timmins, 2006). A significant body of literature examines the information needs of patients and families across the process of diagnosis and treatment and through recovery or end of life (Chelf et al., 2001; Jansen, van Weert, van Dulmen, Heeren, & Bensing, 2007; Rutten, Arora, Bakos, Aziz, & Rowland, 2005; Timmins; Treacy & Mayer, 2000). Techniques for gleaning the information needs of patients include advisory groups, critical incident technique, focus groups, interviews, professional standards, questionnaires, and surveys. To establish priorities for delivery of patient and family education, the clinician begins by focusing on the patient's learning needs. The ONS *Standards of Oncology Education: Patient/Significant Other and Public* (3rd ed.) (Blecher, 2004) and the National Cancer Institute (1998) *Guidelines for Establishing Comprehensive Cancer Patient Education Services* provide APNs with comprehensive guidelines for the development of formal and informal educational programs for patients and their families.

A variety of factors influence patients' information-seeking behaviors and readiness for learning, including coping style, education level, motivation, learning style, health literacy, expectations, values, culture, decision-making preferences, physical and psychological comfort, energy level, developmental stage, and physical, physiologic, and cognitive capabilities. Each of these factors is considered when developing objectives for individual or group education, as well as in the design and evaluation of educational materials. Many commercially prepared educational materials are available for teaching patients. Prepared materials can be used to teach new information and to augment or reinforce previously taught information. Use of prepared materials can be effective and efficient, but these materials must be evaluated for their relevance to learning need, content accuracy, and readability. Some of the factors to consider when developing or evaluating educational materials are listed in Figure 19-6. Language differences between pa-

---

- Is the content accurate, current, and of sufficient breadth and depth?
- Is the content organized logically?
- Are the facts presented in a manner that is balanced and unbiased?
- Does it provide details of additional sources of support and information?
- Does it provide support for shared decision making?
- Does the content achieve the objectives that need to be accomplished?
- Is the material interesting?
- Is the material divided into short sections with good use of titles, subtitles, or headlines?
- Is the level of detail provided fitting to the audience?
- Are the key points emphasized with underlining, bullets, or asterisks?
- Is the material enhanced with illustrations and pictures?
- Is the material visually appealing with font size, layout, and use of white space chosen effectively?
- Is the reading level appropriate?
- Does the material communicate the message using short words and sentences?
- Does the material offer a definition for all technical terms?
- Does it use everyday language, explaining unusual or medical words, abbreviations, and jargon?
- Does the information include a summary?
- Does the document have a designated space in which the reader can make notes?
- Does the document contain contact details for the healthcare services where the reader can receive care or treatment for problems discussed in the document?
- Does the document use generic names for all medications or products instead of or in addition to brand names?
- Is the material written by knowledgeable health professionals?
- Is there any indication of the effectiveness of the materials?
- Are the materials cost effective?

Figure 19-6. Factors to Consider When Developing or Evaluating Educational Materials

---

Note. Based on information from Doak et al., 1996; Frost et al., 1999; Hagopian, 1996; Moult et al., 2004; Rees et al., 2002.

tients and nurses present an obvious obstacle to communication and patient education. Professional interpreters, bilingual professional staff members, and volunteers may facilitate communication. Many prepared materials are available in languages other than English, although these should be similarly evaluated in terms of the dimensions outlined previously.

Staff education: Providing specialty education can enhance provision of competent patient care, improve job satisfaction, and promote recruitment and retention. The format of education delivered to staff nurses and other healthcare team members can range from brief unit-based in-services focusing on a specific aspect of diagnosis or treatment to a formal presentation at a national conference. Creative teaching and learning strategies include case study discussions, journal clubs, computer-assisted instruction, programmed instructional modules, games, and simulation. Demonstrations enhance variety and encourage learning at one's own pace, reinforce content, and build critical-thinking skills. In developing curriculum and evaluating continuing education programs for oncology nurses, the ONS *Standards of Oncology Education: Generalist and Advanced Practice Levels* (3rd ed.) (Jacobs, 2003b) is a useful guide for APNs. Adult learning principles, as summarized in Figure 19-7, can be incorporated into the design, delivery, and evaluation of learning activities. Barriers to staff participation in educational programs are addressed as part of the planning process. APNs can overcome some of these barriers by keeping content relevant to the audience, by considering financial, geographic, and timing issues in program logistics, and by ensuring that educational program faculty members are credible, knowledgeable, experienced, flexible, and skilled.

The development of educational programs is guided by specific and measurable objectives that describe what cognitive, affective, or psychomotor learning will result from the educational program. Objectives describe what the learners are expected to do and how well they must perform, if they have mastered the objective. Table 19-3 provides a taxonomy of educational objectives along with verbs that can be used in developing objectives that reflect each dimension of learning.

- Adult learners must perceive a need for information based on knowledge or skills needed to perform more effectively.
- Learning objectives must be relevant and timely.
- Commitment to the learning experience increases with learner engagement.
- Adults are problem or task oriented. Educational activities need to focus on the resolution of problems or completion of tasks.
- The educator is more of a facilitator and resource person and less of an instructor/transmitter of knowledge; emphasis is on partnership to clearly define learning goals and the means to achieve them.
- Learning activities should recognize and build upon the significant body of experiences that adult learners possess.
- Adult learners have multiple demands on their time. Education therefore should be self-paced, efficient, and self-directed and should allow for flexibility in scheduling.
- The learning environment should be physically and psychologically comfortable, reflect mutual respect, and allow for freedom of expression.
- Feedback is necessary for adult learners, and positive reinforcement can facilitate learning.
- Adults are motivated to learn by both extrinsic (pay, promotion) and intrinsic (self-esteem, personal achievement) rewards.

Figure 19-7. Adult Learning Principles

Note. Based on information from McCorkle et al., 1996.

Table 19-3. Developing Specific and Measurable Educational Objectives

Domain	Level	Definition	Sample Descriptors/ Verbs for Objectives
Cognitive	Knowledge	Recalls previous material	Identifies
	Comprehension	Grasps meaning of material	Describes
			Recognizes
	Application	Applies material in a new situation	Recalls
	Analysis	Breaks down material into components and understands structures	Exemplifies
			Classifies
	Synthesis	Puts components together to form a new whole	Summarizes
			Compares
	Evaluation	Judges the value of material based on defined criteria	Contrasts
			Explains
			Generates
			Plans
			Produces
Affective	Receiving	Aware of and listens to new information	Discusses
	Responding	Actively reacts to a phenomenon	Interprets
	Valuing	Attaches value to a phenomenon or behavior	Expresses
	Organization	Concerned about the relationships between values	Reflects
			Manifests
	Characterization by a value	Holds value system that controls behavior	Behaves in accord with values
Psychomotor	Imitation	Begins crude and imperfect form of skill after observation	Executes
			Implements
	Manipulation	Practices to improve performance	Demonstrates
	Precision	Performs refined, accurate skill	Performs
	Articulation	Efficiently coordinates skill with other activities	Coordinates
	Naturalization	Automatically proficient on cue	

Note. Based on information from Anderson & Krathwohl, 2001; Reilly & Oermann, 1992.

Evaluation strategies, a component of program planning, are chosen to match the learning objectives. Examples of evaluation strategies include tests of knowledge, performance checklists, return demonstrations, peer evaluation, case presentations, and expert review or audit of performance. Evaluation strategies can be formative or summative. Formative evaluation is a method of judging the worth of a program while the program activities are forming or happening. It gives information about the process of learning and what additional information might be needed. In contrast, summative evaluation occurs at the end of a learning activity and is focused on the extent to which the stated objectives or outcomes were achieved. When testing of knowledge or a competency is used for summative evaluation, those tests may be criterion-referenced (i.e., achievement of criterion of 85% of questions correct) or norm-referenced (i.e., achievement is compared with a larger group of learners, for example, with national standardized examinations) (Popham, 1975).

Evaluation of educational programs includes a determination of progress toward meeting the learning objectives (i.e., outcomes evaluation) and how effectively the educational program was delivered (i.e., process evaluation). Process evaluation refers to a systematic method of assessing implementation. The goal of process evaluation is to use data to provide a description of how a program is operating compared with the manner in which the program was intended to operate. Some questions that process evaluations might address include the following: How many nurses attended the educational session? What are their characteristics? How long did it take for participants to complete the program? Were the educational facilities acceptable? Were the objectives met? An outcome evaluation, on the other hand, provides a picture of the results or effectiveness of a program in achieving its intended goals. Depending upon the goals, questions addressed by an outcome evaluation might include the following: Did program participants learn how to effectively perform a particular procedure? Did the educational program result in satisfactory scores on a test of chemotherapy administration knowledge?

Nurses practicing in the field of cancer nursing need to develop and sustain a commitment to lifelong learning. APNs can role-model this for staff in a variety of ways, including demonstrating clinical curiosity, showing responsibility for one's own learning and for the need to remain current with an ever-expanding scientific knowledge base in oncology, actively participating in a professional organization's activities, and regularly reading professional journals.

Researcher

The APN's role in research includes participation in all phases of the research process, research evaluation and critique, research utilization, and the conduct and dissemination of research. McGuire and Harwood (2000) distinguished research competencies of APNs in terms of those that should be present at the time of graduation from those that develop through experience, mentoring, and individual initiative. They identified three levels of research involvement. At level 1, the APN is involved in facilitating clinical research and using research as a foundation for practice. Level 2 competencies focus on evaluating practice using a range of relevant clinical outcomes. At level 3, the APN is involved in generating new knowledge through collaborative and independent research. Table 19-4 shows how the levels are associated with specific research competencies and levels of activity.

Table 19-4. Overview of Research Competencies and Levels of Activity

Competency	Basic Level	Advanced Level
I. Interpretation and use of research	• Incorporate relevant research findings appropriately into own practice • Assist others to incorporate research into individual or unit practice	• Develop programmatic and/or departmental research utilization process
II. Evaluation of practice	• Use existing data to evaluate nursing practice, individual and/or aggregate • Collaborate in conduct of evaluation studies	• Identify and/or develop practice-specific package of outcome criteria • Lead the conduct of evaluation studies
III. Participation in collaborative research	• Identify research problems • Develop study procedures • Assist with recruitment • Participate in interventions • Identify nurse-sensitive outcomes • Collect outcomes data	–

Note. From "Research," by D.B. McGuire and K.V. Harwood in A. Hamric, J. Spross, and C. Hanson (Eds.), *Advanced Nursing Practice: An Integrative Approach* (p. 253), 2000, Philadelphia: Saunders. Copyright 2000 by Saunders. Reprinted with permission.

An understanding of good clinical practices for the conduct of research (American Society of Clinical Oncology [ASCO], 2003) and thorough knowledge of critical appraisal are the core skills needed to achieve level 1 competencies. Also needed are skills in posing a clinical question that is answerable with evidence and the ability to locate and retrieve evidence. At level 2, the APN is engaged in evaluating practice by examining the extent to which desired clinical, system, and fiscal outcomes are achieved. This requires familiarity with the various outcomes that may be measured, as well as an ability to critically assess outcome measurement tools for their reliability, validity, and sensitivity to change. Additional research competencies include the capacity to distinguish research from quality improvement (Thurston, Watson, & Reimer, 1993), knowledge of the principles of the design, conduct, statistical analysis, and interpretation of outcome evaluation research, and effective written and oral presentation skills. APNs prepared at the doctoral level are more likely to have the skills necessary to function at level 2. Other APNs may need some degree of expert consultation in statistical analysis or collaboration with a nurse researcher in selecting an outcome measure, designing the study, and interpreting and disseminating the results (Drenning, 2006).

Goldberg and Moch (1998) described an APN–nurse researcher collaborative model. In this model, the APN offers a strong clinical base in nursing with advanced practice skills and detailed knowledge of the clinical institution. Both of these are necessary to the design and conduct of a clinical research study. The nurse researcher brings a strong theoretical base in nursing, together with skills in research design and statistical analysis and expertise in disseminating findings through publications and presentations. This model is designed to assist APNs to be involved in the generation and dissemination of new knowledge and to receive the additional expert support and coaching necessary to achieve level 2 and 3 competencies without doctoral preparation. These levels are not mutually exclusive, and an APN may function at one or more levels of research participation simultaneously. Collaborative academic-service partnerships between nurses in practice and academic settings (Horns et al., 2007) may be an effective mechanism to establish such APN–nurse researcher collaborations.

Challenges in Advanced Practice Nurse Role Implementation

The process of implementing an APN role is complex, dynamic, and varied. Hardy and Hardy (1988) differentiated role stress, role strain, role conflict, role ambiguity, and role incongruity. *Role stress* is a condition in which role obligations are conflicting, ambiguous, incongruous, excessive, or unpredictable. *Role strain* is the feeling of frustration, tension, or anxiety that results from the experience of role stress. *Role conflict* occurs when the role expectations held by the APN, supervisors, and/or other members of the interdisciplinary team are incompatible. APNs may experience interprofessional role conflicts (e.g., between APNs and physicians) and intraprofessional (e.g., between APNs and other nurses) role conflicts. *Role ambiguity* occurs when a lack of clarity exists regarding the expectations of the APN role or when uncertainty exists about how the APN will meet those expectations. On the other hand, *role incongruity* occurs when a discrepancy exists between the role expectations held by the APN and those held by stakeholders, such as the supervisor or colleagues on the clinical team.

Hardy and Hardy (1988) maintained that role strain accompanies major role transitions and may actually facilitate role transition by increasing awareness of gaps in knowledge and skill. The development of strategies to cope with role stress can minimize role strain. Factors contributing to role stress include role ambiguity, role conflict, and role incongruity (Glen & Waddington, 1998). Role ambiguity results when a lack of clarity about expectations, a blurring of responsibilities, or uncertainty about role implementation exists (Brykczynski, 2000). For many APNs, role ambiguity exists in terms of how to operationalize various roles, who is or should be the primary customer of APN services (patients or staff), where APNs should target their interventions, the amount of autonomy, and a lack of optimal reporting structure. Role conflict develops when role expectations are perceived as contradictory or mutually exclusive. Role conflict may occur between APNs and members of other disciplines and between APNs and other members of the nursing profession. For example, the staff nurse group may perceive that discharge planning is the role of the APN, whereas the APN believes it is the staff nurses' responsibility to coordinate discharge planning and that the APN contribution is as an expert on the team for difficult cases. Role conflict also can develop between the APN and other disciplines, including social workers or physicians. Role incongruity may emerge when a mismatch occurs between one's skills and the obligations of the role. An example of role incongruity is a new APN who has not yet developed strong skills in invasive procedures but is mandated to fulfill this role expectation without sufficient additional training, support, and mentoring. Role incongruity also develops when role expectations are not well matched with strengths, talents, and expected role behaviors. For example, role incongruity can develop if the APN has strong skills in communication and education but must spend most of his or her time developing practice protocols or attending committee meetings.

Characteristics of the work setting (office location, resources available, time pressures, competing objectives, size, complexity, and distribution of patient population) and the administrative structure (structural placement of APNs within the organization, reporting structure, autonomy, consonance between goals and expectations of individual APNs, supervisor, and organization) have a major influence on APN role definition and expectation. A thoroughly developed strategic plan for APN role implementation at both a departmental and corporate level is essential (Cummings & McLennan, 2005). Bryant-Lukosius and DiCenso (2004) offered a framework to guide the development, implementation, utilization, and evaluation of APN roles. They suggested that APN role implementation and utilization should include an examination by all stakeholders of how well the model of care and relationships among team members and services are meeting patients' health needs. Based on an understanding of gaps in met needs, priority problems and goals are identified, and then a revised model of care that notes the APN's role in that model is defined.

Strategies to promote role implementation are tailored to the specific phase of role implementation (Brykczynski, 2000). During role acquisition, APN students benefit from identification with a role model, realistic clinical experiences, and the opportunity to develop competency profiles and gain direct experience with all core skills. Faculty practice, panel discussions, and self and peer evaluation can facilitate role implementation as the APN transitions into practice. As the APN transitions to his or her initial role, a structured, goal-oriented plan for the first two years of role function and identification of a role model are essential. These goals and the structured plan for role implementation ideally are negotiated with the supervisor, and progress is reviewed at each supervisory meeting. Plans for system change should be delayed until the APN is able to fully assess the system and can identify and manage barriers to change. The emphasis in the first phase of role development is on developing role clarity and resolving role incongruity; networking; building effective relationships within the interdisciplinary team and the organization; clinical mastery; and participation in key committees and strategic initiatives (Glen & Waddington, 1998). To minimize role ambiguity and role conflict, it is important to clarify the purpose and multidimensionality of the APN role in terms of expert practice, practice development, education, research, and leadership. Definition of the relationship between the APN role and the role of other care providers and clarification of issues of accountability, autonomy, collaboration, communication, reporting mechanisms, and reimbursement also are important aspects of developing a new APN role (Bryant-Lukosius & DiCenso, 2004).

Once the APN role is established, efforts focus on managing priorities, developing and implementing small-scale projects to demonstrate effectiveness, and gradual broadening of organizational impact. A formal process of goal setting with the supervisor and regular review of progress remain essential to APN success. Development of a support system that allows periodic self-evaluation; a place to manage anger, frustration, or dissatisfaction; and a mechanism to prevent complacency are fundamental to maximize outcomes once the APN role is implemented and integrated within the organization (Brykczynski, 2000; Glen & Waddington, 1998). Mechanisms to ensure continued professional development and sustain clinical competency may be accomplished through continuing education and a network of peer and informational support for management of ongoing role challenges (Lynch et al., 2001; Robison et al., 2004).

Advanced Practice Nurse Skills That Contribute to Improved Outcomes

Evidence-Based Clinical Decision Making, Critical Thinking, and Scholarly Practice

Evidence-based practice is an essential component of quality nursing care and an essential competency for all healthcare professionals. APNs have a fundamental role in building capacity for evidence-based practice in the staff and in promoting the translation of new research into clinical practice. Assisting staff in this process is accomplished by communicating and actively disseminating research findings and promoting system readiness to adopt innovations (DeBourgh, 2001; Profetto-McGrath, Smith, Hugo, Taylor, & El-Hajj, 2007). The process of evidence-based clinical decision making begins by posing an answerable clinical question, searching the literature for relevant information, and then performing a critical appraisal. If change is warranted by the research evidence and fits with clinician skills, resource availability, and patient preferences, the process follows with implementation of the change in practice and outcomes evaluation (Upchurch, Brosnan, & Grimes, 2002).

Translating research evidence into clinical decisions, tools, and programs improves outcomes for patients and staff. This process begins with a critical appraisal of the available literature. The steps in critical appraisal are summarized in Figure 19-8. The goal of critical appraisal is to evaluate the scientific merit and potential clinical applicability of each study's findings. This can be applied to a group of studies covering similar problem areas to determine what findings have a strong enough basis to be used in clinical practice. Users of research need to know how much confidence they can place in the underlying evidence and recommendations. Critical appraisal is balanced and respectful, and if contradictory evidence exists, the full scope of the controversy is con-

- Acquire overall perspective and identify the level of evidence (systematic review, randomized controlled trial, uncontrolled trial, case series, qualitative study, expert opinion).
- Apply critique criteria based on level of evidence:
  - Quantitative
  - Qualitative
  - Guidelines or systematic review.
- Summarize major study elements and findings using a standardized comparative template.
- Identify the strengths and weaknesses.
- Determine the potential applicability of the study to practice.
  - Are setting and sample comparable to your population?
  - Are study findings positive? Equivocal? Negative?
- Is the effect size balanced with potential side effects, cost, feasibility, and patient preferences?
- Determine collective weight of the evidence of this study in comparison to other studies, balancing study quality, findings, and applicability to practice.
- Synthesize the evidence for dissemination to influence practice and improve patient outcomes (protocol, practice standard, policy and procedure, guidelines, patient and family education, integrated review, publication/presentation).

Figure 19-8. Steps in Critical Appraisal of Research

Note. Based on information from DiCenso, Guyatt, et al., 2005; Melnyk & Fineout-Overholt, 2005.

sidered. Critical appraisal is like any other skill: It is learned through practice and dialogue with others. Journal clubs, colleague discussions, problem-based learning, and structured debates (Profetto-McGrath, 2005) are ideal ways to develop skills and discernment in critical appraisal.

The first step in critical appraisal is to determine the level of evidence a particular study represents. Different levels of evidence should be critiqued using somewhat different criteria, and the strength of one's conclusions across studies is influenced by the level of evidence. Figure 19-9 presents an example of an evidence hierarchy, with expert opinion representing the weakest evidence and meta-analysis and systematic reviews of randomized trials representing the strongest evidence. Next, a table is prepared organizing, summarizing, and synthesizing the individual pieces of evidence. This table of evidence or evidence profile highlights what is known, identifies gaps, and gives direction to the application of evidence in clinical practice. An example of a table of evidence is provided in Table 19-5. The next step is to examine the strengths and weaknesses of the study. Guidelines for identifying methodologic weaknesses and limitations of quantitative and qualitative studies are presented in Figures 19-10 and 19-11. In evaluating clinical practice guidelines (Balk, Lau, & Bonis, 2005; Barroso, Sandelowski, & Voils, 2006; Bigby & Williams, 2003; DiCenso, Ciliska, Dobbins, & Guyatt, 2005; Ricci, Celani, & Righetti, 2006; Wimpenny & van Zelm, 2007), one considers why the guideline was developed, the composition (expertise and disciplinary perspective) of the panel that developed the guideline, and the entity of financial sponsorship. The decision-making process (expert opinion, consensus opinion, systematic review of evidence, or some combination) used in developing the guideline is determined. The clinical question for which the guideline was developed to address is verified. Other questions to pose in critically evaluating guidelines include: Were gaps in the evidence explicitly identified? How explicitly is the evidence linked to the recommendations in the guideline? If lower levels of evidence are incorporated (e.g., expert opinion), how explicitly is this labeled? Are the reasons for the inclusion of expert opinion, the line of reasoning, and the strength of extrapolation from other data clearly identified? How are

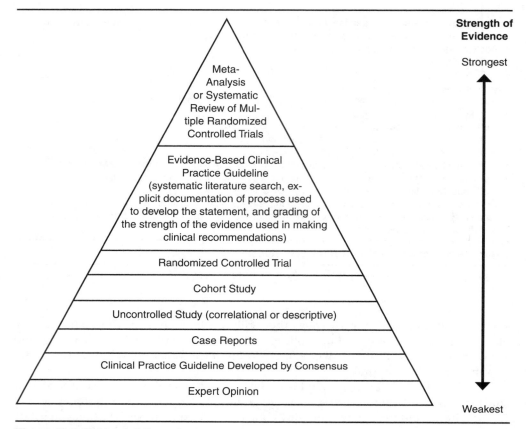

Figure 19-9. Evidence Hierarchy

patient preferences incorporated into the guideline? Is cost effectiveness considered? What is the mechanism and interval for updating the guideline?

Next, the study's potential applicability to practice is determined, taking into consideration several factors. Are the setting and sample comparable to the practice's population? Are study findings positive, equivocal, or negative? Does the effect size (the strength of the relationship between intervention and outcome) balance the potential side effects and costs of the intervention? Is the intervention feasible and consistent with patient preferences? If multiple studies of a given intervention exist, the weight of evidence across studies must be determined, balancing study quality, findings, and the applicability to practice. The last step in the critical appraisal of research is synthesis of the evidence for dissemination in order to influence practice and improve patient outcomes. This can occur through development of a protocol, a practice standard, policy, guidelines, patient and family educational materials, or an integrated review of the literature developed for journal publication.

In summary, oncology APNs make an essential contribution to improved outcomes by role modeling a systematic, evidence-based approach to clinical decision making and through the leadership of initiatives that translate research into practice. With responsibilities for expert practice, education, research, and consultation, the oncology APN

Table 19-5. Example of a Table of Evidence: Advanced Practice Nurse (APN) Interventions and Outcomes

Author	Study Design, Sample, and Setting	APN Description	APN Intervention Provided	Outcome Variables Measured	Selected Findings
Brooten et al., 1994	Randomized controlled trial Designed to evaluate early discharge and home follow-up of women having unplanned cesarean birth Subjects randomized to early discharge with clinical nurse specialist (CNS) follow-up or standardized control group care with no follow-up Data collected from delivery to eight weeks postpartum	CNS	Transitional homecare services Comprehensive discharge planning, instruction, and counseling Daily "on-call" availability Home visit activities such as physical examination of mother and baby; assessment of wound healing, sleeping patterns, emotional status, coping ability to perform child care, home environment Confirmation of follow-up appointments	Maternal and infant length of stay Satisfaction with care Rehospitalizations Acute care visits Anxiety or depression Overall function Costs (rehospitalization, acute care visits)	Earlier discharge group was sent home a mean of 30.3 hours sooner than control. Significantly greater satisfaction with care More timely infant immunizations No statistically significant difference in maternal or neonatal rehospitalization or acute care visits No differences between groups in maternal affect or functional status Conclusion: Nurse specialist transitional care is safe, feasible, and cost effective.

Note. Based on information from Cunningham, 2004.

role is ideally positioned to support clinical staff in identifying, critically appraising, and synthesizing the literature, and to direct organizational initiatives to disseminate evidence and to promote widespread adoption of best practices based on evidence.

Collaboration

Providing quality care often involves partnerships and collaboration. Partnership is a team-based approach to achieving a stated goal. Collaboration is the process of working together within the negotiated framework to achieve the goal of the partnership. In collaboration, values are shared, respect is mutual, and power is shared equally (Hanson, Spross, & Carr, 2000). O'Neill and Krauel (2004) suggested that the building blocks of an effective partnership include a shared agenda and mutually beneficial goals, each partner bringing value and assets to the partnership and demonstrating accountability to each other. Respect for each partner's time commitments, tact, and

Overall Considerations
- Did the study address a clearly focused problem and include specific research questions?
- Can the study be described in terms of its design/level of evidence, participants, the intervention under study, the outcomes being measured, and the comparisons being made?
- What are potential limitations in the sample and setting, study design, outcome measures, intervention, and data analysis, and what might be the impact of these limitations on the applicability of the study?

Sample and Setting
- How were study participants selected? Were all potentially eligible patients approached and screened for participation in the study?
- If participants were self-referred for study participation, to what extent might self-selection to participate in the study play a role in the outcomes?
- Could provider referral biases (e.g., referring less ill patients to a study) have played a role in the research outcomes?
- What criteria were used for inclusion and exclusion?
- How many patients were approached to participate? How many refused? What were reasons for refusal?
- Were refusers different than non-refusers on basic dimensions such as age, gender, education, or disease characteristics?
- Were all subjects who entered the trial accounted for at its conclusion?

Study Design
- Were participants randomly assigned to treatment?
- Did the control group receive a placebo, sham intervention, or attentional intervention (e.g., health education, follow-up phone calls)?
- Were subjects and study personnel "blinded" to treatment assignment and therefore unaware of what intervention the participant received? Approaches to blinding subjects and study personnel:
  - Selective disclosure of the purpose of study or partial information about the expected therapeutic effects
  - Sham treatments, placebo, or attentional control
  - Systematic treatment of expected side effects in both groups
  - Side effects centrally reported
  - External outcome assessors utilized who are unaware of patient group assignment

Outcome Measures
- Are the outcome measures relevant and meaningful? Multifaceted? Valid and reliable? Sensitive to change?
- Were known confounders and prognostic variables measured at baseline and compared across groups?

Intervention
- Did study participants receive treatment (especially supportive care treatment) without parameters being specified within the study design?
- Was the study protocol altered during the trial?
- Were the details of intervention sufficiently described to permit replication?

Data Analysis
- Were data analyses selected correct and sufficiently described?
- If graphical presentation of results, were they accompanied by data to support statistical significance?
- Were one-sided/one-tailed statistical tests used without a directional or a priori hypothesis?

Figure 19-10. Identifying Potential Limitations in the Design, Conduct, Analysis, and Report of Quantitative Research

---

Note. Based on information from DiCenso, Guyatt, et al., 2005; Hadorn et al., 1996; Melnyk & Fineout-Overholt, 2005.

- Report omits methodologic details, such as study purpose, research questions, assumptions, qualitative strategy of inquiry, role of researcher, sampling plan, data gathering strategies, and data analysis strategies.
- Inconsistency exists between qualitative strategy of inquiry and approach to data collection and analysis.
- Role of researcher in possibly introducing bias in data collection and analysis is not explicitly recognized and addressed in study design, conduct, and report.
- Inappropriate approaches were used for gaining access to site or participants.
- Research participants were self-selected and/or recruitment methods were limited rather than selected through extensive recruitment efforts and/or theoretical sampling.
- Data were obtained by a single researcher, during a single interview, or insufficient time was spent in interview/observation to gain familiarity necessary for vivid description.
- Insufficient detail is provided about semistructured interview schedule and follow-up probe questions.
- Insufficient detail is given concerning training and field supervision of interviewers.
- Evidence exists that the presence of the researcher distorted the event being observed or that information provided to researcher may have been shaped by social desirability bias.
- Evidence of sampling until data saturation is not provided.
- If theoretical sampling was utilized, researchers provided insufficient description of rationale for sampling plan.
- Trustworthiness of the data is attenuated by use of field notes rather than verbatim transcripts of tape-recorded data.
- Description of procedures for data analysis, including content analysis and development of thematic categories, is inadequate or absent.
- Decision rules for arriving at ratings or judgments are inadequately developed or absent.
- Insufficient description of process exists for resolving categorization differences.
- Content or thematic analysis was performed by a single researcher.
- Data are insufficiently clear or vivid in written narrative of report.
- Interpretive claims are unsupported or only supported in a limited way by verbatim participant statements.
- Confirmatory interviews with participants were not applied to validate researcher's themes and conclusions.
- Description of investigator triangulation approaches applied is insufficient.
- Insufficient procedures exist for examination of the data for congruence across investigators.
- Insufficient approaches to harmonizing/integrating viewpoints were used.
- Interpretive theoretical statements do not correspond with findings.
- Study conclusions go beyond data collected, analyzed, and presented.
- Fittingness of the study results is not supported by thorough examination of study findings with those of prior research.

Figure 19-11. Identifying Potential Limitations in the Design, Conduct, Analysis, and Report of Qualitative Studies

Note. Based on information from Cresswell, 1998, 2003; Denzin & Lincoln, 2000; Downs, 1999; Lincoln & Guba, 1985; Litva & Jacoby, 2002.

mutual trust also are essential (Plowfield, Wheeler, & Raymond, 2005; Reina, Reina, & Rushton, 2007). APN collaboration with others to improve patient outcomes encompasses collaboration with other members of the nursing team and of other disciplines. Baggs (1994) defined six critical elements for effective collaborative practice: trust, cooperation, assertiveness, shared decision making, communication, and coordination. At the center of intraprofessional and interdisciplinary collaborative practice models are two tenets: (a) patient needs are the foremost priority in the provision of care, and (b) patients require expertise and skills of different types of providers simultaneously during each encounter or hospital admission (King, Parinello, & Baggs, 1995). Collaboration requires developing relationships, building trust, and establishing an atmosphere of candor in communication. Barriers to collaboration include competition, territoriality, defensiveness, withholding of information, unpredictable or inconsistent behaviors, lack of follow-through, devaluing of the contributions, intentions, or integrity of others, and a lack of mutuality in resolving challenges and disappointments (Hanson et al.; Reina et al.).

A certain amount of duplication and role overlap exists among members of the healthcare team, which can result in territorial behaviors among team members. With territoriality, the focus on the patient is displaced, and the professionals' role, knowledge base, or authority becomes the focal point. Simply defining pieces of care provision that individual team members are uniquely trained to provide is not consistent with a focus on the needs of the patient and does not contribute to coordination of care, cooperation, or shared decision making. Collaboration provides opportunities for members of the team to develop a shared purpose, recognize divergent and complementary skills and contributions, and promote effective communication (Hanson et al., 2000). Paradoxically, territoriality may be increased by efforts to artificially define which role components or intervention approaches are the exclusive responsibility or expertise of any one role or one discipline. Establishing credibility often is a matter of time, patience, and the development of mutual respect that evolves as team members share common patient-related experiences. Although successful professional collaboration requires effort, it ultimately enhances continuity and reduces care fragmentation (King & Baggs, 1998; Zwarenstein & Bryant, 2000).

Disch, Walton, and Barnsteiner (2001) proposed that through collaboration with others, APNs not only influence care that patients and families receive, but they also shape the environment of care for patients and families and foster a healthy work environment for staff. These objectives are achieved through forming partnerships with nursing staff, collaborating with the nurse manager, establishing strong interdisciplinary care teams with physicians and other caregivers, and networking with colleagues across the institution, health system, or community. Working as a colleague and a partner, APNs assist staff to develop greater expertise in patient care, strengthen their ability to function effectively as part of the team, frame their work and contributions within the context of the organization, and foster pride in their accomplishments (Disch et al.).

Leadership

To successfully navigate the healthcare system for patients, guide multidisciplinary teams, advocate for practice improvements, strategically manage change, accept risks, garner credibility, inspire others to achieve excellence, and communicate and negotiate effectively, oncology APNs require strong leadership skills. Leadership has been identified as a core competency by NONPF, and in descriptions of the oncology APN role, an emphasis on leadership is prominent.

Leadership is variously defined, however. Rigolosi (2005) suggested that leadership is the use of communication processes to influence the activities of an individual or group toward attainment of a goal. Management theory designates two basic components of leader behavior: a concern for the task and outcomes to be achieved and a concern for the people responsible for the task. A leader's behavioral style is not one component or another but rather a composite of behaviors that provides a balance of the two components. The balance of leader behavior components is illustrated in Figure 19-12. For example, as task behavior decreases, relationship behavior increases. Leadership theory develops these two components further by differentiating transactional leadership

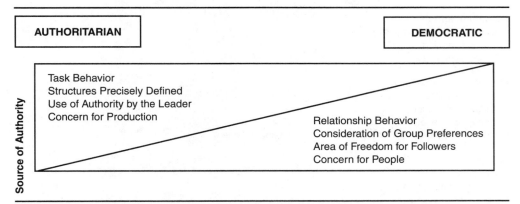

Figure 19-12. Balance of Task Behavior and Relationship Behavior

Note. From "How to Choose a Leadership Pattern," by R. Tannenbaum and W.H. Schmidt, 1958, *Harvard Business Review, 36,* p. 96. Copyright 1958 by Harvard Business School Publishing. Adapted with permission.

(how leaders motivate followers to accomplish goals and solve problems) and transformational leadership (how leaders inspire followers by creating a vision and promoting energetic movement toward making that vision a reality) (Burns, 2003).

Kouzes and Posner (1995) proposed the Leadership Practices Inventory (LPI) based on knowledge gained in extensive leadership research. Oncology APNs can use the LPI in self-assessment and in setting and meeting leadership performance goals. Kouzes and Posner suggested that leadership involves five practices, specifically: (a) challenging the process, (b) inspiring a shared vision, (c) enabling others to act, (d) modeling the way, and (e) encouraging the heart. Leaders search for opportunities to change the status quo and improve the organization. To do this, leaders must experiment and take risks, and this always involves mistakes and failures as well as solutions and successes. Leaders accept disappointments as inevitable and structure those experiences to learn more. Leaders also inspire a shared vision, help others to see exciting possibilities for the future, and encourage others' dreams and goals. Leaders foster collaboration and build spirited teams by enabling others to act and by helping each person on the team to feel trusted, respected, and capable. Leaders also set and consistently role-model high standards for pursing goals and the manner in which others (e.g., colleagues, coworkers, patients, supervisors) should be treated. They recognize the contributions that others make, celebrate accomplishments, and allow all team members to share in the rewards. Lastly, leaders understand that accomplishment of great things is hard work.

Leadership skill development is a lifelong learning process (Judkins & Friedrich-Cuntz, 2007). The list of skills needed for effective APN leadership outlined in Figure 19-13 can be used as a self-evaluation tool to determine areas for goal setting and continued leadership development.

Change Agent

A key skill set and potentially one of the most complex to acquire and refine is that of a change agent. A theoretical framework can be helpful in strategically guiding the process. One of the most frequently applied conceptual frameworks, particularly for

Communication
- Effective verbal and written skills
- Public speaking
- Media speaking
- Negotiation
- Meeting management
- Group facilitation
- Cultural competence
- Conflict management
- Constructive feedback and communication of expectations

Influence
- Credibility
- Change initiation and management
- Risk taking
- Use of data/research for position statements
- Health policy advocate

Critical Thinking
- Decision making
- Project management

Business
- Technology use
- Marketing
- Financial resource management
- Budgeting
- Business plan development
- Process/quality improvement techniques
- Systems approaches
- Team development
- Vision creation
- Organizational commitment

Personal Professionalism
- Personal development plan
- Professional image
- Lifelong learner
- Self-assessment

Figure 19-13. Leadership Skills

Note. Based on information from Gerzon, 2006; Grossman & Valiga, 2005; Rigolosi, 2005; Yoder-Wise & Kowalski, 2006.

change processes that are designed to translate new knowledge into practice, is the diffusion of innovation model proposed by Everett Rogers. Rogers (1995) described five stages in the change process: knowledge (learning about the existence and function of the innovation), persuasion (becoming convinced of its value), decision (committing to the adoption of the innovation), implementation (putting it into practice), and confirmation (accepting the innovation). Change efforts focus on strategies and communication channels specific to each stage in the process of innovation adoption. For example, in the knowledge stage, it is important to publicize the innovation. In the persuasion phase, one-on-one discussion with opinion leaders might be helpful. At the beginning of a change process, two kinds of information are needed: information about current practices and evidence showing why and how current practice could change. At the persuasion stage, when people are starting to think about the pros and cons of a change, gaining the involvement and visible participation of champions and opinion leaders—people who control resources, influence decisions, and have expert and referent power—can be key. In the persuasion stage, it also is important to link the innovation to improvements in outcomes and to address fears, concerns, and barriers. These strategies build a sense of competency and enthusiasm to handle the change. In the decision phase, success is based on the involvement and input of a wide range of stakeholders in making decisions. Decisions may include how to implement the change, how to overcome logistical challenges, and how to define the essential ingredients for success. It is helpful if the stakeholder group includes individuals who are early adopters and strong proponents of organizational change. During implementation, the implementation plan includes the pace and scope of change, who will drive the change (whether from the bottom up or top down), and what support structures are needed for implementation. Throughout implementation, continued communication, involvement, and honesty are necessary, both in providing the reinforcement of the message regarding the need for change and in responding to concerns and resistance. In the last stage, the confirmation stage, it is important to reinforce new behaviors and to capture and disseminate the benefits of the change. An evaluation process can provide data showing that the change is producing the anticipated effects. Acceptance of the innovation and integration into daily practice is enhanced by dissemination efforts—reports to upper management, presentations, newsletter articles, a poster presentation, or a fact sheet can aid in describing the process and outcomes achieved.

Negotiation

Negotiation, an essential skill for APNs, is the mutual discussion and arrangement of the terms of a transaction or agreement. In any negotiation, each party desires basic human needs of security, economic well-being, and a sense of belonging, recognition, and control over one's life (Cornelius, 1998). Negotiation involves analyzing the problem, generating ideas and potential actions that offer a mutually acceptable solution to the problem, understanding the role that each side will play, and identifying criteria that indicate a successful outcome.

Donaldson and Donaldson (1996) divided the negotiating process into six elements: preparing, setting limits and goals, managing emotions, listening, communicating clearly, and closing the deal. Some preparation typically is helpful in conducting a successful negotiation. Before the negotiation, consideration is given to what each party wants from the negotiation. Examine what each party has that the other might want and what each is comfortable giving away. It is important to reflect on what alternatives may exist if agreement is not reached. The past relationship of the parties involved may influence the negotiation. It is helpful to understand what the expected outcomes are, what the results of previous negotiations were, and what, if any, precedents were set. The consequences of winning or losing the negotiation are considered by both parties. Other questions to be considered include: Who has what power in the relationship? Who controls resources? Who stands to lose the most if agreement is not reached? What power does one party have to deliver what the other hopes for? Based on all of these considerations, possible solutions and compromises are identified. In a negotiation that is "win-win," both parties feel positive about the negotiation at its conclusion. This promotes good working relationships afterward. The negotiation itself is a careful exploration of each party's position, with the goal of finding a mutually acceptable compromise. In an ideal situation, one party finds that the other party wants what the first is prepared to trade, and vice versa. Regardless of whether this ideal situation exists, ultimately, both sides feel comfortable with the final solution if the agreement is considered win-win. Win-lose outcomes are considered only if an ongoing relationship with the other party is not required, because having lost, the losing party may be uncooperative or resistant in future mutual endeavors.

When preparing for a negotiation, APNs need to have thorough knowledge of themselves, an understanding of their preferred outcome, and an awareness of their minimally acceptable outcome. This allows them to determine in advance what can and cannot be accepted as an outcome. It may be helpful to discuss this preferred outcome and the minimally acceptable outcome with a mentor or experienced colleague and to benchmark these expectations against others. Donaldson and Donaldson (1996) suggested that on one end of the continuum is the minimally acceptable outcome and at the other end are desired goals and objectives. At each station along that continuum are levels of satisfaction with the deal that is struck.

Three skills are essential for successful negotiation: a clear understanding of the other's perception of the problem, a level of comfort in dealing with highly charged emotions, and communication skills to resolve misunderstandings and maintain a supportive and respectful relationship (Herman, Selph, Knox, Nussbaum, & Franklin, 1998; Rigolosi, 2005). Strong emotions, such as fear, anxiety, anger, frustration, and hurt, often arise during highly charged negotiations. These emotions could interfere with optimal functioning, and thus must be effectively managed. Strong preparation helps to build confidence, which can help with managing emotions. Herman et al. suggested that rehearsing possible scenarios and deciding on a response to each may accomplish emotional and cognitive preparation before a negotiation. This strategy will limit surprises during a negotiation and may assist the development of a thoughtful response. These authors also suggested that remaining aware of emotions and developing strategies during a negotiation to pause the proceedings are needed. Pausing negotiations by acting pensive or using phrases that encourage the other to elaborate further can give additional time for a response. Asking for a break gives time for all parties to have thoughtful reflection on the discussions. Active listening is a communication skill that is essential to obtain the most complete information about the goals and position of the other party. Therapeutic communication techniques, such as restating, paraphrasing, reflecting, and asking for more information, are all essential to effective negotiation.

In any negotiation, the APN must create and sustain mutual respect while at the same time maintaining an attitude of confidence and competence. Selph (1998) called this the "L'Oreal Principle"—the belief that "I am worth it!" Implementation of this principle limits the likelihood that the APN will be placed in a position of weakness or make concessions that undermine his or her personal and professional goals.

Outcomes Evaluation

A number of authors have proposed frameworks for the evaluation of outcomes of APN practice (Kleinpell, 2001; Kleinpell & Gawlinski, 2005; Kleinpell-Nowell & Weiner, 1999; Shah & Sullivan, 1998; Sidani & Irvine, 1999). Although each of these evaluation frameworks varies somewhat in its definition and grouping of variables, most are based on a consideration of structure, process, and patient and family outcome variables. Structure outcomes are contributions of the APN to patient, staff, and organizational system improvements that influence the processes and outcomes of care. Examples of structure outcomes include the number of workshops given for staff and the number of staff who attend each workshop, time spent in each APN role component, patient education resources and critical pathways developed, or the number of patients seen in a nurse-led symptom management clinic. Process outcomes evaluate the human and technical aspects of the APN role, including clinician, educator, researcher, and administrator, and may include staff nurse satisfaction with the APN, peer review, and the degree to which the goals and productivity levels established by the organization with the APN have been met. Evaluation of the direct APN impact on patient and family outcomes may include an evaluation of role impact on symptom distress, functional status, knowledge for self-management, patient satisfaction, adherence, length of stay, hospital admission, prevention of adverse events, resource use, and cost.

The selection of outcome measures for APN practice is problematic, in part because traditional medical outcomes may not fully capture the contribution of the APN (Kleinpell-Nowell & Weiner, 1999). Because patient care is multidisciplinary, isolating the effect of APNs on patient and family outcomes may be challenging. Simultaneously evaluating multiple dimensions of APN functioning, including structure, process, and outcome variables, contributes to describing the full impact of the APN role. APN practice improves the quality, safety, and cost effectiveness of patient care (Fulton & Baldwin, 2004). Initial evaluations of the APN role may focus on outcomes related to acceptance and satisfaction, whereas continued evaluation may emphasize safety, efficacy, and cost savings (Bryant-Lukosius & DiCenso, 2004). Prospective data collection in each domain related to the established goals of the APN is essential in documenting the diversity of the APN's contributions. Data elements may include time spent in each of the role components, number of referrals and types of patients seen, staff programs delivered, standards of practice developed, scholarly presentations and publications, contributions to committees and organizational initiatives, and participation in research (Dayhoff & Lyon, 2001). Activities are linked to specific outcomes, such as the prevention of complications or improvements in staffing patterns, practice quality and consistency, length of stay, readmission, costs, and satisfaction (Bryant-Lukosius & DiCenso). Continued study of APN outcomes to develop a more refined understanding of the roles and cost effectiveness of APNs as providers of quality health care is urgently needed.

Duffy (2002) proposed that APNs are uniquely positioned to provide expertise and leadership in the identification and implementation of nursing-sensitive and multidisciplinary outcome indicator sets. The outcomes that are consistently considered to be sensitive to nursing care across the continuum of healthcare settings include symptom control and management, functional status (including physical and psychosocial functioning and self-care abilities), safety (which includes adverse incidents and complications), and perceptual status (which includes satisfaction with nursing care and with the results of nursing care) (Doran, 2003).

The ONS nursing-sensitive patient outcomes initiative provides helpful tools to identify and measure oncology nursing-sensitive patient outcomes and provides summaries of evidence-based supporting interventions to improve patient and family outcomes (Gobel, Beck, & O'Leary, 2006). Organizations such as the American Nurses Association National Database of Nursing Quality Indicators recommend quality indicators for hospitals and long-term care facilities that are sensitive to the kinds of outcomes affected by nursing care (Gallagher & Rowell, 2003). ASCO is developing a system for measuring the delivery of quality cancer services (Neuss et al., 2005). Also, the Centers for Medicare and Medicaid Services is engaged in new initiatives to identify and measure key indicators of quality of care and to link the achievement of specific quality benchmarks to provider reimbursement incentives (Milgate & Hackbarth, 2005; Rogers, L.M., 2006). Disease-specific standards of care developed by the National Comprehensive Cancer Network and quality measures for breast and colorectal cancer developed by the American College of Surgeons Commission on Cancer (www.facs.org/cancer/qualitymeasures.html) can be used to inform the development of APN outcome measures. No one set of outcome measures is appropriate for all situations.

In selecting and introducing standardized outcome measures, APNs consider immediate and long-term outcomes that are measurable, valued by decision makers, and sensitive to changes in nursing care (Kleinpell, 2007). Valid, reliable, and clinically useful tools for documenting the key aspects of patient care (e.g., pain assessment, prevention and management of oral complications, maintenance of functional status) can be used to promote efficient and systematic documentation of care delivery and retrieval of data that are useful for clinical and programmatic improvements.

Conclusion

Into the future, the challenges and complexity of delivering effective cancer care will continue to grow. Earlier diagnosis and the burgeoning array of effective treatment modalities are transforming cancer into a chronic illness. Patients and their families will have an even greater need for expert guidance and coaching as well as effective case management to support them in making well-informed decisions about treatment options and to optimize their self-management and continuity of care across this extended chronic illness continuum. Moreover, because of the aging of the population, the number of individuals living with cancer is expected to continue to grow. These challenges underscore the importance of the advanced clinical practice role to ensure access to quality cancer care and to optimize clinical and fiscal outcomes. The advent of individualized and customized treatment plans (tailored to individual preferences and increasingly to unique genetic characteristics and biologic disease features) also will require oncology nurses at the bedside to have access to consultative expertise and specialty education programs that oncology APNs are uniquely prepared to offer. Exponential growth in the science of cancer care and in supportive care research emphasizes the essential contribution of oncology APNs' skills in critical appraisal, synthesis, and research translation.

As with all healthcare professionals, oncology APNs will continue to be challenged to measure and describe the outcomes for patients, staff, and system capacity achieved through their activities. Public demand exists for such accountability, and increasingly, reimbursement mechanisms and hospital recognition may be based on a documented achievement of quality outcomes. The knowledge, expertise, broad skill set, flexibility and public credibility of the oncology APN strongly positions this advanced nursing role to lead the continued evolution of cancer care, to address dilemmas surrounding access to care, and to enhance outcomes for patients and families experiencing the diagnosis of cancer.

Case Study

A.S. is a 71-year-old patient admitted two days ago for vertebroplasty and to receive her first cycle of chemotherapy for newly diagnosed stage IIIA IgG kappa multiple myeloma complicated by compression fractures of thoracic vertebrae T4–T8. She has severe bone pain, which is currently well managed with controlled-release long-acting narcotic agents. A staff nurse on the unit mentions in patient care rounds that the patient is quite nauseated, and as the APN is leaving rounds with the nurse, the staff nurse asks whether the patient's nausea is normal, given that the patient has not yet received her chemotherapy treatment.

1. What type of consultation does this represent?
   • Consultation may be formal or informal, may be client or consultee centered, and may focus on patients or on administrative issues. In this situation, the question represents an informal, client-centered, case consultation request.

2. Describe how the APN would proceed in handling this consultation request.
   • In responding to this question, the APN must decide whether the question can be answered immediately or whether additional information is required. In addition, it is not clear whether the nurse is asking for consultative assistance in managing the nausea and exactly what she is seeking from the APN. The APN needs more information about the patient's situation before answering the question, but it is unclear if the nurse wishes to involve the APN in direct evaluation of the patient. More information is needed about the kind of assistance the staff nurse is requesting.
   • The APN responds by saying, "That is interesting, and there are a few different possibilities for her nausea that I can think of—can you tell me more about her status and the other medications she is taking?" The nurse explains that A.S. moves about with the assistance of a walker, has no standing order for antiemetics, and has not had a bowel movement since admission. The nurse admits that she has been too busy to further evaluate the patient.

3. If the nurse chooses to ask the APN to evaluate the patient with her, who is ultimately responsible for the patient's care and outcome?
   • The APN could offer to evaluate the patient with the nurse or could suggest that the nurse evaluate the patient and that they discuss the case further in the afternoon. The first option promotes direct APN consultative involvement in the case, whereas the second option provides the staff nurse with more independence and responsibility. Regardless of which option the nurse chooses, control of the consultation and responsibility for the patient's care must remain with the staff nurse, and the staff nurse must be provided with the opportunity to clarify the kind of assistance she is seeking from the APN.
   • The patient is returning to the community, and her primary nurse consults with the APN because he recognizes that A.S. is at high risk for readmission and has a complex medical regimen to manage at home. The patient is somewhat frail. The consultation request is to help to evaluate the adequacy of the discharge plan.

4. What elements should the APN include in the evaluation and management plan to ensure continuity of care?
   • The plan to ensure continuity of care begins with a comprehensive assessment of patient and family needs and strengths. That assessment addresses three

key questions: (a) What self-care activities are to be performed to maintain or enhance function, comfort, and well-being? (b) Who will perform those activities now, who will perform those over time, and who is the designated alternate? (c) What health teaching, referrals, equipment, devices, or supplies are required? Elements of continuity of care include an interdisciplinary approach to care, comprehensive assessment of patient and family needs and strengths, patient and family education and involvement in decision making, identification and coordination of supplemental resources, integration of care through each transition, and a documented plan of care.

- The APN receives an e-mail from the supervisor that because of shortages in the staff development division, the APN will be required to assist with teaching cardiopulmonary resuscitation (CPR) to staff nurse orientees and with recertifying current staff in CPR. The APN sees this responsibility as inconsistent with her specialty role, perceives that the nurse educators should have primary responsibility for helping staff to meet this basic competency, and worries that to incorporate this responsibility, less time will be devoted to working with the staff in the development of evidence-based care standards for symptom management. The supervisor closed the e-mail by saying that she will discuss this further with the APN at their next regular meeting.

5. Describe how the APN would prepare for this negotiation.
   - Although it is not completely apparent from the e-mail alone that there is room for negotiation on this issue, the fact that the supervisor is willing to discuss it at the next regular meeting suggests that she may be willing to negotiate the scope or the terms of the APN's involvement in CPR training. Negotiation is the mutual discussion and arrangement of the terms of a transaction or agreement and involves analyzing the problem, generating ideas and potential actions that offer a mutually acceptable solution to the problem, understanding the role that each side will play, and identifying criteria that indicate a successful outcome. The APN prepares for the discussion by considering the desired outcome of the negotiation and what the supervisor anticipates. The APN also should consider what the APN and the supervisor each has that the other might want, and what each might be comfortable giving away. Alternatives must be considered if agreement cannot be obtained, as well as the future implications of disagreement. The history of the APN-supervisor relationship is contemplated along with how that history might affect the negotiation. The APN then considers possible solutions and compromises. Were other individuals in the system also recruited to assist with CPR training? Is this a temporary solution until additional educators are recruited to meet the demand? What responsibilities might be shifted from the APN to another team member so that the APN can accommodate this request? If the APN accommodates this request, what resources (e.g., secretarial support, research assistant, equipment, conference attendance, compensatory time off, additional salary support) might be provided to the APN to assist in managing the total workload, to reward teamwork, or to offset the additional time commitment? If the APN agrees to this request, what is the time frame of the commitment to assist with teaching, and when can that commitment be renegotiated? It also may be helpful to discuss the preferred and the minimally acceptable outcomes, as well as the potential solutions and compromises with a colleague or mentor to gain another perspective.

Key Points

- The APN role includes the functions of clinician, consultant, educator, researcher, and coordinator. Essential APN skills include leadership, collaboration, management of change, scholarly practice, mentorship, negotiation, and conflict resolution.
- The educational process begins with a learning needs assessment, followed by development of learning objectives, selection of the method(s) of instruction, and design of the program, and concludes with program evaluation. Learning objectives are specific and measurable with two components: performance and criterion.
- The following adult learning principles may be incorporated into educational programming.
  - Adults are self-directed and require involvement in all stages of the learning process, from planning through evaluation.
  - Adults have significant life experiences and a diverse skill set upon which to base education.
  - Adults like feedback about progress toward goals, learn best in a comfortable environment, and value information that helps them to solve immediate problems.
- The APN's role in research includes participation in research evaluation and critique, research utilization, and the conduct and dissemination of research. APNs have a fundamental responsibility for the translation of research into clinical decisions, tools, and programs to improve patient outcomes.
- Leadership is the use of communication processes to influence the activities of an individual or group toward the attainment of a goal. It includes both concern for the task and outcomes to be achieved and the concerns for the people who are responsible for the task.

Recommended Resources for Oncology Advanced Practice Nurses

- Ambrose, D. (2006). *Making peace with your work: An invitation to find meaning in the madness.* Andover, MN: Expert Publishing.
- Badowski, R. (with Gittines, R.). (2003). *Managing up: How to forge an effective relationship with those above you.* New York: Doubleday.
- Bennis, W., & Goldsmith, J. (1997). *Learning to lead: A workbook on becoming a leader* (2nd ed.). Reading, MA: Perseus Books.
- Berry, C.R. (1989). *When helping you is hurting me: Escaping the Messiah trap.* San Francisco: Harper & Row.
- Bridges, W. (1980). *Transitions: Making sense of life's changes.* Reading, MA: Addison-Wesley.
- De Bono, E. (1985). *Six thinking hats* (1st U.S. ed.). Boston: Little, Brown.
- Edelman, J., & Crain, M.B. (1993). *The Tao of negotiation: How you can prevent, resolve, and transcend conflict in work and everyday life.* New York: HarperBusiness.
- Kritek, P.B. (1994). *Negotiating at an uneven table: A practical approach to working with difference and diversity.* San Francisco: Jossey-Bass.
- Mezey, M.D., McGivern, D.O., & Sullivan-Marx, E.M. (Eds.). (2003). *Nurse practitioners: Evolution of advanced practice* (4th ed.). New York: Springer.

- Stone, D., Patton, B., & Heen, S. (1999). *Difficult conversations: How to discuss what matters most.* New York: Viking Press.

References

Ackerman, M.H., Norsen, L., Martin, B., Wiedrich, J., & Kitzman, H.J. (1996). Development of a model of advanced practice. *American Journal of Critical Care, 5,* 68–73.

Allen, J. (2003). The clinical nurse specialist in gynaecological oncology—the role in vulval cancer. *Best Practice in Research: Clinical Obstetrics and Gynaecology, 17,* 591–607.

American Association of Colleges of Nursing. (2007). *White paper on the education and role of the clinical nurse leader.* Retrieved July 28, 2007, from http://www.aacn.nche.edu/Publications/pdf/2-07CNLWhitePaperf.pdf

American Society of Clinical Oncology. (2003). American Society of Clinical Oncology policy statement: Oversight of clinical research. *Journal of Clinical Oncology, 21,* 2377–2386.

Anderson, L.W., & Krathwohl, D. (Eds.). (2001). *A taxonomy for learning, teaching, and assessing: A revision of Bloom's taxonomy of educational objectives.* New York: Longman.

APRN Joint Dialogue Group. (2008). *Consensus model for APRN regulation: Licensure, accreditation, certification and education.* Retrieved May 7, 2008, from https://www.ncsbn.org/index.htm

Baggs, J.G. (1994). Development of an instrument to measure collaboration and satisfaction about care decisions. *Journal of Advanced Nursing, 20,* 176–182.

Balk, E.M., Lau, J., & Bonis, P.A. (2005). Reading and critically appraising systematic reviews and meta-analyses: A short primer with a focus on hepatology. *Journal of Hepatology, 43,* 729–736.

Barron, A.M., & White, P. (2000). Consultation. In A.B. Hamric, J.A. Spross, & C.M. Hanson (Eds.), *Advanced nursing practice: An integrative approach* (2nd ed., pp. 217–243). Philadelphia: Saunders.

Barroso, J., Sandelowski, M., & Voils, C.I. (2006). Research results have expiration dates: Ensuring timely systematic reviews. *Journal of Evaluation in Clinical Practice, 12,* 454–462.

Beddar, S.M., & Aikin, J.L. (1994). Continuity of care: A challenge for ambulatory oncology nursing. *Seminars in Oncology Nursing, 10,* 254–263.

Belcher, A., & Shurpin, K.M. (1995). Education of the advanced practice nurse in oncology. *Oncology Nursing Forum, 22*(Suppl. 8), 19–24.

Berger, A.M., Eilers, J.G., Heermann, J.A., Warren, J.J., Franco, T., & Triolo, P.K. (1999). State-of-the-art patient care. The impact of doctorally prepared clinical nurses. *Clinical Nurse Specialist, 13,* 259–266.

Berger, A.M., Eilers, J.G., Pattrin, L., Rolf-Fixley, M., Pfeifer, B.A., Rogge, J., et al. (1996). Advanced practice roles for nurses in tomorrow's healthcare systems. *Clinical Nurse Specialist, 10,* 250–255.

Betz, C.L., & Redcay, G. (2005). Dimensions of the transition service coordinator role. *Journal for Specialists in Pediatric Nursing, 10,* 49–59.

Bigby, M., & Williams, H. (2003). Appraising systematic reviews and meta-analyses. *Archives of Dermatology, 139,* 795–798.

Blackburn, K.M. (1998). Roles of advanced practice nurses in oncology. *Oncology, 12,* 591–596.

Blecher, C.S. (Ed.). (2004). *Standards of oncology education: Patient/significant other and public* (3rd ed.). Pittsburgh, PA: Oncology Nursing Society.

Block, P. (1999). *Flawless consulting: A guide to getting your expertise used* (2nd ed.). San Francisco: Pfeiffer & Company.

Bryant-Lukosius, D., & DiCenso, A. (2004). A framework for the introduction and evaluation of advanced practice nursing roles. *Journal of Advanced Nursing, 48,* 530–540.

Brykczynski, K.A. (2000). Role development of the advanced practice nurse. In A.B. Hamric, J.A. Spross, & C.M. Hanson (Eds.), *Advanced nursing practice: An integrative approach* (2nd ed., pp. 107–133). Philadelphia: Saunders.

Buckwalter, K. (1985). Exploring the process of discharge planning: Application to the construct of health. In E. McLelland, K. Kelly, & K. Buckwalter (Eds.), *Continuity of care: Advancing the concept of discharge planning* (pp. 5–10). New York: Grune & Stratton.

Burns, J.M. (2003). *Transforming leadership: A new pursuit of happiness.* New York: Atlantic Monthly Press.

Bush, N.J., & Watters, T. (2001). The emerging role of the oncology nurse practitioner: A collaborative model within the private practice setting. *Oncology Nursing Forum, 28,* 1425–1431.

Callahan, C., & De La Cruz, H. (2004). Central line placement for the pediatric oncology patient: A model of advanced practice nurse collaboration. *Journal of Pediatric Oncology Nursing, 21,* 16–21.

Calzone, K.A., Jenkins, J., & Masny, A. (2002). Core competencies in cancer genetics for advanced practice oncology nurses. *Oncology Nursing Forum, 29,* 1327–1333.

Caplan, G. (1970). *The theory and practice of mental health consultation.* New York: Basic Books.

Carper, E., & Haas, M. (2006). Advanced practice nursing in radiation oncology. *Seminars in Oncology Nursing, 22,* 203–211.

Chachkes, E., & Christ, G. (1996). Cross cultural issues in patient education. *Patient Education and Counseling, 27,* 13–21.

Chase, S.K., & Pruitt, R.H. (2006). The practice doctorate: Innovation or disruption? *Journal of Nursing Education, 45,* 155–161.

Chelf, J.H., Agre, P., Axelrod, A., Chenye, L., Cole, D.D., Conrad, K., et al. (2001). Cancer-related patient education: An overview of the last decade of evaluation and research. *Oncology Nursing Forum, 28,* 1139–1147.

Cohen, E.L., & Cesta, T.G. (2001). *Nursing case management: From essentials to advanced practice applications.* St. Louis, MO: Mosby.

Connors, H. (1993). Impact of care management modalities on curricula. In K. Kelly & M. Maas (Eds.), *Managing nursing care: Promise and pitfalls* (pp. 190–207). St. Louis, MO: Mosby.

Cornelius, H. (1998). *The gentle revolution: Men and women at work, what goes wrong and how to fix it.* New South Wales, Australia: Simon & Schuster.

Cresswell, J.W. (1998). *Qualitative inquiry and research design: Choosing among five traditions.* Thousand Oaks, CA: Sage Publications.

Cresswell, J.W. (2003). *Research design: Qualitative, quantitative, and mixed methods approaches.* Thousand Oaks, CA: Sage Publications.

Cummings, G., & McLennan, M. (2005). Advanced practice nursing: Leadership to effect policy change. *Journal of Nursing Administration, 35,* 61–66.

Cummings, G.G., Fraser, K., & Tarlier, D. (2003). Implementing ANPs in acute care: An evaluation of organizational change. *Journal of Nursing Administration, 33,* 139–145.

Cunningham, R.S. (2004). Advanced practice nursing outcomes: A review of selected empirical literature. *Oncology Nursing Forum, 31,* 219–232.

Dayhoff, N.E., & Lyon, B.L. (2001). Assessing outcomes in clinical nurse specialist practice. In R.M. Kleinpell (Ed.), *Outcome assessment in advanced practice nursing* (pp. 103–130). New York: Springer.

DeBourgh, G.A. (2001). Champions for evidence-based practice: A critical role for advanced practice nurses. *AACN Clinical Issues, 12,* 491–508.

Denzin, N.K., & Lincoln, Y.S. (2000). *Handbook of qualitative research* (2nd ed.). Thousand Oaks, CA: Sage Publications.

DiCenso, A., Ciliska, D., Dobbins, M., & Guyatt, G. (2005). Moving from evidence to action using clinical practice guidelines. In A. DiCenso, G. Guyatt, & D. Ciliska (Eds.), *Evidence-based nursing: A guide to clinical practice* (pp. 154–171). Philadelphia: Elsevier.

DiCenso, A., Guyatt, G., & Ciliska, D. (2005). *Evidence-based nursing: A guide to clinical practice.* St. Louis, MO: Elsevier Mosby.

Disch, J., Walton, M., & Barnsteiner, J. (2001). The role of the clinical nurse specialist in creating a healthy work environment. *AACN Clinical Issues, 12,* 345–355.

Doak, C.C., Doak, L.G., & Root, J.H. (1996). *Teaching patients with low literacy skills* (2nd ed.). Philadelphia: Lippincott.

Donaldson, M.C., & Donaldson, M. (1996). *Negotiating for dummies.* Foster City, CA: IDG Books Worldwide.

Doran, D.M. (2003). *Nursing-sensitive outcomes: State of the science.* Sudbury, MA: Jones and Bartlett.

Downs, F. (1999). *Readings in research methodology* (2nd ed.). Philadelphia: Lippincott.

Dracup, K., Cronenwett, L., Meleis, A.I., & Benner, P.E. (2005). Reflections on the doctorate of nursing practice. *Nursing Outlook, 53,* 177–182.

Drenning, C. (2006). Collaboration among nurses, advanced practice nurses, and nurse researchers to achieve evidence-based practice change. *Journal of Nursing Care Quality, 21,* 298–301.

Duffy, J.R. (2002). The clinical leadership role of the CNS in the identification of nursing-sensitive and multidisciplinary quality indicator sets. *Clinical Nurse Specialist, 16,* 70–76.

Eisenhauer, L., & Bleich, M.R. (2006). The clinical doctorate: Whoa or Go? *Journal of Nursing Education, 45,* 3–4.

Fitch, M.I., & Mings, D. (2003). Cancer nursing in Ontario: Defining nursing roles. *Canadian Oncology Nursing Journal, 13,* 28–44.

Fletcher, R.H., O'Malley, M.S., Fletcher, S.W., Earp, J.A., & Alexander, J.P. (1984). Measuring the continuity and coordination of medical care in a system involving multiple providers. *Medical Care, 22,* 403–411.

Frost, M.H., Thompson, R., & Thiemann, K.B. (1999). Importance of format and design in print patient information. *Cancer Practice, 7,* 22–27.

Fulton, J., & Baldwin, K. (2004). An annotated bibliography reflecting CNS practice and outcomes. *Clinical Nurse Specialist, 18,* 21–39.

Gallagher, R.M., & Rowell, P.A. (2003). Claiming the future of nursing through nursing-sensitive quality indicators. *Nursing Administration Quarterly, 27,* 273–284.

Gardner, G., Chang, A., & Duffield, C. (2007). Making nursing work: Breaking through the role confusion of advanced practice nursing. *Journal of Advanced Nursing, 57,* 382–391.

Gerteis, M. (1993). Coordinating care and integrating services. In M. Gerteis, S. Edgman-Levitan, & J. Dailey (Eds.), *Through the patient's eyes: Understanding and promoting patient-centered care* (pp. 45–71). San Francisco: Jossey-Bass.

Gerzon, M. (2006). *Leading through conflict: How successful leaders transform differences into opportunities.* Boston: Harvard Business School Press.

Glen, S., & Waddington, K. (1998). Role transition from staff nurse to clinical nurse specialist: A case study. *Journal of Clinical Nursing, 7,* 283–290.

Gobel, B.H., Beck, S.L., & O'Leary, C. (2006). Nursing-sensitive patient outcomes: The development of the Putting Evidence Into Practice resources for nursing practice. *Clinical Journal of Oncology Nursing, 10,* 621–624.

Goldberg, N.J., & Moch, S.D. (1998). An advanced practice nurse–nurse researcher collaborative model. *Clinical Nurse Specialist, 12,* 251–255.

Grossman, S.D., & Valiga, T.M. (2005). *The new leadership challenge: Creating the future of nursing.* Philadelphia: F.A. Davis.

Hadorn, D.C., Baker, D., Hodges, J.S., & Hicks, N. (1996). Rating the quality of evidence for clinical practice guidelines. *Journal of Clinical Epidemiology, 49,* 749–754.

Hagopian, G.A. (1996). Patient and family education. In R. McCorkle, M. Grant, M. Frank-Stromborg, & S.B. Baird (Eds.), *Cancer nursing: A comprehensive textbook* (2nd ed., pp. 1223–1234). Philadelphia: Saunders.

Hall, L.M. (2007). Twenty-first-century advanced nursing practice. *Journal of Research in Nursing, 12*(1), 5–6.

Hamric, A.B. (1992). Creating our future: Challenges and opportunities for the clinical nurse specialist. *Oncology Nursing Forum, 19*(Suppl. 1), 11–15.

Hamric, A.B., & Hanson, C.M. (2003). Educating advanced practice nurses for practice reality. *Journal of Professional Nursing, 19,* 262–268.

Hanson, C.M., Spross, J.A., & Carr, D.B. (2000). Collaboration. In A.B. Hamric, J.A. Spross, & C.M. Hanson (Eds.), *Advanced nursing practice: An integrative approach* (2nd ed., pp. 315–347). Philadelphia: Saunders.

Hardy, M.E., & Hardy, W.L. (1988). Role stress and role strain. In M.E. Hardy & M.E. Conway (Eds.), *Role theory: Perspectives for health professionals* (2nd ed., pp. 159–239). Norwalk, CT: Appleton & Lange.

Harris, M.F., & Zwar, N.A. (2007). Care of patients with chronic disease: The challenge for general practice. *Medical Journal of Australia, 187,* 104–107.

Herman, J.A., Selph, A., Knox, M.L., Nussbaum, J.S., & Franklin, R. (1998). Negotiating skills: Empower the acute care nurse practitioner. In R.M. Kleinpell & M.R. Piano (Eds.), *Practice issues for the acute care nurse practitioner* (pp. 79–101). New York: Springer.

Hobbie, W.L., & Hollen, P.J. (1993). Pediatric nurse practitioners specializing with survivors of childhood cancer. *Journal of Pediatric Health Care, 7,* 24–30.

Horns, P.N., Czaplijski, T.J., Engelke, M.K., Marshburn, D., McAuliffe, M., & Baker, S. (2007). Leading through collaboration: A regional academic/service partnership that works. *Nursing Outlook, 55,* 74–78.

Irvine, D., Sidani, S., Porter, H., O'Brien-Pallas, L., Simpson, B., McGillis Hall, L., et al. (2000). Organizational factors influencing nurse practitioners' role implementation in acute care settings. *Canadian Journal of Nursing Leadership, 13*(3), 28–35.

Jacobs, L.A. (Ed.). (2003a). *The master's degree with a specialty in advanced practice oncology nursing* (4th ed.). Pittsburgh, PA: Oncology Nursing Society.

Jacobs, L.A. (Ed.). (2003b). *Standards of oncology nursing education: Generalist and advanced practice levels* (3rd ed.). Pittsburgh, PA: Oncology Nursing Society.

Jacobs, L.A. (Ed.). (2003c). *Statement on the scope and standards of advanced practice nursing in oncology* (3rd ed.). Pittsburgh, PA: Oncology Nursing Society.

Jacobs, L.A., Scarpa, R., Lester, J., & Smith, J. (2004). Oncology nursing as a specialty: The education, scope and standards for advanced practice nursing in oncology. *Oncology Nursing Forum, 31,* 507–509.

Jansen, J., van Weert, J., van Dulmen, S., Heeren, T., & Bensing, J. (2007). Patient education about treatment in cancer care: An overview of the literature on older patients' needs. *Cancer Nursing, 30,* 251–260.

Jones, M.L. (2005). Role development and effective practice in specialist and advanced practice roles in acute hospital settings: Systematic review and meta-synthesis. *Journal of Advanced Nursing, 49,* 191–209.

Judkins, S., & Friedrich-Cuntz, A. (2007). Leadership skills development among nurse practitioners. *American Journal for Nurse Practitioners, 11*(5), 49–57.

Kelvin, J.F., & Moore-Higgs, G.J. (1999). Description of the role of nonphysician practitioners in radiation oncology. *International Journal of Radiation Oncology, Biology, Physics, 45,* 163–169.

Kelvin, J.F., Moore-Higgs, G.J., Maher, K.E., Dubey, A.K., Austin-Seymour, M.M., Daly, N.R., et al. (1999). Non-physician practitioners in radiation oncology: Advanced practice nurses and physician assistants. *International Journal of Radiation Oncology, Biology, Physics, 45,* 255–263.

Kennedy, A., Sloman, F., Douglass, J.A., & Sawyer, S.M. (2007). Young people with chronic illness: The approach to transition. *Internal Medicine Journal, 37,* 555–560.

King, K.B., & Baggs, J.G. (1998). Collaboration: The essence of the acute care nurse practitioner practice. In R.M. Kleinpell & M.R. Piano (Eds.), *Practice issues for the acute care nurse practitioner* (pp. 67–78). New York: Springer.

King, K.B., Parinello, K.A., & Baggs, J.G. (1995). Collaboration and advanced practice nursing. In J.V. Hickey, R.M. Ouimette, & S.L. Venegoni (Eds.), *Advanced practice nursing: Changing roles and clinical applications* (pp. 146–162). Philadelphia: Lippincott.

Kinney, A.Y., Hawkins, R., & Hudmon, K.S. (1997). A descriptive study of the role of the oncology nurse practitioner. *Oncology Nursing Forum, 24,* 811–820.

Kleinpell, R. (2001). *Outcome assessment in advanced practice nursing.* New York: Springer.

Kleinpell, R. (2007). APNs: Invisible champions. *Nursing Management, 38*(5), 18–22.

Kleinpell, R., & Gawlinski A. (2005). Assessing outcomes in advanced practice nursing practice: The use of quality indicators and evidence-based practice. *AACN Clinical Issues, 16,* 43–57.

Kleinpell, R.M., & Hravnak, M.M. (2005). Strategies for success in the acute care nurse practitioner role. *Critical Care Nursing Clinics of North America, 17,* 177–181.

Kleinpell-Nowell, R., & Weiner, T.M. (1999). Measuring advanced practice nursing outcomes. *AACN Clinical Issues, 10,* 356–368.

Kolb Smith, P.C. (2002). The role of the primary care advanced practice nurse in evaluating and monitoring childhood cancer survivors for a second malignant neoplasm. *Journal of Pediatric Oncology Nursing, 19,* 84–96.

Kouzes, J.M., & Posner, B.Z. (1995). *The leadership challenge: How to keep getting extraordinary things done in organizations.* San Francisco: Jossey-Bass.

Kuebler, K.K. (2003). The palliative care advanced practice nurse. *Journal of Palliative Medicine, 6,* 707–714.

Lancaster, J. (2006). Letter from the American Association of Colleges of Nursing to the National Council of State Boards of Nursing (NCSBN) regarding the NCSBN's vision paper. *Journal of Professional Nursing, 22,* 145–149.

Lauria, M. (1991). Continuity of cancer care. *Cancer, 67,* 1759–1766.

Leventhal, H., & Cameron, L. (1987). Behavioral theories and the problem of compliance. *Patient Education and Counseling, 10,* 117–138.

Lin, E.M. (1994). A combined role of clinical nurse specialist and coordinator: Optimizing continuity of care in an autologous bone marrow transplant program. *Clinical Nurse Specialist, 8,* 48–55.

Lincoln, P.E. (2000). Comparing CNS and NP role activities: A replication. *Clinical Nurse Specialist, 14,* 269–277.

Lincoln, Y.S., & Guba, E.G. (1985). *Naturalistic inquiry.* Beverly Hills, CA: Sage.

Lippitt, G., & Lippitt, R. (1986). *The consulting process in action* (2nd ed.). San Diego, CA: University Associates.

Litva, A., & Jacoby, A. (2002). Qualitative research: Critical appraisal. In J.V. Craig & R.L. Smyth (Eds.), *The evidence-based practice manual for nurses* (2nd ed., pp. 154–181). Edinburgh: Elsevier Churchill Livingstone.

Loftus, L.A., & Weston, V. (2001). The development of nurse-led clinics in cancer care. *Journal of Clinical Nursing, 10,* 215–220.

Lynch, M.P., Cope, D.G., & Murphy-Ende, K. (2001). Advanced practice issues: Results of the ONS Advanced Practice Nursing survey. *Oncology Nursing Forum, 28,* 1521–1530.

Macdonald, J.A., Herbert, R., & Thibault, C. (2006). Advanced practice nursing: Unification through a common identity. *Journal of Professional Nursing, 22,* 172–179.

Mahn, V.A., & Spross, J.A. (1996). Nurse case management as an advanced practice role. In A.B. Hamric, J.A. Spross, & C.M. Hanson (Eds.), *Advanced nursing practice: An integrative approach* (pp. 445–465). Philadelphia: Saunders.

Mahn, V.A., & Zazworsky, D.J. (2000). The advanced practice nurse case manager. In A.B. Hamric, J.A. Spross, & C.M. Hanson (Eds.), *Advanced nursing practice: An integrative approach* (2nd ed., pp. 549–606). Philadelphia: Saunders.

Mantzoukas, S., & Watkinson, S. (2006). Review of advanced nursing practice: The international literature and developing the generic features. *Journal of Clinical Nursing, 16,* 28–37.

McCabe, S. (2006). What does it take to make a nurse? Considerations of the CNL and DNP role development. *Perspectives in Psychiatric Care, 42,* 252–255.

McCabe, S., & Burman, M.E. (2006). A tale of two APNs: Addressing blurred practice boundaries in APN practice. *Perspectives in Psychiatric Care, 42,* 3–12.

McCorkle, R., Preston, F., & Volker, D.L. (1996). Cancer nursing education today. In R. McCorkle, M. Grant, M. Frank-Stromborg, & S.B. Baird (Eds.), *Cancer nursing: A comprehensive textbook* (2nd ed., pp. 1247–1260). Philadelphia: Saunders.

McGuire, D.B., & Harwood, K.V. (2000). Research. In A.B. Hamric, J.A. Spross, & C.M. Hanson (Eds.), *Advanced nursing practice: An integrative approach* (2nd ed., pp. 245–278). Philadelphia: Saunders.

McKeehan, K., & Coulton, C. (1985). A systems approach to program development for continuity of care in hospitals. In E. McLelland, K. Kelly, & K. Buckwalter (Eds.), *Continuity of care: Advancing the concept of discharge planning* (pp. 79–92). New York: Grune & Stratton.

McKenney, S.A. (2005). The role of the nurse practitioner in the care of young women with breast cancer. *Breast Disease, 23,* 115–121.

McKinley, M. (2007). *Acute and critical care clinical nurse specialists: Synergy for best practices.* Philadelphia: Saunders.

McMillan, S.C., Small, B.J., Weitzner, M., Schonwetter, R., Tittle, M., Moody, L., et al. (2006). Impact of coping skills intervention with family caregivers of hospice patients with cancer: A randomized clinical trial. *Cancer, 106,* 214–222.

Melnyk, B.M., & Fineout-Overholt, E. (2005). *Evidence-based practice in nursing and healthcare: A guide to best practice.* Philadelphia: Lippincott Williams & Wilkins.

Mick, D.J., & Ackerman, M.H. (2000). Advanced practice nursing role delineation in acute and critical care: Application of the strong model of advanced practice. *Heart and Lung, 29,* 210–221.

Milgate, K., & Hackbarth, G. (2005). Quality in Medicare: From measurement to payment and provider to patient. *Health Care Financing Review, 27,* 91–101.

Mitchell, S.A. (2001). Documentation of service. In E.M. Lin (Ed.), *Advanced practice in oncology nursing* (pp. 401–407). Pittsburgh, PA: Oncology Nursing Society.

Moore, D., & Sweedman, M. (2004). Advanced nurse practice in the oncology setting: A case study. *Australian Journal of Cancer Nursing, 5*(2), 16–24.

Moult, B., Franck, L.S., & Brady, H. (2004). Ensuring quality information for patients: Development and preliminary validation of a new instrument to improve the quality of written health card information. *Health Expectations, 7,* 165–175.

Murphy-Ende, K. (2002). Advanced practice nursing: Reflections on the past, issues for the future. *Oncology Nursing Forum, 29,* 106–112.

National Association of Clinical Nurse Specialists. (2004). *Statement on clinical nurse specialist practice and education.* Harrisburg, PA: Author.

National Association of Clinical Nurse Specialists. (2005). *NACNS update on the clinical nurse leader (CNL), September 2005.* Retrieved July 26, 2007, from http://www.nacns.org/NACNS_Positionstatement_CNL_9_05_3_04.pdf

National Cancer Institute. (1998). *Guidelines for establishing comprehensive cancer patient education services.* Bethesda, MD: Author.

National Organization of Nurse Practitioner Faculties. (2006, March). *Domains and core competencies of nurse practitioner practice.* Retrieved August 28, 2007, from http://www.nonpf.org/NONPF2005/CoreCompsFinal06.pdf

Nelson, R. (2006). NCSBN 'vision paper' ignites controversy. Second licensure exam proposed; clinical nurse specialists excluded from advanced practice model. *American Journal of Nursing, 106*(7), 25–26.

Neuss, M.N., Desch, C.E., McNiff, K.K., Eisenberg, P.D., Gesme, D.H., Jacobson, J.O., et al. (2005). A process for measuring the quality of cancer care: The Quality Oncology Practice Initiative. *Journal of Clinical Oncology, 23,* 6233–6239.

Oncology Nursing Society. (2005). *Position statement on quality cancer care.* Pittsburgh, PA: Author.

Oncology Nursing Society. (2007). *Oncology nurse practitioner competencies.* Pittsburgh, PA: Oncology Nursing Society.

O'Neill, E., & Krauel, P. (2004). Building transformational partnerships in nursing. *Journal of Professional Nursing, 20,* 295–299.

Parkinson, N., & Pratt, H. (2005). Clinical nurse specialists and the psychosexual needs of patients with gynaecological cancer. *Journal of the British Menopause Society, 11,* 33–35.

Piano, M.R., & Zerwic, J.J. (1998). Demonstrating the effectiveness of acute care nurse practitioner: Current and future research. In R.M. Kleinpell & M.R. Piano (Eds.), *Practice issues for the acute care nurse practitioner* (pp. 10–26). New York: Springer.

Plowfield, L., Wheeler, E., & Raymond, J. (2005). Time, tact, talent and trust: Essential ingredients of effective academic-community partnerships. *Nursing Education Perspectives, 26,* 217–220.

Popham, W.J. (1975). *Educational evaluation.* Englewood Cliffs, NJ: Prentice-Hall.

Profetto-McGrath, J. (2005). Critical thinking and evidence-based practice. *Journal of Professional Nursing, 21,* 354–371.

Profetto-McGrath, J., Smith, K.B., Hugo, K., Taylor, M., & El-Hajj, H. (2007). Clinical nurse specialists' use of evidence in practice: A pilot study. *Worldviews on Evidence-Based Nursing, 4,* 86–96.

Rankin, S.H., & Stallings, K.D. (1996). *Patient education: Issues, principles, practices* (3rd ed.). Philadelphia: Lippincott.

Rankin, S.H, Stallings, K.D., & London, F. (2005). *Patient education in health and illness* (5th ed.). Philadelphia: Lippincott Williams & Wilkins.

Rees, C.E., Ford, J.E., & Sheard, C.E. (2002). Evaluating the reliability of DISCERN: A tool for assessing the quality of written patient information on treatment choices. *Patient Education and Counseling, 47,* 273–275.

Reilly, D.E., & Oermann, M.H. (1992). *Clinical teaching in nursing education* (2nd ed.). New York: National League for Nursing.

Reina, M.L., Reina, D.S., & Rushton, C.H. (2007). Trust: The foundation for team collaboration and healthy work environments. *AACN Advanced Critical Care, 18,* 103–108.

Ricci, S., Celani, M.G., & Righetti, E. (2006). Development of clinical guidelines: Methodological and practical issues. *Neurological Science, 27*(Suppl. 3), S228–S230.

Rigolosi, E.L. (2005). *Management and leadership in nursing and health care.* New York: Springer.

Ritz, L.J., Nissen, M.J., Swenson, K.K., Farrell, J.B., Sperduto, P.W., Sladek, M.L., et al. (2000). Effects of advanced nursing care on quality of life and cost outcomes of women diagnosed with breast cancer. *Oncology Nursing Forum, 27,* 923–932.

Robison, J.G., Swan, D., Jolley, C., Robinson, C.B., Simonson, C., Viale, P.H., et al. (2004). Implementing the advanced practice nursing survey results: Report by the online services and education team. *Oncology Nursing Forum, 31,* 881–885.

Rogers, E. (1995). *Diffusion of innovations.* New York: Free Press.

Rogers, J., & Curtis, P. (1980). The concept and measurement of continuity in primary care. *American Journal of Public Health, 70,* 122–127.

Rogers, L.M. (2006). Meeting the Center for Medicare & Medicaid Services requirements for quality assessment and performance improvement: A model for hospitals. *Journal of Nursing Care Quality, 21,* 325–330.

Rutten, L.J., Arora, N.K., Bakos, A.D., Aziz, N., & Rowland, J. (2005). Information needs and sources of information among cancer patients: A systematic review of research (1980–2003). *Patient Education and Counseling, 57,* 250–261.

Saarmann, L., Daugherty, J., & Riegel, B. (2000). Patient teaching to promote behavioral change. *Nursing Outlook, 48,* 281–287.

Scarpa, R. (2004). Advanced practice nursing in head and neck cancer: Implementation of five roles. *Oncology Nursing Forum, 31,* 579–583.

Selph, A.K. (1998). Negotiating an acute care nurse practitioner position. *AACN Clinical Issues, 9,* 269–276.

Shah, H.S., & Sullivan, D.T. (1998). Evaluation of the acute care nurse practitioner's role. In R.M. Kleinpell & M.R. Piano (Eds.), *Practice issues for the acute care nurse practitioner* (pp. 111–143). New York: Springer.

Shepard, N., & Kelvin, J.F. (1999). The nursing role in radiation oncology. *Seminars in Oncology Nursing, 15,* 237–249.

Shortell, S. (1976). Continuity of medical care: Conceptualization and measurement. *Medical Care, 14,* 377–391.

Sidani, S., & Irvine, D. (1999). A conceptual framework for evaluating the nurse practitioner role in acute care settings. *Journal of Advanced Nursing, 30,* 58–66.

Skalla, K.A. (2006). Blended role advanced practice nursing in palliative care of the oncology patient. *Journal of Hospice and Palliative Care Nursing, 8,* 155–163.

Spross, J.A., & Heaney, C.A. (2000). Shaping advanced nursing practice in the new millennium. *Seminars in Oncology Nursing, 16,* 12–24.

Stanley, J.M., Spross, J.A., Hamric, A.B., Hall, G., Minarik, P.A., & Sparacino, P.S. (2004). *Working statement comparing clinical nurse leader and clinical nurse specialist roles: Similarities, differences and complementarities.* Washington, DC: American Association of Colleges of Nursing.

Stanton, M.P., Swanson, M., Sherrod, R.A., & Packa, D.R. (2005). Case management evolution: From basic to advanced practice role. *Lippincott's Case Management, 10,* 274–284.

Starfield, B. (1980). Continuous confusion? *American Journal of Public Health, 70,* 117–119.

Styles, M.M. (1996). Conceptualizations of advanced nursing practice. In A.B. Hamric, J.A. Spross, & C.M. Hanson (Eds.), *Advanced nursing practice: An integrative approach* (pp. 25–41). Philadelphia: Saunders.

Thurston, N.E., Watson, L.A., & Reimer, M.A. (1993). Research or quality improvement? Making the decision. *Journal of Nursing Administration, 23*(7/8), 46–49.

Timmins, F. (2006). Exploring the concept of 'information need'. *International Journal of Nursing Practice, 12,* 375–381.

Treacy, J.T., & Mayer, D.K. (2000). Perspectives on cancer patient education. *Seminars in Oncology Nursing, 16,* 47–56.

Upchurch, S., Brosnan, C.A., & Grimes, D.E. (2002). Teaching research synthesis to advanced practice nurses. *Journal of Nursing Education, 41,* 222–226.

Vaz, F., & Small, S. (2007). The lead cancer nurse—an ill-defined role? *Journal of Nursing Management, 15,* 149–154.

Vogel, W.H. (2003). The advanced practice nursing role in a high-risk breast cancer clinic. *Oncology Nursing Forum, 30,* 115–122.

Volker, D.L., Kahn, D., & Penticuff, J.H. (2004). Patient control and end-of-life care part I: The advanced practice nurse perspective. *Oncology Nursing Forum, 31,* 945–953.

Wimpenny, P., & van Zelm, R. (2007). Appraising and comparing pressure ulcer guidelines. *Worldviews on Evidence-Based Nursing, 4,* 40–50.

Winkler, M.F., Ross, V.M., Piamjariyakul, U., Gajewski, B., & Smith, C.E. (2006). Technology dependence in home care: Impact on patients and their family caregivers. *Nutrition in Clinical Practice, 21,* 544–556.

Yoder-Wise, P.S., & Kowalski, K.E. (2006). *Beyond leading and managing: Nursing administration for the future.* St. Louis, MO: Elsevier Mosby.

Zwarenstein, M., & Bryant, W. (2000). Interventions to promote collaboration between nurses and doctors. *Cochrane Database of Systematic Reviews 2000,* Issue 2, Art No: CD000072. DOI: 10.1002/14651858. CD000072.

CHAPTER 20

Professional Practice of Advanced Practice Nurses

Kathy Sharp, MSN, FNP-BC, AOCNP®

Introduction

This chapter presents a review of the fundamental principles that are part of advanced practice nursing. Demonstration of this knowledge, via successful completion of the Advanced Oncology Certified Nurse Practitioner (AOCNP®) or the Advanced Oncology Certified Clinical Nurse Specialist (AOCNS®) certification examination, is an integral part of the journey to excellence in professional oncology practice (Oncology Nursing Certification Corporation [ONCC], 2007).

Advanced Practice Nursing

Although some authors (Nagelkerk & Ryan, 2003; National Council of State Boards of Nursing [NCSBN], 2006a) have suggested that the roles of the clinical nurse specialist (CNS) and nurse practitioner (NP) should be blended or merged, the Oncology Nursing Society (ONS) acknowledged the unique role of each profession. Rather than follow the suggestion of a national advisory board, such as the NCSBN (2006a), toward merging the roles, ONS recognized that the CNS and NP have unique roles and areas of specialization within the oncology healthcare arena (ONS, 2006). ONS defined each role and, through ONCC, created separate certifications for each. The oncology advanced practice nurse (APN) continues to be defined as a licensed RN with a master's degree in nursing who has completed 500 hours of supervised practice in an advanced practice role in oncology and has passed the certification test for CNSs or NPs (ONCC, 2004).

Regulation of Practice

APN practice is regulated at two levels: licensure, which is at the state level, and certification, which is through national organizations. Other factors that may influence or guide practice are credentialing and privileging, scopes of practice, and standards of practice (Jacobs, 2003b). Agencies, such as the NCSBN, also contribute to regulation of practice. In 1978, the NCSBN was founded to provide a vehicle through which boards of nursing could ensure that nurses in the workforce have the skills and knowledge needed to practice, thus safeguarding the public. In the years since its inception, the NCSBN also has made recommendations regarding APN practice (NCSBN, 2006c).

Registration

Registration is a historical term and was originally used in the early days of nursing when nurses registered with their state boards. In the present time, registration generally is synonymous with licensure. Regardless of and apart from certification requirements, all oncology APNs must be licensed in their state(s) as a registered nurse and are subject to that state's legal regulations for recognition and licensure of advanced practice nursing. Although the American Nurses Association (ANA) and ONS have defined the scope of advanced nursing practice, the state boards of nursing and federal laws are ultimately responsible for regulation (Jacobs, 2003a; Loquist, 2004).

Licensure

Mitchell (2001, p. 395) defined licensure as "the legal permission to practice within a specific scope of practice once educational requirements are met." The NCSBN (2007) defined licensure as "the process by which an agency of state government grants authority to an individual to engage in a given profession upon finding that the applicant has attained the essential degree of competency." The licensing requirements of each state differ according to the state nurse practice act. All states require a license as an RN, and some states require second licensure as an APN (Mitchell, 2001). It is prudent for new APNs to investigate the board of nursing Web site for the state in which they will be practicing prior to graduation. Experienced APNs who may be moving to another state to practice should likewise make use of these Web sites to see if new requirements must be met (NCSBN, 2007). Although it remains controversial, the NCSBN approved a model of mutual recognition for licensure of APNs. This model, known as a multistate compact, would allow compact states to grant reciprocity and recognize the credentials of an APN licensed in another state. Enactment would require legislative approval and implementation. Thus far, Iowa and Utah agreed to mutually recognize APRN licenses. Other states are discussing the ramifications of such a measure (NCSBN, 2006b).

Certification

Unlike the legal scope of practice, which is defined by the laws of each state, certification is not a governmental process. Certification is regulated by a professional agency, such as ONS. Certification is established to determine individual competence based on achievement of specific predetermined criteria. ONS, through ONCC, provides two advanced oncology certifications. Nurses who have the educational preparation to function in the role of CNS and meet the eligibility requirements for testing may receive certification by passing the AOCNS® examination. Successful scores result in awarding of the AOCNS® credential. Likewise, those who are educated in an NP graduate program and meet eligibility requirements for testing may sit for the NP examination. Their awarded credential is AOCNP® (ONCC, 2007).

The separate examinations came about as a result of a role delineation study commissioned by ONCC in 2003. More than 625 APNs participated and rated tasks and knowledge in order of importance to their job. The results provided evidence that although CNSs and NPs needed much core knowledge, definite differences existed in work responsibilities. ONCC also received input about areas of professional development and education that participants desired. As a result, ONCC proceeded to develop the separate certification examinations (ONCC, 2003, 2004).

Also worth noting is that some states grant APN licensure on the basis of national certification but do not specify the type. Generally, states are moving toward certification as a mechanism to grant an APN license. Many states do not specify which type of certification is acceptable, but not all states recognize the AOCNP® or AOCNS® credential. APNs must be thoroughly familiar with the rules and regulations of the state in which they plan to practice (Phillips, 2006).

Credentialing and Privileging

Credentialing is one method of ensuring credibility to and protection of the public (ONS, 2003). It generally is a term that applies to institutional governing bodies, such as those that oversee hospital medical staff, or to insurance providers. Hospitals, managed care organizations, and insurers have the authority to decide if an NP or CNS may be included (i.e., credentialed) on their list of healthcare providers (Buppert, 2005). Credentialing is a way of ensuring that the APN has met all the licensure, certification, and any other federal- or state-mandated regulations for advanced nursing practice. In contrast, *privileging* specifies the service or services the APN can provide and defines the limits of APN practice. The privileges requested may change over time as the APN acquires new skills (Kamajian, Mitchell, & Fruth, 1999; Mitchell, 2001).

Scope of Practice

The scope of practice of oncology APNs integrates both medical and nursing paradigms, which benefits the care of patients with cancer and their families. The oncology APN's scope of practice is defined by federal regulations, state nurse practice acts, ONS guidelines, and practice agreements with the employer. ONS has developed a statement on the scope of practice, which may serve as a guide to both new graduates and APNs with years of experience. It may be utilized to develop a job description and clinical collaborative practice agreement, both of which will affect the practice privileges of APNs in their particular setting (ONS, 2003). The scope of practice may be independent of or in collaboration with a physician, depending on state regulations. Variances of state law may specify physician supervision, delegation, or collaboration with APNs (American College of Nurse Practitioners, n.d.; Phillips, 2006).

Standards

Standards are authoritative statements that define responsibilities of APNs, provide direction and evaluation for APN practice, and reflect the values of advanced practice nursing in oncology. The *Standards of Advanced Practice Nursing in Oncology* may serve as a guide for APNs' self-evaluation and for peer or employer evaluation. Standards also may help the lay public to understand the role of the APN and can provide a resource for health policy makers (Jacobs, 2003b).

Advanced Practice Standards

In 1990, ONS published the *Standards of Advanced Practice in Oncology Nursing*. This document was revised in 1997, retitled as *Statement on the Scope and Standards of Advanced Practice in Oncology Nursing*, and further defined the roles and responsibilities of oncology APNs. A third edition was published in 2003, which describes two types of standards followed by objectives. These are standards of care and standards of professional performance. The standards of care follow the nursing process: assessment, diagnosis, planning, implementation, and evaluation. The standards of professional performance relate to quality of care, self-evaluation, education, leadership ethics, multidisciplinary collaboration, and research. An example of a standard of care is assessment, which has seven measurement criteria. One of those seven criteria states that the APN "orders or recommends relevant diagnostic tests, procedures, and other assessment methods" (Jacobs, 2003b, p. 9). This criterion is measurable by the documentation of orders for the patient and thus provides a benchmark by which APNs or their employer can evaluate performance.

Reimbursement

Effective January 1998, the provisions of the Balanced Budget Act of 1997 expanded to include reimbursement to NPs and CNSs by authorizing them to bill Medicare directly for their services. Reimbursement is set at 85% of the level of physician reimbursement or 80% of the actual charge, whichever is smaller. Prior to 2007, NPs and CNSs had to apply for a Medicare provider number. Starting in 2007, however, all providers must obtain National Provider Identification (NPI) numbers. This number will remain the same no matter where the provider practices. Each practice site also must obtain an NPI number, which is unique to the site. Each APN must go through the credentialing process with each individual commercial insurance company in order to bill for reimbursement. Although many insurance companies follow the Medicare guidelines and provide 85% of physician-level reimbursement for the APN, this may vary from company to company and state to state. Medicare has "incident-to" billing, in which the APN may bill for the full 100% of physician-level reimbursement, but the service provided must follow stringent guidelines as outlined by Medicare. Potential for error or rule misinterpretation exists with the incident-to-billing system, and most experts in reimbursement suggest always billing under the provider number of the APN (Buppert, 2005).

Medicare Standards for Advanced Practice Nurses

Obtaining an NPI number is the first step in being credentialed by Medicare or commercial insurance companies as a provider. The NPI is a unique 10-digit number assigned to each healthcare provider. The use of the NPI officially began in October 2006 and replaced the Medicare Provider Identification number, the Unique Physician Identification Number, and the Medicaid Provider number. As of May 2007, only the NPI is accepted for billing, with the exception of small health plans, which had until May 2008 to make the change. The NPI also replaced identifying numbers that were assigned to the provider by the individual commercial insurers (Buppert, 2006).

APNs may qualify for reimbursement under Medicare Part B if the applicant is
- Legally authorized to provide services in the state where the service is provided
- Licensed as an RN in the state where he or she practices
- Holds a master's degree in a defined clinical area of nursing from an accredited institution
- Certified as an NP or a CNS by a national certifying body that has established standards for NPs or CNSs. Recognized certifying organizations include
  - American Academy of Nurse Practitioners
  - American Nurses Credentialing Center
  - National Certification Corporation for Obstetric, Gynecologic, and Neonatal Nursing
  - National Certification Boards of Pediatric Nurse Practitioners and Nurses
  - ONCC
  - Critical Care Certification Corporation.

Services will be covered if they are comparable to those provided by a medical doctor (MD) or a doctor of osteopathy (DO), furnished in collaboration with the MD or DO as required by state law, and not excluded by Medicare. As of December 2003, Medicare pays for NP services in hospice if the NP is selected as the attending provider. A physician must provide certification of the illness as terminal with a life expectancy of six months or less (Centers for Medicare and Medicaid Services [CMS], 2006a).

To enroll as a Medicare provider, the individual must complete a form provided by CMS. The information requested includes the clinician's name, date of birth, contact information, the location of the practice and address where payments are sent, the year of graduation, and the name of the collaborating or supervising physician. CMS also will request information about the location of patient medical records, practice management organization information, billing agency information, and information about any electronic claims transmissions companies that the APN may use. Any legal actions or judgments previously imposed on the APN must be reported. By signing and submitting the form, the applicant is agreeing to abide by Medicare regulation (Buppert, 2005).

APNs must employ accurate coding and documentation of services in order to receive reimbursement from Medicare and other insurers. Coding is the assignment of a numeric or alphanumeric classification to indicate the diagnosis or procedure. Level I of the Healthcare Common Procedure Coding System (HCPCS) refers to current procedural terminology (CPT) coding and is used to identify procedures, such as paracentesis, biopsy, and injections. Level II HCPCS coding primarily is used to identify products, supplies, and services not included in CPT codes, such as durable medical equipment. The *International Classification of Diseases, Ninth Revision, Clinical Modification (ICD-9-CM)* is used to identify the disease or symptom that is treated (CMS, 2006b).

According to general principles of medical record documentation by Medicare (CMS, 2006c), the following information should be included with each patient encounter.
- Reason(s) for patient visit and relevant history, including appropriate health risks
- Physical examination findings and prior diagnostic test results
- Patient response to previous interventions
- Assessment and diagnosis
- Plan of care, including written or inferred rationale for diagnostic or other services
- Date and identity of provider
- Documentation to substantiate the CPT and ICD-9-CM codes that were reported and billed

Nurse Practitioner Versus Clinical Nurse Specialist Role in Advanced Practice

Delineation and Recognition

In an environment where NP and CNS roles increasingly are being blended under the title of APN, ONS took a firm stance that each of the roles remain separate and distinct entities with unique domains of practice, based on the 2003 role delineation study, which revealed discernable differences in the work responsibilities of NPs and CNSs in oncology. In 2006, ONS further solidified the distinction of each role by dividing the previous certification test with the credential AOCN® (Advanced Oncology Certified Nurse) into two separate examinations, one for NPs and one for CNSs. Although the AOCN examination has been eliminated, people who have received AOCN certification in the past may continue to maintain that title through continuing education (ONCC, 2004).

Scope of Practice Comparison

ONS identified five functional roles for the APN as direct care provider or caregiver, administrator/coordinator, consultant, researcher, and educator (ONS, 2003). Although NPs and CNSs are both recognized as clinical experts, ONS states that the domain of care, the scope of practice, and the spheres of influence distinguish the NP and CNS roles (ONS, 2003).

CNSs' scope of practice includes providing clinical expertise in cancer care, assisting patients and families with symptom and palliative care needs, and serving as a patient advocate. CNSs participate in staff and healthcare team development via education, role modeling, and dissemination of research findings. NPs' "scope of practice includes comprehensive health assessments; differential diagnosis; ordering, supervising, and interpreting diagnostic tests; prescribing pharmacologic and nonpharmacologic treatments in collaboration with a physician partner; and screening to prevent illness and promote wellness" (ONS, 2003).

Spheres of Influence

CNS spheres of influence are multifaceted and currently are organized within three major areas of influence. These are the patient/client sphere, the nurse/nursing sphere, and the organization/system sphere. The patient/client sphere includes demonstration of quality patient outcomes through assessment and intervention by CNSs. The nurse/nursing sphere acknowledges the contributions of CNSs to nurses and nursing through their leadership and staff development activities, including the development of evidence-based policies, procedures, and protocols. The organizational/system sphere recognizes CNSs' contributions to health care via informational, educational, and other activities that involve health team members, communities, and healthcare systems (Moloney-Harmon, 1999).

ONS is developing competencies for oncology CNSs that follow the three spheres of influence (see Table 20-1) (C. Miller-Murphy, personal communication, January 24, 2007). NP competencies have been completed and are available online from ONS at www.ons.org/clinical/professional/qualitycancer/documents/npcompentencies.pdf.

Table 20-1. Clinical Nurse Specialist Competencies

Sphere of Influence	Competency	Description
Patient/client	1. Health assessment 2. Diagnosis of health status and plan of care 3. Intervention 4. Evaluation	Knowledge and skills are used to assess, diagnose, and manage illness and risk behaviors in patients with a past, current, or potential diagnosis of cancer and improve nursing-sensitive outcomes.
Nurse/nursing practice	1. Assessment/definition of problems 2. Diagnosis and outcome identification, and planning 3. Intervention 4. Evaluation 5. Professional role	Nursing practice is advanced and nursing-sensitive patient outcomes are improved by updating and improving norms and standards of oncology nursing practice.
Organization/system	1. Assessment 2. Diagnosis, outcome identification, and plan of care 3. Intervention 4. Evaluation	Competencies in this sphere advocate for professional nursing, provide skill, leadership, knowledge, and behavior to influence changes at the system level, and improve quality cost-effective outcomes.

Note. Based on information from Oncology Nursing Society, in press.

Those pertinent to NPs' professional role are summarized in Table 20-2 (ONS, 2007a).

Generally, NPs have the patient as their primary focus, but they also may have a significant influence on the family and the community at large. Oncology NPs are recognized as clinical experts and provide direct, episodic health care to patients with cancer. This includes acute and chronic problems, symptom management, and palliative care needs. NPs influence the patients' family members, other healthcare providers, nursing staff, hospital and other healthcare systems, and the community through direct and indirect interaction; individual, group, and community education; and legislative and political activism (Jacobs, 2003b; ONS, 2003).

Professional Responsibilities

Healthcare Legislation

ONS standards state that oncology APNs participate in activities that enhance practice, and the arena of healthcare legislation provides multiple opportunities for such participation. APNs should be aware of and promote passage of legislation supporting cancer care and should serve as a liaison to legislative bodies and individuals regarding issues related to oncology nursing and advanced oncology nursing practice (Jacobs, 2003b; Wakefield, 2004).

Oncology APNs may be involved in healthcare legislation by serving as a resource or researcher for specific healthcare issues, especially those involving cancer care. Simply corresponding with policy makers regarding current legislation and providing factual information from the viewpoint of the APN oftentimes can make a positive impact on

Table 20-2. Nurse Practitioner Competencies

Standard	Competency
I. Health promotion, health protection, disease prevention and treatment	Assesses all aspects of patient health, including those for health promotion, health protection, and disease prevention; uses evidence-based clinical practice guidelines to guide screening, health promotion, and counseling
II. Nurse practitioner-patient relationship	Demonstrates personal, collaborative, and therapeutic approaches to patient care
III. Teaching-coaching function	Includes functions such as imparting knowledge to the patient for self-care; coaching involves advocacy, support, and reinforcement.
IV. Professional role	Demonstrates a commitment to the implementation, preservation, and evolution of the oncology nurse practitioner role
V. Negotiating healthcare delivery systems	Oversees and directs the delivery of clinical services within the healthcare system
VI. Monitoring and ensuring quality of healthcare practice	Ensures quality of care via consultation, collaboration, continuing education, certification, and evaluation; engages in interdisciplinary peer and systems review
VII. Caring for diverse populations	Involves provision of culturally competent care with respect to cultural and spiritual beliefs and making healthcare resources available for people from diverse cultures

Note. Based on information from Oncology Nursing Society, 2007.

critical issues. Other ways to engage policy makers is for APNs to invite them to nursing organization meetings or to tour the oncology APN workplace (Wakefield, 2004).

Continuous Quality Improvement

Continuous quality improvement (CQI) may be known by other names, such as quality improvement (QI), quality assurance (QA), or quality improvement process, although some fundamental differences exist in each. The word *continuous* implies an ongoing or constant course of action, unlike QA, which may involve a retrospective review of an event or procedure. The CQI process in a facility such as a hospital usually entails people from different but interactive areas coming together to review a systems process. The end result usually is focused on improving patient care or cost-saving measures and generally is more process oriented than individual oriented (Katz & Green, 1997).

CQI for the APN is a multifaceted process involving self-evaluation, patient evaluation, peer evaluation, systems evaluation, and the use and promotion of evidence-based practice (EBP). The ONS standards of professional performance outline the APN's obligation to be engaged in each level of QI (ONS, 2007a).

Self-evaluation can be achieved by seeking feedback from patients, professional colleagues, members of the healthcare team, and employers and by modifying practice in response to their evaluation. Attainment of professional learning or performance goals can be other measurable self-improvement tools. Finally, a comparison of patient treatment plans to nationally established guidelines may provide valuable feedback for APNs' self-evaluation of performance (i.e., benchmarking) (ONS, 2007a).

Patient evaluation is a continuous process that includes complete patient assessment, diagnosis, planning, and assessment of response to the treatment plan. Measuring patient outcomes and modifying plans according to evidence-based research and benchmarks also are part of patient evaluation and the continuous improvement process (ONS, 2007a).

Peer evaluation involves collaboration with team members to improve self-performance and ultimately patient care. Peer evaluation provides the opportunity for identification of individual strengths as well as behaviors that need to be changed. Honest feedback from peers, although sometimes difficult to absorb and difficult to deliver to others, serves to open avenues for growth and professional excellence (Ishida, 2005).

Several agencies monitor, recommend, and publish standards for healthcare quality. Some of these, along with their mission, are listed in Table 20-3.

Table 20-3. Missions of Agencies Dedicated to Healthcare Quality

Agency	Mission
Agency for Healthcare Research and Quality	Supports research designed to improve healthcare quality, decrease cost, and create more access to essential services
Institute for Healthcare Improvement	Independent, nonprofit organization dedicated to accelerating healthcare system improvement
Institute for Safe Medication Practices	Nonprofit whose mission is providing education for healthcare professionals and consumers regarding safe practices for medications
Institutes of Medicine	Organization whose goal is the reduction of medical errors and improvement of patient safety
Joint Commission on Accreditation of Healthcare Organizations	Agency that provides accreditation for hospitals, managed care entities, and healthcare facilities. Its mission is improved safety and quality of care.
National Association for Healthcare Quality	Organization that supports education and knowledge acquisition for healthcare quality professionals; publishes the *Journal for Healthcare Quality*
National Committee for Quality Assurance	Independent, nonprofit organization whose twofold mission is to improve the quality of health care delivered to consumers and to educate the public to make more informed decisions

Note. Based on information from University of Medicine and Dentistry of New Jersey, 2001.

Evidence-Based Practice

Many definitions exist, but most authors agree that EBP is the appraisal and judicious use of the most current evidence to make decisions regarding the care of patients. As implied, this requires ongoing evaluation of findings from well-designed research or designing and conducting research to supplement evidence that is missing (Krebs, 2005). Standard VII of the standards of professional performance outlined in the *Statement on the Scope and Standards of Advanced Practice Nursing in Oncology* (3rd ed.) (Jacobs, 2003b) mandates that oncology APNs utilize current evidence for decision making and evaluation.

ONS has an Evidence-Based Practice Resource Area available online at http://onsopcontent.ons.org/toolkits/evidence/ to assist APNs in identifying, appraising, and utilizing evidence. The six steps in the EBP process (ONS, n.d.) are

- Problem identification—What is the question to be answered?
- Finding evidence—Where is the evidence?
- Critiquing evidence—How current is the evidence?
- Summarizing evidence—Does all the evidence concur?
- Application to practice—Is it applicable to the situation?
- Evaluation—Was the evidence-based intervention successful?

ONS has categorized evidence into three levels (see Figure 20-1). Level I represents the strongest research-based evidence. Level II includes everything from well-conducted studies without randomization to published practice guidelines. Level III is the weakest evidence, which is not research based. APNs can apply evidence clinically in a multitude of ways. Some of these may include discussing case studies with peers or staff (level III), sharing published guidelines from healthcare agencies such as the National Comprehensive Cancer Network (weaker level II), conducting a case-control study in the workplace (stronger level II), or participating

ONS Levels of Evidence

ONS Level	Level of Evidence Subcategory	Evidence Source	Strength of Evidence
		Research-Based Evidence	
I	1	Meta-analysis or systematic reviews of multiple well-designed, randomized, controlled clinical trials	**Strongest**
	2	Well-controlled, randomized clinical trials with adequate sample size	
	3	Well-designed trial without randomization (single group pre/post, cohort, time series studies)	
II	4	Well-conducted, systematic review of nonexperimental design studies	
	5	Well-conducted case-control study	
	6	Poorly controlled (flawed randomized studies) or uncontrolled studies (correlational descriptive studies)	
	7	Conflicting evidence or meta-analysis showing a trend that did not reach significance	
		National Institutes of Health Consensus Report	
		Published practice guidelines, for example by professional organizations, healthcare organizations, or federal agencies	
		Non-Research Based Evidence	
III	8	Qualitative designs	**Weakest**
		Case studies, opinions of expert authorities, agencies or committees	

Figure 20-1. Oncology Nursing Society (ONS) Levels of Evidence

Note. Based on information from Ropka & Spencer-Cisek, 2001.

in a large, nationwide randomized clinical trial (level I). Several online resources are available for APNs to access nationally recognized guidelines (see Table 20-4). Each of the organizations is committed to quality cancer care and all are composed of experts in oncology.

Table 20-4. Online Resources for Oncology Evidence-Based Guidelines

Agency	Web Address
Agency for Healthcare Research and Quality	www.ahrq.gov
American Society of Clinical Oncology	www.asco.org
National Comprehensive Cancer Network	www.nccn.org
National Oncology Alliance	www.noainc.com/noa/about-noa/index.aspx
Oncology Nursing Society	http://onsopcontent.ons.org/toolkits/evidence

Community Involvement

APNs are in a unique position to support improvement in cancer care through involvement in national organizations focused on cancer, cancer research, or advanced oncology practice. Examples might be the American Cancer Society, ONS, or any of the specialty organizations such as Susan G. Komen for the Cure (www.komen.org), the Leukemia and Lymphoma Society (www.leukemia-lymphoma.org), or the Lance Armstrong Foundation (www.livestrong.org). Involvement may take the form of acting as a resource for factual information or offering to serve on local, community, or national boards.

Media

The media is a great conduit for the distribution of information. By fostering a relationship with local or national media personalities, APNs can open the door of opportunity for disseminating education to the public. That education may be about a disease process, APN practice, or healthcare legislative concerns. Media-savvy APNs have the opportunity to affect public policy and policymakers, as well as heighten awareness of the importance of the APN role (Wakefield, 2004).

Research

Standard VII of the standards of professional practice in the *Statement on the Scope and Standards of Advanced Practice Nursing in Oncology* (Jacobs, 2003b) outlines oncology APNs' involvement in research. An important research obligation of APNs is the dissemination of research to others. This involves ongoing review and analysis of current research reported in the literature, which requires understanding of research design, statistical data analysis, and application of research findings. Notable findings then may be translated into practice through staff education or changing of policies and procedures (Krebs, 2005).

APNs also may be directly involved in performing research through participation in nationally sponsored clinical trials. If so, some of their responsibilities may be the enrollment of patients, the collection of data, education of participants and their families or significant others, and observation of participants for side effects or response to treatment.

Ethics

The Merriam-Webster online dictionary ("Ethics," 2007) defined ethics as a set of principles or values of good or right behavior or as a standard of conduct made by members of a profession. Ethical dilemmas exist when a situation requires a choice about right behavior or conduct between two equal and opposing alternatives. With each patient encounter, APNs incorporate ethical principles and values into their practice. For the purposes of this book, principles and values are identified as separate elements, but one should recognize that much overlap exists. Regardless, they should be used as a guide for individual oncology APN practice. A majority of the time, these principles are such a fundamental part of APN behavior and patient interaction that they are not readily identified as entities unto themselves. However, to understand their importance as an integral part of professional practice, it is necessary to identify and define each principle and value and to understand their specific meaning.

Ethical Principles

Four basic ethical principles exist, although some authors may include more. This chapter will address autonomy, beneficence, nonmaleficence, and justice (Marsee, 1998).

Autonomy describes patients' ability to self-rule and make decisions regarding their care. Each patient has a right to self-determination, including the ability to choose among medically indicated treatments as well as the ability to refuse any unwanted treatments. This principle is the moral basis for obtaining informed consent and accepting informed refusal (Marsee, 1998). Autonomy also is a trait ascribed to the APN, and Gilliss (1996) stated that the development of autonomy is essential to successful role implementation.

Beneficence simply means doing good. Some people may confuse doing good with the intent to do good. All interactions with patients should be based on the intent toward the patient. For instance, chemotherapy is known to have many harmful, painful, or even life-threatening complications; thus, giving chemotherapy might not be considered beneficial in the eyes of some. Although APNs know chemotherapy has negative side effects, it is intended to help rid the patient of cancer cells. The key here is the intent to act in the best interest of the patient while not forgetting that each patient has the autonomy to decide what is good for himself or herself. APNs should not allow internal conflicts to arise because of a paternalistic ideation toward the patient (i.e., deciding what is best for the patient) (Silva & Ludwick, 1999).

Nonmaleficence means to "do no harm." This principle has its origins in the Hippocratic oath and commands that APNs "do not cause injury to patients" (Silva & Ludwick, 1999, p. 2). This term also includes the implication to individually evaluate anticipated treatments to ensure that the potential harm or negative side effects do not outweigh the anticipated benefit (Silva & Ludwick).

Justice is the duty to be fair in all interactions and applies also to the allocation of sometimes meager resources. Institutional or insurance allocation policies may define the benefits dispensed to each person, thus affecting oncology APNs' just actions to the patient. Justice implies that each person will receive what he or she is due. Often, justice is based on need, but in the arena of scarce personnel and fiscal resources, justice may have to be based on the fair distribution of what is available (Silva & Ludwick, 1999).

Ethical Values

In addition to ethical principles, APNs utilize ethical values, including confidentiality, fidelity, compassion, integrity, and veracity, in their professional practice. These ethical values are not unique to oncology practice but should be an integral part of oncology care.

Confidentiality is the respect for patients' private information. The term applies to information shared with the healthcare provider in one-to-one interactions and to information recorded in patients' records. Healthcare Insurance Portability and Accountability Act (HIPAA) regulations spell out how patients' personal information must be handled in order to provide the optimum security. HIPAA laws allow patients to designate which family members, friends, or others may be privy to information contained in their chart. According to these laws, patients also may specify how agencies, such as a hospital billing department, may utilize or share information (HIPAA, 2006; U.S. Department of Health and Human Services, 2006).

Fidelity is the obligation to keep one's promise and commitments, both to others and to oneself. Patients expect APNs to be meticulous in their follow-through and depend on APNs' conscientious attention to detail. Braddock and Snyder (2005) described fidelity as a virtue that supports the patient's trust and confidence and proposed that time spent advocating for the patient with insurance companies and championing healthcare issues are examples of fidelity in action.

Compassion is the ability to be empathetic to the patient's situation and to act in a kind and helpful manner. Sister Simone Roach (2004) stated that the philosophy of caring (which includes compassion) guides interactions with patients, families, and communities and is the very essence of nursing.

Integrity refers to the individual being true to and adhering to a moral set of values, with honesty being among those values. Integrity and veracity overlap to some degree. *Veracity* refers to the duty or obligation to be truthful and honest to the patient. Although it is known that honesty includes telling the truth, Mitchell (n.d.) pointed out that honesty also includes avoiding deception, misrepresentation, and nondisclosure unless the patient indicates a desire to not know certain information. Integrity demands that the patient's informed request to not know certain information must be honored, even if this causes conflict with the oncology APN's sense of values.

Ethical Issues

Informed Consent

Informed consent requires effective communication and represents a joint venture between the patient and the healthcare professional. It is not just an episodic event but rather is a continuous process of information exchange. Informed consent includes disclosure, adequate patient understanding, voluntariness, competence, and recognition of barriers to informed consent. APNs need to recognize that the patient has a right to refuse or withdraw consent at any point in time (Marsee, 1998).

Disclosure is an explanation of the procedure, treatment, or other intervention intended for the patient. Complete disclosure includes all the positive and negative effects associated with the intervention, and it is clearly presented in language that is educationally appropriate for the patient. It also includes the potential outcome without the intended treatment (Ford, 1990).

The patient's understanding may be dependent on many factors, including the type of disclosure, the surroundings in which disclosure takes place, the stress of the individual hearing or presenting the information, the presence of pain or anxiety, the proper education level of the information being presented, and the presence or absence of other individuals, such as family members or extra members of the healthcare team. The presenter must evaluate whether the patient's understanding is adequate. One effective method of doing this may be to have the patient repeat back a summary of what was explained. A signed consent is not always an informed consent. *Voluntariness* refers to the willingness of the patient to give consent without coercion (Scanlon & Glover, 1995).

Competence should not be confused with capacity when referring to the patient's ability to make decisions. *Competence* is a legal term that refers to one's mental ability to understand the information presented and make decisions after weighing the pros and cons of a situation. *Capacity* is only the ability to make a decision and is not necessarily based on competent, rational thought. For instance, a patient with Alzheimer dementia has the capacity to make a decision but not the cognitive prowess to make a competent decision (Marsee, 1998; Pan, 2002). Pan stated that a patient's decision-making capacity is determined by three things: (a) the ability to understand diagnosis and treatment, (b) the ability to deliberate and weigh options, risks, and benefits, and (c) the ability to communicate a choice to another person.

Oncology APNs should be mindful that barriers and exceptions to informed consent exist. Language can be a barrier if the patient and the informer do not speak the same language or if the patient has difficulty understanding or comprehending the informer's language because of education level or because of physical or psychological trauma or illness, such as receptive aphasia. Alterations in level of consciousness from sedation or effects of illness also can be a temporary or permanent barrier. Although often not identified as a barrier, presenting information in a way that implies a bias by the informer can hamper informed consent.

Exceptions for informed consent may be an emergency or the inability to give informed consent because of the presence of mind-altering substances, such as alcohol or drugs. Patients also may waive consent and authorize others to receive information (Scanlon & Glover, 1995).

Do-Not-Resuscitate Orders

Do-not-resuscitate (DNR) orders also may be known as "no code," "no CPR" (cardiopulmonary resuscitation), or the newer term "DNAR" (do not attempt resuscitation). ANA recommends that the DNR decision should be explicitly discussed by patients, family members, and the healthcare team. A designated surrogate or durable power of attorney should also be included in the absence of family or if patients are unable to act in their own best interests. DNR orders should be clearly documented in the patient's record and should not contain implications regarding withdrawal of the care (ANA, 2006c).

Patient Self-Determination Act

The Patient Self-Determination Act became federal law in 1991 and requires healthcare agencies to inform patients about advance directives upon admission. It does not require that patients complete advance directives, only that they are aware of their right to make decisions about these issues (ANA, 2006c).

Advance Directives

Advance directives are mechanisms that provide a way for patients to make their wishes known regarding health care in the event that they lose their decision-making capability. Advance directives may include a legal power of attorney, a durable power of attorney for health care, and a living will (Marsee, 1998). APNs are in a unique position to serve as a patient advocate by educating patients who do not understand advance directives (Basanta, 2002).

Durable Power of Attorney for Health Care

A legal power of attorney also may be called a durable power of attorney, which can cause confusion. No matter what the name, a legal power of attorney or durable power of attorney should not be confused with a durable power of attorney *for health care*. The durable power of attorney for health care also may be known as a healthcare surrogate. The legal power of attorney is a signed and notarized legal document giving an individual, who is appointed by the patient, the authority to conduct the patient's business affairs. In the absence of a durable power of attorney for health care, the legal power of attorney may make healthcare decisions for the patient if the patient becomes unable to make these decisions. The individual who is appointed by the patient to be the durable power of attorney for health care is authorized to make healthcare decisions for the patient if the patient becomes incapable of doing so. The durable power of attorney for health care does not have any authority for legal transactions; this person's job is limited to healthcare decision making. As implied, the durable power of attorney for health care is a legal document and carries no authority unless it is notarized. Notarization is a legal verification that the patient was of a competent mind when the document was signed and that the document was not coerced in any way. A copy of this document should be given to the patient's healthcare provider and to the healthcare facility where the patient may be treated. The patient should keep the original document (Marsee, 1998).

Living Will

A living will is a document written while the patient is competent to make decisions. It may include the patient's preferences about life-prolonging procedures and equipment and whether to withhold treatments. A living will usually specifies the extent of resuscitation efforts and what is included, such as whether to administer defibrillation, CPR, artificial respiration via a ventilator, and so on. A living will may be as specific as the patient desires. Forms are readily available at all healthcare facilities and on the Internet (e.g., the U.S. Living Will Registry at www.uslivingwillregistry.com/forms.shtm). Living wills also can be initiated through an attorney. Although a living will can be a list of handwritten directions by the patient, a typed and notarized document indicating that the patient was competent at the time the document was written is preferable. As with the durable power of attorney for health care, a copy of this document should be given to and discussed with the patient's healthcare provider. A copy should also be filed at the patient's healthcare facility of choice. The patient will keep the original document. Patients have the right to rescind or verbally revise their living will at any time. A written living will never overrides the desires of a competent patient (Marsee, 1998).

Ethical Controversies

Terminating or Withholding Treatment

The decision to terminate or withhold treatment should be directed by the patient if he or she is competent to do so. In the absence of the patient's competence, the patient's living will may provide direction. If no living will exists, a durable power of attorney for health care, if appointed, may make decisions for the patient. Last, the next of kin will be placed in the position of making decisions about treatment based on information provided by the healthcare provider. In cases of conflict about decisions, or if no one is available to make decisions for the patient, APNs can rely on a number of resources. Ethical guidance may be found in the *Code of Ethics for Nurses With Interpretive Statements* from ANA (2005) and the *Ethical and Religious Directives for Catholic Health Care Services* (U.S Conference of Catholic Bishops, 2001). Most hospitals also have ethics committees and ethical experts who can provide consultation for families and healthcare providers. Ethical standards for APNs can be found through ANA (2006a, 2006b) and in the third edition of the *Statement on the Scope and Standards of Advanced Practice Nursing in Oncology* by ONS (Jacobs, 2003b).

Euthanasia

The word *euthanasia* means "good death" (Begley, 1998). The difference between euthanasia and patient-assisted suicide is patient involvement. Euthanasia may take three forms:
• Voluntary—with the consent of the patient
• Nonvoluntary—performed without patient choice in the case of incapacitated patients
• Involuntary—euthanasia against the patient's wishes.
Euthanasia differs from the act of withholding life-sustaining treatment. If life-sustaining treatment is withheld, death occurs as the result of the disease. With euthanasia, death is caused by the physician or other healthcare provider. Voluntary and physician-assisted suicide are alike in that both involve patient choice. Euthanasia is equivalent to homicide in the eyes of the legal system and is illegal in the United States (Walker, 2001).

Healthcare Professional–Assisted Suicide

ONS (2007b) defined *assisted suicide* as "any act that entails making a means of suicide available to a patient with knowledge of the patient's intention." Assisted suicide has been intensely debated in recent years, and physician-assisted suicide has been legalized in the state of Oregon and in the Netherlands. To date, no other state or nation has legalized physician-assisted suicide or euthanasia. Oncology APNs and other nurses have the right to refuse involvement in assisted suicide, either for moral or ethical reasons. ONS's position is that nurses should refrain from using judgmental language in the presence of the patient, family, significant others, and professional colleagues if assisted suicide is requested (ANA, 2006d; ONS, 2007b).

Access to Care

Access to health care has been on the political forefront for many years, and the public regards unequal access to health care as a social injustice. APNs have been given credit for providing health care to rural areas that traditionally have been underserved. Unfortunately, APNs, because of a variety of barriers, may find themselves placed in a position where they cannot provide care because of financial reimbursement issues or restrictions from third-party payers. State scope of practice barriers, physician supervision issues, and prescriptive authority limitations also play a part in access-to-care difficulties for patients. All APNs must be cognizant of state regulations and the presence of access-to-care barriers in the state in which they are employed, as well as in bordering states if appropriate (Wilken, 2004).

Access to hospice care is another end-of-life issue that oncology APNs may encounter. Issues such as insurance coverage, the legal inability of APNs to certify patients for hospice, narrow definitions of eligibility criteria, limitations of hospice care, and discontinuation of hospice have the potential to create barriers and ethical dilemmas for patients and APNs (Bouton, 2005).

Ethical Decision Making

Many models exist to guide or assist in the ethical decision-making process, each with a variety of steps or phases. Most, however, are expanded versions of the nursing process.

The first step is recognition of an ethical dilemma or problem and the need for intervention. Ideally, early recognition and intervention minimizes the severity of the issue (Cohen & Erickson, 2006; Marsee, 1998).

According to Marsee (1998), the second step is to gather relevant information and facts. This stage may include identification of key players. Obviously, the physician or physicians, the oncology APN, and the patient are all primary participants. The patient's family and/or significant others, the primary nurse or nurses, and a durable power of attorney for health care may be members of the discussion group as well (Cohen & Erickson, 2006; Marsee).

Third, a thorough assessment of the problem is required, which includes identification and clarification of the ethical principles and values at stake and a clarification of each key player's viewpoint of the situation. Although input from all affected parties is important, the patient's values and thoughts take top priority. It is important for new oncology APNs to be self-aware regarding ethical dilemmas. Sometimes the dilemma is the oncology APN's response to moral distress. Because the response to conflict is highly individualized, it is always wise to openly discuss the perceived dilemma with peers, other team members, or a more experienced colleague to help to separate individual distress from an actual ethical dilemma involving the patient. APNs also must note that conflicts or dilemmas exist on numerous levels and may involve nurses, other healthcare providers, hospital administration, patients, families, and significant others (Cohen & Erickson, 2006; Marsee, 1998).

Once the conflict is assessed and connected to an ethical value violation, a range of options for resolution are proposed and discussed. At this point, options are only being discussed. If deliberations by all parties do not result in a reasonable set of options, an ethics consult may be needed. Most hospitals have an ethics committee and an ethics consultant available to assist in problem resolution. Ethics committees may comprise people with special training and interest in bioethics, seasoned clinicians with expert decision-making and leadership skills, and people with expertise in conflict mediation. A well-balanced ethics committee contains a mix of people from a wide variety of healthcare and other backgrounds, as well as community members who have been invited because of excellent communication or management skills (Cohen & Erickson, 2006; Marsee, 1998). Ideally, an ethics consultant is available 24 hours a day, seven days a week for crisis situations; however, a formal ethics committee usually will handle the majority of ethical dilemmas.

Steps five and six are synchronous, with the selection of an option and presentation of reasons to support the choice usually occurring in concert. Again, this step may involve the assistance of ethical experts to facilitate selection. Last, as with any problem intervention, the outcome must be evaluated. Questions for review may include the following. Are all the involved parties satisfied with the resolution? Could this dilemma have been avoided, and if so, how? Will this intervention require ongoing intervention as well as evaluation and follow-up? (Cohen & Erickson, 2006; Marsee, 1998; Scanlon & Glover, 1995).

For resources regarding ethics, refer to Table 20-5.

Table 20-5. Ethics Resources

Organization	Resource
American Nurses Association	*Code of Ethics for Nurses With Interpretive Statements* www.nursingworld.org/ethics/code/protected_nwcoe813.htm
	Position Statement on Active Euthanasia and *Position Statement on Assisted Suicide* (available to members) www.nursingworld.org/MainMenuCategories/HealthcareandPolicyIssues /ANAPositionStatements/EthicsandHumanRights.aspx
Ethics Resource Center	www.ethics.org
The Kennedy Institute of Ethics	Academic resources http://kennedyinstitute.georgetown.edu/index.htm
National Hospice and Palliative Care Organization	www.nhpco.org
Oncology Nursing Society	Ethical standards in the *Statement on the Scope and Standards of Advanced Practice Nursing in Oncology* (Jacobs, 2003b)
	Oncology Nursing Society Position on the Nurse's Responsibility to the Patient Requesting Assistance in Hastening Death www.ons.org/publications/positions/AssistedSuicide.shtml

Conclusion

The professional roles, responsibilities, and ethical issues are an integral part of oncology APNs' practice. Oncology APNs must be thoroughly familiar with these concepts and resources if they are to be applied successfully to their practice. The implications of using these concepts will benefit patients as well as oncology APNs.

Case Study

M.S. is a 70-year-old female admitted for febrile neutropenia after one cycle of carboplatin and paclitaxel for stage IV ovarian cancer. The patient had febrile-induced delirium on admission, which resolved as the fever abated. Prior to her diagnosis of ovarian cancer, M.S. was in fair health with controlled hypertension. Her daughter had mentioned some forgetfulness by M.S., and the oncology APN noted this in the chart as questionable early-stage Alzheimer disease. In spite of the severity of her response to the first cycle, M.S. expressed her desire to continue chemotherapy to her daytime nurse. M.S. was not asked about advance directives on admission because of her confused mental status; however, her daughter reported that she is her mother's durable power of attorney for health care. Once the fever resolved and her mental status cleared, M.S. verified that her daughter was indeed her durable power of attorney for health care and denied having any other advance directives. The daughter is an only child and has no other close relatives for emotional support. The daughter wants her mother to discontinue treatment and does not feel that her mother is competent to make decisions regarding her health care. The staff caring for M.S. during her recovery are divided in their opinions about her continuing therapy. They have expressed their views only to each other and the oncology APN, not to the patient or her daughter.

1. How can the oncology APN intervene to assist the patient and family and the healthcare providers?

   Utilizing the steps of the ethical decision-making process, the APN
   - Identifies the problem: Conflict between the patient and her daughter
   - Gathers information (This step may initiate more questions.)
     - The daughter and the physician are questioning the patient's competency.
     - The patient is in reasonable health, but can she physically tolerate more chemotherapy?
     - What is the likelihood of a repeat episode of febrile neutropenia?
     - The nurses are divided in their opinions and have expressed their opinions.

2. What ethical principles and values are affected in this situation?
   - M.S.'s autonomy is paramount in this case. She has the right to self-determination in spite of her daughter's status as durable power of attorney for health care. From the standpoint of the healthcare providers, the principles of nonmaleficence, beneficence, and justice are all important in this situation. The healthcare providers do not want to cause harm to the patient yet want to do good by treating M.S.'s cancer. They realize that their decisions must be fair for all people involved. As part of the information gathering process, the oncology APN talks privately with M.S. and then her daughter to glean an understanding of why each person is approaching the situ-

ation in her particular manner. The oncology APN also meets with the staff to gather their input. The oncology APN realizes from her conversations that M.S. wants treatment because she believes it will improve her chances of survival. Conversely, her daughter believes that her mother may die if she takes more chemotherapy and is more afraid of the chemotherapy than she is of the cancer. The oncology APN also realizes that M.S.'s daughter is frightened of being alone because she has no other living relatives and no emotional support.

- Identifies options: The APN identifies the following needs and interventions.
  - Emotional support for the daughter (i.e., community support group, counseling by a trained professional)
  - Education both for M.S. and her daughter and for the hospital staff regarding National Comprehensive Cancer Network clinical practice guidelines for ovarian cancer, survivorship statistics for patients with ovarian cancer, incidence of febrile neutropenia, and chemotherapy-induced side effects. The APN utilizes her knowledge of learning theory to assess the learning ability of all the parties and how to present the material to each.
  - Through evidence, the oncology APN identifies that an increased risk of febrile neutropenia exists with the current treatment of carboplatin and paclitaxel; however, this may be treated with a colony-stimulating factor such as pegfilgrastim (Neulasta®, Amgen Inc.).
  - Discussion with M.S.'s primary care physician and oncologist regarding the question of mental competency
- Makes a choice: After discussions with the primary care physician and the oncologist and an evaluation of M.S.'s mental status and decision-making capability, all the providers believe M.S. to be quite capable of making an autonomous decision. Following the oncology APN's educational interventions and demonstrations of active listening and compassion, M.S.'s daughter begins to recognize and understand her fears. She also feels hopeful that the colony-stimulating factor will decrease the likelihood of a repeat episode of febrile neutropenia. M.S. and her daughter also understand that ovarian cancer is more of a chronic disease with remissions and relapses, and both decide that treatment really is the best option. The APN also educated the staff and facilitated open discussion of their feelings regarding the situation.
- Identifies reasons to support choices: The oncology APN's excellent oncology education, as well as her knowledge of research findings, has helped to resolve this situation and avert a potentially difficult ethical dilemma.
- Evaluates: The oncology APN is aware that continued evaluation of this situation is needed. If the patient develops febrile neutropenia again, further discussions with the patient and her daughter, as well as with the rest of the healthcare team, will be necessary.

Key Points

Oncology APNs should be familiar with
- Licensing, registration, and certification requirements and scope of practice of the state in which they practice

- Content in the *Statement on the Scope and Standards of Advanced Practice Nursing in Oncology* (Jacobs, 2003b)
- The eight steps to application of EBP guidelines
- The ethical principles and values that are utilized every day to guide interactions with patients, families, healthcare providers, healthcare agencies, suppliers, insurers, and others who may be involved in the provision of patient care
- The ethical issues and purpose of DNR orders, informed consent, patient self-determination, advance directives, and living wills
- Ethical controversies of euthanasia, physician-assisted suicide, termination/withholding of life support, and access-to-care issues
- APN professional practice mandates regarding monitoring of and involvement in healthcare legislation, particularly that which affects the provision of cancer care
- The steps to ethical decision making and how to obtain assistance in decision making.

Recommended Resources for Oncology Advanced Practice Nurses

- Camp-Sorrell, D., & Hawkins, R.A. (Eds.). (2006). *Clinical manual for the oncology advanced practice nurse* (2nd ed.). Pittsburgh, PA: Oncology Nursing Society.
- Individual state Nurse Practice Act information via links on the NCSBN Web site: www.ncsbn.org
- Oncology Nursing Certification Corporation: www.oncc.org
- Oncology Nursing Society: www.ons.org

References

American College of Nurse Practitioners. (n.d.). *Nurse practitioner scope of practice*. Retrieved April 9, 2007, from http://www.acnpweb.org/i4a/pages/index.cfm?pageid=3465

American Nurses Association. (2005). *Code of ethics for nurses with interpretive statements*. Retrieved January 2, 2007, from http://nursingworld.org/ethics/code/protected_nwcoe813.htm

American Nurses Association. (2006a). *Ethics and human rights position statements*. Retrieved January 6, 2007, from http://www.nursingworld.org/MainMenuCategories/HealthcareandPolicyIssues /ANAPositionStatements/EthicsandHumanRights.aspx

American Nurses Association. (2006b). *Ethics and human rights statements: Nursing and the patient self-determination acts*. Retrieved April 6, 2007, from http://www.nursingworld.org/readroom/position/ethics/etsdet.htm

American Nurses Association. (2006c). *Nursing care and do-not-resuscitate (DNR) decisions*. Retrieved January 2, 2007, from http://nursingworld.org/readroom/position/ethics/etdnr.htm

American Nurses Association. (2006d). *Position statement on assisted suicide*. Retrieved January 10, 2007, from http://www.nursingworld.org/ethics/etsuic.htm

Basanta, W.E. (2002). Advance directives and life-sustaining treatment: A legal primer. *Hematology/ Oncology Clinics of North America, 16,* 1381–1396.

Begley, A.M. (1998). Beneficent voluntary active euthanasia: A challenge to professionals caring for terminally ill patients. *Nursing Ethics, 5,* 294–306.

Bouton, B.C. (2005). *Ethical "hot buttons" in hospice care*. Retrieved January 2, 2006, from http://www .medscape.com/viewarticle/505225

Braddock, C.H., & Snyder, L. (2005). The doctor will see you shortly. *Journal of General Internal Medicine, 20,* 1057–1062.

Buppert, C. (2005). *Billing for nurse practitioner services—update 2005: Guidelines for NPs, physicians, employers, and insurers*. Retrieved December 20, 2006, from http://www.medscape.com/viewprogram/4321

Buppert, C. (2006). *How does a nurse practitioner obtain a Medicare/Medicaid number for billing purposes?* Retrieved September 20, 2006, from http://www.medscape.com/viewarticle/544408

Centers for Medicare and Medicaid Services. (2006a). *Advanced practice nursing/physician assistant (APN/PA)*. Retrieved April 20, 2008, from http://www.cms.hhs.gov/MLNProducts/70_APNPA.asp

Centers for Medicare and Medicaid Services. (2006b). *Coding questions*. Retrieved April 20, 2008, from http://www.cms.hhs.gov/MedHCPCSGenInfo/20_HCPCS_Coding_Questions.asp

Centers for Medicare and Medicaid Services. (2006c). *Documentation guidelines for evaluation and management services*. Retrieved April 20, 2008, from http://www.cms.hhs.gov/MLNEdWebGuide/25-EMDOC.asp

Cohen, J.S., & Erickson, J.M. (2006). Ethical dilemmas and moral distress in oncology nursing practice. *Clinical Journal of Oncology Nursing, 10,* 775–794.

Ethics. (2007). *Merriam-Webster online dictionary*. Retrieved July 26, 2007, from http://www.merriam-webster.com/dictionary/ethics

Ford, R.N. (1990). Psychosocial and ethical issues in bone marrow transplantation. In C.A. Kasprisin & E.L. Snyder (Eds.), *Bone marrow transplantation: A nursing perspective*. Arlington, VA: American Association of Blood Banks.

Gilliss, C.L. (1996). Education for advanced practice nursing. In J.V. Hickey, R.M. Ouimette, & S.L. Venegoni (Eds.), *Advanced practice nursing: Changing roles and clinical application* (2nd ed., pp. 34–45). Baltimore: Lippincott.

Health Insurance Portability and Accountability Act. (2006). *HIPAA guidelines 101: Guide to HIPAA compliance, implementation, and privacy*. Retrieved December 20, 2006, from http://www.hipaaguidelines101.com

Ishida, D.N. (2005). Professional issues in cancer care. In J.K. Itano & K.M. Taoka (Eds.), *Core curriculum for oncology nursing* (4th ed., pp. 933–942). St. Louis, MO: Elsevier.

Jacobs, L.A. (Ed.). (2003a). *The master's degree with a specialty in advanced practice oncology nursing* (4th ed.). Pittsburgh, PA: Oncology Nursing Society.

Jacobs, L.A. (Ed.). (2003b). *Statement on the scope and standards of advanced practice nursing in oncology* (3rd ed.). Pittsburgh, PA: Oncology Nursing Society.

Kamajian, M., Mitchell, S.A., & Fruth, R. (1999). Credentialing and privileging of advanced practice nurses. *AACN Clinical Issues, 10,* 316–336.

Katz, J.M., & Green, E. (1997). *Managing quality: A guide to system-wide performance management in health care* (2nd ed.). St. Louis, MO: Mosby.

Krebs, L.U. (2005). Application of the statement on the scope and standards of oncology nursing. In J.K. Itano & K.N. Taoka (Eds.), *Core curriculum for oncology nursing* (4th ed., pp. 877–893). St. Louis, MO: Elsevier.

Loquist, R.S. (2004). Government regulation: Parallel and powerful. In J.A. Milstead (Ed.), *Health policy and politics: A nurse's guide* (2nd ed., pp. 89–128). Sudbury, MA: Jones and Bartlett.

Marsee, V.D. (1998). Ethical perspectives. In C.G. Chernecky & B.J. Berger (Eds.), *Advanced and critical care oncology nursing: Managing primary complications* (pp. 1–16). Philadelphia: Saunders.

Mitchell, H.M. (n.d.). *WV rural health education partnerships. Faculty development committee: Training manual for interdisciplinary session facilitators*. Retrieved December 30, 2006, from http://www.wvrhep.org/ids/manual/IDS-%20Healthcare%20ethics.htm

Mitchell, S.A. (2001). Professional issues. In E.M. Lin (Ed.), *Advanced practice in oncology nursing: Case studies and review* (pp. 395–400). Philadelphia: Saunders.

Moloney-Harmon, P.A. (1999). The synergy model: Contemporary practice of the clinical nurse specialist. *Critical Care Nurse, 19*(2), 101–104.

Nagelkerk, J., & Ryan, M. (2003). The family advanced practice nurse: A blending of the CNS and NP roles. *Advance for Nurse Practitioners, 11*(3), 61–65.

National Council of State Boards of Nursing. (2006a). *Vision paper: The future regulation of advanced practice nursing*. Retrieved April 9, 2007, from http://www.ncsbn.org/Draft_APRN_Vision_Paper.pdf

National Council of State Boards of Nursing. (2006b). *APRN compact*. Retrieved May 4, 2007, from http://www.ncsbn.org/cps/rde/xchg/SID-53EFFC2A-814BE0F0/ncsbn/hs.xsl/917.htm

National Council of State Boards of Nursing. (2006c). *Organizational overview*. Retrieved May 4, 2007, from http://www.ncsbn.org/182.htm

National Council of State Boards of Nursing. (2007). *Licensure*. Retrieved April 9, 2007, from http://www.ncsbn.org/256.htm

Oncology Nursing Certification Corporation. (2003). *Role delineation for advanced oncology certified nurse*. Retrieved April 23, 2008, from http://www.oncc.org/getcertified/testinformation/docs/summaryonly.pdf

Oncology Nursing Certification Corporation. (2004). *Options in advanced oncology nursing certification*. Pittsburgh, PA: Author.

Oncology Nursing Certification Corporation. (2007). *Oncology nursing certification bulletin.* Pittsburgh, PA: Author.

Oncology Nursing Society. (2003). *The role of the advanced practice nurse in oncology care* [Position statement]. Retrieved January 29, 2007, from http://www.ons.org/publications/positions/AdvancePractice .shtml

Oncology Nursing Society. (2006). *Response from the Oncology Nursing Society regarding the National Council of State Boards of Nursing draft vision paper: The future regulation of advanced practice nursing.* Retrieved April 9, 2007, from http://www.ons.org/clinical/professional/QualityCancer/documents /NCSBNresponse.pdf

Oncology Nursing Society. (2007a). *Oncology nurse practitioner competencies.* Retrieved July 26, 2007, from http://www.ons.org/clinical/professional/QualityCancer/documents/NPCompetencies.pdf

Oncology Nursing Society. (2007b). *Oncology Nursing Society position on the nurse's responsibility to the patient requesting assistance in hastening death.* Retrieved January 1, 2007, from http://www.ons.org /publications/positions/AssistedSuicide.shtml

Oncology Nursing Society. (in press). *Oncology clinical nurse specialist competencies.* Pittsburgh, PA: Author.

Oncology Nursing Society. (n.d.). *Evidence-based practice resource area.* Retrieved January 19, 2007, from http://onsopcontent.ons.org/toolkits/evidence/Process/index.shtml

Pan, C.X. (2002). Palliative medicine: Advance directives. *ACP Medicine Online.* Retrieved January 4, 2007, from http://www.medscape.com

Phillips, S.J. (2006). 18th annual legislative update: A comprehensive look at the legislative issues affecting advanced nursing practice. *Nurse Practitioner, 31*(1), 6–38.

Roach, S. (2004). *Caring: The human mode of being: A blueprint for the health professions* (2nd ed.). Ottawa, Ontario, Canada: CHA Press.

Ropka, M.E., & Spencer-Cisek, P. (2001). PRISM: Priority Symptom Management Project Phase I: Assessment. *Oncology Nursing Forum, 28,* 1585–1594.

Scanlon, C., & Glover, J.J. (1995). A professional code of ethics: Providing a moral compass in turbulent times. *Oncology Nursing Forum, 22,* 1515–1521.

Silva, M.C., & Ludwick, R. (1999, July 2). Interstate nursing practice and regulation: Ethical issues for the 21st century. *Online Journal of Issues in Nursing.* Retrieved December 30, 2006, from http://www.nursingworld .org/ojin

University of Medicine and Dentistry of New Jersey. (2001). *Continuous quality improvement—healthcare quality and patient safety.* Retrieved January 19, 2007, from http://www2.umdnj.edu/omcweb/2000 /Continuous%20Quality%20Improvement%20-%20Healthcare%20Quality%20and%20Patient%20 Safety.html

U.S. Conference of Catholic Bishops. (2001). *Ethical and religious directives for Catholic health care services* (4th ed.). Retrieved September 9, 2007, from http://www.usccb.org/bishops/directives.shtml

U.S. Department of Health and Human Services. (2006). *Summary of the HIPAA privacy rule.* Retrieved December 30, 2006, from http://www.hhs.gov/ocr/privacysummary.pdf

Wakefield, M.K. (2004). Government response: Legislation. In J.A. Milstead (Ed.), *Health policy and politics: A nurse's guide* (2nd ed., pp. 67–88). Sudbury, MA: Jones and Bartlett.

Walker, R.M. (2001). Physician-assisted suicide: The legal slippery slope. *Cancer Control, 8,* 25–31.

Wilken, M. (2004). Policy implementation. In J.A. Milstead (Ed.), *Health policy and politics: A nurse's guide* (2nd ed., pp. 161–192). Sudbury, MA: Jones and Bartlett.

CHAPTER 21

Test Questions

Wendy H. Vogel, MSN, FNP, AOCNP®,
Shirley Triest-Robertson, RN, PhD, AOCNS®,
and Barbara Holmes Gobel, RN, MS, AOCN®

1. Which of the following patients is at the highest risk for significant bone marrow suppression?
   a. 70-year-old female with non-small cell carcinoma of the lung, metastatic to the liver with a 10% weight loss prior to diagnosis. Other comorbidities include diabetes and rheumatoid arthritis. Planned treatment with carboplatin, paclitaxel, and bevacizumab.
   b. 22-year-old male with Hodgkin disease, stage II, bulky disease. No comorbidities. Planned treatment with ABVD (doxorubicin, bleomycin, vinblastine, and dacarbazine).
   c. 65-year-old female with breast cancer, stage II. Comorbidities include hypertension. Planned treatment with CMF (cyclophosphamide, methotrexate, and 5-fluorouracil [FU]).
   d. 58-year-old male with colorectal cancer, stage IIIA (Dukes C). Comorbidities include cardiovascular disease with a history of myocardial infarction and hypertension. Planned treatment with FOLFOX (5-FU, leucovorin, and oxaliplatin).

   Answer: A. The risk factors for significant bone marrow suppression in this patient include age, poor nutritional status (indicated by her weight loss prior to diagnosis), her history of rheumatoid arthritis (an autoimmune disease), and diabetes (National Comprehensive Cancer Network [NCCN], 2008). Her chemotherapy also is associated with a greater than 20% risk of febrile neutropenia. In the patient with Hodgkin disease, ABVD has a moderate risk of febrile neutropenia (10%–20%). Age is a risk factor for bone marrow suppression in the patient with breast cancer. FOLFOX has a moderate risk of febrile neutropenia.

2. Which of the following chemotherapeutic agents puts the patient at risk for severe and prolonged myelosuppression?
   a. Cyclophosphamide
   b. Doxorubicin

    c. Carmustine
    d. Paclitaxel

Answer: C. Carmustine is a nitrosourea. This class of drugs is cell cycle nonspecific and has the most potent and prolonged effect on myelosuppression. Carmustine may cause severe myelosuppression that may last up to 85 days. The nadir of carmustine occurs in 26–60 days (Polovich, White, & Kelleher, 2005; Shane & Shelton, 2004). Cyclophosphamide and paclitaxel produce moderate myelosuppression. Although doxorubicin, an alkylating agent, may produce severe myelosuppression, the duration is generally only about 21 days.

3. A patient will begin radiation therapy to marrow-producing fields for about six weeks. The most appropriate time for the advanced practice nurse (APN) to begin assessment for myelosuppression is
    a. Week 3.
    b. Week 4.
    c. Week 6.
    d. One week after radiation.

Answer: A. The APN would assess for myelosuppression beginning at week 3 and continue regularly until bone marrow recovery. Myelosuppression secondary to radiation therapy peaks at week 3. Suppression may occur in all cell lines simultaneously rather than sequentially as seen with chemotherapy. The recovery period also may be less predictable because radiation treatments will be required for several weeks after suppression peaks (Esco et al., 2005; Harrison, Shasha, White, & Ramdeen, 2000).

4. The oncology APN is educating a patient who is neutropenic on strategies to prevent infection. Which of the following strategies to prevent infection during neutropenia has the lowest level of research evidence?
    a. Avoidance of exposure to crowds and small children
    b. Avoidance of fresh flowers in standing water or soil
    c. Compliance with prophylactic antimicrobial therapy
    d. Avoidance of tap water and drinking bottled water only

Answer: D. Drinking only bottled water or processed drinks as a method of avoiding infection during neutropenic episodes has low supporting evidence. The other suggestions all have high supporting evidence and should be encouraged (Zitella et al., 2006).

5. Which of the following patient presentations is the *most* likely to represent a second malignancy caused by treatment of a first malignancy?
    a. Breast cancer presenting in a patient previously treated for Hodgkin disease with chemotherapy and mantle field radiation
    b. Medullary carcinoma of the breast in a patient previously treated for basal carcinoma of the face and upper back treated by resection and topical 5-FU
    c. Prostate cancer in a patient previously treated for lung cancer with radiation to the apex of the left lung
    d. Ovarian cancer in a patient previously treated for adenocarcinoma of the breast with mastectomy and AC (doxorubicin and cyclophosphamide)

Answer: A. Females treated for Hodgkin disease between 10–15 years of age have a great risk for development of secondary malignancies (Jazbec, Todorovski, & Jereb, 2007). Mantle field radiation increases the risk of a subsequent breast or lung cancer. Ovarian cancer occurring in a patient previously diagnosed with breast cancer, regardless of treatment, is more suggestive of a hereditary genetic mutation as the causative factor of the second malignancy rather than the treatment. Medullary breast cancer and prostate cancer in patients previously treated for another cancer do not appear to be second malignancies caused by treatment of the first malignancy.

6. The new APN graduate approaches her mentor because of a conflict with a collaborating physician. Which of the following would be the mentor's best response?
   a. "You would be better off just letting this issue lie, because that physician is difficult to deal with."
   b. "How have you handled conflict with coworkers in the past?"
   c. "I will be happy to intervene for you; I know that physician well."
   d. "Deal with the situation, then come back to me and we will discuss how your method worked."

Answer: B. The new APN graduate is undergoing role acquisition, and a mentor or role model will assist in this process (Brykczynski, 1996). Role acquisition is facilitated by a successful mentor. In asking the new APN how she has handled conflict in the past, the seasoned APN is performing the teacher/coach/trainer role and is assisting the new APN in the evaluation of past conflicts and the success of her previous attempts at resolution. From this evaluation, the seasoned APN can assist the new graduate in formulating a successful response. The APN mentor also can explore the sources of the conflict that have developed between the APN and the physician (e.g., differing expectations, assumptions, priorities, role conflict) that might be intensifying the conflict. Additionally, the mentor could review negotiating strategies with the new APN (Lynch, Cope, & Murphy-Ende, 2001; Robison et al., 2004).

7. Which of the following demonstrates a successful collaborative practice between the APN and a physician?
   a. The physician orders the plan of care, and the APN carries out the order.
   b. The APN has developed protocols based on her previous practice and uses these for her practice.
   c. The physician and APN jointly develop protocols and hold patient conferences weekly.
   d. The physician provides the APN with reference books on which to base APN practice.

Answer: C. Collaboration is the process of working together within the negotiated framework to achieve the goal of the partnership. In collaboration, values are shared, respect is mutual, and power is shared equally (Hanson & Spross, 1998). An effective collaborative partnership includes a shared agenda and mutually beneficial goals (O'Neill & Krauel, 2004). Effective collaborative practice consists of six critical elements: trust, cooperation, assertiveness, shared decision making, communication, and coordination (Baggs, 1994; Mitchell, 2001). The APN and physician developing protocols together demonstrates cooperation, communication, coordination, and shared decision making. By holding weekly patient conferences, information is shared and decisions that are in the patient's best interest may be made.

8. The APN decides to establish a cancer risk consultative practice. What should the APN consider first?
   a. How to write a business plan
   b. Personal strengths and areas of expertise
   c. If insurers will reimburse for this service
   d. Ways to gain community buy-in to the new practice

Answer: B. Many things need to be considered before opening a consultative practice. One of the most important questions is what are the APN's personal strengths and areas of expertise (Aikin, 2001; Block, 1999). It also is important to consider whether cancer risk consultative services are desired by the APN's potential "customers" (patients, administrators, collaborating/referring healthcare providers). Consultation refers to a two-way interaction designed to solicit, provide, and receive help, and the consultant is recognized as having specialized expertise. The nurse also needs to identify areas in which personal growth is needed. The other issues, although important, are secondary to the APN's ability to offer this service. Resistance to change, complacency or apathy, feelings of implied threat or criticism, and unfamiliarity of seeking consultation with an APN can impede development of the consultant role. In every consultative situation, the APN has an opportunity to demonstrate his or her areas of expertise and to provide informal education about the types of cases that are appropriate for future consultations (Lippitt & Lippitt, 1986).

9. Which of the following activities demonstrates to the APN that the staff nurse is functioning at the expert level according to Benner's concepts of practice levels?
   a. The nurse administers appropriate medications at the correct time.
   b. The nurse manages all assigned tasks and copes with unexpected additions of patients to his or her care.
   c. The nurse sets aside time during his or her shift to teach patients about the side effects of their treatment.
   d. The nurse confirms noted subtle changes with full physical examination, finding signs of an oncologic emergency.

Answer: D. Benner's concepts of practice levels (Erickson, 2001) are
• Novice: little or no experience and knowledge; performs rule-governed behaviors
• Advanced beginner: minimal experience; able to integrate guidelines into care but unable to prioritize
• Competent: has mastery of skills and practices with deliberate planning
• Proficient: can perceive the whole situation and anticipates events
• Expert: can intuitively grasp situation and identifies critical areas.
Evaluation of staff proficiency includes using strategies that are specifically chosen to match the learning objectives.

10. Which of the following resources would be the most useful for oncology advanced practice faculty members in planning and evaluating advanced-level education offered in master's programs?
    a. NCCN guidelines for clinical oncology practice
    b. Oncology Nursing Society's (ONS's) *Statement on the Scope and Standards of Advanced Practice Nursing in Oncology*
    c. Comprehensive texts covering oncology diagnosis, management, and follow-up care
    d. ONS's *Standards of Oncology Nursing Education: Generalist and Advanced Practice Levels*

    Answer: D. ONS's *Standards of Oncology Nursing Education: Generalist and Advanced Practice Levels,* in conjunction with the scope and standards of nursing practice, provides educational guidelines for oncology nurse educators to enhance the quality of oncology nursing education, improve the quality of care, and promote the standardization of oncology nursing academic preparation (Jacobs, 2003a, 2003b, 2003c). The standards were developed to reflect the structure, process, and outcomes of educational offerings. Standards are included for faculty, resources, curriculum, the teaching-learning process, and the student.

11. Which of the following is an *accurate* statement regarding cancer risk assessment tools?
    a. The Claus model estimates the risk of breast or ovarian cancer based on age, race, and number of breast biopsies.
    b. The majority of cancers have reliable risk assessment tools, and existing risk assessment tools have weaknesses.
    c. Risk assessment tools enable clinicians to convey a cancer risk estimate to individuals in order to motivate screening activities and behavior changes.
    d. The Gail model, one of the most commonly used breast cancer risk assessment tools, estimates the risk of a genetic mutation that could cause breast cancer.

    Answer: C. Cancer risk assessment tools help to convey cancer risk to patients, hoping to motivate patients to perform screening activities and behavior changes. Most cancers do not have reliable, validated risk assessment tools, and no known existing tool encompasses all known risk factors or is without weaknesses. The Gail model is one of the most commonly used risk assessment tools. It estimates a woman's five-year risk and overall lifetime risk for breast cancer. It does not take into account the age at breast cancer diagnosis in affected family members, history of bilateral breast cancer, second-degree relatives affected with breast cancer, and history of ovarian cancer or lobular carcinoma in situ. It does not evaluate hereditary risk and in fact may be falsely low in people with hereditary breast and ovarian cancer syndrome (Euhus, 2001). The Claus model estimates breast cancer risk based on first- and second-degree relatives with breast or ovarian cancer.

12. Which of the following is an example of primary cancer prevention?
    a. Teaching breast self-examination technique to a 25-year-old female
    b. Ordering a yearly mammogram and performing a yearly clinical breast examination in a 52-year-old woman

    c. Advising a 47-year-old female with a Gail model risk of 2.1% to stop smoking and that taking tamoxifen for five years could lower her breast cancer risk

    d. Ordering carcinoembryonic antigens every three months in an individual following successful treatment for colorectal cancer

Answer: C. Primary cancer prevention aims to reverse or inhibit cancer by modification of a person's environment, behaviors, or through pharmacologic mechanisms (Turini & DuBois, 2002). The APN assists in the achievement of primary cancer prevention by promoting health and wellness and assisting patients to reduce risks known to contribute to cancer development, such as smoking (ONS, 2007).

13. Which of the following studies about cancer risk reduction showed potential for harm by an agent thought to be a candidate for chemoprevention?
    a. The STAR trial (Study of Tamoxifen and Raloxifene)
    b. The SELECT trial (Selenium and Vitamin E Cancer Prevention Trial)
    c. The CARET trial (Beta-Carotene and Retinol Efficacy Trial)
    d. The BCPT trial (Breast Cancer Prevention Trial)

Answer: C. In the CARET study, beta-carotene showed no benefit in men at high risk for lung cancer. In fact, 28% more lung cancers were diagnosed and 17% more deaths occurred in participants taking beta-carotene and vitamin A than in those taking placebos (Clark et al., 1996). The oncology APN must be familiar with current evidence when advising individuals about cancer risk reduction (Jennings-Dozier & Mahon, 2002).

14. Which of the following is not an evidence-based method for promoting tobacco cessation?
    a. Increased tobacco costs and taxes
    b. Use of gum or hard candy as an oral substitute for tobacco
    c. Use of a combination of behavioral counseling and pharmacotherapy
    d. Limits on tobacco advertisements and marketing directed at children and teenagers

Answer: B. All of these methods, with the exception of oral substitutes for tobacco, have evidence that proves effectiveness in decreasing the number of new smokers and increasing smoking cessation rates. Studies show that adolescents are three times more sensitive to tobacco advertising than adults and are more likely to be influenced to smoke by advertisements for cigarettes than by peer pressure (Lindblom & McMahon, 2006), so controlling the marketing of tobacco to children and teenagers will decrease the number of smokers. Increasing the price per pack of cigarettes could reduce the prevalence of smoking among 18-year-olds by 26% (Rivara et al., 2000). Multiple studies have shown that combining behavioral counseling and pharmacotherapy improves smoking cessation rates (Fiore et al., 2000; Rigotti, 2002).

15. The oncology APN is asked to give a lecture about hereditary predisposition testing to a group of medical residents. Which of the following statements would accurately reflect the use of genetic testing in oncology?

a. Genetic testing is now readily and commercially available for most cancers.
b. Genetic testing is best utilized to help individuals at high risk for developing cancer to make good decisions about cancer screening and prevention strategies.
c. Genetic testing could be used in routine population screening because recent scientific advances have decreased costs of testing and insurance policies will readily cover testing.
d. Individuals who have genetic testing require knowledge about the testing process and plan of care following testing, but few negative psychosocial issues have been encountered in clinical practice.

Answer: B. Genetic testing is best utilized to help individuals at high risk for developing cancer to make good decisions about cancer screening and prevention strategies. It is not a tool to be used in routine population screening because most cancers are sporadic and not hereditary in nature. The clinician also must consider the expense of testing and complex counseling needs of these families (Calzone & Tranin, 2003). Individuals with expertise in cancer genetics are necessary to educate those at risk about strengths, limitations, and risks associated with genetic testing. The process of testing can lead to ethical, legal, and social issues, and nurses need to safeguard patients and families from these potential risks.

16. Which of the following best describes germ-line mutations?
    a. Germ-line mutations cause 85% of all cancers.
    b. Primary treatment of cancers often is based on the detection of germ-line mutations.
    c. Germ-line mutations affect one cell line and all subsequent cells derived from that cell division.
    d. Germ-line mutations occur in the sperm or egg cell initially and may be noted in every cell of an individual.

Answer: D. Germ-line mutations occur in hereditary cancer predisposition syndromes, affecting only around 10% of people with cancer. These mutations occur in the egg or sperm and affect every cell in the body and may be passed on to subsequent generations. A common example is a mutation in the *BRCA1* or *BRCA2* gene, which may lead to hereditary breast and ovarian cancer. Detection of a germ-line mutation most often alters prevention and screening strategies (Loescher & Whitesell, 2003).

17. The oncology APN is caring for a patient with a known *MSH2* mutation. Which of the following recommendations would be recommended for cancer prevention or early detection specific for people with this mutation?
    a. Annual mammography beginning at age 35
    b. Annual chest x-rays and sputum cultures
    c. Colonoscopy with prompt removal of polyps annually starting between ages 20–25
    d. Annual full-body skin examination with prompt removal of any suspicious skin lesions

Answer: C. Patients with a mutation in *MLH1* and *MSH2* have an 80% lifetime risk of developing colorectal cancer as compared with a 6% risk in the general population. Women with mutations in these genes have a 60% lifetime risk for developing endometrial cancer and a 12% lifetime risk for developing ovarian cancer (Lindor et al., 2006). Therefore, a biannual pelvic examination beginning at age 25 with transvaginal ultrasound ages 30–35 every 6–12 months would be recommended. A prophylactic hysterectomy with bilateral salpingo-oophorectomy could be discussed when childbearing is complete. Breast cancer risk is not known to increase in people with this mutation.

18. The oncology APN is caring for four different families who are all requesting genetic testing. Which of these families should be counseled that current available genetic tests are not likely to identify a hereditary predisposition?
    a. A family with three members with melanoma and one of whom also has pancreatic cancer
    b. A family with breast cancer in a 65-year-old grandmother, an uncle with prostate cancer diagnosed at age 80, and a son with lung cancer diagnosed at age 48
    c. A family with a grandmother with endometrial cancer diagnosed at age 49, her son with colorectal cancer diagnosed at age 49, and her daughter with renal cancer diagnosed at age 42
    d. A family with a woman who had breast cancer at age 49 and ovarian cancer at age 61. This woman has a paternal cousin with bilateral breast cancer diagnosed at age 50.

    Answer: B. Although several cancers are present in this family, the breast cancer and prostate cancer were both diagnosed after age 50. The first family's history (a) is suggestive of hereditary melanoma because of the incidence of melanoma in three family members as well as the pancreatic cancer, which also can be found in this syndrome (Tsao & Niendorf, 2004). The third family (c) has cancers associated with hereditary nonpolyposis colorectal cancer (HNPCC) syndrome. This family also has cancers diagnosed before age 50 and first-degree relatives affected with an HNPCC cancer (Lynch & de la Chapelle, 2003). The fourth family (d) is suggestive of a hereditary cancer syndrome because of the woman with two primary cancers and an individual with a cancer that is bilateral in a paired organ (Tranin, Masny, & Jenkins, 2003).

19. Which of the following statements regarding performance status is correct?
    a. Performance status has prognostic but not therapeutic implications.
    b. The Karnofsky Performance Status (KPS) scale and the Eastern Cooperative Oncology Group (ECOG) scale, although frequently used, are not yet validated.
    c. Obtaining baseline performance status and then monitoring periodically is not an accurate assessment of changes resulting from disease and thus making treatment modifications based on this would be inappropriate.
    d. The ECOG performance scale has five levels to evaluate patients and their behaviors, from fully ambulatory and functional to fully bedridden and nonfunctional (0–5).

    Answer: D. The ECOG performance scale was developed by ECOG and has five levels (0–5), with level 0 indicating fully ambulatory and functional and level 4 indicating fully bedridden and nonfunctional (Mor, Laliberle, & Wiemann, 1984). The ECOG and KPS scales are the most frequently used, validated measurement tools for performance status both in clinical practice and in clinical trials. By obtaining a baseline score, and then periodic assessments of performance status, the clinician can predict the initial impact of disease upon the patient, tolerance of treatment, and the progression or regression of disease burden. The information gleaned from this assessment will influence initial and ongoing therapeutic interventions.

20. For which patient would a plain radiograph (x-ray) be most appropriate?
    a. An obese male with a suspected sacral tumor
    b. A 55-year-old female with multiple myeloma
    c. An obese patient with a suspected intestinal obstruction
    d. Assessment of progression of a scapular lesion

Answer: B. Plain radiographs still play a significant role in cancer diagnosis by demonstrating suspicious areas in two-dimensional imaging. They also have the advantage of being relatively quick and inexpensive. Purely lytic bone metastases, such as in multiple myeloma, are best evaluated by plain bone films (skeletal surveys), so the 55-year-old female with multiple myeloma could be evaluated by x-ray. In a patient with a peripheral lung lesion, x-ray is ideal for evaluation and also is excellent for pneumonias and intestinal obstructions. Radiographs of the chest can provide information regarding the size of lesions in the lung, the presence or absence of calcifications, and the growth rate of lung nodules (Ost, Fein, & Feinsilver, 2003). Radiography may be limited by obesity because of reduced contrast imaging. Interpretation of x-rays can be hindered because of location, particularly in areas such as the sacrum, sternum, and scapula, which have obscured views (Shaffer, 1996).

21. In which of the following is the choice of diagnostic scanning most appropriate?
    a. Positron-emission tomography (PET) scan for staging in renal cancer
    b. Magnetic resonance imaging (MRI) evaluation of an upper abdominal lesion
    c. Computed tomography (CT) scan to evaluate a musculoskeletal malignancy
    d. PET scan in the work-up of a solitary pulmonary nodule

Answer: D. PET scanning involves the injection of a positron-labeled (radioactive) tracer, usually glucose (F-fluorodeoxyglucose). Metabolically active areas, such as tumors, will take up the glucose and will show up as "hot" spots on images produced by gamma camera tomography (Bhalla, 2002). Certain tissues, such as kidney and brain, take up glucose, limiting evaluation by PET scanning. PET scanning is considered the gold standard for evaluating a solitary pulmonary nodule or mass (Schrevens, Lorent, Dooms, & Vansteenkiste, 2004). CT scanning for evaluating musculoskeletal malignancies can be difficult because the CT may produce image artifact where cortical bone is present (Cothran & Helms, 2006). MRI can be limited in chest and upper abdominal scanning because of respiratory motion artifact.

22. The OctreoScan® (Mallinckrodt Inc.) would be appropriate to evaluate which of the following malignancies?
    a. Breast cancer

    b. Osteosarcoma
    c. Carcinoid tumor
    d. Brain metastases from a small cell lung primary

Answer: C. The OctreoScan can visualize somatostatin receptors on a variety of neuroendocrine tumors that express somatostatin receptors (Coleman, 2006). It is specifically designed to evaluate carcinoid tumors and also may be used for pancreatic endocrine and medullary carcinoma of the thyroid.

23. The pathology report on a 42-year-old female postlumpectomy reveals the following: 2.5 cm tumor, estrogen receptor/progesterone receptor negative, HER2/neu 2+ by immunohistochemistry, 1 of 15 lymph nodes positive. The oncology APN recognizes that the next appropriate step is to
    a. Recommend referral for chemotherapy.
    b. Order repeat testing to ensure that the tumor is not hormonally reactive.
    c. Order further testing by fluorescent in situ hybridization (FISH) on the tumor to reassess HER2/neu status.
    d. Recommend proceeding with mastectomy because of the aggressiveness of the tumor.

Answer: C. IHC testing of HER2/neu reported at 2+ is considered equivocal; therefore, further testing by FISH is indicated to detect overexpression. FISH is the more accurate test to assess for HER2/neu status (Kakar et al., 2000).

24. Which of the following is a risk factor for postoperative nausea and vomiting?
    a. Older age
    b. Male sex
    c. Surgical procedure involving the ear
    d. Short duration of surgery

Answer: C. Male sex, shorter surgery, and age are not considered to be risk factors for postoperative nausea and vomiting. Female sex, surgeries of longer duration, and surgical procedures involving the ear do increase the risk of postoperative nausea and vomiting. Other risk factors might include ingesting food too quickly following surgery; surgeries of the nose, throat, or breast; long duration of surgery; and a pediatric patient (Iverson & Lynch, 2006).

25. Which of the following statements about surgical biopsy is accurate?
    a. An incisional biopsy removes the entire nonvisible mass.
    b. An excisional biopsy removes a visible mass in its entirety.
    c. A negative core needle biopsy reading ensures a benign lesion.
    d. The disadvantage of needle biopsy is difficult access to tumor.

Answer: B. An excisional biopsy removes a visible mass in its entirety. An incisional biopsy removes part of a visible mass. A negative biopsy reading obtained via a fine or core needle does not ensure a benign lesion. If a lesion is highly suspect for malignancy and a needle biopsy yields negative or inconclusive results, an open biopsy is necessary to obtain enough tissue to verify a diagnosis (Sabel, 2007). In the case of precursor neoplastic findings, as in lobular carcinoma in situ of the breast, a needle biopsy is insufficient for diagnosis and/or management. A follow-up surgical excision removes additional tissue for pathologic examination to exclude adjacent malignant cells (Elsheikh & Silverman, 2005). Needle biopsies have the advantage of easy access, minimal or no scarring, and minimal discomfort.

26. Each of the following comorbid conditions increases the risk for intraoperative or postoperative complications except
  a. Personal history of congestive heart failure.
  b. Personal history of gastroesophageal reflux.
  c. Obesity.
  d. Recent personal history of herpes zoster infection.

Answer: D. All of the comorbid conditions listed have a potential for causing intraoperative or postoperative complications, except for a personal history of herpes zoster infection. A personal history of congestive heart failure infers a 12% increase in hospital stay. Obesity increases the risk for intraoperative and postoperative respiratory events by fourfold, and a history of uncontrolled reflux allows for an eight-time increase in intubation events including aspiration (Backman, Bondy, Deschamps, Moore, & Schricker, 2006).

27. All of the following presurgical conditions would increase the risk of postsurgical infection except
  a. Malnutrition.
  b. Being a current smoker.
  c. Uncontrolled diabetes.
  d. Past personal history of hepatitis.

Answer: D. A past personal history of hepatitis is not known to increase the risk of postoperative infection. Abstinence from smoking for as little as one week before surgery can make a positive impact on tissue oxygenation. Suboptimal nutritional states increase the risk of infection. Nutritional supplements or enteral feedings may be necessary to ready the body for surgery and improve nitrogen balance and protein stores (Mirtallo & Ezzone, 2006). Tight control of serum blood sugars with sliding scale insulin may improve the infection threshold (Meakins & Masterson, 2006).

28. The oncology APN is performing a preoperative assessment. The assessment reveals that the patient is on the following medications. Which of these medications should be discontinued more than 24 hours preoperatively?
  a. St. John's wort
  b. Benazepril
  c. Lorazepam
  d. Sertraline

Answer: A. St. John's wort is an herbal preparation with reported uses for anxiety, depression, and insomnia. The concentration of active ingredients in herbal products varies widely between preparations. Adverse reactions of St. John's wort include an antiplatelet affect. Abrupt cessation of this alternative medication may initiate withdrawal symptoms. Therefore, it is recommended that St. John's wort be discontinued two weeks before surgery (Pass & Simpson, 2004). Sertraline, lorazepam, and benazepril should not be discontinued more than 24 hours preoperatively (Backman et al., 2006).

29. All of the following statements accurately define breakthrough pain except
    a. Breakthrough pain may be somatic, visceral, neuropathic, or a combination of these types of pain.
    b. The definition of breakthrough pain is a transitory pain that "breaks through" a well-controlled pain plan.
    c. Breakthrough pain is quantified easily, is of limited duration, has an identifiable cause, and functions to warn and protect from tissue damage.
    d. Breakthrough pain may occur without stimulus or as a result of certain activities or biologic events and is associated with decreased quality of life and increased cost and hospitalizations.

Answer: C. Breakthrough pain is defined as transitory pain that "breaks through" a well-controlled pain plan (Portenoy, Payne, & Jacobsen, 1999). It may be somatic, visceral, neuropathic, or a combination of these. It results from certain activities or biologic events or may occur without a precipitating factor. Breakthrough pain is associated with decreased quality of life and increased cost and hospitalizations (Fortner, Okon, & Portenoy, 2002). However, breakthrough pain is not easily quantified and, unlike acute pain, does not function to warn of or protect from tissue damage.

30. Which of the following is associated with genetic, psychological, and environmental factors and causes a state of dependency upon some substance?
    a. Addiction
    b. Tolerance
    c. Pseudoaddiction
    d. Physical dependence

Answer: A. Addiction is a disease that has genetic, psychosocial, and environmental influences causing a state of dependence upon some substance, and it is caused by habitual use of this substance for nonmedical reasons. Addiction is associated with deviant behavior, such as inadequate self-control over drug use, continued use despite harm, drug craving, and drug-seeking behaviors (Colleau & Joranson, 1998). Opioid addiction is rare among patients with cancer (American Cancer Society, 2007).

31. A patient with chronic pain is currently taking acetaminophen 325 mg and oxycodone 5 mg, two tablets every four hours. The patient's pain rating is 7, which is unacceptable to him. During the work-up for the increase in pain, the APN should
    a. Consider the use of an interventional strategy such as nerve block or neurostimulation.
    b. Consider the addition of a neuropathic agent such as an antidepressant, anticonvulsant, or topical anesthetic.
    c. Instruct the patient to increase the acetaminophen and oxycodone combination to three tablets every four hours for up to a week.

    d. Calculate the 24-hour analgesic dose and increase by 50%; administer equi-analgesic dose in controlled-release form, using oxycodone-acetaminophen for breakthrough.

Answer: D. According to the NCCN guidelines, when pain intensity is rated at a 4–6 or 7–10, the total 24-hour dose should be calculated. The new scheduled dose is determined by the previous total 24-hour dose and is increased by 50%. If the patient has reached the maximum daily limit of the nonsteroidal anti-inflammatory drug, then consider a sustained-release medication. A new breakthrough dose is calculated at 10%–20% of this new 24-hour dose and is given every one hour as needed (NCCN, 2007a). Increasing the acetaminophen and oxycodone combination to three tablets every four hours would give the patient an acetaminophen dose of 5,850 mg per 24 hours, which is over the recommended 4 g/day maximum dose. Although an interventional strategy or addition of a neuropathic agent might eventually be helpful, until the cause of the increased pain is determined, neither of these is appropriate.

32. The incidence of fatigue subjectively reported in patients with cancer undergoing active treatment is estimated to be
    a. 25%.
    b. 75%.
    c. 100%.
    d. 25%–50%.

Answer: C. Subjective reports of fatigue in patients with cancer approach 100% in patients receiving chemotherapy, radiation therapy, stem cell transplant, or biologic therapy (Lawrence, Kupelnick, Miller, Devine, & Lau, 2004).

33. Which of the following pharmacologic interventions is approved by the U.S. Food and Drug Administration for the treatment of chemotherapy-associated cognitive dysfunction?
    a. Erythropoietin
    b. Modafinil
    c. Methylphenidate
    d. No approved treatments are available.

Answer: D. No treatment is currently approved to prevent or decrease any of the cognitive symptoms associated with chemotherapy (Barton & Loprinzi, 2002). Various treatments are proposed based on potential etiologies and are under study. The passage of time may relieve cognitive dysfunction (Wefel, Lenzi, Theriault, Davis, & Meyers, 2004).

34. A patient with non-small cell lung cancer is in the second week of combination therapy with gemcitabine and radiation. The patient is reporting symptoms of "heartburn" pain in the upper chest. Which of the following interventions would be most appropriate for this patient?
    a. Rule out grade 3 or 4 esophagitis, and consider treatment delay until esophagitis resolves.
    b. Order a chest x-ray to rule out other causes of the heartburn, and follow with a recommendation of antacids.

    c. Administer antacids to counter the heartburn symptoms, and follow up with this patient within the next two weeks.

    d. No intervention is warranted, as this is an expected side effect of gemcitabine when given concurrently with radiation therapy.

Answer: A. According to the package insert, esophagitis and pneumonitis occurred when gemcitabine was given concurrently or less than or equal to seven days apart from radiation therapy in patients with non-small cell lung cancer. It usually was observed when patients received large doses of radiation therapy and also was dose dependent for the gemcitabine. Esophagitis can be severe (grade 3 or 4) and potentially lethal, thus requiring treatment delays until diagnosed and treated. This is an expected side effect, but an intervention is warranted. Antacids may or may not be helpful depending on the grade of the esophagitis toxicity. Chest x-rays and pulmonary function tests may give helpful information, but the priority is on ruling out a severe grade of esophagitis and supporting the patient through the toxicity, which may include a treatment delay (Eli Lilly and Co., 2007).

35. A patient with metastatic breast cancer consults the APN regarding treatment with paclitaxel rather than paclitaxel protein-bound particles. The patient has experienced peripheral neuropathy with past treatment and has read that paclitaxel causes less peripheral neuropathy. The APN's best response is

    a. Neurotoxicity with paclitaxel protein-bound particles will reverse itself in three to six months.

    b. The incidence of peripheral neuropathies is equal in paclitaxel and paclitaxel protein-bound particles.

    c. The incidence with arthralgias is equal for both drugs, but protein-bound paclitaxel neuropathies are more quickly reversible.

    d. Paclitaxel protein-bound particles is not approved for metastatic breast cancer and is not a choice at this time.

Answer: C. Paclitaxel protein-bound particles does not use Cremophor® (BASF Corp.) to deliver the drug to the cancer cell, which increases the neurotoxicity. However, the higher incidence of neurotoxicity with paclitaxel protein-bound particles occurs because higher doses (71% versus 56%) can be used. This side effect is more quickly reversible, but if the toxicity exceeds grade 3, dose interruption is required. Paclitaxel protein-bound particles is approved for metastatic breast cancer (Abraxis Oncology, 2007).

36. After the third cycle of an irinotecan-containing protocol for colon cancer, the patient presents with grade 3 diarrhea and incontinence and requires IV fluids for more than 24 hours. The APN recommends

    a. IV atropine.

    b. Oral hydration and IVs.

    c. Octreotide.

    d. Standard regimen of loperamide.

Answer: C. IV atropine is recommended for early-onset and grade 1 or 2 diarrhea caused by irinotecan. Aggressive loperamide is used to prevent late-onset diarrhea. Oral hydration is not aggressive enough to treat grade 3 or 4 diarrhea. IVs also will be indicated, but octreotide is used to treat grade 3 or 4 secretory diarrhea (Novartis Pharmaceuticals Corp., 2005).

37. Which monoclonal antibody would be more likely to cause a hypersensitivity reaction when administered?
    a. Cetuximab
    b. Alemtuzumab
    c. Panitumumab
    d. Ibritumomab tiuxetan

Answer: D. Monoclonal antibodies are made to be totally human (human, suffix -umab), mostly human and only a small part mouse (humanized, suffix -zumab), some mouse and some human (chimeric, suffix -ximab), or entirely mouse protein (murine, suffix -momab). The more mouse protein a monoclonal antibody contains, the greater the risk of hypersensitivity reactions when administered (Muehlbauer, Cusack, & Morris, 2006).

38. After completing her first infusion of rituximab, the patient informs the APN of difficulty breathing. The O_2 saturation on room air is 90% (baseline 99%). Physical assessment reveals crackles in the bases of both lungs. The APN's priority intervention would be to
    a. Initiate emergency medical system response.
    b. Obtain an electrocardiogram to rule out myocardial infarction.
    c. Order blood gases to determine the cause of dyspnea.
    d. Obtain a chest x-ray to rule out capillary leak syndrome.

Answer: A. Most recently, the drug has been implicated in rare sudden death within 24 hours of receiving the drug (symptom constellation includes hypoxia, pulmonary infiltrates, acute respiratory distress syndrome, myocardial infarction, ventricular fibrillation, or cardiogenic shock); 80% of fatal reactions occur after the first infusion. If symptoms appear, the drug must be stopped and life-saving treatment begun. Because this is potentially an emergency situation, the patient should be supported through an emergency response approach until her symptoms stabilize (Genentech, Inc., 2008b).

39. The APN notes that a patient is taking St. John's wort for depression. She is currently receiving irinotecan for metastatic colorectal cancer. The APN's best response is to
    a. Recommend that the patient stop taking St. John's wort, as it is not a scientifically supported treatment for depression.
    b. Allow the patient to continue taking St. John's wort, as it is a relatively harmless complementary therapy.
    c. Tell the patient to not alter the dose of St. John's wort, so that the effectiveness of the chemotherapy will not change.
    d. Recommend an alternative drug because St. John's wort may decrease the effectiveness of chemotherapy.

Answer: D. Strong evidence shows that St. John's wort may have some effectiveness in relieving mild to moderate depression. But multiple side effects are possible, including gastrointestinal distress, skin reactions, fatigue, sedation, restlessness, anxiety, sexual dysfunction, dizziness, headache, dry mouth, weight loss, and increased thyroid levels. It also is metabolized by the cytochrome P450 systems and therefore interacts with many drugs, including warfarin, digoxin, antidepressants, antibiotics, loperamide, and irinotecan. St. John's wort decreases the effectiveness of the active metabolite SN-38 of irinotecan by almost 50% (Natural Standard, n.d.).

40. The APN gathers the following information from a new patient: highly educated white female, former smoker, existing comorbidities, and newly diagnosed lung cancer. Family history reveals that the mother died of breast cancer after receiving multiple chemotherapy protocols. The patient is reluctant to receive conventional therapy or prescription medication. The APN recognizes the patient is at high risk for
    a. Depression and anxiety disorders.
    b. Addiction to opioids and benzodiazepines.
    c. Suicide from lack of coping skills.
    d. Taking complementary and alternative medications.

Answer: D. Information from several studies has begun to describe the characteristics of people who would be more likely to use complementary and alternative medicine (CAM). These characteristics include higher educated women who have taken CAM previously; have recent hospitalization; have family who failed conventional medication; are former smokers (as opposed to current smokers or those who never smoked); suffer from conditions like back or neck pain, colds, joint pain and stiffness, anxiety, and depression; and have strong beliefs in CAM and the values of mind-body healing (Ashikaga, Bosompra, O'Brien, & Nelson, 2002; Barnes, Powell-Griner, McFann, & Nahin, 2004; Kozachik, Wyatt, Given, & Given, 2006; Maskarinec, Shumay, Kakai, & Gotay, 2000; Richardson, Sanders, Palmer, Greisinger, & Singletary, 2000; Sparber et al., 2000; Swisher et al., 2002; Verhoef & White, 2002).

41. Which of the following bests describes the Dietary Supplement Health and Education Act (DSHEA) of 1994?
    a. It is voluntary for all supplements, herbals, other botanicals, vitamins, and minerals.
    b. It verifies the accuracy of the individual ingredients listed within each supplement.
    c. It verifies that claims are not made regarding diagnosis, prevention, treatment, or cure.
    d. It prohibits the use of literature that describes the use of and outcome of using supplements.

Answer: C. Claims must not be made about the diagnosis, prevention, treatment, or cure for a specific disease. This is not a voluntary process. If the DSHEA determines that unfounded claims have been made, the manufacturer is liable. Literature that explains the use of the supplement and their outcomes is allowed but is monitored. Manufacturers of supplements may say, for example, that a supplement improves the respiratory status, but not that it prevents colds (Kinsel & Straus, 2003).

42. The Federation of State Medical Boards approved the "Model Guidelines for the Use of CAM in Medical Practice," of which the major emphasis was to
    a. Encourage the use of only CAM with level 1–based evidence such as meta-analyses.
    b. Discourage the use of non–scientifically supported interventions that may harm the patient.
    c. Encourage APNs to recommend scientifically supported CAM therapy to their patients.
    d. Balance evidence-based practice with compassion and respect for the autonomy and dignity of the patient.

    Answer: D. The Federation of State Medical Boards approved the "Model Guidelines for the Use of CAM in Medical Practice." This model is used in educating and regulating physicians and those who comanage patients, such as APNs, who use CAM in their practices and may not be currently licensed by a governing body with licensed or state-regulated CAM providers. The guidelines affirm that all healthcare providers have a duty to avoid harm and a duty to act in a patient's best interest. The initiative encourages the medical community to adopt clinically responsible and ethically appropriate standards that promote public safety, and at the same time educates healthcare providers on safeguards to ensure that services are provided within professional practice boundaries (Institute of Medicine, 2005).

43. Which of the following statements reflects the most significant contribution to the further success of CAM therapy?
    a. Most CAM therapy has an established billing code to obtain reimbursement.
    b. Safe and effective CAM modalities exist for some common conditions.
    c. Acupuncturists, naturopaths, and massage therapists are licensed in every state.
    d. Many certification programs exist for APN practitioners in the area of CAM.

    Answer: B. Evidence exists for safe and effective CAM modalities for several medical conditions. However, very few established billing codes exist, which necessitates out-of-pocket expenses for most patients who participate in CAM. Licensure for specific people who practice CAM is the responsibility of each individual state, and not all states choose to license acupuncturists, naturopaths, and other CAM practitioners ("ABC Coding Solutions—Alternative Link," n.d.; American Holistic Nurses' Certification Corporation, 2007; Eisenberg et al., 1998).

44. A patient presents to the APN with edema, muscle and joint aches, pruritus, ecchymosis, headache, and low-grade fever. The patient has completed chemotherapy for breast cancer and has been on tamoxifen for more than six months. Which laboratory test would the APN expect to be abnormal?
    a. Complete blood count
    b. Alanine aminotransferase, aspartate aminotransferase
    c. Albumin
    d. Creatinine

    Answer: B. The most common presenting signs and symptoms of drug-induced liver injury include edema, pruritus, jaundice, malaise, headache, anorexia, ecchymosis, low-grade fever, muscle and joint aches, and urine and stool color changes. Hepatotoxicity is influenced by the chemical property of the drug, such as with tamoxifen; individual genetics, such as obesity and diabetes, which are common in women with breast cancer; and environmental factors. And because most liver test abnormalities occur 5–90 days after drug ingestion, the patient must be considered for drug-induced liver injury. Abnormal serum aminotransferases, alanine aminotransferase and aspartate aminotransferase, would be most frequently elevated with liver damage. Serum albumin and coagulation factors detect abnormalities of liver metabolism and synthesis. A decrease in serum albumin is seen in patients with cirrhosis and ascites. Serum albumin levels typically are normal in viral hepatitis, drug-induced liver injury, and obstructive jaundice (Astegiano et al., 2004; Ryder & Beckingham, 2001).

45. A patient diagnosed with colon cancer postchemotherapy presents with complaints of abdominal fullness, fatigue, and anorexia. The symptoms have increased since completing therapy. Which diagnostic would yield the most information for the APN?
    a. MRI
    b. CT scan
    c. Liver biopsy
    d. Abdominal ultrasound

Answer: A. Abdominal ultrasounds are used for dimensions of the hepatobiliary tree and to view intra- or extrahepatic lesions and gallstones but are difficult to perform in obese patients or those with excess bowel air. A CT scan will delineate dilated bile ducts and soft abdominal masses, pancreatic lesions, or any other space-occupying lesions and will determine vertical liver span and overall size. The MRI is more sensitive than CT scan for determining metastasis, and this patient is describing potential signs of liver metastasis. Liver biopsy can determine the etiology of the hepatotoxicity and the pathology of masses or lesions identified after imaging. Liver biopsy can prove to be definitive, especially if clinical signs of hepatotoxicity are present but serologic, autoimmune, metabolic, and other measures fail to yield diagnostic information. Biopsy also is used to verify drug-induced liver injury and to rule out hepatocellular carcinoma, infiltrative disorders, cirrhosis, and viral hepatitis. Cultures may be obtained on liver biopsy tissue to determine success of therapy for metabolic or viral liver disease. Liver biopsy is contraindicated if the patient has coagulopathy abnormalities, suspected hemangioma, ascites, or pleural effusion (Bryant, 2006; Gopal & Rosen, 2000).

46. Which of the following should be included in post-treatment surveillance for patients with breast cancer?
    a. Complete blood count and liver function tests
    b. Chest x-ray, bone scan, MRI, PET scan
    c. Mammogram within six months after radiation therapy
    d. Close follow-up at three- to six-month intervals for at least three years

Answer: D. According to the American Society of Clinical Oncology "2006 Update of the Breast Cancer Follow-Up and Management Guideline in the Adjuvant Setting" (Khatcheressian et al., 2006) summary of recommendations, the only recommended breast cancer surveillance of the available answer choices is a history and physical examination every 3–6 months for the first three years after primary therapy; every 6–12 months for years 4 and 5; and then annually. Other recommendation schedules are given for breast self-examination, mammography at least six months after radiation therapy and preferably one year after the initial diagnostic mammogram, and regular pelvic examinations (Khatcheressian et al.).

47. Which of the following would be a comprehensive resource that examines the medical and psychosocial issues that adult cancer survivors face with recommendations to improve health care and quality of life?
   a. *National Action Plan for Cancer Survivorship*
   b. *Living Beyond Cancer: Finding a New Balance*
   c. *From Cancer Patient to Cancer Survivor: Lost in Transition*
   d. "Seasons of Survival: Reflections of a Physician With Cancer"

   Answer: C. Two reports, the *National Action Plan for Cancer Survivorship* published in 2003 by the U.S. Department of Health and Human Services, the Centers for Disease Control and Prevention, and the Lance Armstrong Foundation, and *Living Beyond Cancer: Finding a New Balance* published in 2004 by the President's Cancer Panel, outlined the issues of cancer survivorship and set out specific national goals. The Institute of Medicine (IOM) of the National Academies of Science established a committee in 2005 to examine the range of medical and psychosocial issues faced by adult cancer survivors and to make recommendations to improve their health care and quality of life. This resulted in the comprehensive publication *From Cancer Patient to Cancer Survivor: Lost in Transition* (Hewitt, Greenfield, & Stovall, 2006).

48. A 35-year-old patient is seen in the follow-up clinic. The patient received radiation therapy to the chest for Hodgkin lymphoma 10 years ago. The surveillance test the APN would order during this visit is
   a. Bone scan.
   b. Brain scan.
   c. Mammogram/MRI.
   d. Bone marrow biopsy.

   Answer: C. The risk of breast cancer is increased in those treated with chest radiation before age 30 and increases with age at the end of follow-up, time since diagnosis, and radiation dose. These projections are based on older regimens associated with greater risk; more modern treatment approaches include limited-field radiation and chemotherapy with less effect on ovarian function (Travis et al., 2005). Still, monitoring for breast cancer as a late effect of chest radiation is recommended in the NCCN guidelines beginning five to eight years after treatment using MRI and mammography for women receiving chest radiation between ages 10–30 years. This screening should be initiated 8–10 years after radiation or at age 40, whichever occurs first (NCCN, 2007b). In particular, those surviving Hodgkin disease are at greatest risk of second primary cancers, with the degree of risk associated with the age at which treatment was delivered. Solid tumors are more prevalent after treatment at a younger age, and leukemia is more frequent in those treated at an older age (Kattlove & Winn, 2003; NCCN, 2007b; Travis et al.).

49. Which of the following generalizations is most consistent with the research on psychosocial effects in cancer survivors?
    a. The type of cancer according to organ of involvement was the strongest predictor of depression.
    b. Less than 10% of older, long-term survivors continue to worry about recurrence, a second cancer, and the symptoms they experience as a sign of cancer.
    c. Risks factors for poor adjustment and functional limitations include treatment with chemotherapy, social isolation or conflict, and expectancies for low control and negative outcomes.
    d. Survivors' needs and concerns improve over time as external sources of support increase with time.

Answer: C. Stanton (2006) identifies risk and protective factors related to psychological adjustment outcomes. Risks factors for poor adjustment and functional limitations include treatment with chemotherapy, social isolation or conflict, expectancies for low control and negative outcomes, and concerted attempts to avoid feelings surrounding cancer. Persistent cancer-related symptoms were the strongest predictors of depression and the post-traumatic stress disorder subdimension of hyperarousal (Deimling, Kahana, Bowman, & Schaefer, 2002). A survey of the cancer-related health worries and related distress of older, long-term survivors in another study revealed that one-third continue to worry about recurrence, a second cancer, and symptoms they experience as a sign of cancer. These worries were significant predictors of anxiety and depression and occurred least commonly among African Americans (Deimling, Bowman, Sterns, Wagner, & Kahana, 2006). Survivors' needs and concerns shift over time, and evidence has shown that external sources of support erode, particularly for those most distressed and of older age (Deimling, Bowman, et al.; Deimling et al., 2002; Deimling, Wagner, et al., 2006; Stanton).

50. Which statistical procedure is used to determine the time until an event occurs?
    a. Blinding
    b. Survival analysis
    c. Analysis of variance
    d. Statistical significance

Answer: B. Survival analysis is the collection of statistics that deal with analyzing the time until an event occurs. Examples of events include duration of response or survival. Blinding is a process by which the patient, and sometimes the researcher, is unaware of which treatment is being administered. Analysis of variance is a method to statistically compare means of several groups or observations. Statistical significance refers to the probability that the results of research could have occurred by chance (Chan, 2004).

51. Which principle of risk/benefit analysis ensures that benefits are maximized and harm is minimized during clinical trial research?
    a. Justice: Declaration of Helsinki
    b. Beneficence: The Belmont Report
    c. Voluntary consent: Nuremberg Code
    d. Protection of Human Subjects: Code of Federal Regulations

Answer: B. The Belmont Report actually covers three basic ethical principles: respect, beneficence, and justice (National Commission for the Protection of Human Subjects of Biomedical and Behavioral Research, 1979). *Beneficence* describes the principle of doing no harm and maximizing benefits while minimizing harm. *Justice* means giving each person an equal share and according to need, individual effort, societal contribution, or merit. *Respect* describes the need to treat individuals and their decisions as autonomous and, if that autonomy is compromised, the obligation to protect that individual. The Declaration of Helsinki contains the recommendations for the process of clinical research (World Medical Association, n.d.). The Nuremberg Code established voluntary consent and required justification for research (National Institutes of Health Office of Human Subjects Research, n.d.). The *Code of Federal Regulations* contains guidelines for the conduct of institutional review boards (U.S. Department of Health and Human Services, 2005).

52. The participant's signature on the informed consent form for a clinical trial signifies
    a. The individual's agreement to participate in this clinical research based on the treatment group to which he or she is randomized.
    b. If it is a phase III clinical trial, the realization that no other acceptable treatment is available.
    c. That the participant has agreed to release the investigator, sponsor, institution, and its agents from liability for negligence.
    d. Acknowledgment that the consenting process was adequate for the participant to make a decision to participate in the clinical research.

Answer: D. The informed consent process begins the first time that clinical research is mentioned to potential research participants. The process continues beyond the signing of the informed consent document to the formalization or documentation that the consenting process has been adequate for the person to make a decision to participate in the clinical research. Participants are discouraged from beginning participation in a clinical trial if they are likely to withdraw based on the arm to which they are randomized. Phase III clinical trials usually are randomized controlled trials that compare the outcomes of the usual standard of care to the research treatment. The patient can be randomized to an acceptable standard of care or research treatment. One of the requirements of informed consent is that it must not release or appear to release the investigator, sponsor, institution, or its agents from liability for negligence (U.S. Food and Drug Administration, 2007).

53. The International Committee of Medical Journal Editors (ICMJE) will only consider publishing clinical trial results if the clinical trial is
    a. Conducted through a national oncology study group.
    b. Registered before enrolling the first human subject.
    c. Powered for detecting a significant difference at 80%.
    d. At least a phase II clinical trial with significant results.

Answer: B. The ICMJE is interested in providing clinical trial information for all potential participants that will increase their access to medical information and contribute to their decision making. This includes but is not limited to phase III clinical trials (DeAngelis et al., 2005). The goal of the ICMJE is to provide full knowledge of and access to clinical trials for potential participants. Additionally, the ICMJE supports the publication of both negative and positive clinical trial results in the spirit of full disclosure to the scientific and public community.

54. Which of the following has the strongest level of evidence when conducted with multiple randomized controlled clinical trials?
   a. Correlational descriptive study
   b. Well conducted case-control study
   c. Expert opinions from an international group
   d. Meta-analysis of randomized controlled studies

   Answer: D. Although meta-analyses may be conducted with studies having similar hypotheses or variables, they have the strongest level of evidence when conducted with multiple randomized controlled clinical trials. Meta-analysis of studies with small samples or poorly designed studies does not provide the same level of evidence as that of meta-analysis of randomized controlled studies. Correlational descriptive studies and case-control studies provide mid-level evidence. Expert opinion is the weakest level of evidence (ONS, n.d.).

55. Which two levels regulate APN practice?
   a. Licensure and certification
   b. Credentialing and privileging
   c. Certification and credentialing
   d. Scope of practice and standards of practice

   Answer: A. Licensure, which is at the state level, and certification, which is given by national organizations, provide APN regulation. Other factors that may influence or guide practice in individual settings of care are credentialing and privileging, scopes of practice, and standards of practice. Credentialing is one method of ensuring credibility to and protection of the public. The oncology APN's scope of practice is defined by federal regulations, state nurse practice acts, ONS guidelines, and practice agreements with the employer. ONS has developed a statement on the scope of practice, which may serve as a guide to both new graduates and APNs with years of experience. Standards are authoritative statements that define responsibilities of APNs, provide direction and evaluation for APN practice, and reflect the values of advanced practice in oncology (Jacobs, 2003c).

56. One of the qualifications required by APNs to obtain Medicare Part B reimbursement is to
   a. Hold a minimum of a bachelor's degree in nursing.
   b. Provide a service included by Medicare or secondary insurance.
   c. Provide service in collaboration with the medical doctor (MD) or doctor of osteopathy (DO) as required by state law.
   d. Be certified in specialty area of oncology such as advanced oncology certified clinical nurse specialist (AOCNS®) or advanced oncology certified nurse practitioner (AOCNP®).

Answer: C. APNs may qualify for reimbursement under Medicare Part B if applicants meet the following requirements: legally authorized to provide services in the state where the service is provided; licensed as an RN in the state where they practice; hold a master's degree in a defined clinical area of nursing from an accredited institution; and certified as an nurse practitioner (NP) or a clinical nurse specialist (CNS) by a national certifying body that has established standards for NPs or CNSs. Recognized certifying organizations include the American Academy of Nurse Practitioners; the American Nurses Credentialing Center; the National Certification Corporation for Obstetric, Gynecologic, and Neonatal Nursing; National Certification Boards of Pediatric Nurse Practitioners and Nurses; Oncology Nursing Certification Corporation; and AACN Certification Corporation. Services will be covered if they are comparable to those provided by an MD or DO, furnished in collaboration with the MD or DO as required by state law, and not excluded by Medicare (Centers for Medicare and Medicaid Services, 2006).

57. The sphere of influence in which the CNS contributes to the development of evidence-based nurse care policies is
    a. Patient/client.
    b. Nurse/nursing.
    c. Patient/family.
    d. Organizational/systems.

Answer: B. The nurse/nursing sphere acknowledges the contributions of CNSs to nurses and nursing through their leadership and staff development activities, including the development of evidence-based policies, procedures, and protocols. The organizational/systems sphere recognizes CNS contributions to health care via informational, educational, and other activities that involve healthcare team members, communities, and healthcare systems (Mooney-Harmon, 1999).

58. The APN observes that the bed rest instruction to patients after intrathecal methotrexate administration is different among practitioners. The APN intends to gather and document information on the current practice. This is an example of
    a. Benchmarking.
    b. Quality assurance.
    c. Evidence-based practice.
    d. Quality improvement.

Answer: B. All of these answers are examples of continuous quality improvement and imply an ongoing or constant course of action, but quality assurance usually involves a retrospective review of an event or procedure. Quality improvement in a facility such as a hospital usually entails people from different but interactive areas coming together to review a systems process. The end result usually is focused on improving patient care or cost-saving measures and generally is more process-oriented than individual-oriented (Katz & Green, 1997). Continuous quality improvement for the APN is a multifaceted process involving self-evaluation, patient evaluation, peer evaluation, systems evaluation, and the use and promotion of evidence-based practice (Katz & Green).

59. What does the Patient Self-Determination Act require hospitals to do?
    a. Require a patient to complete a living will
    b. Inform patients about advance directives
    c. Require patients to complete an advance directive
    d. Inform patients about a durable power of attorney for health care

Answer: B. The Patient Self-Determination Act became federal law in 1991 and requires healthcare agencies to inform patients about advance directives upon admission. It does not require patients to fill out advance directives, only to be aware of their right to make decisions about these issues (American Nurses Association, 2006).

60. A patient diagnosed with colon cancer is on a continuous infusion of fluorouracil. The patient calls to report symptoms of chest pain. Past medical history includes arteriosclerotic disease with associated renal and cardiac compromise. The APN recognizes the chest pain is most likely caused by
    a. Congestive heart failure.
    b. Ventricular arrhythmias.
    c. Arterial vasocontractions.
    d. Decreased left ventricular ejection fraction.

Answer: C. Fluorouracil is known to produce arterial vasocontractions that could produce chest pain. In addition, risk factors for the development of cardiotoxicity identified in a group of 668 patients receiving fluorouracil or capecitabine included preexisting cardiac and renal disease. When cardiotoxicity from 5-FU does occur, it most frequently is associated with the continuous infusion of the drug (Jensen & Sorensen, 2006; Schimmel, Richel, van den Brink, & Guchelaar, 2004; Sudhoff et al., 2004).

61. Which of the following best describes heart disease risk for patients who received radiation to the left breast?
    a. Is no greater in women who received radiation therapy to the right breast
    b. Continues to rise each year after treatment has ended for the patient's entire lifetime
    c. Continues to decrease annually reaching equal risk as having radiation therapy to the right breast
    d. Remains greater than for women who had radiation therapy to the right breast at 20 years after treatment

Answer: D. Even 20 years after treatment, the risk of heart disease appears to be greater in women who received radiation to the left breast as compared to the right breast (Harris et al., 2006).

62. A patient with cancer is experiencing acute diarrhea that the APN recognizes as osmotic diarrhea. The APN recommends that the patient
    a. Increase fiber.
    b. Take a multivitamin.
    c. Avoid sugar-free foods.
    d. Take loperamide.

Answer: C. When experiencing osmotic diarrhea, the patient should not consume foods labeled "sugar free," as these contain sweeteners that act like osmotic laxatives and worsen diarrhea. The diet is modified to eliminate food items that worsen diarrhea, such as fiber, most dairy products (especially milk), caffeine, and fatty foods that may increase intestinal motility (Harris et al., 2006; Osterlund et al., 2004; Stern & Ippoliti, 2003). Acute diarrhea, such as may occur within 24 hours of irinotecan infusion, is cholinergic in origin and responds to atropine (Lomotil®, Pfizer Inc.) 0.25–1 mg IV or SC (Wilkes & Barton-Burke, 2007). Late diarrhea (as may occur 24 hours or more after irinotecan) is secretory and is treated with aggressive loperamide (Imodium® AD, McNeil Consumer & Specialty Pharmaceuticals; Kaopectate® II, Pfizer Inc.).

63. A patient presents to the APN with a headache, confusion, and some visual and neurologic disturbances. The patient has colon cancer and is currently being treated with bevacizumab, irinotecan, leucovorin, and fluorouracil. The most appropriate diagnostic test for the APN to order is
    a. A CT scan.
    b. An MRI.
    c. An EEG.
    d. A lumbar puncture.

Answer: B. Reversible posterior leukoencephalopathy syndrome (RPLS) has been reported to occur < 0.1%. The signs of RPLS include headache, seizure, lethargy, confusion, blindness, and other visual and neurologic disturbances. Mild to severe hypertension may be present but is not necessary. MRI is used to confirm a diagnosis. Symptoms have been reported to begin from 16 hours to one year after start of bevacizumab. If RPLS occurs, discontinue bevacizumab and treat hypertension, if present. Symptoms usually resolve or improve within days, but patients may experience ongoing neurologic sequelae. No data exist that demonstrate safety of reinitiating bevacizumab therapy in patients previously experiencing RPLS (Allen, Adlakha, & Bergethon, 2006; Genentech, Inc., 2008a).

64. A woman with breast cancer is being treated with weekly docetaxel and is nearing a cumulative dose of 400 mg/m². The patient describes constant tearing in her right eye for the last several days. After a baseline ophthalmic examination is completed, the APN must rule out
    a. Canalicular inflammation, and begin treatment with topical antibiotics and steroids.
    b. Conjunctivitis from a compromised immune system, and order topical antibiotics.
    c. A blocked tear duct, and surgical removal of the canalicular and nasolacrimal ducts may be necessary.
    d. Trichomegaly irritating the cornea, and recommend trimming of the eyelashes.

Answer: A. For patients who are going to undergo weekly docetaxel therapy (Taxotere®, Sanofi-Aventis U.S. LLC), epiphora is an expected side effect and is seen at median doses of 400 mg/m². Docetaxel is secreted in tears, causing irritation of the eye, and may cause canalicular inflammation and blockage of tear ducts with epiphora. Weekly docetaxel is associated with a 64% incidence rate of patients developing epiphora and canalicular stenosis. Erosive conjunctivitis may be reversible, but punctal stenosis may not be reversible. Patients on weekly docetaxel should be seen by an ophthalmologist at baseline and then every four to six weeks or more often as needed. Assess patients for excess tearing at baseline and prior to each dose. Topical antibiotics and dexamethasone may be useful. Surgery with silicone intubation of canalicular and nasolacrimal ducts may be needed to manage stenosis. Docetaxel may need to be discontinued. If the patient is still tearing, it is doubtful that the tear duct is blocked, but treatment is necessary to minimize the occurrence of this side effect (Burstein et al., 2000; Esmaeli et al., 2003).

65. A patient with small cell lung cancer comes into the office with complaints of cough, dyspnea, and a feeling of fullness in the head that is worse in the morning. The APN recognizes the symptoms may indicate
    a. Pleural effusion.
    b. Cardiac tamponade.
    c. Spinal cord compression.
    d. Superior vena cava syndrome.

    Answer: D. The most common signs and symptoms related to superior vena cava syndrome (SVCS) include face or neck swelling (82%), upper extremity swelling (68%), dyspnea (66%), cough (50%), and dilated chest vein collaterals (38%) (Rice, Rodriguez, & Light, 2006). Symptoms related to SVCS frequently are worse in the morning because the patient has been lying supine during the night.

66. A new graduate nurse asks the APN when a patient with cancer may experience the resolution of symptoms of SVCS after radiation therapy has been initiated. The APN's most appropriate response is
    a. Within three weeks.
    b. Within 24 hours.
    c. Within two months.
    d. Within three to four days.

    Answer: A. Although patients may notice improvement in venous congestion within three to four days following the initiation of radiation therapy for the management of SVCS, maximum symptom relief generally is seen in three weeks in 70%–95% of the patients treated with radiation therapy (Nicholson, Ettles, & Arnold, 1997).

67. The most common symptom of cardiac tamponade is
    a. Cough.
    b. Dyspnea.
    c. Chest pain.
    d. Hoarseness.

    Answer: B. Symptoms of cardiac tamponade can include cough, chest pain, and hoarseness, but the most common symptom of cardiac tamponade is dyspnea (Rice et al., 2006).

68. A patient with cancer complains of pain in the lower back that radiates around to the chest and a heaviness of the legs. The most appropriate test for the APN to order is
    a. Plain film x-rays.
    b. A lumbar puncture.
    c. An electromyelography.
    d. An MRI.

    Answer: D. Pain and weakness are two of the most common symptoms related to spinal cord compression (SCC). MRI currently is the gold standard to evaluate for SCC. MRI allows visualization of the extent of the lesion and anatomy, detects paraspinal masses, and can image multiple levels to assess for areas of disease that are not clinically apparent (Baehring, 2005b).

69. A patient newly diagnosed with acute promyelocytic leukemia complains of a headache and experiences vomiting unrelated to food intake. The APN recognizes these symptoms as
    a. Hypercalcemia.
    b. Superior vena cava syndrome.
    c. Increased intracranial pressure.
    d. Disseminated intravascular coagulation.

    Answer: C. Patients with acute promyelocytic leukemia often have a high blast cell count on diagnosis and are at risk for increased intracranial pressure (ICP). Increased ICP associated with leukemia also may be a result of hemorrhage caused by coagulopathy or thrombocytopenia (Baehring, 2005a).

70. What is the most important strategy in treating a patient for disseminated intravascular coagulation (DIC)?
    a. Treat the clotting.
    b. Treat the bleeding.
    c. Treat the underlying cause.
    d. Treat the electrolyte imbalance.

    Answer: C. The first priority in managing DIC is to treat the underlying disorder. All other treatments will provide only temporary relief of the symptoms associated with DIC (see Chapter 14).

71. The characteristic metabolic disturbances associated with tumor lysis syndrome include
    a. Hyperkalemia, hyperuricemia, hypophosphatemia, and hypocalcemia.
    b. Hypokalemia, hyperuricemia, hyperphosphatemia, and hypercalcemia.
    c. Hyperkalemia, hyperuricemia, hyperphosphatemia, and hypocalcemia.
    d. Hyperkalemia, hyperuricemia, hyperphosphatemia, and hypercalcemia.

    Answer: C. When a cell is lysed as a result of chemotherapy or other precipitating factors, intracellular contents are released into the vascular system. These intracellular contents include potassium, nucleic acids (which are converted into uric acid in the kidneys), and phosphorus. The phosphorus binds to calcium in the circulation, which causes hypocalcemia (Kaplow, 2002).

72. Which of the following patients has the greatest risk for the development of tumor lysis syndrome?
    a. A patient with stage I breast cancer
    b. A patient with stage IIB colon cancer
    c. A patient with acute promyelocytic leukemia
    d. A patient with chronic myeloid leukemia

    Answer: C. Tumor lysis syndrome occurs most frequently in patients with lymphoproliferative malignancies or in patients with elevated white blood cell counts, such as high-grade lymphomas or acute leukemias (Krishnan & Hammad, 2006; Secola, 2006).

73. A patient is admitted to the hospital for treatment of a newly diagnosed Burkitt lymphoma. The patient has a large mediastinal tumor and positive retroperitoneal nodes. Which of the following medications is most important to order?
    a. Allopurinol
    b. Rasburicase
    c. Fluconazole
    d. Itraconazole

    Answer: A. Allopurinol helps to prevent uric acid nephropathy by inhibiting the conversion of the enzyme hypoxanthine, in the presence of xanthine oxidase, to xanthine and then uric acid in the kidneys (Gobel, 2002). By blocking the formation of uric acid and crystals, renal insufficiency and renal failure may be prevented.

74. A patient with metastatic breast cancer is admitted to the hospital with weakness, confusion, and serum calcium of 13.5 mg/dl. What nonpharmacologic interventions are appropriate for this patient?
    a. Encourage fluid intake, and put the patient on strict fall precautions.
    b. Encourage fluid intake, and do not allow the patient to get out of bed.
    c. Encourage fluid intake, and put the patient on standard fall precautions.
    d. Encourage fluid intake, and allow the patient to walk without assistance.

    Answer: A. The management of hypercalcemia requires improved renal calcium excretion that may be enhanced by good fluid intake (Kaplan, 2006). Neurologic manifestations of hypercalcemia that include weakness and confusion can progress to coma and obtundation; thus, it is critical to provide for safety by instituting measures such as strict fall precautions.

75. Fifteen minutes into an infusion of asparaginase for the treatment of acute lymphocytic leukemia, the patient experiences flushing, dyspnea, wheezing, hypotension, and flank pain. The APN recognizes the symptoms as
    a. Sepsis.
    b. Anaphylaxis.
    c. Tumor lysis syndrome.
    d. Disseminated intravascular coagulation.

    Answer: B. The symptoms of flushing, dyspnea, wheezing, hypotension, and flank pain are indicative of anaphylaxis (Tang, 2003). Hypersensitivity reactions to the drug asparaginase are common.

76. A patient is in need of an allogeneic stem cell transplant, but a related human leukocyte antigen (HLA) match has not been found. The patient expresses fear that an unrelated donor transplant will not be effective. The most appropriate response to the patient is
    a. "Overall survival rates of related donor versus unrelated donor stem cell transplants are similar."
    b. "Overall survival rates of unrelated donor transplants are much higher than with related donor stem cell transplants."
    c. "Overall survival rates of unrelated donor versus related donor stem cell transplants are not as good, but there is a better chance of developing graft-versus-host disease."
    d. "It doesn't really matter which type of matching is the most effective, as you do not have a related donor match."

    Answer: A. According to the International Bone Marrow Transplant Registry/Autologous Blood and Marrow Transplant Registry, overall survival outcomes of related versus unrelated hematopoietic stem cell transplants are similar (Loberiza, 2003).

77. How long must a transplant recipient be monitored for a delayed immune hemolysis response after receiving marrow from an ABO-mismatched donor?
    a. The rest of the patient's life
    b. For one year after the transplant
    c. The first 100 days after transplant
    d. Approximately four months after transplant

    Answer: D. Because the life span of the red blood cells is approximately 120 days, the patient who has received marrow from an ABO mismatched donor should be monitored for delayed immune hemolysis for approximately four months following transplant (see Chapter 7).

78. Graft-versus-host disease is best defined as
    a. A histocompatibility reaction that occurs between the recipient cells and the donor HLA cells
    b. An immune reaction that occurs between the recipient cells and the immunologically competent donor eosinophils
    c. An immune reaction that occurs between the recipient cells and the immunologically competent donor T lymphocytes
    d. An immune reaction that occurs between the recipient cells and the immunologically competent donor B lymphocytes

    Answer: C. Graft-versus-host disease is an immune reaction that occurs between the recipient cells and the immunologically competent donor T lymphocytes (Erlich, Oelz, & Hansen, 2001).

79. The most common virus associated with oral mucositis in a patient who has received stem cells is
    a. Cytomegalovirus.

    b. Epstein-Barr virus.

    c. Herpes simplex virus.

    d. Human immunodeficiency virus-6.

Answer: C. The most common virus associated with oral mucositis in the stem cell recipient is herpes simplex virus (Johnson & Quiett, 2004).

80. Sulfonamides are used prophylactically in patients undergoing stem cell transplant to prevent

    a. *Aspergillus.*

    b. *Varicella zoster.*

    c. *Clostridium difficile.*

    d. *Pneumocystis carinii* pneumonia.

Answer: D. The prophylactic administration of sulfonamides (e.g., pentamidine, dapsone) is used in the patient undergoing stem cell transplantation to prevent *Pneumocystis carinii* pneumonia (Johnson & Quiett, 2004).

81. A patient who had undergone breast-conserving treatment (BCT) with a lumpectomy informs the APN that she does not intend to have follow-up radiation therapy because the daily treatments will be too disruptive for her. The APN's most appropriate response to this patient is

    a. "That is fine. The radiation therapy is not necessary when you have a lumpectomy."

    b. "You must have radiation therapy following a lumpectomy because that is the way that we always treat patients."

    c. "Recent studies have demonstrated that women who underwent BCT and radiation therapy had a significantly lower risk of death compared to women who were treated with BCT alone."

    d. "I can't tell you whether you are making a good decision, as the studies that have looked at women who underwent BCT and radiation therapy compared to women who were treated with BCT alone are inconclusive."

Answer: C. A recent study by Joslyn (2006) found that women who underwent BCT and radiation therapy had a significantly lower risk of death compared to women who were treated with BCT alone. Another recent study (Bijker et al., 2006) demonstrated that at 10-year follow-up, women who underwent local excision versus those who received local excision plus radiation therapy were more likely to have a local recurrence.

82. Which of the following are considered the common side effects related to radiation therapy for breast cancer?

    a. Fatigue and infection

    b. Fatigue and skin reaction

    c. Alopecia and pancytopenia

    d. Anemia and thrombocytopenia

Answer: B. The two most common acute side effects related to radiation therapy for breast cancer are fatigue and skin reaction (dermatitis) (Mock et al., 1997).

Significant amounts of bone marrow are not included in the fields for radiation therapy for breast cancer; thus, low blood counts and infection are not common side effects.

83. A patient with colorectal cancer is receiving concomitant fluorouracil and radiation therapy. Which of the following is an important teaching strategy to explain to this patient?
    a. Diarrhea typically occurs toward the end of treatment and generally is not a problem for most patients.
    b. Constipation typically occurs toward the end of treatment and generally is not a problem for most patients.
    c. Diarrhea typically occurs one to two weeks into treatment, and the amount and duration of diarrhea should be assessed routinely.
    d. Constipation typically occurs one to two weeks into treatment, and the patient should contact the healthcare provider, as it often can be serious.

    Answer: C. Diarrhea typically occurs one to two weeks into treatment, and the amount and duration of diarrhea should be assessed routinely, as it can be serious (Hauer-Jensen, Wang, & Denham, 2003).

84. Late effects of radiation therapy to the colorectal area include
    a. Fatigue and skin reactions.
    b. Fatigue and sexuality issues.
    c. Enteritis and sexuality issues.
    d. Enteritis and delayed immunosuppression.

    Answer: C. Late effects in this population may include enteritis and sexuality issues. Enteritis is characterized by dysmotility and malabsorption (Hauer-Jensen et al., 2003). Sexuality issues include dyspareunia, vaginal dryness, and vaginal stenosis in women, and weakened orgasm and erectile dysfunction in men.

85. An important teaching strategy for a woman receiving radiation therapy to the breast is that the patient will
    a. Have the entire breast exposed during the radiation therapy.
    b. Need to be completely exposed during the radiation therapy.
    c. Be able to be covered by a patient gown during the radiation therapy.
    d. Have the entire breast exposed during the radiation therapy, but no one will see the patient during this time.

    Answer: A. Because it can cause emotional distress, women must understand that during the radiation treatments to the breast, the entire breast will be exposed (see Chapter 6). They also need to know that a camera and microphone will be present in the treatment area so that the radiation therapy technician can see the patient and know that the patient is safe.

86. Which of the following assessment criteria takes priority when caring for a patient with cancer and depression?
    a. Anger
    b. Delirium

   c. Suicidal ideation
   d. Unrelenting pain

Answer: C. Too often, healthcare professionals assume that psychological distress is *normal* for the patient with cancer and overlook its significant impact. Patients with cancer have a higher rate of depression than the general public, and depressive states place patients at a higher risk for suicide (Albright & Valente, 2006).

87. Which of the following factors places a patient with cancer at the highest risk for major depression?
    a. Male gender
    b. Lack of social support
    c. Family history of alcoholism
    d. Personal history of depression

Answer: D. A personal history of major depression significantly increases the risk of recurrent depression (Agency for Health Care Policy and Research, 1993), although a lack of social support and alcoholism are contributing factors. Depression rates are higher in women than men.

88. A patient appears anxious and inquires about the next doctor's visit for the patient's first chemotherapy treatment. Which response by the APN would be most appropriate to help to alleviate the patient's fears?
    a. "Didn't the doctor already review the treatment with you?"
    b. "Chemotherapy is not your enemy; it is to try and cure you."
    c. "Everyone is scared of chemotherapy, but everyone survives."
    d. "It is normal to feel anxious about chemotherapy. Let me tell you what to expect."

Answer: D. Fear and anxiety result from a perceived threat or apprehension regarding the unknown. Educating the patient about what to expect when undergoing tests, procedures, or a new treatment such as chemotherapy helps the patient to regain a sense of control over his or her cancer and cancer treatment (Stephenson, 2006). A high level of anxiety at the start of treatment has been shown to negatively affect overall quality of life, and studies have shown that psychological distress does not decrease over the course of treatment (Schreier & Williams, 2004).

89. Which of the following symptoms differentiates delirium from dementia?
    a. Risk of wandering
    b. Acute onset of confusion
    c. Impairment in personality
    d. Progressive onset of cognitive decline

Answer: B. Delirium is characterized by an acute onset of confusion with symptoms of agitation, restlessness, and fluctuating changes in cognition (Bond, Neelon, & Belyea, 2006; Caeiro, Ferro, Albuquerque, & Figueria, 2004). Dementia is characterized by a progressive change in cognition with symptoms of impaired personality, memory, and behavior, including the risk of wandering (Smith & Buckwalter, 2005).

90. Which of the following statements regarding sexuality is true?
    a. A person is considered asexual if he or she is not able to engage in intercourse.
    b. External changes in body image changes are the only predictors of sexual self-image.
    c. The emotional responses to body image changes such as mastectomy are consistent among all patients.
    d. Emotions such as fear, anxiety, and depression can exacerbate feelings of loss related to changes in body image.

    Answer: D. Emotional responses to body image changes are personal: What is normal for one person may be considered abnormal for another (Anastasia, 2006). Many factors influence the emotional responses to body image changes, including the patient's values, cultural and religious norms, and past and present life experiences.

91. A patient informs the APN that she feels uncomfortable undressing in front of her husband since her mastectomy six months ago. The APN's most appropriate response is
    a. "Maybe with time you will feel better."
    b. "It really isn't my position to discuss sexual issues with patients."
    c. "Then you must not have felt comfortable before the mastectomy."
    d. "Has the cancer affected the way you feel about yourself as a woman?"

    Answer: D. According to Wilmoth (2006), one of the four key processes that nurses must address to enable them to carry out sexual assessments is to hone their effective communication skills. Answer choice D is an open-ended question that allows the patient to identify how the mastectomy has changed her feelings about her sexuality.

92. Which of the following factors has been shown to positively affect coping?
    a. Marital status
    b. Social support
    c. Age and gender
    d. Culture and ethnicity

    Answer: B. Social support such as family, friends, and community and religious resources, as well as the healthcare team, can positively affect the patient's coping responses by changing the person's appraisal of the event or their emotional response to it (Hudek-Knezevic, Kardum, & Pahljina, 2002). Variables such as marital status, age, gender, and culture and ethnicity do not directly affect coping styles.

93. A patient with metastatic lung cancer is actively dying and expresses fear that he will not go to heaven when he dies. The APN's most appropriate response to the patient is
    a. "What's done is done."
    b. "Don't worry about those things; it will all work out."
    c. "Do you want to share with me why you feel this way?"
    d. "Should I ask a chaplain to come and discuss this concern with you?"

Answer: C. Spiritual care is a vital component of oncology nursing care, and the nurse can provide spiritual care through empathic listening and by helping patients to process the meaning of their illness as it relates to their beliefs, life experiences, and religious beliefs (Kemp, 2006). One outcome of a spiritual assessment may be to have a chaplain see the patient.

94. Which of the following is considered best for treatment of depression in patients with cancer because of a low side effect profile and low risk of overdose?
    a. Benzodiazepines
    b. Psychostimulants
    c. Tricyclic antidepressants
    d. Selective serotonin reuptake inhibitors

Answer: D. Selective serotonin reuptake inhibitors affect only one neurotransmitter (serotonin) and, as such, have a low side effect profile and a low risk of overdose potential (Stahl, 1998; Van Fleet, 2006).

95. Which of the following characterizes care provided to those with life-threatening illness not amenable to long-term survival?
    a. Hospice care
    b. Intensive care
    c. Palliative care
    d. Supportive care

Answer: C. Palliative care is the overriding construct that characterizes care provided to those with life-threatening illness not amenable to long-term survival (Kuebler, Lynn, & von Rohen, 2005). Palliative care uses interventions to provide symptom management to patients.

96. An important nursing strategy in the management of cluster symptoms is to
    a. Assess the symptoms with one assessment scale.
    b. Assess the symptoms using multiple assessment approaches.
    c. Treat each symptom one by one to effect a positive response.
    d. Treat the symptom that the patient identifies as the most burdensome.

Answer: B. An important nursing strategy related to the management of symptoms in clusters is to assess the symptoms using multiple assessment approaches according to their complexity (LaCasse & Beck, 2007). Effecting an outcome related to only one symptom may not make a positive impact on another symptom.

97. The unit of care in palliative care is
    a. The family.
    b. The patient.
    c. The healthcare team.
    d. The patient and the healthcare team.

Answer: A. The family is the unit of care in palliative care. The family is expected to provide "hands on" care and may experience more deleterious effects of caregiving during the time of advanced disease (Cameron, Franche, Cheung, & Stewart, 2002).

98. The wife of a patient being cared for by hospice tells the APN, "I just can't take this anymore. I am exhausted and can't take care of my husband anymore." The APN's most appropriate response to the wife is
    a. "You are the only one who is able to take care of your husband."
    b. "We will have to change your husband's benefits so that he can go back in the hospital."
    c. "Tell me more about how you are feeling, and let's try to identify ways that we can get you more support."
    d. "Your comments are very selfish. I am sure that your husband would have taken care of you if you were dying."

Answer: C. Recognition of family caregiver vulnerability has become a well-acknowledged aspect of palliative care (Davies, 2006; Pasacreta & McCorkle, 2000). Family members often are responsible for decision making about palliative care services, completing household tasks, working outside of the home, and intervening with multiple healthcare providers (Houldin, 2007). These demands may impart considerable challenges onto an existing stressful situation. Family members caring for patients who are dying require significant support and guidance in their role as caregiver.

99. A patient with lung cancer receiving radiation therapy for two weeks presents with the following vital signs: a temperature of 101.5°F (38.6°C), a blood pressure of 90/50, pulse of 116, and respirations of 24. What is the most likely cause of the patient's change in vital signs?
    a. Sepsis
    b. Infection
    c. Radiation fibrosis
    d. Radiation pneumonitis

Answer: B. Based on the time the patient has been receiving radiation therapy, infection is the most likely cause of the change in vital signs. Sepsis would be ruled out by observing the patient's response to fluids and antimicrobial therapy. Radiation pneumonitis generally occurs within 12 weeks after thoracic radiotherapy. The threshold dose of radiotherapy to the lung is about 6 Gy (Srinivas, Agarwal, & Aggarwal, 2007). Symptoms related to radiation pneumonitis include mild cough, mild to progressive dyspnea, nonproductive cough, and low-grade fever (generally less than 101°F [38.3°C]). Radiation fibrosis occurs 6–24 months after the completion of radiation therapy (Srinivas et al.).

100. The primary risk factor for the development of radiation-induced pulmonary fibrosis is
    a. Older age.
    b. Smoking history.
    c. Underlying disease.
    d. History of radiation pneumonitis.

Answer: D. The primary risk factor related to the development of radiation-induced pulmonary fibrosis is a history of radiation pneumonitis. Older age and smoking history are risk factors for the development of radiation pneumonitis (Lind et al., 2002; Rancati, Ceresoli, Gagliardi, Schipani, & Cattaneo, 2003).

References

ABC coding solutions—alternative link. (n.d.). Retrieved January 15, 2007, from http://www.alternativelink.com/ali/home/

Abraxis Oncology. (2007). Abraxane (paclitaxel protein-bound particles) [Package insert]. Los Angeles: Author.

Agency for Health Care Policy and Research. (1993). *Depression in primary care: Detection, diagnosis, and treatment* [AHCPR Publication No. 93-0552]. Rockville, MD: Author.

Aikin, J. (2001). Consultation. In E.M. Lin (Ed.), *Advanced practice in oncology nursing: Case studies and review* (pp. 413–421). Philadelphia: Saunders.

Albright, A.V., & Valente, S.M. (2006). Depression and suicide. In R.M. Carroll-Johnson, L.M. Gorman, & N.J. Bush (Eds.), *Psychosocial nursing care along the cancer continuum* (2nd ed., pp. 241–260). Pittsburgh, PA: Oncology Nursing Society.

Allen, J.A., Adlakha, A., & Bergethon, P.R. (2006). Reversible posterior leukoencephalopathy syndrome after bevacizumab/FOLFIRI regimen for metastatic colorectal cancer. *Archives of Neurology, 63,* 1475–1478.

American Cancer Society. (2007). *Cancer facts and figures, 2007.* Atlanta, GA: Author.

American Holistic Nurses' Certification Corporation. (2007). *The school endorsement program.* Retrieved January 23, 2007, from http://www.ahncc.org/pages/1/index.htm

American Nurses Association. (2006). *Nursing care and do-not-resuscitate (DNR) decisions.* Retrieved January 2, 2007, from http://nursingworld.org/readroom/position/ethics/etdnr.htm

Anastasia, P.J. (2006). Altered sexuality. In R.M. Carroll-Johnson, L.M. Gorman, & N.J. Bush (Eds.), *Psychosocial nursing care along the cancer continuum* (2nd ed., pp. 327–350). Pittsburgh, PA: Oncology Nursing Society.

Ashikaga, T., Bosompra, K., O'Brien, P., & Nelson, L. (2002). Use of complimentary and alternative medicine by breast cancer patients: Prevalence, patterns and communication with physicians. *Supportive Care in Cancer, 10,* 542–548.

Astegiano, M., Sapone, N., Demarchi, B., Rossetti, S., Bonardi, R., & Rizzetto, M. (2004). Laboratory evaluation of the patient with liver disease. *European Review for Medical and Pharmacological Sciences, 8,* 3–9.

Backman, S.B., Bondy, R.M., Deschamps, A., Moore, A., & Schricker, T. (2006). Perioperative consideration for anesthesia. In W.W. Souba, M.P. Fink, G.J. Jurkovich, L.R. Kaiser, W.H. Pearce, J.H. Pemberton, et al. (Eds.), *ACS surgery: Principles and practice 2006* (pp. 46–59). New York: WebMD Professional Publishing.

Baehring, J.M. (2005a). Oncologic emergencies: Increased intracranial pressure. In V.T. DeVita, Jr., S. Hellman, & S.A. Rosenberg (Eds.), *Cancer: Principles and practice of oncology* (7th ed., pp. 2281–2287). Philadelphia: Lippincott Williams & Wilkins.

Baehring, J.M. (2005b). Oncologic emergencies: Spinal cord compression. In V.T. DeVita, Jr., S. Hellman, & S.A. Rosenberg (Eds.), *Cancer: Principles and practice of oncology* (7th ed., pp. 2287–2292). Philadelphia: Lippincott Williams & Wilkins.

Baggs, J.G. (1994). Development of an instrument to measure collaboration and satisfaction about care decisions. *Journal of Advanced Nursing, 20,* 176–182.

Barnes, P.M., Powell-Griner, E., McFann, K., & Nahin, R.L. (2004). *Complementary and alternative medicine using among adults: United States, 2002* [DHHS Publication No. PHS 2004-1250 04-0342]. Hyattsville, MD: Centers for Disease Control and Prevention, National Center for Health Statistics.

Barton, D., & Loprinzi, C. (2002). Novel approaches to preventing chemotherapy-induced cognitive dysfunction in breast cancer: The art of the possible. *Clinical Breast Cancer, 3*(Suppl. 3), S121–S127.

Bhalla, S. (2002). Oncologic imaging. In R. Govindan & M. Arquette (Eds.), *The Washington manual of oncology* (pp. 533–541). Philadelphia: Lippincott Williams & Wilkins.

Bijker, N., Meijnen, O., Peterse, J.L., Bogaerts, J., Van Hoorebeck, I., Julien, J.P., et al. (2006). Breast-conserving treatment with or without radiotherapy in ductal carcinoma-in-situ: Ten-year results of

European Organisation for Research and Treatment of Cancer randomized phase III trial 10853—a study by the EORTC Breast Cancer Cooperative Group and EORTC Radiotherapy Group. *Journal of Clinical Oncology, 24,* 3381–3387.

Block, P. (1999). *Flawless consulting: A guide to getting your expertise used* (2nd ed.). San Francisco: Pfeiffer & Company.

Bond, S.M., Neelon, V.J., & Belyea, M.J. (2006). Delirium in hospitalized older patients with cancer. *Oncology Nursing Forum, 33,* 1075–1083.

Bryant, G. (2006). Hepatotoxicity. In D. Camp-Sorrell & R.A. Hawkins (Eds.), *Clinical manual for the oncology advance practice nurse* (2nd ed., pp. 553–565). Pittsburgh, PA: Oncology Nursing Society.

Brykczynski, K.A. (1996). Role development of the advanced practice nurse. In A. Hamric, J. Spross, & C. Hanson (Eds.), *Advanced nursing practice: An integrative approach* (pp. 81–105). Philadelphia: Saunders.

Burstein, H.J., Manola, J., Younger, J., Parker, L.M., Bunnell, C.A., Scheib, R., et al. (2000). Docetaxel administered on a weekly basis for metastatic breast cancer. *Journal of Clinical Oncology, 18,* 1212–1219.

Caeiro, L., Ferro, J.M., Albuquerque, R., & Figueria, M.L. (2004). Delirium in the first days of acute stroke. *Journal of Neurology, 251,* 171–178.

Calzone, K.A., & Tranin, A.S. (2003). The scope of cancer genetics nursing practice. In A.S. Tranin, A. Masny, & J. Jenkins (Eds.), *Genetics in oncology practice: Cancer risk assessment* (pp. 13–22). Pittsburgh, PA: Oncology Nursing Society.

Cameron, J.I., Franche, R.L., Cheung, A.M., & Stewart, D.E. (2002). Lifestyle interference and emotional distress in family caregivers of advanced cancer patients. *Cancer, 94,* 521–527.

Centers for Medicare and Medicaid Services. (2006). *Documentation guidelines for evaluation and management services.* Retrieved July 26, 2007, from http://www.cms.hhs.gov/MLNEdWebGuide/25-EMDOC.asp

Chan, Y.H. (2004). Biostatistics 203. Survival analysis. *Singapore Medicine Journal, 45,* 249–256.

Clark, L.C., Combs, G.F., Turnbull, B.W., Slate, E.H., Chalker, D.K., Chow, J., et al. (1996). Effects of selenium supplementation for cancer prevention in patients with carcinoma of the skin: A randomized controlled trial. *JAMA, 276,* 1957–1963.

Coleman, R.E. (2006). Radionuclide imaging in cancer medicine. In D.W. Kufe, R.C. Bast, Jr., W.N. Hait, W.K. Hong, R.E. Pollack, R.R. Weichselbaum, et al. (Eds.), *Cancer medicine 7* (pp. 488–491). Hamilton, Canada: BC Decker.

Colleau, S., & Joranson, D. (1998). Tolerance, physical dependence, and addiction: Definitions, clinical relevance and perceptions. *Cancer Pain Release, 11*(3). Retrieved July 1, 2007, from http://www.whocancerpain.wisc.edu/eng/11_3/tpda.html

Cothran, R.L., & Helms, C.A. (2006). Imaging of musculoskeletal neoplasms. In D.W. Kufe, R.C. Bast Jr., W.N. Hait, W.K. Hong, R.E. Pollack, R.R. Weichselbaum, et al. (Eds.), *Cancer medicine 7* (pp. 479–481). Hamilton, Canada: BC Decker.

Davies, B. (2006). Supporting families in palliative care. In B. Ferrell & N. Coyle (Eds.), *Textbook of palliative nursing* (2nd ed., pp. 545–560). New York: Oxford University Press.

DeAngelis, C., Drazen, J.M., Frizelle, F.A., Haug, C., Hoey, J., Horton, R., et al. (2005). Is this clinical trial fully registered? A statement from the International Committee of Medical Journal Editors. *JAMA, 293,* 2927–2929.

Deimling, G.T., Bowman, K.F., Sterns, S., Wagner, L.J., & Kahana, B. (2006). Cancer-related health worries and psychological distress among older adult, long-term cancer survivors. *Psycho-Oncology, 15,* 306–320.

Deimling, G.T., Kahana, B., Bowman, K.F., & Schaefer, M.L. (2002). Cancer survivorship and psychological distress in later life. *Psycho-Oncology, 11,* 479–494.

Deimling, G.T., Wagner, L.J., Bowman, K.F., Sterns, S., Kercher, K., & Kahana, B. (2006). Coping among older, long-term cancer survivors. *Psycho-Oncology, 15,* 143–159.

Eisenberg, D.M., Davis, R.B., Ettner, S.L., Appel, S., Wilkey, S., Van Rompay, M., et al. (1998). Trends in alternative medicine use in the United States, 1990–1997: Results of a follow-up national survey. *JAMA, 280,* 1569–1575.

Eli Lilly and Co. (2007). Gemzar (gemcitabine HCl) [Package insert]. Indianapolis, IN: Author.

Elsheikh, T.M., & Silverman, J.F. (2005). Follow-up surgical excision is indicated when breast core needle biopsies show atypical lobular hyperplasia or lobular carcinoma in situ. *American Journal of Surgical Pathology, 29,* 534–543.

Erickson, J. (2001). Educator role. In E.M. Lin (Ed.), *Advanced practice in oncology nursing: Case studies and review* (pp. 444–455). Philadelphia: Saunders.

Erlich, H.A., Oelz, G., & Hansen, J. (2001). HLA DNA typing and transplantation. *Immunity, 14,* 347–356.

Esco, B.R., Valencia, J.J., Polo, J.S., Bascon, S.N., Velilla, M.C., & Lopez, M.M. (2005). Hemoglobin levels and acute radiotherapy-induced toxicity. *Tumori, 91,* 40–45.

Esmaeli, B., Hidaji, L., Adinin, R.B., Faustina, M., Coats, C., Arbuckle, R., et al. (2003). Blockage of the lacrimal drainage apparatus as a side effect of docetaxel therapy. *Cancer, 98,* 504–507.

Euhus, D.M. (2001). Understanding mathematical models for breast cancer risk assessment and counseling. *Breast Journal, 7,* 224–232.

Fiore, M.C., Bailey, W.C., Cohen, S.J., Dorfman, S.F., Goldstein, M.G., Gritz, E.R., et al. (2000). *Treating tobacco use and dependence: Clinical practice guideline.* Rockville, MD: U.S. Department of Health and Human Services.

Fortner, B.V., Okon, T.A., & Portenoy, R.K. (2002). A survey of pain-related hospitalizations, emergency department visits, and physician office visits reported by cancer patients with and without history of breakthrough pain. *Journal of Pain, 3,* 38–44.

Genentech, Inc. (2008a). Avastin [Package insert]. South San Francisco, CA: Author.

Genentech, Inc. (2008b). Rituxan [Package insert]. South San Francisco, CA: Author.

Gobel, B.H. (2002). Management of tumor lysis syndrome: Prevention and treatment. *Seminars in Oncology Nursing, 18*(Suppl. 3), 12–16.

Gopal, D.V., & Rosen, H.R. (2000). Abnormal findings on liver function tests. *Postgraduate Medicine, 107,* 100–114.

Hanson, C.M., & Spross, J.A. (1998). Collaboration. In A. Hamric, J. Spross, & C. Hanson (Eds.), *Advanced nursing practice: An integrative approach* (pp. 229–248). Philadelphia: Saunders.

Harris, E.E.R., Correa, C., Hwang, W.-T., Liao, J., Litt, H.I., Gerrari, V.A., et al. (2006). Late cardiac mortality and morbidity in early-stage breast cancer patients after breast-conservation treatment. *Journal of Clinical Oncology, 25,* 4100–4106.

Harrison, L.B., Shasha, D., White, C., & Ramdeen, B. (2000). Radiotherapy-associated anemia: The scope of the problem. *Oncologist, 5*(Suppl. 2), 1–7.

Hauer-Jensen, M., Wang, J., & Denham, J.W. (2003). Bowel injury: Current and evolving management strategies. *Seminars in Radiation Oncology, 13,* 357–371.

Hewitt, M., Greenfield, S., & Stovall, E. (Eds.). (2006). *From cancer patient to cancer survivor: Lost in transition.* Washington, DC: National Academies Press.

Houldin, A.D. (2007). A qualitative study of caregivers' experiences with newly diagnosed advanced colorectal cancer. *Oncology Nursing Forum, 34,* 323–330.

Hudek-Knezevic, J., Kardum, I., & Pahljina, R. (2002). Relations among social support, coping, and negative affect in hospitalized and nonhospitalized cancer patients. *Journal of Psychosocial Oncology, 20*(2), 45–63.

Institute of Medicine. (2005). *Complementary and alternative medicine in the United States.* Washington, DC: National Academies Press.

Iverson, R.E., & Lynch, D.J. (2006). Practice advisory on pain management and prevention of postoperative nausea and vomiting. *Plastic and Reconstructive Surgery Journal, 118,* 1060–1069.

Jacobs, L.A. (Ed.). (2003a). *The master's degree with a specialty in advanced practice oncology nursing* (4th ed.). Pittsburgh, PA: Oncology Nursing Society.

Jacobs, L.A (Ed.). (2003b). *Standards of oncology nursing education: Generalist and advanced practice levels* (3rd ed.). Pittsburgh, PA: Oncology Nursing Society.

Jacobs, L.A. (Ed.). (2003c). *Statement on the scope and standards of advanced practice nursing in oncology* (3rd ed.). Pittsburgh, PA: Oncology Nursing Society.

Jazbec, J., Todorovski, L., & Jereb, B. (2007, February 2). Classification tree analysis of second neoplasms in survivors of childhood cancer. *BMC Cancer,* pp. 7–27.

Jennings-Dozier, K., & Mahon, S. (Eds.). (2002). *Cancer prevention, detection, and control: A nursing perspective.* Pittsburgh, PA: Oncology Nursing Society.

Jensen, S.A., & Sorensen, J.B. (2006). Risk factors and prevention of cardiotoxicity induced by 5-fluorouracil or capecitabine. *Cancer Chemotherapy and Pharmacology, 58,* 487–493.

Johnson, G.B., & Quiett, K. (2004). Hematologic effects. In S.E. Ezzone (Ed.), *Hematopoietic stem cell transplantation: A manual for nursing practice* (pp. 133–145). Pittsburgh, PA: Oncology Nursing Society.

Joslyn, S.A. (2006). Ductal carcinoma in situ: Trends in geographic, temporal, and demographic patterns of care and survival. *Breast Journal, 12,* 20–27.

Kakar, S., Puangsuvan, N., Stevens, J.M., Serenas, R., Mangan, G., Sahai, S., et al. (2000). HER-2/neu assessment in breast cancer by immunohistochemistry and fluorescence in situ hybridization: Comparison of results and correlation with survival. *Molecular Diagnosis, 5,* 199–207.

Kaplan, M. (2006). Hypercalcemia of malignancy. In M. Kaplan (Ed.), *Understanding and managing oncologic emergencies: A resource for nurses* (pp. 51–97). Pittsburgh, PA: Oncology Nursing Society.

Kaplow, R. (2002). Pathophysiology, signs, and symptoms of acute tumor lysis syndrome. *Seminars in Oncology Nursing, 18*(Suppl. 3), 6–11.

Kattlove, H., & Winn, R.J. (2003). Ongoing care of patients after primary treatment for their cancer. *CA: A Cancer Journal for Clinicians, 53,* 172–196.

Katz, J.M., & Green, E. (1997). *Managing quality: A guide to system-wide performance management in health care* (2nd ed.). St. Louis, MO: Mosby.

Kemp, C. (2006). Spiritual care interventions. In B.R. Ferrell & N. Coyle (Eds.), *Textbook of palliative nursing* (2nd ed., pp. 595–604). New York: Oxford University Press.

Khatcheressian, J.L., Wolff, A.C., Smith, T.J., Grunfeld, E., Muss, H.B., Vogel, V.G., et al. (2006). ASCO 2006 update of the breast cancer follow-up and management guideline in the adjuvant setting. *Journal of Clinical Oncology, 24,* 5091–5097.

Kinsel, J.F., & Straus, S.E. (2003). Complementary and alternative therapeutics: Rigorous research is needed to support claims. *Annual Review of Pharmacology and Toxicology, 43,* 463–484.

Kozachik, S.L., Wyatt, G., Given, C.W., & Given, B.A. (2006). Patterns of use of complementary therapies among cancer patients and their family caregivers. *Cancer Nursing, 29,* 84–94.

Krishnan, K., & Hammad, A. (2006, December). *Tumor lysis syndrome.* Retrieved December 28, 2006, from http://www.emedicine.com/med/topic2327.htm

Kuebler, K.K., Lynn, J., & Von Rohen, J. (2005). Perspectives in palliative care. *Seminars in Oncology Nursing, 21,* 2–10.

LaCasse, C., & Beck, S.L. (2007). Clinical assessment of symptom clusters. *Seminars in Oncology Nursing, 23,* 106–112.

Lawrence, D.P., Kupelnick, B., Miller, K., Devine, D., & Lau, J. (2004). Evidence report on the occurrence, assessment, and treatment of fatigue in cancer patients. *Journal of the National Cancer Institute Monographs, 2004*(32), 40–50.

Lind, P.A., Marks, L.B., Hollis, D., Fan, M., Zhou, S.M., Munley, M.T., et al. (2002). Receiver operating characteristic curves to assess predictors of radiation-induced symptomatic lung injury. *International Journal of Radiation Oncology, Biology, Physics, 54,* 340–347.

Lindblom, E., & McMahon, K. (2006, October 30). *Toll of tobacco in the United States of America.* Retrieved January 8, 2007, from http://tobaccofreekids.org/research/factsheets/index.php?CategoryID=1

Lindor, N.M., Petersen, G.M., Hadley, D.W., Kinney, A.Y., Miesfeldt, S., Lu, K.H., et al. (2006). Recommendations for the care of individuals with an inherited predisposition to Lynch syndrome: A systematic review. *JAMA, 296,* 1507–1517.

Lippitt, G., & Lippitt, R. (1986). *The consulting process in action* (2nd ed.). San Diego, CA: University Associates.

Loberiza, F. (2003). Report on state of the art in blood and marrow transplantation—part 1 of the IBMTR/ABMTR summary slides with guide. *IBMTR/ABMTR Newsletter, 10*(1), 7–10.

Loescher, L.J., & Whitesell, L. (2003). The biology of cancer. In A.S. Tranin, A. Masny, & J. Jenkins (Eds.), *Genetics in oncology practice: Cancer risk assessment* (pp. 23–56). Pittsburgh, PA: Oncology Nursing Society.

Lynch, H.T., & de la Chapelle, A. (2003). Genomic medicine: Hereditary colorectal cancer. *New England Journal of Medicine, 348,* 919–932.

Lynch, M.P., Cope, D.G., & Murphy-Ende, K. (2001). Advanced practice issues: Results of the ONS advanced practice nursing survey. *Oncology Nursing Forum, 28,* 1521–1530.

Maskarinec, G., Shumay, D.M., Kakai, H., & Gotay, C.C. (2000). Ethnic differences in complementary and alternative medicine use among cancer patients. *Journal of Alternative and Complementary Medicine, 6,* 531–538.

Meakins, J.L., & Masterson, B.J. (2006). Prevention of postoperative infection. In W.W. Souba, M.P. Fink, G.J. Jurkovich, L.R. Kaiser, W.H. Pearce, J.H. Pemberton, et al. (Eds.), *ACS surgery: Principles and practice 2006* (pp. 27–45). New York: WebMD Professional Publishing.

Mirtallo, J.M., & Ezzone, S.A. (2006). Total parenteral nutrition ordering and monitoring. In D. Camp-Sorrell & R.A. Hawkins (Eds.), *Clinical manual for the oncology advanced practice nurse* (2nd ed., pp. 1137–1143). Pittsburgh, PA: Oncology Nursing Society.

Mitchell, S. (2001). Professional issues. In E.M. Lin (Ed.), *Advanced practice in oncology nursing: Case studies and review* (pp. 395–400). Philadelphia: Saunders.

Mock, V., Dow, K.H., Meares, C.J., Grimm, P.M., Dienemann, J.A., Haisfield-Wolfe, M.E., et al. (1997). Effects of exercise on fatigue, physical functioning, and emotional distress during radiation therapy for breast cancer. *Oncology Nursing Forum, 24,* 991–1000.

Mooney-Harmon, P. (1999). *The synergy model: Contemporary practice of the clinical nurse specialist.* Retrieved from http://www.aacn.org

Mor, V., Laliberle, L., & Wiemann, M. (1984). The Karnofsky performance status scale: An examination of its reliability and validity in a research setting. *Cancer, 53,* 2002–2007.

Muehlbauer, P.M., Cusack, G., & Morris, J.C. (2006). Monoclonal antibodies and side-effect management. *Oncology (Nurse Edition), 20*(10, Suppl. 7), 11–27.

National Commission for the Protection of Human Subjects of Biomedical and Behavioral Research. (1979). *The Belmont report: Ethical principles and guidelines for the protection of human subjects of research.* Retrieved March 10, 2008, from http://ohsr.od.nih.gov/guidelines/belmont.html

National Comprehensive Cancer Network. (2007a). *NCCN clinical practice guidelines in oncology: Adult cancer pain, version 1.2007.* Retrieved June 10, 2007, from http://www.nccn.org/professionals/physician_gls/PDF/pain.pdf

National Comprehensive Cancer Network. (2007b). *NCCN clinical practice guidelines in oncology: Hodgkin's disease/lymphoma, version 1.2007.* Retrieved September 2, 2007, from http://www.nccn.org/professionals/physician_gls/PDF/hodgkins.pdf

National Comprehensive Cancer Network. (2008). *NCCN clinical practice guidelines in oncology: Myeloid growth factors, version 1.2008.* Retrieved March 8, 2008, from http://www.nccn.org/professionals/physician_gls/PDF/myeloid_growth.pdf

National Institutes of Health Office of Human Subjects Research. (n.d.). *Directives for human experimentation: Nuremberg code.* Retrieved March 10, 2008, from http://ohsr.od.nih.gov/guidelines/nuremberg.html

Natural Standard. (n.d.). *Natural Standard databases.* Retrieved March 9, 2008, from http://www.naturalstandard.com

Nicholson, A.A., Ettles, D.F., & Arnold, A. (1997). Treatment of malignant superior vena cava obstruction: Metal stents or radiation therapy? *Journal of Vascular Interventional Radiology, 8,* 781–788.

Novartis Pharmaceuticals Corp. (2005). Sandostatin [Package insert]. East Hanover, NJ: Author.

Oncology Nursing Society. (2007, March). *Prevention and early detection of cancer in the United States* [Position statement]. Retrieved May 12, 2008, from http://www.ons.org/publications/positions/PreventionDetection.shtml

Oncology Nursing Society. (n.d.). *EBP process: Critique: Levels of evidence.* Retrieved March 10, 2008, from http://onsopcontent.ons.org/toolkits/evidence/Process/levels.shtml#table

O'Neill, E., & Krauel, P. (2004). Building transformational partnerships in nursing. *Journal of Professional Nursing, 20,* 295–299.

Ost, D., Fein, A.M., & Feinsilver, S.H. (2003). Clinical practice. The solitary pulmonary nodule. *New England Journal of Medicine, 348,* 2535–2542.

Osterlund, P., Ruotsalainen, T., Peuhkuri, K., Korpela, R., Ollus, A., Ikonen, M., et al. (2004). Lactose intolerance associated with adjuvant 5-fluorouracil-based chemotherapy for colorectal cancer. *Clinical Gastroenterology and Hepatology, 2,* 696–703.

Pasacreta, J.V., & McCorkle, R. (2000). Cancer care: Impact of interventions on caregiver outcomes. *Annual Review of Nursing Research, 18,* 127–148.

Pass, S.E., & Simpson, R.W. (2004). Discontinuation and reinstitution of medications during the perioperative period. *American Journal of Health-System Pharmacy, 61,* 899–912.

Polovich, M., White, J.M., & Kelleher, L.O. (Eds.). (2005). *Chemotherapy and biotherapy guidelines and recommendations for practice* (2nd ed.). Pittsburgh, PA: Oncology Nursing Society.

Portenoy, R., Payne, D., & Jacobsen, P. (1999). Breakthrough pain: Characteristics and impact in patients with cancer pain. *Pain, 81,* 129–134.

Rancati, T., Ceresoli, G.L., Gagliardi, G., Schipani, S., & Cattaneo, G.M. (2003). Factors predicting radiation pneumonitis in lung cancer patients: A retrospective study. *Radiotherapy and Oncology, 67,* 275–283.

Rice, T.W., Rodriguez, R.M., & Light, R.W. (2006). The superior vena cava syndrome: Clinical characteristics and evolving etiology. *Medicine, 85,* 37–42.

Richardson, M.A., Sanders, T., Palmer, J.L., Greisinger, A., & Singletary, S.E. (2000). Complementary/alternative medicine use in a comprehensive cancer center and the implications for oncology. *Journal of Clinical Oncology, 18,* 2505–2514.

Rigotti, N. (2002). Treatment of tobacco use and dependence. *New England Journal of Medicine, 346,* 506–512.

Rivara, F.P., Ebel, B.E., Garrison, M.M., Christakis, D.A., Wiche, S.E., & Levy, D.T. (2004). Prevention of smoking-related deaths in the United States. *American Journal of Preventive Medicine, 27,* 118–125.

Robison, J.G., Swan, D., Jolley, C., Robinson, C.B., Simonson, C., Viale, P.H., et al. (2004). Implementing the advanced practice nursing survey results: Report by the online services and education team. *Oncology Nursing Forum, 31,* 881–885.

Ryder, S.D., & Beckingham, I.J. (2001). ABC of disease of liver, pancreas, and biliary system. *BMJ, 322,* 290–292.

Sabel, M.S. (2007). Principles of surgical therapy. In M.S. Sabel, V.K. Sondak, & J.J. Sussman (Eds.), *Surgical foundations: Essentials of surgical oncology* (pp. 39–64). Philadelphia: Elsevier Mosby.

Schimmel, K.J.M., Richel, D.J., van den Brink, R.B.A., & Guchelaar, H.-J. (2004). Cardiotoxicity of cytotoxic drugs. *Cancer Treatment Reviews, 30,* 181–191.

Schreier, A.M., & Williams, S.A. (2004). Anxiety and quality of life of women who receive radiation or chemotherapy for breast cancer. *Oncology Nursing Forum, 31,* 127–130.

Schrevens, L., Lorent, N., Dooms, C., & Vansteenkiste, J. (2004). The role of PET scan in diagnosis, staging, and management of non-small cell lung cancer. *Oncologist, 9,* 633–643.

Secola, R. (2006). Tumor lysis syndrome: Nursing management and new therapeutic options. *Advanced Studies in Nursing, 3,* 41–48.

Shaffer, K. (1996). Radiologic evaluation of cancer. In A.T. Skarin (Ed.), *Atlas of diagnostic oncology* (2nd ed., pp. 5–25). London: Mosby-Wolfe.

Shane, K., & Shelton, B.K. (2004). Myelosuppression. In B.K. Shelton, C.R. Ziegfeld, & M.M. Olsen (Eds.), *Manual of cancer nursing* (pp. 309–352). Philadelphia: Lippincott Williams & Wilkins.

Smith, M., & Buckwalter, K. (2005). Behaviors associated with dementia: Whether resisting care or exhibiting apathy, an older adult with dementia is attempting communication. Nurses and other caregivers must learn to 'hear' this language. *American Journal of Nursing, 105*(7), 40–52.

Sparber, A., Bauer, L., Curt, G., Eisenberg, D., Levin, T., Parks, S., et al. (2000). Use of complementary medicine by adult patients participating in cancer clinical trials. *Oncology Nursing Forum, 27,* 623–630.

Srinivas, R., Agarwal, R., & Aggarwal, A.N. (2007). A deferred dilemma. *American Journal of Medicine, 120,* 594–597.

Stahl, S.M. (1998). Selecting an antidepressant by using mechanism of action to enhance efficacy and avoid side effects. *Journal of Clinical Psychiatry, 59*(Suppl. 18), 23–29.

Stanton, A.L. (2006). Psychosocial concerns and interventions for cancer survivors. *Journal of Clinical Oncology, 24,* 5132–5137.

Stephenson, P.L. (2006). Before the teaching begins: Managing patient anxiety prior to providing education. *Clinical Journal of Oncology Nursing, 10,* 241–245.

Stern, J., & Ippoliti, C. (2003). Management of acute cancer treatment-induced diarrhea. *Seminars in Oncology Nursing, 19*(4, Suppl. 3), 11–16.

Sudhoff, T., Enderle, M.-D., Pahlke, M., Petz, C., Teschendorf, C., Graeven, U., et al. (2004). 5-fluorouracil induces arterial vasocontractions. *Annals of Oncology, 15,* 661–664.

Swisher, E.M., Cohn, D.E., Goff, B.A., Parham, J., Herzog, T.J., Rader, J.S., et al. (2002). Use of complementary and alternative medicine among women with gynecologic cancers. *Gynecologic Oncology, 84,* 363–367.

Tang, A.W. (2003). A practical guide to anaphylaxis. *American Family Physician, 68,* 1325–1332, 1339–1340.

Tranin, A., Masny, A., & Jenkins, J. (Eds.). (2003). *Genetics in oncology practice: Cancer risk assessment.* Pittsburgh, PA: Oncology Nursing Society.

Travis, L.B., Hill, D., Dores, G.M., Gospodarowicz, M., van Leeuwen, F.E., Holowaty, E., et al. (2005). Cumulative absolute breast cancer risk for young women treated for Hodgkin lymphoma. *Journal of the National Cancer Institute, 97,* 1428–1437.

Tsao, H., & Niendorf, K. (2004). Genetic testing in hereditary melanoma. *Journal of the American Academy of Dermatology, 51,* 803–808.

Turini, M., & DuBois, R. (2002). Primary prevention: Phytoprevention and chemoprevention of colorectal cancer. *Hematology/Oncology Clinics of North America, 16,* 811–840.

U.S. Department of Health and Human Services. (2005). *Title 45: Public welfare. Department of Health and Human Services. Part 46: Protection of human subjects. Code of Federal Regulations.* Retrieved March 10, 2008, from http://www.hhs.gov/ohrp/humansubjects/guidance/45cfr46.htm

U.S. Food and Drug Administration. (2007). *Title 21—Food and Drugs—Chapter I—Food and Drug Administration Department of Health and Human Services. Subchapter A—General. Part 50. Sec. 50.25: Elements of informed consent.* Retrieved May 12, 2008, from http://www.accessdata.fda.gov/scripts/cdrh/cfdocs/cfcfr/CFRSearch.cfm?FR=50.25

Van Fleet, S. (2006). Assessment and pharmacotherapy of depression. *Clinical Journal of Oncology Nursing, 10,* 158–161.

Verhoef, M.J., & White, M.A. (2002). Factors in making the decision to forgo conventional cancer treatment. *Cancer Practice, 10,* 201–207.

Wefel, J.S., Lenzi, R., Theriault, R.L., Davis, R.N., & Meyers, C.A. (2004). The cognitive sequelae of standard-dose adjuvant chemotherapy in women with breast carcinoma: Results of a prospective, randomized, longitudinal trial. *Cancer, 100,* 2292–2299.

Wilkes, G., & Barton-Burke, M. (2007). *Oncology nursing drug handbook* (7th ed.). Sudbury, MA: Jones and Bartlett.

Wilmoth, M.C. (2006). Life after cancer: What *does* sexuality have to do with it? *Oncology Nursing Forum, 33,* 905–910.

World Medical Association. (n.d.). *Declaration of Helsinki: Recommendation for conduct of clinical research.* Retrieved March 10, 2008, from http://www.bioscience.org/guides/declhels.htm

Zitella, L.J., Friese, C.R., Hauser, J., Gobel, B.H., Woolery, M., O'Leary, C., et al. (2006). Putting evidence into practice: Prevention of infection. *Clinical Journal of Oncology Nursing, 10,* 739–750.

Index

The letter f after a page number indicates that relevant content appears in a figure; the letter t, in a table.

A